Further enhance your Clinical Reasoning with the additional resources below.
For more information and purchasing options visit **www.mypearsonstore.com.**

Thinking Like a Nurse in Clinical

REAL Nursing SKILLS

Real Nursing Skills 2.0 for the RN offers students the complete foundation for competency in performing clinical nursing skills. Visit www.realnursingskills.com

Thinking Like a Nurse in Clinical

Clinical references across the nursing curriculum available.

Thinking Like a Nurse for NCLEX-RN® Success

ALWAYS LEARNING

PEARSON

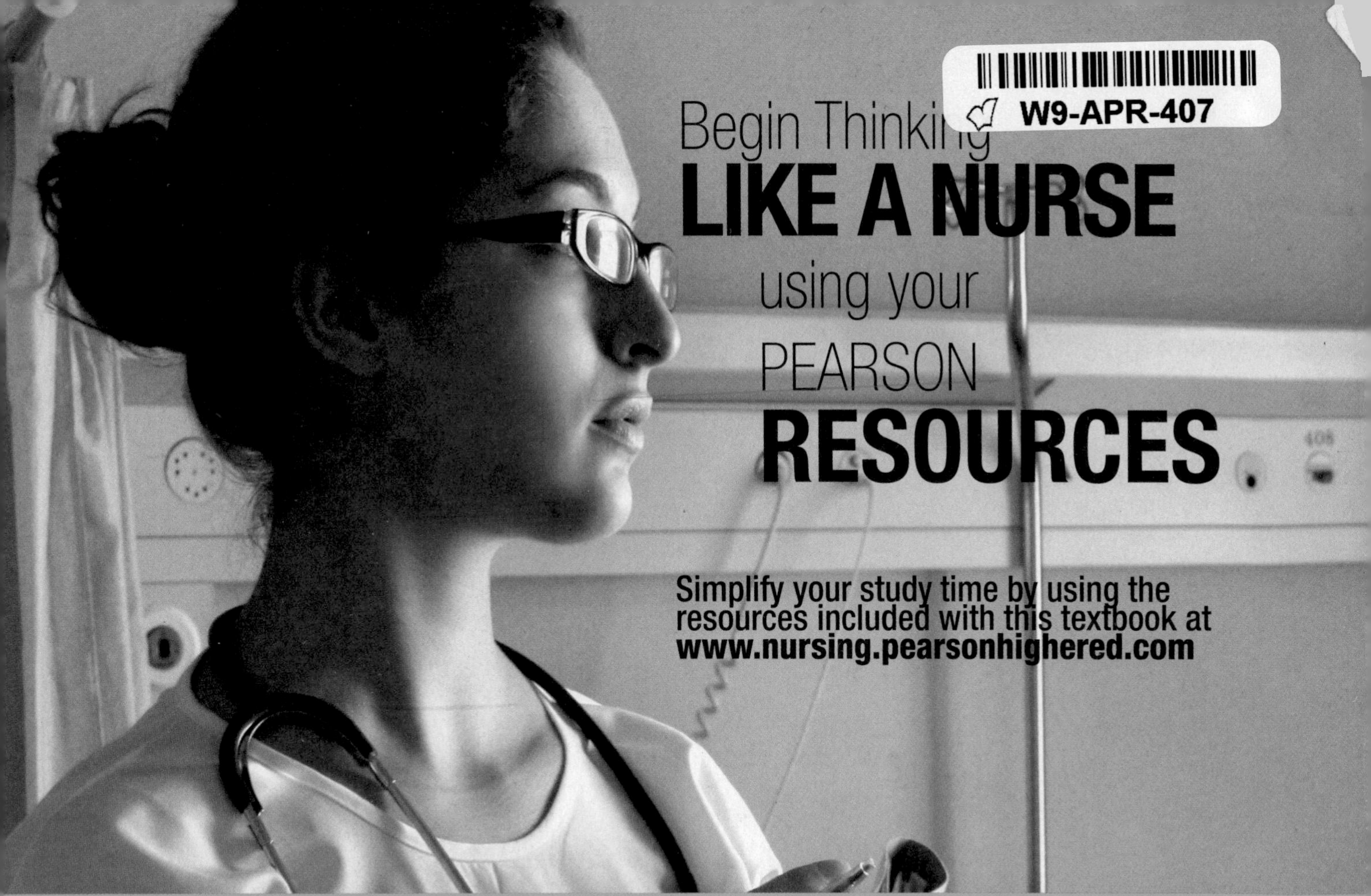

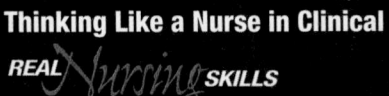

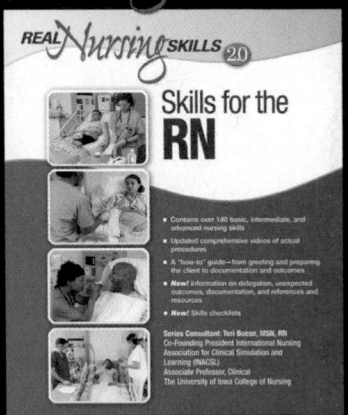

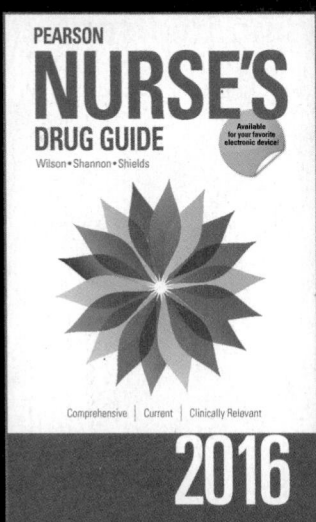

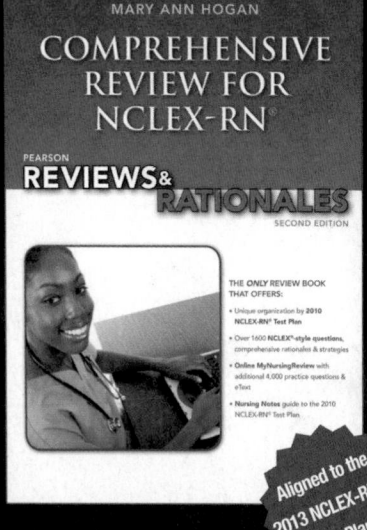

myPEARSONstore

www.mypearsonstore.com
Find your textbook and everything
that goes with it.

www.realnursingskills.com
Real Nursing Skills contains the
complete foundation for competency
in performing clinical nursing skills.

www.nursing.pearsonhighered.com
Find everything you need to simplify your
study time by using the resources on our site.

SKILLS in CLINICAL NURSING

EIGHTH EDITION

Audrey Berman, PhD, RN
Professor, Dean of Nursing
Samuel Merritt University
Oakland, California

Shirlee J. Snyder, EdD, RN
Former Dean and Professor, Nursing
Nevada State College
Henderson, Nevada

PEARSON

Boston   Columbus   Indianapolis   New York   San Francisco   Hoboken
Amsterdam   Cape Town   Dubai   London   Madrid   Milan   Munich   Paris   Montréal   Toronto
Delhi   Mexico City   São Paulo   Sydney   Hong Kong   Seoul   Singapore   Taipei   Tokyo

Publisher: Julie Levin Alexander
Executive Editor: Kelly Trakalo
Program Manager: Melissa Bashe
Editorial Assistant: Kevin Wilson
Development Editor: Teri Zak
Project Manager: Michael Giacobbe
Production Editor: Lynn Steines, S4Carlisle Publishing Services
Manufacturing Buyer: Maura Zaldivar-Garcia
Art Director/Cover and Interior Design: Mary Siener

Senior Product Marketing Manager: Phoenix Harvey
Field Marketing Manager: Debi Doyle
Marketing Specialist: Michael Sirinides
Director, Product Management Services: Etain O'Dea
Project Management, Team Lead: Cynthia Zonneveld
Composition: S4Carlisle Publishing Services
Printer/Binder: Courier Kendallville
Cover Printer: Courier Kendallville
Cover Image: ISebyl

Notice: Care has been taken to confirm the accuracy of information presented in this book. The authors, editors, and the publisher, however, cannot accept any responsibility for errors or omissions or for consequences from application of the information in this book and make no warranty, express or implied, with respect to its contents.

The authors and publisher have exerted every effort to ensure that drug selections and dosages set forth in this text are in accord with current recommendations and practice at time of publication. However, in view of ongoing research, changes in government regulations, and the constant flow of information relating to drug therapy and drug reactions, the reader is urged to check the package inserts of all drugs for any change in indications of dosage and for added warnings and precautions. This is particularly important when the recommended agent is a new and/or infrequently employed drug.

Library of Congress Cataloging-in-Publication Data
Berman, Audrey, author.
  Skills in clinical nursing / Audrey Berman and Shirlee Snyder. — Eighth edition.
    p.; cm.
  Includes bibliographical references and index.
  ISBN-13: 978-0-13-399743-9
  ISBN-10: 0-13-399743-X
  I. Snyder, Shirlee, author.   II. Title.
  [DNLM: 1. Nursing Care—Handbooks.   2. Nursing Process—Handbooks.   WY 49]
  RT41
  610.73—dc23
                                                                            2014043489

10 9 8 7 6 5 4 3 2 1

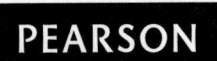

ISBN-13: 978-0-13-399743-9
ISBN-10:   0-13-399743-X

Dedication

Audrey again dedicates this book to her daughter, Jordanna Elise MacIntyre, who has evolved and matured just as has the book itself. Also like the book, she seeks to—and will—make the world a healthier and better place.

Shirlee again dedicates this book to her husband, Terry J. Schnitter, for his continual love and support, and also to the Nevada State College nursing students and nursing faculty. It was a genuine honor to work with all of them.

Acknowledgments

Special thanks to those without whom this edition would not have been possible:

- **Teri Zak**, Development Editor, whose unfailing energy, intelligence, memory, experience, and professionalism supported each aspect of the book's creation.

- **Kelly Trakalo**, Nursing Editor, without whose support for enhancing and marketing this book, it would never have come to be the quality production it is.
- **Lynn Steines**, and the rest of the **S4Carlisle** team, who always go above and beyond to ensure a quality and timely production.
- The reviewers, who provided many helpful comments.

Thank You

We extend thanks to our contributors from previous editions, who gave their time, effort, and expertise to the development and writing of chapters and resources that helped foster our goal of preparing student nurses for clinical practice.

Contributors to the Seventh Edition

Janet Adams, MSN, RT (AART), RN
Southeast Missouri State University
Cape Girardeau, MO

Betty M. L. Bedner, RN, MSN/Ed
University of Pittsburgh Bradford
Pittsburgh, PA

Annette Gunderman, DEd, MSN, RN
Associate Professor of Nursing
Bloomsburg University
Bloomsburg, PA

Kathleen Kunkler, MS, BSN
Capital University
Columbus, OH

Lora McDonald McGuire, MS, BSN
Joliet Junior College
Joliet, IL

Gail Rattigan, MSN, RN, FNP-BC
Nevada State College School of Nursing
Henderson, NV

Janice L. Reilly, EdD, MSN, RN-BC
Immaculata University
Immaculata, PA

Melissa Schmidt, PhD, MSN, BSN
Tompkins Cortland Community College
Dryden, NY

Ruby Wertz, MSHA, BSN, RN
Nevada State College School of Nursing
Henderson, NV

Reviewers of the Eighth Edition

We would like to express our sincere thanks to the educators who reviewed chapters of this text. Their insights, comments, suggestions, criticisms, and encouragement contributed to making this a more useful and relevant tool for students.

Barbara Celia, EdD, RN
Drexel University
Philadelphia, PA

Kathleen Fraley, MSN, RN
St. Clair County Community College
Port Huron, MI

Elizabeth Long, DNP, APRN, GNP-BC
Lamar University
Beaumont, TX

Colleen Marzilli, DNP, MBA, RN
University of Texas at Tyler
Tyler, TX

Alnisa Shabazz, MS, RN
Bronx Community College
New York, NY

Laura Warner, MSN, RN
Ivy Tech Community College
Greenfield, IN

Clinical Reviewers of the Eighth Edition

Patti Christy, APRN, FNP-BC
Primary Physician's Care, LLC
Lake Charles, LA

Katherine Houle, RN, BSN, MSN
Gillette Children's Specialty Healthcare
St. Paul, MN

Cheryl Tveit, RN, MSN, CAPA
Gillette Children's Specialty Healthcare
St. Paul, MN

Preface

The skills performed by nurses exemplify the integration of knowledge, psychomotor dexterity, attitude, and critical thinking necessary for effective clinical practice in the 21st century. The eighth edition of *Skills in Clinical Nursing* has been revised, and updated to reflect the changes in practice that have occurred since the previous edition. It includes:

- The 166 most important skills performed by nurses, including all common variations, organized from the simple to the more complex. All skills have been revised to reflect current clinical practice.
- More than 800 illustrations. *Skills in Clinical Nursing* is intended as a primary textbook for nursing education programs and as a reference for practicing nurses. Content was selected based on feedback from reviewers of previous editions, market surveys, and the extensive teaching and practice experience of the authors.

All content was reviewed by practicing clinical nurses who provided invaluable firsthand knowledge of current practice.

FORMAT

Each chapter contains concise introductory material, placing the skills in perspective to client anatomy, physiology, and pathophysiology, and provides an overview of the rationale and purpose of the skills. The presentation of each skill follows the steps of the nursing process:

- A review of the **assessment** data required before performing the skill.
- During **diagnosing**, the second phase of the nursing process, the nurse uses critical thinking skills to interpret specific assessment data and identify the client's strengths and problems. The authors did not include this step of the nursing process for the skills in this book because the focus is on the skill and no specific client assessment data are included. Application of nursing diagnoses is reflected in each end-of-unit feature on the nursing process.

- As a component of the **planning** phase, information about when it is and is not appropriate to delegate each skill to unlicensed assistive personnel (UAP).
- **Implementation** steps, including client teaching, observation of standard infection prevention precautions, and client record documentation. Rationales are indicated by italic type.
- Considerations in **evaluation** of the skill, focusing on steps indicated for follow-up and communication with other members of the health care team.

NEW TO THE 8TH EDITION

- **Emphasis on QSEN!** The delivery of high-quality and safe nursing practice is imperative for every nurse. This edition has incorporated QSEN competencies and specified expectations in special QSEN features. These features highlight relevant information in patient-centered care, teamwork and collaboration, and safety.
  - Culturally Responsive Care
  - Ambulatory and Community Settings
  - Safety Alert
- **Updated art!** More than 150 new photos/drawings.
- **New! Interprofessional Practice** sections where relevant in specific skills. This feature reinforces to the student how other members of the health care team may be involved.
- Current CDC and WHO definitions and guidelines
- 2014 National Patient Safety Goals (NPSGs) for hospitals and long-term care
- 2013 CMS guidelines for use of restraints
- *Healthy People 2020* objectives for cholesterol, hypertension, and diabetes
- Updated Infusion Nurses Society guidelines
- Updated nursing standards and references (ANA, NPSG, etc.)

Features

Skills in Clinical Nursing continues to be a definitive resource for the most commonly performed nursing skills. This skills book is designed as an easy reference for both the classroom and clinical practice!

Skills are organized in a nursing process framework and include **step-by-step instructions**.

Critical steps are **visually represented** with full-color photos and illustrations.

Easy-to-find **rationales** provide a better understanding of why critical steps are performed.

●○● **NURSING PROCESS: DISCONTINUING INFUSIONS**

Discontinuing Infusion Devices

SKILL 18-6

ASSESSMENT
Assess:
• Appearance of the venipuncture site.
• Any bleeding from the infusion site.
• Amount of fluid infused.
• Appearance of IV catheter.

PLANNING
Review the client record regarding the primary care provider's orders. Note if there are any previous infusions and if there were any complications and how they were managed.

In many states, an LPN/LVN with special IV therapy training may discontinue IV infusions. Check the applicable state's nurse practice act.

DELEGATION

In some states and agencies, removal of a peripheral IV catheter may be delegated to UAP. In others, removal of IV infusions or devices is not delegated to UAP. In any case, the nurse must ensure that the UAP knows what complications or adverse signs following removal should be reported to the nurse.

Equipment
• Clean gloves
• Linen-saver pad
• Small sterile dressing and tape

IMPLEMENTATION
Performance
1. Prior to performing the procedure, introduce self and verify the client's identity using agency protocol. Explain to the client what you are going to do, why it is necessary, and how he or she can participate. Explain the reason for discontinuing the IV and that the procedure should cause no discomfort other than that associated with removing the tape.
2. Perform hand hygiene and observe other appropriate infection prevention procedures.
3. Assist the client to a comfortable position, either sitting or lying. Expose the IV site but provide for client privacy. Place a linen-saver pad under the extremity that has the IV.
4. Prepare the equipment.
   • Clamp the infusion tubing. **Rationale:** *Clamping the tubing prevents the fluid from flowing out of the IV catheter onto the client or bed.*
   • Apply clean gloves.
   • Remove the dressing, stabilization device, and tape at the venipuncture site while holding the IV catheter firmly and applying countertraction to the skin. ❶ **Rationale:** *Movement of the IV catheter can injure the vein and cause discomfort to the client.* Countertraction prevents pulling the ...mfort.

... site. **Rationale:** *Assess for signs of*

... above the venipuncture site. Only ... ortion of the gauze pad and maintain ...ttom) portion that is in contact with ...

... the vein.

...y pulling it out along the line of the ... ing it out in line with the vein avoids ...ein. Do not press down on the sterile ... ng the catheter.

... pressure to the site, using sterile ...es. **Rationale:** *Pressure helps stop* ...nts hematoma formation.

...ve heart level if any bleeding persists. ...mb decreases blood flow to the area. ...m the nurse if the site begins to ...client notes any other abnormalities

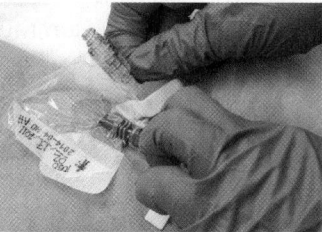

❶ Remove the dressing, stabilization device, and tape while holding the IV catheter firmly.

❷ Withdraw the IV catheter from the vein. Do not apply pressure on the sterile gauze pad until the catheter is completely removed.

Working with Implanted Vascular Access Devices—continued

SKILL 18-10

IMPLEMENTATION
Preparation
• Assemble the equipment.
• Attach the IV tubing to the infusion or transfusion container.
• Prime the infusion tubing with fluid.
• Prepare and label syringes of normal saline and heparinized saline. Connect the first of these to be used to the Huber needle. Saline followed by heparinized saline is used to flush the device before and after medications or periodically if not in use (check agency policy). **Rationale:** *Heparinized saline may help prevent clotting. There is also some risk of heparin-induced thrombocytopenia so that heparin is not used without clear policy.*

Performance
1. Prior to performing the procedure, introduce self and verify the client's identity using agency protocol. Explain to the client what you are going to do, why it is necessary, and how he or she can participate.
2. Perform hand hygiene and observe other appropriate infection prevention procedures.
3. Provide for client privacy and prepare the client.
   • Assist the client to a comfortable position, either sitting or lying. Expose the IVAD site but provide for client privacy.
4. Prepare the site.
   • Locate the IVAD device and its septum, the disk at the center of the port where the needle will be inserted.
   • Prepare the skin in accordance with agency policy and let the area dry after applying solutions.
   • Apply sterile gloves and mask.
   • *Optional:* Inject 2% lidocaine subcutaneously over the needle insertion site. **Rationale:** *This anesthetizes the area for injection.* It may be ordered during the first few weeks after the implant surgery, when the area is tender and swollen and more pain from the needle puncture is felt. Other topical anesthetics may be used.
   • An ice pack may be placed over the site for several minutes to reduce discomfort from the needle puncture.
5. Insert the Huber needle.
   • Grasp the base of the IVAD device between two fingers of your nondominant hand to stabilize it. IVADs may have top entry or side entry ports, depending on the design.

• Infuse the saline flush. There should be no discomfort or sign of subcutaneous infiltration with infusion of the flush.
6. Prevent manipulation or dislodgment of the needle.
   • If the needle will remain in place for longer than needed to withdraw a blood sample or flush an unused port, secure the needle.
   • Support the Huber needle with 2×2 dressings and apply an occlusive transparent dressing to the needle site. Some manufacturers' devices include a safety lock to decrease accidental needlesticks and a client comfort pad that sits between the needle hub and the skin.
   • Loop and tape the tubing. **Rationale:** *Looping prevents tension on the needle.*
7. Attach infusion tubing or an intermittent infusion access cap to the Huber needle.
   • A Huber needle can remain in place for 1 week before it needs to be changed.
8. After use, perform a final flush with heparinized saline.
   • When flushing, maintain positive pressure, and clamp the tubing immediately before the flush is finished. **Rationale:** *These actions avoid reflux of the heparinized saline.*

Variation: Obtaining a Blood Specimen
To obtain a blood specimen:
• Withdraw 10 mL of blood (or an amount according to agency policy) and discard it. **Rationale:** *This initial specimen may be diluted with saline and heparin from previous flushes.*
• Draw up the required amount of blood and transfer it to the appropriate containers.
• Slowly instill 10 mL of normal saline, according to agency policy. **Rationale:** *This thoroughly flushes the catheter of blood.*
• Inject 5 mL of heparin flush solution to prevent clotting.
9. Remove and discard gloves.
   • Perform hand hygiene.
10. Document all relevant information.
    • Record the appearance of the IVAD site, any difficulty accessing the port and interventions used, presence of drainage, the type of dressing applied, infusions given, and client complaints or concerns. Note any clinical signs indicating venous thrombosis (pain in the neck, arm, and/or

Variations present alternative methods of performing certain skills.

DELEGATION

Due to the need for sterile technique and technical complexity, use of infusion devices is not delegated to UAP. UAP may care for clients with such devices, and the nurse must ensure that the UAP knows how to perform routine tasks such as positioning and changing gowns when a device is in place. The UAP should also know what complications or adverse signs, such as alarms, should be reported to the nurse. In many states, an LPN/LVN with special IV therapy training may manage infusions. Check the state's nurse practice act.

NEW!
Interprofessional Practice reinforces interactions with other members of the health care team.

INTERPROFESSIONAL PRACTICE

Sterile fields and procedures may be within the scope of practice for many health care providers. These providers may perform the procedure independently or with a nurse or other provider. Although these providers may verbally communicate about the procedure to the health care team members, the nurse must also know where to locate their documentation in the client's medical record.

Delegation highlights guidelines of when it is appropriate and how to delegate skills to unlicensed assistive personnel (UAP).

INCLUDES CLINICALLY RELEVANT INFORMATION!

QSEN features provide guidance on maintaining safety and quality of nursing care.

Culturally Responsive Care | PATIENT-CENTERED CARE

Ethnopharmacology

Drug response can be affected by ancestry. Until recently, clinical drug research was conducted on Caucasian males even when the health disorder being studied was prevalent in other ethnic groups. Research has shown that one size does *not* fit all.

IMPLICATIONS FOR NURSING INTERVENTIONS

- Remember that there may be differences in medication responses among different ethnic groups and differences *within* ethnic groups.
- Avoid profiling and stereotyping.
- Ask about health beliefs, values, and customs/practices.
- Be accepting of differences in cultural beliefs and practices.

- Conduct a cultural assessment with each client.
- Learn about drug effects (including adverse effects) that are related to ancestry.
- Ask the client direct, specific questions to reveal the presence or absence of potential adverse effects of medications.
- Monitor the client and document findings carefully, because it may be possible to maintain therapeutic benefit at a lower dosage of a given drug.
- Implement a treatment plan with the client and family that is consistent with their cultural and traditional beliefs while incorporating the necessary modern treatments.
- Keep cultural context in mind when planning education for clients and families.

Culturally Responsive Care boxes focus on approaches and techniques for a diverse client population.

Ambulatory and Community Settings provide information about performing skills in different health care settings.

Ambulatory and Community Settings   **Administering Medications** | PATIENT-CENTERED CARE

The nurse should instruct the client to:

- Learn the names of the medications as well as their actions and possible adverse effects. Carry a complete list of all prescriptions, OTC medications, and home remedies at all times.
- Keep all medications out of reach of children and pets.
- If using a syringe to administer the medication to an infant or child, remove and dispose of the plastic cap that fits on the end of the syringe. Infants and small children have been known to choke on these caps.
- Take the medications only as prescribed. Know which medications need to be taken on an empty stomach and which can be taken with food/meals. Immediately consult the nurse, pharmacist, or primary care provider about any problems with the medication.
- Always check the medication label to make sure the correct medication is being taken.
- Request labels printed with larger type on medication containers if there is difficulty reading the label.
- Check the expiration date and discard outdated medications. Previously, most people discarded old medicines by flushing them down the toilet. The Environmental Protection Agency (EPA) no longer recommends this. Inform clients to check with their local government. Many cities and towns have household

hazardous waste facilities where they can take their old medicines. The expired medications may be placed in the trash if the following precautions are used: Keep the medication in the original container and mark out the person's name. Add a nontoxic but bad tasting product (e.g., cayenne pepper, mustard) to the container to keep individuals or animals from eating it. Place in a sturdy container, tape the container shut, and have this container be the last thing put in the garbage can.

- Ask the pharmacist to substitute childproof caps with ones that are more easily opened, as necessary.
- If a dose or more is missed, do not take two or more doses; ask the pharmacist or primary care provider for directions.
- Do not crush or cut a tablet or capsule without first checking with the primary care provider or pharmacist. Doing so may affect the medication's absorption.
- Never stop taking the medication without first discussing it with the primary care provider.
- Always check with the pharmacist before taking any nonprescription medications. Some OTC medications can interact with the prescribed medication.

Additionally, the nurse can set up a medication plan to assist clients and family members to remember a schedule. Weekly pill containers (available at pharmacies) or a written plan may be helpful.

SAFETY ALERT! | SAFETY

2014 The Joint Commission National Patient Safety Goals (2013a)

GOAL 3: MAINTAIN AND COMMUNICATE ACCURATE CLIENT MEDICATION INFORMATION.

Rationale: *There is evidence that medication discrepancies can affect client outcomes.* Medication reconciliation is intended to identify and resolve discrepancies—it is a process of comparing the medications a client is taking (and should be taking) with newly ordered medications. The comparison addresses duplication, omissions, and interactions, and the need to continue current medications.

Safety Alerts correlate to the National Patient Safety Goals and identify other crucial safety information.

CLINICAL MANIFESTATIONS

Fever

- Increased heart rate
- Increased respiratory rate and depth
- Shivering
- Pallid, cold skin (during onset)
- Complaints of feeling cold (during onset)
- "Gooseflesh" appearance of the skin (during onset)
- Glassy-eyed appearance
- Flushed, warm skin
- Sweating

Clinical Manifestations outline the signs and symptoms nurses will encounter in clinical practice.

Dermatologic Medication Administration

POWDER

Make sure the skin surface is dry. Spread apart any skinfolds, and sprinkle the site until the area is covered with a fine *thin* layer. Cover the site with a dressing if ordered.

SUSPENSION-BASED LOTION

Shake the container before use to distribute suspended particles. Put a little lotion on a small gauze dressing or pad, and apply the lotion to the skin by stroking it evenly in the direction of the hair growth.

CREAMS, OINTMENTS, PASTES, AND OIL-BASED LOTIONS

Warm and soften the preparation in gloved hands to make it easier to apply and to prevent chilling (if a large area is to be treated). Smear it evenly over the skin using long strokes that follow the direction of the hair growth. Explain that the skin may feel somewhat greasy after application. Apply a sterile dressing if ordered by the primary care provider.

AEROSOL SPRAY

Shake the container well to mix the contents. Hold the spray container at the recommended distance from the area (usually about 15 to 30 cm [6 to 12 in.] but check the label). Cover the client's face with a towel if the upper chest or neck is to be sprayed. Spray the medication over the specified area.

TRANSDERMAL PATCHES

Select a clean, dry area that is free of hair and matches the manufacturer's recommendations. Remove the patch from its protective covering, holding it without touching the adhesive edges, and apply it by pressing firmly with the palm of the hand for about 10 seconds. Advise the client to avoid using a heating pad over the area to prevent an increase in circulation and the rate of absorption. Remove the patch at the appropriate time, folding it so that the sticky, medicated sides are together. Some patches contain nonvisible metal in their backing. This may cause burning in the area of the patch. Inform clients to tell MRI personnel that they are wearing a transdermal patch (MRIsafety.com, 2012).

Practice Guidelines provide instant access summaries of common procedures and clinical practice.

Client Teaching Considerations give tips and tools to help clients facilitate self-care and wellness.

Infection Prevention

Describe ways to manipulate the bed, the room, and other household facilities to prevent injury or to contain possible cross contamination.

- Instruct to clean obviously soiled linen separately from other laundry. Wash in hot water if possible, adding a cup of bleach or phenol-based disinfectant such as Lysol concentrate to the wash, and rinse in cold water.
- Based on assessment of client and family knowledge, teach proper hand hygiene (e.g., before handling foods, before eating, after toileting, before and after any required home care treatment, and after touching any body substances such as wound drainage) and related hygienic measures to all family members.
- Promote nail care. Keep fingernails short, clean, and well manicured to eliminate rough edges or hangnails, which can harbor microorganisms.
- Instruct not to share personal care items such as toothbrushes or used washcloths and towels. Describe how infections can be transmitted from shared personal items.
- Discuss antimicrobial soaps and effective disinfectants.
- Discuss the relationship between hygiene, rest, activity, and nutrition in the chain of infection.

- Instruct about cleaning reusable equipment and supplies. Use soap and water, and disinfect with a chlorine bleach solution.
- Teach the client and family members the signs and symptoms of infection, and when to contact a health care provider. Determine by verbal questions the level of understanding of the topic after each teaching session.
- Teach the client and family members how to avoid infections.
- Suggest techniques for safe food preservation and preparation (e.g., wash raw fruits and vegetables before eating them, refrigerate all opened and unpackaged foods).
- Remind to avoid coughing, sneezing, or breathing directly on others. Cover the mouth and nose to prevent the transmission of airborne microorganisms.
- Inform of the importance of maintaining sufficient fluid intake to promote urine production and output. This helps flush the bladder and urethra of microorganisms.
- Emphasize the need for proper immunizations of all family members.

Lifespan Considerations present age-related content to alert you to differences in caring for clients.

INFANTS/CHILDREN

- Assess risk for falls (age, mental status, medications, physical and mental impairments).
- Encourage parents to change the infant's diaper on a soft towel placed on the floor.
- Use changing tables and cribs with properly padded sides and rails.
- Use home safety devices, such as guards on windows that are above ground level, stair gates, and guard rails to help keep an active child from taking a dangerous fall.

OLDER ADULTS

- Assess for potential personal causes of falls: hypotension, unsteady gait, altered mental responsiveness (such as from medications), poor vision, foot pathology, unsafe footwear (loose, poorly fitting, slippery bottoms, high heels, rough edges), cognitive changes, and fear.

- In the home or community setting, assess for potential environmental causes of falls:
  - *Lighting:* inadequate amount, inaccessible or inconvenient switches
  - *Floors:* presence of electrical cords, loose rugs, clutter, slippery surfaces
  - *Stairs:* absent or unsteady railings, uneven step height or surfaces
  - *Furniture:* unsteady base, lack of armrests, cabinets too high or too low
  - *Bathroom:* inappropriate toilet height, slippery floors or tub, absence of grab bars.
- In the home, consider alternatives to a hospital or regular bed if the client is extremely prone to falling out of bed:
  - Place the mattress directly onto the floor.
  - Use a water mattress.
  - Place padding on the floor next to the bed or between the client and side rails.

Clinical Alerts highlight important information such as high risk situations.

Normal saline must always be used when giving a blood transfusion. If the client has an infusion of any other IV solution, stop that infusion and flush the line with saline prior to initiating the transfusion, or establish IV access through an additional site. Solutions other than saline can cause damage to the blood components.

FOCUS ON CLINICAL THINKING!

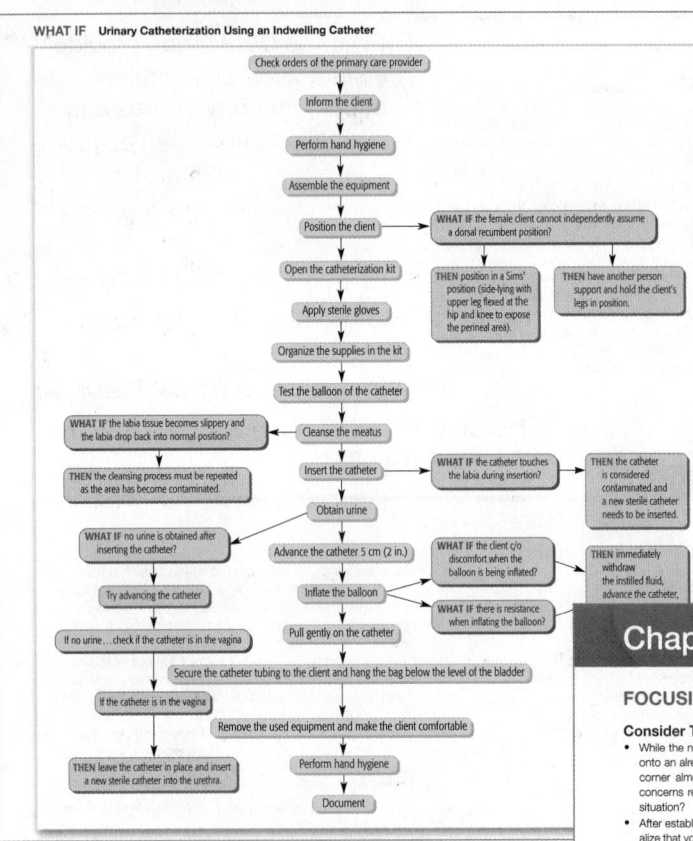

WHAT IF Urinary Catheterization Using an Indwelling Catheter

Check orders of the primary care provider
→ Inform the client
→ Perform hand hygiene
→ Assemble the equipment
→ Position the client

WHAT IF the female client cannot independently assume a dorsal recumbent position?

THEN position in a Sims' position (side-lying with upper leg flexed at the hip and knee to expose the perineal area).

THEN have another person support and hold the client's legs in position.

→ Open the catheterization kit
→ Apply sterile gloves
→ Organize the supplies in the kit
→ Test the balloon of the catheter

WHAT IF the labia tissue becomes slippery and the labia drop back into normal position?

THEN the cleansing process must be repeated as the area has become contaminated.

→ Cleanse the meatus
→ Insert the catheter

WHAT IF the catheter touches the labia during insertion?

THEN the catheter is considered contaminated and a new sterile catheter needs to be inserted.

→ Obtain urine

WHAT IF no urine is obtained after inserting the catheter?

→ Try advancing the catheter

→ Advance the catheter 5 cm (2 in.)

WHAT IF the client c/o discomfort when the balloon is being inflated?

THEN immediately withdraw the instilled fluid, advance the catheter,

→ Inflate the balloon

WHAT IF there is resistance when inflating the balloon?

If no urine…check if the catheter is in the vagina
→ Pull gently on the catheter
→ Secure the catheter tubing to the client and hang the bag below the level of the bladder

If the catheter is in the vagina
→ Remove the used equipment and make the client comfortable

THEN leave the catheter in place and insert a new sterile catheter into the urethra.

→ Perform hand hygiene
→ Document

UNIQUE! What If … concept maps visually represent the flow of a skill and present options for unexpected outcomes.

Focusing on Clinical Thinking at the end of every chapter promotes critical thinking with application-oriented scenarios and questions.

Chapter **7** Review

FOCUSING ON CLINICAL THINKING

Consider This
- While the nurse is dropping commercially packaged sterile gauze onto an already established sterile field, the gauze lands with one corner almost off the edge of the field. Does this present any concerns regarding its sterility? If so, how would you handle the situation?
- After establishing a sterile field and applying sterile gloves, you realize that you have forgotten to open the bottle of saline that needs to be poured into a bowl on the field. The bottle is not sterile on the outside. What are two ways you could solve this dilemma?

- A client is being admitted to the hospital with a diagnosis of severe diarrhea, unknown origin. What infection prevention precautions would be appropriate at this time?
- You are assigned to care for a client who has a disseminated herpes zoster infection (shingles). In reviewing the agency infection prevention manual, you learn that individuals who have not had chickenpox should not enter this client's room. Individuals who have had chickenpox or a blood titer indicating immunity to chickenpox may interact with the client. Explain why this is the case.

See Focusing on Clinical Thinking answers on student resource website.

TEST YOUR KNOWLEDGE

1. The nurse knows that any substance can serve as an intermediate means to transport and introduce an infectious agent into a susceptible host through a suitable portal of entry. Which term best describes this type of transmission?
   1. Direct transmission
   2. Vehicle-borne transmission
   3. Airborne transmission
   4. Vector-borne transmission
2. Which statement, if made by a nurse, indicates the need for further teaching about the six links in the chain of infection?
   1. "The goal of infection prevention measures is to break the chain whenever and wherever possible so that disease is not [spread] from one person to another."
   [2. Transm]ission can occur through touching, biting, [sex]ual intercourse."
   [3. Tran]smission may involve droplets or dust."
   [4. Transm]ission can be either vehicle-borne or [...]
   [...trin]g to establish a sterile field. Which technique, [...]se, could compromise the maintenance of the

4. Which technique of applying sterile gloves indicates a good understanding of this technique? Select all that apply.
   1. Place the package of gloves on a clean, dry surface.
   2. Open the outer package without contaminating the gloves or the inner package.
   3. Put the first glove on the nondominant hand.
   4. Pick up the other glove with the sterile gloved hand, inserting the gloved fingers under the cuff and holding the gloved thumb close to the gloved palm.
   5. Once both gloves are on, unroll any portion of the cuff that had been caught during application.
5. A nurse is caring for a client with tuberculosis. The transmission-based precautions used are in addition to standard precautions. Which of the following would the nurse use and be consistent with infection prevention guidelines? Select all that apply.
   1. A surgical mask at all times while in the client's room
   2. An N95 respirator mask when within 1 m (3 ft) of the client
   3. Gloves for all contact with the client
   4. Hand hygiene before applying and after removing gloves
   5. A gown when performing a physical examination of the client
6. A nurse is assigned to care for a client on contact precautions.

Test Your Knowledge helps you prepare for the NCLEX-RN® exam. Alternate-style questions are included.

UNIT 6

Applying the Nursing Process

This unit explores skills related to nutrition and elimination. Meeting the client's nutritional needs is essential to promoting health, preventing illness, and enhancing recovery from injury and disease. Urinary and bowel elimination are basic human needs that can be affected by illness, injury, medications, and treatments. The nurse plays an important role in assessing and maintaining nutrition and elimination when providing client care in any setting.

Client: Michael   AGE: 78 Years   CURRENT MEDICAL DIAGNOSIS: Cerebrovascular Accident, Hypertension, Chronic Renal Failure

Medical History: Michael, 78 years old, is an African American who emigrated from Sierra Leone 12 years ago. He was diagnosed with hypertension at age 35 and was intermittently compliant with his treatment plan, often choosing to stop taking his antihypertensive medication because he "felt fine" and didn't think he needed it. He was diagnosed with chronic renal failure 10 years ago, and his kidney function has steadily declined. Two weeks ago while playing cards at home he suddenly lost sensation and function on the left side of his body. He was rushed to the emergency department where he was diagnosed with a cerebrovascular accident (stroke). When his condition stabilized he was transferred to a rehabilitation facility where he receives occupational and physical therapy as well as assistance with meeting his self-care needs. He takes hydrochlorothiazide 50 mg and atenolol 100 mg PO daily to control his hypertension, and furosemide 40 mg PO daily to improve urine output. Michael has developed dysphagia, constipation, and occasional urinary incontinence.

Personal and Social History: Michael is married and has four grown children and 10 grandchildren. Two of his children live nearby. His wife is anxious for him to recover enough to return home. They live in a two-story detached home.

Questions

Assessment
1. What assessment data will the nurse collect related to the client's nutritional and elimination status?

Analysis
2. List two possible nursing diagnoses that can be identified from the medical/personal history and assessment data above related to nutrition and/or elimination.

Planning
3. Based on the assessment data and nursing diagnoses, identify one desired outcome.
4. Identify the action verb, measurable criteria, and time line for the outcome.

Implementation
5. What interventions can the nurse provide to improve Michael's ability to meet nutritional requirements?
6. What interventions can the nurse provide to treat Michael's constipation?
7. Suggest interventions to reduce urinary incontinence.

Evaluation
8. What data might the nurse collect to indicate the desired outcome has been met?

See Applying the Nursing Process suggested answers on student resource website.

End-of-Unit **Applying the Nursing Process** activities provide the opportunity to think through themes and competencies presented across chapters in a unit and think critically to link theory to nursing practice.

Contents

Introduction

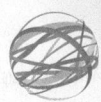

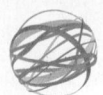 # 1 Foundational Skills

LEARNING OUTCOMES

At the completion of this chapter, the student will be able to:

1. Define the key terms used in foundational skills and equipment that protect nurses and clients.
2. Recognize when it is appropriate to delegate skills to unlicensed assistive personnel.
3. Identify indications for standard precautions and hand hygiene.
4. Describe factors that affect the use of personal protective equipment such as gloves, gowns, masks, and eyewear.
5. Verbalize the steps used in:
   a. Using standard precautions.
   b. Performing hand hygiene.
   c. Applying and removing personal protective equipment (gown, mask, eyewear, gloves).
   d. Assisting with invasive procedures.
6. Demonstrate appropriate disposal of equipment and supplies.
7. Demonstrate appropriate documentation and recording of foundational skills.

SKILLS

Skill 1–1 Using Standard Precautions
Skill 1–2 Performing Hand Washing

Skill 1–3 Applying and Removing Personal Protective Equipment (Gown, Mask, Eyewear, Gloves)
Skill 1–4 Assisting with Invasive Procedures

KEY TERMS

bloodborne pathogens, 5
delegation, 3
documenting, 15
health care–associated infections (HAIs), 6
nosocomial infections, 6

personal protective equipment (PPE), 4
positive affirmation, 7
respiratory hygiene/cough etiquette, 5
self-care, 2

Situation, Background, Assessment, and Recommendation (SBAR) process, 15
standard precautions (SP), 4
therapeutic presence, 2

unlicensed assistive personnel (UAP), 3

This chapter introduces the skills that are fundamental to all nursing care. Because nursing is both art and science, attention is given to a variety of skills that create healing environments for clients. A caring approach to any and all nurse–client encounters is a foundational skill. The holistic caring process involves attention to the body–mind–spirit nature of self and client, the environment around and within individuals, and relationships with clients and colleagues that facilitate healing.

CREATING AND MAINTAINING THE HEALING ENVIRONMENT

Creating environments in which clients can experience healing takes a great deal of skill. Nurses provide sustenance, comfort, and safety. Therefore, nurses are instruments of healing and must stay "in tune" in order to be maximally effective. This requires nurses to attend to their own **self-care** on a daily basis. Engaging in a regular movement or exercise discipline, paying attention to healthy nutrition, practicing clear communication, cultivating positive relationships, and taking regular meal and rest breaks while on the job are examples of self-care. The more time nurses give to self-care, the more they will cultivate their ability to be mindful and therapeutically present to their clients.

Florence Nightingale addressed the concept of **therapeutic presence** in her writings for nurses when she emphasized deep listening, compassion, focus, self-awareness, finding meaning, and using the imagination (Dossey, 2009). Nurse theorist Jean Watson (2013) described therapeutic presence as using caring intentions, intuitive and loving connections, self-awareness, and a centered, mindful focus. To be mindful is to be fully focused in the present moment. Mindful presence on the nurse's part amplifies the therapeutic effects of nursing skills offered to clients. The use of deep breathing and positive imagery facilitates mindfulness.

Holistic nursing care embraces the whole nature of clients by offering skills that address the body–mind–spirit interconnectedness of individuals. The psychosocial, emotional, and spiritual issues that arise in clients who have any kind of disruption in physical or mental health must be taken into account during each client encounter. To ignore this totality can lead to an objectification of the client and a mechanized style of nursing care—a "doing to" approach rather than a therapeutic, "doing with" partnership. This focus on the quality of the nurse–client relationship is a hallmark of holistic practice. In such a caring relationship, emphasis on respect and ethical practice is essential. This is the art of nursing, and it takes a great deal of skill.

Clinical skills such as the ones included in this book can be offered in ways that are holistic. The attitude and intention of the nurse offering the skill make a critical difference. Though nurses may have performed any given skill many times, it may be the first time for the client. The client will most likely feel threatened and anxious to some degree. Technical competence alone, though reassuring, will not facilitate healing unless it is delivered with kindness and compassion. Therapeutic communication skills enable nurses to offer technical skills in ways that will facilitate healing. *Holistic Nursing: A Handbook for Clinical Practice* (Dossey & Keegan, 2013) is an excellent resource for therapeutic communication processes and skills.

Touch therapies, mind–body skills, and spiritual care are basic skills that all nurses should be prepared to offer. Indeed, The Joint Commission, the organization that accredits hospitals, specifies that a spiritual assessment should be conducted on all clients. Guided imagery, massage, and progressive muscle relaxation skills are detailed in Chapter 9 ∞ of this text, and many more skills can be learned and practiced at the nurse's discretion to facilitate healing. To focus on body parts or disease processes may facilitate curing, but will not facilitate whole-person healing. Many organizations, including the World Health Organization (WHO), American Nurses Association (ANA), International Council of Nurses, and American Association of Colleges of Nursing, specify the importance of spiritual care.

CLINICAL ALERT!

All nurses must learn to provide culturally and spiritually responsive care.

Some nursing skills are performed directly—the nurse provides the care to the client. Other nursing care is indirect—the care is provided to the client by another nurse or by **unlicensed assistive personnel (UAP)**, such as nursing assistants. Indirect care may be entrusted (delegated) to others only if certain conditions exist; the process of delegating nursing care is described in this chapter. The quality of the relationships among members of the health care team directly affects the quality of care provided. As team leaders, nurses can attend to building environments where the worth and value of each provider are affirmed, where continuing education and curiosity are encouraged, and where accountability is fostered. The interpersonal skills of the nurse are foundational to the provision of effective, safe nursing care.

At the same time as health care team member communication is encouraged, client confidentiality must be protected at all times. This is essential not only because of Health Insurance Portability and Accountability Act (HIPAA) privacy regulations, but because it is the ethical and respectful way to practice nursing.

ALERT! | SAFETY

Respectful, clear, and thorough communication increases safety in clinical environments.

Florence Nightingale wrote extensively about promoting innate healing ability within each client by attending to the environment. By ensuring proper light, fresh air, quiet, wholesome nutrition, and soothing interactions, she believed that individuals would be put in

---

Culturally Responsive Care | **PATIENT-CENTERED CARE**

Cultural Considerations in Health Care

It is imperative for nurses to remember the unfamiliar and overwhelming nature of health care settings. Most clients are uncomfortable in a clinical environment, especially when they are undergoing procedures, hearing unfamiliar terminology, and receiving care from people who may be wearing masks and gloves. In addition, what if English is not a client's primary language or if the client is deaf? In these types of situations, the challenges to the client's psychoemotional and even physical safety increase. When clarity of communication is compromised, therapeutic efficacy and client safety are compromised. It is essential to clarify all aspects of care with clients, and to provide trained interpreters whenever necessary. It is also necessary for members of the health care team to make sure that they understand each other, because English may not be the primary language of every nurse, UAP, physician, or other health care provider. Asking for clarification frequently and not making assumptions are two habits that can help prevent clinical care errors. When in doubt, ask.

When it comes to cultural diversity, it is especially important to ask the client about nutritional and exercise patterns, health and healing practices, family organization and roles, social support network, spiritual and religious beliefs and practices, communication styles, gender relation patterns, and attitudes toward individuals in authority. Personal space issues, time orientation, and the client's explanation of his or her health status are also important to explore.

For essential resources regarding cultural considerations in health care environments, search the Internet for culturally and linguistically appropriate services (CLAS) for health care settings. *Holistic nursing: A handbook for clinical practice* (Dossey & Keegan, 2013) also includes resources and cultural assessments for nurses to incorporate into their admissions and clinical care processes.

---

the best position for nature to assist in the healing process (Dossey, 2009). She even wrote about the benefits of pet-assisted therapy, music, color, nature, and spiritual care.

DELEGATION

Delegation is the transfer of responsibility and authority for an activity to a competent individual. RNs increasingly delegate components of nursing care to other health care workers, especially UAP. These "nurse extenders" may be individuals identified as certified nursing aides/assistants, home health aides, client care technicians, orderlies, surgical technicians, or a variety of other titles. They have diverse degrees of training and experience. They are employees and do not include family members or friends who provide some client care. Each state nurse practice act specifies which actions constitute the legal practice of nursing, which actions are the purview only of nurses, and which actions may be delegated to others. In nursing, delegation refers to indirect care—the intended outcome is achieved through the work of someone supervised by a nurse.

It is not possible to generate an exhaustive list of exactly which actions may or may not be delegated to UAP. Examples of tasks that may and may not be delegated are enumerated in Box 1–1. A statement regarding delegation is included with the steps for each skill in this book.

The unlicensed person may not delegate tasks to another person. Principles guiding the nurse's decision to delegate ensure the

BOX 1–1	Examples of Tasks That May and May Not Be Delegated to Unlicensed Assistive Personnel

TASKS THAT *MAY* BE DELEGATED TO UNLICENSED ASSISTIVE PERSONNEL	TASKS THAT *MAY NOT* BE DELEGATED TO UNLICENSED ASSISTIVE PERSONNEL
• Taking of vital signs • Measuring and recording intake and output • Client transfers and ambulation • Postmortem care • Bathing • Feeding • Gastrostomy feedings in established systems • Attending to safety • Weighing • Performing simple dressing changes • Suctioning of chronic tracheostomies • Performing basic life support (CPR)	• Assessment • Interpretation of data • Making a nursing diagnosis • Creation of a nursing care plan • Evaluation of care effectiveness • Care of invasive lines • Administering parenteral medications • Insertion of nasogastric tubes • Client education • Performing triage • Giving telephone advice

safety and quality of outcomes (Box 1–2). Once the decision has been made to delegate, the nurse must communicate clearly to the UAP and verify that the UAP understands:

- The specific tasks to be done for each client.
- When each task is to be done.
- The expected outcomes for each task, including parameters outside of which the unlicensed person must immediately report to the nurse (and any action that must urgently be taken).
- Who is available to serve as a resource if needed.
- When and in what format (written or verbal) a report on the tasks is expected.

A specific task that can be delegated to one UAP may not be appropriate for a different UAP, depending on the UAP's experience and individual skill sets. Also, a task that is appropriate for the UAP to perform with one client may not be appropriate with a different client or the same client under altered circumstances. For example, routine vital signs may be delegated to the UAP for a client in stable condition but would not be delegated for the same client who has become unstable.

It is important to note that the nurse is not held legally responsible for the acts of the unlicensed person, but is always accountable for the quality of the act of delegation and has the ultimate responsibility for ensuring that proper care is provided. Delegation can be an extremely useful strategy in providing thorough and effective nursing care. Skill in delegation, however, must be learned and developed over time. The ANA website includes reference materials addressing RN

delegation to UAP and LPN/LVN staff. The nurse should not hesitate to consult with others regarding the appropriateness of delegation.

STANDARD PRECAUTIONS

Preventing the transmission of potentially infective organisms among the nurse, the client, and other individuals is a priority. Prevention begins with implementation of **standard precautions (SP)**. SP include (a) hand hygiene; (b) use of **personal protective equipment (PPE)**, which includes gloves, gowns, eyewear, and masks; (c) safe injection practices; (d) safe handling of potentially contaminated equipment or surfaces in the client environment; and (e) respiratory hygiene/cough etiquette. This chapter focuses on the use of standard infection precautions, the practice of proper hand hygiene, and the use of PPE, which are fundamental skills and are used with all clients. Further information about caring for clients who are known to have infections is found in Chapter 7 ∞.

Microorganisms occur normally in various locations of the human body such as the surface of the skin and the gastrointestinal tract. Usually, they do not cause infection in the client. When the microorganisms enter a different part of the client's body, or the client's immune system is suppressed, infection may occur. Also, these same microorganisms could cause infection in another person. Because it is not always possible to know which clients may have infectious organisms, guidelines have been established by the Centers for Disease Control and Prevention (CDC), Occupational Safety and Health Administration

BOX 1–2	Principles Used by the Nurse to Determine Delegation to Unlicensed Assistive Personnel

1. The nurse must assess the individual client prior to delegating tasks.
2. The client must be medically stable or in a chronic condition and not fragile.
3. The task must be considered routine for this client.
4. The task must not require a substantial amount of scientific knowledge or technical skill.
5. The task must be considered safe for this client.
6. The task must have a predictable outcome.
7. Learn the agency's procedures and policies regarding delegation.
8. Know the scope of practice and the customary knowledge, skills, and job description for each health care discipline represented on your team.
9. Be aware of individual variations in work abilities. Each individual has different experiences and may not be capable of performing every task cited in the job description.
10. When unsure about an assistant's abilities to perform a task, observe while the person performs it, or demonstrate it to the person and get a return demonstration before allowing the person to perform it independently.
11. Clarify reporting expectations to ensure the task is completed.
12. Create an atmosphere that fosters communication, teaching, and learning. For example, encourage staff to ask questions, listen carefully to their concerns, and make use of every opportunity to teach.
13. Know your state's regulations regarding UAP practice and the legal aspects of nurse supervision of UAP.

(OSHA), and other organizations outlining steps all health care workers must follow to reduce the chances that potentially infectious organisms in blood (**bloodborne pathogens**) and from other body tissues will be transmitted from the client to other individuals. The guidelines contain a two-tiered approach. The most basic approach is standard precautions. Some agencies may use an earlier term—universal precautions—reflecting their applicability in all client care situations. If the client is known to have an infection, transmission-based precautions are used to protect the nurse and others from acquiring the infectious organism (see Skill 7–3 in Chapter 7 ∞).

The CDC publishes recommendations for hospitals that reinforce the need for effective hand hygiene, PPE, and environmental controls. These include **respiratory hygiene/cough etiquette**, which calls for covering the mouth and nose when sneezing or coughing, proper disposal of tissues, and separating potentially infected individuals from others by at least 1 m (3 ft) or having them wear a surgical mask. Health care professionals use SP when providing care to all clients (Skill 1–1). That is, the risk of caregiver exposure to client body tissues and fluids rather than the suspected presence or absence of infectious organisms determines the use of clean gloves, gowns, masks, and eye protection.

●○○● NURSING PROCESS: STANDARD PRECAUTIONS

Using Standard Precautions

SKILL 1–1

ASSESSMENT
- All health care providers use SP with all clients.
- SP apply when the provider could come into contact with (a) blood; (b) all body fluids, excretions, and secretions except sweat; (c) nonintact (broken) skin; and (d) mucous membranes.

PLANNING
Consider the procedures about to be performed and determine which aspects require SP. Gather all necessary equipment. Review the steps of SP as indicated.

DELEGATION

The technique of using SP is identical for all health care providers, including UAP. All health care team members must be aware and accountable so that appropriate SPs are implemented in all health care situations.

INTERPROFESSIONAL PRACTICE

The use of SP is an essential skill for all health care providers. In some states, failure to follow infection prevention practices is a violation of the practice act for nurses and other health care providers. OSHA's Whistleblower Protection Program protects the rights of providers who report another provider for violation of workplace safety mandates such as SP from any form of retaliation.

Equipment
Depending on the specific aspects of the procedures, have available PPE:
- Clean gloves
- Waterproof gown
- Eye protection/goggles
- Mask (Surgical masks are generally adequate. However, for clients suspected of having certain conditions such as tuberculosis or H1N1 influenza, an N95 particulate respirator mask may be required. N95 masks must be tested on each individual nurse to ensure that they are fitted and adjusted correctly.)

IMPLEMENTATION
Performance
1. Remove or secure all loose items such as name tags or jewelry.
2. If PPE will be used, explain to the client why this is necessary and that SP are performed with all clients. **Rationale:** *Clients may feel alienated, fearful, or even ashamed when staff members use this equipment. Masks block facial expressions, and being touched by gloved hands feels different. It will help clients to understand that SPs are used to protect both clients and health care workers.*
3. Perform hand hygiene before applying PPE.
4. Wear gloves during contact that could involve blood, body fluids, secretions, excretions, and contaminated objects. See Skill 1–3.
5. Perform hand hygiene after contact with blood, body fluids, secretions, excretions, and contaminated objects (linens, dressings, instruments, or any other items that have come in contact with potentially infective material) whether or not gloves are worn. Always cleanse hands after the removal of PPE. **Rationale:** *Gloves can develop invisible holes during use. Moisture that collects on hands under gloves promotes the growth of microorganisms.*
6. Wear a mask, eye protection, or a face shield and a clean, waterproof gown during client care that could involve splashes or sprays of blood, body fluids, secretions, or excretions. See Skill 1–3.
7. Ensure that objects that have come in contact with blood, body fluids, secretions, or excretions are disposed of or cleaned properly. Check labels and/or institutional procedure manuals for details regarding proper disposal or decontamination.
8. Place used needles and other "sharps" directly into puncture-resistant containers as soon as their use is completed. Do not attempt to recap needles or place sharps back in their sheaths using two hands. **Rationale:** *Recapping can result in a needlestick/puncture injury if the nurse accidentally misses the cover.*
9. Handle all soiled linen as little as possible. Do not shake it. Bundle it up with the clean side out and dirty side in, and hold it away from yourself so that your uniform or clothing is not contaminated (soiled).
10. Place all human tissue and laboratory specimens in leakproof containers. If the outside of the container becomes contaminated, place the container inside another sealable container prior to transport.

Continued on page 6

Using Standard Precautions—*continued*

EVALUATION

Health care workers can be exposed to potentially infective materials through puncture wounds, direct contact with broken skin or wounds, or mucous membrane contact. Contact between potentially infective material and intact skin is not normally considered a risk for transmission of infection. If there is concern that the exposure has a significant risk for transmission of bloodborne pathogens such as hepatitis or human immunodeficiency virus (HIV) due to the large volume of material or percutaneous (through the skin) exposure, the nurse should follow the steps in the accompanying Practice Guidelines.

PRACTICE GUIDELINES

Steps to Follow After Exposure to Bloodborne Pathogens

- Report the incident immediately to appropriate personnel within the agency.
- Complete an incident report.
- Seek appropriate evaluation and follow-up. This includes:
  - Identification and documentation of the source individual when feasible and legal.
  - Testing of the source individual's blood for hepatitis B, hepatitis C, and HIV when feasible and consent is given.
  - Making results of the test available to the source individual's health care provider.
  - Testing of blood of the exposed nurse (with consent) for hepatitis B, hepatitis C, and HIV.
  - Postexposure prophylaxis if medically indicated (see below).
  - Medical and psychological counseling regarding personal risk of infection or risk of infecting others.
- For a puncture/laceration:
  - Wash/clean the area with soap and water.
  - Initiate first aid and seek treatment if indicated.
- For a mucous membrane exposure (eyes, nose, mouth), saline or water flush for 5 to 10 minutes.

POSTEXPOSURE PROTOCOL (PEP)

- Treatment should begin as soon as possible, preferably within hours of exposure, and may be less effective when started more than 24 hours after exposure. Starting treatment after a longer period (e.g., 1 week) should be considered for high-risk exposures previously untreated.

- Offer pregnancy counseling to all women of childbearing age not already known to be pregnant.

HIV

- For high-risk exposure (high blood volume *and* source with a high HIV titer): Three-drug treatment is recommended.
- For increased-risk exposure (high blood volume *or* source with a high HIV titer): Three-drug treatment is recommended.
- For low-risk exposure (neither high blood volume *nor* source with a high HIV titer): Two-drug treatment is considered.
- Drug prophylaxis continues for 4 weeks. If the source is determined to be HIV negative, PEP should be discontinued.
- Drug regimens vary, and new drugs and regimens are continuously being developed.
- HIV tests should be done shortly after exposure (baseline), and 6 weeks, 3 months, and 6 months afterward.

HEPATITIS B

- Hepatitis B surface antigen blood testing 1 to 2 months after last vaccine dose.
- Receipt of hepatitis B immune globulin and/or hepatitis B vaccine within 1 to 7 days following exposure for nonimmune workers.

HEPATITIS C

- Hepatitis C antigen and alanine aminotransferase blood testing at baseline and 4 to 6 months after exposure.
- Perform HCV RNA test at 4 to 6 weeks if earlier diagnosis of HCV is needed.

HAND HYGIENE

Any client may harbor microorganisms that are currently harmless to the client yet potentially harmful to another person or to the same client if they find a portal of entry to a different part of the body. Hand hygiene is important in every setting where people are cared for, including hospitals and home settings. It is considered the most effective measure of controlling **health care–associated infections (HAIs)** (those that may have originated in any health care setting) and **nosocomial infections** (those that originate in the hospital). The Joint Commission (2013) has listed reduction of HAIs as one of their national patient safety goals since 2004, currently mandating compliance with either the CDC or WHO hand hygiene guidelines. This goal reflects the increasing frequency of HAIs, particularly multidrug-resistant infections, central line–associated bloodstream infections, surgical site infections, and catheter-associated urinary tract infections. Much research has been conducted to examine adherence rates and barriers to and promoters of adequate hand hygiene.

Factors include the availability of hand cleansing supplies, knowledge of which practices are indicated in different situations, and organizational skills. As with many nursing practices, hand hygiene must become an essential component of every nurse's routine—all of the time.

Hand hygiene consists of a vigorous rubbing together of hands using soap or other cleansing agent. The use of adequate friction, allowing enough time to cleanse all surfaces of the hands and in between fingers, and proper drying are essential to effectiveness. The goal of hand hygiene is to remove transient microorganisms that might be transmitted to the nurse, clients, visitors, or other health care personnel. Box 1–3 lists times when nurses should perform hand hygiene.

SAFETY ALERT! | SAFETY

Opportunities for contamination occur even during brief encounters with clients. Practice hand hygiene before and after each client encounter.

BOX 1–3	Times for Hand Hygiene

BEFORE
- Giving care of any kind to any client
- Invasive procedures
- Caring for susceptible individuals such as newborns and immunocompromised clients
- Handling wounds
- Serving or consuming food
- Handling medications

AFTER
- Caring for any client
- Using the bathroom
- Contact with any body fluids
- Handling wounds
- Handling contaminated items such as bedpans or wet linens
- Removing PPE (including gloves)

BETWEEN
- Caring for individual clients

Note: Vigorous overwashing with soaps and detergents more than several times per hour damages the skin and can increase transmission of microorganisms. Following hand hygiene guidelines provides sufficient infection prevention without causing skin damage.

Because hand hygiene is performed so frequently, it provides a good opportunity for the nurse to take a moment to breathe and prepare for the next client encounter. By allowing a full, quiet breath in and a slow, complete exhalation, along with a quick **positive affirmation** (a positive statement) such as "I am focused and caring" or a brief prayer, the nurse can focus his or her attention and intention to remain mindful. This mindful attitude enhances the nurse's therapeutic presence. This attitude also increases the effectiveness and safety of care.

For routine client care, hand washing under a stream of water for 15 to 20 seconds using granular soap, soap-filled sheets, or liquid soap at the beginning of the nurse's shift, when hands are visibly soiled, and after using the toilet is recommended (WHO, 2009). Antimicrobial soaps are usually provided in high-risk areas (e.g., the newborn nursery). In the following situations, the CDC recommends antimicrobial hand hygiene agents:

- When there are known multiple resistant bacteria
- Before invasive procedures
- In special care units, such as nurseries and intensive care units (ICUs)
- Before caring for severely immunocompromised clients.

CLINICAL ALERT!

Cases of methicillin-resistant *Staphylococcus aureus* (MRSA) are increasing dramatically in hospital and community settings. Nurses must be vigilant about hand hygiene to reduce this threat.

Hand washing with soap and water may be inadequate to sufficiently remove pathogens, particularly because health care personnel tend to not wash thoroughly. After the initial soap and water hand washing, the CDC recommends the use of alcohol-based antiseptic hand rubs (rinses, gels, or foams) before and after each direct client contact. If there is visible dirt or matter, or if *Clostridium difficile* (*C. difficile*) may be present, alcohol-based rubs will not be sufficient, and soap and water washing is necessary (WHO, 2009). Even if soap and water or alcohol-based rubs are used appropriately, gloves are still required in some situations such as when caring for clients with *C. difficile* ("Hand washing ineffective," 2013).

Proper use of alcohol-based products includes following these steps:

- Apply a palmful of product into a cupped hand—enough to cover all surfaces of both hands.
- Rub palm against palm.
- Interlace fingers palm to palm.
- Rub palms to back of hands.
- Rub all surfaces of each finger with opposite hand.
- Continue until product is dry—about 20 to 30 seconds.

The CDC promotes the use of alcohol-based hand rubs (foam or gel) because:

- They kill more effectively and more quickly than hand washing with soap and water.
- They are less damaging to skin than soap and water, resulting in less dryness and irritation.
- They require less time than hand washing with soap and water.
- Bottles/dispensers can be placed at the point of care so they are more accessible.

Skill 1–2 describes the process of hand hygiene when washing with soap and water.

CLINICAL ALERT!

Although some religions prohibit drinking alcohol, all accept the value of using alcohol-based hand rubs in health care settings (Longtin, Sax, Allegranzi, Schneider, & Pittet, 2011).

●○● NURSING PROCESS: HAND HYGIENE

Performing Hand Washing

ASSESSMENT

Determine the client's:
- Risk for acquiring an infection including current or recent taking of immunosuppressive medications.
- Recent diagnostic procedures or treatments that penetrated the skin or a body cavity.
- Current nutritional status.

- Signs and symptoms indicating the presence of an infection:
  - *Localized signs:* swelling, redness, pain or tenderness with palpation or movement, palpable heat at site, loss of function of affected body part, presence of exudate.
  - *Systemic indications:* fever, increased pulse and respiratory rates, lack of energy, anorexia, enlarged lymph nodes.

Continued on page 8

SKILL 1–2

Performing Hand Washing—*continued*

PLANNING

Determine the location of sinks/running water and soap or soap substitutes.

DELEGATION

The skill of hand hygiene is identical for all health care providers, including UAP. Health care team members are accountable for themselves and others in implementing appropriate hand hygiene procedures.

IMPLEMENTATION

Preparation

Assess the hands:

- Nails should be kept short. Most agencies do not permit health care workers in direct contact with clients to have any form of artificial nails. The CDC guidelines prohibit artificial nails in caring for high-risk clients, and the WHO guidelines prohibit artificial nails in all settings. **Rationale:** *Short, natural nails are less likely to harbor microorganisms, scratch a client, or puncture gloves.*
- Removal of jewelry is recommended. **Rationale:** *Although the research is controversial (WHO, 2009), microorganisms can lodge in the settings of jewelry and under rings. Removal facilitates proper cleaning of the hands and arms.*
- Check hands for breaks in the skin, such as hangnails or cuts. **Rationale:** *A nurse who has open sores may require a work assignment with decreased risk for transmission of infectious organisms due to the chance of acquiring or passing on an infection.*

Performance

1. If you are washing your hands where the client can observe you, introduce yourself and explain to the client what you are going to do and why it is necessary.
2. Turn on the water and adjust the flow.
   - There are five common types of faucet controls:
     a. Hand-operated handles.
     b. Knee levers. Move these with the knee to regulate flow and temperature.
     c. Foot pedals. Press these with the foot to regulate flow and temperature.
     d. Elbow controls. Move these with the elbows instead of the hands.
     e. Infrared control. Motion in front of the sensor causes water to start and stop flowing automatically.
   - Adjust the flow so that the water is warm. **Rationale:** *Warm water removes less of the protective oil of the skin than hot water.*
3. Wet the hands thoroughly by holding them under the running water and apply soap to the hands.
   - Hold the hands lower than the elbows so that the water flows from the arms to the fingertips. **Rationale:** *The water should flow from the least contaminated to the most contaminated area; the hands are generally considered more contaminated than the lower arms. Note that this is a different skill than is used when performing surgical hand hygiene (see Skill 33–2).*
   - If the soap is liquid, apply 4 to 5 mL (1 tsp). If it is granules or sheets, rub them firmly between the hands.
4. Thoroughly wash and rinse the hands.
   - Use firm, rubbing, and circular movements to wash the palm, back, and wrist of each hand. Be sure to include the heel of the hand. Interlace the fingers and thumbs, and move the hands back and forth. ❶ The WHO recommends these steps:
     a. Right palm over left dorsum with interlaced fingers and vice versa (Figure ❶ *A*)

INTERPROFESSIONAL PRACTICE

Hand washing is an essential skill for all health care providers.

Equipment

- Soap
- Warm running water
- Paper towels

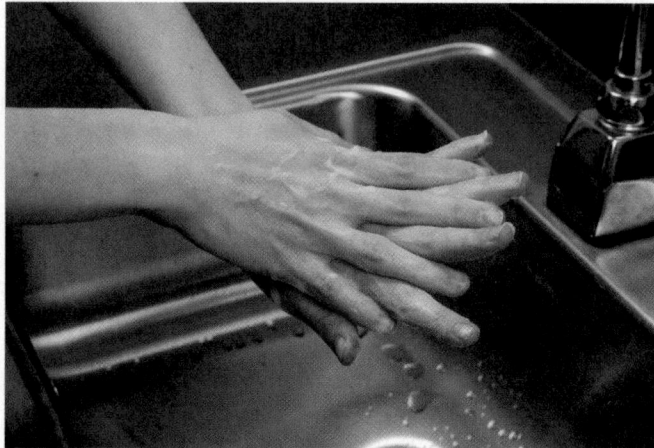

A

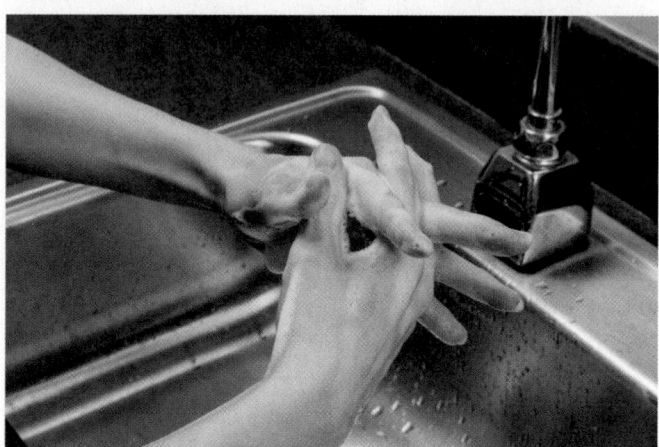

B

❶ Hand washing steps.

   b. Palm to palm with fingers interlaced (Figure ❶ *B*)
   c. Backs of fingers to opposing palms with fingers interlocked (Figure ❶ *C*)
   d. Rotational rubbing of left thumb clasped in right palm and vice versa (Figure ❶ *D*).
- Continue these motions for about 30 seconds (WHO, 2009). **Rationale:** *The circular action creates friction that helps remove microorganisms mechanically. Interlacing the fingers and thumbs cleans the interdigital spaces.*
- Rub the fingertips against the palm of the opposite hand. **Rationale:** *The nails and fingertips are commonly missed during hand hygiene.*
- Rinse the hands.

SKILL 1–2

Performing Hand Washing—*continued*

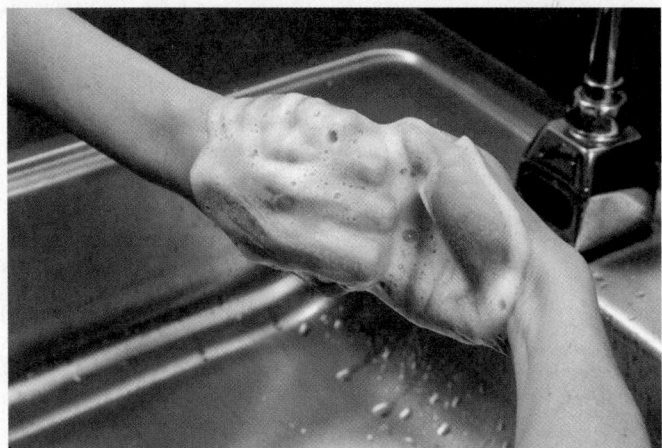

C

❷ Using a paper towel to grasp the handle of a hand-operated faucet.

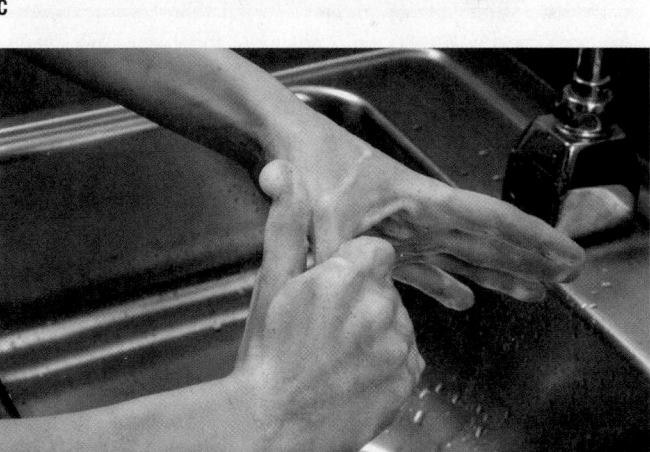

D
❶ Hand washing steps (*continued*)

5. Thoroughly pat dry the hands and arms.
   • Dry hands and arms thoroughly with a paper towel without scrubbing. **Rationale:** *Moist skin becomes chapped readily as does dry skin that is rubbed vigorously; chapping may produce lesions.*
   • Discard the paper towel in the appropriate container.

6. Turn off the water.
   • Use a new paper towel to grasp a hand-operated control. **❷ Rationale:** *This prevents the nurse from picking up microorganisms from the faucet handles.*
7. Hand lotions are important to prevent skin dryness and irritation. Use only agency-approved hand lotions and dispensers. Other lotions may make hand hygiene less effective, cause breakdown of latex gloves, and become contaminated with bacteria if dispensers are refilled.

Variation: Hand Washing Before Performing Sterile Skills
• Apply the soap and wash as described in step 4, but hold the hands higher than the elbows during this hand wash. Wet the hands and forearms under the running water, letting it run from the fingertips to the elbows so that the hands become cleaner than the elbows. In this way, the water runs from the area that has the fewest microorganisms to areas with a relatively greater number of pathogens.
• After washing and rinsing, use a towel to dry one hand thoroughly in a rotating motion from the fingers to the elbow. Use a new towel to dry the other hand and arm. **Rationale:** *A clean towel prevents the transfer of microorganisms from one elbow (least clean area) to the other hand (cleanest area).*
• Apply sterile gloves before touching any unsterile items (see Skill 7–2).

EVALUATION

There is no traditional evaluation of the effectiveness of the individual nurse's hand washing techniques. Institutional quality control departments monitor the occurrence of client infections and investigate those situations in which health care providers are implicated in the transmission of infectious organisms. Research has repeatedly shown the positive impact of careful hand hygiene on client health associated with prevention of infection (see the Readings and References section at the end of this chapter). However, studies also show that hand hygiene is not performed as frequently as it should be. Recently, researchers have been focusing on the relationship between quality of hand hygiene products (gentle, nondrying, aromatic) and care provider adherence to recommended protocols. *Note:* In some agencies, clients are encouraged to ask the provider if they have cleansed their hands before allowing them to perform procedures (McGuckin & Govednik, 2013).

Ambulatory and Community Settings | **Safety**

Hand Hygiene
When making a home visit:
• Keep fingernails clean, short, and well trimmed.
• Perform hand hygiene carefully before and after any hands-on care.

• If there is no running water, use commercially available hand hygiene agents that require no water.
• You may wish to bring your own alcohol-based rub or bactericidal soap and paper towels for use when performing hand hygiene.
• Always turn the water off with a dry paper towel.

PERSONAL PROTECTIVE EQUIPMENT

All health care providers must apply PPE (clean or sterile gloves, gowns, masks, and protective eyewear) according to the risk of exposure to potentially infective materials.

Gloves

Disposable clean gloves are worn to protect the hands when the nurse is likely to come in contact with any potentially infective objects or materials (e.g., blood, urine, feces, sputum, mucous membranes, nonintact skin, and used equipment). Gloves also reduce the likelihood of the nurse's transmitting any potentially infectious organisms to clients. Nurses who have open sores or cuts on the hands should wear gloves for protection. In addition, gloves reduce the chance of transmitting organisms from one client or object to another client. Hand hygiene is performed before applying gloves. Gloves must be changed between client contacts. Hand hygiene must also be performed after removing gloves because gloves may have holes, allowing microorganisms in, or hands may become contaminated during removal of gloves. Sterile gloves are used when the hands will come in contact with sterile equipment or wounds (see Chapter 7 ∞).

Many types of gloves contain latex rubber. Increasingly, both clients and health care workers are developing allergies to latex. Ask clients if they have had any adverse reactions to items such as balloons, condoms, or dishwashing or utility gloves. Those with other allergic conditions as well as those who have had frequent or long-term exposure to latex are at highest risk for the allergy. Latex gloves lubricated by cornstarch or powder are particularly allergenic because the latex allergen adheres to the lubricant and is aerosolized and inhaled during use. A newer formulation of latex, aluminum hydroxide–modified natural rubber latex, has been developed that reduces the antigenic protein content while preserving the durability, comfort, fit, tactile sensitivity, and high resistance to puncture and tear for which latex is known (Doyle, 2011). Nurses may see these latex gloves in use.

If either the client or the nurse is known to have a latex sensitivity, nonlatex gloves must be used. Most hospitals have eliminated latex products wherever possible and aim for a "latex-free environment." Alternatives to latex gloves include both vinyl and nitrile. Due to the high failure rate of vinyl gloves, nitrile gloves are preferable for clinical procedures that require manual dexterity and/or involve more than brief client contact.

Gowns

Impervious (waterproof or solid enough to prevent microorganisms from moving through it even when wet) gowns or plastic aprons are worn when the nurse's uniform may become soiled. Sterile gowns may be indicated when the nurse changes the dressings of a client with extensive wounds (e.g., burns). Using a gown only once before discarding or laundering it is the usual practice in hospitals.

CLINICAL ALERT!

Wearing a client hospital gown over your uniform serves **no** infection prevention purpose.

Face Masks, Face Shields, Eyewear

In SP, masks are worn to prevent potentially infective material from entering the nurse's mouth, nose, or eyes during procedures in which blood or droplets of other body fluids may splash or become airborne near the nurse's face. A one-piece unit consisting of a paper mask with a clear plastic shield rising from the mask to protect the eyes is commonly used. If the nurse wears prescription eyeglasses, goggles or a shield must still be worn over the glasses to provide shielding around the sides of the glasses. Remember the feelings of strangeness, alienation, fear, or even shame these protective measures may engender in clients who must look at people wearing masks and receive touch from gloved hands. Sensitivity, warmth, caring eye contact, and compassionate intention on the part of staff are very important.

●○○● NURSING PROCESS: PERSONAL PROTECTIVE EQUIPMENT

Applying and Removing Personal Protective Equipment (Gown, Mask, Eyewear, Gloves)

SKILL 1-3

ASSESSMENT
Consider which activities will be required while the nurse is in the client's room at this time. **Rationale:** *This will determine which equipment is required.*

PLANNING
- Application and removal of PPE can be time consuming. Prioritize care and arrange for personnel to care for your other clients if indicated.
- Determine which supplies are present within the client's room and which must be brought to the room.
- Consider whether special handling is indicated for removal of any specimens or other materials from the room.

DELEGATION

Use of PPE is identical for all health care providers. Clients whose care requires use of PPE may be delegated to UAP. Health care team members are accountable for proper implementation of these procedures by themselves and others.

INTERPROFESSIONAL PRACTICE

Proper use of PPE is an essential skill for all health care providers.

Equipment
As indicated according to the activities that will be performed, ensure that extra supplies are easily available.
- Gown
- Mask
- Eyewear
- Clean gloves

Applying and Removing Personal Protective Equipment—*continued*

IMPLEMENTATION

Preparation
Remove or secure all loose items such as name tags or jewelry.

Performance
1. Prior to performing the procedure, introduce self and verify the client's identity using agency protocol. Explain to the client what you are going to do, why it is necessary, and how he or she can participate.
2. Perform hand hygiene.
3. Apply a clean gown.
   - Pick up a clean gown, and allow it to unfold in front of you without allowing it to touch any area soiled with body substances.
   - Slide the arms and the hands through the sleeves.
   - Fasten the ties at the neck to keep the gown in place.
   - Overlap the gown at the back as much as possible and fasten the waist ties or belt. ❶ **Rationale:** *Overlapping securely covers the uniform at the back. Waist ties keep the gown from falling away from the body, which can lead to inadvertent soiling of the exposed uniform.*
4. Apply the face mask. ❷
   - Locate the top edge of the mask. The mask usually has a narrow metal strip along the edge.
   - Hold the mask by the top two strings or loops.
   - Place the upper edge of the mask over the bridge of the nose, and tie the upper ties at the back of the head or secure the loops around the ears. If glasses are worn, fit the upper edge of the mask under the glasses. **Rationale:** *With the edge of the mask under the glasses, clouding of the glasses is less likely to occur.*
   - Secure the lower edge of the mask under the chin, and tie the lower ties at the nape of the neck. **Rationale:** *To be effective, a mask must cover both the nose and the mouth, because air moves in and out of both.*
   - If the mask has a metal strip, adjust this firmly over the bridge of the nose. **Rationale:** *A secure fit prevents both the escape and the inhalation of microorganisms around the edges of the mask and the fogging of eyeglasses.*
   - Wear the mask only once, and do not wear any mask longer than the manufacturer recommends or once it becomes wet. **Rationale:** *A mask should be used only once because it becomes ineffective when moist.*
   - Do not leave a used face mask hanging around the neck.

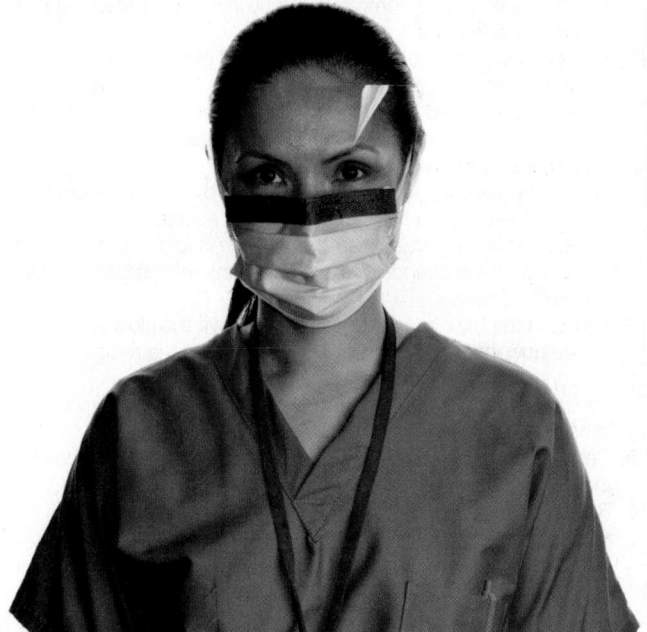

❷ A face mask and eye protection covering the nose, mouth, and eyes.
Custom Medical Stock Photo/Custom Medical Stock Photo.

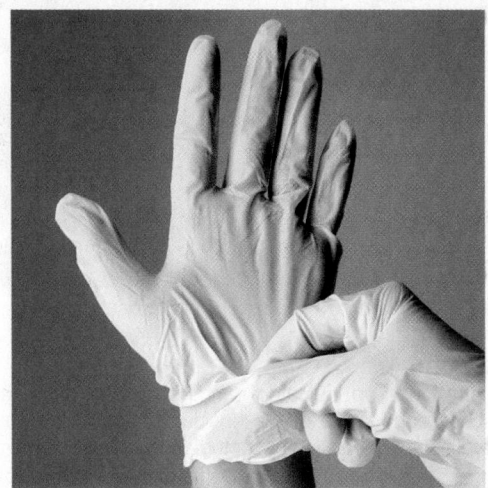

❸ Plucking the palmar surface of a contaminated glove.

5. Apply protective eyewear if it is not combined with the face mask.
6. Apply clean gloves.
   - No special technique is required.
   - If wearing a gown, pull the gloves up to cover the cuffs of the gown. If not wearing a gown, pull the gloves up to cover the wrists.
7. To remove soiled PPE, remove the gloves first since they are the most soiled.
   - If wearing a gown that is tied at the waist in front, undo the ties before removing gloves.
   - Remove the first glove by grasping it on its palmar surface, taking care to touch only glove to glove. ❸ **Rationale:** *This keeps the soiled parts of the used gloves from touching the skin of the wrist or hand.*

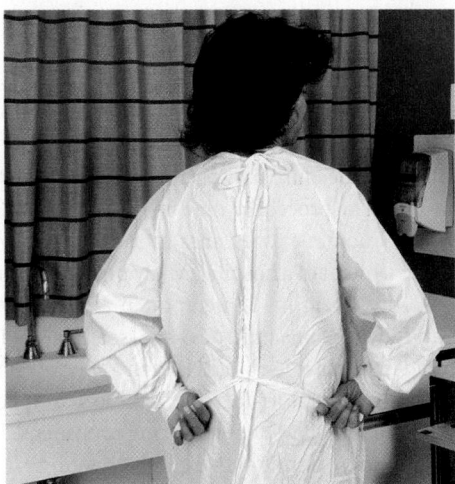

❶ Overlapping the gown at the back to cover the nurse's uniform.

Continued on page 12

SKILL 1-3

Applying and Removing Personal Protective Equipment—*continued*

- Pull the first glove completely off by inverting or rolling the glove inside out.
- Continue to hold the inverted removed glove by the fingers of the remaining gloved hand. Place the first two fingers of the bare hand inside the cuff of the second glove. ❹ **Rationale:** *Touching the outside of the second soiled glove with the bare hand is avoided.*
- Pull the second glove off to the fingers by turning it inside out. This pulls the first glove inside the second glove. **Rationale:** *The soiled part of the glove is folded to the inside to reduce the chance of transferring any microorganisms by direct contact.*
- Using the bare hand, continue to remove the gloves, which are now inside out, and dispose of them in the refuse container. ❺

8. Perform hand hygiene. **Rationale:** *Contact with microorganisms may occur while removing PPE.*
9. Remove protective eyewear and dispose of properly or place in the appropriate receptacle for cleaning.
10. Remove the gown when preparing to leave the room.
    - Avoid touching soiled parts on the outside of the gown, if possible. **Rationale:** *The top part of the gown may be soiled, for example, if you have been holding an infant with a respiratory infection.*
    - Grasp the gown along the inside of the neck and pull down over the shoulders. Do not shake the gown.
    - Roll up the gown with the soiled part inside, and discard it in the appropriate container.
11. Remove the mask.
    - Remove the mask at the doorway to the client's room. If using a respirator mask, remove it after leaving the room and closing the door.
    - If using a mask with strings, first untie the *lower* strings of the mask. **Rationale:** *This prevents the top part of the mask from falling onto the chest.*
    - Untie the top strings and, while holding the ties securely, remove the mask from the face. If side loops are present, lift the side loops up and away from the ears and face. Do not touch the front of the mask. **Rationale:** *The front of the mask through which the nurse has been breathing is contaminated.*
    - Discard a disposable mask in the waste container.
    - Perform hand hygiene again.

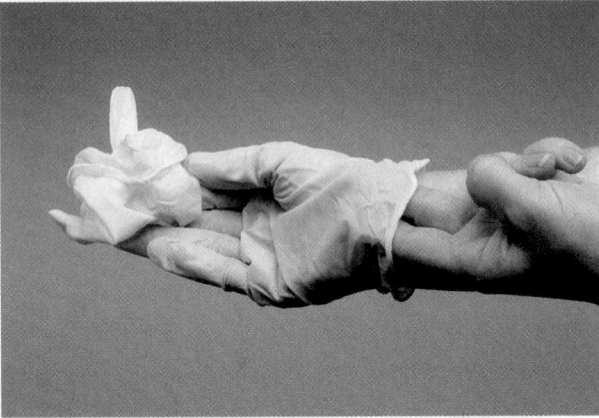

❹ Inserting fingers to remove the second contaminated glove.

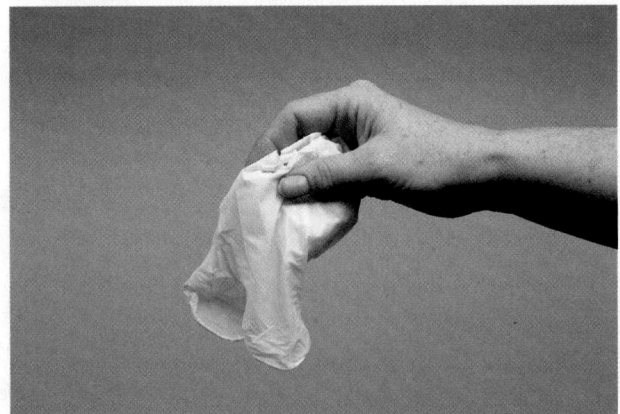

❺ Holding contaminated gloves, which are inside out when properly removed.

EVALUATION
Conduct any follow-up indicated during your care of the client. If there has been any failure of the equipment and exposure to potentially infective materials is suspected, follow the procedure given earlier in Practice Guidelines: Steps to Follow After Exposure to Bloodborne Pathogens.

Ensure that an adequate supply of equipment is available for the next health care provider.

Ambulatory and Community Settings | **Safety**

Standard Precautions and Personal Protective Equipment
- All aspects of SP apply equally in the clinic, home, or long-term care setting.
- Ensure that the supply of gloves, gowns, masks, and eyewear is adequate.
- Ensure that procedures are in place for removal and disposal of used materials.
- Teach the client and family appropriate aspects of SP.

ASSISTING WITH PROCEDURES
When procedures are performed by the physician or other health care provider, the nurse may be asked to participate in a number of different ways: preparing the client and/or the support persons, monitoring and assisting the client during the procedure, caring for the client after the procedure, and documenting the client's response to the procedure. The procedure may be performed at the bedside, in an examining room, or sometimes in the emergency or special procedures department of a hospital. Many procedures are invasive, involving insertion of an instrument, often a needle, through the skin and withdrawing some fluid or tissue (see Table 1–1 for examples). The fluid or tissue is usually placed in a special container and sent to the hospital laboratory for examination. Complications can occur with each of the techniques for taking specimens. The knowledge and skill of the assisting nurse can help minimize complications and maximize the therapeutic value of the procedure.

Skill 1–4 describes assisting with invasive procedures.

TABLE 1–1	Common Studies Involving Removal of Body Fluid or Tissue		
Name	**Type of Specimen**	**Source**	**Common Tests**
Lumbar puncture	Spinal fluid	Subarachnoid space of the spinal canal	Pressure, appearance, sugar, protein, cell count, bacteria
Abdominal paracentesis	Ascitic fluid	Peritoneal cavity	Cell count, cytology, specific gravity, protein
Thoracentesis	Pleural fluid	Pleural cavity	Cell count, cytology, protein
Bone marrow biopsy/aspiration	Bone marrow	Iliac crest, posterior superior iliac spine, or sternum	Cytology, iron
Liver biopsy	Liver tissue	Liver	Cytology, iron, copper
Amniocentesis	Amniotic fluid	Amniotic sac	Fetal maturity, genetic abnormalities
Vaginal examination	Cells, secretions	Cervical os or vaginal floor	Papanicolaou test, culture

●○● NURSING PROCESS: ASSISTING WITH PROCEDURES

Assisting with Invasive Procedures

ASSESSMENT
- Review the primary care provider's order for the procedure, if available. Note carefully the time and place of the planned procedure, any medications or techniques to be performed prior to the procedure (e.g., giving enemas, starting an intravenous [IV] infusion, administering eyedrops), and any documents that must be signed (e.g., a consent for the procedure) or available. Determine if more than one nurse or assistant will be needed.
- Determine if the client has had this procedure performed previously. If so, obtain the client's knowledge of the procedure and ability to participate, how it was performed, and the client's reactions to the procedure. **Rationale:** *This information helps the nurse determine what teaching or precautions are needed.*
- Assess for pertinent health factors, for example, the presence of dyspnea or any drug allergies, particularly allergies to drugs contained in local anesthetics and skin antiseptics, which could present a problem during the procedure.
- Measure vital signs before the procedure. **Rationale:** *This provides baseline data against which vital signs during or after the procedure can be compared.*

PLANNING
Carefully review the procedure that will be performed. Reflect on the sequence of events, how long it will take, and what may be required of the client and the nurse at each step. Check with the person performing the procedure to determine the best time for opening supplies. Arrange for someone to care for your other clients if necessary.

DELEGATION

Unlicensed personnel may be delegated the task of assisting the nurse or other health care provider with some skills. However, if these activities require the assistant to perform skills not generally expected of unlicensed personnel, such as sterile technique, they may not be delegated to the UAP. As always, the nurse must verify the individual UAP's abilities and experience, verify the individual client's needs, and be knowledgeable about agency and individual state regulatory policies and procedures.

INTERPROFESSIONAL PRACTICE

Assisting with procedures may be within the scope of practice for many health care providers. Although the other providers may verbally communicate their findings and plan to the health care team members, the nurse must know where to locate their documentation in the client's medical record.

Equipment
- Varies according to the procedure.
- Always have extra gloves and other common supplies available.

IMPLEMENTATION
Preparation
- Ensure that the results of relevant laboratory tests are available.
- Determine if a consent form has been signed. Some agencies require a signed consent from the client for special procedures.
- Coordinate the services of personnel from other departments who are involved in the procedure.

Performance
1. Prior to performing the procedure, introduce self and verify the client's identity using agency protocol. Explain to the client what you and any other health care providers are going to do, why it is necessary, and how he or she can participate. Discuss how the results will be used in planning further care or treatments.
2. Perform hand hygiene and observe other appropriate infection prevention procedures.
3. Provide for client privacy and safety.
4. Prepare the client.
   - Have the client empty the bladder and bowels prior to the procedure. **Rationale:** *This prevents discomfort resulting from a need to use the bathroom during the procedure.*
   - Position the client as required for the procedure.
   - Drape the client to expose only the necessary area.

Continued on page 14

SKILL 1–4

SKILL 1–4

Assisting with Invasive Procedures—*continued*

5. Open any sterile trays or equipment that is needed. Fill in labels and laboratory slips with the client's identification data.

6. Prepare and provide equipment and medications needed during the procedure.
  • Maintain sterility of dressings, needles, syringes, specimen containers, and other equipment (see Chapter 7 ∞).
  • Draw up or pour medications or solutions as needed. If another practitioner is wearing sterile gloves and will be drawing the medication from a vial that you are holding (nonsterile outside), show the practitioner the label and say the name and concentration of the fluid before it is aspirated. For example, show the label while you say "Heparin one thousand units per milliliter" or "Xylocaine one percent without epinephrine" and then tilt the vial top so the practitioner can access it. ❶

7. Support the client during the procedure.
  • If you are not needed to handle equipment or supplies for the practitioner, position yourself where you can observe and reassure the client.
  • Observe the client closely for signs of distress, for example, abnormal pulse, respirations, or blood pressure; altered level of consciousness; or change in skin color.

8. Label any specimens and arrange for them to be sent immediately to the laboratory. **Rationale:** *Incorrect identification of specimens can lead to subsequent error of diagnosis or therapy for the client.*

9. Provide required nursing care after the procedure.
  • Assist the client to a comfortable position.

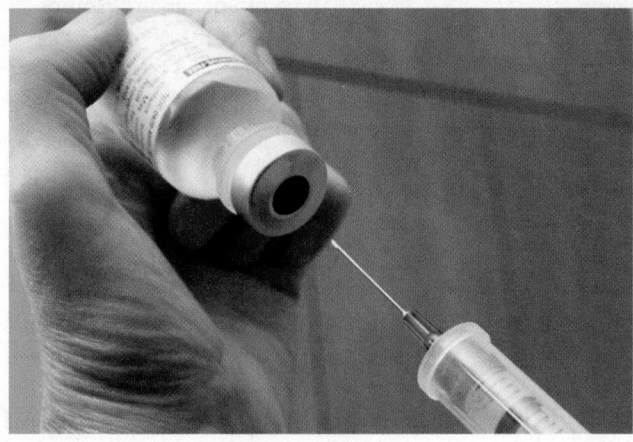

❶ Holding a vial.

  • Measure vital signs and compare with baseline; continue to monitor as indicated.
  • Wash off any excess antiseptic or other product applied to the skin.
  • Observe the insertion site for swelling or bleeding.
  • Apply a bandage or other covering as indicated.

10. Document the procedure and findings in the client record using forms or checklists supplemented by narrative notes when appropriate.

EVALUATION
  • Perform follow-up care based on findings that deviated from expected or normal for the client. Relate findings to previous assessment data if available.

  • Report significant deviations from normal to the primary care provider.

DISPOSAL OF SOILED EQUIPMENT AND SUPPLIES

Many pieces of equipment are supplied for single use only and are disposed of after use. Some items, however, are reusable. Agencies have specific policies and procedures for handling soiled equipment (e.g., disposal, cleaning, disinfecting, and sterilizing); the nurse needs to become familiar with these practices in the employing agency. Appropriate handling of soiled equipment and supplies is essential for these reasons:

  • To prevent inadvertent exposure of health care workers to articles contaminated with body substances.
  • To prevent contamination of the environment.

Bagging

Articles contaminated, or likely to have been contaminated, with infective material such as pus, blood, body fluids, feces, or respiratory secretions need to be enclosed in a sturdy bag that is impervious to microorganisms before they are removed from the client's room. Some agencies use labels or bags of a particular color that designate them as infective wastes. Biohazardous waste is placed in a container with special labeling such as that shown in Figure 1–1 ■.

CDC guidelines recommend the following methods:

  • Use of a single bag is acceptable if it is sturdy and impervious to microorganisms and if the contaminated articles can be placed in the bag without soiling or contaminating its outside.
  • Use double-bagging if the above conditions are not met.

Follow agency protocol, or use the following CDC guidelines to handle and bag soiled items:

  • Place *disposable sharps* instruments such as scalpels, needles, and lancets directly into a hard plastic sharps container.
  • Place garbage and soiled *disposable nonsharps* equipment, including dressings and tissues, in the plastic bag that lines the waste

Figure 1–1 ■ Biohazard alert symbol.

container and tie the bag. If the bag is sturdy and impervious, a single bag is adequate. If not, place the first bag inside another impermeable bag. Some agencies have a particular location where such garbage is to be placed, and some use bags of a particular color (e.g., red) to indicate potentially infective waste. Some also separate dry and wet waste material and incinerate dry items, such as paper towels and disposable items.

- Place *nondisposable* or *reusable* equipment that is visibly soiled in a labeled bag before removing it, and send it to a central processing area for decontamination. Some agencies may require that glass bottles or jars and metal items be placed in separate bags from rubber and plastic items. Glass and metal can be sterilized in an autoclave, but rubber and plastic are damaged by this process and must be cleaned by other methods, such as gas sterilization.
- Disassemble special procedure trays into component parts. Some components are disposable; others need to be sent to the laundry or central services for cleaning and decontaminating.

Linens

Handle soiled linen as little as possible, hold it away from your body, and with the least agitation possible place it in the laundry hamper bag. This prevents gross microbial contamination of the air and individuals handling the linen. Close the bag before sending it to the laundry in accordance with agency practice. Detergent and warm water safely inactivate microorganisms. Place soiled clothing in an impervious bag before sending it home.

Laboratory Specimens

Laboratory specimens, if placed in a leakproof container with a secure lid and a biohazard label, need no special precautions. Use care when collecting specimens to avoid contaminating the outside of the container. Containers that are contaminated on the outside (and, in some agencies, all specimen containers) should be placed inside a sealable plastic bag with a biohazard label before sending them to the laboratory. This prevents personnel from having hand contact with potentially infective material.

Dishes

Dishes require no special precautions. Soiling of dishes can largely be prevented by assisting clients to cleanse their hands before eating. Detergent and warm water safely remove microorganisms. Some agencies use paper dishes for convenience, which are disposed of in the refuse container.

Blood Pressure Equipment

Blood pressure equipment needs no special precautions unless it becomes contaminated with infective material. If it does become contaminated, follow agency policy for decontamination. Cleaning procedures vary according to whether it is a wall or portable unit. In some agencies, a disposable cuff is used for clients placed on isolation precautions or even for all clients. Stethoscopes should be cleaned frequently and between clients to remove gross contamination. Dedicated stethoscopes are used when a client is in isolation.

Thermometers

Nondisposable used thermometers are generally disinfected after each use. Check agency policy.

Disposable Needles, Syringes, and Sharps

Place needles, syringes, and sharps (e.g., lancets, scalpels, and broken glass) into a puncture-resistant container. To avoid puncture wounds, use approved safety or needleless systems and do not detach needles from the syringe or recap the needle before disposal. The ANA website has a needlestick prevention guide available for download. See Chapter 17 ∞ for ways to prevent needlestick injuries.

DOCUMENTATION

There are several reasons why it is critically important for all client care activities to be documented in the medical record. These include facilitating continuity of care through ongoing communication among health care providers, promoting effective care through the ability to examine results of previous care and care plans, meeting legal and accreditation requirements, and providing data for research and reimbursement. One of The Joint Commission's national patient safety goals (2013) is to improve the effectiveness of communication among caregivers.

SAFETY ALERT! | SAFETY

2014 The Joint Commission National Patient Safety Goals (2013)
Although many of the national patient safety goals (NPSGs) reference the need for health care providers to communicate more effectively, the goal cited below is specifically focused on this objective.

GOAL 2: IMPROVE THE EFFECTIVENESS OF COMMUNICATION AMONG CAREGIVERS.
NPSG.02.03.01: Report critical results of tests and diagnostic procedures on a timely basis. **Rationale:** *Critical results of tests and diagnostic procedures fall significantly outside the normal range and may indicate a life-threatening situation. The objective is to provide the responsible licensed caregiver these results within an established time frame so that the patient can be promptly treated.*

A variety of documentation formats, such as the problem-oriented medical record and source-oriented record, are used in different agencies. Records may be written or electronic. The process of making an entry in a client record is called recording, charting, or **documenting**. In most cases, care is documented through a combination of checklists, forms, and narrative notes. Notations should be carefully dated, timed, and signed. Any changes/additions should be correctly dated, timed, and signed as an addendum after the fact, with no attempt to alter an existing note. No matter what format is used, key requirements of documenting procedures are the same (Box 1–4).

The **Situation, Background, Assessment, and Recommendation (SBAR) process** is an approach to documentation that can enhance safety in situations where nurses communicate with primary care providers and other nurses about client status. Change of shift, transferring a client to another unit, and contacting primary care providers regarding a change in client condition are examples of when this system can be most helpful in structuring clear, complete

---

BOX 1–4   **Documenting Procedures**

As with all documentation, be objective, use approved abbreviations only, be timely, and sign with your name and title. Health care records are confidential documents, and HIPAA privacy regulations must be observed at all times. Remember that clients may have access to their own health records and information regarding their health care status. If using paper records, write legibly in ink. For each procedure, include:

- Date and time it was performed, using the agency preference for 12- or 24-hour clock times
- First initial, last name, and title (e.g., RN, MD) of the health care provider who performed the procedure
- The exact procedure performed (e.g., right subclavian IV inserted; bone marrow biopsy, left iliac crest)
- Number, color, character, and amount of any specimens, fluid, or tissue obtained
- Any measurements or other readings (including vital signs) taken
- Client teaching done prior to, during, and following the procedure
- Client's reaction to and tolerance of the procedure
- Any unusual incidents or omitted treatments
- Safety precautions you took to protect the client
- Nurse's interventions and care following the procedure.

Do not leave anything blank or leave out any information about the procedure.

Sample Recording: Lumbar Puncture

DATE	TIME	NOTES
5/24/15	1500	Lumbar puncture performed by Dr. Guido. Four 2-mL specimens of cloudy serous CSF sent to lab. Initial pressure 130 mm. Closing pressure 100 mm. No apparent discomfort. Resting ——————— B. Snyder, RN

Sample Recording: Soap Suds Enema

Date	Time	Notes
10/02/15	0830	600 mL soap suds enema delivered and retained by client for 15 minutes. Client assisted to commode. Returned large amount dark brown, soft stool. C/o mild abdominal cramping during procedure, relieved after passing stool. Returned to bed with rails up, call light in reach. Client verbalizes awareness of need to increase fluid and fiber intake to promote bowel regularity. ——————— L. Roberts, RN

---

communication. Because it includes background, assessment, and nurse recommendations, it encourages critical evaluation and holistic input on the part of the nurse.

Examples of content under each of the four steps include:

S = Situation:
- Identify yourself, your location, and the client about whom you are speaking.
- What has prompted this communication (e.g., a change in client condition or report of laboratory results)?
- How do you know this information? Did you directly assess the client?

B = Background:
- Has this happened previously? What was the client's condition prior to what has prompted this communication?

- Also provide medical history and current care plan information as appropriate if the provider is not familiar with the client.

A = Assessment:
- What is the trend that concerns you? What do you think the assessment indicates?

R = Recommendation:
- Is there an order you need from the provider?
- What standard protocol or procedures will you be following?
- When will the two of you next be communicating about the situation?
- Be sure to repeat back any orders the care provider gives.

Chapter 1 Review

FOCUSING ON CLINICAL THINKING

Consider This

1. You are preparing to measure the blood pressure of a client who has been experiencing explosive vomiting and diarrhea. What specific precautions (gown, gloves, mask, eyewear) would you take?

2. After caring for a client who has a bloodborne pathogen infection, upon removing your gown you notice that you have blood on your arm. What would you do?

3. Although you have assisted physicians with several invasive procedures such as a thoracentesis, this will be the first time you

assist with a liver biopsy. How will you prepare and what will you tell the physician about your abilities?

4. You observe a nursing assistant bathing and changing the linens of a client who has been incontinent of stool. The assistant is not wearing gloves or any other personal protective equipment. How would you respond?

5. You are considering asking the UAP to assist with a recent new admission. The client has been admitted with a fractured hip. Which tasks of the admission may you delegate to UAP? Explain how you reached that conclusion.

See Focusing on Clinical Thinking answers on student resource website.

TEST YOUR KNOWLEDGE

1. Which steps are appropriate when utilizing an alcohol-based hand hygiene product? Select all that apply.
   1. Apply a palmful of product into a cupped hand—enough to cover all surfaces of both hands.
   2. Rub palm against palm.
   3. Interface fingers palm to palm.
   4. Rub palms to back of hands.
   5. Rub all surfaces of each finger with the opposite hand.
   6. Continue for about 10 to 15 seconds.

2. A nurse is receiving a manicure. What directions given to the manicurist are acceptable? Select all that apply.
   1. Short polished nails
   2. Unpolished artificial nails
   3. Squarely filed nails
   4. Intact cuticles

3. A nurse is performing hand washing after administering intravenous medications. Which action is *inconsistent* with proper technique?
   1. The use of warm water to wash
   2. The use of firm, rubbing, and circular movements to wash
   3. The use of a paper towel to vigorously scrub hands dry
   4. The use of a new paper towel to turn the faucet off

4. In which instance would the nurse *not* need to use standard precautions?
   1. Caring for a client with oozing leg edema
   2. Performing oral care on a client
   3. Caring for a diaphoretic client with chest pain
   4. Performing a dressing change on a client with diabetes

5. A student nurse is describing different forms of personal protective equipment. Which statement, if made by the student nurse, indicates the need for further teaching?
   1. "I will wear clean gloves to protect my hands when I handle any potentially infective material."
   2. "Since I wear prescription glasses at work, I do not need to wear goggles."
   3. "I will wear a sterile gown when I change the dressing of a client with burns."
   4. "Even though I wear gloves, I still cleanse my hands after removing my gloves because my hands may have become contaminated."

6. A nurse is preparing to assist with a chest tube insertion on a client. Which nursing action demonstrates that further teaching regarding safety measures is indicated?
   1. The nurse reviews the primary care provider's order for the procedure.
   2. The nurse measures and records vital signs before the procedure.
   3. The nurse arranges for someone to care for the other assigned clients.
   4. The nurse delegates setup of the sterile field to the unlicensed assistive personnel.

7. A nurse has just finished assisting a physician with a procedure. Which elements should be included in the nurse's documentation? Select all that apply.
   1. Exact procedure, including date and time
   2. Client response to the procedure
   3. Vital signs before and after the procedure, including pain assessment
   4. Method of disposing of used supplies
   5. Any client teaching that was offered

8. A nurse is preparing to enter a room where full personal protective equipment is required. Which technique, if done by the nurse, indicates a good understanding of infection prevention principles?
   1. The nurse pulls the gloves up to cover the cuffs of the gown.
   2. The nurse's mask covers the mouth but not the nose.
   3. The nurse fastens the ties on the gown without overlapping the gown edges.
   4. The nurse applies a mask that has been used no more than once before.

9. When the nurse returns for follow-up with a home care client 2 days after the insertion of an indwelling catheter, the client has cloudy urine, has a low-grade fever, and complains of lower abdominal discomfort. The nurse recognizes the client most likely has developed a urinary tract infection and that it is what type of infection?
   1. Nosocomial
   2. Health care–associated
   3. Viral
   4. Fungal

10. While dressing for work, the nurse discovers all of her favorite uniforms are dirty. The nurse's best strategy would be to:
    1. Wear one of the dirty uniforms again as long as there are no stains and it smells clean.
    2. Spray a dirty uniform with a disinfectant spray prior to wearing it.
    3. Wear the pants of a dirty uniform and the top of a clean, less favorite uniform.
    4. Wear a clean uniform even if it is not a favorite.

See Answers to Test Your Knowledge in Appendix A.

READINGS AND REFERENCES

References

Dossey, B. M. (2009). *Florence Nightingale: Mystic, visionary, healer.* Philadelphia, PA: F.A. Davis.

Dossey, B. M., & Keegan, L. (2013). *Holistic nursing: A handbook for clinical practice* (6th ed.). Burlington, MA: Jones & Bartlett.

Doyle, W. (2011). A new generation of latex gloves. *Occupational Health & Safety, 80*(4), 18–19.

Hand washing ineffective, gloves must be used. (2013). *Hospital Infection Control & Prevention, 40*(4), 42–44.

The Joint Commission. (2013). *Hospital: 2014 national patient safety goals.* Retrieved from http://www.jointcommission.org/assets/1/6/HAP_NPSG_Chapter_2014.pdf

Longtin, Y., Sax, H., Allegranzi, B., Schneider, F., & Pittet, D. (2011). Videos in clinical medicine: Hand hygiene. *New England Journal of Medicine, 364*(13), e24. doi:10.1056/NEJMvcm0903599

McGuckin, M., & Govednik, J. (2013). Patient empowerment and hand hygiene, 1997–2012. *Journal of Hospital Infection, 84,* 191–199. doi:10.1016/j.jhin.2013.01.014

Watson, J. (2013). *Transpersonal caring and the caring moment defined.* Retrieved from http://watsoncaringscience.org/about-us/caring-science-definitions-processes-theory

World Health Organization. (2009). *WHO guidelines on hand hygiene in health care.* Geneva, Switzerland: Author.

Selected Bibliography

Aziz, A. (2013). How better availability of materials improved hand-hygiene compliance. *British Journal of Nursing, 22,* 458–463.

Berman, A., Snyder, S., & Frandsen, G. (2016). Kozier & Erb's fundamentals of nursing: Concepts, process, and practice (10th ed.). Upper Saddle River, NJ: Pearson.

Casanova, L. M., Rutala, W. A., Weber, D. J., & Sobsey, M. D. (2012). Effect of single-versus double-gloving on virus transfer to health care workers' skin and clothing during removal of personal protective equipment. *American Journal of Infection Control, 40,* 369–374. doi:10.1016/j.ajic.2011.04.324

Centers for Disease Control and Prevention. (2011). *Guide to infection prevention for outpatient settings: Minimum expectations for safe care.* Retrieved from http://www.cdc.gov/HAI/settings/outpatient/outpatient-care-guidelines.html

Davis, R., Anderson, O., Vincent, C., Miles, K., & Sevdalis, N. (2012). Predictors of hospitalized patients' intentions to prevent healthcare harm: A cross sectional survey. *International Journal of Nursing Studies, 49,* 407–415. doi:10.1016/j.ijnurstu.2011.10.013

Fitzgerald, G., Moore, G., & Wilson, A. P. (2013). Hand hygiene after touching a patient's surroundings: The opportunities most commonly missed. *Journal of Hospital Infection, 84*(1), 27–31. doi:10.1016/j.jhin.2013.01.008

Harding, A. D., Almquist, L. J., & Hashemi, S. (2011). The use and need for standard precautions and transmission-based precautions in the emergency department. *Journal of Emergency Nursing, 37,* 367–373. doi:10.1016/j.jen.2010.11.017

Helder, O., van den Hoogen, A., de Boer, C., van Goudoever, J., Verboon-Maciolek, M., & Kornelisse, R. (2013). Effectiveness of non-pharmacological interventions for the prevention of bloodstream infections in infants admitted to a neonatal intensive care unit: A systematic review. *International Journal of Nursing Studies, 50,* 819–831. doi:10.1016/j.ijnurstu.2012.02.009

Lebovic, G., Siddiqui, N., & Muller, M. P. (2013). Predictors of hand hygiene compliance in the era of alcohol-based hand rinse. *Journal of Hospital Infection, 83,* 276–283. doi:10.1016/j.jhin.2013.01.001

Miller, S., Yardley, L., & Little, P. (2012). Development of an intervention to reduce transmission of respiratory infections and pandemic flu: Measuring and predicting hand-washing intentions. *Psychology, Health & Medicine, 17,* 59–81. doi:10.1080/13548506.2011.564188

Neo, F., Edward, K., & Mills, C. (2012). Current evidence regarding non-compliance with personal protective equipment: An integrative review to illuminate implications for nursing practice. *ACORN: The Journal of Perioperative Nursing in Australia, 25*(4), 22–30.

Occupational Safety and Health Administration. (2008). *Latex allergy.* Retrieved from http://www.osha.gov/SLTC/latexallergy

Ottum, A., Sethi, A. K., Jacobs, E. A., Zerbel, S., Gaines, M. E., & Safdar, N. (2012). Do patients feel comfortable asking healthcare workers to wash their hands? *Infection Control and Hospital Epidemiology, 33,* 1282–1284. doi:10.1086/668419

Siegel, J. D., Rhinehart, E., Jackson, M., Chiarello, L., & Healthcare Infection Control Practices Advisory Committee. (2007). *Guidelines for isolation precautions: Preventing transmission of infectious agents in healthcare settings 2007.* Retrieved from http://www.cdc.gov/hicpac/pdf/isolation/Isolation2007.pdf

Turner, S., McNamee, R., Agius, R., Wilkinson, S., Carder, M., & Stocks, S. (2012). Evaluating interventions aimed at reducing occupational exposure to latex and rubber glove allergens. *Occupational & Environmental Medicine, 69,* 925–931. doi:10.1136/oemed-2012-100754

UNIT

1

Applying the Nursing Process

This unit looks at foundational skills including hand hygiene, standard precautions, and assisting with invasive procedures. Infection prevention skills are used when performing many procedures and are basic but essential to maintaining the health of the client. Nurses are responsible for both performance of the skills and supervision of other health care team members to ensure that they correctly perform these skills.

CLIENT: Rhonda   AGE: 19 Years   CURRENT MEDICAL DIAGNOSIS: Meningococcal Meningitis

Medical History: Rhonda is admitted through the emergency department and is diagnosed with meningococcal meningitis. She is placed in a private room and started on IV antibiotics. She has no history of past medical or surgical problems. On initial examination, vital signs are 38.8°C (101.8°F) orally, pulse 104 beats/min, respirations 24/min, and blood pressure 102/54 mmHg in her left arm. She reports a severe persistent headache, neck stiffness, nausea, photophobia, and joint pain in her arms and legs. She has a fine purple rash on her legs from below the ankles to midthigh.

Personal and Social History: Rhonda is a college freshman living in a dormitory 63 miles from her parents' home. She tells the nurse her roommate went home sick 2 days ago, but she does not know what she was diagnosed with.

Questions

Assessment
1. How might the nurse verify the client's subjective symptoms gathered during the interview?

Analysis
2. List two possible nursing diagnoses that can be identified from the medical/personal history and assessment data above.

Planning
3. Based on the assessment data and nursing diagnoses, identify one desired outcome.
4. How will the nurse share the desired outcomes with other members of the health care team?

Implementation
5. What personal protective equipment will the nurse wear when caring for this client?
6. What is the nurse's role when assisting the provider with performance of invasive procedures such as placement of a central venous access device?

Evaluation
7. How will the nurse know if the expected outcome has been achieved?

See Applying the Nursing Process suggested answers on student resource website.

Health Assessment

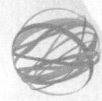

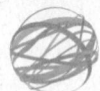

2 Vital Signs

LEARNING OUTCOMES

At the completion of this chapter, the student will be able to:

1. Define the key terms used in the skills of measuring vital signs.
2. Identify the indications for measuring and assessing:
   a. Temperature.
   b. Pulse.
   c. Respirations.
   d. Blood pressure.
   e. Oxygen saturation.
3. Recognize when it is appropriate to delegate measurement of vital signs to unlicensed assistive personnel.
4. Verbalize the steps used to measure:
   a. Temperature.
   b. Pulse.
   c. Respirations.
   d. Blood pressure.
   e. Oxygen saturation.
5. Describe factors that affect the measurement of:
   a. Temperature.
   b. Pulse.
   c. Respirations.
   d. Blood pressure.
   e. Oxygen saturation.

6. Predict the variations in vital signs that occur from infancy to old age.
7. Identify the normal range for:
   a. Temperature.
   b. Pulse.
   c. Respirations.
   d. Blood pressure.
   e. Oxygen saturation.
8. Describe the advantages and disadvantages of the various routes of measuring body temperature (e.g., oral, rectal, axillary, tympanic, temporal artery).
9. List nine anatomic sites commonly used to assess the pulse, and state the reasons for their use.
10. Explain the characteristics that should be included when assessing pulses.
11. Describe assessment of the rate, depth, rhythm, and characteristics of respirations.
12. Demonstrate appropriate documentation and reporting of vital signs.

SKILLS

Skill 2–1   Assessing Body Temperature
Skill 2–2   Assessing Peripheral Pulses
Skill 2–3   Assessing an Apical Pulse
Skill 2–4   Assessing an Apical-Radial Pulse

Skill 2–5   Assessing Respirations
Skill 2–6   Assessing Blood Pressure
Skill 2–7   Assessing Oxygen Saturation (Pulse Oximeter)

KEY TERMS

apical pulse, *29*
apical-radial pulse, *36*
arrhythmias, *30*
auscultatory gap, *41*
core temperature, *22*
costal (thoracic) breathing, *37*
diaphragmatic (abdominal)
    breathing, *37*
diastolic, *40*

exhalation, *37*
expiration, *37*
febrile, *22*
fever, *22*
hyperpyrexia, *22*
hypertension, *40*
hyperthermia, *22*
hyperventilation, *37*
hypotension, *40*

hypothermia, *22*
hypoventilation, *37*
inhalation, *37*
inspiration, *37*
Korotkoff's sounds, *40*
mean arterial pressure (MAP), *40*
oxygen saturation (SaO$_2$), *46*
peripheral pulse, *29*
pulse deficit, *36*

pulse oximeter, *46*
pulse pressure, *40*
pyrexia, *22*
respiration, *37*
sphygmomanometer, *40*
systolic, *40*
ventilation, *37*
vital signs, *21*

The traditional **vital signs** are body temperature, pulse, respirations, and blood pressure. Many agencies such as the Veterans Administration, the American Pain Society, and The Joint Commission have designated pain as a fifth vital sign. Pain assessment is covered in Chapter 9 ∞. In addition, the effectiveness of respirations and circulation is commonly measured noninvasively through pulse oximetry at the same time as other vital signs. These signs, which should be looked at both individually and collectively, enable nurses to monitor the functions of the body. Vital signs reflect changes that otherwise might not be observed. Monitoring a client's vital signs should not be an automatic or routine procedure; it should be a thoughtful, scientific assessment. Vital signs should be evaluated with reference to the client's present and prior health status and compared to accepted standards. If findings appear inconsistent with those anticipated, they

- On admission to a health care agency to obtain baseline data
- When a client has a change in health status or reports symptoms such as chest pain or feeling hot or faint
- Before and after surgery or an invasive procedure
- Before and/or after the administration of a medication that could affect the respiratory or cardiovascular systems; for example, before giving a digitalis preparation
- Before and after any nursing intervention that could affect the vital signs (e.g., ambulating a client who has been on bed rest)

should immediately be rechecked. Some of the vital signs that are confirmed to vary from expected values will require a nursing care plan, and a few represent medical emergencies.

When and how often to assess a specific client's vital signs are chiefly nursing judgments, depending on the client's health status. Some agencies have policies about the frequency of measuring vital signs, and primary care providers may specifically order assessment of a vital sign, for example, "Blood pressure q2h." Ordered assessments, however, should be considered the minimum; nurses should measure clients' vital signs more often if their health status requires it. Examples of times to assess vital signs are listed in Box 2–1.

When assessing vital signs, the nurse invades the client's personal space. A gentle, caring approach is essential, and offering brief explanations to make sure a client understands what you are about to do will ensure a smoother process. When entering a client's room, remind yourself that you are entering into a sacred encounter with someone who is on a healing journey. The person has come to the hospital to literally experience "hospitality." Carefully choosing thoughtful words such as "I'd like to measure your vital signs now" conveys respect and does not assume permission. Remember, it is a whole person who has specific vital signs. So, it is not the "hypertensive in Room 255," but rather a human being with biologic, psychological, and social attributes who is experiencing elevated blood pressure.

BODY TEMPERATURE

Body temperature is the balance between the heat produced by the body and the heat lost from the body. There are two kinds of body temperature: core temperature and surface temperature. **Core temperature** is the temperature of the deep tissues of the body, for example, the abdominal cavity and pelvic cavity. The normal core body temperature is not an exact point on a scale but a range of temperatures. When measured orally, the average body temperature of an adult is between 36°C and 37.5°C (96.8°F and 99.5°F). See Figure 2–1 ■. The surface temperature is the temperature of the skin, the subcutaneous tissue, and fat. Surface temperature rises and falls in response to the environment.

Factors Affecting Body Temperature

Nurses should be aware of factors that can affect a client's body temperature so that they can recognize normal temperature variations and understand the significance of body temperatures that deviate from normal. Normally, a person's temperature can vary as much as 1.0°C (1.8°F) from early morning to late afternoon. Exercise and stress increase body temperature temporarily. Older adults' temperatures

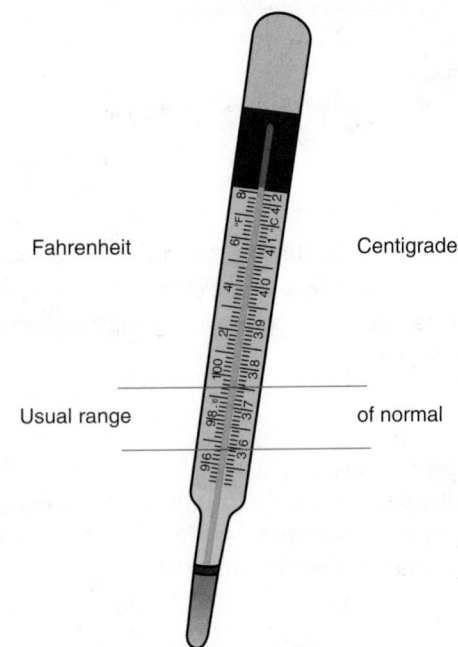

Figure 2–1 ■ Estimated ranges of body temperatures in normal adults.

are often lower than those of middle-age adults, although some research has shown that temperatures for older adults are significantly influenced by ambient temperature (e.g., summer versus winter) (Marigold, Arias, Vassallo, Allen, & Kwan, 2011).

Alterations in Body Temperature

There are two primary alterations in body temperature: pyrexia and hypothermia.

PYREXIA

A body temperature above the usual range is called **pyrexia**, **hyperthermia**, or (in lay terms) **fever**. A very high fever—for example, 41°C (105.8°F)—is called **hyperpyrexia**. Signs of fever the nurse may assess are shown in Clinical Manifestations: Fever. A client with a fever is said to be **febrile**.

HYPOTHERMIA

Hypothermia is a core body temperature below the lower limit of normal. Death usually occurs when the temperature falls

CLINICAL MANIFESTATIONS

Fever

- Increased heart rate
- Increased respiratory rate and depth
- Shivering
- Pallid, cold skin (during onset)
- Complaints of feeling cold (during onset)
- "Gooseflesh" appearance of the skin (during onset)
- Glassy-eyed appearance
- Flushed, warm skin
- Sweating

CLINICAL MANIFESTATIONS

Hypothermia

- Severe shivering (initially)
- Feelings of cold and chills
- Pale, cool, waxy skin
- Hypotension
- Decreased urinary output
- Lack of muscle coordination
- Disorientation
- Drowsiness progressing to coma

below 34°C (93.2°F). With severe hypothermia, sleepiness and even coma are likely to develop, which depress the activity of heat control mechanisms further and prevent shivering. Clinical signs of hypothermia are shown in Clinical Manifestations: Hypothermia.

Body Temperature Assessment Sites

A number of body sites are used for measuring body temperature. The most common are oral, rectal, axillary, tympanic membrane, and temporal artery. Each of the sites has advantages and disadvantages (Table 2–1). Under normal circumstances, the temperature should be measured consistently in the single best site for the client based on his or her specific circumstances.

The body temperature may be measured *orally*. If a client has been taking cold or hot food or fluids or smoking, the nurse should wait 30 minutes before taking the temperature orally to ensure that the temperature of the mouth is not affected by the temperature of the food, fluid, or warm smoke.

Rectal temperature readings are considered to be very accurate. Rectal temperatures are contraindicated for clients who are undergoing rectal surgery, have diarrhea or diseases of the rectum, are immunosuppressed, have a clotting disorder, or have significant hemorrhoids.

The *axilla* is often the preferred site for measuring temperature in newborns because it is accessible and safe. Research indicates that the axillary temperature correlates acceptably with other temperature

sites (Barringer et al., 2011). Adult clients for whom the axillary method of temperature assessment is appropriate generally include those for whom other temperature sites are contraindicated.

The *tympanic membrane*, or nearby tissue in the ear canal, is a frequent site for estimating core body temperature. However, tympanic temperature measurements have been shown to be imprecise (Rubia-Rubia, Arias, Sierra, & Aguirre-Jaime, 2011). If the probe fits too loosely in the ear canal, the reading can be lower than the true value. Electronic tympanic thermometers are found extensively in both inpatient and ambulatory care settings.

The temperature can also be measured on the forehead using a chemical thermometer or a *temporal artery* thermometer. Forehead temperature measurements are most useful for infants and children where a more invasive measurement is not necessary. However, temporal artery temperature measurements have shown inconsistent reliability (Penning, van der Linden, Tibboel, & Evenhuis, 2011; Rubia-Rubia et al., 2011).

Types of Thermometers

New thermometers are constantly being developed that are faster, more accurate, and easier to use than the earlier ones. The nurse uses thermometers as only one indicator of the client's condition, however, because the accuracy of some types of thermometers varies.

Traditionally, body temperatures were measured using mercury-in-glass thermometers. However, glass thermometers can be hazardous due to exposure to broken glass should the thermometer crack or break. Also, the mercury inside is toxic to humans. Hospitals no longer use mercury-in-glass thermometers, and the manufacture and sale of them is being banned. However, the nurse may still encounter this type of thermometer, especially in the community setting. In some cases, plastics have replaced glass and safer chemicals have replaced mercury in modern versions of the thermometer.

Although the amount of mercury in a thermometer (or in a fluorescent light bulb) is minimal, should it break, cleanup involves several "dos and don'ts." Keep children and pets away from the area. Wearing rubber gloves, wipe mercury beads off clothing, skin, or disposable items with a paper towel. Place the paper towel

TABLE 2–1	Advantages and Disadvantages of Sites for Body Temperature Measurement	
Site	**Advantages**	**Disadvantages**
Oral	Accessible and convenient	Thermometers can break if bitten. Inaccurate if client has just ingested hot or cold food or fluid or smoked. Could injure the mouth following oral surgery.
Rectal	Reliable measurement	Inconvenient and more unpleasant for clients; difficult for client who cannot turn to the side. Could injure the rectum. Presence of stool may interfere with thermometer placement.
Axillary	Safe and noninvasive	The thermometer may need to be left in place a long time to obtain an accurate measurement.
Tympanic membrane	Readily accessible; reflects the core temperature; very fast	Can be uncomfortable and involves risk of injuring the membrane if the probe is inserted too far. Repeated measurements may vary. Right and left measurements can differ. Presence of cerumen can affect the reading.
Temporal artery	Safe and noninvasive; very fast	Requires electronic equipment that may be expensive or unavailable. Variation in technique needed if the client has perspiration on the forehead.

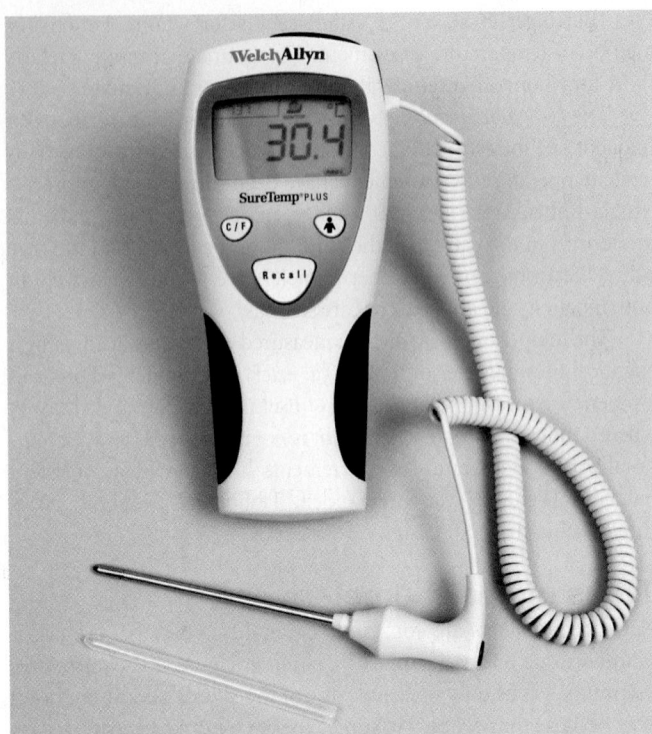

Figure 2–2 ■ An electronic thermometer. Note the probe and probe cover.

immediately into a plastic bag and discard the bag. If the spill is on a porous material that cannot be discarded (e.g., carpet), a contractor trained in mercury disposal may be needed. If the mercury is on a hard surface, use folded stiff cardboard to slowly gather the beads and pour them into a wide-mouthed container. Use a flashlight to search for the beads since the light will reflect off the mercury. Dispose of all items used in the cleanup in a plastic bag that is sealed with tape. Shower or wash well. Keep the area well ventilated for several days. Do not use any type of vacuum cleaner or broom because these will disperse the mercury and be contaminated. Do not pour the mercury down a toilet or drain and do not wash or reuse contaminated materials.

SAFETY ALERT!

SAFETY

Whenever mercury-in-glass thermometers are encountered, the nurse should recommend their immediate replacement with less hazardous thermometers and their safe disposal.

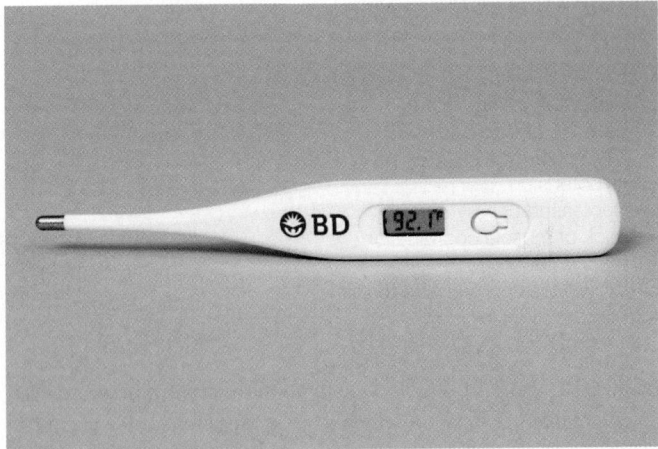

Figure 2–3 ■ One-piece home electronic thermometer.

Electronic thermometers can provide a reading in only 2 to 60 seconds, depending on the model. The equipment typically used in a health care setting consists of an electronic base, a probe, and a probe cover, which is usually disposable (Figure 2–2 ■). Some institutional models have different probes for oral and rectal measurement. Electronic oral thermometers for home use generally consist of a single piece (Figure 2–3 ■).

Chemical disposable thermometers are also used to measure body temperatures. Chemical thermometers have liquid crystal dots or bars that change color to indicate temperature. Some of these are single use, and others may be reused several times. One type that has small chemical dots at one end is shown in Figure 2–4 ■. To read the temperature, the nurse notes the highest reading among the dots that have changed color. These thermometers can be used orally, in the axilla, or rectally.

Temperature-sensitive tape may also be used to obtain a general indication of body surface temperature. It does not indicate the core temperature. The tape contains liquid crystals that change color according to temperature. When applied to the skin, usually of the forehead or abdomen, the temperature digits on the tape respond by changing color (Figure 2–5 ■). The skin area should be dry. After the length of time specified by the manufacturer (e.g., 15 seconds), a color appears on the tape. This method is particularly useful at home and for infants whose temperatures are to be monitored.

Infrared thermometers sense body heat in the form of infrared energy given off by a heat source, which in the ear canal is primarily the tympanic membrane (Figure 2–6 ■). The infrared thermometer makes no contact with the tympanic membrane.

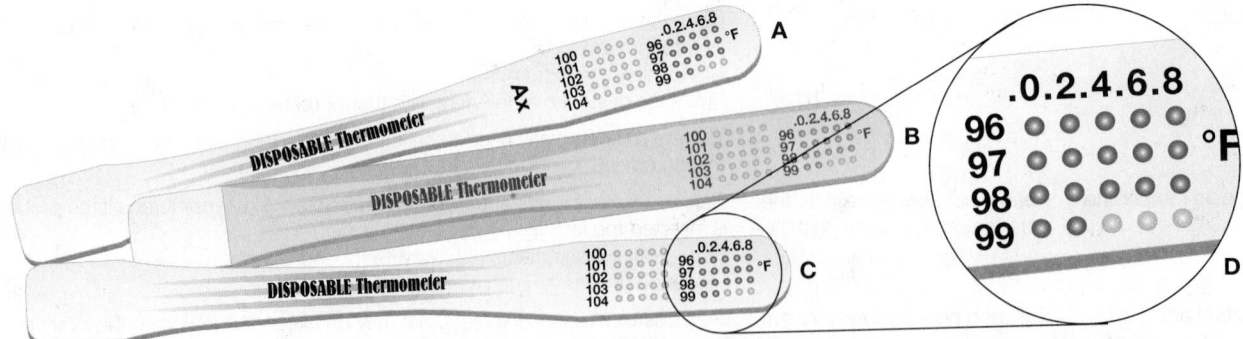

Figure 2–4 ■ Chemical dot thermometers: *A,* axillary (note the "Ax" on the stem); *B,* rectal (note the plastic cover); *C,* oral; *D,* an enlargement showing a reading of 99.2°F.

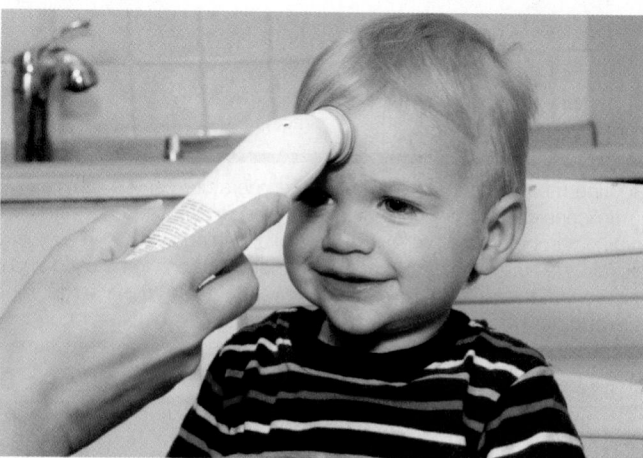

Figure 2–5 ■ A temperature-sensitive skin tape.

Figure 2–7 ■ A temporal artery thermometer.
© A. Wilson / Custom Medical Stock Photo.

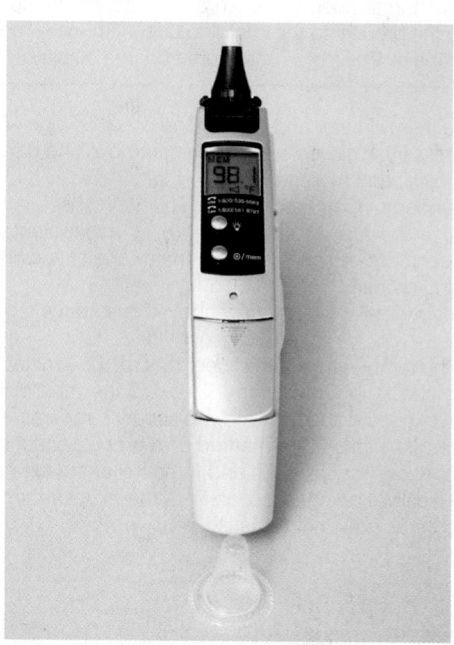

Figure 2–6 ■ An infrared tympanic thermometer used to measure the tympanic membrane temperature.

Temporal artery thermometers determine temperature using a scanning infrared thermometer that compares arterial temperature in the temporal artery of the forehead to the temperature in the room and calculates the heat balance to approximate the core temperature of the blood in the pulmonary artery. The probe is placed in the middle of the forehead and is then drawn laterally to the hairline (Figure 2–7 ■). If the client has perspiration on the forehead, the probe is also touched behind the earlobe so the thermometer can compensate for evaporative cooling.

●○● NURSING PROCESS: ASSESSING BODY TEMPERATURE

Assessing Body Temperature

ASSESSMENT
- Based on the purpose of taking the temperature and the client's age and condition, determine the most appropriate site and method of measuring the client's temperature.
- Consider the purpose of assessing the temperature. Is the temperature being taken as part of a routine examination or for assessment of a current illness?
  - If fever or hypothermia is suspected, the most accurate measurement possible should be obtained.

- If fever or hypothermia is suspected, know what the last temperature reading was. In this way, you can estimate if the temperature reading you obtain is likely to be accurate.

SKILL 2-1

Continued on page 26

SKILL 2–1

Assessing Body Temperature—*continued*

PLANNING
DELEGATION

Routine measurement of the client's temperature can be delegated to unlicensed assistive personnel (UAP), or it can be performed by family members/caregivers in nonhospital settings. The nurse must explain the appropriate type of thermometer and site to be used and ensure that the person knows when to report an abnormal temperature and how to record the finding. The interpretation of an abnormal temperature and determination of appropriate responses are done by the nurse.

INTERPROFESSIONAL PRACTICE

Measuring the temperature may be within the scope of practice for many health care providers. Although these providers may verbally communicate their findings and plan to the other health care team members, the nurse must also know where to locate their documentation in the client's medical record.

Equipment
- Thermometer
- Thermometer sheath or cover
- Water-soluble lubricant for a rectal temperature
- Clean gloves for a rectal temperature
- Towel for axillary temperature
- Tissues/wipes

IMPLEMENTATION
Preparation
Check that all equipment is functioning normally.

Performance
1. Prior to performing the procedure, introduce self and verify the client's identity using agency protocol. Explain to the client what you are going to do, why it is necessary, and how he or she can participate. Discuss how the results will be used in planning further care or treatments.
2. Perform hand hygiene and observe other appropriate infection prevention procedures. Apply gloves if measuring a rectal temperature.
3. Provide for client privacy.
4. Place the client in the appropriate position (e.g., lateral or Sims' position for inserting a rectal thermometer).
5. Place the thermometer (see Box 2–2 on page 27).
   - Apply a protective sheath or probe cover if appropriate.
   - Lubricate a rectal thermometer.
6. Wait the appropriate amount of time. Electronic and tympanic thermometers will indicate that the reading is complete by means of a light or tone. Check package instructions for length of time to wait prior to reading chemical dot or tape thermometers.

CLINICAL ALERT!

Be sure to record the temperature from an electronic thermometer before replacing the probe into the charging unit. With many models, replacing the probe erases the temperature from the display.

7. Remove the thermometer and discard the cover or wipe with a tissue if necessary. If gloves were applied, remove and discard gloves. Perform hand hygiene.
8. Read the temperature and record it on your worksheet. If the temperature is obviously too high, too low, or inconsistent with the client's condition, recheck it with a thermometer known to be functioning properly.
9. Wash the thermometer if necessary and return it to the storage location.
10. Document the temperature in the client record. ❶ A rectal temperature may be recorded with an "R" next to the value or with the mark on a graphic sheet circled. An axillary temperature may be recorded with "AX" or marked on a graphic sheet with an X. Abbreviations for tympanic and temporal artery temperatures vary. Usually, if no route is identified, the temperature is assumed to be an oral one. Consult agency policy.

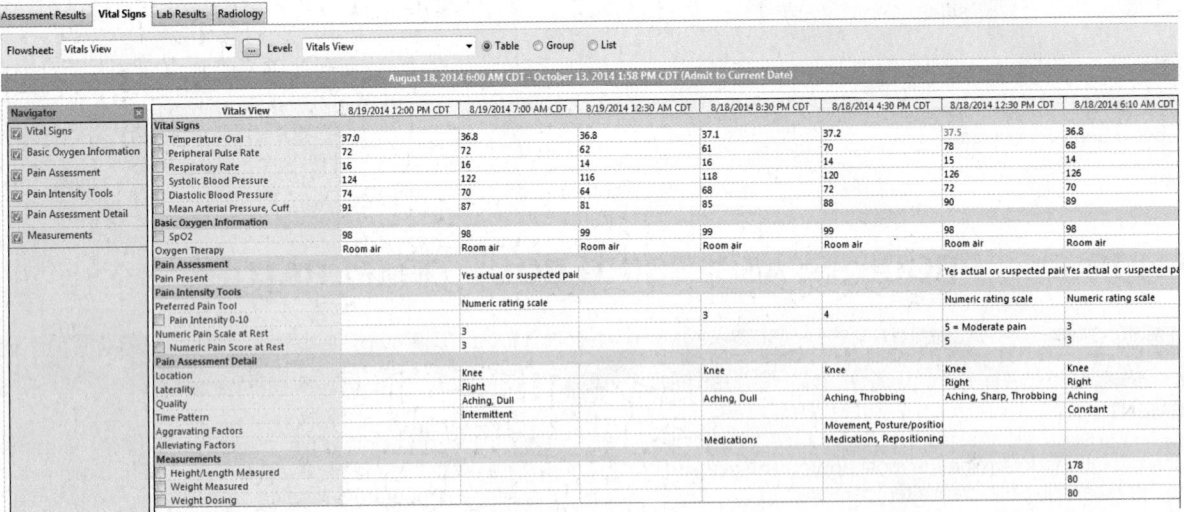

❶ Vital signs record.

"Vital signs record" from Cerner Electronic Health Record. Copyright © by Cerner Corporation. Used by permission of Cerner Corporation.

Assessing Body Temperature—*continued*

EVALUATION

- Compare the temperature measurement to baseline data, normal range for age of client, and client's previous temperatures. Analyze considering time of day and any additional influencing factors and other vital signs.
- Conduct appropriate follow-up such as notifying the primary care provider if a temperature is outside of a specific range or is

not responding to interventions, giving a medication, or altering the client's environment. This includes teaching the client how to lower an elevated temperature through actions such as increasing fluid intake, coughing and deep breathing, cool compresses, or removing heavy coverings. Interventions for hypothermia include intake of warm fluids and use of warm or electric blankets.

BOX 2–2 | **Thermometer Placement**

ORAL

- Place the tip on either side of the frenulum. ❶

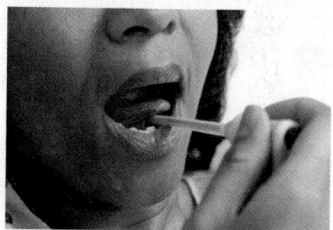

❶ Oral thermometer placement.

RECTAL

- Apply clean gloves.
- Instruct the client to take a slow deep breath during insertion. ❷
- Never force the thermometer if resistance is felt.
- Insert 3.5 cm (1.5 in.) in adults.

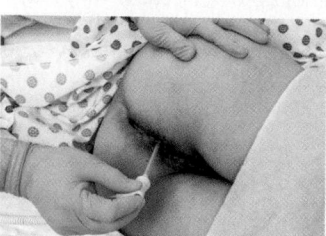

❷ Inserting a rectal thermometer.

AXILLARY

- Pat the axilla dry if very moist.
- Place the tip in the center of the axilla. ❸

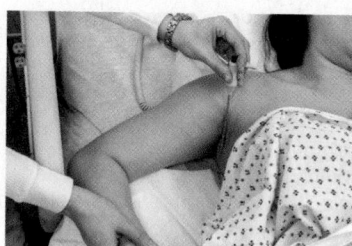

❸ Placing the tip of the thermometer in the center of the axilla.

TYMPANIC MEMBRANE

- Pull the pinna slightly upward and backward.
- Point the probe slightly anteriorly, toward the eardrum.
- Insert the probe slowly using a circular motion until snug. ❹

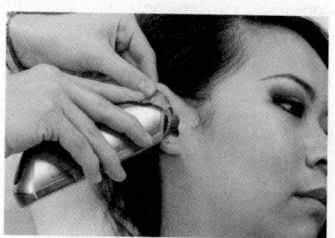

❹ Pull the pinna of the ear up and back for an adult while inserting the tympanic thermometer.

TEMPORAL ARTERY

- Brush hair aside if covering the temporal artery area. With the probe flush on the center of the forehead, depress the red button; keep depressed. Slowly slide the probe midline across the forehead to the hairline, not down the side of the face. Lift the probe from the forehead and touch on the neck just behind the earlobe. Release the button. ❺

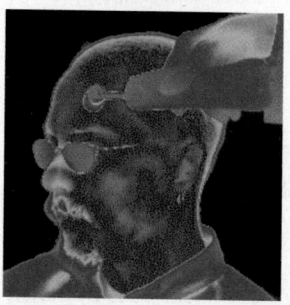
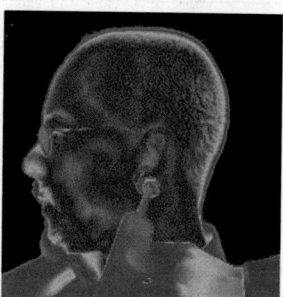

❺ Positioning a temporal artery thermometer.

LIFESPAN CONSIDERATIONS Temperature

INFANTS

- The body temperature of newborns is extremely labile (changeable), and newborns must be kept warm and dry to prevent hypothermia.
- Using the axillary site, you need to hold the infant's arm against the chest to keep the thermometer in place.
- The axillary route may not be as accurate as other routes for detecting fevers in children.
- The tympanic route is fast and convenient. Place the infant supine and stabilize the head. Pull the pinna straight back and slightly downward. Remember that the pinna is pulled upward for children over 3 years of age and adults but downward for children younger than 3. Direct the probe tip anteriorly, and insert far enough to seal the canal. The tip will not touch the tympanic membrane.
- Avoid the tympanic route in a child with active ear infections or tympanic membrane drainage tubes.
- The tympanic membrane route may be more accurate in determining temperature in febrile infants.
- When using a temporal artery thermometer, touching only the forehead or behind the ear is needed.
- The rectal route is least desirable in infants.

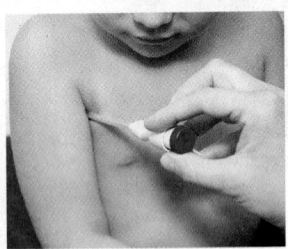

Axillary thermometer placement for a child.

CHILDREN

- Tympanic or temporal artery sites are preferred.
- For the tympanic route, have an adult hold the child in his or her lap with the child's head held gently against the adult for support. Pull the pinna straight back and upward for children over age 3.

- Avoid the tympanic route in a child with active ear infections or tympanic membrane drainage tubes.
- The oral route may be used for children over age 3, but nonbreakable, electronic thermometers are recommended.
- For a rectal temperature, place the child prone across your lap or in a side-lying position with the knees flexed. Insert the thermometer 2.5 cm (1 in.) into the rectum.

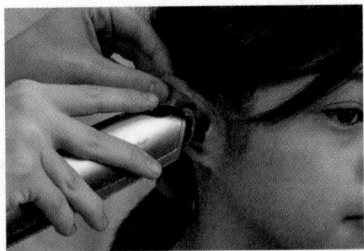

Pull the pinna of the ear back and up for placement of a tympanic thermometer in a child over 3 years of age; back and down for children under age 3.

OLDER ADULTS

- Temperatures tend to be lower than those of middle-aged adults.
- Temperatures are strongly influenced by both environmental and internal temperature changes. Their thermoregulation control processes are not as efficient as when they were younger, and they are at higher risk for both hypothermia and hyperthermia.
- Significant buildup of ear cerumen can develop and interfere with tympanic thermometer readings.
- Hemorrhoids are more likely to occur. Inspect the anus before taking a rectal temperature.
- Older adults' temperatures may not be a valid indication of the seriousness of the pathology of a disease. They may have pneumonia or a urinary tract infection and have only a slight temperature elevation. Other symptoms, such as confusion and restlessness, may be displayed and need follow-up to determine if there is an underlying process.

CLIENT TEACHING CONSIDERATIONS

Temperature

- Teach the client accurate use and reading of the type of thermometer to be used. Examine the thermometer used by the client in the home for safety and proper functioning. Facilitate the replacement of mercury thermometers with nonmercury ones. Instructions regarding management of a broken mercury thermometer are given on page 24.
- Observe the client or caregiver taking and reading a temperature. Reinforce the importance of reporting the site and type of thermometer used and the value of using the same thermometer consistently.

- Discuss means of keeping the thermometer clean, such as warm water and soap, and avoiding cross contamination.
- Instruct the client or family member to notify the health care provider if the temperature is higher than a specified level, for example, 38.5°C (101.3°F).
- Check that the client knows how to record the temperature. Provide a recording chart/table if indicated.
- Discuss environmental control modifications that should be taken during illness or extreme climate conditions (e.g., heating, air conditioning, appropriate clothing and bedding).

Ambulatory and Community Settings **Temperature**

- Ensure that the client has water-soluble lubricant if using a rectal thermometer.
- When making a home visit, take a thermometer with you in case the client does not own a functional thermometer.
- Consider whether environmental conditions, such as lack of heat or air conditioning, are affecting the client's temperature or temperature measurement.
- Pacifier thermometers are being used more in the home setting for children under age 2. The manufacturer's instructions must be followed carefully since many require adding 0.5°F in order to estimate rectal temperature.

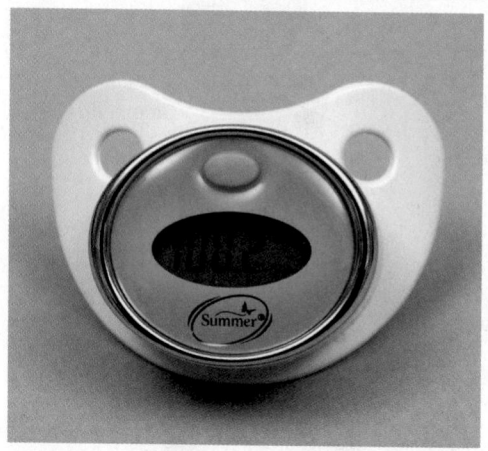

A pacifier thermometer.

PULSE

Pulse is the term used to describe the rate, rhythm, and volume of the heartbeat as it is assessed at either central or peripheral locations. The pulse is a wave of blood created by contraction of the left ventricle of the heart. Generally, the pulse wave represents the volume output by each cardiac contraction and the compliance of the arteries. Compliance of the arteries refers to the distensibility of the arteries; that is, their ability to contract and expand. The rate of the pulse is expressed in beats per minute (beats/min).

In a healthy person, the pulse reflects the heartbeat; that is, the pulse rate is the same as the rate of the ventricular contractions of the heart. However, in some types of cardiovascular disease, the heartbeat and pulse rates can differ. For example, a client's heart may produce very weak or small pulse waves that are not easily palpable in a peripheral pulse. In these instances, the nurse should assess the heartbeat (apical pulse) and the peripheral pulse. See the section on assessing the apical pulse later in this chapter. A **peripheral pulse** is a pulse located in the periphery of the body, for example, in the foot, hand, or neck, and is assessed by palpation (feeling). The **apical pulse** is a central pulse located at the apex of the heart and is assessed by auscultation (listening).

Factors Affecting Pulse Rate

- *Age.* As age increases, the pulse rate gradually decreases. See Table 2–2 for specific variations in pulse rates from birth to adulthood.
- *Sex.* After puberty, the average male's pulse rate is slightly lower than the female's.
- *Exercise.* The pulse rate normally increases with activity. Both the resting pulse and rate of increase in exercising athletes may be less than those of the average person because of greater cardiac size, strength, and efficiency.

TABLE 2–2	Variations in Pulse and Respirations by Age	
Age	**Pulse Average (and Ranges)**	**Respiration Average (and Ranges)**
Newborns	130 (80–180)	35 (30–60)
1 year	120 (80–140)	30 (20–40)
5–8 years	100 (75–120)	20 (15–25)
10 years	70 (50–90)	19 (15–25)
Teen	75 (50–90)	18 (15–20)
Adult	80 (60–100)	16 (12–20)
Older adult	70 (60–100)	16 (15–20)

- *Fever.* The pulse rate increases (a) in response to the lowered blood pressure that results from peripheral vasodilation associated with elevated body temperature and also (b) because of the increased metabolic rate.
- *Medications.* Some medications decrease the pulse rate, and others increase it. For example, cardiotonics (e.g., digitalis preparations) decrease the heart rate, whereas epinephrine increases it.
- *Hypovolemia/dehydration.* Loss of fluid from the vascular system increases the pulse rate.
- *Stress.* In response to stress, sympathetic nervous stimulation increases the overall activity of the heart. Stress increases the rate as well as the force of the heartbeat. Fear and anxiety as well as the perception of severe pain stimulate the sympathetic system.
- *Position.* When a person is sitting or standing, blood pools in dependent vessels of the venous system. Pooling results in a transient decrease in the venous blood return to the heart and a subsequent reduction in blood pressure, increasing cardiac rate.

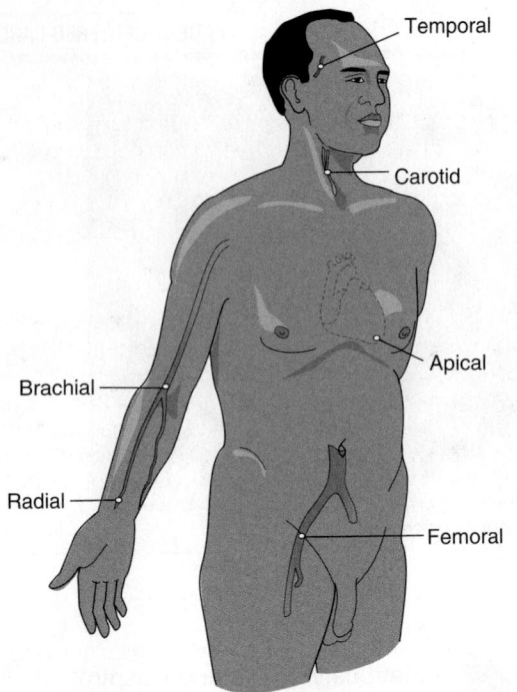

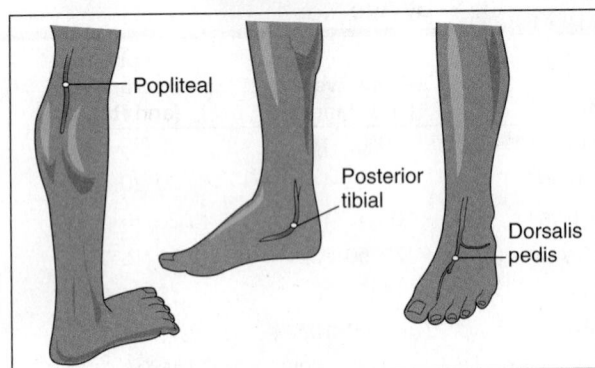

Figure 2–8 ■ Nine sites for assessing pulse.

Pulse Assessment Sites

The pulse is commonly taken in nine sites (Figure 2–8 ■):

1. Temporal, where the temporal artery passes over the temporal bone of the head. The site is superior (above) and lateral to (away from the midline of) the eye.
2. Carotid, in the mid-neck, where the carotid artery runs between the trachea and the sternocleidomastoid muscle.

CLINICAL ALERT!

Never press both carotids at the same time because this can cause a reflex drop in blood pressure or pulse rate.

3. Apical, at the apex of the heart. In an adult, this is located on the left side of the chest, about 8 cm (3 in.) left of the sternum (breastbone) at the fifth intercostal space.
4. Brachial, at the inner aspect of the biceps muscle of the arm or medially in the antecubital space.
5. Radial, where the radial artery runs along the radial bone, on the thumb side of the inner aspect of the wrist.
6. Femoral, where the femoral artery passes alongside the inguinal ligament.
7. Popliteal, where the popliteal artery passes behind the knee.
8. Posterior tibial, on the medial surface of the ankle where the posterior tibial artery passes behind the medial malleolus.
9. Pedal (dorsalis pedis), where the dorsalis pedis artery passes over the bones of the foot. This artery can be palpated by feeling the dorsum of the foot on an imaginary line from the middle of the ankle to the space between the big and second toe.

Some reasons for use of each site are given in Table 2–3.

TABLE 2–3	Reasons for Using a Specific Pulse Site
Pulse Site	**Reasons for Use**
Radial	Readily accessible
Temporal	Used when radial pulse is not accessible
Carotid	Used during cardiac arrest/shock in adults Used to determine circulation to the brain
Apical	Routinely used for infants and children up to 3 years of age Used to determine discrepancies with radial pulse Used in conjunction with some medications
Brachial	Used to measure blood pressure Used during cardiac arrest for infants
Femoral	Used in cases of cardiac arrest/shock Used to determine circulation to a leg
Popliteal	Used to determine circulation to the lower leg
Posterior tibial	Used to determine circulation to the foot
Dorsalis pedis	Used to determine circulation to the foot

●○● NURSING PROCESS: ASSESSING PERIPHERAL PULSES

Assessing Peripheral Pulses

SKILL 2–2

ASSESSMENT
- Peripheral pulses may be assessed as an indicator either of cardiac function or of vascular integrity. As an indicator of cardiac function, the peripheral pulse is used to:
  - Provide baseline data for subsequent evaluation.
  - Identify whether the pulse rate is within normal range.
  - Determine whether the pulse rhythm is regular.

- Monitor and assess changes in the client's health status.
- Monitor clients at risk for pulse alterations such as those with a history of heart disease or cardiac **arrhythmias** (irregular heart rhythms), hemorrhage, acute pain, infusion of large volumes of fluids, or fever.

Assessing Peripheral Pulses—*continued*

- As an indicator of vascular integrity, the peripheral pulse is used to:
  - Determine whether the pulse volume is normal.
  - Compare the equality of corresponding peripheral pulses on each side of the body.
  - Determine the adequacy of blood flow to a particular part of the body.

- To provide a complete picture of the client's cardiovascular health, also assess for clinical signs of cardiovascular alterations such as dyspnea (difficult respirations), fatigue, pallor, cyanosis (bluish discoloration of skin and mucous membranes), palpitations, syncope (fainting), or impaired peripheral tissue perfusion as evidenced by skin discoloration and cool temperature.

PLANNING
DELEGATION

Measurement of the client's radial or brachial pulse can be delegated to UAP, or be performed by the client/family members/caregivers in nonhospital settings. Reports of abnormal pulse rates or rhythms require reassessment by the nurse, who also determines appropriate action if the abnormality is confirmed. UAP are generally not delegated these techniques due to the skill required in locating and interpreting peripheral pulses other than the radial or brachial artery and in using Doppler ultrasound devices.

INTERPROFESSIONAL PRACTICE

Assessing a peripheral pulse may be within the scope of practice for many health care providers. For example, in addition to nurses, both physical therapists and respiratory therapists may check the client's pulse before, during, and after treatment. Although the therapists may verbally communicate their findings and plan to the health care team members, the nurse must also know where to locate their documentation in the client's medical record.

Equipment
- Clock or watch with a sweep second hand or digital seconds indicator
- If using a Doppler ultrasound stethoscope (DUS), the transducer probe, the stethoscope headset (some models), transmission gel, and tissues/wipes

IMPLEMENTATION
Preparation
If using the DUS, check that the equipment is functioning normally.

Performance
1. Prior to performing the procedure, introduce self and verify the client's identity using agency protocol. Explain to the client what you are going to do, why it is necessary, and how he or she can participate. Discuss how the results will be used in planning further care or treatments.
2. Perform hand hygiene and observe appropriate infection prevention procedures.
3. Provide for client privacy.
4. Select the pulse point. Normally, the radial pulse is taken, unless it cannot be exposed or circulation to another body area is to be assessed.
5. Assist the client to a comfortable resting position. When the radial pulse is assessed, with the palm facing downward, the client's arm can rest alongside the body or the forearm can rest at a 90° angle across the chest. For the client who can sit, the forearm can rest across the thigh, with the palm of the hand facing downward or inward.
6. Palpate and count the pulse. Place two or three middle fingertips lightly and squarely over the pulse point. ❶

Rationale: *Using the thumb is contraindicated because the nurse's thumb has a pulse that could be mistaken for the client's pulse.*
- Count for 15 seconds and multiply by 4. Record the pulse in beats per minute on your worksheet. If taking a client's pulse for the first time, when obtaining baseline data, or if the pulse is irregular, count for a full minute. If an irregular pulse is found, also take the apical pulse.
7. Assess the pulse rhythm and volume.
- Assess the pulse rhythm by noting the pattern of the intervals between the beats. A normal pulse has equal time periods between beats. If this is an initial assessment, assess for 1 minute.
- Assess the pulse volume. A normal pulse can be felt with moderate pressure, and the pressure is equal with each beat. A forceful pulse volume is full; an easily obliterated pulse is weak. Record the rhythm and volume on your worksheet.
8. Document the pulse rate, rhythm, and volume and your actions in the client record (see Figure ❶ in Skill 2–1). Also record in the nurse's notes pertinent related data such as variation in pulse rate compared to normal for the client and abnormal skin color and skin temperature.

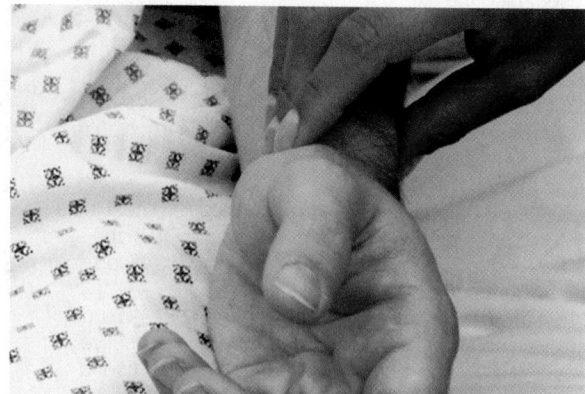

Assessing the pulses: ❶ *A, Radial*

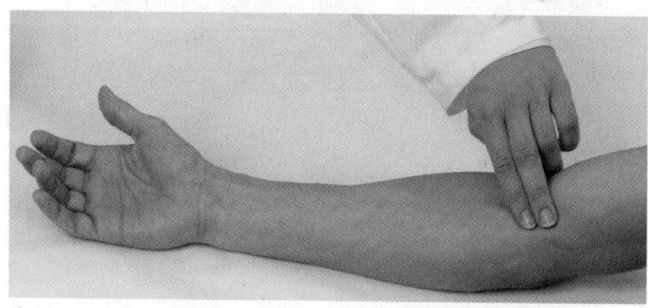

❶ *B, Brachial*

Continued on page 32

Assessing Peripheral Pulses—*continued*

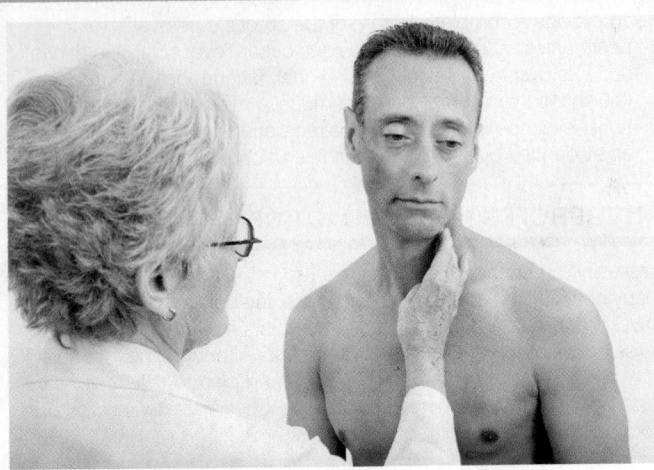

① *C,* Carotid

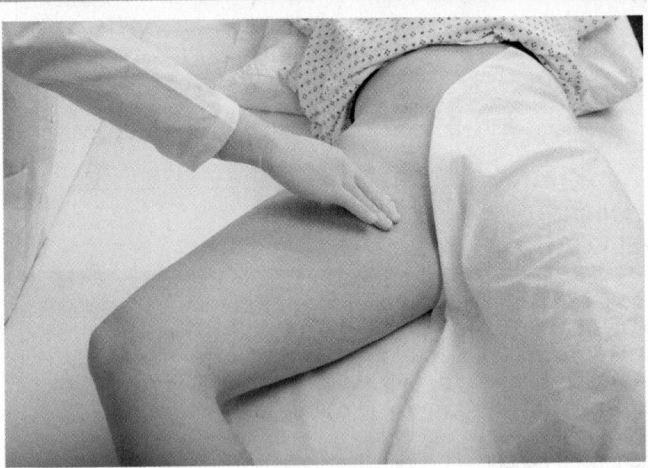

① *D,* Femoral

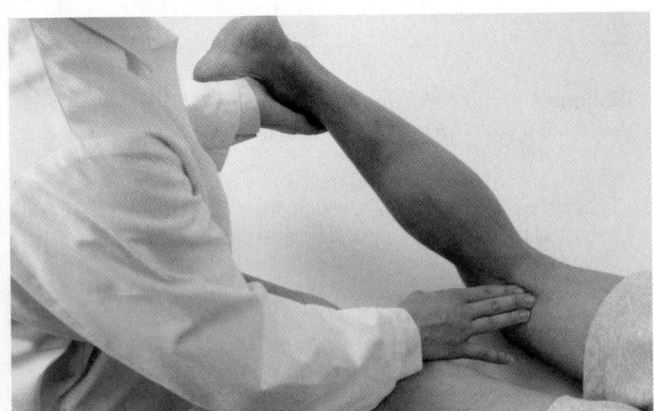

① *E,* Popliteal

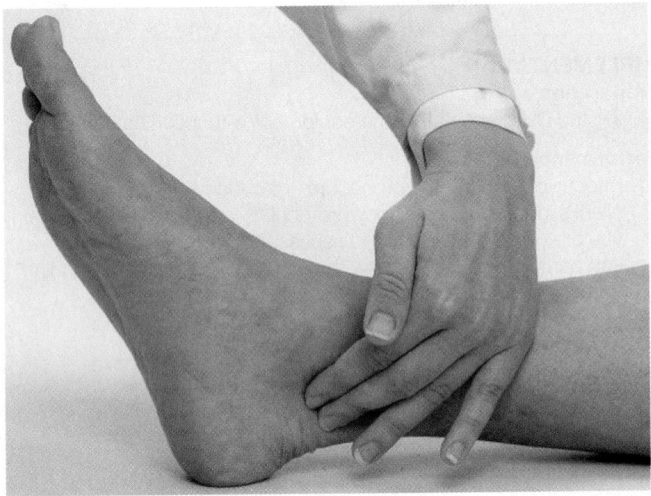

① *F,* Posterior tibial

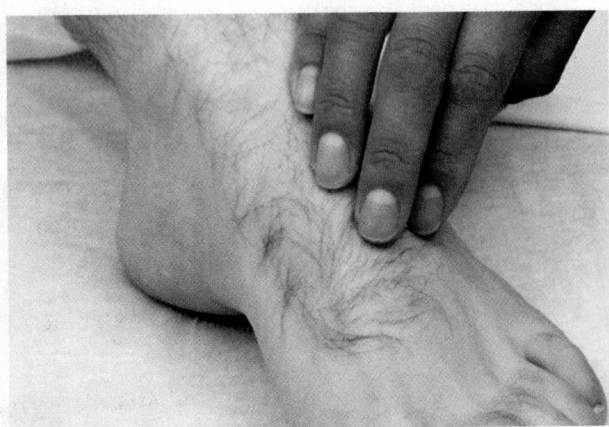

① *G,* Dorsalis pedis

Variation: Using a DUS ❷

- If used, plug the stethoscope headset into the output jack located next to the volume control.
- Apply transmission gel either to the probe at the narrow end of the plastic case housing the transducer, or to the client's skin. **Rationale:** *Ultrasound beams do not travel well through air. The gel makes an airtight seal, which then promotes optimal ultrasound wave transmission.*
- Press the "on" button.
- Hold the probe against the skin over the pulse site. Use a light pressure, and keep the probe in contact with the skin. ❸ **Rationale:** *Too much pressure can stop the blood flow and obliterate the signal.*
- Adjust the volume if necessary. Distinguish artery sounds from vein sounds. The artery sound (signal) is distinctively pulsating and has a pumping quality. The venous sound

Assessing Peripheral Pulses—*continued*

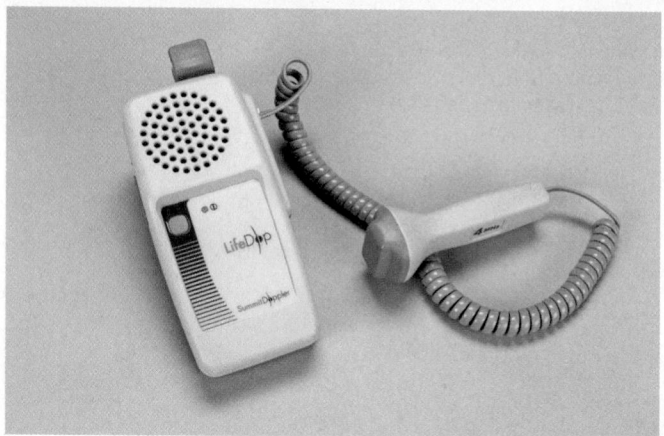

❷ A Doppler ultrasound stethoscope (DUS).

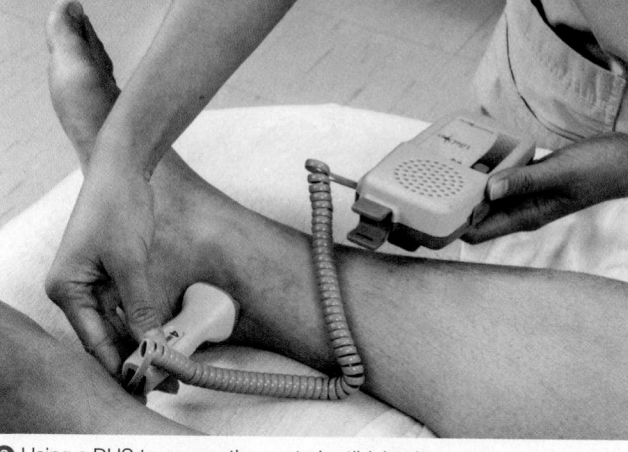

❸ Using a DUS to assess the posterior tibial pulse.

is intermittent and varies with respirations. Both artery and vein sounds are heard simultaneously through the DUS because major arteries and veins are situated close together throughout the body. If arterial sounds cannot be easily heard, reposition the probe.

- After assessing the pulse, remove all gel from the probe to prevent damage to the surface. Clean the transducer with a water-based solution. **Rationale:** *Alcohol or other disinfectants may damage the face of the transducer.* Remove all gel from the client.

EVALUATION
- Compare the pulse rate to baseline data or normal range for age of client.
- Relate pulse rate and volume to other vital signs; relate pulse rhythm and volume to baseline data and health status.
- If assessing peripheral pulses, evaluate equality, rate, and volume in corresponding extremities.

- Conduct appropriate follow-up such as notifying the primary care provider or giving medication. A pulse of less than 45 or greater than 140 beats/min is considered extremely serious, and the nurse should consider taking immediate action or calling for assistance.

●○● NURSING PROCESS: ASSESSING AN APICAL PULSE

Assessing an Apical Pulse

ASSESSMENT
- Assess the apical pulse of an adult with an irregular peripheral pulse, clients with cardiac disease, and clients receiving medications to improve heart action.
- To provide a complete picture of the client's cardiovascular health, also assess for clinical signs of cardiovascular alterations

such as dyspnea (difficult respirations), fatigue, pallor, cyanosis (bluish discoloration of skin and mucous membranes), palpitations, syncope (fainting), or impaired peripheral tissue perfusion as evidenced by skin discoloration and cool temperature.

PLANNING
DELEGATION

Due to the degree of skill and knowledge required, UAP are generally not responsible for assessing apical pulses.

INTERPROFESSIONAL PRACTICE

Assessing an apical pulse may be within the scope of practice for many health care providers. For example, in addition to nurses, respiratory therapists may check the client's apical pulse before, during, and after treatment and physicians often check the apical pulse when assessing the chest during examinations. Although the providers may verbally communicate their findings and plan to other health care team members, the nurse must also know where to locate their documentation in the client's medical record.

Continued on page 34

Assessing an Apical Pulse—*continued*

Equipment

- Clock or watch with a sweep second hand or digital seconds indicator
- Stethoscope
- Antiseptic wipes
- If using a DUS, the transducer probe, the stethoscope headset, transmission gel, and tissues/wipes

IMPLEMENTATION

Preparation

If using the DUS, check that the equipment is functioning normally.

Performance

1. Prior to performing the procedure, introduce self and verify the client's identity using agency protocol. Explain to the client what you are going to do, why it is necessary, and how he or she can participate. Discuss how the results will be used in planning further care or treatments.
2. Perform hand hygiene and observe other appropriate infection prevention procedures.
3. Provide for client privacy.
4. Position the client appropriately in a comfortable supine position or in a sitting position. Expose the area of the chest over the apex of the heart.
5. Locate the apical impulse. This is the point over the apex of the heart where the apical pulse can be most clearly heard.
   - Palpate the angle of Louis (the angle between the manubrium, the top of the sternum, and the body of the sternum). It is palpated just below the suprasternal notch and is felt as a prominence. ❶
   - Slide your index finger just to the left of the sternum, and palpate the second intercostal space. ❷

CLINICAL ALERT!

When "left" and "right" are used in describing the nurse's hand placement on the client, the terms refer to the client's right or left side, not the nurse's.

- Place your middle or next finger in the third intercostal space, ❸ and continue palpating downward until you locate the fifth intercostal space.
- Move your index finger laterally along the fifth intercostal space toward the midclavicular line (MCL). ❹ Normally, the apical impulse is palpable at or just medial to the MCL (see Figure ❶).

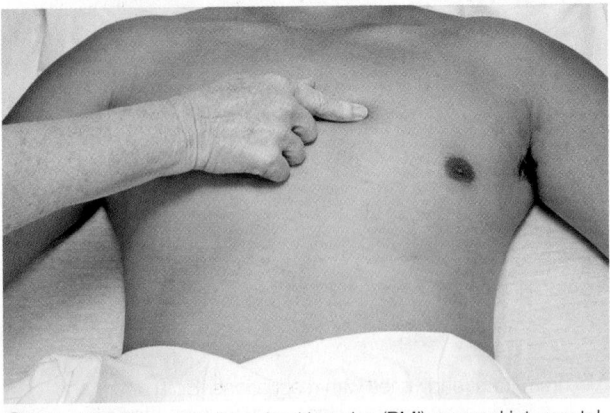

❷ Palpating the point of maximal impulse (PMI): second intercostal space.

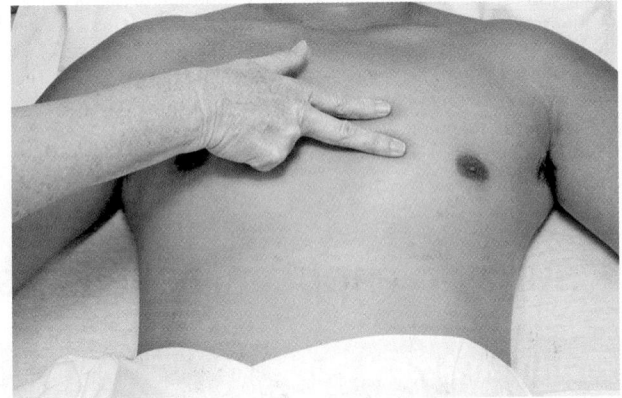

❸ Third intercostal space.

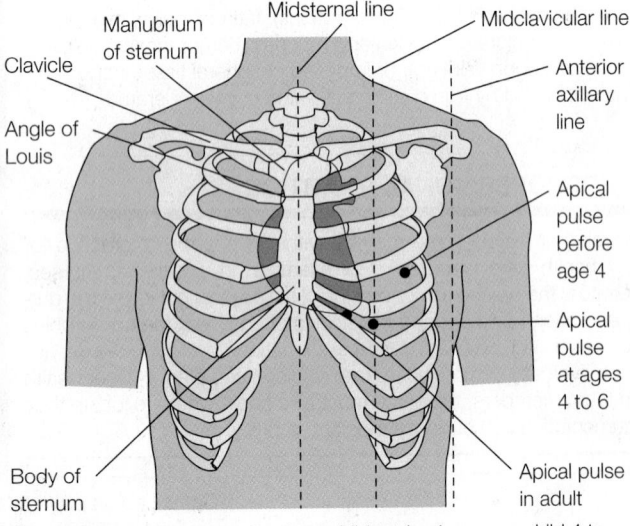

Manubrium of sternum — Midsternal line — Midclavicular line

Clavicle

Angle of Louis

Anterior axillary line

Apical pulse before age 4

Apical pulse at ages 4 to 6

Body of sternum

Apical pulse in adult

❶ Location of the apical pulse for a child under 4 years, a child 4 to 6 years, and an adult.

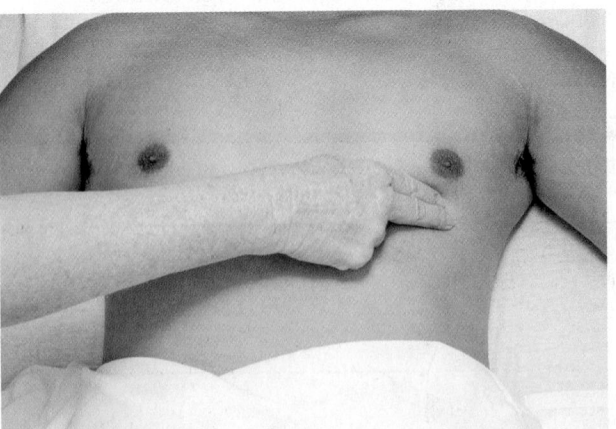

❹ Fifth intercostal space: MCL.

Assessing an Apical Pulse—*continued*

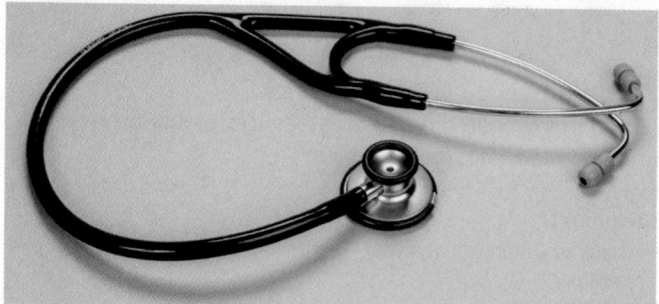

⑤ *A,* Stethoscope with both a bell and a diaphragm.

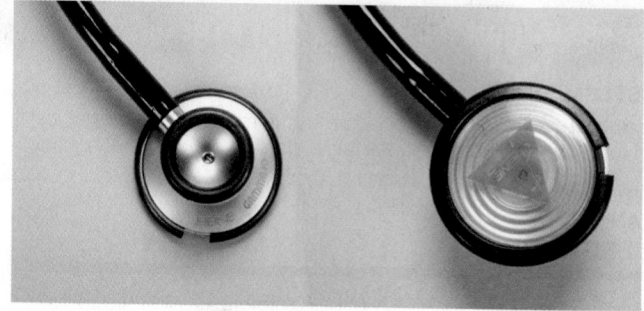

⑤ *B,* Close-up of a bell (left) and a diaphragm (right).

6. Auscultate and count heartbeats.
   - Use antiseptic wipes to clean the earpieces and diaphragm of the stethoscope if their cleanliness is in doubt. **Rationale:** *The diaphragm needs to be cleaned and disinfected if soiled with body substances. Both earpieces and diaphragms have been shown to harbor pathogenic bacteria (Muniz, Sethi, Zaghi, Ziniel, & Sandora, 2012).*
   - Warm the diaphragm of the stethoscope by holding it in the palm of the hand for a moment. **Rationale:** *The metal of the diaphragm is usually cold and can startle the client when placed immediately on the chest.*
   - Insert the earpieces of the stethoscope into your ears in the direction of the ear canals, or slightly forward, to facilitate hearing.
   - Tap your finger lightly on the diaphragm. **Rationale:** *This is to be sure it is the active side of the stethoscope head.* If necessary, rotate the head to select the diaphragm side. ⑤
   - Place the diaphragm of the stethoscope over the apical impulse and listen for the normal S_1 and S_2 heart sounds, which are heard as "lub-dub." ⑥ **Rationale:** *The heartbeat is normally loudest over the apex of the heart.* Each lub-dub is counted as one heartbeat. **Rationale:** *The two heart sounds are produced by closure of the heart valves.* The S_1 heart sound (lub) occurs when the atrioventricular valves close after the ventricles have been sufficiently filled. The S_2 heart sound (dub) occurs when the semilunar valves close after the ventricles empty.
   - If you have difficulty hearing the apical pulse, ask the supine client to roll onto the left side or ask the sitting client to lean slightly forward. **Rationale:** *This positioning moves the apex of the heart closer to the chest wall.*
   - If the rhythm is regular, count the heartbeats for 30 seconds and multiply by 2. If the rhythm is irregular or for giving certain medications such as digoxin, count the beats for 60 seconds. **Rationale:** *A 60-second count provides a more accurate assessment of an irregular pulse than a 30-second count.*

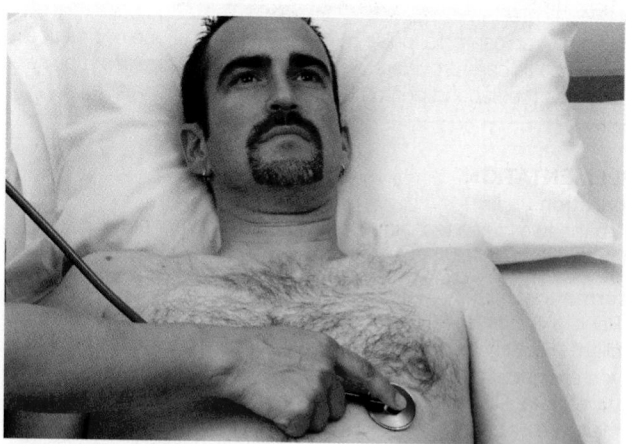

⑥ Taking an apical pulse using the flat-disc stethoscope. Note how the amplifier is held against the chest.

7. Assess the rhythm and the strength of the heartbeat.
   - Assess the rhythm of the heartbeat by noting the pattern of intervals between the beats. A normal pulse has equal time periods between beats.
   - Assess the strength (volume) of the heartbeat. Normally, the heartbeats are equal in strength and can be described as strong or weak.
8. Document the apical pulse rate and rhythm and nursing actions in the client record. Also record pertinent related data such as variation in pulse rate compared to normal for the client and abnormal skin color and skin temperature.

SAMPLE DOCUMENTATION

2/24/15 1000 Radial pulse 116 & irregular. Had been 82 & regular at 0600. T, R, & BP within client's usual range. C/o slight dizziness. Skin warm & dry. Apical pulse 120, irregular, with slight pause after q 3rd beat. MD notified & ECG ordered. ————— G. Chapman, RN

EVALUATION
- Relate pulse rate to other vital signs; relate pulse rhythm to baseline data and health status.
- Report to the primary care provider any abnormal findings such as irregular rhythm, reduced ability to hear the heartbeat, pallor, cyanosis, dyspnea, tachycardia, or bradycardia.

- Conduct appropriate follow-up such as administering medication ordered based on apical heart rate.

●○● NURSING PROCESS: ASSESSING AN APICAL-RADIAL PULSE

SKILL 2–4

Assessing an Apical-Radial Pulse

ASSESSMENT

An **apical-radial pulse** involves measurement of both the apical and radial pulse simultaneously. This is done to determine adequacy of peripheral circulation or presence of a discrepancy between the apical and radial rates (**pulse deficit**).

PLANNING
DELEGATION

UAP are generally not responsible for assessing apical-radial pulses.

INTERPROFESSIONAL PRACTICE

Assessing an apical-radial pulse may be within the scope of practice for many health care providers. Any provider who assesses a pulse can serve as the second person in the two-person technique.

Equipment

- Clock or watch with a sweep second hand or digital seconds indicator
- Stethoscope
- Antiseptic wipes

IMPLEMENTATION
Preparation

If using the two-nurse technique, ensure that the other nurse is available at this time.

Performance

1. Prior to performing the procedure, introduce self and verify the client's identity using agency protocol. Explain to the client what you are going to do, why it is necessary, and how he or she can participate. Discuss how the results will be used in planning further care or treatments.
2. Perform hand hygiene and observe other appropriate infection prevention procedures.
3. Provide for client privacy.
4. Position the client appropriately. Assist the client to a comfortable supine or sitting position. Expose the area of the chest over the apex of the heart. If previous measurements were taken, determine what position the client assumed, and use the same position. **Rationale:** *This ensures an accurate comparative measurement.*
5. Locate the apical and radial pulse sites. In the two-nurse technique, one nurse locates the apical impulse with the stethoscope while the other nurse palpates the radial pulse site (see Skills 2–2 and 2–3).
6. Count the apical and radial pulse rates.

   #### Two-Nurse Technique
   - Place the clock or watch where both nurses can see it. The nurse who is taking the radial pulse may hold the watch.
   - Decide on a time to begin counting. A time when the second hand is on 12, 3, 6, or 9, or an even number on digital clocks is usually selected. The nurse taking the radial pulse says "Start." **Rationale:** *This ensures that simultaneous counts are taken.*
   - Each nurse counts the pulse rate for 60 seconds. Both nurses end the count when the nurse taking the radial pulse says, "Stop." **Rationale:** *A full 60-second count is necessary for accurate assessment of any discrepancies between the two pulse sites.*
   - The nurse who assesses the apical rate also assesses the apical pulse rhythm and volume (i.e., whether the heartbeat is strong or weak). If the pulse is irregular, note whether the irregular beats come at random or at predictable times.
   - The nurse assessing the radial pulse rate also assesses the radial pulse rhythm and volume.

   #### One-Nurse Technique
   Within a few minutes,
   - Assess the apical pulse for 60 seconds.

   and

   - Assess the radial pulse for 60 seconds.

7. Document the apical and radial (AR) pulse rates, rhythm, volume, and any pulse deficit in the client record. Also record related data such as variation in pulse rate compared to normal for the client and other pertinent observations, such as pallor, cyanosis, or dyspnea.

EVALUATION

- Relate pulse rate and rhythm to other vital signs, to baseline data, and to general health status.
- Report to the primary care provider any changes from previous measurements or any discrepancy between the two pulse rates.
- Conduct appropriate follow-up such as administering medication or other actions to be taken for a discrepancy in the AR pulse rates.

INFANTS

- Use the apical pulse for the heart rate of newborns, infants, and children 2 to 3 years old to establish baseline data for subsequent evaluation, to determine whether the cardiac rate is within normal range, and to determine if the rhythm is regular.
- Place a baby in a supine position, and offer a pacifier if the baby is crying or restless. Crying and physical activity will increase the pulse rate. For this reason, take the resting apical pulse rate of infants and small children before assessing body temperature.
- Locate the apical pulse in the left fourth intercostal space, lateral to the midclavicular line during infancy.
- Brachial, popliteal, and femoral pulses may be palpated. Due to a normally low blood pressure and rapid heart rate, infants' other distal pulses may be difficult to feel.
- Newborn infants may have heart murmurs that are not pathologic, but reflect functional incomplete closure of fetal heart structures (ductus arteriosus or foramen ovale).

CHILDREN

- To take a peripheral pulse, position the child comfortably in the adult's arms, or have the adult remain close by. This may decrease anxiety and yield more accurate results.
- To assess the apical pulse, assist a young child to a comfortable supine or sitting position.

- Demonstrate the procedure to the child using a stuffed animal or doll, and allow the child to handle the stethoscope before beginning the procedure. This will decrease anxiety and promote cooperation.
- The apex of the heart is normally located in the left fourth intercostal space in young children; it is located in the fifth intercostal space in children 7 years of age and over, between the MCL and the anterior axillary line (see Skill 2–3, Figure ❶, on page 34).
- Count the pulse prior to other uncomfortable procedures so that the rate is not artificially elevated by the discomfort.

OLDER ADULTS

- If the client has severe hand or arm tremors, the radial pulse may be difficult to count.
- Cardiac changes in older adults, such as decrease in cardiac output, sclerotic changes to heart valves, and dysrhythmias, may suggest that obtaining an apical pulse will be more accurate than a peripheral pulse.
- Older adults often have decreased peripheral circulation. To detect it, check pedal pulses for regularity, volume, and symmetry.
- The pulse returns to baseline after exercise more slowly than with other age groups.

Pulse

- Teach the client/family to monitor the pulse prior to taking medications that affect the heart rate. Tell them to report any notable changes in heart rate or rhythm (regularity) to the health care provider.

- Inform the client/family of activities known to significantly affect pulse rate such as emotional stress, exercise, ingesting caffeine, and sleep. Clients sensitive to pulse rate changes should consider whether any of these activities should be modified in order to stabilize the pulse.

- Ensure that all users are familiar with using an electronic pulse-measuring device if indicated.
- Some clients require lengthy monitoring of the pulse and cardiac pattern (electrocardiogram). A special device, often referred to as a Holter monitor, is used for this type of monitoring. It is usually applied in an office or clinic setting, and the

client wears the portable recorder for 24 hours. Other portable devices used for recording episodic arrhythmias include cardiac event monitors. The client activates the device during times when symptoms appear and then the recorded data can be transmitted to a central location through a telephone.

RESPIRATIONS

Respiration is the act of breathing. It includes the intake of oxygen and the output of carbon dioxide. The term **inhalation** or **inspiration** refers to the intake of air into the lungs. **Exhalation** or **expiration** refers to breathing out or the movement of gases from the lungs to the atmosphere. **Ventilation** is another word that is used to refer to the movement of air in and out of the lungs. **Hyperventilation** refers to very deep, rapid respirations. **Hypoventilation** refers to very shallow respirations.

Nurses observe two types of breathing: costal breathing and diaphragmatic breathing. **Costal (thoracic) breathing** can be observed by the movement of the chest upward and outward. **Diaphragmatic (abdominal) breathing** is observed by the movement of the abdomen, which occurs as a result of the diaphragm's contraction and downward movement.

Factors Affecting Respirations

- *Age.* As age increases, the respiratory rate gradually decreases. See Table 2–2 on page 29.
- *Exercise.* Respirations increase in rate and depth with exercise.
- *Fever.* The respiratory rate will be faster in clients with an elevated temperature.
- *Medications.* Narcotics and other central nervous system depressants often slow the respiratory rate.
- *Stress.* Anxiety and pain are likely to increase respiratory rate and depth, although in some individuals with pain, respirations may become shallow.

Assessing Respirations

The rate, depth, rhythm, and special characteristics of respirations should be assessed. *Respiratory rate* is described in breaths per minute. A healthy adult normally takes between 12 and 20 breaths per minute.

CLINICAL ALERT!

An adult sleeping client's respirations can fall to fewer than 10 shallow breaths per minute. Use other vital signs to validate the sleeping client's condition.

The *depth* of a person's respirations can be established by watching the movement of the chest. Respiratory depth is generally described as normal, deep, or shallow. *Deep respirations* are those in which a large volume of air is inhaled and exhaled, inflating most of the lungs. *Shallow respirations* involve the exchange of a small volume of air and often the minimal use of lung tissue. During a normal inspiration and expiration, an adult takes in about 500 mL of air.

Respiratory rhythm or *pattern* refers to the regularity of the expirations and the inspirations. Normally, respirations are evenly spaced. Respiratory rhythm can be described as *regular* or *irregular*. An infant's respiratory rhythm may be less regular than an adult's.

Respiratory quality or *character* refers to those aspects of breathing that are different from normal, effortless breathing. Normal breathing is silent, but a number of abnormal sounds such as a wheeze are obvious to the nurse's ear. Many sounds occur as a result of the presence of fluid in the lungs and are most clearly heard with a stethoscope. See Chapter 3 ∞ for auscultation and percussion methods used to assess lung sounds. Additional terms used to describe respirations are listed in Box 2–3.

BOX 2–3 Altered Breathing Patterns and Sounds

BREATHING PATTERNS

Rate
- Tachypnea—quick, shallow breaths
- Bradypnea—abnormally slow breathing
- Apnea—cessation of breathing

Volume
- Hyperventilation—overexpansion of the lungs, characterized by rapid and deep breaths
- Hypoventilation—underexpansion of the lungs, characterized by shallow respirations

Rhythm
- Cheyne-Stokes breathing—rhythmic waxing and waning of respirations, from very deep to very shallow breathing and temporary apnea

Ease or Effort
- Dyspnea—difficult and labored breathing during which the individual has a persistent, unsatisfied need for air and feels distressed
- Orthopnea—ability to breathe only in upright sitting or standing positions

BREATH SOUNDS

Audible Without Amplification
- Stridor—a shrill, harsh sound heard during inspiration with laryngeal obstruction
- Stertor—snoring or sonorous respiration, usually due to a partial obstruction of the upper airway
- Wheeze—continuous, high-pitched musical squeak or whistling sound occurring on expiration and sometimes on inspiration when air moves through a narrowed or partially obstructed airway
- Bubbling—gurgling sounds heard as air passes through moist secretions in the respiratory tract

CHEST MOVEMENTS
- Intercostal retraction—indrawing between the ribs
- Substernal retraction—indrawing beneath the breastbone
- Suprasternal retraction—indrawing above the clavicles

SECRETIONS AND COUGHING
- Hemoptysis—the presence of blood in the sputum
- Productive cough—a cough accompanied by expectorated secretions
- Nonproductive cough—a dry, harsh cough without secretions

●○○● NURSING PROCESS: ASSESSING RESPIRATIONS

Assessing Respirations

SKILL 2–5

ASSESSMENT
- Measurement of the rate, rhythm, and character of respirations is used to:
  - Acquire baseline data against which future measurements can be compared.
  - Monitor abnormal respirations and respiratory patterns and identify changes.
  - Assess respirations before or after the administration of a medication that can depress respirations (an abnormally slow respiratory rate may warrant withholding the medication).
  - Monitor clients at risk for respiratory alterations (e.g., those with fever, pain, acute anxiety, chronic obstructive pulmonary disease, respiratory infection, pulmonary edema or emboli, chest trauma or constriction, or brainstem injury).
- To assess the client's general pulmonary health, examine skin and mucous membrane color (e.g., cyanosis or pallor), position assumed for breathing (e.g., use of orthopneic position), signs of cerebral anoxia (e.g., irritability, restlessness, drowsiness, or loss of consciousness), chest movements (e.g., retractions between the ribs or above or below the sternum), activity tolerance, chest pain, dyspnea, and medications affecting respiratory rate.

Assessing Respirations—*continued*

PLANNING
DELEGATION

Counting and observing respirations may be delegated to UAP. The follow-up assessment, interpretation of abnormal respirations, and determination of appropriate responses are done by the nurse.

INTERPROFESSIONAL PRACTICE

Assessing respirations may be within the scope of practice for many health care providers. For example, in addition to nurses, respiratory therapists will check the client's breathing before, during, and after treatment. Although the therapists may verbally communicate their findings and plan to the health care team members, the nurse must also know where to locate their documentation in the client's medical record.

Equipment
- Clock or watch with a sweep second hand or digital seconds indicator

IMPLEMENTATION
Preparation

For a routine assessment of respirations, determine the client's activity schedule and choose a suitable time to monitor the respirations. A client who has been exercising will need to rest for a few minutes to permit the accelerated respiratory rate to return to normal.

Performance
1. Prior to performing the procedure, introduce self and verify the client's identity using agency protocol. Explain to the client what you are going to do, why it is necessary, and how he or she can participate. Discuss how the results will be used in planning further care or treatments.
2. Perform hand hygiene and observe other appropriate infection prevention procedures.
3. Provide for client privacy.
4. Observe or palpate and count the respiratory rate.
   - The client's awareness that the nurse is counting the respiratory rate could cause the client to alter the respiratory pattern. If you anticipate this, place a hand against the client's chest to feel the chest movements with breathing, or place the client's arm across the chest and observe the chest movements while supposedly taking the radial pulse.
   - Count the respiratory rate for 30 seconds if the respirations are regular. Count for 60 seconds if they are irregular. An inhalation and an exhalation count as one respiration.

5. Observe the depth, rhythm, and character of respirations.
   - Observe the respirations for depth by watching the movement of the chest. **Rationale:** *During deep respirations, a large volume of air is exchanged; during shallow respirations, a small volume is exchanged.*
   - Observe the respirations for regular or irregular rhythm. **Rationale:** *Normally, respirations are evenly spaced except for the occasional normal sigh.*
   - Observe the character of respirations—the sound they produce and the effort they require. **Rationale:** *Normally, respirations are silent and effortless.*
6. Document the respiratory rate, depth, rhythm, and character on the appropriate record.

SAMPLE DOCUMENTATION

5/17/15 1320 Respirations irregular, from 18–34/min in past hour. Shallower respirations during tachypnea. Slight wheezing noted. Respiratory therapist called to provide treatment. ———— D. Katano, RN

EVALUATION
- Relate respiratory rate to other vital signs, in particular pulse rate; relate respiratory rhythm and depth to baseline data and health status.
- Report to the primary care provider a respiratory rate significantly above or below the normal range and any notable change in respirations from previous assessments; irregular respiratory rhythm; inadequate respiratory depth; abnormal character of breathing (orthopnea, wheezing, stridor, or bubbling); and any complaints of dyspnea.
- Conduct appropriate follow-up such as administering oxygen or other appropriate medications or treatments, positioning the client to ease breathing, and requesting involvement of other members of the health care team such as the respiratory therapist.

LIFESPAN CONSIDERATIONS | Respirations

INFANTS AND CHILDREN
- An infant or child who is crying will have an abnormal respiratory rate and rhythm and needs to be quieted before respirations can be accurately assessed.
- Infants use their diaphragms for inhalation and exhalation. If necessary, place your hand gently on the infant's abdomen to feel the rapid rise and fall during respirations.
- Most newborns are complete nose breathers, and nasal obstruction can be life threatening.
- Some newborns display "periodic breathing" in which they pause for a few seconds between respirations. This condition can be normal, but parents should be alert to prolonged or frequent pauses (apnea) that require medical attention.

- Compared to adults, infants have fewer alveoli and their airways have a smaller diameter. As a result, infants' respiratory rate and effort of breathing will increase with respiratory infections.
- Count respirations prior to uncomfortable procedures so that the respiratory rate is not artificially elevated by the discomfort.

OLDER ADULTS
- Ask the client to remain quiet, or count respirations after taking the pulse.
- Older adults experience anatomic and physiological changes that cause the respiratory system to be less efficient. Any changes in rate or type of breathing should be reported immediately.

BLOOD PRESSURE

Arterial blood pressure is a measure of the pressure exerted by blood as it pulsates through the arteries. Because blood moves in waves, there are two blood pressure measures: the **systolic** pressure, the pressure of the blood as a result of contraction of the ventricles (i.e., the pressure of the height of the blood wave), and the **diastolic** pressure, the pressure when the ventricles are at rest. Diastolic pressure, then, is the lower pressure, present at all times within the arteries. The difference between the diastolic and systolic pressures is called the **pulse pressure**. Sometimes, it is useful to also determine the **mean arterial pressure (MAP)** because it represents the pressure actually delivered to the body organs. The MAP can be calculated in several different ways, one of which is to add two-thirds of the diastolic pressure to one-third of the systolic pressure. A normal MAP is 70 to 110 mmHg.

When the blood pressure exceeds a certain range, it is referred to as **hypertension**; when it is lower than the usual range, it is called **hypotension**. The categories of hypertension are officially determined by federal agencies and are revised periodically (Table 2–4).

Factors Affecting Blood Pressure

- *Age.* Systolic and diastolic pressures rise gradually with age until adulthood. In older adults, the arteries are more rigid and less yielding to the pressure of the blood. This produces an elevated systolic pressure. Because the walls no longer retract as flexibly with decreased pressure, the diastolic pressure is also higher.
- *Sex.* Women usually have lower blood pressures than men of the same age, most likely due to hormonal variations. After menopause, women generally have higher blood pressures than before.
- *Exercise.* Physical activity increases blood pressure. For reliable assessment of resting blood pressure, wait 20 to 30 minutes following exercise.

TABLE 2–4 Classification of Blood Pressure

Category	Systolic BP (mmHG)		Diastolic BP (mmHG)
Normal	<120	and	<80
Prehypertension	120–139	or	80–89
Hypertension, stage 1	140–159	or	90–99
Hypertension, stage 2	>160	or	>100

From *The Seventh Report of the Joint National Committee for the Detection, Evaluation, and Treatment of High Blood Pressure*, National Institutes of Health, National Heart, Lung, and Blood Institute, 2004.

- *Medications.* Many medications may increase or decrease the blood pressure.
- *Stress.* Stimulation of the sympathetic nervous system increases cardiac output and vasoconstriction of the arterioles, thus increasing the blood pressure reading. However, severe pain can produce vasodilation and decrease blood pressure greatly.
- *Race.* African Americans over 35 years of age tend to have higher blood pressures than European Americans of the same age (Covelli, Wood, & Yarandi, 2012).
- *Obesity.* Both childhood and adult obesity predispose individuals to hypertension.
- *Medical conditions.* Both type 1 and type 2 diabetes can result in arterial disease and hypertension.
- *Diurnal variations.* Blood pressure is usually lowest early in the morning, when the metabolic rate is lowest, then rises throughout the day and peaks in the late afternoon or early evening.
- *Temperature.* Because of increased metabolic rate, fever can increase blood pressure. However, external heat causes vasodilation and decreased blood pressure. Cold causes vasoconstriction and elevates blood pressure.
- *Miscellaneous.* Smoking and caffeine raise the blood pressure through vasoconstriction and increased pulse rate. Heavy alcohol consumption is associated with hypertension.

Blood Pressure Assessment Sites

Blood pressure is usually assessed in the client's arm using the brachial artery and a standard stethoscope.

Blood pressure is *not* measured on a particular client's arm in the following situations:

- The shoulder, arm, or hand is injured or diseased.
- A cast or bulky bandage is on any part of the limb.
- The client has had surgical removal of a breast or axillary lymph nodes on that side.
- The client has an intravenous infusion or a blood transfusion in that limb.
- The client has an arteriovenous fistula (e.g., for renal dialysis) in that limb.

Assessing the blood pressure on a client's thigh using the popliteal artery is usually indicated in these situations:

- The blood pressure cannot be measured on either arm.
- The blood pressure in one thigh is to be compared with the blood pressure in the other thigh.

Measuring Blood Pressure

Blood pressure can be assessed directly or indirectly. Direct (invasive monitoring) measurement involves the insertion of a catheter into the brachial, radial, or femoral artery. Arterial pressure is represented as wavelike forms displayed on a monitor. With correct placement, this pressure reading is highly accurate.

Two common *noninvasive indirect methods* of measuring blood pressure are the auscultatory and palpatory methods. The *auscultatory method* is commonly used in hospitals, clinics, and homes. External pressure is applied to a superficial artery and the nurse reads the pressure from the **sphygmomanometer** (blood pressure measuring device consisting of a cuff and gauge) while listening through a stethoscope for the five phases of sounds called **Korotkoff's sounds** (Figure 2–9 ■ and Box 2–4).

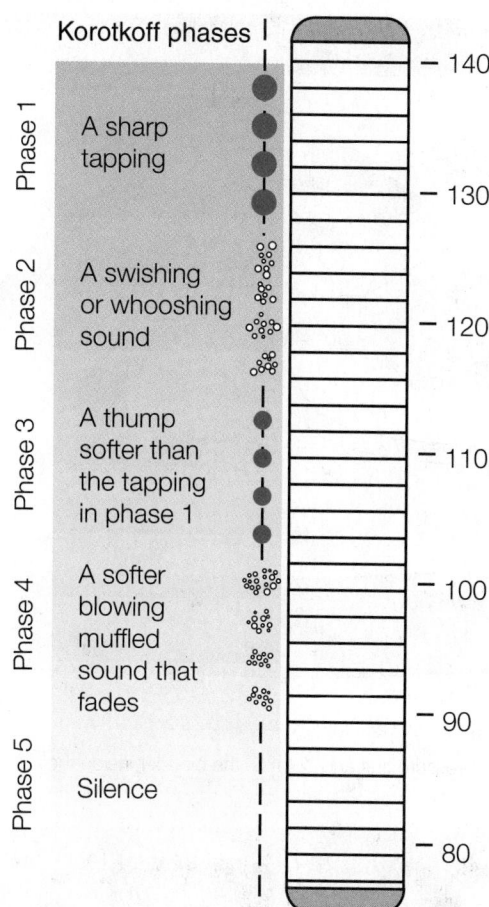

Korotkoff phases

Phase 1 — A sharp tapping

Phase 2 — A swishing or whooshing sound

Phase 3 — A thump softer than the tapping in phase 1

Phase 4 — A softer blowing muffled sound that fades

Phase 5 — Silence

140 — 130 — 120 — 110 — 100 — 90 — 80

Figure 2–9 ■ Korotkoff's sounds can be differentiated into five phases. In the illustration, the blood pressure is 138/90 or 138/102/90 mmHg.

BOX 2–4   **Korotkoff's Sounds**

- *Phase 1:* The pressure level at which the first faint, clear tapping or thumping sounds are heard. These sounds gradually become more intense. To ensure that they are not extraneous sounds, the nurse should identify at least two consecutive tapping sounds. The first tapping sound heard during deflation of the cuff is the systolic blood pressure.
- *Phase 2:* The period during deflation when the sounds have a muffled, whooshing, or swishing quality.
- *Phase 3:* The period during which the blood flows freely through an increasingly open artery and the sounds become crisper and more intense and again assume a thumping quality but softer than in phase 1.
- *Phase 4:* The time when the sounds become muffled and have a soft, blowing quality.
- *Phase 5:* The pressure level when the last sound is heard. This is followed by a period of silence. The pressure at which the last sound is heard is the diastolic blood pressure in adults.*

*In agencies where the fourth phase is considered the diastolic pressure, three measures are recommended (systolic pressure, diastolic pressure, and phase 5). These may be referred to as systolic, first diastolic, and second diastolic pressures. The phase 5 (second diastolic pressure) reading may be zero; that is, the muffled sounds are heard even when there is no air pressure in the blood pressure cuff. In some instances, muffled sounds are never heard, in which case a dash is inserted where the reading would normally be recorded (e.g., /–/110).

The systolic pressure is the point where the first tapping sound is heard (phase 1). In adults, the diastolic pressure is the point where the sounds become inaudible (phase 5). The phase 5 reading may be zero; that is, the muffled sounds are heard even when there is no air pressure in the blood pressure cuff. For complete accuracy, the phase 4 and 5 readings should be recorded.

The *palpatory method* is sometimes used when Korotkoff's sounds cannot be heard and electronic equipment to amplify the sounds is not available. The nurse palpates the pulsations of the artery as the pressure in the cuff is released. The systolic pressure is read from the sphygmomanometer when the first pulsation is felt. A single whiplike vibration, felt in addition to the pulsations, identifies the point at which the pressure in the cuff nears the diastolic pressure. This vibration is no longer felt when the cuff pressure is below the diastolic pressure. If recorded in the client record, the nurse clearly indicates that this is a palpated blood pressure since it is not as accurate as other methods.

The nurse palpates the blood pressure prior to auscultation to avoid being caught in the auscultatory gap. An **auscultatory gap**, which occurs particularly in clients with hypertension, is the temporary disappearance of sounds normally heard over the brachial artery when the cuff pressure is high, followed by the reappearance of the sounds at a lower level. This temporary disappearance of sounds occurs in the latter part of phase 1 and may cover a range of 40 mmHg. If a palpated estimation of the systolic pressure is not made prior to auscultation, the nurse may begin listening in the middle of this range and underestimate the systolic pressure.

●○● NURSING PROCESS: ASSESSING BLOOD PRESSURE

Assessing Blood Pressure

ASSESSMENT
- Blood pressure readings are used to:
  - Provide a baseline measure of arterial blood pressure for subsequent evaluation.
  - Determine the client's hemodynamic status (e.g., cardiac output and blood vessel resistance).
  - Identify and monitor changes in blood pressure resulting from a disease process or medical therapy (e.g., cardiovascular disease, renal disease, circulatory shock, or acute pain; rapid infusion of fluids or blood products).
  - Determine the client's safety in performing activity such as arising after extended bed rest or recovery from anesthesia.

- To assess the client's general health, examine for signs and symptoms of:
  - Hypertension (e.g., headache, ringing in the ears, flushing of face, nosebleeds, fatigue)
  - Hypotension (e.g., tachycardia, dizziness, mental confusion, restlessness, cool and clammy skin, pale or cyanotic skin)
  - Factors affecting blood pressure (e.g., activity, emotional stress, pain, and time the client last smoked or ingested caffeine).
- Some blood pressure cuffs contain latex. Assess the client for latex allergy and use a latex-free cuff if indicated.

SKILL 2–6

Continued on page 42

Assessing Blood Pressure—*continued*

PLANNING
DELEGATION

Blood pressure measurement may be delegated to UAP. The interpretation of abnormal blood pressure readings and determination of appropriate responses are done by the nurse.

INTERPROFESSIONAL PRACTICE

Measurement of blood pressure is within the scope of practice for many health care providers. For example, in addition to nurses, therapists may check the client's blood pressure before, during, and after treatment. Although the therapists may verbally communicate their findings and plan to the health care team members, the nurse must also know where to locate their documentation in the client's medical record.

Equipment

* Stethoscope or DUS
* Blood pressure cuff

    The blood pressure cuff consists of a bag that can be inflated with air called a bladder. ❶ It is covered with cloth and has two tubes attached to it. One tube connects to a bulb that inflates the bladder. A small valve on the side of this bulb traps and releases the air in the bladder. The other tube is attached to a sphygmomanometer.

    Blood pressure cuffs come in various sizes (newborn, infant, child, small adult, adult, large adult, thigh) because the bladder must be the correct width and length for the client's arm. ❷ The width should be 40% of the circumference, or 20% wider than the diameter of the midpoint of the limb on which it is used. The arm circumference, not the age of the client, should always be used to determine bladder size. Lay the cuff lengthwise at the midpoint of the upper arm, and hold the outermost side of the bladder edge laterally on the arm. With the other hand, wrap the width of the cuff around the arm, and ensure that the width is 40% of the arm circumference. ❸

    The length of the bladder also affects the accuracy of measurement. The bladder should be sufficiently long to cover at least two thirds of the limb's circumference. For obese clients, a standard sized bladder in an extra-long cuff may be the most appropriate (McFarlane, 2012).

* Blood pressure cuffs are made of nondistensible material so that an even pressure is exerted around the limb. Most cuffs are held in place by hooks, snaps, or hook-and-loop fabric. Others have a cloth bandage that is long enough to encircle the limb several times; this type is closed by tucking the end of the bandage into one of the bandage folds.

* Sphygmomanometer

    The sphygmomanometer indicates the pressure of the air within the bladder. The aneroid sphygmomanometer is a calibrated dial with a needle that points to the calibrations. ❹

    The pumping action to inflate the blood pressure cuff can be used as a prompt for self-care. As the nurse inflates a manual cuff, taking a few slow and complete breaths will help the nurse to remain calm and focused, and to really tune in to the whole person as vital signs are accessed.

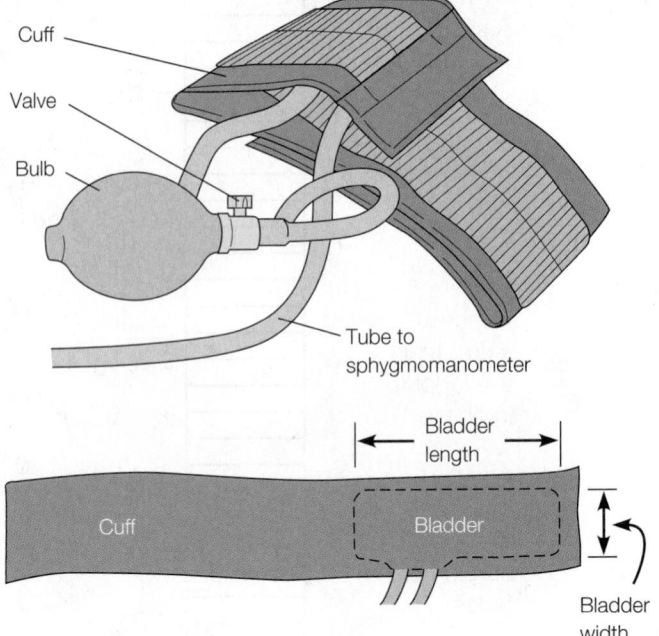

❶ *A,* Blood pressure cuff and bulb; *B,* the bladder inside the cuff.

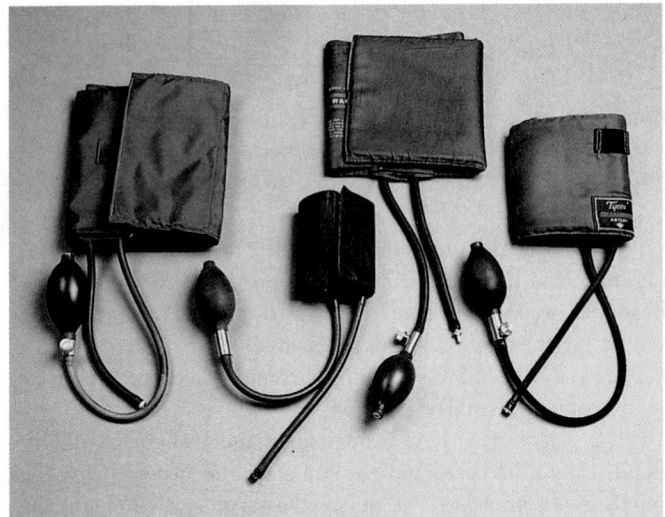

❷ Standard cuff sizes: smaller cuffs are used for infants, small children, or frail adults; midsize cuffs are used for most adults; and larger cuffs are used for measuring the blood pressure on the leg or arm of an adult who is obese.

Many agencies use digital (electronic) sphygmomanometers, ❺ which eliminate the need to listen for the sounds of the client's systolic and diastolic blood pressures through a stethoscope. Electronic blood pressure devices should be calibrated periodically to check accuracy. All health care facilities should have manual blood pressure equipment available as backup.

Assessing Blood Pressure—*continued*

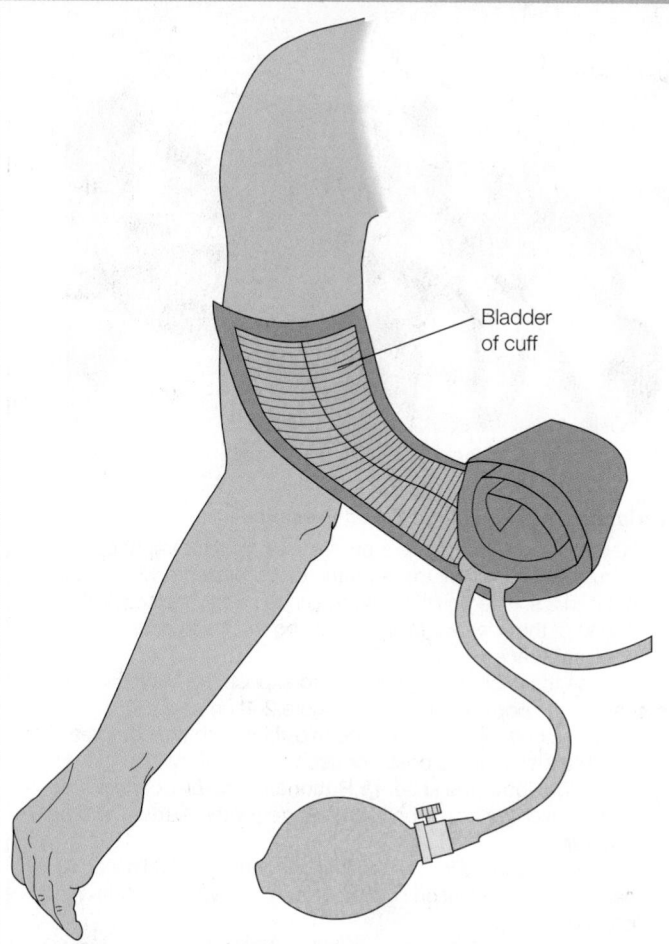

Bladder
of cuff

❸ Determining that the bladder of a blood pressure cuff is 40% of the arm circumference or 20% wider than the diameter of the midpoint of the limb.

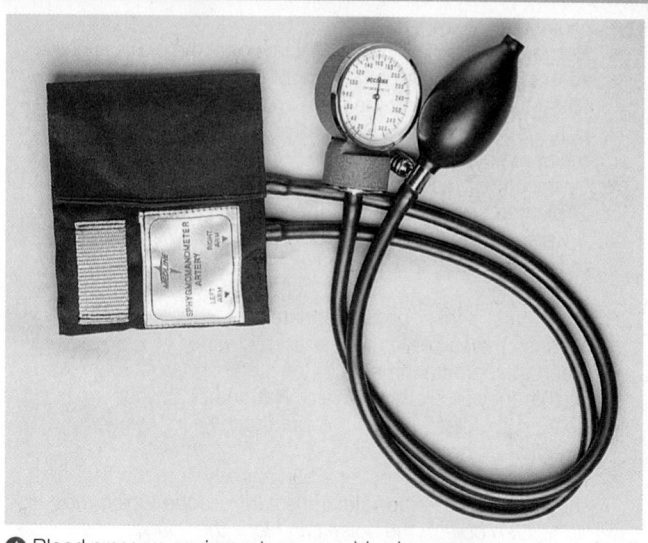

❹ Blood pressure equipment: an aneroid sphygmomanometer and cuff.

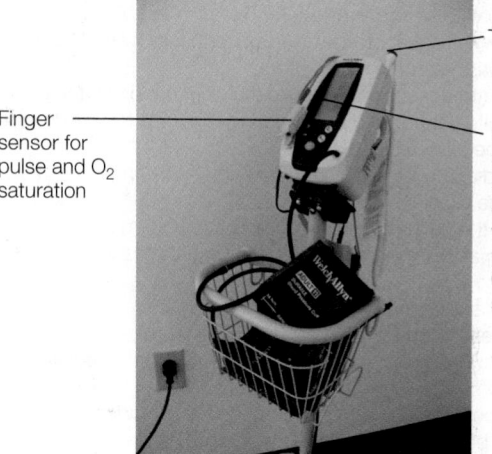

Thermometer

Finger
sensor for
pulse and O₂
saturation

Digital
display of
systolic and
diastolic BP,
temperature,
pulse, and
O₂
saturation

❺ Electronic blood pressure monitors register blood pressures.

IMPLEMENTATION

Preparation

- Ensure that the equipment is intact and functioning properly. Check for leaks in the tubing of the sphygmomanometer.
- Make sure that the client has not smoked or ingested caffeine within 30 minutes prior to measurement. **Rationale:** *Smoking constricts blood vessels, and caffeine increases the pulse rate. Both of these cause a temporary increase in blood pressure.*

Performance

1. Prior to performing the procedure, introduce self and verify the client's identity using agency protocol. Explain to the client what you are going to do, why it is necessary, and how he or she can participate. Discuss how the results will be used in planning further care or treatments.
2. Perform hand hygiene and observe other appropriate infection prevention procedures.
3. Provide for client privacy.
4. Position the client appropriately.
   - The adult client should be sitting unless otherwise specified. Both feet should be flat on the floor. **Rationale:** *Legs crossed at the knee result in elevated systolic and diastolic blood pressures (Pinar, Ataalkin, & Watson, 2010).*

- The elbow should be slightly flexed with the palm of the hand facing up and the forearm supported at heart level. Readings in any other position should be specified. The blood pressure is normally similar in sitting, standing, and lying positions, but it can vary significantly by position in certain individuals. See Table 2–5.
- Expose the upper arm.
5. Wrap the deflated cuff evenly around the upper arm. Locate the brachial artery (see Figure 2–8 on page 30). Apply the center of the bladder directly over the artery. **Rationale:** *The bladder inside the cuff must be directly over the artery to be compressed if the reading is to be accurate.*
   - For an adult, place the lower border of the cuff approximately 2.5 cm (1 in.) above the antecubital space.
6. If this is the client's initial examination, perform a preliminary palpatory determination of systolic pressure. **Rationale:** *The initial estimate tells the nurse the maximal pressure to which the sphygmomanometer needs to be elevated in subsequent determinations. It also prevents underestimation of the systolic pressure or overestimation of the diastolic pressure should an auscultatory gap occur.*
   - Palpate the brachial artery with the fingertips.

Continued on page 44

SKILL 2–6

Assessing Blood Pressure—*continued*

- Close the valve on the bulb.
- Pump up the cuff until you no longer feel the brachial pulse. At that pressure the blood cannot flow through the artery. Note the pressure on the sphygmomanometer at which the pulse is no longer felt. **Rationale:** *This gives an estimate of the systolic pressure.*
- Release the pressure completely in the cuff, and wait 1 to 2 minutes before making further measurements. **Rationale:** *A waiting period gives the blood trapped in the veins time to be released. Otherwise, false high systolic readings will occur.*

7. Position the stethoscope appropriately.
   - Cleanse the earpieces with antiseptic wipe.
   - Insert the ear attachments of the stethoscope in your ears so that they tilt slightly forward. **Rationale:** *Sounds are heard more clearly when the ear attachments follow the direction of the ear canal.*
   - Ensure that the stethoscope hangs freely from the ears to the diaphragm. **Rationale:** *If the stethoscope tubing rubs against an object, the noise can block the sounds of the blood within the artery.*
   - Place the bell side of the diaphragm of the stethoscope over the brachial pulse site. **Rationale:** *Because the blood pressure is a low-frequency sound, it is best heard with the bell-shaped diaphragm.*
   - Place the stethoscope directly on the skin, not on clothing over the site. **Rationale:** *This is to avoid noise made from rubbing the amplifier against cloth.*
   - Hold the diaphragm with the thumb and index finger.

8. Auscultate the client's blood pressure.
   - Pump up the cuff until the sphygmomanometer reads 30 mmHg above the point where the brachial pulse disappeared.
   - Release the valve on the cuff carefully so that the pressure decreases at the rate of 2 to 3 mmHg per second. **Rationale:** *If the rate is faster or slower, an error in measurement may occur.*
   - As the pressure falls, identify the manometer reading at Korotkoff phases 1, 4, and 5. **Rationale:** *There is no clinical significance to phases 2 and 3.*
   - Deflate the cuff rapidly and completely.
   - Wait 1 to 2 minutes before taking additional readings. **Rationale:** *This permits blood trapped in the veins to be released.*
   - Repeat the above steps to confirm the accuracy of the reading—especially if it falls outside the normal range (although this may not be routine procedure for hospitalized or well clients). If there is greater than a 5 mmHg difference between the two readings, additional measurements may be taken and the results averaged.

9. If this is the client's initial examination, repeat the procedure on the client's other arm. There should be a difference of no more than 10 mmHg between the arms. The arm found to have the higher pressure should be used for subsequent examinations (Fonseca-Reyes, Forsyth-Macquarrie, & Garcia de Alba-Garcia, 2012).

Variation: Obtaining a Blood Pressure by the Palpation Method

If it is not possible to use a stethoscope to obtain the blood pressure or if Korotkoff's sounds cannot be heard, palpate the radial or brachial pulse site as the cuff pressure is released. The manometer reading at the point where the pulse reappears is an estimate of the systolic blood pressure.

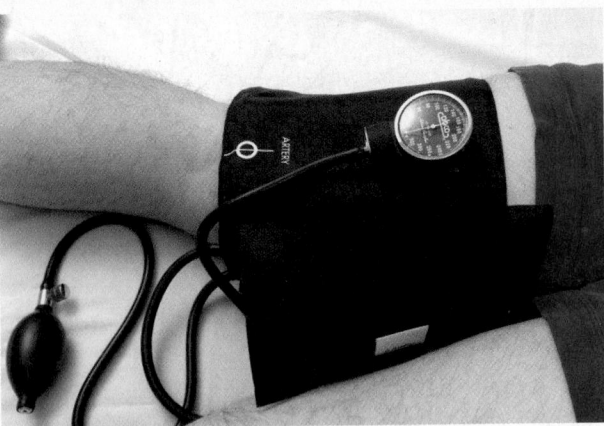

⑥ Measuring blood pressure in the client's thigh.

Variation: Taking a Thigh Blood Pressure

- Help the client to assume a prone position. If the client cannot assume this position, measure the blood pressure while the client is in a supine position with the knee slightly flexed. Slight flexing of the knee will facilitate placing the stethoscope on the popliteal space.
- Expose the thigh, taking care not to expose the client unduly.
- Locate the popliteal artery (see Figure 2–8 on page 30).
- Wrap the cuff evenly around the mid-thigh with the compression bladder over the posterior aspect of the thigh and the bottom edge above the knee. **⑥ Rationale:** *The bladder must be directly over the posterior popliteal artery if the reading is to be accurate.*
- If this is the client's initial examination, perform a preliminary palpatory determination of systolic pressure while palpating the popliteal artery.
- In adults, the systolic pressure in the popliteal artery is often 20 to 30 mmHg higher than that in the brachial artery; the diastolic pressure is usually the same.

Variation: Using an Electronic Blood Pressure Monitoring Device (see Figure ⑤ on page 43.)

- Place the blood pressure cuff on the extremity according to the manufacturer's guidelines.
- Turn on the blood pressure switch.
- If appropriate, set the device for the desired number of minutes between blood pressure determinations.
- When the device has determined the blood pressure reading, note the digital results.
- Electronic/automatic blood pressure cuffs can be left in place for many hours. Remove the cuff and check skin condition periodically.

10. Remove the cuff from the client's arm.
11. Wipe the cuff with an approved disinfectant. **Rationale:** *Cuffs can become significantly contaminated.* Many institutions use disposable blood pressure cuffs. The client uses it for the length of stay and then it is discarded. **Rationale:** *This decreases the risk of spreading infection by sharing cuffs.*
12. Document and report pertinent assessment data according to agency policy. Record two pressures in the form "130/80" where "130" is the systolic (phase 1) and "80" is the diastolic (phase 5) pressure. Record three pressures in the form "130/90/0," where "130" is the systolic, "90" is the first diastolic (phase 4), and sounds are audible even after the cuff is completely deflated. Use the abbreviations RA or RL for right arm or right leg and LA or LL for left arm or left leg.

Assessing Blood Pressure—*continued*

EVALUATION

- Relate blood pressure to other vital signs, to baseline data, and to health status. If the findings are significantly different from previous values without obvious reasons, consider possible causes (see Table 2–5).
- Report any significant change in the client's blood pressure. Also report these findings if they are consistent over time:
  - Systolic blood pressure (of an adult) above 140 mmHg.
  - Diastolic blood pressure (of an adult) above 90 mmHg.
- Systolic blood pressure (of an adult) below 100 mmHg.
- Conduct appropriate follow-up such as administration of medication. If the blood pressure is significantly higher or lower than usual, implement appropriate safety precautions. A systolic blood pressure less than 80 or greater than 180 mmHg is considered extremely serious, and the nurse should consider taking immediate action or calling for assistance.

TABLE 2–5 Selected Sources of Error in Blood Pressure Assessment

Error	Effect
Bladder cuff too narrow	Erroneously high
Bladder cuff too wide	Erroneously low
Arm unsupported	Erroneously high
Insufficient rest before the assessment	Erroneously high
Repeating assessment too quickly	Erroneously high systolic or low diastolic readings
Cuff wrapped too loosely or unevenly	Erroneously high
Deflating cuff too quickly	Erroneously low systolic and high diastolic readings
Deflating cuff too slowly	Erroneously high diastolic reading
Failure to use the same arm consistently	Inconsistent measurements
Arm above level of the heart	Erroneously low
Arm below heart level	Erroneously high
Assessing immediately after a meal or while client smokes or has pain	Erroneously high
Failure to identify auscultatory gap	Erroneously low systolic pressure and erroneously low diastolic pressure

---

LIFESPAN CONSIDERATIONS Blood Pressure

INFANTS

- Use a pediatric stethoscope with a small diaphragm.
- The lower edge of the blood pressure cuff can be closer to the antecubital space of an infant.
- Use the palpation method if auscultation with a stethoscope or DUS is unsuccessful.
- Arm and thigh pressures are equivalent in children under 1 year of age.
- The systolic blood pressure of a newborn averages around 75 mmHg (D'Amico & Barbarito, 2012).
- Use only the first and fifth Korotkoff sounds for children ages 1 to 26 months.

CHILDREN

- Blood pressure should be measured in all children over 3 years of age and in children less than 3 years of age with certain medical conditions (e.g., congenital heart disease, renal malformation, medications that affect blood pressure).
- Explain each step of the process and what it will feel like. Demonstrate on a doll.
- Use the palpation technique for children under 3 years old.
- Cuff bladder width should be 40% and length should be 80% to 100% of the arm circumference.
- Take the blood pressure prior to other uncomfortable procedures so that the blood pressure is not artificially elevated by the discomfort.

- In children, the diastolic pressure is considered to be the onset of phase 4, where the sounds become muffled.
- In children, the thigh pressure is about 10 mmHg higher than the arm.
- One quick way to determine the normal systolic blood pressure of a child is to use the following formula:

Normal systolic BP = 80 + (2 × child's age in years)

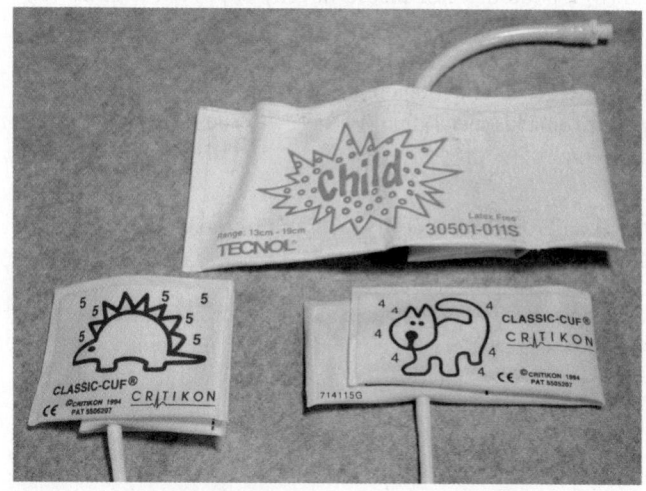

Pediatric blood pressure cuffs.

Continued on page 46

OXYGEN SATURATION

A **pulse oximeter** is a noninvasive device that estimates a client's arterial blood **oxygen saturation (SaO₂)** by means of a sensor attached to the client's finger (Figure 2–10 ■), toe, nose, earlobe, or forehead (or around the hand or foot of a neonate). Because the sensor estimates this value indirectly at a peripheral site, the oximeter displays the measurement as SpO_2. The pulse oximeter can detect hypoxemia before clinical signs and symptoms, such as dusky skin color and dusky nail bed color, develop.

The pulse oximeter's *sensor* has two parts: (a) two light-emitting diodes (LEDs)—one red, the other infrared—that transmit light through nails, tissue, venous blood, and arterial blood; and (b) a photodetector placed directly opposite the LEDs (e.g., the other side of the finger, toe, or nose). The photodetector measures the amount of red and infrared light absorbed by oxygenated and deoxygenated hemoglobin in arterial blood and reports it as SpO_2. Normal oxygen saturation is 95% to 100%. Below 70% is life threatening.

Factors Affecting Oxygen Saturation Readings

- *Hemoglobin.* If the hemoglobin is fully saturated with oxygen, the SpO_2 will appear normal even if the total hemoglobin level is low. Thus, the client could be severely anemic and have inadequate oxygen to supply the tissues but the pulse oximeter would return a normal value.

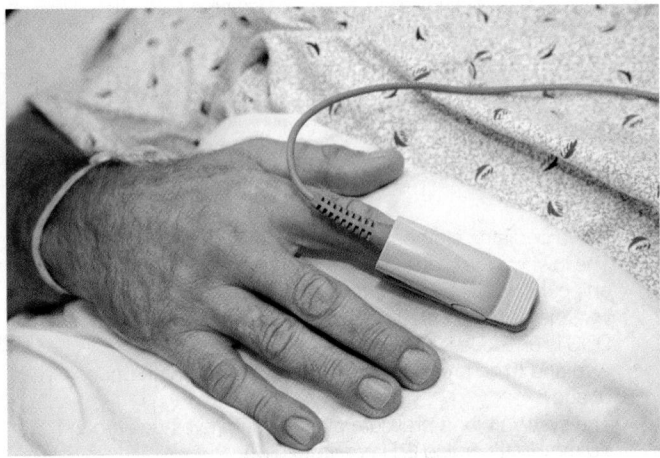

Figure 2–10 ■ Fingertip oximeter sensor (adult).

- *Circulation.* The oximeter will not return an accurate reading if the area under the sensor has impaired circulation. If no other site can be used, the area will need to be warmed so that there is adequate circulation for the device to work properly.
- *Activity.* Shivering or excessive movement of the sensor site may interfere with accurate readings.
- *Carbon monoxide poisoning.* Pulse oximeters cannot discriminate between hemoglobin saturated with carbon monoxide versus oxygen. In this case, other measures of oxygenation are needed.

●○○● NURSING PROCESS: ASSESSING OXYGEN SATURATION

Assessing Oxygen Saturation (Pulse Oximeter)

ASSESSMENT

- Based on the client's age and physical condition, determine the best location for a pulse oximeter sensor. Unless contraindicated, the finger is usually selected for adults.
- Consider the client's overall condition including risk factors for development of hypoxemia (e.g., respiratory or cardiac disease) and hemoglobin level.
- Determine vital signs, skin and nail bed color, and tissue perfusion of extremities as baseline data.
- Assess for allergy to adhesive.

PLANNING

Many hospitals and clinics have pulse oximeters readily available for use with other vital signs equipment (or even as an integrated part of the electronic blood pressure device). Other facilities may have a limited supply of oximeters, and the nurse may need to request one from the central supply department.

DELEGATION

Application of the pulse oximeter sensor and recording of the SpO_2 value may be delegated to UAP. The interpretation of the oxygen saturation value and determination of appropriate responses are done by the nurse.

INTERPROFESSIONAL PRACTICE

Measuring oxygen saturation may be within the scope of practice for many health care providers. For example, in addition to nurses, respiratory therapists may check the client's oxygen saturation before, during, and after treatment. Although the therapists may verbally communicate their findings and plan to the health care team members, the nurse must also know where to locate their documentation in the client's medical record.

Equipment

- Nail polish remover as needed
- Alcohol wipe
- Sheet or towel
- Pulse oximeter

Pulse oximeters with various types of sensors are available from several manufacturers. The *oximeter unit* consists of an inlet connection for the sensor cable, and a faceplate that indicates (a) the oxygen saturation measurement (expressed as a percentage) and (b) the pulse rate. Cordless units are also available. ❶ A preset alarm system signals high and low SpO_2 measurements and a high and low pulse rate. The high and low SpO_2 levels are generally preset at 100% and 85%, respectively, for adults. The high and low pulse rate alarms are usually preset at 140 and 50 beats/min for adults. These alarm limits can, however, be changed according to the manufacturer's directions.

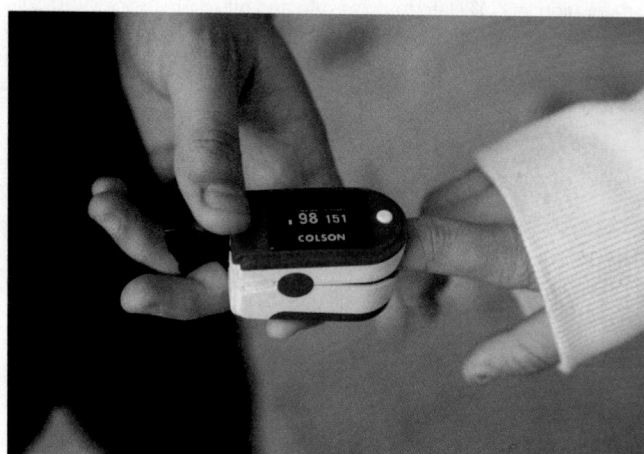

❶ Fingertip oximeter sensor (cordless).
Amelie-Benoist/BSIP/Alamy.

IMPLEMENTATION

Preparation
Check that the oximeter equipment is functioning normally.

Performance
1. Prior to performing the procedure, introduce self and verify the client's identity using agency protocol. Explain to the client what you are going to do, why it is necessary, and how he or she can participate. Discuss how the results will be used in planning further care or treatments.
2. Perform hand hygiene and observe other appropriate infection prevention procedures.
3. Provide for client privacy.
4. Choose a sensor appropriate for the client's weight, size, and desired location. Because weight limits of sensors overlap, a pediatric sensor could be used for a small adult.
   - If the client is allergic to adhesive, use a clip or sensor without adhesive.
   - If using an extremity, apply the sensor only if the proximal pulse and capillary refill at the point closest to the site are present. If the client has low tissue perfusion due to peripheral vascular disease or therapy using vasoconstrictive

medications, use a nasal sensor or a reflectance sensor on the forehead. Avoid using lower extremities that have compromised circulation and extremities that are used for infusions or other invasive monitoring.
   - If the same sensor is used on multiple clients, cleanse the sensor with alcohol or as specified by the manufacturer.
5. Prepare the site.
   - If visibly soiled, clean the site with an alcohol wipe before applying the sensor.
   - It may be necessary to remove a female client's dark nail polish. **Rationale:** *Dark polish may interfere with accurate measurements although the data about this are inconsistent.*
   - Alternatively, position the sensor on the side of the finger rather than perpendicular to the nail bed.
6. Apply the sensor, and connect it to the pulse oximeter.
   - Make sure the LED and photodetector are accurately aligned, that is, opposite each other on either side of the finger, toe, nose, or earlobe. Many sensors have markings to facilitate correct alignment of the LEDs and photodetector.

Continued on page 48

SKILL 2–7

Assessing Oxygen Saturation (Pulse Oximeter)—*continued*

- Attach the sensor cable to the connection outlet on the oximeter. Turn on the machine according to the manufacturer's directions. Appropriate connection will be confirmed by an audible beep indicating each arterial pulsation. Some devices have a wheel that can be turned clockwise to increase the volume and counterclockwise to decrease it.
- Ensure that the bar of light or waveform on the face of the oximeter fluctuates with each pulsation.

7. Set and turn on the alarm when using continuous monitoring.
   - Check the preset alarm limits for high and low oxygen saturation and high and low pulse rates. Change these alarm limits according to the manufacturer's directions as indicated. Ensure that the audio and visual alarms are on before you leave the client. A tone will be heard and a number will blink on the faceplate.

8. Ensure client safety.
   - Inspect and/or move or change the location of an adhesive toe or finger sensor every 4 hours and a spring-tension sensor every 2 hours.

- Inspect the sensor site tissues for irritation from adhesive sensors.

9. Ensure the accuracy of measurement.
   - Minimize motion artifacts by using an adhesive sensor, or immobilize the client's monitoring site. **Rationale:** *Movement of the client's finger or toe may be misinterpreted by the oximeter as arterial pulsations.*
   - If indicated, cover the sensor with a sheet or towel to block large amounts of light from external sources (e.g., sunlight, procedure lamps, or bilirubin lights in the nursery). **Rationale:** *Bright room light may be sensed by the photodetector and alter the SpO$_2$ value.*
   - Compare the pulse rate indicated by the oximeter to the radial pulse periodically. **Rationale:** *A large discrepancy between the two values may indicate oximeter malfunction.*

10. Document the oxygen saturation on the appropriate record at designated intervals.

EVALUATION

- Compare the oxygen saturation to the client's previous oxygen saturation level. Relate to pulse rate and other vital signs.
- Conduct appropriate follow-up such as notifying the primary care provider, adjusting oxygen therapy, or providing breathing

treatments. An oxygen saturation of less than 90%, especially if also associated with a respiratory rate less than 8 or greater than 30, is considered extremely serious. The nurse should consider taking immediate action or calling for assistance.

LIFESPAN CONSIDERATIONS   Pulse Oximetry

INFANTS
- If an appropriate-sized finger or toe sensor is not available, consider using an earlobe or forehead sensor.
- The high and low SpO$_2$ alarm levels are generally preset at 95% and 80% for neonates.
- The high and low pulse rate alarms are usually preset at 200 and 100 for neonates.
- The oximeter may need to be taped, wrapped with an elastic bandage, or covered by a stocking to keep it in place.

CHILDREN
- Instruct the child that the sensor does not hurt. Disconnect the probe whenever possible to allow for movement.

OLDER ADULTS
- Use of vasoconstrictive medications, poor circulation, or thickened nails may make finger or toe sensors inaccurate.
- Use a forehead or earlobe sensor if indicated.

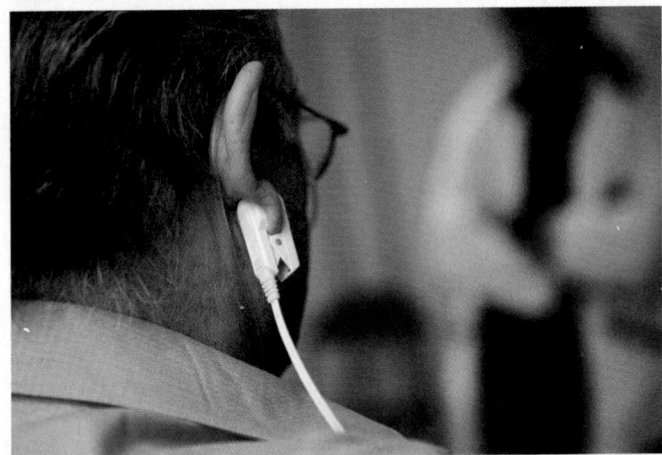

Earlobe oximeter sensor.

Ambulatory and Community Settings   Pulse Oximetry

PATIENT-CENTERED CARE

- Pulse oximetry is a quick, inexpensive, noninvasive method of assessing oxygenation. Like an automatic blood pressure cuff, it also provides a pulse rate reading. Use in the ambulatory or home setting whenever indicated.

- If the client requires frequent or continuous home monitoring, teach the client and family how to apply and maintain the equipment. Remind them to rotate the site periodically and assess for skin trauma.

FOCUSING ON CLINICAL THINKING

Consider This

1. What should you do if the client has been eating or smoking within the past 30 minutes and you wish to take the temperature?
2. How should you proceed if the client is not cooperative or able to understand your instructions regarding the use of an oral thermometer?
3. Why is it important to know by what route the last temperature reading was taken, when, and what the resultant temperature reading was? Give several reasons.
4. In an emergency, the radial pulse may not be accessible or palpable. What other two sites are useful in such situations?
5. When assessing pulses in the foot, what is the next action to take if neither the posterior tibial nor dorsalis pedis pulse can be felt?
6. While you are counting respirations after counting the client's pulse, the client asks why it is taking so long. What would be an appropriate response?
7. While you are releasing the cuff and auscultating the blood pressure, the client coughs loudly and jerks the arm, resulting in your inability to accurately hear Korotkoff's sounds. In detail, how should you proceed?
8. The pulse oximeter on the client's finger reads 85%. The client's skin is warm and has normal color. The client is awake and oriented, temperature is 37.1°C (98.8°F), apical pulse is 78 beats/min, and blood pressure is 136/84 mmHg. What would be your next actions?

See Focusing on Clinical Thinking answers on student resource website.

TEST YOUR KNOWLEDGE

1. Which of the following tasks can be delegated to unlicensed assistive personnel (UAP)? Select all that apply.
   1. Vital signs for a client just admitted to the floor from a nursing home
   2. A client who needs an apical pulse checked prior to medication administration
   3. Vital signs for a client just returned to the floor from dialysis
   4. A client who needs a tympanic temperature taken
   5. Blood pressure for a client whose last two BPs were 98/72 and 85/60 mmHg

2. The nurse is assessing the student's skill set in taking blood pressures. Which observation, if made by the nurse, requires intervention so that the student takes proper measurements?
   1. The student nurse has the client hold his arm out from his body at shoulder level while taking the reading.
   2. The student nurse has the client place his arm at the level of the heart while taking the reading.
   3. The student nurse allows 1 to 2 minutes between readings if unsure of the numbers.
   4. The student nurse allows the client to rest after finishing eating before taking a blood pressure.

3. A nurse is teaching a group of nursing students the differences in pulse and respiration readings across the life span. Which statement, if made by a nursing student, indicates the need for further teaching?
   1. "An average pulse rate for a teenager is 100 beats per minute."
   2. "An average range of respirations for a newborn is 30 to 80 breaths per minute."
   3. "An average pulse range for a 1-year-old is 80 to 140 beats per minute."
   4. "An average respiration rate for an older adult is 16 breaths per minute."

4. A client's blood pressure reading is 144/96 mmHg. In which classification does this blood pressure reading qualify?
   1. Normal
   2. Prehypertension
   3. Hypertension, stage 1
   4. Hypertension, stage 2

5. A nurse is considering the different sites for body temperature measurement. Which statement regarding site choice for body temperature measurement requires further instruction or clarification?
   1. "Although oral temperatures are accessible and convenient, they are inaccurate if the client has just smoked or eaten."
   2. "Rectal thermometers are a reliable measurement even in the presence of stool."
   3. "Temporal artery measurements are safe, noninvasive, and very fast."
   4. "Tympanic membrane readings are readily accessible, reflect the core temperature, and are very fast."

6. The nurse is preparing to take a pulse on a client who is receiving digoxin (Lanoxin), which affects the heart rate. This assessment needs to be completed prior to medication administration. Which skill is correct when assessing the pulse of this client?
   1. A radial pulse taken for 15 seconds
   2. A femoral pulse taken for 30 seconds
   3. A carotid pulse taken for a full minute
   4. An apical pulse taken for a full minute

7. A client presents with quick shallow breaths, indrawing between the ribs, and bloody sputum. Upon auscultation, the client is found to have a shrill harsh sound heard during inspiration. Which assessments most accurately describe this client?
   1. Bradypnea, intercostal retractions, productive cough, and wheezing
   2. Bradypnea, substernal retractions, hemoptysis, and stridor
   3. Tachypnea, intercostal retractions, hemoptysis, and stridor
   4. Tachypnea, substernal retractions, productive cough, and wheezing

8. The nurse is teaching a nursing student about blood pressure measurement. Which statement, if made by the nursing student, demonstrates the need for further teaching?
   1. "If the client is sitting in a chair, I should make sure that both feet are flat on the floor."
   2. "After I locate the brachial artery, I should wrap the deflated cuff evenly around the upper arm."
   3. "I should pump up the cuff until the sphygmomanometer reads 30 mmHg above the point where the brachial pulse disappeared."
   4. "After I hear the first heart sound, I should release the valve on the cuff rapidly so as not to injure the client."

9. Which action performed by the nurse demonstrates proper measurement of oxygen saturation?
    1. The nurse ensures that the LED and photodetector face each other.
    2. The nurse uses the finger for a pulse oximetry reading on a client with dark nail polish.
    3. The nurse moves the spring sensor on the client's finger every 12 hours.
    4. The nurse documents the pulse rate daily using only the oximeter.

10. A nurse is documenting the respiratory assessment on a client who has just undergone a bronchoscopy. In addition to the respiratory rate, which components should be included in the nurse's note?
    1. Character of respirations
    2. Depth, rhythm, and character of respirations
    3. Rhythm of respirations
    4. Arterial blood gases, rhythm and depth of respirations

See Answers to Test Your Knowledge in Appendix A.

READINGS AND REFERENCES

References

Barringer, L. B., Evans, C. W., Ingram, L. L., Tisdale, P. P., Watson, S. P., & Janken, J. K. (2011). Agreement between temporal artery, oral, and axillary temperature measurements in the perioperative period. *Journal of Perianesthesia Nursing, 26*(3), 143–150. doi:10.1016/j.jopan.2011.03.010

Covelli, M., Wood, C., & Yarandi, H. (2012). Biologic measures as epidemiological indicators of risk for the development of hypertension in an African American adolescent population. *Journal of Cardiovascular Nursing, 27,* 476–484. doi:10.1097/JCN.0b013e31822f7971

D'Amico, D., & Barbarito, C. (2012). *Health and physical assessment in nursing* (2nd ed.). Upper Saddle River, NJ: Pearson.

Fonseca-Reyes, S., Forsyth-Macquarrie, A., & Garcia de Alba-Garcia, J. E. (2012). Simultaneous blood pressure measurement in both arms in hypertensive and nonhypertensive adult patients. *Blood Pressure Monitoring, 17*(4), 149–154. doi:10.1097/MBP.0b013e32835681e2

Marigold, J., Arias, M., Vassallo, M., Allen, S., & Kwan, J. (2011). Autonomic dysfunction in older people. *Reviews in Clinical Gerontology, 21*(1), 28–44. doi:10.1017/S0959259810000286

McFarlane, J. (2012). Blood pressure measurement in obese patients. *Critical Care Nurse, 32*(6), 70–73. doi:10.4037/ccn2012489

Muniz, J., Sethi, R. K., Zaghi, J., Ziniel, S. I., & Sandora, T. J. (2012). Predictors of stethoscope disinfection among pediatric health care providers. *American Journal of Infection Control, 40,* 922–925. doi:10.1016/j.ajic.2011.11.021

National Institutes of Health, National Heart, Lung, and Blood Institute. (2004). *The seventh report of the Joint National Committee on Prevention, Detection, Evaluation, and Treatment of High Blood Pressure* (NIH Publication No. 04–5230). Retrieved from http://www.nhlbi.nih.gov/guidelines/hypertension/jnc7full.htm

Penning, C., van der Linden, J. H., Tibboel, D., & Evenhuis, H. (2011). Is the temporal artery thermometer a reliable instrument for detecting fever in children? *Journal of Clinical Nursing, 20,* 1632–1639. doi:10.1111/j.1365-2702.2010.03568.x

Pinar, R., Ataalkin, S., & Watson, R. (2010). The effect of crossing legs on blood pressure in hypertensive patients. *Journal of Clinical Nursing, 19,* 1284–1288. doi:10.1111/j.1365-2702.2009.03148.x

Rubia-Rubia, J., Arias, A., Sierra, A., & Aguirre-Jaime, A. (2011). Measurement of body temperature in adult patients: Comparative study of accuracy, reliability and validity of different devices. *International Journal of Nursing Studies, 48,* 872–880. doi:10.1016/j.ijnurstu.2010.11.003

Selected Bibliography

Akpolat, T., Aydogdu, T., Erdem, E., & Karatas, A. (2011). Inaccuracy of home sphygmomanometers: A perspective from clinical practice. *Blood Pressure Monitoring, 16,* 168–171. doi:10.1097/MBP.0b013e328348ca52

Batra, P., & Goyal, S. (2013). Comparison of rectal, axillary, tympanic, and temporal artery thermometry in the pediatric emergency room. *Pediatric Emergency Care, 29*(1), 63–66. doi:10.1097/PEC.0b013e31827b5427

Berman, A., Snyder, S., & Frandsen, G. (2016). *Kozier & Erb's fundamentals of nursing: Concepts, process, and practice* (10th ed.). Upper Saddle River, NJ: Pearson.

Cacciolati, C., Hanon, O., Dufouil, C., Alpérovitch, A., & Tzourio, C. (2013). Categories of hypertension in the elderly and their 1-year evolution. The Three-City Study. *Journal of Hypertension, 31,* 680–689. doi:10.1097/HJH.0b013e32835ee0ca

Casey, G. (2011). Pulse oximetry—What are we really measuring? *Kai Tiaki Nursing New Zealand, 17*(3), 24–29.

James, P. A., Oparil, S., Carter, B. L., Cushman, W. C., Dennison-Himmelfarb, C., Handler, J., . . . Ortiz, E. (2014). 2014 Evidence-based guideline for the management of high blood pressure in adults: Report from the panel members appointed to the Eighth Joint National Committee (JNC 8). *Journal of the American Medical Association, 311,* 507–520. doi:10.1001/jama.2013.284427

Khoshdel, A. R., Carney, S., & Gillies, A. (2010). The impact of arm position and pulse pressure on the validation of a wrist-cuff blood pressure measurement device in a high risk population. *International Journal of General Medicine, 3,* 119–125.

Klein, M., & DeWitt, T. G. (2010). Reliability of parent-measured axillary temperatures. *Clinical Pediatrics, 49,* 271–273. doi:10.1177/0009922809350215

Korhan, E. A., Yönt, G. H., & Khorshid, L. (2011). Comparison of oxygen saturation values obtained from fingers on physically restrained or unrestrained sides of the body. *Clinical Nurse Specialist, 25*(2), 71–74. doi:10.1097/NUR.0b013e31820aeff2

Mager, D. R. (2012) Orthostatic hypotension: Pathophysiology, problems, and prevention. *Home Healthcare Nurse, 30,* 525–530. doi:10.1097/NHH.0b013e31826a6805

Non, A. L., Gravlee, C. C., & Mulligan, C. J. (2012). Education, genetic ancestry, and blood pressure in African Americans and Whites. *American Journal of Public Health, 102,* 1559–1565. doi:10.2105/AJPH.2011.300448

Pak, J. G., & Park, K. H. (2012). Advanced pulse oximetry system for remote monitoring and management. *Journal of Biomedicine and Biotechnology, 2012,* Article ID 930582, 1–8. doi:10.1155/2012/930582

Schell, K., Morse, K., & Waterhouse, J. K. (2010). Forearm and upper-arm oscillometric blood pressure comparison in acutely ill adults. *Western Journal of Nursing Research, 32,* 322–340. doi:10.1177/0193945909351887

Storm-Versloot, M. N., Verweij, L., Lucas, J., Ludikhuiae, J., Goslings, J. C., Legemate, D. A., & Vermeulen, H. (2014). Clinical relevance of routinely measured vital signs in hospitalized patients: A systematic review. *Journal of Nursing Scholarship, 46,* 39–49. doi:10.1111/jnu.12048

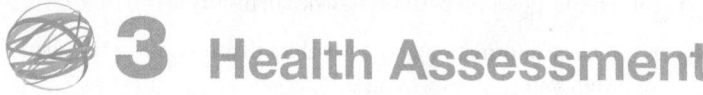

3 Health Assessment

LEARNING OUTCOMES

At the completion of this chapter, the student will be able to:

1. Define the key terms used in the skills of health assessment.
2. Describe the components of a nursing health history.
3. Perform the four examination techniques: inspection, palpation, percussion, and auscultation.
4. Recognize when it is appropriate to delegate assessment skills to unlicensed assistive personnel.
5. Verbalize the steps used in performing selected assessment skills:
   a. Assessing appearance and mental status.
   b. Assessing the skin.
   c. Assessing the hair.
   d. Assessing the nails.
   e. Assessing the skull and face.
   f. Assessing the eye structures and visual acuity.
   g. Assessing the ears and hearing.
   h. Assessing the nose and sinuses.
   i. Assessing the mouth and oropharynx.
   j. Assessing the neck.
   k. Assessing the thorax and lungs.
   l. Assessing the heart and central vessels.
   m. Assessing the peripheral vascular system.
   n. Assessing the breasts and axillae.
   o. Assessing the abdomen.
   p. Assessing the musculoskeletal system.
   q. Assessing the neurologic system.
   r. Assessing the female genitals and inguinal area.
   s. Assessing the male genitals and inguinal area.
   t. Assessing the anus.
   u. Assessing intake and output.
6. Discuss variations in assessment techniques appropriate for clients across the life span.
7. Predict the variations in health assessment findings of clients across the life span.
8. Demonstrate appropriate documentation and reporting of health assessment findings.
9. Describe sequencing to conduct an abbreviated screening assessment in an orderly fashion.
10. Describe variations in the depth and breadth of performing a health assessment according to the client circumstances.

SKILLS

KEY TERMS

Health assessment, the collection and interpretation of data regarding the client's previous and current health status, is one of the most important professional responsibilities of the registered nurse. Vigilance in performing relevant assessment techniques, determining the meaning of the findings, and taking appropriate action based on the evaluation of the data are central aspects of effective nursing care and cannot be delegated to those without the requisite skills and knowledge.

In order for the process of assessment to be more client focused than nurse focused, we must guide our intentions. Rather than viewing this process as simply gathering information and data, the nurse should view assessment as a process of discovery in which the nurse and client identify patterns, accessing what is already known to the client. The nurse uses listening skills to hear clients' stories and beliefs about what is going on inside their bodies and to seek clarification and verification. The nurse may also use intuitive skills to enhance the pattern recognition process.

The nurse is able to perform a comprehensive assessment of each individual body system. In practice, however, the generalist nurse performs a brief initial screening assessment of all systems (sometimes referred to as a head-to-toe assessment) and then more detailed focused assessments of particular systems as indicated by the client's condition. Independent clinical judgment drives the selection of those components for which an assessment is indicated. Box 3–1 presents the order generally followed when performing a head-to-toe assessment. This order provides a systematic approach and includes all vital areas to assess while minimizing positioning changes for both nurse and client. Advanced practice nurses such as nurse practitioners may perform much more in-depth assessments of selected systems.

NURSING HEALTH HISTORY
The nursing health history interview is the first part of the assessment of the client's health status and is usually carried out before the physical examination. This is a structured interview designed to collect specific health data and to obtain a detailed health record of the client. The purposes for performing a health history are:

- To elicit information about variables that may affect the client's health status.
- To obtain data that help the nurse understand and appreciate the client's life experiences.
- To initiate a nonjudgmental, trusting interpersonal relationship with the client.

The nurse uses the data obtained in collaboration with the client to develop individualized care. Components of the nursing history include (a) biographic data, (b) chief complaint or reason for visit, (c) history of present illness (current health status), (d) past history, (e) family history of illness, (f) lifestyle, (g) social data, (h) psychological data, and (i) patterns of health care. Content of each of these components is described in Box 3–2. In addition, a review of systems (also called a screening interview) may be done. This involves a brief review of the essential functioning of each body part or physiological system. While collecting historical data, the nurse applies knowledge of the variations in verbal and nonverbal communication styles among individuals of different cultures. See the accompanying Culturally Responsive Care feature on page 54.

PHYSICAL HEALTH EXAMINATION
A complete health assessment varies in many ways according to the age of the individual, the severity of the illness, the preferences of the nurse, and the agency's priorities and procedures. Regardless of what procedure is used, the assessment is conducted in a systematic and efficient manner that conserves energy and time and requires the fewest position changes for the client.

The nurse should prepare the client by introducing self and explaining the procedure, the reasons for the examination, and what the client can expect. Prepare the environment by obtaining all necessary equipment, including adequate lighting and drapes for privacy, and

---

BOX 3–1 Head-to-Toe Framework

GENERAL SURVEY INCLUDING VITAL SIGNS
Areas below are assessed including determination of current complaints and inspection. Palpation, percussion, and auscultation are used if indicated.

- Head
  - Hair, scalp, and face
  - Eyes and vision
  - Ears and hearing
  - Nose
  - Mouth and oropharynx
- Neck
  - Muscles
  - Lymph nodes
  - Trachea
  - Thyroid gland
  - Carotid arteries
  - Neck veins
- Upper extremities
  - Skin and nails
  - Muscle strength and tone
  - Joint range of motion

- Brachial and radial pulses
- Sensation
- Chest and back
  - Skin
  - Thorax shape and size
  - Lungs
  - Heart
  - Spinal column
  - Breasts and axillae
- Abdomen
  - Skin
  - Abdominal sounds
  - Femoral pulses
- External genitals
- Anus
- Lower extremities
  - Skin and toenails
  - Gait and balance
  - Joint range of motion
  - Popliteal, posterior tibial, and dorsalis pedis pulses

BOX 3–2 Components of a Nursing Health History

BIOGRAPHIC DATA

Client's name, address, age, sex, marital or partnered status, occupation, religious preference, health care financing, and usual source of medical care.

CHIEF COMPLAINT OR REASON FOR VISIT

The answer given to the question "What is troubling you?" or "Can you tell me the reason you came to the hospital or clinic today?" The chief complaint should be recorded in the client's own words.

HISTORY OF PRESENT ILLNESS

- When the symptoms started
- Whether the onset of symptoms was sudden or gradual
- How often the symptoms occur
- Exact location of the symptoms
- Character of the symptoms (e.g., intensity of pain or quality of sputum, emesis, or discharge)
- Activity in which the client was involved when the symptoms first occurred
- Phenomena or other signs associated with the chief complaint
- Factors that aggravate or alleviate the symptoms

PAST HISTORY

- Childhood illnesses, such as chickenpox, mumps, measles, rubella (German measles), rubeola (red measles), streptococcal infections, scarlet fever, rheumatic fever, and other significant illnesses
- Childhood immunizations and the dates of the last tetanus shot and adult immunizations
- Allergies to drugs, animals, insects, or other environmental agents, the type of reaction that occurs, and how the reaction is treated
- Accidents and injuries: how, when, and where the incident occurred, type of injury, treatment received, and any complications
- Hospitalization for serious illnesses: reasons for the hospitalization, dates, surgery performed, course of recovery, and any complications
- History of major illnesses or conditions, such as hepatitis, heart disease, HIV disease, tuberculosis, or osteoporosis
- Medications: all currently used prescription and over-the-counter medications, such as aspirin, nasal spray, herbal remedies, dietary supplements such as vitamins, or laxatives

FAMILY HISTORY OF ILLNESS

To determine risk factors for certain diseases, the ages of siblings, parents, and grandparents and their current state of health or, if they are deceased, the cause of death are obtained. Particular attention should be given to disorders such as heart disease, cancer, diabetes, hypertension, obesity, allergies, arthritis, tuberculosis, bleeding, alcoholism, and any mental health disorders.

LIFESTYLE

- *Personal habits:* the amount, frequency, and duration of substance use (tobacco, alcohol, coffee, cola, tea, and illicit or recreational drugs). See Box 3–3 for screening guidelines.
- *Diet:* description of a typical diet on a normal day or any special diet, number of meals and snacks per day, who cooks and shops for food, ethnically distinct food patterns, and allergies

- *Sleep/rest patterns:* usual daily sleep/wake times, difficulties sleeping, and remedies used for difficulties
- *Activities of daily living (ADLs):* any difficulties experienced in the basic activities of eating, grooming, dressing, elimination, and locomotion
- *Instrumental ADLs:* any difficulties experienced in food preparation, shopping, transportation, housekeeping, laundry, and ability to use the telephone, handle finances, and manage medications
- *Recreation/hobbies:* exercise activity and tolerance, hobbies and other interests, and vacations

SOCIAL DATA

- *Family relationships/friendships:* the client's support system in times of stress (who helps in time of need?), what effect the client's illness has on the family, and whether any family problems are affecting the client
- *Ethnic affiliation:* health customs and beliefs; cultural practices that may affect health care and recovery
- *Educational history:* data about the client's highest level of education attained and any past difficulties with learning
- *Occupational history:* current employment status, the number of days missed from work because of illness, any history of accidents on the job, any occupational hazards with a potential for future disease or accident, the client's need to change jobs because of past illness, the employment status of spouses or partners and the way child care is handled, and the client's overall satisfaction with work
- *Economic status:* information about how the client is paying for medical care (including what kind of medical and hospitalization coverage the client has), and whether the client's illness presents financial concerns
- *Home and neighborhood conditions:* home safety measures and adjustments in physical facilities that may be required to help the client manage a physical disability, activity intolerance, and ADLs; the availability of neighborhood and community services to meet the client's needs

PSYCHOLOGICAL DATA

- Major stressors experienced and the client's perception of them
- Usual coping pattern with a serious problem or a high level of stress
- Communication style: ability to verbalize appropriate emotion; nonverbal communication, such as eye movements, gestures, use of touch, and posture; interactions with support persons; and the congruence of verbal and nonverbal behavior

PATTERNS OF HEALTH CARE

All health care resources the client is currently using and has used in the past. These include the primary care provider, medical specialists (e.g., ophthalmologist or gynecologist), dentist, chiropractor, folk practitioners (e.g., herbalist or curandero), health clinic or health center, mental health practitioners (e.g., psychologist or social worker), or alternative health practitioners (e.g., massage therapist or aromatherapist); whether the client considers the care being provided adequate; and whether access to health care is a problem.

Culturally Responsive Care

Cultural Norms Relevant to Health Assessment

Here are a few examples of different cultural norms in nonverbal communication. Cultural norms will vary within a culture, and from generation to generation. Therefore, it is extremely important to observe carefully, ask your client about preferences, and not make assumptions. Your assessment and care will benefit greatly from this awareness of differences.

EYE CONTACT
Keep in Mind—Eye contact and the handshake have different meanings for different cultures. For example, some Native American communities consider direct eye contact an invasion of privacy and a firm handshake aggressive. Many Asian cultures avoid eye contact as a sign of respect for the other individual. The nurse of Western European descent might believe that a client who avoids direct eye contact is somewhat suspicious, and that a weak handshake signifies disinterest. In some Middle Eastern and Latin countries, direct eye contact is common and accepted.

Nursing Implications—Be careful not to assume things about your client based on the norms for your own cultural group. For example, if you value eye contact as a sign of interest, you may incorrectly assume your client is disinterested if he or she does not maintain eye contact. In fact, the client may be trying to show respect for you. Observing your client with family and other individuals is a helpful way to learn about his or her usual pattern of eye contact.

TOUCH AND PERSONAL SPACE
Keep in Mind—Americans tend to keep a certain amount of space between themselves and others, typically 3 feet, and use touch sparingly. French people typically feel comfortable standing very close to others and are comfortable touching. Cultural groups such as Orthodox Jews and Chinese Americans may consider excessive touching, especially from someone of the opposite sex, offensive.

Nursing Implications—Note patterns of touch between family members, or individuals of the same culture. Just as with eye contact, it may be difficult for you to change your habits of touch and personal space. However, if you sense unease in your clients, reevaluate your actions to be more sensitive to their comfort level. When in doubt, ask your client if he or she feels comfortable in the situation.

USE OF BODY LANGUAGE
Keep in Mind—Body language can easily be misinterpreted during the assessment, so pay careful attention to the assumptions you are making based on your own cultural norms. For example, many North Americans typically nod to indicate agreement or approval. Asian people may nod to be polite, but this may not actually indicate agreement.

Nursing Implications—Make sure that you are not relying solely on nonverbal clues to determine if your client understands or agrees with you. Instead of asking, "Did you understand how we will test your blood?" and relying on a nod for affirmation, you might ask, "Can you explain how we will test your blood?" In addition, follow up on your questions so that you actually hear a verbal "yes" or "no" response.

BOX 3–3 Screening for Alcohol and Drug Problems

There are many different instruments nurses can use to help identify clients with problems related to the unsafe use of alcohol and drugs. One of the most common is the CAGE Questionnaire Adapted to Include Drugs (CAGE-AID). The four questions to ask clients are:

1. Have you felt you ought to cut down on your drinking or drug use?
2. Have people annoyed you by criticizing your drinking or drug use?
3. Have you felt bad or guilty about your drinking or drug use?
4. Have you ever had a drink or used drugs first thing in the morning to steady your nerves or to get rid of a hangover (eye-opener)?

A score of 2/4 or greater is a "positive CAGE" and further evaluation is indicated (Bowman, Eiserman, Beletsky, Stancliff, & Bruce, 2013). Refer to a health professional qualified to conduct this evaluation.

---

adjusting the room temperature. Equipment commonly used in performing an examination is shown in Table 3–1 on page 55.

Examination Techniques

Four primary techniques are used in the physical examination: inspection, palpation, percussion, and auscultation.

INSPECTION

Inspection is visual examination, which is assessing by using the sense of sight. The nurse inspects with the naked eye and with a lighted instrument such as an **otoscope** (used to view the ear). Use of the senses of hearing and smell may also be considered part of inspection. Inspection should be systematic, so that nothing is missed.

PALPATION

Palpation is the examination of the body using the sense of touch. The pads of the fingers are used because their concentration of nerve endings makes them highly sensitive to tactile discrimination.

Palpation is used to determine (a) texture (e.g., of the hair); (b) temperature (e.g., of a skin area); (c) vibration (e.g., of a joint); (d) position, size, consistency, and mobility of organs or masses; (e) distention (e.g., of the urinary bladder); (f) presence and rate of peripheral pulses; and (g) tenderness or pain.

There are two types of palpation: light and deep. Light (superficial) palpation should always precede deep palpation, because heavy pressure on the fingertips can dull the sense of touch. For light palpation, the nurse extends dominant hand fingers parallel to the skin surface and presses gently downward while moving the hand in a circular fashion (Figure 3–1 ■).

Deep palpation is usually not done during a routine examination and requires significant practitioner skill. It is performed with extreme caution because pressure can damage internal organs. It is usually not indicated in clients who have acute abdominal pain or enlarged abdominal organs such as the liver or spleen.

There are two methods of performing deep palpation: with two hands (bimanually) or one hand. In deep bimanual palpation, the

TABLE 3–1 Equipment and Supplies Used for a Health Examination

Equipment/Supplies		Purpose
Flashlight or penlight		To assist viewing of the pharynx or to determine the reactions of the pupils of the eye
Ophthalmoscope		A lighted instrument to visualize the interior of the eye
Otoscope		A lighted instrument to visualize the eardrum and external auditory canal (a nasal speculum may be attached to the otoscope to inspect the nasal cavities)
Percussion (reflex) hammer		An instrument with a rubber head to test reflexes
Tuning fork		A two-pronged metal instrument used to test hearing acuity and vibratory sense
Cotton applicators		To obtain specimens
Gloves		To protect the nurse
Tongue blades (depressors)		To depress the tongue during assessment of the mouth and pharynx

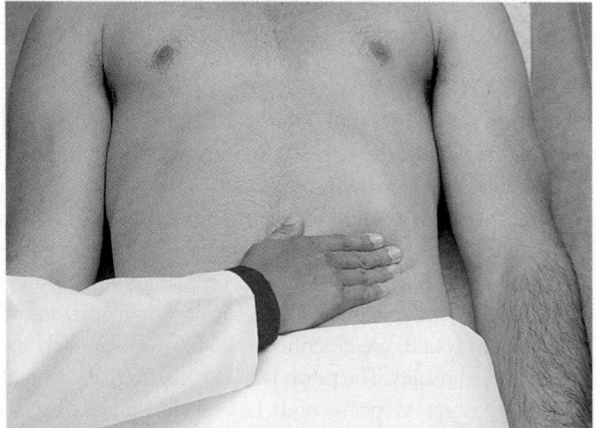

Figure 3–1 ■ The position of the hand for light palpation.

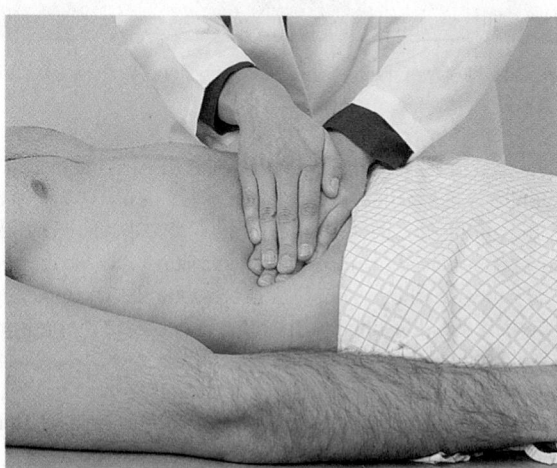

Figure 3–2 ■ The position of the hands for deep bimanual palpation.

nurse extends the dominant hand as for light palpation, then places the finger pads of the nondominant hand on the dorsal surfaces of the distal interphalangeal joint of the middle three fingers of the dominant hand (Figure 3–2 ■). The nondominant hand applies pressure while the dominant hand remains relaxed to perceive the tactile sensations.

For deep palpation using one hand, the finger pads of the dominant hand press over the area to be palpated. Often, the other hand is used to support from below (Figure 3–3 ■).

PERCUSSION

In **percussion**, the body surface is struck to elicit sounds that can be heard or vibrations that can be felt. The two types of percussion are direct and indirect. In direct percussion, the nurse strikes the area to be percussed directly with the pads of two, three, or four fingers or with the pad of the middle finger. The strikes are rapid, and the movement is from the wrist. This technique is useful in percussing an adult's sinuses (Figure 3–4 ■).

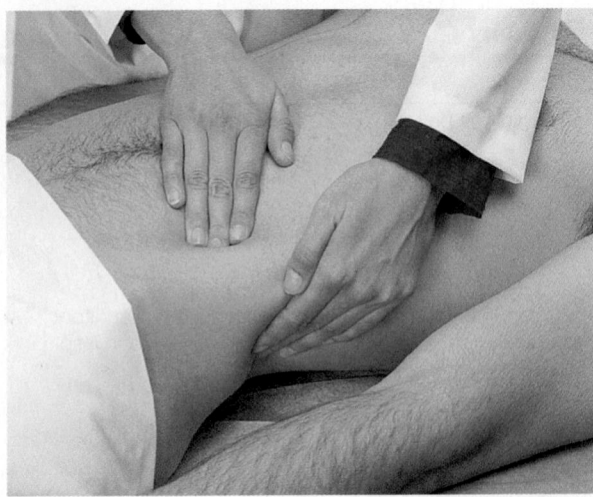

Figure 3–3 ■ Deep palpation using the lower hand to support the body while the upper hand palpates the organ.

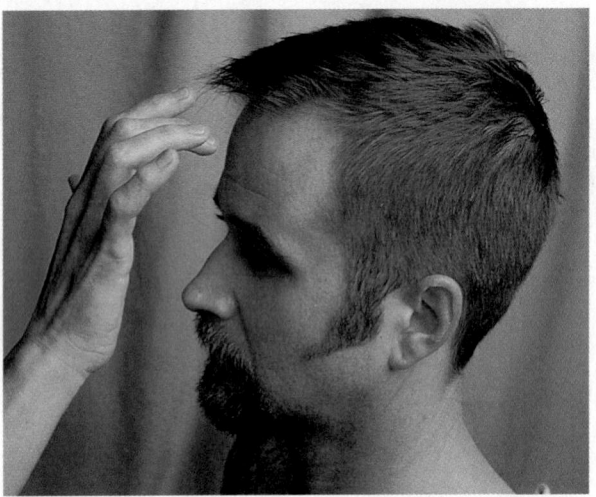

Figure 3–4 ■ Direct percussion. Using one hand to strike the surface of the body.

The second type, indirect percussion, is the striking of an object (e.g., a finger) held against the body area to be examined. In this technique, the middle finger of the nondominant hand, referred to as the **pleximeter**, is placed firmly on the client's skin. Only the distal phalanx and joint of this finger should be in contact with the skin. Using the tip of the flexed middle finger of the other hand, called the **plexor**, the nurse strikes the pleximeter, usually at the distal interphalangeal joint or a point between the distal and proximal joints (Figure 3–5 ■). The striking motion comes from the wrist; the forearm remains stationary.

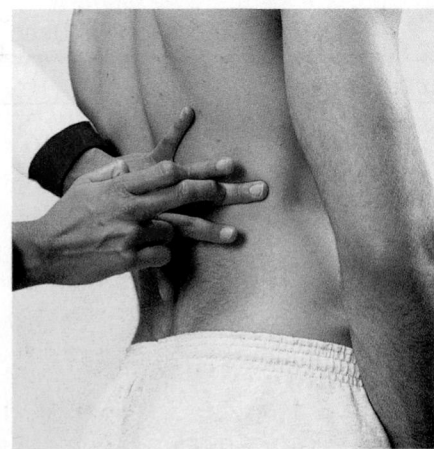

Figure 3–5 ■ Indirect percussion. Using the finger of one hand to tap the finger of the other hand.

The angle between the plexor and the pleximeter should be 90°, and the blows must be firm, rapid, and short to obtain a clear sound.

Percussion is used to determine the size and shape of internal organs by establishing their borders. It indicates whether tissue is fluid filled, air filled, or solid. Percussion elicits five types of sound: flatness, dullness, resonance, hyperresonance, and tympany. **Flatness** is an extremely dull sound heard when percussing over very dense tissue, such as muscle or bone. **Dullness** is a thudlike sound heard with percussion over dense tissue such as the liver, spleen, or heart. **Resonance** is a hollow sound such as that elicited over lungs filled with air. Percussion does not produce **hyperresonance** in the normal body. It is described as booming and can be heard over an emphysematous lung. **Tympany** is a musical or drumlike sound produced when percussing an air-filled organ such as the stomach. On a continuum, flatness reflects the most dense tissue (the least amount of air) and tympany reflects the least dense tissue (the greatest amount of air). See Table 3–2 for characteristics of the sounds and examples of where they may be heard.

AUSCULTATION

Auscultation is the process of listening to sounds produced within the body, such as with the use of a stethoscope that amplifies the sounds and conveys them to the nurse's ears. The stethoscope should be 30 to 35 cm (12 to 14 in.) long, with both a flat-disk and a bell-shaped diaphragm. (See ❺ in Skill 2–3 on page 35.) The diaphragm best transmits high-pitched sounds (e.g., bronchial sounds), and the bell best transmits low-pitched sounds, such as some heart sounds.

Auscultated sounds are described according to their pitch, intensity, duration, and quality. The **pitch** is the frequency of the vibrations (the number of vibrations per second). Low-pitched sounds (e.g., some

TABLE 3–2	Percussion Sounds and Tones					
Sound	**Intensity**	**Pitch**	**Duration**	**Quality**	**Example of Location**
Flatness	Soft	High	Short	Extremely dull	Muscle, bone
Dullness	Medium	Medium	Moderate	Thudlike	Liver, heart
Resonance	Loud	Low	Long	Hollow	Normal lung
Hyperresonance	Very loud	Very low	Very long	Booming	Emphysematous lung
Tympany	Loud	High (distinguished mainly by musical timbre)			
Moderate	Musical	Stomach filled with gas (air)			

heart sounds) have fewer vibrations per second than high-pitched sounds (e.g., bronchial sounds). The **intensity** (amplitude) refers to the loudness or softness of a sound. Some body sounds are loud (e.g., bronchial sounds heard over the trachea), whereas others are soft (e.g., normal breath sounds heard in the lungs). The **duration** of a sound is its length (long or short). The **quality** of a sound is a subjective description (e.g., whistling, gurgling, or snapping). By simply closing the eyes while auscultating and picturing the inner workings of the body, the nurse can enhance accuracy of assessment. This mindful focus can also bring new awareness and insights into what might be going on inside the client.

GENERAL SURVEY

Health assessment begins with a general survey that includes observation of the client's general appearance, mental status, vital signs, height, and weight. Many of the components of the general survey, such as body build, posture, hygiene, and mental status, are observed while completing the client's health history.

General Appearance and Mental Status

The general appearance and behavior of an individual must be assessed in terms of culture, educational level, socioeconomic status, and current circumstances. For example, an individual who has recently experienced a personal loss may appropriately appear depressed. Also, the client's age, sex, and race are useful factors in interpreting findings that suggest increased risk for known conditions.

CLINICAL ALERT!

Review the agency charting form before beginning your assessment to ensure that you know all the data you will need to collect, have all of the equipment you require, and know how to perform the assessment using a systematic approach.

Vital Signs

Vital signs are measured to establish baseline data against which to compare future measurements and to detect actual or potential health problems. See Chapter 2 ∞ for measurements of temperature, pulse, respirations, blood pressure, and oxygen saturation. See Chapter 9 ∞ for pain assessment.

Height and Weight

In adults, the ratio of weight to height provides a general measure of health. By asking clients about their height and weight before actually measuring them, the nurse gains some insight into their self-image. Excessive discrepancies between the client's verbal responses and the measurements may provide clues to actual or potential problems in self-concept. Note any unintentional weight gains or losses lasting or progressing over several weeks.

The nurse measures height with a measuring stick attached to a weight scale or to a wall. The client removes the shoes and stands erect, with heels together; buttocks, shoulders, and head against the measuring stick; and eyes looking straight ahead. The nurse raises the L-shaped sliding arm until it rests on top of the client's head, or places a small flat object, such as a ruler or book, on the client's head. The edge of the ruler should abut the measuring guide.

Weight is usually measured when a client is admitted to a health care agency, and then regularly, for example, each morning before breakfast in the hospital or weekly in a long-term facility. Most scales

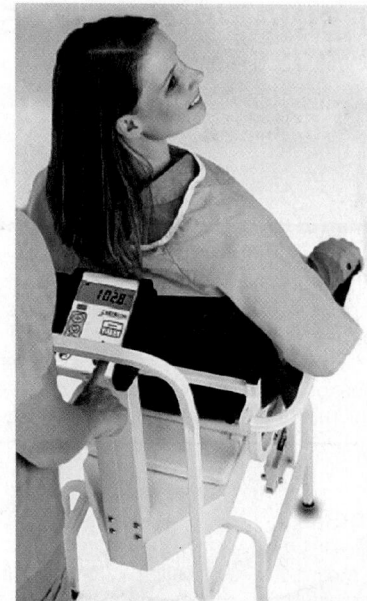

Figure 3–6 ■ Chair scale.
Courtesy DETECTO Scale.

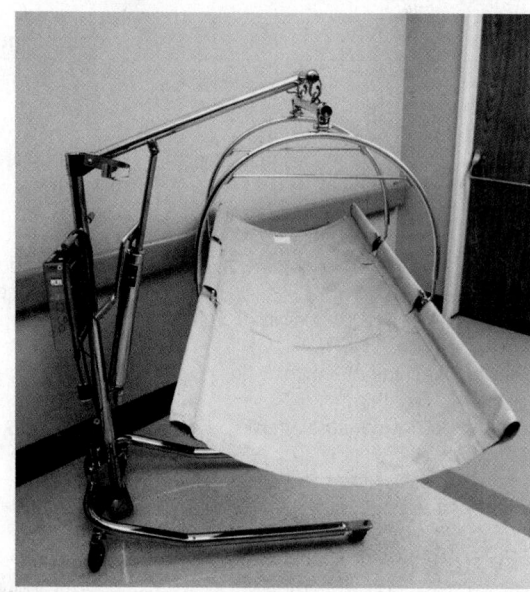

Figure 3–7 ■ Bed scale.

can measure in pounds (lb) or kilograms (kg). The nurse should be able to convert between pounds and kilograms. One kilogram is equal to 2.2 pounds. When accuracy is essential, the nurse should use the same scale each time (because every scale weighs slightly differently), take the measurements at the same time each day, and ensure the client has on a similar amount of clothing and no footwear. If the client's absolute weight must be known, the clothing must be weighed separately and subtracted from the weight indicated on the scale. This situation may exist, for example, when a medication dose must be calculated based on the client's exact weight.

Weight is read from a digital display panel or a balancing arm on the scale. It is important to check that the scale reads zero prior to placing the client on the scale. Clients who cannot stand can be weighed using a chair (Figure 3–6 ■) or bed scale. The bed scale (Figure 3–7 ■) has a canvas strap or a stretcher-like apparatus to support the client. The machine lifts the client above the bed, and the weight is reflected either on a digital display panel or on a balance arm. Newer hospital beds have built-in scales.

●○● NURSING PROCESS: ASSESSING APPEARANCE AND MENTAL STATUS

Assessing Appearance and Mental Status

PLANNING
DELEGATION

Due to the substantial knowledge and skill required, assessment of general appearance and mental status is not delegated to unlicensed assistive personnel (UAP) such as nursing or medical assistants. UAP may collect data but are not qualified to perform assessments nor analyze the data. However, many aspects of a client's condition are observed during usual care and may be recorded by UAPs. Abnormal findings must be validated and interpreted by the nurse.

INTERPROFESSIONAL PRACTICE

Assessing appearance and mental status is also within the scope of practice of many health care providers other than nurses before, during, and after their treatments. Although these providers may verbally communicate their findings and plan to other health care team members, the nurse must also know where to locate their documentation in the client's medical record.

Equipment
None

IMPLEMENTATION
Performance

1. Prior to conducting the examination, introduce self and verify the client's identity using agency protocol. Explain to the client what you are going to do, the reason for the examination, and how he or she can participate. Discuss how the findings will be used in planning further care or treatments.

2. Perform hand hygiene and observe other appropriate infection prevention procedures.
3. Provide for client privacy.

Assessment	Normal Findings	Deviations from Normal
4. Observe body build, height, and weight in relation to the client's age, lifestyle, and health.	Proportionate, varies with lifestyle	Excessively thin or obese
5. Observe client's posture and gait, standing, sitting, and walking.	Relaxed, erect posture; coordinated movement	Tense, slouched, bent posture; uncoordinated movement; tremors, unbalanced gait
6. Observe client's overall hygiene and grooming.	Clean, neat	Dirty, unkempt
7. Note body and breath odor in relation to activity level.	No body odor or minor body odor relative to work or exercise; no breath odor	Foul body odor; ammonia odor; acetone breath odor; foul breath
8. Observe for signs of distress in posture or facial expression.	No apparent distress	Bending over because of abdominal pain, wincing, frowning, or labored breathing
9. Note obvious signs of health or illness (e.g., skin color or breathing).	Well developed, well nourished, intact skin, easy breathing	**Pallor** (paleness), weakness, lesions, cough
10. Assess the client's attitude (frame of mind).	Cooperative, able to follow instructions	Negative, hostile, withdrawn, anxious
11. Note the client's affect/mood; assess the appropriateness of the client's responses.	Appropriate to situation	Inappropriate to situation, sudden mood changes, paranoia
12. Listen for speech quantity (amount and pace) and quality (loudness, clarity, inflection).	Understandable, moderate pace; clear tone and inflection	Rapid or slow pace; overly loud or soft
13. Listen for relevance and organization of thoughts.	Logical sequence, relevant answers, has sense of reality	Illogical sequence, flight of ideas, confusion, generalizations, vague

14. Document findings in the client record using handwritten or electronic forms and checklists supplemented by narrative notes when appropriate. ❶

EVALUATION
- Relate findings to previous assessment data if available. Perform a detailed system-specific follow-up examination based on findings that deviated from those expected.

- Report deviations from expected findings to the primary care provider.

Assessing Appearance and Mental Status—*continued*

P Adult Admission Assessment - Sweda, Katherine

✓ ■ ⊘ ✎ ⊞ ↑ ↓ | ▭ ▤ ▨

*Performed on: 08/21/2014 ▲▼ ▾ 0655 ▲▼ CDT   By: Border, Cathy

Vital Signs	
Height/Weight	
Height/Weight - English Calc	
Subjective	
Pain Assessment	
Pain Associated Behaviors/PA	
Additional Pain	
Pain Interventions	
Comfort Measures	
Cardiovascular	
CV Detailed	
Respiratory	
Resp Detailed	
Mental Status	
Orientation Memory Concentra	
Neurological	
Neuro Detailed	
Glasgow Coma	
Musculoskeletal	
Functional Assessment	
MS Detailed	
Gastrointestinal	
GI Detailed	
Genitourinary	
GU Detailed	
Integumentary	
Incision/Wound Detailed	
Peripheral IV	
Central Line	
Drains/Tubes	
Meds/Immunizations	
Suicide Risk Assessment	
Social Habits	
Education	
Education History	
Faculty Review	

Subjective

Assess symptoms relative to any new medications administered for the first time. Evaluate the need to notify the physician for dosage adjustments, discontinuation of the medication, or other interventions.

Pain Present

○ Unable to assess
○ No actual or suspected pain
○ Yes actual or suspected pain

General Symptoms

☐ Activity intolerance   ☐ Edema   ☐ Nausea
☐ Anorexia   ☐ Faintness   ☐ Weakness
☐ Confusion/Disorientation ☐ Fatigue   ☐ Other:
☐ Dizziness   ☐ Heartburn
☐ Drooling   ☐ Itching

Documentation of Activity Intolerance, Confusion/Disorientation, Dizziness, Faintness or Weakness will create an order for Morse Fall Risk Assessment if not done within the last 24 hours

Activity Tolerance

○ Dyspnea/Fatigue at levels limiting normal person   ○ Dyspnea/Fatigue at rest
○ Dyspnea/Fatigue with ordinary activity
○ Dyspnea/Fatigue with less than ordinary activity

Respiratory Symptoms

☐ Cough   ☐ Other:
☐ Denies shortness of breath at rest
☐ Denies shortness of breath with usual activity
☐ Drooling
☐ Shortness of breath

Any of the above symptoms may indicate a problem of Activity Intolerance

Cardiovascular Symptoms

☐ Chest pain/pressure at rest   ☐ Dizziness   ☐ Fluid retention
☐ Chest pain/pressure with activity ☐ Edema   ☐ Palpitations
☐ Claudication   ☐ Fatigue   ☐ Other:

Any of the above symptoms may indicate a problem of Activity Intolerance

Gastrointestinal Symptoms

☐ Abdominal tenderness ☐ Constipation ☐ Flatulence ☐ Impaction   ☐ Stools, black/bloody ☐ Other:
☐ Anorexia   ☐ Cramping   ☐ Heartburn ☐ Incontinence ☐ Vomiting

In Progress

❶ Nursing assessment form.

"Nursing Assessment Form" from Cerner Electronic Health Record. Copyright © by Cerner Corporation. Used by permission of Cerner Corporation.

LIFESPAN CONSIDERATIONS   General Survey

INFANTS
- Observation of children's behavior can provide important data for the general survey, including physical development, neuromuscular function, and social and interactional skills.
- It may be helpful to have parents hold older infants and very young children for part of the assessment.
- Measure height of children under age 2 in the supine position with knees fully extended.
- Weigh without clothing.
- Include measurement of head circumference until age 2. Standardized growth charts include head circumference up to age 3.

CHILDREN
- Anxiety in preschool-age children can be decreased by letting them handle and become familiar with examination equipment.

- School-age children may be very modest and shy about exposing parts of the body.
- Adolescents should be examined without parents present unless the adolescent requests their presence.
- Weigh children without shoes and with as little clothing as possible.

OLDER ADULTS (OVER AGE 65)
- Allow extra time for clients to answer questions.
- Adapt questioning techniques as appropriate for clients with hearing or visual limitations.
- Older adults can lose several inches in height. Be sure to document height and ask if they are aware of becoming shorter.
- When asking about weight loss, be specific about amount and time frame, for example, "Have you lost more than five pounds in the last two months?"

Ambulatory and Community Settings   General Survey

PATIENT-CENTERED CARE

- Assess the client in private whenever possible. If a family member is needed to assist with recall of events or translation, obtain the client's permission to have the family member present.

- Use your own equipment when possible in measuring vital signs. Bring a tape measure for measuring height. Recognize that the client's home scale for measuring weight may not be accurate.

INTEGUMENT

The integument includes the skin, hair, and nails. The examination begins with a generalized inspection using a good source of lighting, preferably indirect natural daylight.

Skin

Assessment of the skin involves inspection and palpation. In addition, the nurse may detect unusual skin odors, usually most evident in the skinfolds, groin, or axillae. Pungent body odor is frequently related to poor hygiene, hyperhidrosis (excessive perspiration), or bromhidrosis (foul-smelling perspiration).

Hyperpigmentation (increased pigmentation) and **hypopigmentation** (decreased pigmentation) may result from changes in the distribution of melanin (the dark pigment) in the epidermis. **Vitiligo**

presents as patches of hypopigmented skin, whereas albinism is the complete or partial lack of melanin in the skin, hair, and eyes. Dark-skinned clients normally have areas of lighter pigmentation. These areas include the palms, lips, and nail beds.

Other localized color changes may indicate an abnormality. **Edema**, the presence of excess interstitial fluid, makes skin appear swollen, shiny, and taut, and tends to blanch skin color. Color variations may appear differently as a result of the clients' underlying skin color (Table 3–3).

A skin lesion is an alteration in a client's normal skin appearance. Primary skin lesions appear initially in response to a change in the external or internal environment of the skin (Figure 3–8 ■, ❶–❽). Secondary skin lesions result from modifications such as chronicity, trauma, or infection of a primary lesion. For example, a vesicle or

TABLE 3–3   Variations in Skin Color

Color	Common Location	Cultural Variation
Pallor (paleness)	Buccal mucosa; in people with light skin color, may also be evident in the face, the conjunctiva of the eyes, and the nails	Absence of underlying red tones in very dark-skinned individuals. In black-skinned clients, may appear ashen gray. In brown-skinned clients, may appear as a yellowish brown tinge.
Cyanosis (a bluish tinge)	Nail beds, lips, and buccal mucosa	In dark-skinned clients, conjunctiva and palms and soles may also show cyanosis.
Jaundice (a yellowish tinge)	Sclera of the eyes; mucous membranes; skin	Do not confuse jaundice with the normal yellow pigmentation in the sclera of a dark-skinned or African American client. If jaundice is suspected, the posterior part of the hard palate should also be inspected for a yellowish color tone.
Erythema (redness)	Skin	May not be visible in very dark skin.

Macule, Patch Flat, unelevated change in color. Macules are 1 mm to 1 cm (0.04 to 0.4 in.) in size and circumscribed. Examples: freckles, measles, petechiae, flat moles. Patches are larger than 1 cm (0.4 in.) and may have an irregular shape. Examples: port wine birthmark, vitiligo (white patches), rubella. ❶

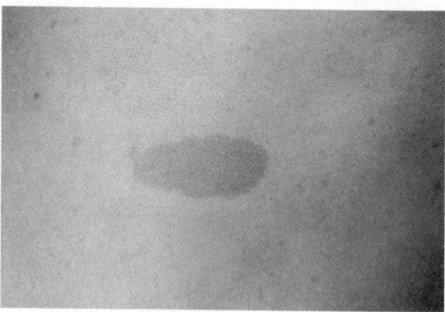

❶ A café-au-lait macule

Papule Circumscribed, solid elevation of skin. Papules are less than 1 cm (0.4 in.). Examples: warts, acne, pimples, elevated moles. ❷

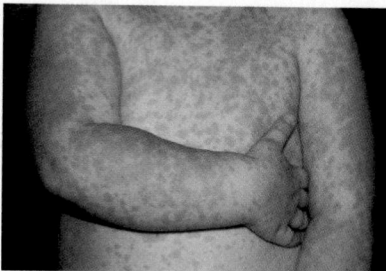

❷ Papular drug eruption

Plaque Plaques are larger than 1 cm (0.4 in.). Examples: psoriasis, rubeola. ❸

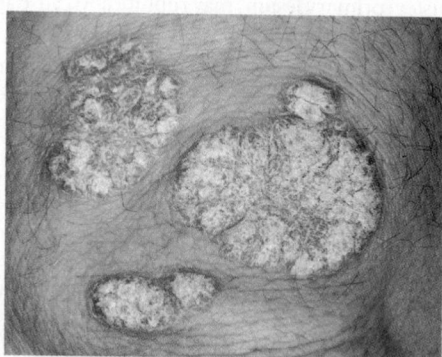

❸ Psoriasis

Nodule, Tumor Elevated, solid, hard mass that extends deeper into the dermis than a papule. Nodules have a circumscribed border and are 0.5 to 2 cm (0.2 to 0.8 in.). Examples: squamous cell carcinoma, fibroma. Tumors are larger than 2 cm (0.8 in.) and may have an irregular border. Examples: malignant melanoma, hemangioma. ❹

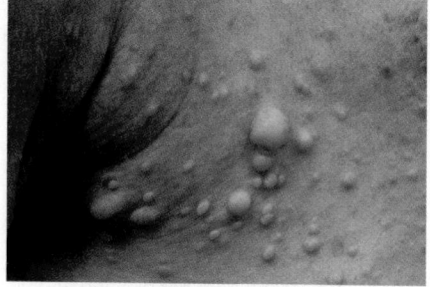

❹ Nodules from Recklinghausen's Disease

Pustule Vesicle or bulla filled with pus. Examples: acne vulgaris, impetigo. ❺

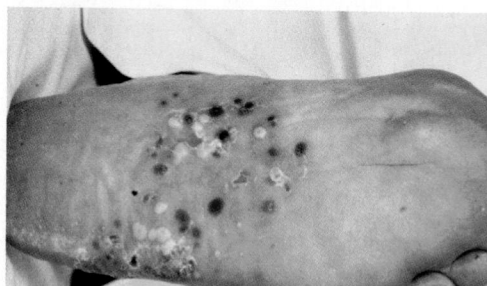

❺ White pustules along with darker healing areas

Vesicle, Bulla A circumscribed, round or oval, thin translucent mass filled with serous fluid or blood. Vesicles are less than 0.5 cm (0.2 in.). Examples: herpes simplex, early chicken pox, small burn blister. Bullae are larger than 0.5 cm (0.2 in.). Examples: large blister, second-degree burn, herpes simplex. ❻

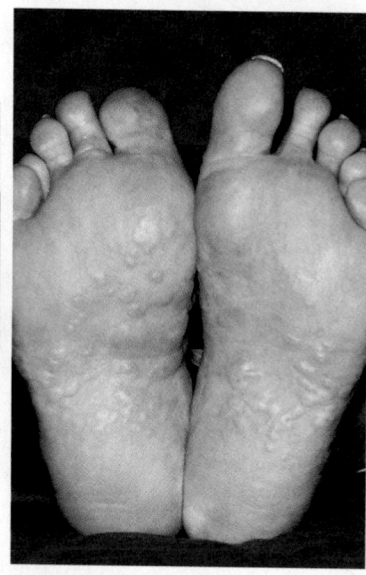

❻ Bullous pemphigoid

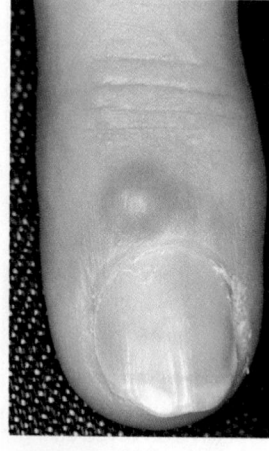

❼ Digital mucous cyst

Cyst A 1-cm (0.4 in.) or larger, elevated, encapsulated, fluid-filled or semisolid mass arising from the subcutaneous tissue or dermis. Examples: sebaceous and epidermoid cysts, chalazion of the eyelid. ❼

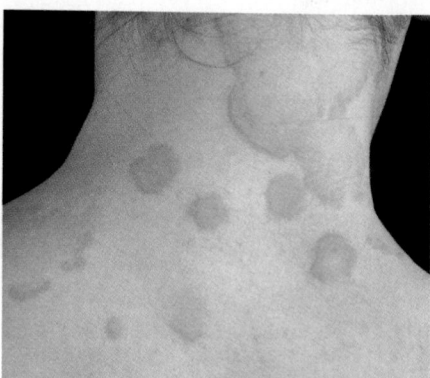

❽ Allergic wheals, urticaria

Wheal A reddened, localized collection of edema fluid; irregular in shape. Size varies. Examples: hives, mosquito bites. ❽

Figure 3–8 ■ Primary skin lesions.
Source: Figures ❶ Dr. P. Marazzi/Science Source; ❷ Scott Camazine/Alamy; ❸, ❽ Mediscan/Alamy; ❹ BSIP SA/Alamy; ❺–❻ Wellcome Image Library/Custom Medical Stock Photo; ❼ Hercules Robinson/Alamy.

blister (primary lesion) may rupture and cause an erosion (secondary lesion). Table 3–4 illustrates secondary lesions. Treatment of a secondary lesion may vary from that of its primary lesion. Nurses are responsible for describing skin lesions accurately in terms of location (e.g., face), distribution (e.g., scattered on forehead and left cheek), configuration (the arrangement or position of several lesions), and color, shape, size, firmness, texture, and characteristics of individual lesions.

TABLE 3–4 Secondary Skin Lesions

Atrophy

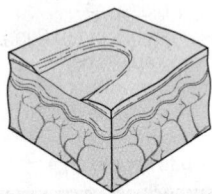

A translucent, dry, paper-like, sometimes wrinkled skin surface resulting from thinning or wasting of the skin due to loss of collagen and elastin.

Examples: Striae, aged skin

Ulcer

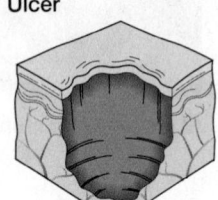

Deep, irregularly shaped area of skin loss extending into the dermis or subcutaneous tissue. May bleed. May leave scar.

Examples: Pressure ulcers, stasis ulcers, chancres

Erosion

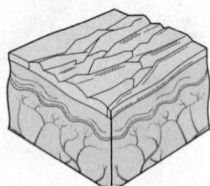

Wearing away of the superficial epidermis causing a moist, shallow depression. Because erosions do not extend into the dermis, they heal without scarring.

Examples: Scratch marks, ruptured vesicles

Fissure

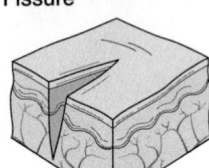

Linear crack with sharp edges, extending into the dermis.

Examples: Cracks at the corners of the mouth or in the hands, athlete's foot

Lichenification

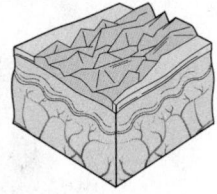

Rough, thickened, hardened area of epidermis resulting from chronic irritation such as scratching or rubbing.

Example: Chronic dermatitis

Scar

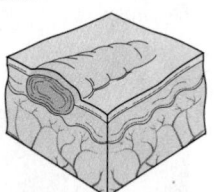

Flat, irregular area of connective tissue left after a lesion or wound has healed. New scars may be red or purple; older scars may be silvery or white.

Examples: Healed surgical wound or injury, healed acne

Scales

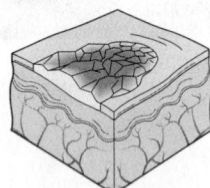

Shedding flakes of greasy, keratinized skin tissue. Color may be white, gray, or silver. Texture may vary from fine to thick.

Examples: Dry skin, dandruff, psoriasis, and eczema

Keloid

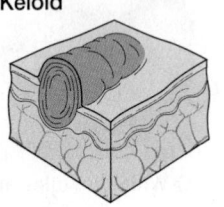

Elevated, irregular, darkened area of excess scar tissue caused by excessive collagen formation during healing. Extends beyond the site of the original injury. Higher incidence in people of African descent.

Examples: Keloid from ear piercing or surgery

Crust

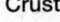

Dry blood, serum, or pus left on the skin surface when vesicles or pustules burst. Can be red-brown, orange, or yellow. Large crusts that adhere to the skin surface are called scabs.

Examples: Eczema, impetigo, herpes, or scabs following abrasion

Excoriation

Linear erosion.

Examples: Scratches, some chemical burns

●○● NURSING PROCESS: ASSESSING THE SKIN

Assessing the Skin

PLANNING
Review characteristics of primary and secondary skin lesions if necessary (see Figure 3–8 and Table 3–4). Ensure that adequate lighting is available.

DELEGATION

Due to the substantial knowledge and skill required, assessment of the skin is not delegated to UAP. However, the skin is observed during usual care and UAPs should record their findings. Abnormal findings must be validated and interpreted by the nurse.

SKILL 3–2

Assessing the Skin—*continued*

INTERPROFESSIONAL PRACTICE

Assessing the skin may be within the scope of practice of many health care providers. For example, physical therapists and occupational therapists may notice edema or skin lesions during treatment. Although these providers may verbally communicate their findings and plan to other health care team members, the nurse must also know where to locate their documentation in the client's medical record.

Equipment
- Millimeter ruler
- Clean gloves
- Magnifying glass

IMPLEMENTATION
Performance

1. Prior to conducting the examination, introduce self and verify the client's identity using agency protocol. Explain to the client what you are going to do, the reason for the examination, and how he or she can participate. Discuss how the findings will be used in planning further care or treatments.
2. Perform hand hygiene and observe other appropriate infection prevention procedures.
3. Provide for client privacy.

4. Inquire if the client has any history of the following: pain or itching; presence and spread of lesions, bruises, abrasions, or pigmented spots; previous experience with skin problems; family history of skin problems; related systemic conditions; use of medications, lotions, or home remedies; excessively dry or moist feel to the skin; tendency to bruise easily; association of the problem with season of year, stress, occupation, medications, recent travel, housing, and so on; or recent contact with allergens (e.g., metal paint).

Assessment	Normal Findings	Deviations from Normal
5. Inspect skin color, including areas not usually exposed to the sun. It is best to use natural light for the inspection.	Skin color varies from light to deep brown or black; from light pink to ruddy pink; from yellow overtones to olive	Pallor, cyanosis, jaundice, erythema
6. Inspect uniformity of skin color.	Generally uniform in color except in areas exposed to the sun; areas of lighter pigmentation (palms, lips, nail beds) in dark-skinned people	Areas of either hyperpigmentation or hypopigmentation
7. Assess for the presence of edema. If present, note the location, color, temperature, and shape of the skin, and the degree to which the skin remains indented or pitted when pressed by a finger. Measure the circumference of the extremity in millimeters with a nonstretchable tape measure.	No edema	See the scale for describing edema. ❶
8. Inspect, palpate, and describe skin lesions. Apply gloves if lesions are open or draining. Palpate lesions to determine shape and texture. Describe lesions according to location, distribution, color, configuration, size, shape, type, or structure (Box 3–4). Use the millimeter ruler to measure lesions. If gloves were applied, remove and discard gloves. • Perform hand hygiene.	Freckles, pigmented birthmarks that have not changed since childhood, and some long-standing vascular birthmarks such as strawberry or port-wine hemangiomas, some flat and raised nevi (moles); no abrasions or other lesions	Various interruptions in skin integrity; irregular, multicolored, or raised nevi; some pigmented birthmarks such as melanocystic nevi; and some vascular birthmarks such as cavernous hemangiomas. Even these deviations from normal may not be dangerous or require treatment. Assessment by an advanced-level practitioner is required.

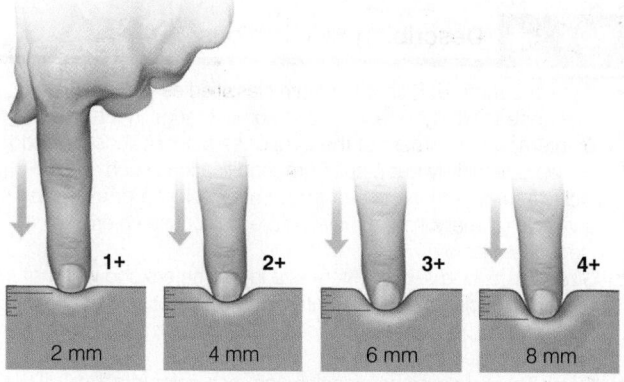

❶ Scale for grading edema.

Continued on page 64

Assessing the Skin—*continued*

Assessment	Normal Findings	Deviations from Normal
9. Observe and palpate skin moisture.	Moisture in skinfolds and the axillae (varies with environmental temperature and humidity, body temperature, and activity)	Excessive moisture (e.g., in hyperthermia); excessive dryness (e.g., in dehydration)
10. Palpate skin temperature. Compare the extremities using the backs of your fingers.	Uniform; within normal range	Generalized hyperthermia (e.g., in fever); generalized hypothermia (e.g., in shock); localized hyperthermia (e.g., in infection); localized hypothermia (e.g., in arteriosclerosis)
11. Note skin turgor (fullness or elasticity) by lifting and grasping the skin below the clavicle or on the forearm.	When grasped, skin springs back to previous state; may be slower in older adults	Skin stays pinched or tented or moves back slowly (e.g., in dehydration); count in seconds how long the skin remains tented; there is no widely accepted time span distinguishing normal from abnormal skin turgor (de Vries Feyens & de Jager, 2011)

12. Document findings in the client record using forms or checklists supplemented by narrative notes when appropriate. Draw location of skin lesions on body surface diagrams. ❷

CLINICAL ALERT!

If agency policy permits and the client agrees (follow agency privacy policies), take a digital or instant photograph of significant skin lesions for the client record. Include a measuring guide (ruler or tape) in the picture to demonstrate lesion size.

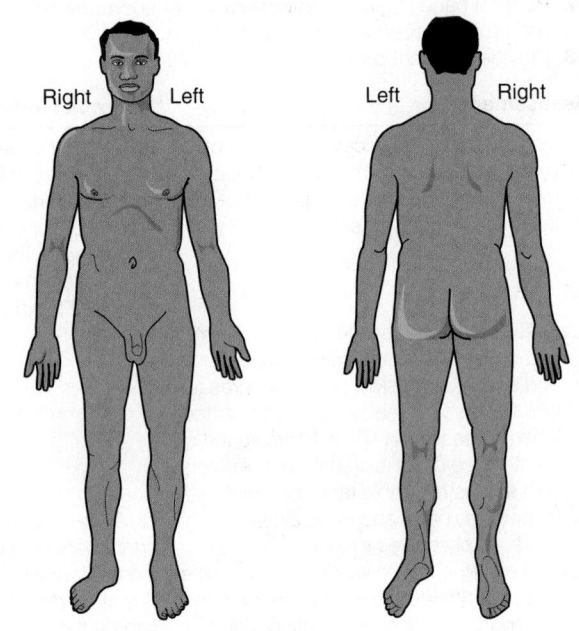

Right Left   Left Right

❷ Diagram for charting skin lesions.

EVALUATION

- Compare findings to previous skin assessment data if available to determine if lesions or abnormalities are changing.
- Report deviations from expected findings to the primary care provider.

BOX 3–4 | **Describing Skin Lesions**

- *Type or structure.* Skin lesions are classified as primary (those that appear initially in response to some change in the external or internal environment of the skin) or secondary (those that do not appear initially but result from modifications such as chronicity, trauma, or infection of the primary lesion). For example, a vesicle (primary lesion) may rupture and cause an erosion (secondary lesion).
- *Size, shape, and texture.* Note size in millimeters and whether the lesion is circumscribed or irregular; round or oval shaped; flat, elevated, or depressed; solid, soft, or hard; rough or thickened; fluid filled or has flakes.
- *Color.* There may be no discoloration, one color (e.g., red, brown, or black), or several colors, as with ecchymosis (a

bruise), in which an initial dark red or blue color fades to a yellow color. When color changes are limited to the edges of a lesion, they are described as *circumscribed*; when spread over a large area, they are described as *diffuse*.
- *Distribution.* Distribution is described according to the location of the lesions on the body and symmetry or asymmetry of findings in comparable body areas.
- *Configuration.* Configuration refers to the arrangement of lesions in relation to each other. Configurations of lesions may be annular (arranged in a circle), clustered together (grouped), linear (arranged in a line), arc or bow shaped, merged together (indiscrete), or meshed in the form of a network, or they may follow the course of cutaneous nerves.

LIFESPAN CONSIDERATIONS | Assessing the Skin

INFANTS

- Physiological jaundice may appear in newborns 2 to 3 days after birth and usually lasts about 1 week. This jaundice can last longer in breast-fed newborns. Pathologic jaundice, or that which indicates a disease, appears within 24 hours of birth and may last more than 8 days.
- Newborns may have milia (whiteheads), tiny white nodules over the nose and face, and vernix caseosa (white cheesy, greasy material on the skin).
- Premature infants may have lanugo, a fine downy hair covering their shoulders and back.
- In dark-skinned infants, areas of hyperpigmentation may be found especially on the back, in the sacral area.
- Diaper dermatitis (a rash in the groin area) may be seen.
- If a rash is present, inquire in detail about immunization history.
- Assess skin turgor by grasping the skin on the abdomen.

CHILDREN

- Children normally have minor skin lesions (e.g., bruising or abrasions) on arms and legs due to their high activity level. Lesions on other parts of the body may be signs of disease or abuse, and a thorough history should be taken.
- Secondary skin lesions may occur frequently as children scratch or expose a primary lesion to microbes.
- With puberty, oil glands become more productive, and children may develop acne. Most individuals 12 to 24 years have some acne.
- In dark-skinned children, areas of hyperpigmentation may be found especially on the back, in the sacral area.
- If a rash is present, inquire in detail about immunization history.

OLDER ADULTS

- Changes in light skin occur at an earlier age than in dark skin.

- The skin loses its elasticity and develops wrinkles. Wrinkles first appear on the face and neck, which are abundant in collagen and elastic fibers.
- The skin appears thin and translucent because of loss of dermis and subcutaneous fat.
- The skin is dry and flaky because sebaceous and sweat glands are less active. Dry skin is more prominent over the extremities.
- The skin takes longer to return to its natural shape after being pinched between the thumb and finger. This is called tenting.
- Due to the normal loss of peripheral skin turgor in older adults, assess for hydration by checking skin turgor over the sternum or clavicle.
- Flat tan- to brown-colored macules, referred to as senile lentigines or melanotic freckles, are normally apparent on the back of the hand and other skin areas that are exposed to the sun. These macules may be as large as 1 to 2 cm.
- Warty lesions (seborrheic keratosis) with irregularly shaped borders and a scaly surface often occur on the face, shoulders, and trunk. These benign lesions begin as yellowish to tan and progress to a dark brown or black.
- Vitiligo becomes more common with age and is thought to result from an autoimmune response.
- Cutaneous tags (acrochordons) are most commonly seen in the neck and axillary regions. These skin lesions vary in size and are soft, often flesh colored, and pedicled.
- Visible, bright red, fine dilated blood vessels commonly occur as a result of the thinning of the dermis and the loss of support for the blood vessel walls.
- Pink to slightly red lesions with indistinct borders (actinic keratoses) may appear at about age 50, often on the face, ears, backs of the hands, and arms. They may become malignant if untreated.

Ambulatory and Community Settings | Assessing the Skin | PATIENT-CENTERED CARE

- When making a home visit, take a penlight or examination lamp with you in case the home has inadequate lighting.
- If skin lesions are suggestive of physical abuse, follow governmental and agency regulations for follow-up and reporting. Signs of abuse may include a pattern of bruises, unusual location of burns, or lesions that are not easily explainable. If lesions are present in adults or verbal-age children, conduct the interview and assessment in private.
- Document lesions in the health record by taking a photo if the client consents and it is permitted by institutional policy. Because digital cameras are common (including on cell phones

and tablet computers), the client can be encouraged to take pictures of their own lesions in order to check changes over time or to send to the health care provider.
- Another method that can be used to record lesion size and shape is to lay clean double-thick clear plastic (such as a grocery bag) over the lesion or wound and trace the shape with a permanent marker. Cut away and dispose of the bottom layer that came in contact with the client and place the top layer in the client record. Use this method only if contact with the plastic does not contaminate the wound.

Hair

Assessing a client's hair includes inspecting the hair, considering developmental changes, and determining the individual's hair care practices and the factors influencing them. Much of the information about hair can be obtained when interviewing the client.

Normal hair is resilient and evenly distributed on the scalp. Some disease processes cause the hair to be more coarse or thinner.

An example of this condition is individuals with a severe protein deficiency (kwashiorkor). The hair color is faded and appears reddish or bleached, and the texture is coarse and dry. **Alopecia** (scalp or body hair loss) may occur as an adverse effect of drug therapies and radiation treatments, as well as certain diseases. Renal disease, hepatic disease, blood disorders, hormonal abnormalities, advanced age, and some psychiatric conditions may also alter the client's hair.

●○● NURSING PROCESS: ASSESSING THE HAIR

Assessing the Hair

PLANNING
DELEGATION

Assessment of the hair is not delegated to UAP. However, many aspects are observed during usual care and may be recorded by individuals other than the nurse. Abnormal findings must be validated and interpreted by the nurse.

INTERPROFESSIONAL PRACTICE

Assessing the hair is within the scope of practice of many health care providers. Although the providers may verbally communicate their findings and plan to other health care team members, the nurse must also know where to locate their documentation in the client's medical record.

Equipment
• Clean gloves

IMPLEMENTATION
Performance

1. Prior to conducting the examination, introduce self and verify the client's identity using agency protocol. Explain to the client what you are going to do, the reason for the examination, and how he or she can participate. Discuss how the findings will be used in planning further care or treatments.
2. Perform hand hygiene, apply gloves, and observe other appropriate infection prevention procedures.
3. Provide for client privacy.
4. Inquire if the client has any history of the following: recent use of hair dyes, rinses, or curling or straightening preparations; chemotherapy; and the presence of acute or chronic conditions.

Assessment	Normal Findings	Deviations from Normal
5. Inspect the evenness of growth over the scalp.	Evenly distributed hair	Patches of hair loss (i.e., alopecia)
6. Inspect hair thickness or thinness.	Thick hair	Very thin hair
7. Inspect hair texture and oiliness.	Silky, resilient hair	Brittle hair, excessively oily or dry hair
8. Note presence of infections or parasite infestations by parting the hair in several areas, checking behind the ears and along the hairline at the neck.	No infection or infestation	Flaking, sores, lice, nits (louse eggs), and ringworm
9. Inspect amount of body hair.	Variable	Hirsutism (abnormal hairiness); naturally absent or sparse leg hair

10. Remove and discard gloves.
    • Perform hand hygiene.
11. Document findings in the client record using forms or checklists supplemented by narrative notes when appropriate.

EVALUATION

• Relate findings to previous assessment data if available. Perform a detailed system-specific follow-up examination based on findings that deviated from those expected.

• Report deviations from expected findings to the primary care provider.

LIFESPAN CONSIDERATIONS Assessing the Hair

INFANTS
• There is a wide variation of normal hair distribution in infants, which can range from very little or none to a great deal of body and scalp hair.

CHILDREN
• As puberty approaches, axillary and pubic hair will appear (see Box 3–8 later in this chapter).

OLDER ADULTS
• Older adults may experience a loss of scalp, pubic, and axillary hair.
• Hairs of the eyebrows, ears, and nostrils become bristle-like and coarse.

Ambulatory and Community Settings   Assessing the Hair

PATIENT-CENTERED CARE

• When making a home visit, ask to see the products the client usually uses on the hair. Assist the client to determine if the products are appropriate for the client's type of hair and scalp (e.g., for dry or oily hair). Provide education regarding hygiene of the hair and scalp.

• When making a home visit, examine the equipment that the client uses on the hair. Provide client teaching regarding appropriate combs and brushes and regarding safety in using electric hair styling appliances such as hair dryers.

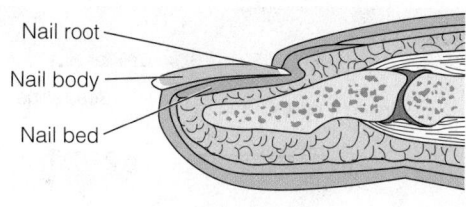
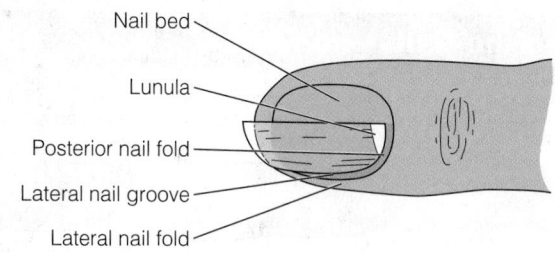

Figure 3–9 ■ The parts of a nail.

Nails

Parts of the nail are shown in Figure 3–9 ■. Nails are inspected for nail plate shape, angle between the nail and nail bed, nail texture, nail bed color, and the intactness of the tissues around the nails.

●○● NURSING PROCESS: ASSESSING THE NAILS

Assessing the Nails

PLANNING
DELEGATION

Due to the substantial knowledge required, assessment of the nails is not delegated to UAP. However, many nail characteristics are observed during usual care and may be recorded by individuals other than the nurse. Abnormal findings must be validated and interpreted by the nurse.

INTERPROFESSIONAL PRACTICE

Assessing the nails is within the scope of practice of many health care providers. Although these providers may verbally communicate their findings and plan to other health care team members, the nurse must also know where to locate their documentation in the client's medical record.

Equipment
None

IMPLEMENTATION
Performance

1. Prior to conducting the examination, introduce self and verify the client's identity using agency protocol. Explain to the client what you are going to do, the reason for the examination, and how he or she can participate. Discuss how the findings will be used in planning further care or treatments. In most situations, clients with artificial nails or polish on fingernails or toenails are not required to remove these for assessment. If the assessment cannot be conducted due to the presence of polish or artificial nails, document this in the record.

2. Perform hand hygiene and observe other appropriate infection prevention procedures.
3. Provide for client privacy.
4. Inquire if the client has any history of the following: presence of diabetes mellitus, peripheral circulatory disease, previous injury, or severe illness.

Assessment	Normal Findings	Deviations from Normal
5. Inspect fingernail plate shape to determine the curvature and angle.	Convex curvature; angle of nail plate about 160° ❶ *A*	Spoon-shaped nail ❶ *B*; clubbing (180° or greater) ❶ *C* and *D*
6. Inspect fingernail and toenail texture.	Smooth texture	Excessive thickness or thinness or presence of grooves or furrows; Beau's lines ❶ *E;* discolored or detached nail
7. Inspect fingernail and toenail bed color.	Highly vascular and pink in light-skinned clients; dark-skinned clients may have brown or black pigmentation in longitudinal streaks	Bluish or purplish tint (may reflect cyanosis); pallor (may reflect poor arterial circulation)
8. Inspect tissues surrounding nails.	Intact epidermis	Hangnails; paronychia (inflammation)
9. Perform blanch test to determine capillary refill. Press the nail between your thumb and index finger; look for blanching and return of color to nail bed. Count in seconds the time for the color to return completely. Perform on at least one nail on each hand and foot.	Prompt return of usual color (generally less than 2 seconds)	Delayed return of usual color (may indicate circulatory impairment)

10. Document findings in the client record using forms or checklists supplemented by narrative notes when appropriate.

SKILL 3–4

Continued on page 68

Assessing the Nails—*continued*

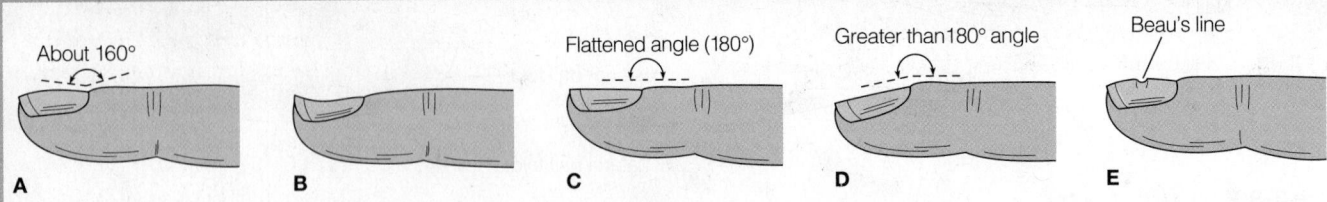

About 160°   A   B   Flattened angle (180°)   C   Greater than180° angle   D   Beau's line   E

❶ *A,* A normal nail, showing the convex shape and the nail plate angle of about 160°; *B,* a spoon-shaped nail, which may be seen in clients with iron deficiency anemia; *C,* early clubbing; *D,* late clubbing (may be caused by long-term oxygen deficit); *E,* Beau's line on nail (may result from severe injury or illness).

EVALUATION

- Relate findings to previous assessment data if available. Perform a detailed system-specific follow-up examination based on findings that deviated from those expected.

- Report deviations from expected findings to the primary care provider.

LIFESPAN CONSIDERATIONS | **Assessing the Nails**

INFANTS
- Newborns' nails grow very quickly, are extremely thin, and tear easily.

CHILDREN
- Bent, bruised, or ingrown toenails may indicate that shoes are too tight.
- Nail biting should be discussed with an adult family member because it may be a symptom of stress.

OLDER ADULTS
- The nails grow more slowly and thicken.
- Longitudinal bands commonly develop, and the nails tend to split.
- Bands across the nails may indicate protein deficiency; white spots, zinc deficiency; and spoon-shaped nails, iron deficiency.
- Toenail fungus is more common and difficult to eliminate (although not dangerous to health).

Ambulatory and Community Settings | **Assessing the Nails**   **PATIENT-CENTERED CARE**

- If indicated, teach the client or family member about proper nail care including how to trim and shape the nails to avoid paronychia. To avoid cutting the skin accidentally, file infant nails instead of clipping.

- If eyesight, fine motor control, or cognition prevents the client from safely trimming the nails, refer the client to a podiatrist or manicurist.

HEAD

During an examination of the head, the nurse often inspects and palpates simultaneously. The nurse examines the skull, face, eyes, ears, nose, sinuses, mouth, and oropharynx.

Skull and Face

There is a large range of normal shapes of skulls. A normal head size and shape is referred to as **normocephalic**. If head size appears to be outside of the normal range, the circumference can be compared to standard size tables. Measurements more than two standard deviations from the norm for the age, sex, and race of the client are abnormal and should be reported to the primary care provider. Names of areas of the head are derived from names of the underlying bones: frontal, parietal, occipital, mastoid process, mandible, maxilla, and zygomatic (Figure 3–10 ■).

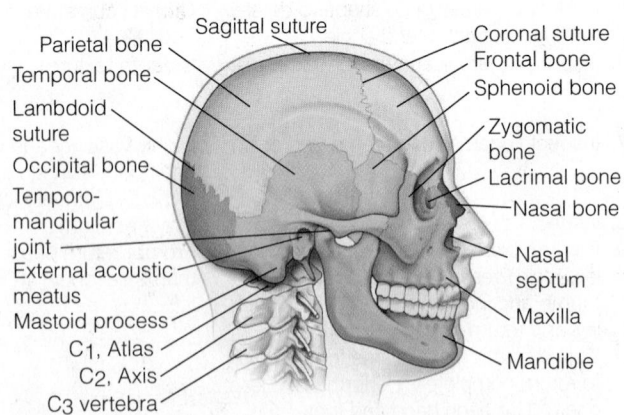

Sagittal suture — Parietal bone — Temporal bone — Lambdoid suture — Occipital bone — Temporo-mandibular joint — External acoustic meatus — Mastoid process — C₁, Atlas — C₂, Axis — C₃ vertebra — Coronal suture — Frontal bone — Sphenoid bone — Zygomatic bone — Lacrimal bone — Nasal bone — Nasal septum — Maxilla — Mandible

Figure 3–10 ■ Bones of the head.

Many disorders cause a change in facial shape or condition. Kidney or cardiac disease can cause edema of the eyelids. Hyperthyroidism can cause **exophthalmos**, a protrusion of the eyeballs with elevation of the upper eyelids off the iris, resulting in a startled or staring expression. Hypothyroidism, or myxedema, can cause a dry, puffy face with dry skin and coarse features and thinning of scalp hair and eyebrows. Increased adrenal hormone production or administration of steroids can cause a round face with reddened cheeks, referred to as moon face, and excessive hair growth on the upper lips, chin, and sideburn areas. Prolonged illness, starvation, and dehydration can result in sunken eyes, cheeks, and temples.

●○● NURSING PROCESS: ASSESSING THE SKULL AND FACE

Assessing the Skull and Face

SKILL 3–5

PLANNING
DELEGATION

Due to the substantial knowledge and skill required, assessment of the skull and face is not delegated to UAP. However, many aspects of the skull and face are observed during usual care and may be recorded by individuals other than the nurse. Abnormal findings must be validated and interpreted by the nurse.

INTERPROFESSIONAL PRACTICE

Assessing the skull and face is within the scope of practice of many health care providers. Although these providers may verbally communicate their findings and plan to other health care team members, the nurse must also know where to locate their documentation in the client's medical record.

Equipment
None

IMPLEMENTATION
Performance

1. Prior to conducting the examination, introduce self and verify the client's identity using agency protocol. Explain to the client what you are going to do, the reason for the examination, and how he or she can participate. Discuss how the findings will be used in planning further care or treatments.
2. Perform hand hygiene and observe other appropriate infection prevention procedures.
3. Provide for client privacy.

4. Inquire if the client has any history of the following: past problems with lumps or bumps, itching, scaling, or dandruff; history of loss of consciousness, dizziness, seizures, headache, facial pain, or injury; when and how any lumps occurred; length of time any other problem existed; any known cause of problem; and associated symptoms, treatment, and recurrences.

Assessment	Normal Findings	Deviations from Normal
5. Inspect the skull for size, shape, and symmetry.	Rounded (normocephalic and symmetric, with frontal, parietal, and occipital prominences); smooth skull contour	Lack of symmetry; increased skull size with more prominent nose and forehead; longer mandible (may indicate excessive growth hormone or increased bone thickness)
6. Inspect the facial features (e.g., symmetry of structures and of the distribution of hair).	Symmetric or slightly asymmetric facial features, palpebral fissures equal in size, symmetric nasolabial folds	Increased facial hair, low hairline, thinning of eyebrows, asymmetric features, exophthalmos, myxedema facies, moon face
7. Inspect the eyes for edema or hollowness.	No edema	Periorbital edema; sunken eyes
8. Note symmetry of facial movements. Ask the client to elevate the eyebrows, frown or lower the eyebrows, close the eyes tightly, puff the cheeks, and smile and show the teeth.	Symmetric facial movements	Asymmetric facial movements (e.g., eye on affected side cannot close completely); drooping of lower eyelid and mouth; involuntary facial movements (i.e., tics or tremors)

9. Document findings in the client record using forms or checklists supplemented by narrative notes when appropriate.

EVALUATION

- Relate findings to previous assessment data if available. Perform a detailed system-specific follow-up examination based on findings that deviated from those expected.
- Report deviations from expected findings to the primary care provider.

LIFESPAN CONSIDERATIONS Assessing the Skull and Face

INFANTS
- Newborns delivered vaginally can have elongated, molded heads, which take on more rounded shapes after a week or two. Infants born by cesarean section tend to have smooth, rounded heads.
- The posterior fontanel (soft spot) is about 1 cm (0.4 in.) in size and usually closes by 8 weeks. The anterior fontanel is larger,

about 2 to 3 cm (0.8 to 1.2 in.) in size. It closes by 18 to 24 months.
- Newborns can lift their heads slightly and turn them from side to side. Voluntary head control is well established by 4 to 6 months.

Eyes and Vision

It is recommended that people under age 40 have their eyes tested every 3 to 5 years, or more frequently if there is a family history of diabetes, hypertension, blood dyscrasia, or eye disease (e.g., glaucoma). After age 40, an eye examination is recommended every 2 years. Examination of the eyes commonly includes assessment of **visual acuity** (the degree of detail the eye can discern in an image), ocular movement, **visual field** (the area an individual can see when looking straight ahead), and external structures. For the anatomic structures of the eye, see Figures 3–11 ■ and 3–12 ■.

Many people wear eyeglasses or contact lenses to correct common refractive errors of the lens of the eye: **myopia** (nearsightedness), **hyperopia** (farsightedness), and **presbyopia** (loss of elasticity of the lens and thus loss of ability to see close objects). **Astigmatism**, an uneven curvature of the cornea that prevents horizontal and vertical rays from focusing on the retina, is a common problem that may occur in conjunction with myopia and hyperopia. Three types of eye charts are available to test visual acuity (Figure 3–13 ■). People with denominators of 40 or more on the Snellen chart with or without corrective lenses should be referred to an optometrist or ophthalmologist.

Common inflammatory visual problems that nurses may encounter in clients include conjunctivitis, dacryocystitis, hordeolum, iritis, and contusions or hematomas of the eyelids and surrounding structures. **Conjunctivitis** is an inflammatory process of the bulbar and palpebral conjunctiva, resulting from foreign bodies, chemicals, allergenic agents, bacteria, or viruses. Redness, itching, tearing, and mucopurulent discharge are common manifestations. During sleep, the eyelids may become encrusted and matted together. Dacryocystitis (inflammation of the lacrimal sac) is manifested by tearing and a discharge from the nasolacrimal duct. **Hordeolum** (sty) is redness, swelling, and tenderness of the hair follicle and glands that empty at the edge of the eyelids. **Iritis** (inflammation of the iris) may be caused by local or systemic infections and results in pain, tearing, and photophobia (sensitivity to light). A **hematoma** or **contusion**, commonly called a "black eye," results from injury.

Cataracts tend to occur in those over 65 years old, although they may be present at any age. This opacity of the lens or its capsule, which blocks light rays, is frequently corrected by surgery. Cataracts may also occur in infants—possibly due to a malformation of the lens if the mother contracted rubella in the first trimester of pregnancy. **Glaucoma** is a disturbance in the circulation of aqueous fluid, which causes an increase in intraocular pressure. It is the most

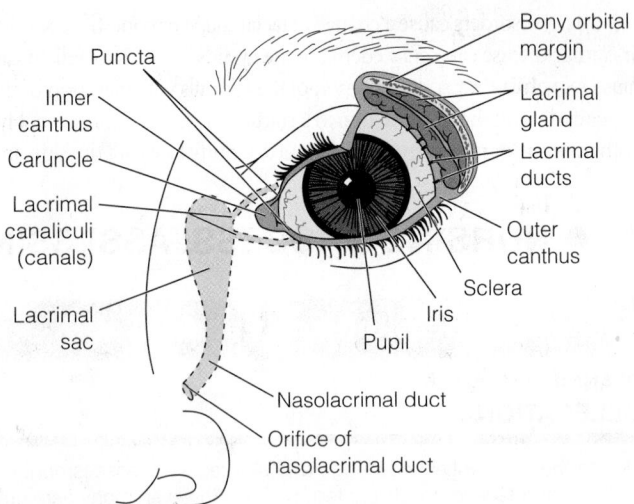

Figure 3–11 ■ The external structures and lacrimal apparatus of the left eye.

frequent cause of blindness in people over age 40 although it can occur at younger ages. It can be controlled if diagnosed early. Danger signs of glaucoma include blurred or foggy vision, loss of peripheral vision, difficulty focusing on close objects, difficulty adjusting to dark rooms, and seeing rainbow-colored rings around lights.

Upper eyelids that lie at or below the pupil margin are referred to as ptosis. Ptosis is usually associated with aging, edema from drug allergy or systemic disease (e.g., kidney disease), congenital lid muscle dysfunction, neuromuscular disease (e.g., myasthenia gravis), or third cranial nerve impairment. Eversion, an outturning of the eyelid, is called ectropion; inversion, an inturning of the lid, is called entropion. These abnormalities are often associated with scarring injuries or the aging process.

Pupils are normally black and equal in size, usually measure 3 to 7 mm in diameter, and have round, smooth borders. Cloudy pupils are often indicative of cataracts. **Mydriasis**, known as enlarged pupils, may indicate injury or glaucoma or result from certain drugs (e.g., atropine, cocaine, amphetamines). **Miosis** (constricted pupils) may indicate an inflammation of the iris or result from such drugs as morphine/heroin and other narcotics, barbiturates, or pilocarpine. Unequal pupils (*anisocoria*) may result from a central nervous system disorder; however, slight variations may be normal. The iris is normally flat and round. A bulging toward the cornea can indicate increased intraocular pressure.

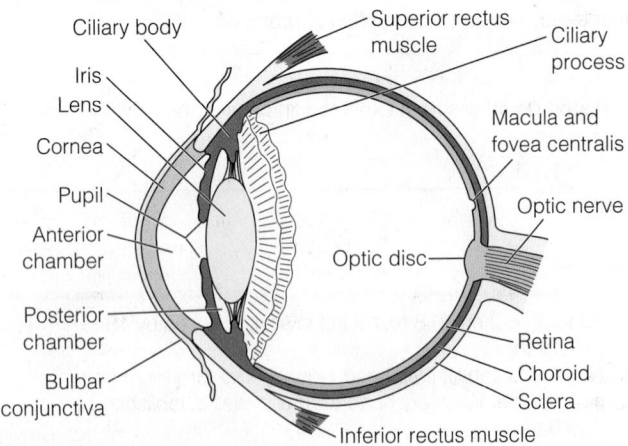

Figure 3–12 ■ Anatomic structures of the right eye, lateral view.

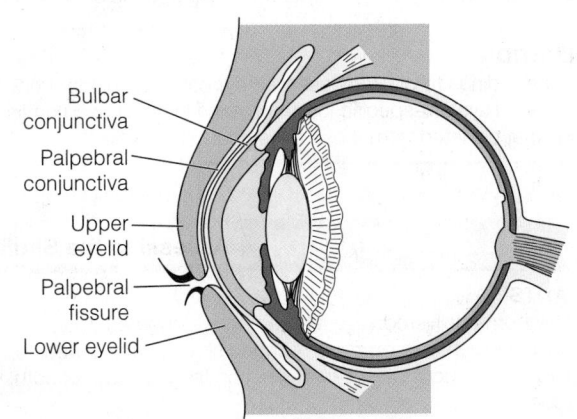

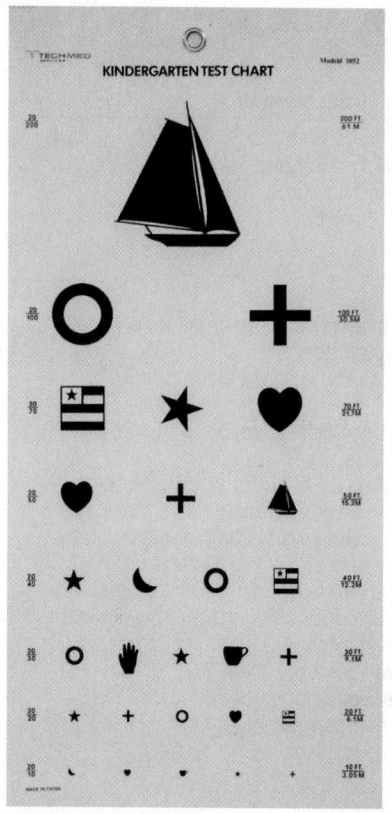 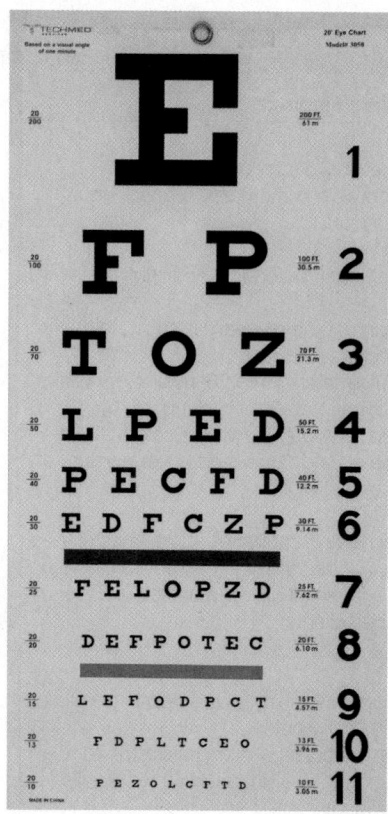 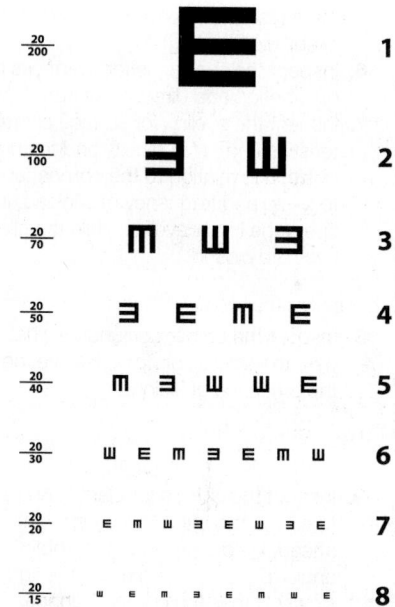

Figure 3–13 ■ Three types of eye charts: *left,* the preschool children's chart; *center,* the Snellen standard chart; *right,* the Snellen E chart for clients unable to read.
right, Roman Sotola/Shutterstock.

●○● NURSING PROCESS: ASSESSING THE EYES AND VISION

Assessing the Eye Structures and Visual Acuity

PLANNING
Place the client in an appropriate room for assessing the eyes and vision. The nurse must be able to control natural and overhead lighting during some portions of the examination.

DELEGATION

Due to the substantial knowledge and skill required, assessment of the eyes and vision is not delegated to UAP. However, many aspects of eye function are observed during usual care and may be recorded by individuals other than the nurse. Abnormal findings must be validated and interpreted by the nurse.

INTERPROFESSIONAL PRACTICE

Assessing the eyes and vision may be within the scope of practice of other health care providers. Although these providers may verbally communicate their findings and plan to other health care team members, the nurse must also know where to locate their documentation in the client's medical record.

Equipment
- Millimeter ruler
- Penlight
- Snellen standard or E chart
- Opaque card

IMPLEMENTATION
Performance
1. Prior to conducting the examination, introduce self and verify the client's identity using agency protocol. Explain to the client what you are going to do, the reason for the examination, and how he or she can participate. Discuss how the findings will be used in planning further care or treatments.
2. Perform hand hygiene and observe other appropriate infection prevention procedures.
3. Provide for client privacy.
4. Inquire if the client has any history of the following: family history of diabetes, hypertension, blood dyscrasia, or eye disease, injury, or surgery; client's last visit to an ophthalmologist; current use of eye medications; use of contact lenses or eyeglasses; hygienic practices for corrective lenses; and current symptoms of eye problems (e.g., changes in visual acuity, blurring of vision, tearing, spots, photophobia, itching, or pain).

Continued on page 72

SKILL 3–6

Assessing the Eye Structures and Visual Acuity—*continued*

Assessment	Normal Findings	Deviations from Normal
EXTERNAL EYE STRUCTURES		
5. Inspect the eyebrows for hair distribution, alignment, skin quality, and movement (ask client to raise and lower the eyebrows).	Hair evenly distributed; skin intact Eyebrows symmetrically aligned; equal movement	Loss of hair; scaling and flakiness of skin Unequal alignment and movement of eyebrows
6. Inspect the eyelashes for evenness of distribution and direction of curl.	Equally distributed; curled slightly outward	Turned inward
7. Inspect the eyelids for surface characteristics (e.g., skin quality and texture), position in relation to the cornea, ability to blink, and frequency of blinking. Inspect the lower eyelids while the client's eyes are closed.	Skin intact; no discharge; no discoloration Lids close symmetrically Approximately 15 to 20 involuntary blinks per minute; bilateral blinking When lids open, no visible sclera above corneas, and upper and lower borders of cornea are slightly covered	Redness, swelling, flaking, crusting, plaques, discharge, nodules, lesions Lids close asymmetrically, incompletely, or painfully Rapid, monocular, absent, or infrequent blinking Ptosis, ectropion, or entropion; rim of sclera visible between lid and iris
8. Inspect the bulbar conjunctiva (that lying over the sclera) for color, texture, and the presence of lesions.	Transparent; capillaries sometimes evident; sclera appears white (darker or yellowish and with small brown macules in dark-skinned clients)	Jaundiced sclera (e.g., in liver disease); excessively pale sclera (e.g., in anemia); reddened sclera (e.g., marijuana use, rheumatoid disease); lesions or nodules (may indicate damage by mechanical, chemical, allergenic, or bacterial agents)
9. Inspect the cornea for clarity and texture. Ask the client to look straight ahead. Hold a penlight at an oblique angle to the eye, and move the light slowly across the corneal surface.	Transparent, shiny, and smooth; details of the iris are visible In older people, a thin, grayish white ring around the margin, called arcus senilis, may be evident	Opaque; surface not smooth (may be the result of trauma or abrasion) Arcus senilis in clients under age 40
10. Inspect the pupils for color, shape, and symmetry of size. Pupil charts are available in some agencies. See ❶ for variations in pupil diameters.	Black in color; equal in size; normally 3 to 7 mm in diameter; round, smooth border, iris flat and round	Cloudiness, mydriasis, miosis, anisocoria; bulging of iris toward cornea

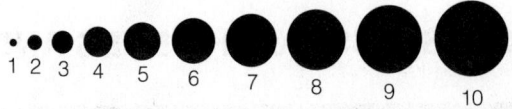

1 2 3 4 5 6 7 8 9 10

❶ Variations in pupil diameters in millimeters.

11. Assess each pupil's direct and consensual reaction to light to determine the function of the third (oculomotor) cranial nerve. • Partially darken the room. • Ask the client to look straight ahead. • Using a penlight and, approaching from the side, shine a light on the pupil. • Observe the response of the illuminated pupil. It should constrict (direct response). • Shine the light on the pupil again, and observe the response of the other pupil. It should also constrict (consensual response).	Illuminated pupil constricts (direct response) Nonilluminated pupil constricts (consensual response) Response is brisk	Neither pupil constricts Unequal responses Absent or sluggish responses

Assessing the Eye Structures and Visual Acuity—*continued*

SKILL 3-6

Assessment	Normal Findings	Deviations from Normal
12. Assess each pupil's reaction to accommodation. • Hold an object (a penlight or pencil) about 10 cm (4 in.) from the bridge of the client's nose. • Ask the client to look first at the top of the object and then at a distant object (e.g., the far wall) behind the penlight. Alternate the gaze from the near to the far object. • Observe the pupil response. • Next, ask the client to look at the near object, and then move the penlight or pencil toward the client's nose.	Pupils constrict when looking at near object; pupils dilate when looking at far object; pupils converge when near object is moved toward nose To record normal assessment of the pupils, use the abbreviation **PERRLA** (pupils equally round and react to light and accommodation)	One or both pupils fail to constrict, dilate, or converge
VISUAL FIELDS		
13. Assess peripheral visual fields to determine function of the retina and neuronal visual pathways to the brain and second (optic) cranial nerve. • Have the client sit directly facing you at a distance of 60 to 90 cm (2 to 3 ft). • Ask the client to cover the right eye with a card and look directly at your nose. • Cover or close your eye directly opposite the client's covered eye (i.e., your left eye), and look directly at the client's nose. • Hold an object (e.g., a penlight or pencil) in your fingers, extend your arm, and move the object into the visual field from various points in the periphery. The object should be at an equal distance from the client and yourself. Ask the client to tell you when the moving object is first spotted.	When looking straight ahead, client can see objects in the periphery	Visual field smaller than normal (possible glaucoma); one-half vision in one or both eyes (possible nerve damage)
a. To test the temporal field of the left eye, extend and move your right arm in from the client's right periphery.	Temporally, peripheral objects can be seen at right angles (90°) to the central point of vision	
b. To test the upward field of the left eye, extend and move the right arm down from the upward periphery.	The upward field of vision is normally 50° because the orbital ridge is in the way	
c. To test the downward field of the left eye, extend and move the right arm up from the lower periphery.	The downward field of vision is normally 70° because the cheekbone is in the way	
d. To test the nasal field of the left eye, extend and move your left arm in from the periphery. ❷	The nasal field of vision is normally 50° away from the central point of vision because the nose is in the way	
• Repeat the above steps for the right eye, reversing the process.		

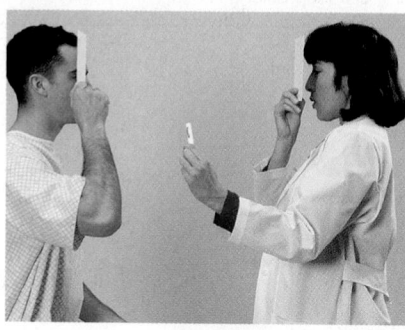

❷ Assessing the client's left peripheral vision field.

Continued on page 74

Assessing the Eye Structures and Visual Acuity—*continued*

Assessment	Normal Findings	Deviations from Normal
EXTRAOCULAR MUSCLE TESTS	Both eyes coordinated, move in unison, with parallel alignment	Eye movements not coordinated or parallel; one or both eyes fail to follow a penlight in specific directions, e.g., **strabismus** (cross-eye) **Nystagmus** (rapid involuntary rhythmic eye movement) other than at end point may indicate neurologic impairment

14. Assess six ocular movements to determine eye alignment and coordination.
  • Stand directly in front of the client and hold the penlight at a comfortable distance, such as 30 cm (1 ft) in front of the client's eyes.
  • Ask the client to hold the head in a fixed position facing you and to follow the movements of the penlight with the eyes only.
  • Move the penlight in a slow, orderly manner through the six cardinal fields of gaze, that is, from the center of the eye along the lines of the arrows in ❸ and back to the center.
  • Stop the movement of the penlight periodically so that nystagmus can be detected.

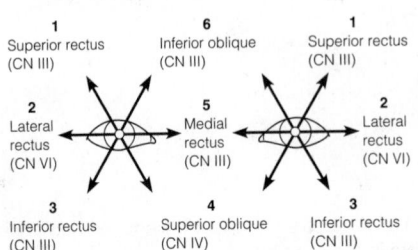

❸ The six muscles that govern eye movement.

15. Assess for location of the corneal light reflex by shining the penlight on the pupil in the corneal surface (Hirschberg test).

Light falls symmetrically (e.g., at "6 o'clock" on both pupils)

Light falls off center on one eye

16. Have the client fixate on a near or far object. Cover one eye and observe for movement in the uncovered eye (cover test).

Uncovered eye does not move

If misalignment is present, when dominant eye is covered, the uncovered eye will move to focus on object

VISUAL ACUITY

17. If the client can read, assess near vision by providing adequate lighting and asking the client to read from a magazine or newspaper held at a distance of 36 cm (14 in.). If the client normally wears corrective lenses, the glasses or lenses should be worn during the test. The document must be in a language the client can read.

Able to read newsprint

Difficulty reading newsprint unless due to aging process

18. Assess distance vision by asking the client to wear corrective lenses, unless they are used for reading only, i.e., for distances of only 36 cm (14 in.).
  • Ask the client to stand or sit 6 m (20 ft) from a Snellen or character chart, ❹ cover the eye not being tested, and identify the letters or characters on the chart.
  • Take three readings: right eye, left eye, both eyes.
  • Record the readings of each eye and both eyes (i.e., the smallest line from which the person is able to read one half or more of the letters).

20/20 vision on Snellen-type chart

Denominator of 40 or more on Snellen-type chart with corrective lenses

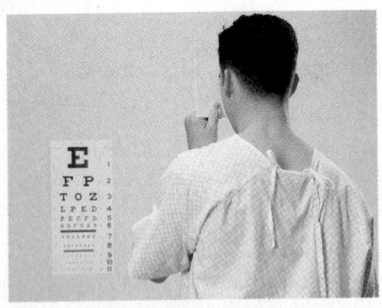
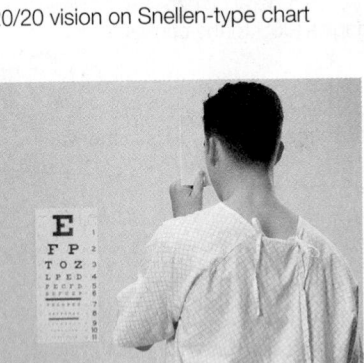

❹ Testing distance vision.

Assessing the Eye Structures and Visual Acuity—continued

Assessment	Normal Findings	Deviations from Normal
At the end of each line of the chart are standardized numbers (fractions). The top line is 20/200. The numerator (top number) is always 20, the distance the person stands from the chart. The denominator (bottom number) is the distance from which the normal eye can read the chart. Therefore, a person who has 20/40 vision can see at 20 feet from the chart what a normal-sighted person can see at 40 feet from the chart. Visual acuity is recorded as "s̄–c" (without correction), or "c̄–c" (with correction). You can also indicate how many letters were misread in the line, e.g., "visual acuity 20/40-2 c̄–c" indicates that two letters were misread in the 20/40 line by a client wearing corrective lenses.		
19. If the client is unable to see even the top line (20/200) of the Snellen-type chart, perform one or more of the following vision tests.		Limited vision only (e.g., light perception, hand movements, counting fingers at 30 cm [1 ft])

LIGHT PERCEPTION
Shine a penlight into the client's eye from a lateral position, and then turn the light off. Ask the client to tell you when the light is on or off.

HAND MOVEMENTS
Hold your hand 30 cm (1 ft) from the client's face and move it slowly back and forth, stopping it periodically. Ask the client to tell you when your hand stops moving.

COUNTING FINGERS
Hold up some of your fingers 30 cm (1 ft) from the client's face, and ask the client to count your fingers.

20. Document findings in the client record using forms or checklists supplemented by narrative notes when appropriate.

EVALUATION
- Relate findings to previous assessment data if available. Perform a detailed system-specific follow-up examination based on findings that deviated from those expected.
- Report deviations from expected findings to the primary care provider. Individuals with denominators of 40 or more on the Snellen or character chart, with or without corrective lenses, may need to be referred to an optometrist or ophthalmologist.

LIFESPAN CONSIDERATIONS   Assessing the Eyes and Vision

INFANTS
- Infants 4 weeks of age should gaze at and follow objects.
- Ability to focus with both eyes should be present by 6 months of age.
- Infants do not have tears until about 3 months of age.
- Visual acuity is about 20/300 at 4 months and progressively improves.

CHILDREN
- Epicanthal folds, common in individuals of Asian heredity, may cover the medial canthus and cause eyes to appear misaligned. Epicanthal folds may also be seen in young children of any race before the bridge of the nose begins to elevate.
- Preschool children's acuity can be checked with picture cards or the E chart. Acuity should approach 20/20 by 6 years of age.

Continued on page 76

- Always perform the acuity test with glasses on if a child has prescription lenses.
- Children should be tested for color vision deficit. From 8% to 10% of Caucasian males and from 0.5% to 1% of Caucasian females have this deficit; it is much less common in non-Caucasian children. The Ishihara or Hardy-Rand-Rittler test can be used.

OLDER ADULTS
Visual Acuity
- Visual acuity decreases as the lens of the eye ages and becomes more opaque and loses elasticity.
- The ability of the iris to accommodate to darkness and dim light diminishes.
- Peripheral vision diminishes.
- The adaptation to light (glare) and dark decreases.
- Accommodation to far objects often improves, but accommodation to near objects decreases.
- Color vision declines; older people are less able to perceive purple colors and to discriminate pastel colors.
- Many older adults wear corrective lenses; they are most likely to have hyperopia. Visual changes are due to loss of elasticity (presbyopia) and diminishing transparency of the lens.

External Eye Structures
- The skin around the orbit of the eye may darken.
- The eyeball may appear sunken because of the decrease in orbital fat.
- Skinfolds of the upper lids may seem more prominent, and the lower lids may sag.
- The eyes may appear dry and dull because of the decrease in tear production from the lacrimal glands.
- A thin, grayish white arc or ring (arcus senilis) appears around part or all of the cornea. It results from an accumulation of a lipid substance on the cornea. The cornea tends to cloud with age.
- The iris may appear pale with brown discolorations as a result of pigment degeneration.
- The conjunctiva of the eye may appear paler than that of younger adults and may take on a slightly yellow appearance because of the deposition of fat.
- Pupil reaction to light and accommodation is normally symmetrically equal but may be less brisk.
- The pupils can appear smaller in size, unequal, and irregular in shape because of sclerotic changes in the iris.

- When making a home visit, take your equipment and charts with you. Also, include a tape measure to lay out the 20 feet for distance vision testing.
- Use the assessment as an opportunity to reinforce proper eye care and the need for regular vision testing.

Ears and Hearing

Nursing assessment of the ear includes direct inspection and palpation of the external ear, inspection of the internal parts of the ear by an otoscope, and determination of auditory acuity. Audiometric evaluations, conducted by an audiometrist, measure hearing at various decibels and are recommended for older adults or other individuals with suspected hearing loss. An audiologist interprets the evaluation and recommends a care plan.

To inspect the external ear canal and tympanic membrane, the nurse inserts an otoscope into the external auditory canal. In some practice settings, the generalist nurse does not perform otoscopic examinations.

●○● NURSING PROCESS: ASSESSING THE EARS AND HEARING

Assessing the Ears and Hearing

PLANNING
It is important to conduct the ear and hearing examination in an area that is quiet. In addition, the location should allow the client to be positioned sitting or standing at the same level as the nurse.

DELEGATION

Due to the substantial knowledge and skill required, assessment of the ears and hearing is not delegated to UAP. However, many aspects of ear function are observed during usual care and may be recorded by individuals other than the nurse. Abnormal findings must be validated and interpreted by the nurse.

INTERPROFESSIONAL PRACTICE

Assessing the ears and hearing is within the scope of practice of many health care providers. For example, audiologists and physician assistants may check the client's hearing. Although these providers may verbally communicate their findings and plan to other health care team members, the nurse must also know where to locate their documentation in the client's medical record.

Equipment
- Otoscope with several sizes of ear specula
- Tuning fork

Assessing the Ears and Hearing—*continued*

IMPLEMENTATION
Performance

1. Prior to conducting the examination, introduce self and verify the client's identity using agency protocol. Explain to the client what you are going to do, the reason for the examination, and how he or she can participate. Discuss how the findings will be used in planning further care or treatments.
2. Perform hand hygiene and observe other appropriate infection prevention procedures.
3. Provide for client privacy.
4. Inquire if the client has any history of the following: family history of hearing problems or loss; presence of ear problems or pain; medication history, especially if there are complaints of ringing in ears (tinnitus); hearing difficulty (its onset, factors contributing to it, and how it interferes with ADLs) or use of a corrective hearing device (when and from whom it was obtained).
5. Position the client comfortably, seated if possible.

Assessment	Normal Findings	Deviations from Normal
AURICLES		
6. Inspect the auricles for color, symmetry of size, and position. To inspect position, note the level at which the superior aspect of the auricle attaches to the head in relation to the eye.	Color same as facial skin Symmetrical Auricle aligned with outer canthus of eye, about 10° from vertical 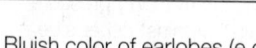	Bluish color of earlobes (e.g., cyanosis); pallor (e.g., frostbite); excessive redness (inflammation or fever) Asymmetry Low-set ears (associated with a congenital abnormality, such as Down syndrome)

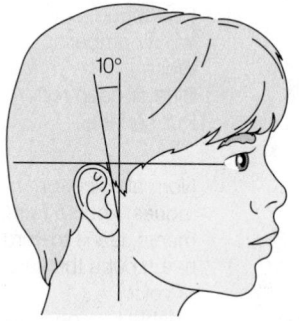

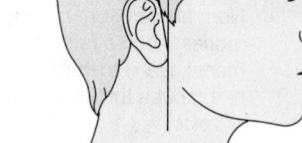

❶ Alignment of ears.　　Normal alignment　　　　Low-set ears and deviation in alignment

7. Palpate the auricles for texture, elasticity, and areas of tenderness. • Gently pull the auricle upward, downward, and backward. • Fold the pinna forward (it should recoil). • Push in on the tragus. • Apply pressure to the mastoid process.	Mobile, firm, and not tender; pinna recoils after it is folded	Lesions (e.g., cysts); flaky, scaly skin (e.g., seborrhea); tenderness when moved or pressed (may indicate inflammation or infection of external ear)
EXTERNAL EAR CANAL AND TYMPANIC MEMBRANE		
8. Inspect the external ear canal for cerumen, skin lesions, pus, and blood.	Distal third contains hair follicles and glands Dry cerumen, grayish tan color; or sticky, wet cerumen in various shades of brown	Redness and discharge Scaling Excessive cerumen obstructing canal
9. Visualize the tympanic membrane using an otoscope. • Attach a speculum to the otoscope. Use the largest diameter that will fit the ear canal without causing discomfort. **Rationale:** *This achieves maximum vision of the entire ear canal and tympanic membrane.* • Tip the client's head away from you, and straighten the ear canal. For an adult, straighten the ear canal by pulling the pinna up and back. **Rationale:** *Straightening the ear canal facilitates vision of the ear canal and the tympanic membrane.*		

Continued on page 78

SKILL 3-7

Assessing the Ears and Hearing—*continued*

Assessment	Normal Findings	Deviations from Normal

- Hold the otoscope either (a) right side up, with your fingers between the otoscope handle and the client's head, or (b) upside down, with your fingers and the ulnar surface of your hand against the client's head. ❷ **Rationale:** *These positions stabilize the head and protect the eardrum and canal from injury if a quick head movement occurs.*
- Gently insert the tip of the otoscope into the ear canal, avoiding pressure by the speculum against either side of the ear canal. **Rationale:** *The inner two thirds of the ear canal is bony; if the speculum is pressed against either side, the client will experience discomfort.*

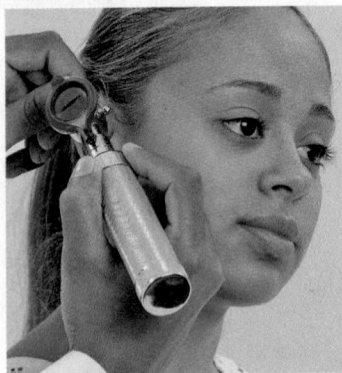

❷ Inserting an otoscope.

- Inspect the tympanic membrane for color and gloss.

Pearly gray color, semitransparent

Pink to red, some opacity
Yellow-amber
White
Blue or deep red
Dull surface

GROSS HEARING ACUITY TESTS

10. Assess the client's response to normal voice tones. If the client has difficulty hearing the normal voice, proceed with the following tests.

Normal voice tones audible

Normal voice tones not audible (e.g., requests nurse to repeat words or statements, leans toward the speaker, turns the head, cups the ears, or speaks in loud tone of voice)

10A. *Whisper test.* Perform the whisper test to assess high-frequency hearing.
- Have the client occlude one ear. Out of the client's sight, at a distance of 0.3 to 0.6 m (1 to 2 ft.), whisper a simple phrase such as "The weather is hot today."
- Ask the client to repeat the phrases.
- Repeat with the other ear using a different phrase.

Able to repeat the phrases correctly in both ears

Unable to repeat the phrases correctly in one or both ears

10B. *Tuning fork tests.* Perform Weber's test to assess bone conduction by examining the lateralization (sideward transmission) of sounds.
- Hold the tuning fork at its base. Activate it by tapping the fork gently against the back of your hand near the knuckles or by stroking the fork between your thumb and index fingers. It should be made to ring softly.
- Place the base of the vibrating fork on top of the client's head ❸ and ask where the client hears the noise.
- Conduct the Rinne test to compare air conduction to bone conduction.

Sound is heard in both ears or is localized at the center of the head (Weber negative)
Air-conducted (AC) hearing is greater than bone-conducted (BC) hearing, i.e., AC > BC (positive Rinne)

Sound is heard better in impaired ear, indicating a bone-conductive hearing loss; or sound is heard better in ear without a problem, indicating a sensorineural disturbance (Weber positive)
Bone conduction time is equal to or longer than the air conduction time, i.e., BC > AC or BC = AC (negative Rinne; indicates a conductive hearing loss)

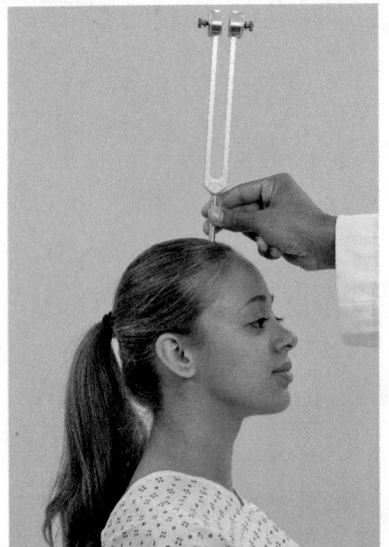

❸ Placing the base of the tuning fork on the client's skull (Weber's test).

Assessing the Ears and Hearing—*continued*

Assessment	Normal Findings	Deviations from Normal
• Hold the handle of the activated tuning fork on the mastoid process of one ear ❹ *A* until the client states that the vibration can no longer be heard. • Immediately, hold the still vibrating fork prongs in front of the client's ear canal. ❹ *B* Push aside the client's hair if necessary. Ask whether the client now hears the sound. Sound conducted by air is heard more readily than sound conducted by bone. The tuning fork vibrations conducted by air are normally heard longer. **11.** Document findings in the client record using forms or checklists supplemented by narrative notes when appropriate.	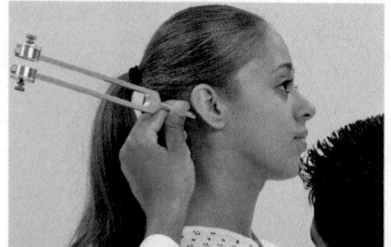 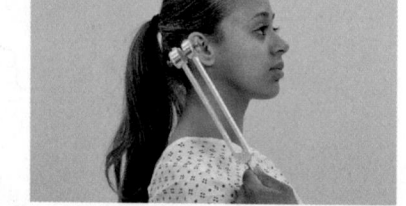 ❹ Rinne test tuning fork placement: *A*, base of the tuning fork on the mastoid process; *B*, tuning fork prongs placed in front of the client's ear.	

EVALUATION

• Relate findings to previous assessment data if available. Perform a detailed system-specific follow-up examination based on findings that deviated from those expected.

• Report deviations from expected findings to the primary care provider.

LIFESPAN CONSIDERATIONS | Assessing the Ears and Hearing

INFANTS

• To assess gross hearing, ring a bell from behind the infant or have the parent call the child's name to check for a response. Newborns will quiet to the sound and may open their eyes wider. By 3 to 4 months of age, the child will turn head and eyes toward the sound.

• All newborns should be assessed for hearing prior to discharge from the hospital. Most states and many countries have a law or regulation requiring universal newborn hearing screening.

CHILDREN

• To inspect the external canal and tympanic membrane in children less than 3 years old, pull the pinna down and back. Insert the otoscopic speculum only 0.64 to 1.27 cm (0.25 to 0.50 in.).

• Perform routine hearing checks and follow up on abnormal results. In addition to congenital or infection-related causes of hearing loss, noise-induced hearing loss is becoming more common in adolescents and young adults as a result of exposure to extremely loud music and prolonged use of headsets at loud volumes (Weichbold, Holzer, Newesely, & Stephan, 2012).

Teach that music loud enough to prevent hearing a normal conversation can damage hearing.

OLDER ADULTS

• The skin of the ear may appear dry and be less resilient because of the loss of connective tissue.

• Increased coarse and wire-like hair growth occurs along the helix, antihelix, and tragus.

• The pinna increases in both width and length, and the earlobe elongates.

• Earwax is drier.

• The tympanic membrane is more translucent and less flexible. The intensity of the light reflex may diminish slightly.

• Sensorineural hearing loss occurs.

• Generalized hearing loss (**presbycusis**) occurs in all frequencies, although the first symptom is the loss of high-frequency sounds: the *f, s, sh,* and *ph* sounds. To such individuals, conversation can be distorted and result in what appears to be inappropriate or confused behavior.

Ambulatory and Community Settings | Assessing the Ears and Hearing | **PATIENT-CENTERED CARE**

• Ensure that the examination is conducted in a quiet place. In particular, older adults will have difficulty accurately reporting results of hearing tests if there is excessive outside noise.

• If necessary, ask the adult present with an infant or child to assist in holding the child still during the examination.

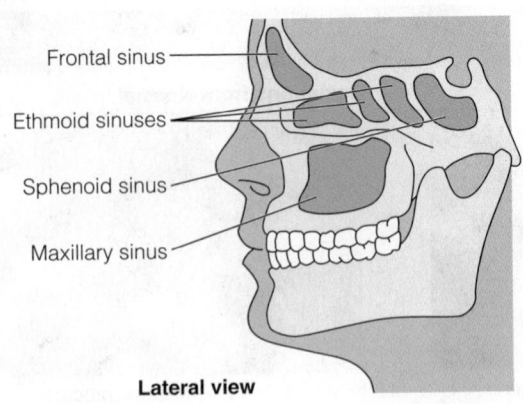

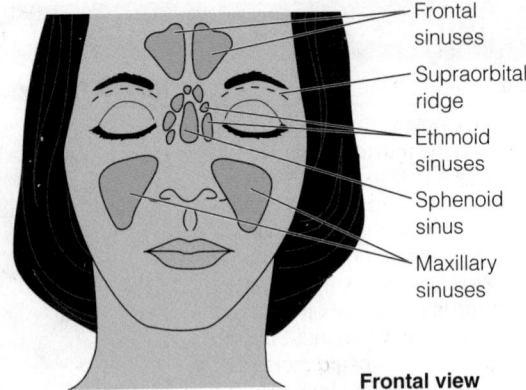

Figure 3–14 ■ The facial sinuses.

Nose and Sinuses

A nurse can inspect the nasal passages very simply with a flashlight. However, a nasal speculum and a penlight, or an otoscope with a nasal attachment, facilitates examination of the nasal chambers.

Assessment of the nose includes inspection and palpation of the external nose (the upper third of the nose is bone; the remainder is cartilage); patency of the nasal cavities; and inspection of the nasal cavities. The nurse also palpates the facial sinuses (Figure 3–14 ■).

●○● NURSING PROCESS: ASSESSING THE NOSE AND SINUSES

Assessing the Nose and Sinuses

SKILL 3–8

PLANNING
DELEGATION

Due to the substantial knowledge and skill required, assessment of the nose and sinuses is not delegated to UAP. However, many aspects of nasal function are observed during usual care and may be recorded by individuals other than the nurse. Abnormal findings must be validated and interpreted by the nurse.

INTERPROFESSIONAL PRACTICE

Assessing the nose and sinuses may be within the scope of practice of several health care providers, such as physician assistants. Although these providers may verbally communicate their findings and plan to other health care team members, the nurse must also know where to locate their documentation in the client's medical record.

Equipment
• Nasal speculum
• Flashlight/penlight

IMPLEMENTATION
Performance

1. Prior to conducting the examination, introduce self and verify the client's identity using agency protocol. Explain to the client what you are going to do, the reason for the examination, and how he or she can participate. Discuss how the findings will be used in planning further care or treatments.
2. Perform hand hygiene and observe other appropriate infection prevention procedures.
3. Provide for client privacy.
4. Inquire if the client has any history of the following: allergies, difficulty breathing through the nose, sinus infections, injuries to nose or face, nosebleeds, medications taken, or changes in sense of smell.
5. Position the client comfortably, seated if possible.

Assessment	Normal Findings	Deviations from Normal
NOSE		
6. Inspect the external nose for any deviations in shape, size, or color and flaring or discharge from the nares.	Symmetric and straight No discharge or flaring Uniform color	Asymmetric Discharge from nares Localized areas of redness or presence of skin lesions
7. Lightly palpate the external nose to determine any areas of tenderness, masses, and displacements of bone and cartilage.	Not tender; no lesions	Tenderness on palpation; presence of lesions

Assessing the Nose and Sinuses—*continued*

Assessment	Normal Findings	Deviations from Normal
8. Determine patency of both nasal cavities. Ask the client to close the mouth, exert pressure on one naris, and breathe through the opposite naris. Repeat the procedure to assess patency of the opposite naris.	Air moves freely as the client breathes through the nares	Air movement is restricted in one or both nares
9. Inspect the nasal cavities using a flashlight or a nasal speculum. <ul><li>Hold the speculum in your right hand to inspect the client's left nostril and your left hand to inspect the client's right nostril.</li><li>Tip the client's head back.</li><li>Facing the client, insert the tip of the speculum about 1 cm (0.4 in.). Care must be taken to avoid pressure on the sensitive nasal septum.</li><li>Inspect the lining of the nares and the integrity and the position of the nasal septum. ❶</li></ul>		
10. Observe for the presence of redness, swelling, growths, and discharge.	Mucosa pink Clear, watery discharge No lesions	Mucosa red, edematous Abnormal discharge (e.g., pus) Presence of lesions (e.g., polyps)
11. Inspect the nasal septum between the nasal chambers.	Nasal septum intact and in midline	Septum deviated to the right or to the left or septum eroded
FACIAL SINUSES		
12. Palpate the maxillary and frontal sinuses for tenderness.	Not tender	Tenderness in one or more sinuses
13. Document findings in the client record using forms or checklists supplemented by narrative notes when appropriate.		

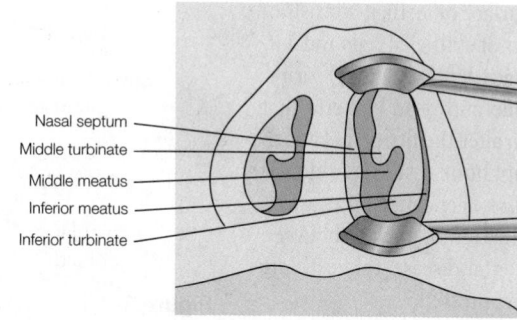

Nasal septum
Middle turbinate
Middle meatus
Inferior meatus
Inferior turbinate

❶ The nasal septum, inferior and middle turbinates of the nasal passage.

EVALUATION

- Relate findings to previous assessment data if available. Perform a detailed system-specific follow-up examination based on findings that deviated from expected or normal for the client.
- Report deviations from expected findings to the primary care provider.

LIFESPAN CONSIDERATIONS | Assessing the Nose and Sinuses

INFANTS
- A speculum is usually not necessary to examine the septum, turbinates, and vestibule. Instead, push the tip of the nose upward with the thumb and shine a light into the nares.
- Ethmoid and maxillary sinuses are present at birth; frontal sinuses begin to develop by 1 to 2 years of age; and sphenoid sinuses develop later in childhood. Infants and young children have fewer sinus problems than older children and adolescents.

CHILDREN
- A speculum is usually not necessary to examine the septum, turbinates, and vestibule, and it might cause the child to be apprehensive. Instead, push the tip of the nose upward with the thumb and shine a light into the nares.

- Ethmoid sinuses continue to develop until age 12.
- Cough and runny nose are the most common signs of sinusitis in preadolescent children.
- Adolescents may have headaches, facial tenderness, and swelling, similar to the signs of sinusitis seen in adults.

OLDER ADULTS
- The sense of smell markedly diminishes because of a decrease in the number of olfactory nerve fibers and atrophy of the remaining fibers. Older adults are less able to identify and discriminate odors.
- Nosebleeds may result from hypertensive disease, blood disorders, or other arterial vessel changes.

Mouth and Oropharynx

Assessment of the mouth and oropharynx includes a number of structures: lips, inner and buccal mucosa, the tongue and floor of the mouth, teeth and gums, hard and soft palates, uvula, salivary glands, tonsillar pillars, and tonsils (Figure 3–15 ■).

Dental caries (cavities) and periodontal disease (pyorrhea) are two problems that most frequently affect the teeth. Both are commonly associated with plaque and tartar deposits. **Plaque** is an invisible soft film that adheres to the enamel surface of teeth; it consists of bacteria, molecules of saliva, and remnants of epithelial cells and leukocytes. When plaque is unchecked, tartar (dental calculus) forms. **Tartar** is a visible, hard deposit of plaque and dead bacteria that forms at the gum lines. Tartar buildup can alter the fibers that attach the teeth to the gum and eventually disrupt bone tissue. Periodontal disease is characterized by **gingivitis** (red, swollen gingiva, i.e., gum), bleeding, receding gum lines, and the formation of pockets between the teeth and gums. In advanced periodontal disease, the teeth are loose, and pus is evident when the gums are pressed.

Other problems nurses may see are **glossitis** (inflammation of the tongue), **stomatitis** (inflammation of the oral mucosa), and **parotitis** (inflammation of the parotid salivary gland). The accumulation of foul matter (food, microorganisms, and epithelial elements) on the teeth and gums is referred to as **sordes**.

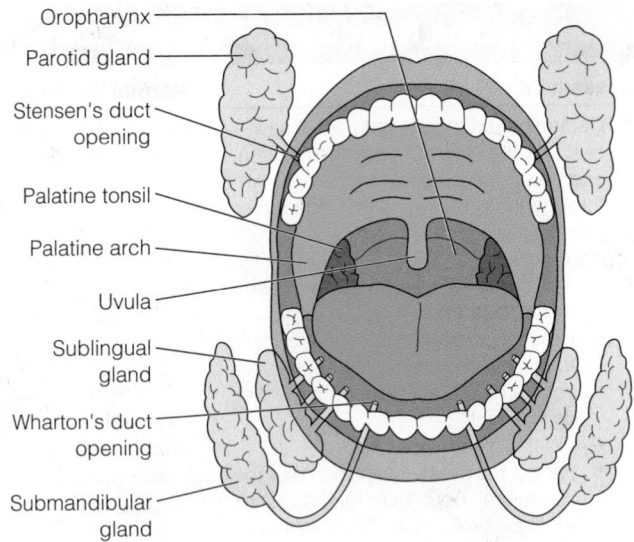

Oropharynx
Parotid gland
Stensen's duct opening
Palatine tonsil
Palatine arch
Uvula
Sublingual gland
Wharton's duct opening
Submandibular gland

Figure 3–15 ■ Anatomic structures of the mouth.

●○● NURSING PROCESS: ASSESSING THE MOUTH AND OROPHARYNX

Assessing the Mouth and Oropharynx

SKILL 3-9

PLANNING

If possible, arrange for the client to sit with the head against a firm surface such as a headrest or examination table. This makes it easier for the client to hold the head still during the examination.

DELEGATION

Due to the substantial knowledge and skill required, assessment of the mouth and oropharynx is not delegated to UAP. However, many aspects of mouth function are observed during usual care and may be recorded by individuals other than the nurse. Abnormal findings must be validated and interpreted by the nurse.

INTERPROFESSIONAL PRACTICE

Assessing the mouth and oropharynx is within the scope of practice of many health care providers, such as physician assistants. Although these providers may verbally communicate their findings and plan to other health care team members, the nurse must also know where to locate their documentation in the client's medical record.

Equipment
- Clean gloves
- Tongue depressor
- 2×2 gauze pads
- Penlight

IMPLEMENTATION

Performance
1. Prior to conducting the examination, introduce self and verify the client's identity using agency protocol. Explain to the client what you are going to do, the reason for the examination, and how he or she can participate. Discuss how the findings will be used in planning further care or treatments.
2. Perform hand hygiene and observe other appropriate infection prevention procedures.
3. Provide for client privacy.
4. Inquire if the client has any of the following: routine pattern of dental care, last visit to dentist; length of time ulcers or other lesions have been present; denture discomfort; medications the client is receiving.
5. Position the client comfortably, seated if possible.

Assessing the Mouth and Oropharynx—*continued*

Assessment	Normal Findings	Deviations from Normal
LIPS AND BUCCAL MUCOSA **6.** Inspect the outer lips for symmetry of contour, color, and texture. Ask the client to purse the lips as if to whistle.	Uniform pink color (darker, e.g., bluish hue, in Mediterranean groups and dark-skinned clients) Soft, moist, smooth texture Symmetry of contour Ability to purse lips	Pallor; cyanosis Blisters; generalized or localized swelling; fissures, crusts, or scales (may result from excessive moisture, nutritional deficiency, or fluid deficit) Inability to purse lips (may indicate facial nerve damage) Pallor; leukoplakia (white patches), red, bleeding Excessive dryness Mucosal cysts; irritations from dentures; abrasions, ulcerations; nodules
7. Inspect the inner lips and buccal mucosa for color, moisture, texture, and the presence of lesions. • Apply clean gloves. • Ask the client to relax the mouth, and, for better visualization, pull the lip outward and away from the teeth. • Grasp the lip on each side between the thumb and index finger. ❶	Uniform pink color (freckled brown pigmentation in dark-skinned clients) Moist, smooth, soft, glistening, and elastic texture (drier oral mucosa in older adults due to decreased salivation)	

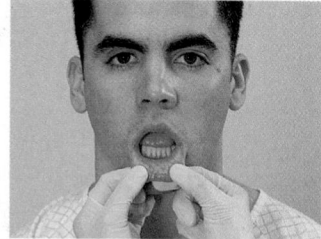
❶ Inspecting the mucosa of the lower lip.

Assessment	Normal Findings	Deviations from Normal
TEETH AND GUMS **8.** Inspect the teeth and gums while examining the inner lips and buccal mucosa. • Ask the client to open the mouth. Using a tongue depressor, retract the cheek. ❷ View the surface buccal mucosa from top to bottom and back to front. A flashlight or penlight will help illuminate the surface. Repeat the procedure for the other side. • Examine the back teeth. For proper vision of the molars, use the index fingers of both hands to retract the cheek. ❸ Ask the client to relax the lips and first close, then open, the jaw. **Rationale:** *Closing the jaw assists in observation of tooth alignment and loss of teeth; opening the jaw assists in observation of dental fillings and caries.* • Observe the number of teeth, tooth color, the state of fillings, dental caries, and tartar along the base of the teeth. Note the presence and fit of partial or complete dentures. • Inspect the gums around the molars. Observe for bleeding, color, retraction (pulling away from the teeth), edema, and lesions.	32 adult teeth Smooth, white, shiny tooth enamel Pink gums (bluish or brown patches in dark-skinned clients) Moist, firm texture to gums No retraction of gums (pulling away from the teeth)	Missing teeth; ill-fitting dentures Brown or black discoloration of the enamel (may indicate staining or the presence of caries) Excessively red gums Spongy texture; bleeding; tenderness (may indicate periodontal disease) Receding, atrophied gums; swelling that partially covers the teeth

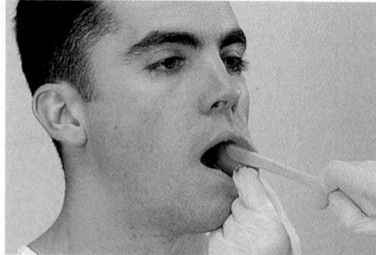
❷ Inspecting the buccal mucosa using a tongue depressor.

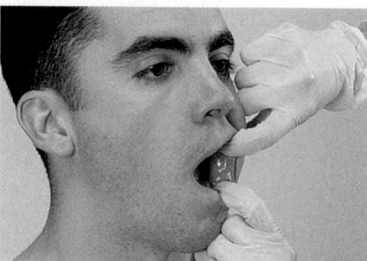
❸ Inspecting the back teeth.

Continued on page 84

SKILL 3-9

Assessing the Mouth and Oropharynx—*continued*

Assessment	Normal Findings	Deviations from Normal
9. Inspect the dentures. Ask the client to remove complete or partial dentures. Inspect their fit and condition, noting in particular broken or worn areas.	Smooth, intact dentures	Ill-fitting dentures; irritated and excoriated area under dentures
TONGUE/FLOOR OF THE MOUTH		
10. Inspect the surface of the tongue for position, color, and texture. Ask the client to protrude the tongue.	Central position Pink color (some brown pigmentation on tongue borders in dark-skinned clients); moist; slightly rough; thin whitish coating Smooth, lateral margins; no lesions Raised papillae (taste buds)	Deviated from center (may indicate damage to hypoglossal [12th cranial] nerve); excessive trembling Smooth red tongue (may indicate iron, vitamin B_{12}, or vitamin B_3 deficiency) Dry, furry tongue (associated with fluid deficit), white coating (may be oral yeast infection) Nodes, ulcerations, discolorations (white or red areas); areas of tenderness
11. Inspect tongue movement. Ask the client to roll the tongue upward and move it from side to side.	Moves freely; no tenderness	Restricted mobility
12. Inspect the base of the tongue, the mouth floor, and the frenulum. Ask the client to place the tip of the tongue against the roof of the mouth.	Smooth tongue base with prominent veins	Swelling, ulceration
PALATES AND UVULA		
13. Inspect the hard and soft palate for color, shape, texture, and the presence of bony prominences. Ask the client to open the mouth wide and tilt the head backward. Then, depress the tongue with a tongue depressor as necessary, and use a penlight for appropriate visualization.	Light pink, smooth, soft palate Lighter pink hard palate, more irregular texture	Discoloration (e.g., jaundice or pallor) Palates the same color Irritations Exostoses (bony growths) growing from the hard palate
14. Inspect the uvula for position and mobility while examining the palates. To observe the uvula, ask the client to say "ah" so that the soft palate rises.	Positioned in midline of soft palate	Deviation to one side from tumor or trauma; immobility (may indicate damage to trigeminal [5th cranial] nerve or vagus [10th cranial] nerve)
OROPHARYNX AND TONSILS		
15. Inspect the oropharynx for color and texture. Inspect one side at a time to avoid eliciting the gag response. To expose one side of the oropharynx, press a tongue depressor against the tongue on the same side about halfway back while the client tilts the head back and opens the mouth wide. Use a penlight for illumination, if needed.	Pink and smooth posterior wall	Reddened or edematous; presence of lesions, plaques, or drainage
16. Inspect the tonsils (behind the fauces [throat]) for color, discharge, and size.	Pink and smooth No discharge Of normal size or not visible • *Grade 1 (normal):* The tonsils are behind the tonsillar pillars (the soft structures supporting the soft palate)	Inflamed Presence of discharge Swollen • *Grade 2:* The tonsils are between the pillars and the uvula • *Grade 3:* The tonsils touch the uvula • *Grade 4:* One or both tonsils extend to the midline of the oropharynx
17. Remove and discard gloves. • Perform hand hygiene.		
18. Document findings in the client record using forms or checklists supplemented by narrative notes when appropriate.		

EVALUATION

• Relate findings to previous assessment data if available. Perform a detailed system-specific follow-up examination based on findings that deviated from those expected.

• Report deviations from expected findings to the primary care provider.

LIFESPAN CONSIDERATIONS Assessing the Mouth and Oropharynx

INFANTS

- Inspect the palate and uvula for a cleft. A bifid (forked) uvula may indicate an undetected cleft palate (i.e., a cleft in the cartilage that is covered by skin).
- Newborns may have a pearly white nodule on their gums, which resolves without treatment.
- The first teeth erupt at about 6 to 7 months of age. Assess for dental hygiene; parents should cleanse the infant's teeth daily with a soft cloth or soft toothbrush.
- Fluoride supplements should be given by 6 months if the child's drinking water contains less than 0.3 parts per million (ppm) of fluoride.
- Children should see a dentist by 1 year of age.

CHILDREN

- Tooth development should be appropriate for age.
- White spots on the teeth may indicate excessive fluoride ingestion.
- Drooling is common up to 2 years of age.
- The tonsils are normally larger in children than in adults and commonly extend beyond the palatine arch until the age of 11 or 12 years.

OLDER ADULTS

- The oral mucosa may be drier than that of younger individuals because of decreased salivary gland activity. Decreased salivation occurs in older adults taking prescribed medications such as antidepressants, antihistamines, decongestants, diuretics, antihypertensives, tranquilizers, antispasmodics, and antineoplastics. Extreme dryness is associated with dehydration.
- Some receding of the gums occurs, giving an appearance of increased toothiness.
- Taste sensations diminish. Sweet and salty tastes are lost first. Older adults may add more salt and sugar to food than they did when they were younger. Diminished taste sensation is due to atrophy of the taste buds and a decreased sense of smell. It indicates diminished function of the fifth and seventh cranial nerves.
- Tiny purple or bluish black swollen areas (varicosities) under the tongue, known as *caviar spots*, are not uncommon.
- The teeth may show signs of staining, erosion, chipping, and abrasions due to loss of dentin. Medicare does not cover dental cleanings or treatments, so older adults with limited incomes may delay or avoid professional dental care.
- Tooth loss occurs as a result of dental disease but is preventable with good dental hygiene.
- Check that full or removable partial dentures fit properly. Bone loss and weight loss or gain can change the way these prosthetics fit.
- The gag response may be slightly sluggish.
- Older adults who are homebound or are in long-term care facilities often have teeth or dentures in need of repair, due to the difficulty of obtaining dental care in these situations. Do a thorough assessment of missing teeth and those in need of repair, whether they are natural teeth or dentures.

CLIENT TEACHING CONSIDERATIONS

Assessing the Mouth and Oropharynx

- Although clients may be sensitive to discussion of their personal hygiene practices, use the assessment as an opportunity to provide teaching regarding appropriate oral and dental care for the entire family. Refer clients to a dentist if indicated.

NECK

Examination of the neck may include assessment of the muscles, lymph nodes, trachea, thyroid gland, carotid arteries, and jugular veins. Generalist nurses usually only inspect the thyroid. Advanced practice nurses may also palpate the thyroid gland. In this text, assessment of the carotid arteries and jugular veins is described in Skill 3–12, *Assessing the Heart and Central Vessels*. Areas of the neck are defined by the sternocleidomastoid muscles, which divide each side of the neck into two triangles: the anterior and posterior (Figure 3–16 ■). The trachea, thyroid gland, anterior cervical nodes, and carotid artery lie within the anterior triangle (the carotid artery runs parallel and anterior to the sternocleidomastoid muscle) (Figure 3–17 ■). The supraclavicular and posterior cervical lymph nodes lie within the posterior triangle (Figure 3–18 ■).

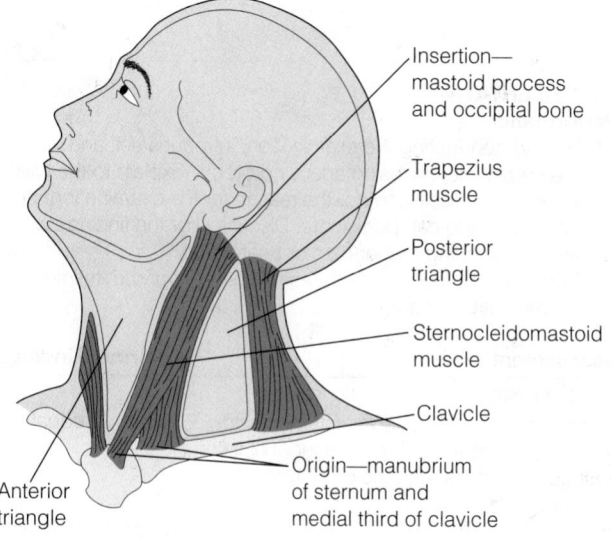

Insertion—mastoid process and occipital bone

Trapezius muscle

Posterior triangle

Sternocleidomastoid muscle

Clavicle

Origin—manubrium of sternum and medial third of clavicle

Anterior triangle

Figure 3–16 ■ Major muscles of the neck.

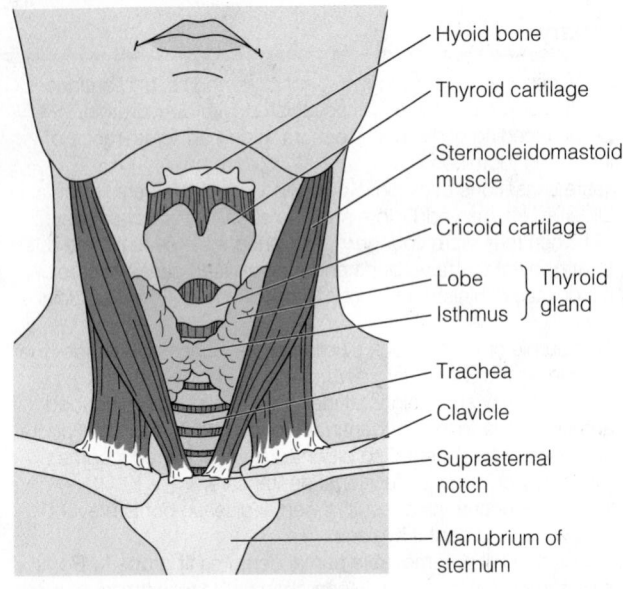

Figure 3–17 ■ Structures of the neck.

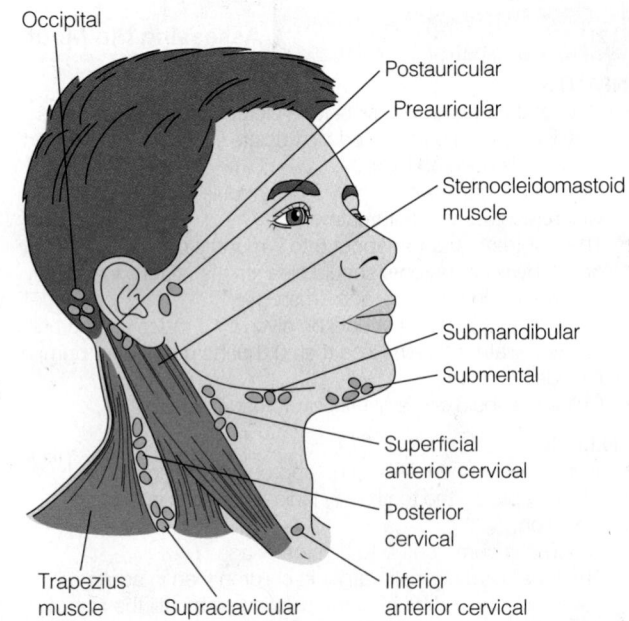

Figure 3–18 ■ Lymph nodes of the neck.

●○●● NURSING PROCESS: ASSESSING THE NECK

SKILL 3-10

Assessing the Neck

PLANNING
DELEGATION

Due to the substantial knowledge and skill required, assessment of the neck is not delegated to UAP. However, many aspects of the neck are observed during usual care and may be recorded by individuals other than the nurse. Abnormal findings must be validated and interpreted by the nurse.

INTERPROFESSIONAL PRACTICE

Assessing the neck is within the scope of practice of many health care providers, such as physician assistants and physical therapists. Although these providers may verbally communicate their findings and plan to other health care team members, the nurse must also know where to locate their documentation in the client's medical record

Equipment
None

IMPLEMENTATION
Performance

1. Prior to conducting the examination, introduce self and verify the client's identity using agency protocol. Explain to the client what you are going to do, the reason for the examination, and how he or she can participate. Discuss how the findings will be used in planning further care or treatments.
2. Perform hand hygiene and observe other appropriate infection prevention procedures.
3. Provide for client privacy.
4. Inquire if the client has any history of the following: problems with neck lumps, neck pain or stiffness, when and how any lumps occurred, previous diagnoses of thyroid problems, and any treatments provided (e.g., surgery, radiation).

Assessment	Normal Findings	Deviations from Normal
NECK MUSCLES		
5. Inspect the neck muscles (sternocleidomastoid and trapezius) for abnormal swellings or masses. Ask the client to hold the head erect.	Muscles equal in size; head centered	Unilateral neck swelling; head tilted to one side (indicates presence of masses, injury, muscle weakness, shortening of sternocleidomastoid muscle, scars)

Assessing the Neck—*continued*

Assessment	Normal Findings	Deviations from Normal
6. Observe head movement. Ask the client to: • Move the chin to the chest. **Rationale:** *This determines function of the sternocleidomastoid muscle.*	Coordinated, smooth movements with no discomfort Head flexes 45°	Muscle tremor, spasm, or stiffness Limited range of motion; painful movements; involuntary movements (e.g., up-and-down nodding movements associated with Parkinson's disease)
• Move the head back so that the chin points upward. **Rationale:** *This determines function of the trapezius muscle.*	Head hyperextends 60°	Head hyperextends less than 60°
• Move the head so that the ear is moved toward the shoulder on each side. **Rationale:** *This determines function of the sternocleidomastoid muscle.*	Head laterally flexes 40°	Head laterally flexes less than 40°
• Turn the head to the right and to the left. **Rationale:** *This determines function of the sternocleidomastoid muscle.*	Head laterally rotates 70°	Head laterally rotates less than 70°
7. Assess muscle strength. • Ask the client to turn the head to one side against the resistance of your hand. Repeat with the other side. **Rationale:** *This determines the strength of the sternocleidomastoid muscle.*	Equal strength	Unequal strength
• Ask the client to shrug the shoulders against the resistance of your hands. **Rationale:** *This determines the strength of the trapezius muscles.*	Equal strength	Unequal strength

LYMPH NODES

8. Palpate the entire neck for enlarged lymph nodes. • Face the client, and bend the client's head forward slightly or toward the side being examined. **Rationale:** *This relaxes the soft tissue and muscles.* • Palpate the nodes using the pads of the fingers. Move the fingertips in a gentle rotating motion. • When examining the submental and submandibular nodes, place the fingertips under the mandible on the side nearest the palpating hand, and pull the skin and subcutaneous tissue laterally over the mandibular surface so that the tissue rolls over the nodes.	Not palpable	Enlarged, palpable, possibly tender (associated with infection and tumors)

• When palpating the supraclavicular nodes, have the client bend the head forward to relax the tissues of the anterior neck and to relax the shoulders so that the clavicles drop. Use your hand nearest the side to be examined when facing the client (i.e., your left hand for the client's right nodes). Use your free hand to flex the client's head forward if necessary. Hook your index and third fingers over the clavicle lateral to the sternocleidomastoid muscle. ❶

• When palpating the anterior cervical nodes and posterior cervical nodes, move your fingertips slowly in a forward circular motion against the sternocleidomastoid and trapezius muscles, respectively.

• To palpate the deep cervical nodes, bend or hook your fingers around the sternocleidomastoid muscle.

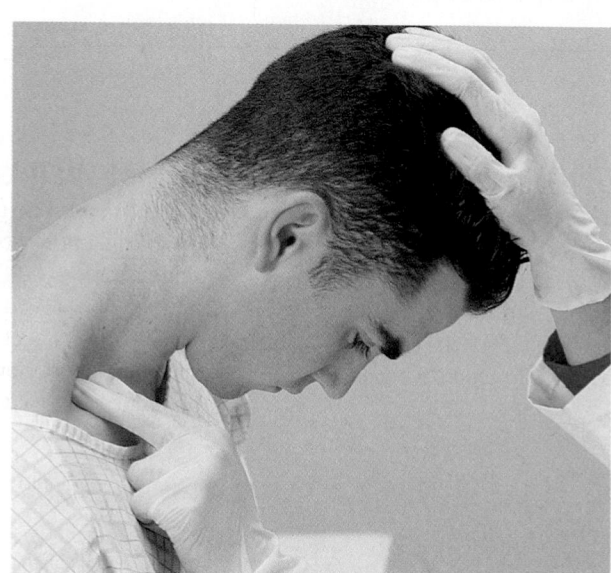
❶ Palpating the supraclavicular lymph nodes.

Continued on page 88

SKILL 3-10

Assessing the Neck—*continued*

Assessment	Normal Findings	Deviations from Normal
TRACHEA 9. Palpate the trachea for lateral deviation. Place your fingertip or thumb on the trachea in the suprasternal notch (see Figure 3–17, earlier), and then move your finger laterally to the left and the right in spaces bordered by the clavicle, the anterior aspect of the sternocleidomastoid muscle, and the trachea.	Central placement in midline of neck; spaces are equal on both sides	Deviation to one side, indicating possible neck tumor; thyroid enlargement; enlarged lymph nodes
THYROID GLAND 10. Inspect the thyroid gland. Stand in front of the client. • Observe the lower half of the neck overlying the thyroid gland for symmetry and visible masses.	Not visible on inspection	Visible diffuseness or local enlargement
• Ask the client to extend the head and swallow. If necessary, offer a glass of water to make it easier for the client to swallow. **Rationale:** *This action determines how the thyroid and cricoid cartilages move and whether swallowing causes a bulging of the gland.* 11. Document findings in the client record using forms or checklists supplemented by narrative notes when appropriate.	Gland ascends during swallowing	Gland is not fully movable with swallowing

EVALUATION

- Relate findings to previous assessment data if available. Perform a detailed system-specific follow-up examination based on findings that deviated from those expected.
- Report deviations from expected findings to the primary care provider.

LIFESPAN CONSIDERATIONS   Assessing the Neck

INFANTS AND CHILDREN
- Examine the neck while the infant or child is lying supine. Lift the head and turn it from side to side to determine neck mobility.

- An infant's neck is normally short, lengthening by about age 3 years. This makes palpation of the trachea difficult.

THORAX AND LUNGS

Assessing the thorax and lungs is critical when evaluating the client's oxygen and respiratory status or any other concerns related to the thorax. The client's posture is important to note. Some people with chronic respiratory problems tend to bend forward or even prop their arms on a support to elevate their clavicles. This posture is an attempt to expand the thorax fully and thus breathe with less effort.

Chest Wall Landmarks

The nurse must be familiar with a series of imaginary lines on the chest wall and be able to locate the position of each rib and some spinous processes. These landmarks help the nurse to identify the position of underlying organs (e.g., lobes of the lung) and document accurate assessment findings. Figure 3–19 ■ shows the anterior, lateral, and posterior series of lines. Figure 3–20 ■ shows anterior, posterior, and right and left lateral views of the chest and underlying

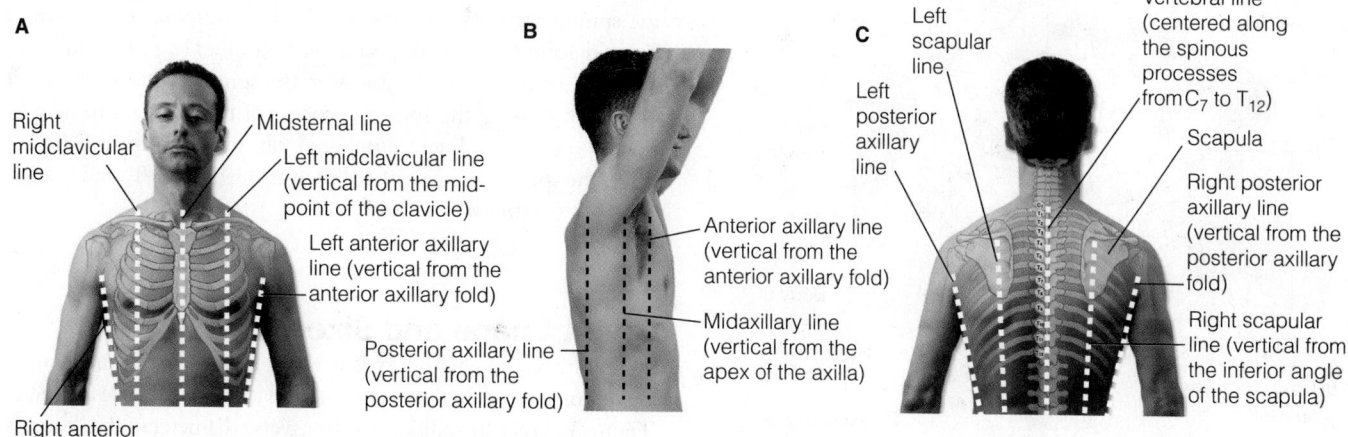

Figure 3–19 ■ Chest wall landmarks: *A,* anterior chest; *B,* lateral chest; *C,* posterior chest.

lungs. Each lung is first divided into the upper and lower lobes by an oblique fissure that runs from the level of the spinous process of the third thoracic vertebra (T_3) to the level of the sixth rib at the midclavicular line. The right upper lobe is abbreviated RUL; the right lower lobe, RLL. Similarly, the left upper lobe is abbreviated LUL; the left lower lobe, LLL. The right lung is further divided by a minor fissure into the right upper lobe and right middle lobe (RML). This fissure runs anteriorly from the right midaxillary line at the level of the fifth rib to the level of the fourth rib.

These specific landmarks (i.e., T_3 and the fourth, fifth, and sixth ribs) are located as follows: The starting point for locating the

ribs anteriorly is the angle of Louis, the junction between the body of the sternum and the manubrium (the handle-like superior part of the sternum that joins with the clavicles). The superior border of the second rib attaches to the sternum at this manubriosternal junction (Figure 3–21 ■). The nurse can identify the manubrium by first palpating the clavicle and following its course to its attachment at the manubrium. The nurse then palpates and counts distal ribs and intercostal spaces (ICSs) from the second rib. It is important to note that an ICS is numbered according to the number of the rib immediately above the space. When palpating for rib identification, the nurse should palpate along the midclavicular line rather than the sternal

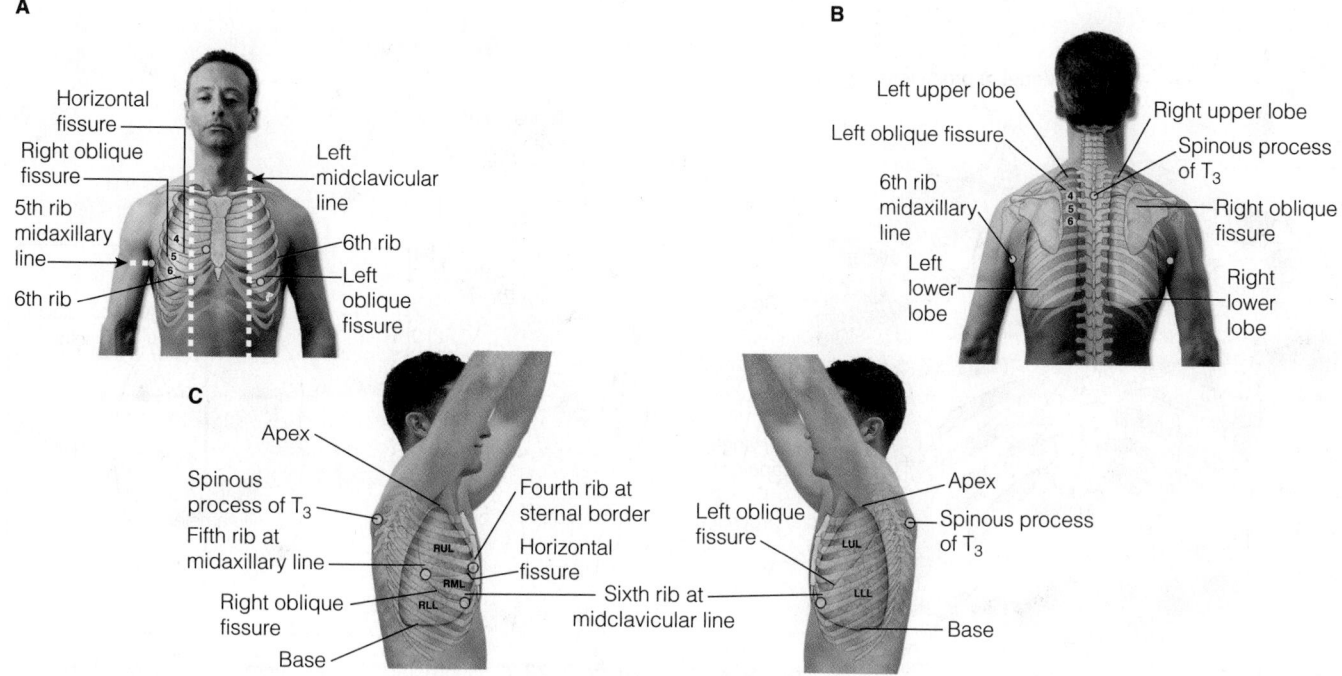

Figure 3–20 ■ Chest landmarks and underlying lungs: *A,* anterior chest; *B,* posterior chest; *C,* lateral chest.

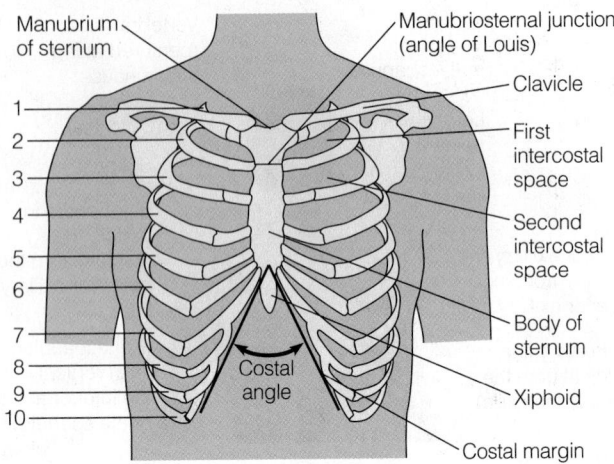

Figure 3–21 ■ Location of the anterior ribs, the angle of Louis, and the sternum.

border, because the rib cartilages are very close at the sternum. Only the first seven ribs attach directly to the sternum.

The counting of ribs is more challenging on the posterior thorax than on the anterior thorax. For identifying underlying lung lobes, the pertinent landmark is T_3. The starting point for locating T_3 is the spinous process of the seventh cervical vertebra (C_7), also referred to as the vertebra prominens (Figure 3–22 ■). When the client flexes the neck anteriorly, a prominent process can be observed and palpated. This is the spinous process of the seventh cervical vertebra. If two spinous processes are observed, the superior one is C_7, and the inferior one is the spinous process of the

first thoracic vertebra (T_1). The nurse then palpates and counts the spinous processes from C_7 to T_3. Each spinous process up to T_4 is adjacent to the corresponding rib number (e.g., T_3 is adjacent to the third rib). After T_4, however, the spinous processes project obliquely, causing the spinous process of the vertebra to lie, not over its correspondingly numbered rib, but over the rib below. Thus, the spinous process of T_5 lies over the body of T_6 and is adjacent to the sixth rib.

Chest Shape and Size

In healthy adults, the thorax is oval. Its diameter measured in the anteroposterior direction is smaller than its transverse diameter (Figure 3–23 ■). In addition, the transverse diameter of the thorax is smaller at the top than at the base.

There are several abnormal shapes of the chest (Figure 3–24 ■). Pigeon chest (pectus carinatum), a permanent change, may be caused by rickets (abnormal bone formation due to lack of dietary calcium). A narrow transverse diameter, an increased anteroposterior diameter, and a protruding sternum characterize pigeon chest. A funnel chest (pectus excavatum), a congenital defect, is the opposite of pigeon chest in that the sternum is depressed, narrowing the anteroposterior diameter. Because the sternum points posteriorly in clients with a funnel chest, abnormal pressure on the heart may result in altered function. A barrel chest, in which the ratio of the anteroposterior to transverse diameter is 1 to 1, is seen in clients with thoracic kyphosis (excessive convex curvature of the thoracic spine) and emphysema (chronic pulmonary condition in which the air sacs, or alveoli, are dilated and distended). Scoliosis is a lateral deviation of the spine.

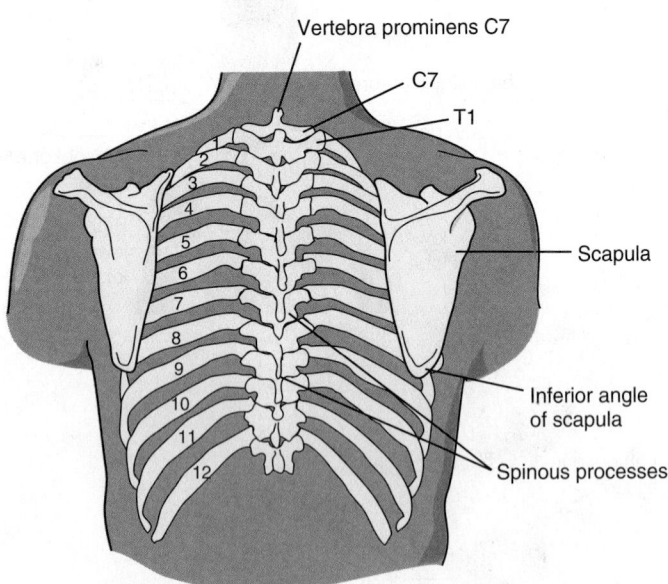

Figure 3–22 ■ Location of the posterior ribs in relation to the spinous processes.

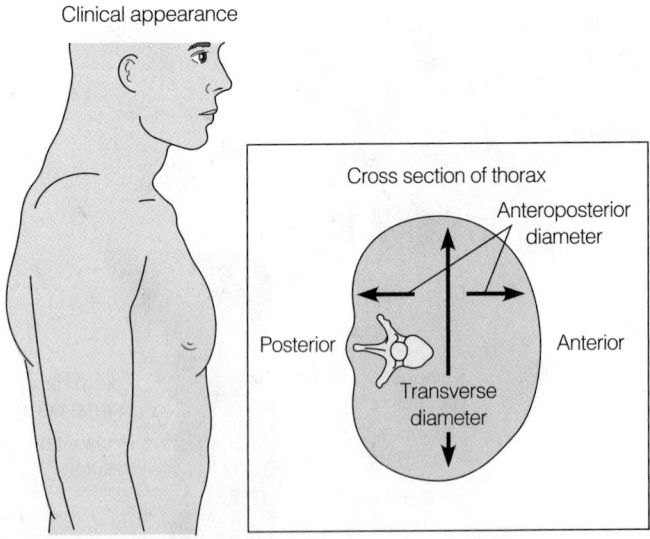

Figure 3–23 ■ Configurations of the thorax showing oval shape, anteroposterior diameter, and transverse diameter.

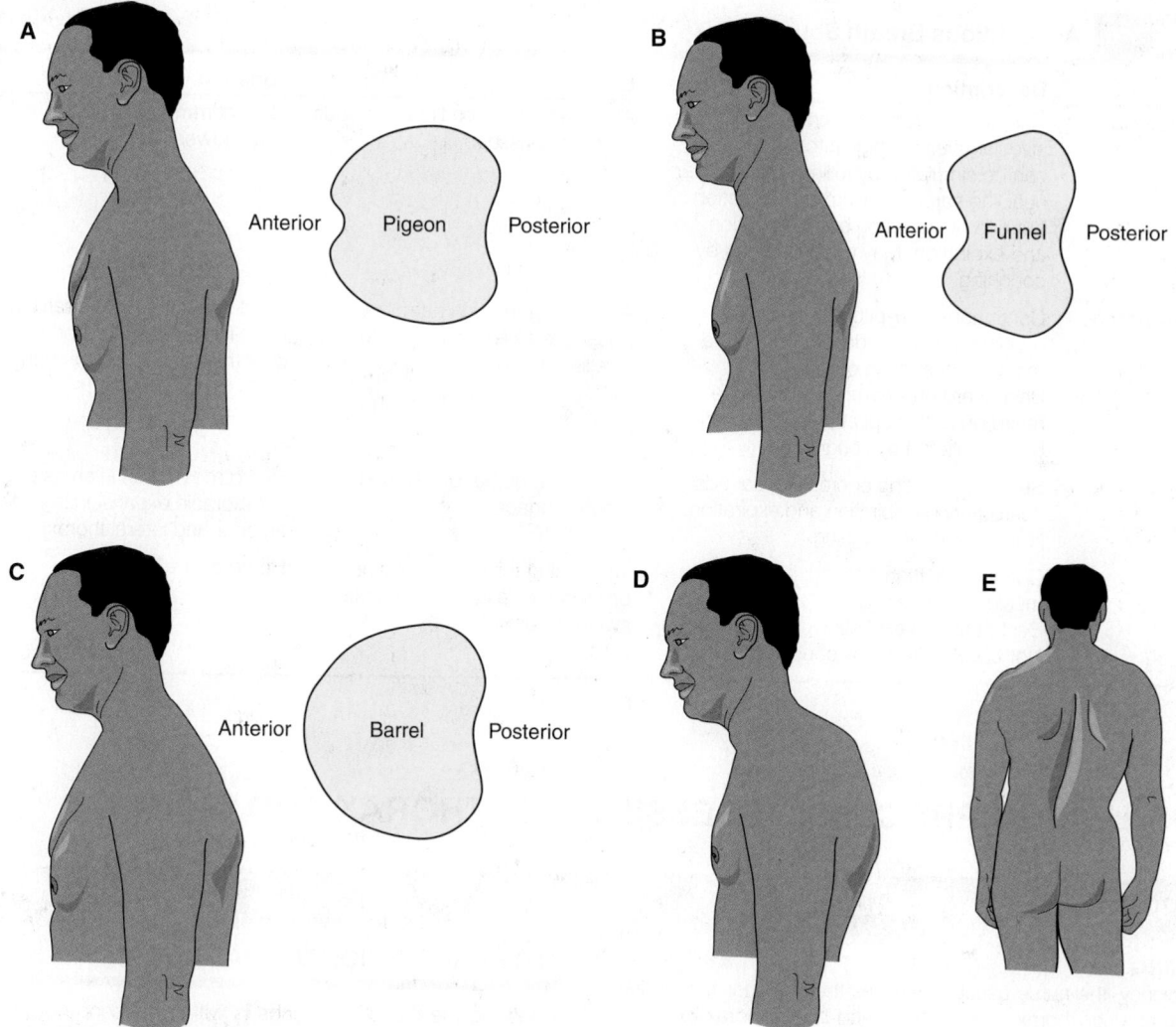

Figure 3–24 ■ Chest deformities: *A,* pigeon chest; *B,* funnel chest; *C,* barrel chest; *D,* kyphosis; *E,* scoliosis.

Breath Sounds

Assessment of the lungs and thorax includes all methods of examination: inspection, palpation, percussion, and auscultation. Abnormal or **adventitious breath sounds** occur when air passes through narrowed airways or airways filled with fluid or mucus, or when pleural linings are inflamed. See Table 3–5 for normal breath sounds. Adventitious sounds are often superimposed over normal sounds (Table 3–6).

TABLE 3–5 Normal Breath Sounds

Type	Description	Location	Characteristics
Vesicular	Soft-intensity, low-pitched, "gentle sighing" sounds created by air moving through smaller airways (bronchioles and alveoli)	Over peripheral lung; best heard at base of lungs	Best heard on inspiration, which is about 2.5 times longer than the expiratory phase (5:2 ratio)
Bronchovesicular	Moderate-intensity and moderate-pitched "blowing" sounds created by air moving through larger airways (bronchi)	Between the scapulae and lateral to the sternum at the first and second intercostal spaces	Equal inspiratory and expiratory phases (1:1 ratio)
Bronchial (tubular)	High-pitched, loud, "harsh" sounds created by air moving through the trachea	Anteriorly over the trachea; not normally heard over lung tissue	Louder than vesicular sounds; have a short inspiratory phase and long expiratory phase (1:2 ratio)

TABLE 3–6	Adventitious Breath Sounds		
Name	**Description**	**Cause**	**Location**
Crackles (rales)	Fine, short, interrupted crackling sounds; alveolar rales are high pitched. Sound can be simulated by rolling a lock of hair near the ear. Best heard on inspiration but can be heard on both inspiration and expiration. May not be cleared by coughing.	Air passing through fluid or mucus in any air passage	Most commonly heard in the bases of the lower lung lobes
Gurgles (rhonchi)	Continuous, low-pitched, coarse, gurgling, harsh, louder sounds with a moaning or snoring quality. Best heard on expiration but can be heard on both inspiration and expiration. May be altered by coughing.	Air passing through narrowed air passages as a result of secretions, swelling, tumors	Loud sounds can be heard over most lung areas but predominate over the trachea and bronchi
Friction rub	Superficial grating or creaking sounds heard during inspiration and expiration. Not relieved by coughing.	Rubbing together of inflamed pleural surfaces	Heard most often in areas of greatest thoracic expansion (e.g., lower anterior and lateral thorax)
Wheeze	Continuous, high-pitched, squeaky musical sounds. Best heard on expiration. Not usually altered by coughing.	Air passing through a constricted bronchus as a result of secretions, swelling, tumors	Heard over all lung fields

●○● NURSING PROCESS: ASSESSING THE THORAX AND LUNGS

Assessing the Thorax and Lungs

PLANNING

For efficiency, the nurse usually examines the posterior thorax first, then the anterior thorax. For posterior and lateral thorax examinations, the client is uncovered to the waist and in a sitting position. A sitting or lying position may be used for anterior thorax examination. The sitting position is preferred because it maximizes expansion. Good lighting is essential, especially for thorax inspection.

DELEGATION

Due to the substantial knowledge and skill required, assessment of the thorax and lungs is not delegated to UAP. However, many aspects of breathing are observed during usual care and may be recorded by individuals other than the nurse. Abnormal findings must be validated and interpreted by the nurse.

INTERPROFESSIONAL PRACTICE

Assessing the thorax and lungs is within the scope of practice of many health care providers before, during, and after their treatments. For example, both physician assistants and respiratory therapists may check the client's lungs. Although these providers may verbally communicate their findings and plan to other health care team members, the nurse must also know where to locate their documentation in the client's medical record.

Equipment
- Stethoscope

IMPLEMENTATION
Performance
1. Prior to conducting the examination, introduce self and verify the client's identity using agency protocol. Explain to the client what you are going to do, the reason for the examination, and how he or she can participate. Discuss how the findings will be used in planning further care or treatments.
2. Perform hand hygiene and observe other appropriate infection prevention procedures.
3. Provide for client privacy. In women, drape the anterior thorax when it is not being examined.
4. Inquire if the client has any of the following: family history of illness, including cancer, allergies, tuberculosis; lifestyle habits such as smoking and occupational hazards (e.g., inhaling fumes); medications being taken; and current problems (e.g., swellings, coughs, wheezing, pain).

Assessing the Thorax and Lungs—*continued*

Assessment	Normal Findings	Deviations from Normal
POSTERIOR THORAX		
5. Inspect the shape and symmetry of the thorax from posterior and lateral views. Compare the anteroposterior diameter to the transverse diameter.	Anteroposterior to transverse diameter in ratio of 1:2 Thorax asymmetric	Barrel chest; increased anteroposterior to transverse diameter Thorax symmetric
6. Inspect the spinal alignment for deformities if the client can stand. From a lateral position, observe the three normal curvatures: cervical, thoracic, and lumbar.	Spine vertically aligned	Exaggerated spinal curvatures (kyphosis, lordosis)
• To assess for lateral deviation of the spine (scoliosis), observe the standing client from the rear. Have the client bend forward at the waist and observe from behind.	Spinal column is straight, right and left shoulders and hips are at same height	Spinal column deviates to one side, often accentuated when bending over; shoulders or hips not even (level)
7. Palpate the posterior thorax.		
• Assess the temperature and integrity of all thorax skin.	Skin intact; uniform temperature	Skin lesions; areas of hyperthermia
• For clients who have respiratory complaints, palpate all areas for bulges, tenderness, or abnormal movements. Avoid deep palpation for painful areas, especially if a fractured rib is suspected. In such a case, deep palpation could lead to displacement of the bone fragment against the lungs.	Thorax intact; no tenderness; no masses	Lumps, bulges; depressions; areas of tenderness; movable structures (e.g., rib)
8. Palpate the posterior thorax for respiratory excursion (thoracic expansion). Place the palms of both your hands over the lower thorax with your thumbs adjacent to the spine and your fingers stretched laterally. ❶ Ask the client to take a deep breath while you observe the movement of your hands and any lag in movement.	Full and symmetric thorax expansion (i.e., when the client takes a deep breath, your thumbs should move apart an equal distance and at the same time; normally the thumbs separate 3 to 5 cm [1 1/2 to 2 in.] during deep inspiration)	Asymmetric and/or decreased thorax expansion

❶ Position of the nurse's hands when assessing posterior respiratory excursion on the posterior thorax.

Assessment	Normal Findings	Deviations from Normal
9. Palpate the thorax for vocal (tactile) **fremitus**, the faintly perceptible vibration felt through the chest wall when the client speaks.	Bilateral symmetry of vocal fremitus Fremitus is heard most clearly at the apex of the lungs	Decreased or absent fremitus (associated with pneumothorax) Increased fremitus (associated with consolidated lung tissue, as in pneumonia)

SKILL 3-11

Continued on page 94

Assessing the Thorax and Lungs—*continued*

SKILL 3-11

Assessment	Normal Findings	Deviations from Normal
• Place the palmar surfaces of your fingertips or the ulnar aspect of your hand or closed fist on the posterior thorax, starting near the apex of the lungs, ❷ position A. • Ask the client to repeat such words as "blue moon" or "one, two, three." • Repeat the two steps, moving your hands sequentially to the base of the lungs, through positions B–E in ❷. • Compare the fremitus on both lungs and between the apex and the base of each lung, using either one hand and moving it from one side of the client to the corresponding area on the other side *or* using two hands that are placed simultaneously on the corresponding areas of each side of the thorax.	Low-pitched voices of males are more readily palpated than higher pitched voices of females 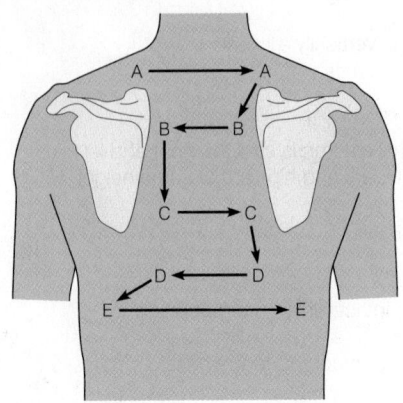 ❷ Areas and sequence for palpating tactile fremitus on the posterior thorax.	
10. Percuss the thorax. Percussion of the thorax is performed to determine whether underlying lung tissue is filled with air, liquid, or solid material and to determine the positions and boundaries of certain organs. Because percussion penetrates to a depth of 5 to 7 cm (2 to 3 in.), it detects superficial rather than deep lesions. See ❸ and Table 3–2, earlier. • Ask the client to bend the head and fold the arms forward across the chest. **Rationale:** *This separates the scapula and exposes more lung tissue to percussion.* • Percuss in the intercostal spaces at about 5-cm (2-in.) intervals in a systematic sequence. ❹ • Compare one side of the lung with the other. • Percuss the lateral thorax every few inches, starting at the axilla and working down to the eighth rib.	Percussion notes resonate, except over scapula Lowest point of resonance is at the diaphragm (i.e., at the level of the 8th to 10th rib posteriorly) *Note:* Percussion on a rib normally elicits dullness. 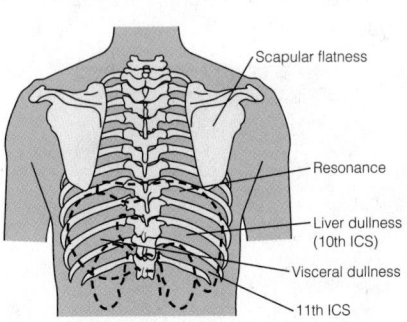 ❸ Normal percussion sounds on the posterior thorax.	Asymmetry in percussion notes Areas of dullness or flatness over lung tissue (associated with fluid, consolidation of lung tissue, or a mass) 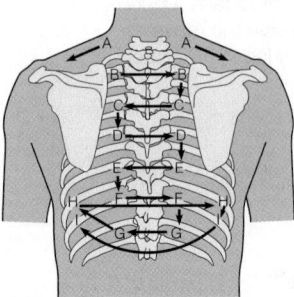 ❹ Sequence for posterior thorax percussion.
11. Auscultate the thorax using the diaphragm of the stethoscope. **Rationale:** *The diaphragm of the stethoscope is best for transmitting the high-pitched breath sounds.* • Use the systematic zigzag procedure used in percussion. • Ask the client to take slow, deep breaths through the mouth. Listen at each point to the breath sounds during a complete inspiration and expiration. • Compare findings at each point with the corresponding point on the opposite side of the thorax.	Vesicular and bronchovesicular breath sounds (see Table 3–5)	Adventitious breath sounds (e.g., crackles, gurgles, friction rub, wheeze; see Table 3–6) Absence of breath sounds
12. Inspect breathing patterns (e.g., respiratory rate and rhythm).	Quiet, rhythmic, and effortless respirations (see Chapter 2 ∞, page 38)	See Chapter 2 ∞, Box 2–3, page 38, for altered breathing patterns and sounds

Assessing the Thorax and Lungs—*continued*

Assessment	Normal Findings	Deviations from Normal
13. Inspect the costal angle (angle formed by the intersection of the costal margins) and the angle at which the ribs enter the spine.	Costal angle is less than 90°, and the ribs insert into the spine at approximately a 45° angle (see Figure 3–21, earlier)	Costal angle is widened (associated with chronic obstructive pulmonary disease)
14. Palpate the anterior thorax (see posterior thorax palpation, steps 7–9 above).		
15. Palpate the anterior thorax for respiratory excursion. • Place the palms of both your hands on the lower thorax, with your fingers laterally along the lower rib cage and your thumbs along the costal margins. ❺ • Ask the client to take a deep breath while you observe the movement of your hands.	Full symmetric excursion; thumbs normally separate 3 to 5 cm (1.5 to 2 in.)	Asymmetric and/or decreased respiratory excursion

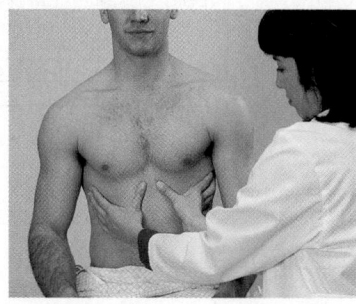

❺ Position of the nurse's hands when assessing respiratory excursion on the anterior thorax.

Assessment	Normal Findings	Deviations from Normal
16. Palpate tactile fremitus in the same manner as for the posterior thorax and using the sequence shown in ❻. If the breasts are large and cannot be retracted adequately for palpation, this part of the examination is usually omitted.	Same as posterior vocal fremitus; fremitus is normally decreased over heart and breast tissue	Same as posterior fremitus

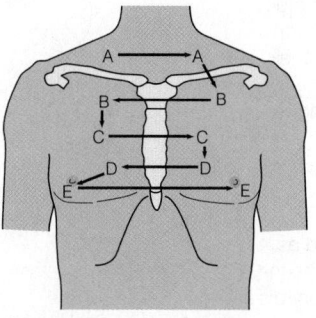

❻ Areas and sequence for palpating tactile fremitus on the anterior thorax.

Assessment	Normal Findings	Deviations from Normal
17. Percuss the anterior thorax systematically. • Begin above the clavicles in the supra-clavicular space, and proceed down-ward to the diaphragm. ❼ • Compare the lung on one side to the lung on the other side. • Lift the breasts as needed to facilitate percussion of the lungs.	Percussion notes resonate down to the sixth rib at the level of the diaphragm but are flat over areas of heavy muscle and bone, dull on areas over the heart and the liver, and tympanic over the underlying stomach ❽	Asymmetry in percussion notes Areas of dullness or flatness over lung tissue

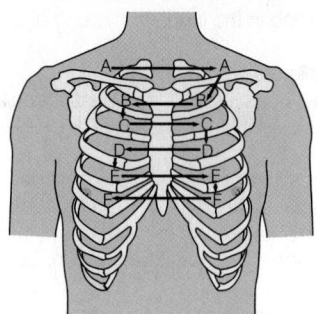

❼ Sequence for anterior thorax percussion.

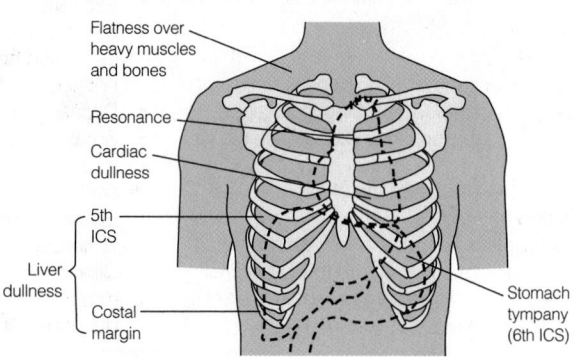

Flatness over heavy muscles and bones
Resonance
Cardiac dullness
5th ICS
Liver dullness
Costal margin
Stomach tympany (6th ICS)

❽ Normal percussion sounds on the anterior thorax.

Continued on page 96

SKILL 3–11

Assessing the Thorax and Lungs—*continued*

Assessment	Normal Findings	Deviations from Normal
18. Auscultate the trachea.	Bronchial and tubular breath sounds (see Table 3–5 on page 91)	Adventitious breath sounds (see Table 3–6 on page 92)
19. Auscultate the anterior thorax. Use the sequence used in percussion (see ❼), beginning over the bronchi between the sternum and the clavicles.	Bronchovesicular and vesicular breath sounds (see Table 3–5)	Adventitious breath sounds (see Table 3–6)
20. Document findings in the client record using forms or checklists supplemented by narrative notes when appropriate.		

SAMPLE DOCUMENTATION

6/10/2015 0830 Lungs clear to auscultation except for fine crackles both posterior lower lobes, partially cleared after coughing. Only moves in bed when repositioned every 2 hours. Assisted to a chair. Reviewed deep breathing exercises. Effective return demonstration.
—— N. Schmidt, RN

EVALUATION

- Relate findings to previous assessment data if available. Perform a detailed system-specific follow-up examination based on findings that deviated from those expected.
- Report deviations from expected findings to the primary care provider.

LIFESPAN CONSIDERATIONS | Assessing the Thorax and Lungs

INFANTS

- The thorax is rounded; that is, the diameter from the front to the back (anteroposterior) is equal to the transverse diameter. It is also cylindrical, having a nearly equal diameter at the top and the base. This makes it harder for infants to expand their thoracic space.
- To assess tactile fremitus, place your hand over the crying infant's thorax.
- Infants tend to breathe using the diaphragm; assess rate and rhythm by watching the abdomen, rather than the thorax, rise and fall.
- The right bronchial branch is short and angles downward as it leaves the trachea, making it easy for small objects to be inhaled. Sudden onset of cough or other signs of respiratory distress may indicate that the infant has inhaled a foreign object.

CHILDREN

- By about 6 years of age, the anteroposterior diameter has decreased in proportion to the transverse diameter, with a 1:2 ratio present.
- Children tend to breathe more abdominally than thoracically up to age 6.
- During the rapid growth spurts of adolescence, spinal curvature and rotation (scoliosis) may appear. Children should be assessed for scoliosis by age 12 and annually until their growth slows. Curvature greater than 10% should be referred for further medical evaluation.

OLDER ADULTS

- The thoracic curvature may be accentuated (kyphosis) because of osteoporosis and changes in cartilage, resulting in collapse of the vertebrae. This can also compromise and decrease normal respiratory effort.
- Kyphosis and osteoporosis alter the size of the chest cavity as the ribs move downward and forward.
- The anteroposterior diameter of the thorax widens, giving the person a barrel-chested appearance. This is due to loss of skeletal muscle strength in the thorax and diaphragm and constant lung inflation from excessive expiratory pressure on the alveoli.

Clinical appearance

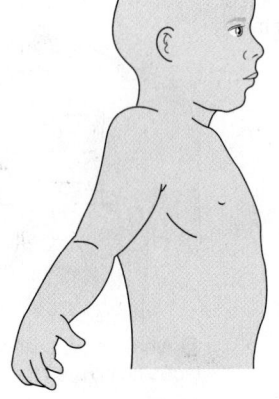 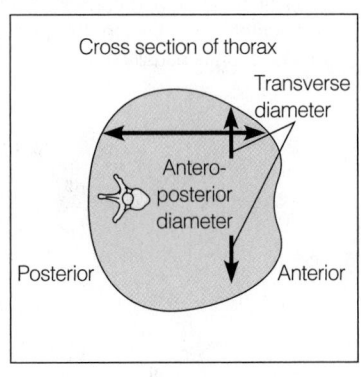

Cross section of thorax

Configuration of the infant's thorax showing anteroposterior diameter and transverse diameter.

- Breathing rate and rhythm are unchanged at rest; the rate normally increases with exercise but may take longer to return to the preexercise rate.
- Inspiratory muscles become less powerful, and the inspiratory reserve volume decreases. A decrease in depth of respiration is therefore apparent.
- Expiration may require the use of accessory muscles. The expiratory reserve volume significantly increases because of the increased amount of air remaining in the lungs at the end of a normal breath.
- Deflation of the lung is incomplete.
- Small airways lose their cartilaginous support and elastic recoil; as a result, they tend to close, particularly in basal or dependent portions of the lung.
- Elastic tissue of the alveoli loses its stretchability and changes to fibrous tissue. Exertional capacity decreases.
- Cilia in the airways decrease in number and are less effective in removing mucus; older clients are therefore at greater risk for pulmonary infections.

THE CARDIOVASCULAR AND PERIPHERAL VASCULAR SYSTEMS

The cardiovascular system consists of the heart and the central blood vessels (primarily the pulmonary, coronary, and neck arteries and veins). The peripheral vascular system includes those arteries and veins distal to the central vessels, extending all the way to the brain and to the extremities.

Heart

Heart function is assessed by findings in the history, symptoms such as shortness of breath, the client's general appearance (e.g., cyanosis and edema of the legs suggest impaired heart function), and pulse rate, rhythm, and quality. In addition, nurses assess heart functions through inspection, palpation, and auscultation, in that sequence. Auscultation is more meaningful when other data are obtained first.

The nurse must determine the heart's exact location. In the average adult, most of the heart lies behind and to the left of the sternum. A small portion (the right atrium) extends to the right of the sternum. The upper portion of the heart (both atria), referred to as its base, lies toward the back. The lower portion (the ventricles), referred to as its apex, points forward. The apex of the left ventricle actually touches the anterior chest wall at or medial to the left midclavicular line (MCL) and at or near the fifth ICS, which is slightly below the left nipple (see ❷ on page 99). The point where the apex touches the anterior chest wall and heart movements are most easily observed and palpated is known as the **point of maximal impulse (PMI)**.

CLINICAL ALERT!

Remember that the base of the lungs is the lower (inferior) portion, and the base of the heart is the upper (superior) portion.

The precordium, the area of the chest overlying the heart, is inspected and palpated simultaneously for the presence of abnormal pulsations. Several heart sounds can be heard by auscultation. The first heart sound, S_1, occurs when the atrioventricular (AV) valves close. Although the right and left AV valves do not close simultaneously, the closures occur closely enough to be heard as one sound (S_1), a dull, low-pitched sound described as "lub." After this, the semilunar

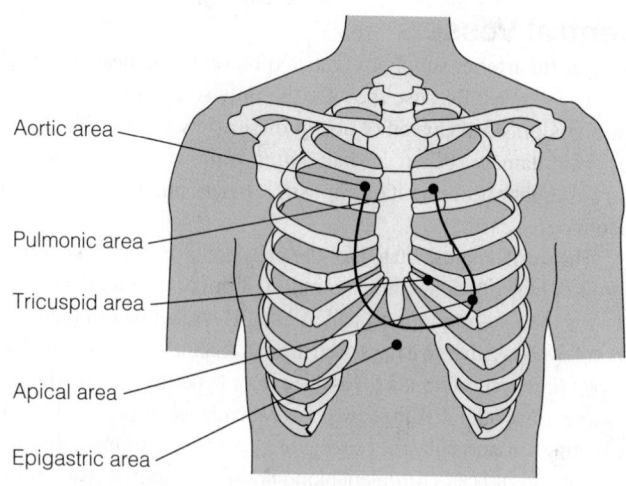

valves close, producing the second heart sound, S_2, described as "dub." The S_2 sound has a higher pitch than S_1 and is also shorter. These two sounds, S_1 and S_2 ("lub-dub"), occur within 1 second or less, depending on the heart rate.

The two heart sounds are best heard over the aortic, pulmonic, tricuspid, and apical areas associated with the closure of the corresponding valves (Figure 3–25 ■). Associated with these sounds are systole and diastole. Systole is the period in which the ventricles contract. It begins with the first heart sound and ends at the second heart sound. Systole is normally shorter than diastole. Diastole is the period in which the ventricles relax. It starts with the second sound and ends at the subsequent first sound. Normally, no sounds are audible during these periods. The experienced nurse, however, may auscultate extra heart sounds (S_3 and S_4) during diastole. Both sounds are low in pitch and heard best at the apical site, with the bell of the stethoscope, and with the client lying on the left side. The S_3 sound (ventricular gallop) occurs early in diastole right after S_2 and sounds like "lub-dub-ee" (S_1, S_2, S_3) or "Kentuc-ky." It often disappears when the client sits up. An S_3 sound is normal in children and young adults. In older adults, it may indicate heart failure. The S_4 sound (atrial gallop) occurs near the very end of diastole just before S_1 and creates the sound of "dee-lub-dub" (S_4, S_1, S_2) or "Ten-nessee." The S_4 sound may be heard in older clients and can be a sign of hypertension. Normal heart sounds are summarized in Table 3–7.

Figure 3–25 ■ Anatomic sites of the precordium.

TABLE 3–7 Normal Heart Sounds

Sound or Phase	Description	Aortic	Pulmonic	Area Tricuspid	Apical
S_1	Dull, low pitched, and longer than S_2; sounds like "lub"	Less intensity than S_2	Less intensity than S_2	Louder than or equal to S_2	Louder than or equal to S_2
Systole	Normally silent interval between S_1 and S_2				
S_2	Higher pitch than S_1; sounds like "dub"	Louder than S_1	Louder than S_1; abnormal if louder than the aortic S_2 in adults over 40 years of age	Less intense than or equal to S_1	Less intense than or equal to S_1
Diastole	Normally silent interval between S_2 and next S_1				

Central Vessels

The carotid arteries supply oxygenated blood to the head and neck (Figure 3–26 ■). Because they are the only source of blood to the brain, prolonged occlusion of one of these arteries can result in serious brain damage. When cardiac output is diminished, the peripheral pulses may be difficult or impossible to feel, but the carotid pulse should be felt easily.

The carotid is auscultated for the presence of an abnormal sound: a bruit (a blowing or swishing sound). If a bruit is found, the carotid artery is then palpated for a thrill. A bruit is created by turbulence of blood flow due either to a narrowed arterial channel (common in older people) or to a condition, such as anemia or hyperthyroidism, that increases cardiac output. A thrill, which frequently accompanies a bruit, is a vibrating sensation like the purring of a cat or water running through a hose. It, too, indicates turbulent blood flow due to arterial obstruction.

The jugular veins drain blood from the head and neck directly into the superior vena cava and right side of the heart (see Figure 3–26). The external jugular veins are superficial and may be visible above the clavicle. The internal jugular veins lie deeper along the carotid artery and may transmit pulsations onto the skin of the neck. Normally, external neck veins are distended and visible when a person lies down; they are flat and not as visible when a person stands up, because gravity encourages venous drainage. Bilateral jugular vein distention (JVD) may indicate right-sided heart failure.

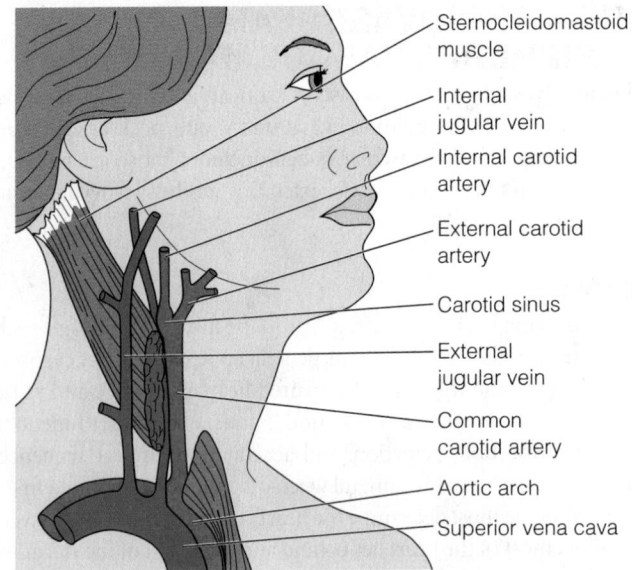

Figure 3–26 ■ Arteries and veins of the right side of the neck.

Labels: Sternocleidomastoid muscle; Internal jugular vein; Internal carotid artery; External carotid artery; Carotid sinus; External jugular vein; Common carotid artery; Aortic arch; Superior vena cava

●○● NURSING PROCESS: ASSESSING THE HEART AND CENTRAL VESSELS

Assessing the Heart and Central Vessels

SKILL 3-12

PLANNING

Heart examinations are usually performed while the client is in a semireclined position. The practitioner stands at the client's right side, facilitating palpation of the cardiac area and allowing optimal inspection.

DELEGATION

Due to the substantial knowledge and skill required, assessment of the heart and central vessels is not delegated to UAP. However, many aspects of cardiac function are observed during usual care and may be recorded by individuals other than the nurse. Abnormal findings must be validated and interpreted by the nurse.

INTERPROFESSIONAL PRACTICE

Assessing the heart and central vessels is within the scope of practice of many health care providers. For example, physician assistants may assess the heart and central vessels before, during, and after treatment. Although these providers may verbally communicate their findings and plan to other health care team members, the nurse must also know where to locate their documentation in the client's medical record.

Equipment
- Stethoscope
- Centimeter ruler

IMPLEMENTATION
Performance

1. Prior to conducting the examination, introduce self and verify the client's identity using agency protocol. Explain to the client what you are going to do, the reason for the examination, and how he or she can participate. Discuss how the findings will be used in planning further care or treatments.
2. Perform hand hygiene and observe other appropriate infection prevention procedures.
3. Provide for client privacy.
4. Inquire if the client has any of the following: family history of incidence of heart disease, high cholesterol levels, high blood pressure, stroke, obesity, congenital heart disease, arterial disease, hypertension, and rheumatic fever and age at which event occurred; client's past history of rheumatic fever, heart murmur, heart attack, varicosities, or heart failure; present symptoms indicative of heart disease (e.g., fatigue, dyspnea, orthopnea, edema, cough, chest pain, palpitations, syncope, hypertension, wheezing, hemoptysis); presence of diseases that affect the heart (e.g., obesity, diabetes, lung disease, endocrine disorders); or lifestyle habits that are risk factors for cardiac disease (e.g., smoking, alcohol intake, eating and exercise patterns, areas and degree of stress perceived).

Assessing the Heart and Central Vessels—*continued*

Assessment	Normal Findings	Deviations from Normal

5. Simultaneously inspect and palpate the precordium for the presence of abnormal pulsations, lifts, or heaves. Locate the valve areas of the heart:
- Locate the angle of Louis. It is felt as a prominence on the sternum.
- Move your fingertips down each side of the angle until you can feel the second intercostal spaces. The client's right second intercostal space is the aortic area, and the left second intercostal space is the pulmonic area. ❶
- From the pulmonic area, move your fingertips down three left intercostal spaces along the side of the sternum. The left fifth intercostal space close to the sternum is the tricuspid or right ventricular area.
- From the tricuspid area, move your fingertips laterally 5 to 7 cm (2 to 3 in.) to the left MCL. ❷ This is the apical or mitral area, or PMI. If you have difficulty locating the PMI, have the client roll onto the left side to move the apex closer to the chest wall.

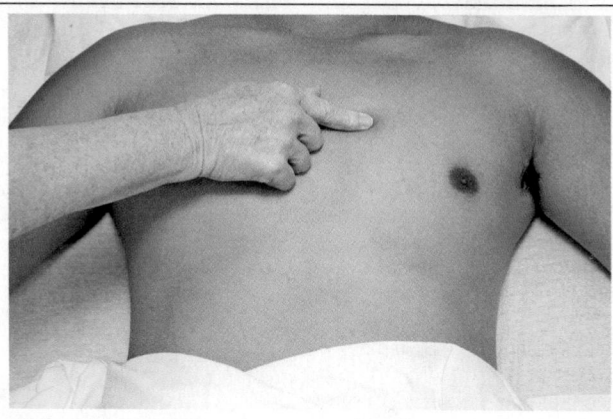

❶ Second intercostal space.

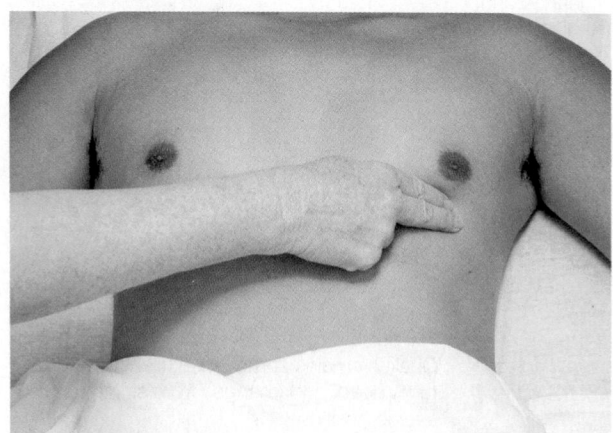

❷ Fifth intercostal space, MCL.

- Inspect and palpate the aortic and pulmonic areas, observing them at an angle and to the side, to note the presence or absence of pulsations. Observing these areas at an angle increases the likelihood of seeing pulsations.

- Inspect and palpate the tricuspid area for pulsations and heaves or lifts.

No pulsations
No lift or heave

Pulsations
Diffuse lift or heave, indicating enlarged or overactive right ventricle

- Inspect and palpate the apical area for pulsation, noting its specific location (it may be displaced laterally or lower) and diameter. If displaced laterally, record the distance between the apex and the MCL in centimeters.

Pulsations visible in 50% of adults and palpable in most
PMI in fifth left ICS at or medial to MCL
Diameter of 1 to 2 cm (1/3 to 1/2 in.)
No lift or heave

PMI displaced laterally or lower (indicates enlarged heart)
Diameter over 2 cm (1/2 in.); indicates enlarged heart or aneurysm
Diffuse lift or heave lateral to apex; indicates enlargement or overactivity of left ventricle

- Inspect and palpate the epigastric area at the base of the sternum for abdominal aortic pulsations.

Aortic pulsations

Bounding abdominal pulsations (e.g., aortic aneurysm)

Continued on page 100

SKILL 3-12

Assessing the Heart and Central Vessels—*continued*

Assessment	Normal Findings	Deviations from Normal
6. Auscultate the heart in all four anatomic sites: aortic, pulmonic, tricuspid, and apical (mitral). Auscultation need not be limited to these areas; the nurse may need to move the stethoscope to find the most audible sounds for each client.	S_1: Usually heard at all sites Usually louder at apical area S_2: Usually heard at all sites Usually louder at base of heart	Increased or decreased intensity Varying intensity with different beats Increased intensity at aortic area Increased intensity at pulmonic area
• Eliminate all sources of room noise. **Rationale:** *Heart sounds are of low intensity, and other noise hinders the nurse's ability to hear them.*	*Systole:* silent interval; slightly shorter duration than diastole at normal heart rate (60 to 90 beats/min) *Diastole:* silent interval; slightly longer duration than systole at normal heart rates S_3 in children and young adults S_4 in many older adults	Sharp-sounding ejection clicks S_3 in older adults S_4 may be a sign of hypertension
• Keep the client in a supine position with head elevated 30° to 45°.		
• In every area of auscultation, distinguish both S_1 and S_2 sounds.		
• When auscultating, concentrate on one particular sound at a time in each area: the first heart sound, followed by systole, then the second heart sound, then diastole. Systole and diastole are normally silent intervals.		
• Use both the diaphragm and the bell to listen to all areas.		
• Later, reexamine the heart while the client is in the upright sitting position. **Rationale:** *Certain sounds are more audible in certain positions.*		
CAROTID ARTERIES		
7. Palpate the carotid artery, using extreme caution.	Symmetric pulse volumes	Asymmetric volumes (possible stenosis or thrombosis)
• Palpate only one carotid artery at a time. **Rationale:** *This ensures adequate blood flow through the other artery to the brain.*	Full pulsations, thrusting quality Quality remains same when client breathes, turns head, and changes from sitting to supine position	Decreased pulsations (may indicate impaired left cardiac output) Increased pulsations
• Avoid exerting too much pressure or massaging the area. **Rationale:** *Pressure can occlude the artery, and carotid sinus massage can precipitate bradycardia. The carotid sinus is a small dilation at the beginning of the internal carotid artery just above the bifurcation of the common carotid artery, in the upper third of the neck.*		
• Ask the client to turn the head slightly toward the side being examined. This makes the carotid artery more accessible.	Elastic arterial wall	Thickening, hard, rigid, beaded, inelastic walls (indicate arteriosclerosis)
8. Auscultate the carotid artery.	No sound heard on auscultation	Presence of bruit in one or both arteries (suggests occlusive artery disease)
• Turn the client's head slightly away from the side being examined. **Rationale:** *This facilitates the placement of the stethoscope.*		
• Auscultate the carotid artery on one side and then the other.		
• Listen for the presence of a bruit. If you hear a bruit, gently palpate the artery to determine the presence of a thrill.		

Assessing the Heart and Central Vessels—*continued*

Assessment	Normal Findings	Deviations from Normal
JUGULAR VEINS		
9. Inspect the jugular veins for distention while the client is placed in a semi-Fowler's position (15° to 45° angle), with the head supported on a small pillow.	Veins not visible (indicating right side of heart is functioning normally)	Veins visibly distended (indicating advanced cardiopulmonary disease)
10. If jugular distention is present, assess the jugular venous pressure (JVP). <ul><li>Locate the highest visible point of distention of the internal jugular vein. Although either the internal or the external jugular vein can be used, the internal jugular vein is more reliable. **Rationale:** *The external jugular vein is more easily affected by obstruction or kinking at the base of the neck.*</li><li>Measure the vertical height of this point in centimeters from the sternal angle, the point at which the clavicles meet. ❸</li><li>Repeat the preceding steps on the other side.</li></ul>		Bilateral measurements above 3 to 4 cm (1.2 to 1.6 in.) are considered elevated (may indicate right-sided heart failure) Unilateral distention (may be caused by local obstruction)
11. Document findings in the client record using forms or checklists supplemented by narrative notes when appropriate.		

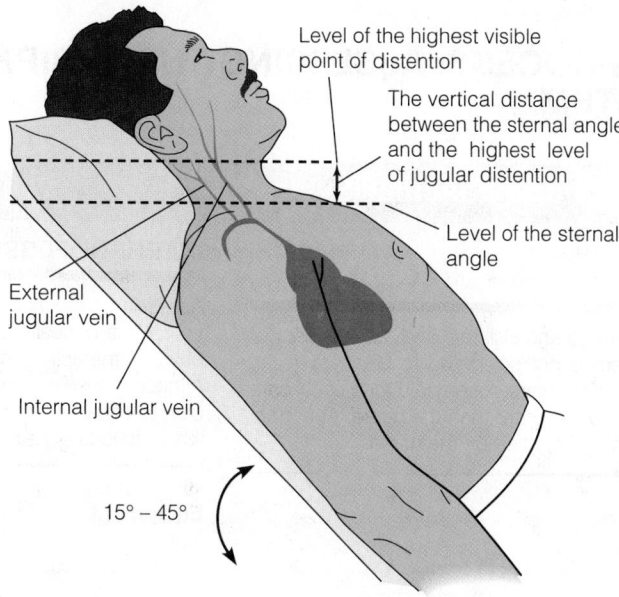

❸ Assessing the highest point of distention of the jugular vein.

Labels:
- Level of the highest visible point of distention
- The vertical distance between the sternal angle and the highest level of jugular distention
- Level of the sternal angle
- External jugular vein
- Internal jugular vein
- 15° – 45°

EVALUATION

- Relate findings to previous assessment data if available. Perform a detailed system-specific follow-up examination based on findings that deviated from those expected.
- Report deviations from expected findings to the primary care provider.

LIFESPAN CONSIDERATIONS Assessing the Heart and Central Vessels

INFANTS

- Physiological splitting of the second heart sound (S_2) may be heard when the child takes a deep breath and the aortic valve closes a split second before the pulmonic valve. If splitting of S_2 is heard during normal respirations, it is abnormal and may indicate an atrial-septal defect, pulmonary stenosis, or another heart problem.
- Sinus arrhythmia related to respiration is common in infants and children. The heart rate slows during expiration and increases when the child breathes in.

- Murmurs may be heard in newborns before the structures of fetal circulation, especially the ductus arteriosus, close.

CHILDREN

- Heart sounds may be louder because of the thinner chest wall.
- A third heart sound (S_3), caused as the ventricles fill, is best heard at the apex, and is present in about one third of all children.
- The PMI is higher and more medial in children under 8 years old.

OLDER ADULTS
- If no disease is present, heart size remains the same size throughout life.
- Cardiac output and strength of contraction decrease, thus lessening the older person's activity tolerance.
- The heart rate returns to its resting rate more slowly after exertion than it did when the individual was younger.

- S_4 heart sound is considered normal in older adults.
- Extra systoles (premature ventricular contractions) are common in older adults. However, if an individual has 10 or more extra systoles per minute, this is considered abnormal.
- Sudden emotional and physical stress may result in cardiac arrhythmias and heart failure.

Peripheral Vascular System

Assessment of the peripheral vascular system includes measurement of the blood pressure, palpation of peripheral pulses, inspection of the peripheral veins, and inspection of the skin and tissues to determine perfusion to the extremities. (Pulse sites and pulse assessments are described in Chapter 2 ∞. Figure 2–8 illustrates the sites for palpating the peripheral pulses.)

●○● NURSING PROCESS: ASSESSING THE PERIPHERAL VASCULAR SYSTEM

Assessing the Peripheral Vascular System

SKILL 3–13

PLANNING
DELEGATION

Due to the substantial knowledge and skill required, assessment of the peripheral vascular system is not delegated to UAP. However, many aspects of the vascular system are observed during usual care and may be recorded by individuals other than the nurse. Abnormal findings must be validated and interpreted by the nurse.

INTERPROFESSIONAL PRACTICE

Assessing the peripheral vascular system is within the scope of practice of many health care providers. For example, occupational and physical therapists may check the client's pulses before treatment. Although these providers may verbally communicate their findings and plan to other health care team members, the nurse must also know where to locate their documentation in the client's medical record.

Equipment
None

IMPLEMENTATION
Performance
1. Prior to conducting the examination, introduce self and verify the client's identity using agency protocol. Explain to the client what you are going to do, the reason for the examination, and how he or she can participate. Discuss how the findings will be used in planning further care or treatments.
2. Perform hand hygiene and observe other appropriate infection prevention procedures.

3. Provide for client privacy.
4. Inquire if the client has any of the following: past history of heart disorders, varicosities, arterial disease, and hypertension; lifestyle habits such as exercise patterns, activity patterns and tolerance, smoking, and use of alcohol.

Assessment	Normal Findings	Deviations from Normal
PERIPHERAL PULSES 5. Palpate the peripheral pulses on both sides of the client's body individually, simultaneously (except the carotid pulse), and systematically to determine the symmetry of the pulses. If you have difficulty palpating some of the peripheral pulses, use a Doppler ultrasound probe.	Symmetric pulse volumes Full pulsations	Asymmetric volumes (indicate impaired circulation) Absence of pulsation (indicates arterial spasm or occlusion) Decreased, weak, thready pulsations (indicate impaired cardiac output) Increased pulse volume (may indicate hypertension, high cardiac output, or circulatory overload)

Assessing the Peripheral Vascular System—*continued*

Assessment	Normal Findings	Deviations from Normal
6. Inspect the peripheral veins in the arms and legs for the presence and/or appearance of superficial veins when limbs are dependent and when limbs are elevated.	In dependent position, presence of distention and nodular bulges at calves When limbs elevated, veins collapse (veins may appear tortuous or distended in older people)	Distended veins in the thigh and/or lower leg or on posterolateral part of calf from knee to ankle
7. Assess the peripheral leg veins for signs of phlebitis. • Inspect the calves for redness and swelling over vein sites • Palpate the calves for firmness or tension of the muscles, the presence of edema over the dorsum of the foot, and areas of localized warmth. **Rationale:** *Palpation augments inspection findings, particularly for darker pigmented people in whom redness may not be visible.* • Push the calves from side to side to test for tenderness. • Firmly dorsiflex the client's foot while supporting the entire leg in extension (Homans' test), or have the person stand or walk.	Limbs not tender Symmetric in size	Tenderness on palpation Pain in calf muscles with forceful dorsiflexion of the foot (positive Homans' test) Warmth and redness over vein Swelling of one calf or leg No one sign or symptom consistently confirms or excludes presence of phlebitis or a deep venous thrombosis. Homans' sign has been found to give inconsistent results (D'Amico & Barbarito, 2012)
PERIPHERAL PERFUSION		
8. Inspect the skin of the hands and feet for color, temperature, edema, and skin changes.	Skin color pink Skin temperature not excessively warm or cold No edema Skin texture resilient and moist	Cyanotic (venous insufficiency) Pallor that increases with limb elevation Dependent rubor, a dusky red color when limb is lowered (arterial insufficiency) Brown pigmentation around ankles (arterial or chronic venous insufficiency) Cool skin (arterial insufficiency) Marked edema (venous insufficiency) Mild edema (arterial insufficiency) Skin thin and shiny or thick, waxy, shiny, and fragile, with reduced hair and/or ulceration (venous or arterial insufficiency)
9. Assess the adequacy of arterial flow if arterial insufficiency is suspected.		
CAPILLARY REFILL TEST • Press at least one nail on each hand and foot between your thumb and index finger sufficiently to cause blanching (about 5 seconds). • Release the pressure, and observe how quickly normal color returns.	Immediate return of color (less than 2 seconds)	Delayed return of color (arterial insufficiency)
OTHER ASSESSMENTS • Inspect the fingernails for changes indicative of circulatory impairment. See the section on assessment of nails, earlier in this chapter. • See also peripheral pulse assessment, earlier.		

Continued on page 104

SKILL 3–13

Assessing the Peripheral Vascular System—*continued*

Assessment	Normal Findings	Deviations from Normal
10. Document findings in the client record using forms or checklists supplemented by narrative notes when appropriate.		**SAMPLE DOCUMENTATION** 6/10/2015 0830 Legs mottled red bilaterally toes to mid-calf. States "actually looks a bit better." Capillary refill 4 seconds in toes on both feet. Pedal pulses present but weak. Homans' test negative. c/o pain in calves after walking 100 feet. ———————— N. Schmidt, RN

EVALUATION

- Relate findings to previous assessment data if available. Perform a detailed system-specific follow-up examination based on findings that deviated from those expected.

- Report deviations from expected findings to the primary care provider.

LIFESPAN CONSIDERATIONS | Assessing the Peripheral Vascular System

INFANTS

- Screen for coarctation of the aorta by palpating the peripheral pulses and comparing the strength of the femoral pulses with the radial pulses and apical pulse. If coarctation is present, femoral pulses will be diminished and radial pulses will be stronger. There may also be increased upper extremity blood pressure although this is seen more commonly in older children.

CHILDREN

- Changes in the peripheral vasculature, such as bruising, petechiae, and purpura, can indicate serious systemic diseases in children (e.g., leukemia, meningococcemia).

OLDER ADULTS

- The overall efficiency of blood vessels decreases as smooth muscle cells are replaced by connective tissue. The lower extremities are more likely to show signs of arterial and venous impairment because of the more distal and dependent position.
- Peripheral vascular assessment should always include upper and lower extremities' temperature, color, pulses, edema, skin integrity, and sensation. Any differences in symmetry of these findings should be noted.
- Proximal arteries become thinner and dilate.
- Peripheral arteries become thicker and dilate less effectively because of arteriosclerotic changes in the vessel walls.
- Blood vessels lengthen and become more tortuous and prominent. Varicosities occur more frequently.
- In some instances, arteries may be palpated more easily because of the loss of supportive surrounding tissues. Often, however, the most distal pulses of the lower extremities are more difficult to palpate because of decreased arterial perfusion.
- Systolic and diastolic blood pressures increase, but the increase in the systolic pressure is greater. As a result, the pulse pressure widens. Any client with a blood pressure reading above 140/90 mmHg should be referred for follow-up assessments.
- Peripheral edema is frequently observed and is most commonly the result of chronic venous insufficiency or low protein levels in the blood (hypoproteinemia).

CLIENT TEACHING CONSIDERATIONS

Assessing the Peripheral Vascular System

- Use the assessment as an opportunity to provide teaching regarding appropriate care of the extremities in those at high risk for or with actual vascular impairment. Educate clients and families regarding skin and nail care, exercise, and positioning to promote circulation.

BREASTS AND AXILLAE

The breasts of men and women need to be inspected and palpated. Glandular tissue, a potential site for malignancy, is present throughout the breast in women and beneath the nipples in men. The largest portion of glandular breast tissue is in the upper outer quadrant of each breast, including the axillary tail of Spence (Figure 3–27 ■). During assessment, the nurse can localize specific findings by dividing the breast into quadrants and the axillary tail.

Clients need to be aware of breast health guidelines (Box 3–5).

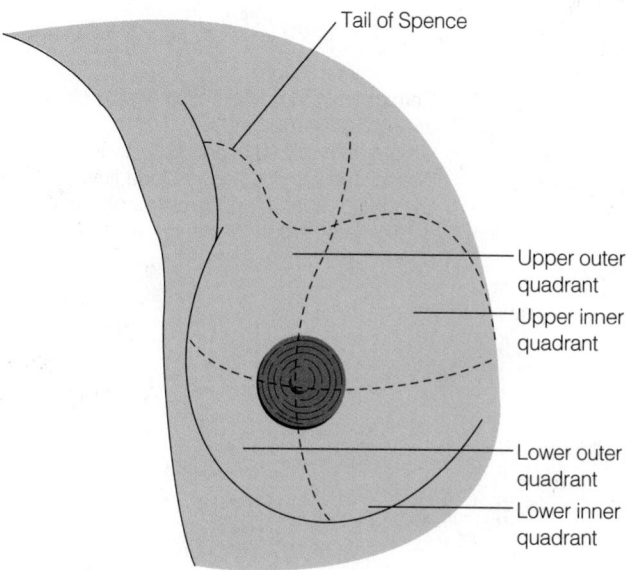

Figure 3–27 ■ The four breast quadrants and the axillary tail of Spence.

BOX 3–5 Breast Health Guidelines

Not all organizations and providers agree about the age and frequency of **breast self-examination (BSE)**, clinical breast exams, and mammography. BSE is a systematic procedure for palpating one's own breast tissues in search of abnormal lumps.

BREAST SELF-EXAMINATION
The American Cancer Society (Smith et al., 2014) recommends BSE be introduced at age 20. The advantages, disadvantages, and technique should be reviewed with the client regularly.

The U.S. Preventive Services Task Force (USPSTF) (2009) does not recommend BSE at any age.

CLINICAL BREAST EXAMINATION BY A HEALTH CARE PROFESSIONAL
- ACS: clinical breast exam by a health professional every 3 years between ages 20 and 40, every year after age 40
- USPSTF: does not recommend clinical breast examination

MAMMOGRAPHY
- ACS: yearly starting at age 40
- USPSTF: every 2 years for ages 50 to 74

WOMEN AT INCREASED RISK
- Magnetic resonance imaging (MRI) yearly or as advised by the primary care provider

Women at increased risk are identified by the American Cancer Society as those who:
- Have a known *BRCA1* or *BRCA2* gene mutation.
- Have a first-degree relative (mother, father, brother, sister, or child) with a *BRCA1* or *BRCA2* gene mutation, and have not had genetic testing themselves.
- Had radiation therapy to the chest when they were between the ages of 10 and 30 years.
- Have Li-Fraumeni syndrome, Cowden syndrome, or Bannayan-Riley-Ruvalcaba syndrome, or have one of these syndromes in first-degree relatives.
- Have a personal history of breast cancer, ductal carcinoma in situ (DCIS), lobular carcinoma in situ (LCIS), atypical ductal hyperplasia (ADH), or atypical lobular hyperplasia (ALH).
- Have extremely dense breasts or unevenly dense breasts when viewed by mammograms.

●○● NURSING PROCESS: ASSESSING THE BREASTS AND AXILLAE

Assessing the Breasts and Axillae

PLANNING
DELEGATION

Due to the substantial knowledge and skill required, assessment of the breasts and axillae is not delegated to UAP. However, individuals other than the nurse may record aspects observed during usual care. Abnormal findings must be validated and interpreted by the nurse.

INTERPROFESSIONAL PRACTICE

Assessing the breasts and axillae is within the scope of practice of a few health care providers. For example, physician assistants may check the client's breasts during their health assessment. Although these providers may verbally communicate their findings and plan to other health care team members, the nurse must also know where to locate their documentation in the client's medical record.

Equipment
- Centimeter ruler

IMPLEMENTATION
Performance
1. Prior to conducting the examination, introduce self and verify the client's identity using agency protocol. Explain to the client what you are going to do, the reason for the examination, and how he or she can participate. Inquire whether the client has ever had a clinical breast exam previously. Discuss how the results will be used in planning further care or treatments.

Continued on page 106

SKILL 3-14

Assessing the Breasts and Axillae—*continued*

2. Perform hand hygiene and observe other appropriate infection prevention procedures.
3. Provide for client privacy.
4. Inquire if the client has any of the following: history of breast masses and what was done about them; pain or tenderness in the breasts and relation to the woman's menstrual cycle; discharge from the nipple; medication history (some medications, e.g., oral contraceptives, steroids, digitalis, and diuretics, may cause nipple discharge; estrogen replacement therapy may be associated with the development of cysts or cancer); risk factors that may be associated with development of breast cancer (e.g., mother, sister, aunt with breast cancer; alcohol consumption, high-fat diet, obesity, use of oral contraceptives, menarche before age 12, menopause after age 55, age 30 or more at first pregnancy). Inquire if the client performs breast self-examination, technique used, and when performed in relation to the menstrual cycle.

Assessment	Normal Findings	Deviations from Normal
5. Inspect the breasts for size, symmetry, and contour or shape while the client is in a sitting position.	*Females:* rounded shape; slightly unequal in size; generally symmetric *Males:* breasts even with the chest wall; if obese, may be similar in shape to female breasts	Recent change in breast size; swellings; marked asymmetry
6. Inspect the skin of the breast for localized discolorations or hyperpigmentation, retraction or dimpling, localized hypervascular areas, swelling, or edema. ❶	Skin uniform in color (similar to skin of abdomen if not tanned) Skin smooth and intact Diffuse symmetric horizontal or vertical vascular pattern in light-skinned people Striae (stretch marks); moles and nevi	Localized discolorations or hyperpigmentation Retraction or dimpling (result of scar tissue or an invasive tumor) Unilateral, localized hypervascular areas (associated with increased blood flow) Swelling or edema appearing as pig skin or orange peel due to exaggeration of the pores

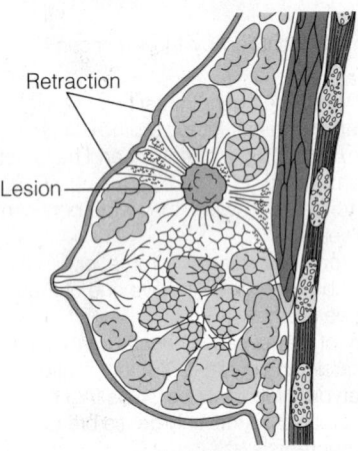

Retraction

Lesion

❶ A lesion causing retraction of the skin.

7. Emphasize any retraction by having the client:
   • Raise the arms above the head.
   • Push the hands together, with elbows flexed. ❷
   • Press the hands down on the hips. ❸

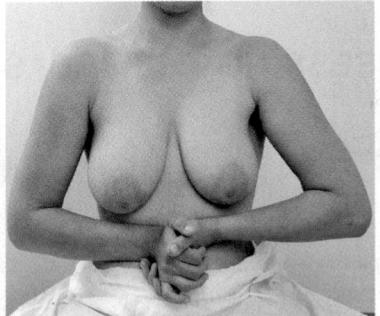

❷ Pushing the hands together to accentuate retraction of breast tissue.

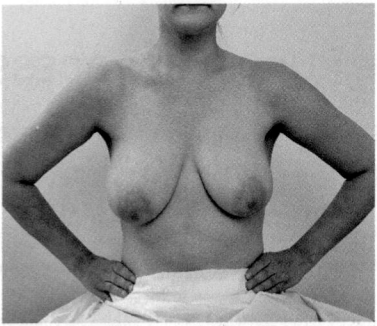

❸ Pressing the hands down on the hips to accentuate retraction of breast tissue.

8. Inspect the areola area for size, shape, symmetry, color, surface characteristics, and any masses or lesions.	Round or oval and bilaterally the same Color varies widely, from light pink to dark brown Irregular placement of sebaceous glands on the surface of the areola (Montgomery's tubercles)	Any asymmetry, mass, or lesion

Assessing the Breasts and Axillae—*continued*

Assessment	Normal Findings	Deviations from Normal
9. Inspect the nipples for size, shape, position, color, discharge, and lesions.	Round, everted, and equal in size; similar in color; soft and smooth; both nipples point in same direction (out in young women and men, downward in older women) No discharge, except from pregnant or breast-feeding females Inversion of one or both nipples that is present from puberty	Asymmetrical size and color Presence of discharge, crusts, or cracks Recent inversion of one or both nipples
10. Palpate the axillary, subclavicular, and supraclavicular lymph nodes ❹ while the client sits with the arms abducted and supported on the nurse's forearm. For palpation of clavicular lymph nodes, see page 87. Use the flat surfaces of all fingertips to palpate the four areas of the axilla: • The edge of the greater pectoral muscle along the anterior axillary line • The thoracic wall in the midaxillary area • The upper part of the humerus • The anterior edge of the latissimus dorsi muscle along the posterior axillary line.	No tenderness, masses, or nodules	Tenderness, masses, or nodules

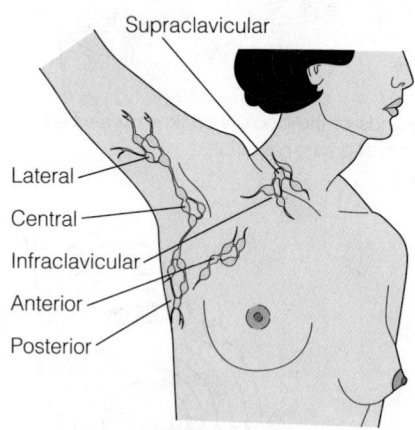

Supraclavicular

Lateral

Central

Infraclavicular

Anterior

Posterior

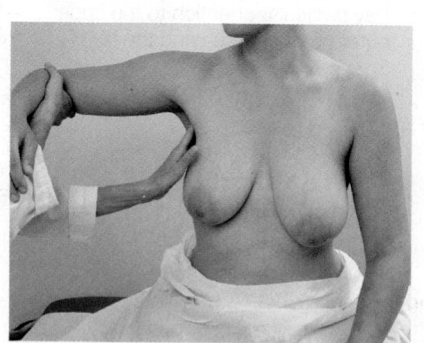

❹ Location and palpation of the lymph nodes that drain the lateral breast: *A,* lymph nodes; *B,* palpating the axilla.

Assessment	Normal Findings	Deviations from Normal
11. Palpate the breast for masses, tenderness, and any discharge from the nipples. Palpation of the breast is generally performed while the client is supine. **Rationale:** *In the supine position, the breasts flatten evenly against the chest wall, facilitating palpation.* For clients who have a past history of breast masses, who are at high risk for breast cancer, or who have pendulous breasts, examination in both a supine and a sitting position is recommended. • If the client reports a breast lump, start with the "normal" breast to obtain baseline data that will serve as a comparison to the involved breast. • To enhance flattening of the breast, instruct the client to abduct the arm and place her hand behind her head. Then place a small pillow or rolled towel under the client's shoulder.	No tenderness, masses, nodules, or nipple discharge	Tenderness, masses, nodules, or nipple discharge If you detect a mass, record the following data: • *Location:* the exact location relative to the quadrants and axillary tail, or the clock and the distance from the nipple in centimeters • *Size:* the length, width, and thickness of the mass in centimeters (If you are able to determine the discrete edges, record this fact.) • *Shape:* whether the mass is round, oval, lobulated, indistinct, or irregular • *Consistency:* whether the mass is hard or soft • *Mobility:* whether the mass is movable or fixed • *Skin over the lump:* whether it is reddened, dimpled, or retracted • *Nipple:* whether it is displaced or retracted • *Tenderness:* whether palpation is painful

Continued on page 108

SKILL 3–14

Assessing the Breasts and Axillae—*continued*

Assessment	Normal Findings	Deviations from Normal
• For palpation, use the palmar surface of the middle three fingertips (held together) and make a gentle rotary motion on the breast. • Choose one of three patterns for palpation: a. Hands-of-the-clock or spokes-on-a-wheel ❺ b. Concentric circles ❻ c. Vertical strips pattern. ❼ • Start at one point for palpation, and move systematically to the end point to ensure that all breast surfaces are assessed. • Pay particular attention to the upper outer quadrant area and the tail of Spence.		

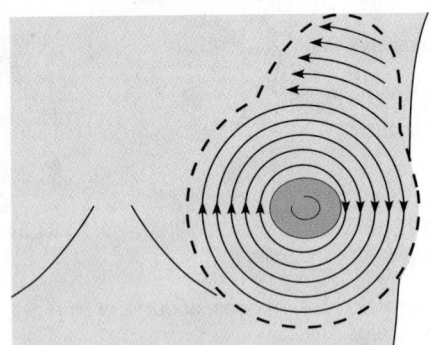

❺ Hands-of-the-clock or spokes-on-a-wheel pattern of breast palpation.

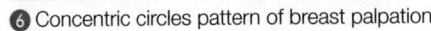

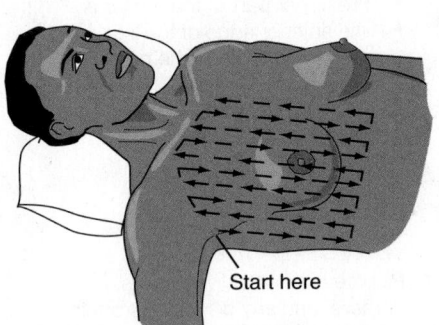

❻ Concentric circles pattern of breast palpation. ❼ Vertical strips pattern of breast palpation.

Assessment	Normal Findings	Deviations from Normal
12. Palpate the areolae and the nipples for masses. Compress each nipple to determine the presence of any discharge. If discharge is present, milk the breast along its radius to identify the discharge-producing lobe. Assess any discharge for amount, color, consistency, and odor. Note also any tenderness on palpation. **13.** If the client wishes, teach the client the technique of BSE. See Client Teaching Considerations. **14.** Document findings in the client record using forms or checklists supplemented by narrative notes when appropriate.	No tenderness, masses, nodules, or nipple discharge	Tenderness, masses, nodules, or nipple discharge

EVALUATION
• Relate findings to previous assessment data if available. Perform a detailed system-specific follow-up examination based on findings that deviated from those expected.

• Report deviations from expected findings to the primary care provider.

LIFESPAN CONSIDERATIONS | Assessing the Breasts and Axillae

INFANTS
- Newborns up to 2 weeks of age, both boys and girls, may have breast enlargement and white discharge from the nipples (witch's milk).
- Supernumerary ("extra") nipples infrequently are present along the mammary chain; these may be associated with renal anomalies.

CHILDREN
- Female breast development begins between 9 and 13 years of age and occurs in five stages (Tanner stages). One breast may develop more rapidly than the other, but at the end of development, they are more or less the same size.
  Stage 1: Prepubertal with no noticeable change
  Stage 2: Breast bud with elevation of nipple and enlargement of the areola
  Stage 3: Enlargement of the breast and areola with no separation of contour
  Stage 4: Projection of the areola and nipple
  Stage 5: Recession of the areola by about age 14 or 15, leaving only the nipple projecting
- Boys may develop breast buds and have slight enlargement of the areola in early adolescence. Further enlargement of breast tissue (gynecomastia) can occur. This growth is transient,

usually lasting about 2 years, resolving completely by late puberty.
- Axillary hair usually appears in Tanner stages 3 or 4 and is related to adrenal rather than gonadal changes.

PREGNANT FEMALES
- Breast, areola, and nipple size increase.
- The areolae and nipples darken; nipples may become more erect; areolae contain small, scattered, elevated Montgomery's glands.
- Superficial veins become more prominent, and jagged linear stretch marks may develop.
- A thick yellow fluid (colostrum) may be expressed from the nipples after the first trimester.

OLDER ADULTS
- In the postmenopausal female, breasts change in shape and often appear pendulous or flaccid; they lack the firmness they had in younger years.
- The presence of breast lesions may be detected more readily because of the decrease in connective tissue.
- General breast size remains the same. Although glandular tissue atrophies, the amount of fat in breasts (predominantly in the lower quadrants) increases in most women.

CLIENT TEACHING CONSIDERATIONS

Breast Self-Examination

Instruct the client to perform the following steps.

INSPECTION BEFORE A MIRROR
Look for any change in size or shape; lumps or thickenings; any rashes or other skin irritations; dimpled or puckered skin; any discharge or change in the nipples (e.g., position or asymmetry). Inspect the breasts in all of the following positions:

- Stand and face the mirror with your arms relaxed at your sides or hands resting on the hips; then turn to the right and the left for a side view (look for any flattening in the side view).
- Bend forward from the waist with arms raised over the head.
- Stand straight with the arms raised over the head and move the arms slowly up and down at the sides. (Look for free movement of the breasts over the chest wall.)
- Press your hands firmly together at chin level while the elbows are raised to shoulder level.

PALPATION: LYING POSITION
- Place a pillow under your right shoulder and place the right hand behind your head. This position distributes breast tissue more evenly on the chest.

- Use the finger pads (tips) of the three middle fingers (held together) on your left hand to feel for lumps.
- Press the breast tissue against the chest wall firmly enough to know how your breast feels. A ridge of firm tissue in the lower curve of each breast is normal.
- Use small circular motions along one arrow in your chosen pattern (**5**, **6**, or **7** on page 108). Then move your fingers about 2 cm (3/4 in.) and feel along the next arrow. Repeat this action as many times as necessary until the entire breast is covered.
- Bring your arm down to your side and feel under your armpit, where breast tissue is also located.
- Repeat the exam on your left breast, using the finger pads of your right hand.

PALPATION: STANDING OR SITTING
- Repeat the examination of both breasts while upright with one arm behind your head. This position makes it easier to check the area where a large percentage of breast cancers are found, the upper outer part of the breast and toward the armpit.
- *Optional:* Do the upright BSE in the shower. Soapy hands glide more easily over wet skin.

Report any changes to your health care provider promptly.

ABDOMEN

The nurse locates and describes abdominal findings by using two common methods of subdividing the abdomen: quadrants and nine regions. To divide the abdomen into quadrants, the nurse imagines two lines: a vertical line from the xiphoid process to the pubic symphysis, and a horizontal line across the umbilicus (Figure 3–28 ■). These quadrants are labeled right upper quadrant, left upper quadrant, right lower quadrant, and left lower quadrant. Using the second

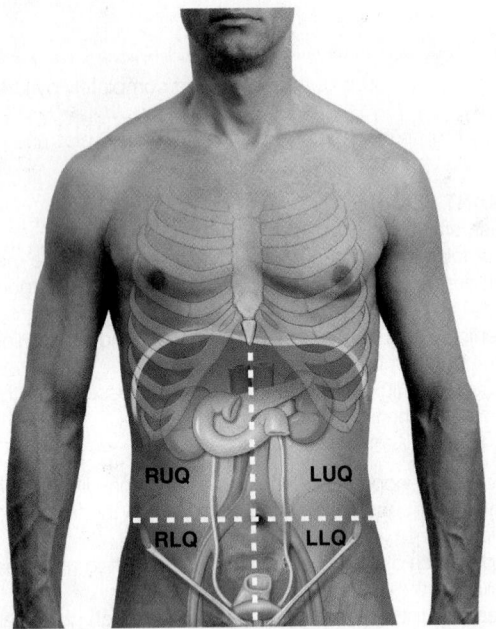

Figure 3–28 ■ The four abdominal quadrants and underlying organs. RUQ, right upper quadrant; LUQ, left upper quadrant; RLQ, right lower quadrant; LLQ, left lower quadrant.

method, division into nine regions, the nurse imagines two vertical lines that extend superiorly from the midpoints of the inguinal ligaments, and two horizontal lines, one at the level of the edge of the lower ribs and the other at the level of the iliac crests (Figure 3–29 ■). Specific organs or parts of organs lie in each abdominal region (Boxes 3–6 and 3–7).

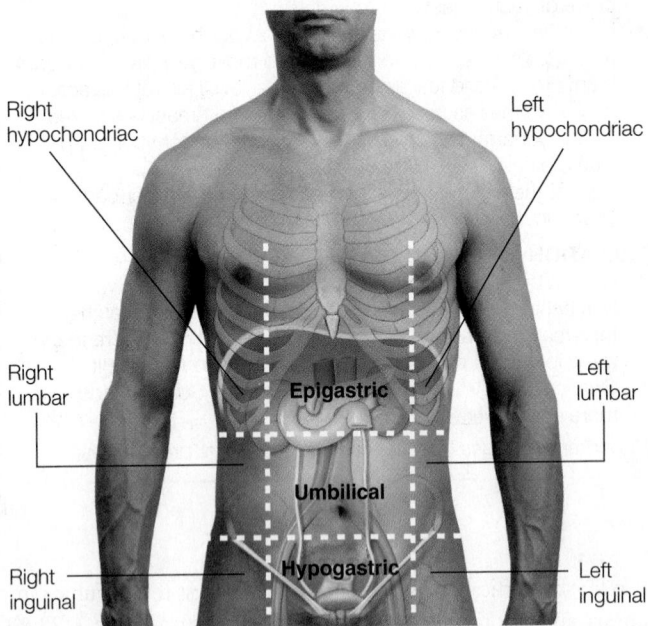

Figure 3–29 ■ The nine abdominal regions: epigastric; left and right hypochondriac; umbilical; left and right lumbar; hypogastric; left and right inguinal or iliac.

BOX 3–6 Organs in the Four Abdominal Quadrants

RIGHT UPPER QUADRANT
Liver
Gallbladder
Duodenum
Head of pancreas
Right adrenal gland
Upper lobe of right kidney
Hepatic flexure of colon
Section of ascending colon
Section of transverse colon

LEFT UPPER QUADRANT
Left lobe of liver
Stomach
Spleen
Upper lobe of left kidney
Pancreas
Left adrenal gland
Splenic flexure of colon
Section of transverse colon
Section of descending colon

RIGHT LOWER QUADRANT
Lower lobe of right kidney
Cecum
Appendix
Section of ascending colon
Right ovary
Right fallopian tube
Right ureter
Right spermatic cord
Part of uterus

LEFT LOWER QUADRANT
Lower lobe of left kidney
Sigmoid colon
Section of descending colon
Left ovary
Left fallopian tube
Left ureter
Left spermatic cord
Part of uterus

In addition, practitioners use landmarks to locate abdominal signs and symptoms. These are the xiphoid process of the sternum, the costal margins, the midline (a line drawn from the tip of the sternum through the umbilicus to the pubic symphysis), the

---

BOX 3–7 Organs in the Nine Abdominal Regions

RIGHT HYPOCHONDRIAC
Right lobe of liver
Gallbladder
Part of duodenum
Hepatic flexure of colon
Upper half of right kidney
Suprarenal gland

RIGHT LUMBAR
Ascending colon
Lower half of right kidney
Part of duodenum
    and jejunum

RIGHT INGUINAL
Cecum
Appendix
Lower end of ileum
Right ureter
Right spermatic cord
Right ovary

EPIGASTRIC
Aorta
Pyloric end of stomach
Part of duodenum
Pancreas
Part of liver

UMBILICAL
Omentum
Mesentery
Lower part of duodenum
Part of jejunum and ileum

HYPOGASTRIC (PUBIC)
Ileum
Bladder
Uterus

LEFT HYPOCHONDRIAC
Stomach
Spleen
Tail of pancreas
Splenic flexure of colon
Upper half of left kidney
Suprarenal gland

LEFT LUMBAR
Descending colon
Lower half of left kidney
Part of jejunum and ileum

LEFT INGUINAL
Sigmoid colon
Left ureter
Left spermatic cord
Left ovary

anterosuperior iliac spine, the inguinal ligaments, and the superior margin of the pubic symphysis (Figure 3–30 ■).

Assessment of the abdomen involves inspection, auscultation, palpation, and percussion. The nurse performs inspection first, followed by auscultation, palpation, and/or percussion. Auscultation is done before palpation and percussion because palpation and percussion cause movement or stimulation of the bowel, which can increase bowel motility and thus heighten bowel sounds, creating false results.

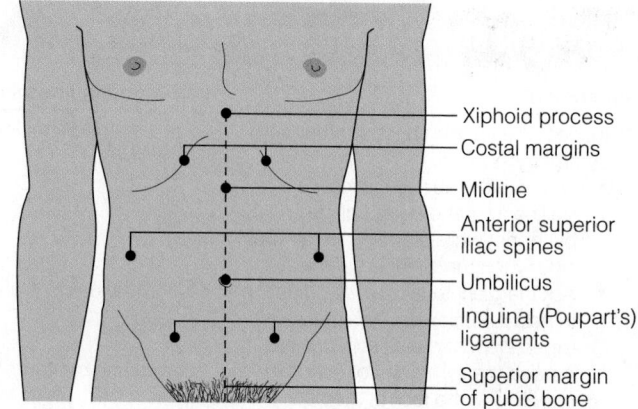

Figure 3–30 ■ Landmarks commonly used to identify abdominal areas.

Labels:
- Xiphoid process
- Costal margins
- Midline
- Anterior superior iliac spines
- Umbilicus
- Inguinal (Poupart's) ligaments
- Superior margin of pubic bone

●○●● NURSING PROCESS: ASSESSING THE ABDOMEN

Assessing the Abdomen

SKILL 3-15

PLANNING

- Ask the client to urinate since an empty bladder makes the assessment more comfortable.
- Ensure that the room is warm since the client will be exposed.

DELEGATION

Due to the substantial knowledge and skill required, assessment of the abdomen is not delegated to UAP. However, signs and symptoms of problems may be observed during usual care and should be recorded by those individuals. Abnormal findings must be validated and interpreted by the nurse.

INTERPROFESSIONAL PRACTICE

Assessing the abdomen is within the scope of practice of many health care providers. For example, both physician assistants and nutritionists may check the client's abdomen. Although these providers may verbally communicate their findings and plan to other health care team members, the nurse must also know where to locate their documentation in the client's medical record.

Equipment

- Examining light
- Tape measure (metal or unstretchable cloth)
- Water-soluble skin-marking pencil
- Stethoscope

IMPLEMENTATION

Performance

1. Prior to conducting the examination, introduce self and verify the client's identity using agency protocol. Explain to the client what you are going to do, the reason for the examination, and how he or she can participate. Discuss how the findings will be used in planning further care or treatments.
2. Perform hand hygiene and observe other appropriate infection prevention procedures.
3. Provide for client privacy.
4. Inquire if the client has any of the following: incidence of abdominal pain; its location, onset, sequence, and chronology; its quality (description); its frequency; associated symptoms (e.g., nausea, vomiting, diarrhea); incidence of constipation or diarrhea (have client describe what client means by these terms);

change in appetite, food intolerances, and foods ingested in last 24 hours; specific signs and symptoms (e.g., heartburn, flatulence and/or belching, difficulty swallowing, hematemesis [vomiting blood], blood or mucus in stools, and aggravating and alleviating factors); and previous problems and treatment (e.g., stomach ulcer, gallbladder surgery, history of jaundice).

5. Assist the client to a supine position, with the arms placed comfortably at the sides. Place small pillows beneath the knees and the head to reduce tension in the abdominal muscles. Expose the client's abdomen only from the chest to the pubic area to avoid chilling and shivering, which can tense the abdominal muscles.

Assessment	Normal Findings	Deviations from Normal
INSPECTION OF THE ABDOMEN		
6. Inspect the abdomen for skin integrity (refer to the discussion of skin assessment earlier in this chapter).	Unblemished skin Uniform color	Presence of rash or other lesions Tense, glistening skin (may indicate ascites, edema)
	Silver-white striae (stretch marks) or surgical scars	Purple striae (associated with Cushing's disease or rapid weight gain and loss)

Continued on page 112

Assessing the Abdomen—*continued*

Assessment	Normal Findings	Deviations from Normal
7. Inspect the abdomen for contour and symmetry: • Observe the abdominal contour (profile line from the rib margin to the pubic bone) while standing at the client's side when the client is supine. • Ask the client to take a deep breath and to hold it. **Rationale:** *This makes an enlarged liver or spleen more obvious.* • Assess the symmetry of contour while standing at the foot of the bed. • If distention is present, measure the abdominal girth by placing a tape measure around the abdomen at the level of the umbilicus. ❶ If girth will be measured repeatedly, use an indelible skin marker to outline the upper and lower margins of the tape placement for consistency of future measurements.	Flat, rounded (convex), or scaphoid (concave) No evidence of enlargement of liver or spleen Symmetric contour	Distended Evidence of enlargement of liver or spleen Asymmetric contour, e.g., localized protrusions around umbilicus, inguinal ligaments, or scars (possible hernia or tumor)

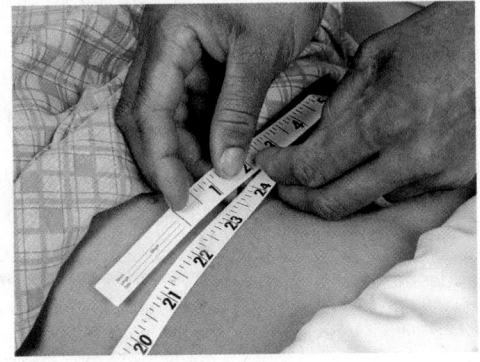

❶ Measuring abdominal girth.

Assessment	Normal Findings	Deviations from Normal
8. Observe abdominal movements associated with respiration, peristalsis, or aortic pulsations.	Symmetric movements caused by respiration Visible peristalsis in very lean people Aortic pulsations in thin individuals at epigastric area	Limited movement due to pain or disease process Visible peristalsis in nonlean clients (possible bowel obstruction) Marked aortic pulsations
9. Observe the vascular pattern.	No visible vascular pattern	Visible venous pattern (dilated veins) is associated with liver disease, ascites, and venocaval obstruction

AUSCULTATION OF THE ABDOMEN

10. Auscultate the abdomen for bowel sounds, vascular sounds, and peritoneal friction rubs. ❷ Warm the hands and the stethoscope diaphragm and bell. **Rationale:** *Cold hands and a cold stethoscope may cause the client to contract the abdominal muscles, and these contractions may be heard during auscultation.*

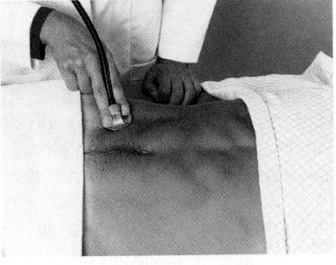

❷ Auscultating the abdomen for bowel sounds.

For Bowel Sounds

Assessment	Normal Findings	Deviations from Normal
• Use the diaphragm. **Rationale:** *Intestinal sounds are relatively high pitched and best transmitted by the diaphragm.* Light pressure with the stethoscope is adequate. • Ask when the client last ate. **Rationale:** *Shortly after or long after eating, bowel sounds may increase.* They are loudest when a meal is long overdue. Four to 7 hours after a meal, bowel sounds may be heard continuously over the ileocecal valve area (right lower quadrant) while the digestive contents from the small intestine empty through the valve into the large intestine.	Audible bowel sounds	Hypoactive, i.e., extremely soft and infrequent (e.g., one per minute); hypoactive sounds indicate decreased motility and are usually associated with manipulation of the bowel during surgery, inflammation, paralytic ileus, or late bowel obstruction Hyperactive/increased, i.e., high-pitched, loud, rushing sounds that occur frequently (e.g., every 3 seconds); also known as borborygmi Hyperactive sounds indicate increased intestinal motility and are usually associated with diarrhea, an early bowel obstruction, or the use of laxatives True absence of sounds (none heard in 3 to 5 minutes) indicates a cessation of intestinal motility

Assessing the Abdomen—*continued*

Assessment	Normal Findings	Deviations from Normal
• Place diaphragm of the stethoscope in each of the four quadrants of the abdomen. • Listen for active bowel sounds—irregular gurgling noises occurring about every 5 to 20 seconds. The duration of a single sound may range from less than a second to more than several seconds.	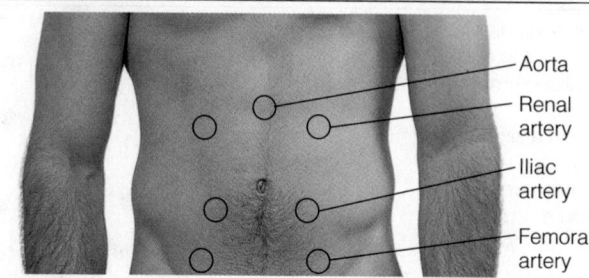 ❸ Sites for auscultating vascular sounds.	

For Vascular Sounds

• Use the bell of the stethoscope over the aorta, renal arteries, iliac arteries, and femoral arteries. ❸ • Listen for bruits.	Absence of bruits	Loud bruit over aortic area (possible aneurysm) Bruit over renal or iliac arteries

Peritoneal Friction Rubs

• Peritoneal friction rubs are rough, grating sounds like two pieces of leather rubbing together. Friction rubs may be caused by inflammation, infection, or abnormal growths.	Absence of friction rub	Friction rub

Percussion of the Abdomen

11. Percuss several areas in each of the four quadrants to determine presence of tympany (sound indicating gas in stomach and intestines) and dullness (decrease, absence, or flatness of resonance over solid masses or fluid). Use a systematic pattern: Begin in the lower right quadrant, proceed to the upper right quadrant, the upper left quadrant, and the lower left quadrant. ❹	Tympany over the stomach and gas-filled bowels; dullness, especially over the liver and spleen, or a full bladder 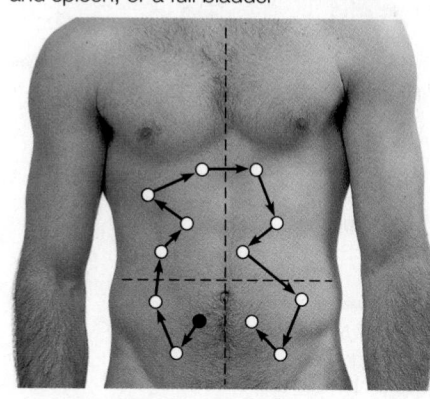	Large dull areas (associated with presence of fluid or a tumor) ❹ Systematic percussion sites for all four abdominal quadrants.

Palpation of the Abdomen

12. Perform light palpation to detect areas of tenderness and/or muscle guarding. Systematically explore all four quadrants. Ensure that the client's position is appropriate for relaxation of the abdominal muscles, and warm the hands. **Rationale:** *Cold hands can elicit muscle tension and thus impede palpatory evaluation.*	No tenderness; relaxed abdomen with smooth, consistent tension	Tenderness and hypersensitivity Superficial masses Localized areas of increased tension

Light Palpation

• Hold the palm of your hand slightly above the client's abdomen, with your fingers parallel to the abdomen.

Continued on page 114

SKILL 3–15

Assessing the Abdomen—*continued*

Assessment	Normal Findings	Deviations from Normal
• Depress the abdominal wall lightly, about 1 cm (0.4 in.) or to the depth of the subcutaneous tissue, with the pads of your fingers. ❺ • Move the finger pads in a slight circular motion. • Note areas of tenderness or superficial pain, masses, and muscle guarding. To determine areas of tenderness, ask the client to tell you about them and watch for changes in the client's facial expressions. • If the client is excessively ticklish, begin by pressing your hand on top of the client's hand while pressing lightly. Then slide your hand off the client's and onto the abdomen to continue the examination.	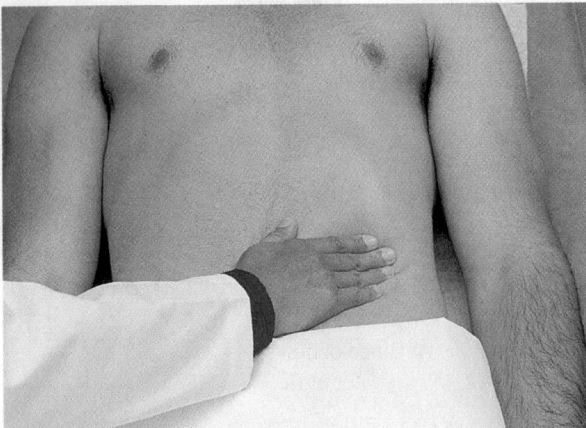 ❺ Light palpation of the abdomen.	
Palpation of the Bladder **13.** Palpate the area above the pubic symphysis if the client's history indicates possible urinary retention. ❻ **14.** Document findings in the client record using forms or checklists supplemented by narrative notes when appropriate.	Not palpable 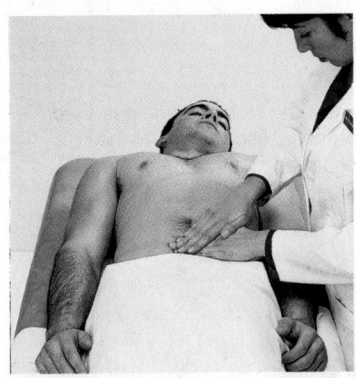 ❻ Palpating the bladder.	Distended and palpable as smooth, round, tense mass (indicates urinary retention)

SAMPLE DOCUMENTATION

6/10/2015 0945 c/o "gassy" pain lower right quadrant. No bowel movement x 48 hrs. Ate 75% regular diet yesterday. Abdomen flat. Active bowel sounds all 4 quadrants. Tympany above umbilicus, dull below. No masses felt on palpation. 30 mL Milk of Magnesia given.
— N. Schmidt, RN

EVALUATION

• Relate findings to previous assessment data if available. Perform a detailed system-specific follow-up examination based on findings that deviated from those expected.

• Report deviations from expected findings to the primary care provider.

LIFESPAN CONSIDERATIONS   Assessing the Abdomen

INFANTS
• Internal organs of newborns and infants are proportionately larger than those of older children and adults, so their abdomens are rounded and tend to protrude.
• Umbilical hernias may be present at birth and should resolve by the age of 3 without intervention.

CHILDREN
• Toddlers have a characteristic "pot belly" appearance, which can persist until age 3 to 4 years.
• Late preschool and school-age children are leaner than toddlers and have a flat abdomen.
• Peristaltic waves may be more visible than in adults.

LIFESPAN CONSIDERATIONS Assessing the Abdomen—*continued*

- Children may not be able to pinpoint areas of tenderness; by observing facial expressions the examiner can determine areas of maximum tenderness.
- If the child is ticklish, guarding, or fearful, use a task that requires concentration (such as squeezing the hands together) to distract the child, or have the child place his or her hands on yours as you palpate the abdomen, "helping" you to do the exam.

OLDER ADULTS

- The rounded abdomens of older adults are due to an increase in adipose tissue and a decrease in muscle tone.
- The abdominal wall is slacker and thinner, making palpation easier and more accurate than in younger clients. Muscle wasting and loss of fibroconnective tissue occur.
- The pain threshold in older adults is often higher; major abdominal problems such as appendicitis or other acute emergencies may therefore go undetected.
- Gastrointestinal pain needs to be differentiated from cardiac pain. Gastrointestinal pain may be located in the thorax or abdomen, whereas cardiac pain is usually located in the thorax. However, these relationships are not absolute because cardiac abnormalities may present as gastrointestinal complaints, especially in women. Factors aggravating gastrointestinal pain are usually related to either ingestion or lack of food intake;

gastrointestinal pain is usually relieved by antacids, food, or assuming an upright position. Common factors that can aggravate cardiac pain are activity or anxiety. Rest or nitroglycerin relieves cardiac pain.
- Stool passes through the intestines at a slower rate in older adults, and the perception of stimuli that produce the urge to defecate often diminishes.
- Fecal incontinence may occur in older adults who are confused or neurologically impaired.
- Many older adults believe that the absence of a daily bowel movement signifies constipation. When assessing for constipation, the nurse must consider the client's diet, activity, medications, and characteristics and ease of passage of feces as well as the frequency of bowel movements.
- The incidence of colon cancer is higher among older adults than younger adults. Symptoms include a change in bowel function, rectal bleeding, and weight loss. Changes in bowel function, however, are associated with many factors, such as diet, exercise, and medications.
- Decreased absorption of oral medications often occurs with aging.
- In the liver, impaired metabolism of some drugs may occur with aging.

Ambulatory and Community Settings Assessing the Abdomen

PATIENT-CENTERED CARE

- Be sure you have the required equipment on a home visit, including a tape measure and skin-marking pen.
- Use pillows to position the client.

- Undressing the client to perform a complete abdominal examination may not be necessary. Focus the assessment on areas indicated by the history and present complaint.

MUSCULOSKELETAL SYSTEM

The musculoskeletal system encompasses the muscles, bones, and joints. The nurse assesses the musculoskeletal system for muscle strength, tone, size and symmetry of muscle development, and fasciculations and tremors. A **fasciculation** is an abnormal contraction of a bundle of muscle fibers that appears as a twitch. A **tremor** is an involuntary trembling of a limb or body part. An intention tremor

becomes more apparent when an individual attempts a voluntary movement (e.g., holding a cup of coffee). A resting tremor is more apparent when the client is relaxed and diminishes with activity.

Bones are assessed for normalcy of form. Joints are assessed for tenderness, swelling, thickening, crepitation (a crackling, grating sound), and range of motion. Body posture is assessed for normalcy in standing and sitting positions.

●○● NURSING PROCESS: ASSESSING THE MUSCULOSKELETAL SYSTEM

Assessing the Musculoskeletal System

SKILL 3-16

PLANNING
DELEGATION

Due to the substantial knowledge and skill required, assessment of the musculoskeletal system is not delegated to UAP. However, many aspects of its functioning are observed during usual care and may be recorded by persons other than the nurse. Abnormal findings must be validated and interpreted by the nurse.

INTERPROFESSIONAL PRACTICE

Assessing the musculoskeletal system is within the scope of practice of many health care providers. For example, both physical therapists and occupational therapists assess the musculoskeletal system as an integral part of their work. Although these providers may verbally communicate their findings and plan to other health care team members, the nurse must also know where to locate their documentation in the client's medical record.

Equipment
- Goniometer
- Tape measure

Continued on page 116

SKILL 3-16

Assessing the Musculoskeletal System—*continued*

IMPLEMENTATION
Performance

1. Prior to conducting the examination, introduce self and verify the client's identity using agency protocol. Explain to the client what you are going to do, the reason for the examination, and how he or she can participate. Discuss how the findings will be used in planning further care or treatments.
2. Perform hand hygiene and observe other appropriate infection prevention procedures.

3. Provide for client privacy.
4. Inquire if the client has any history of the following: muscle or joint pain; onset, location, character, associated phenomena (e.g., redness and swelling of joints), and aggravating and alleviating factors; limitations to movement or inability to perform ADLs; previous sports injuries; or loss of function without pain.

Assessment	Normal Findings	Deviations from Normal
MUSCLES		
5. Inspect the muscles for size. Compare the muscles on one side of the body (e.g., of the arm, thigh, and calf) to the same muscle on the other side. For any discrepancies, measure the muscles with a tape.	Equal size on both sides of body	Atrophy (a decrease in size) or hypertrophy (an increase in size), asymmetry
6. Inspect the muscles and tendons for contractures (shortening).	No contractures	Malposition of body part, e.g., foot drop (foot flexed downward)
7. Inspect the muscles for tremors, for example, by having the client hold the arms out in front of the body.	No tremors	Presence of tremor
8. Test muscle strength. Compare the right side with the left side. *Sternocleidomastoid:* Client turns the head to one side against the resistance of your hand. Repeat with the other side. *Trapezius:* Client shrugs the shoulders against the resistance of your hands. *Deltoid:* Client holds arm up and resists while you try to push it down. *Biceps:* Client fully extends each arm and tries to flex it while you attempt to hold arm in extension. *Triceps:* Client flexes each arm and then tries to extend it against your attempt to keep arm in flexion. *Wrist and finger muscles:* Client spreads the fingers and resists as you attempt to push the fingers together. *Grip strength:* Client grasps your index and middle fingers while you try to pull the fingers out. *Hip muscles:* Client is supine, both legs extended; client raises one leg at a time while you attempt to hold it down. *Hip abduction:* Client is supine, both legs extended. Place your hands on the lateral surface of each knee; client spreads the legs apart against your resistance. *Hip adduction:* Client is in same position as for hip abduction. Place your hands between the knees; client brings the legs together against your resistance. *Hamstrings:* Client is supine, both knees bent. Client resists while you attempt to straighten the legs.	Equal strength on each body side	25% or less of normal strength **Grading Muscle Strength** **0:** 0% of normal strength; complete paralysis **1:** 10% of normal strength; no movement, contraction of muscle is palpable or visible **2:** 25% of normal strength; full muscle movement against gravity, with support **3:** 50% of normal strength; normal movement against gravity **4:** 75% of normal strength; normal full movement against gravity and against minimal resistance **5:** 100% of normal strength; normal full movement against gravity and against full resistance

Assessing the Musculoskeletal System—*continued*

Assessment	Normal Findings	Deviations from Normal
Quadriceps: Client is supine, knee partially extended; client resists while you attempt to flex the knee. *Muscles of the ankles and feet:* Client resists while you attempt to dorsiflex the foot and again resists while you attempt to flex the foot.		

BONES

9. Inspect the skeleton for structure.	No deformities	Bones misaligned
10. Palpate the bones to locate any areas of edema or tenderness.	No tenderness or swelling	Presence of tenderness or swelling (may indicate fracture, neoplasms, or osteoporosis)

JOINTS

11. Inspect the joints for swelling. Palpate each joint for tenderness, smoothness of movement, swelling, crepitation, and presence of nodules.	No swelling No tenderness, swelling, crepitation, or nodules Joints move smoothly	One or more swollen joints Presence of tenderness, swelling, crepitation, or nodules
12. Assess joint range of motion. See Chapter 13 ∞ for the types of joint movements. • Ask the client to move selected body parts. The range of joint movement can be measured by a **goniometer**, a device that measures the angle of the joint movement in degrees. ❶	Varies to some degree in accordance with person's genetic makeup and degree of physical activity	Limited range of motion in one or more joints

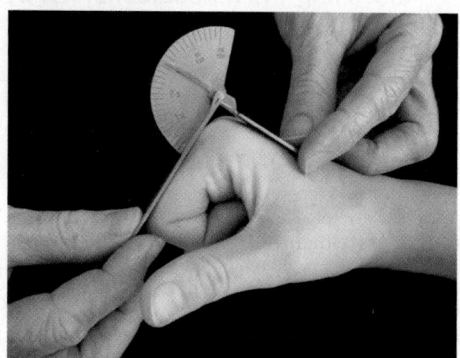

❶ A goniometer is used to measure joint angle.

13. Document findings in the client record using forms or checklists supplemented by narrative notes when appropriate.

EVALUATION

• Relate findings to previous assessment data if available. Perform a detailed system-specific follow-up examination based on findings that deviated from those expected.

• Report deviations from expected findings to the primary care provider.

LIFESPAN CONSIDERATIONS Assessing the Musculoskeletal System

INFANTS

• Palpate the clavicles of newborns. A mass and crepitus may indicate a fracture experienced during vaginal delivery. The newborn may also have limited movement of the arm and shoulder on the affected side.
• When the arms and legs of newborns are pulled to extension and released, newborns naturally return to the flexed fetal position.
• Check muscle strength by holding the infant lightly under the arms with feet placed lightly on a table. Infants should not fall

through the hands and should be able to bear body weight on their legs if normal muscle strength is present.
• Check infants for developmental dysplasia of the hip (congenital dislocation) by examining for asymmetric gluteal folds, asymmetric abduction of the legs (Ortolani and Barlow tests), or apparent shortening of the femur.
• Infants should be able to sit without support by 8 months of age, crawl by 7 to 10 months, and walk by 12 to 15 months.
• Observe for symmetry of muscle mass, strength, and function.

Continued on page 118

LIFESPAN CONSIDERATIONS   Assessing the Musculoskeletal System—*continued*

CHILDREN

- Pronation and "toeing in" of the feet are common in children between 12 and 30 months of age.
- Genu varum (bowleg) is normal in children for about 1 year after beginning to walk.
- Genu valgus (knock-knee) is normal in preschool and early school-age children.
- Lordosis (swayback) is common in children before age 5.
- Observe the child in normal activities to determine motor function.
- During the rapid growth spurts of adolescence, spinal curvature and rotation (scoliosis) may appear. Children should be assessed for scoliosis by age 12 and annually until their growth slows. Curvature greater than 10% should be referred for further medical evaluation.
- Muscle mass increases in adolescence, especially as children engage in strenuous physical activity, and requires increased nutritional intake.
- Children are at risk for injury related to physical activity and should be assessed for nutritional status, physical conditioning, and safety precautions in order to prevent injury.

- Adolescent girls who participate extensively in strenuous athletic activities are at risk for delayed menses, osteoporosis, and eating disorders; assessment should include a history of these factors.

OLDER ADULTS

- Muscle mass decreases progressively with age, but there are wide variations among different individuals.
- The decrease in speed, strength, resistance to fatigue, reaction time, and coordination in the older person is due to a decrease in nerve conduction and muscle tone.
- The bones become more fragile, and osteoporosis leads to a loss of total bone mass. As a result, older adults are predisposed to fractures and compressed vertebrae.
- In most older adults, osteoarthritic changes in the joints can be observed.
- Note any surgical scars from joint replacement surgeries.

Ambulatory and Community Settings   Assessing the Musculoskeletal System   PATIENT-CENTERED CARE

- When making a home visit, observe the client in natural movement around the living area. To assess children, have them remove their clothes down to the underwear.

- A complete examination of joints, bones, and muscles may not be necessary. Focus the assessment on areas indicated by the history and present complaint.

NEUROLOGIC SYSTEM

Examination of the neurologic system includes assessment of (a) mental status, (b) level of consciousness, (c) the cranial nerves, (d) reflexes, (e) motor function, and (f) sensory function. A thorough neurologic examination may take 1 to 3 hours; however, routine screening tests are usually done first. If the results of these screening tests are questionable, more extensive evaluations are made.

To determine the extent of the neurologic exam that is needed, the nurse considers three major factors: (1) the client's chief complaints; (2) the client's physical condition such as **level of consciousness**

(LOC), which is the degree of alertness or awareness, and ability to ambulate because many parts of the exam require coordination of the extremities; and (3) the client's willingness to participate and cooperate. Parts of the neurologic assessment are performed throughout the health examination. For example, the nurse performs a large part of the mental status assessment during the taking of the history and when observing the client's general appearance. The nurse also assesses the function of cranial nerves. Cranial nerves II, III, IV, V, and VI (ophthalmic branch) are assessed with the eyes and vision, and cranial nerve VIII (cochlear branch) is assessed with the ears and hearing.

●○● NURSING PROCESS: ASSESSING THE NEUROLOGIC SYSTEM

Assessing the Neurologic System

SKILL 3–17

PLANNING

If possible, determine whether a screening or full neurologic examination is indicated. This will affect preparation of the client, equipment, and timing.

DELEGATION

Due to the substantial knowledge and skill required, assessment of the neurologic system is not delegated to UAP. However, many aspects of neurologic behavior are observed during usual care and may be recorded by persons other than the nurse. Abnormal findings must be validated and interpreted by the nurse.

INTERPROFESSIONAL PRACTICE

Assessing the neurologic system is within the scope of practice of many health care providers. For example, physical therapists, occupational therapists, and physician assistants will assess those aspects of the client's neurologic functioning relevant to their plan of care. Although these providers may verbally communicate their findings and plan to other health care team members, the nurse must also know where to locate their documentation in the client's medical record.

Equipment (Depending on Components of Examination)

- Percussion hammer
- Wisps of cotton to assess light-touch sensation
- Sterile safety pin for tactile discrimination

Assessing the Neurologic System—*continued*

IMPLEMENTATION

Performance

1. Prior to conducting the examination, introduce self and verify the client's identity using agency protocol. Explain to the client what you are going to do, the reason for the examination, and how he or she can participate. Discuss how the findings will be used in planning further care or treatments.
2. Perform hand hygiene and observe other appropriate infection prevention procedures.
3. Provide for client privacy.
4. Inquire if the client has any of the following: presence of pain in the head, back, or extremities, as well as onset and aggravating and alleviating factors; disorientation to time, place, or person; speech disorder; history of loss of consciousness, fainting, convulsions, trauma, tingling or numbness, tremors or tics, limping, paralysis, uncontrolled muscle movements, loss of memory, mood swings, or problems with smell, vision, taste, touch, or hearing.

CLINICAL ALERT!

All questions and tests used in a neurologic examination must be age, language, education level, and culturally appropriate. Individualize questions and tests before using them.

Language

5. If the client displays difficulty speaking:
   - Point to common objects and ask if the client can name them.
   - If the client can read, ask the client to match written words naming objects with their pictures.
   - Ask the client to respond to simple verbal and written commands, for example, "point to your toes" or "raise your left arm."

Orientation

6. Determine the client's orientation to *time*, *place*, and *person* by tactful questioning. Ask the client the time of day, date, day of the week, duration of illness, city and state of residence, and names of family members. Orientation is lost gradually, and early disorientation may be very subtle. Ask the client the reason he or she is seeing a health care provider. "Why" questions may elicit a more accurate clinical picture of the client's orientation status than questions directed to time, place, and person. If possible, avoid actual use of the word *why* because it can be perceived as threatening. To evaluate the responses, you must know the correct answers.

   More direct questioning may be necessary for some people, for example, "Where are you now?" "What day is it today?" Most people readily accept these questions if initially the nurse asks, "Do you get confused at times?" If the client cannot answer these questions regarding place and time accurately, also include assessment of the *self* by asking the client to state his or her full name.

Memory

7. Listen for lapses in memory. Ask the client about difficulty with memory. If lapses are apparent, three categories of memory are tested: immediate recall, recent memory, and remote memory.

   To assess immediate recall:
   - Ask the client to repeat a series of three digits (e.g., 7–4–3), spoken slowly.
   - Gradually increase the number of digits (e.g., 7–4–3–5, 7–4–3–5–6, and 7–4–3–5–6–7), until the client fails to repeat the series correctly.
   - Start again with a series of three digits, but this time ask the client to repeat them backward. The average person can repeat a series of five to eight digits in sequence and four to six digits in reverse order.

   To assess recent memory:
   - Ask the client to recall the recent events of the day, such as how the client got to the clinic. This information must be validated, however.
   - Ask the client to recall information given early in the interview (e.g., the name of a doctor).
   - Provide the client with three facts to recall (e.g., a color, an object, and an address), and ask the client to repeat all three. Later in the interview, ask the client to recall all three items.

   To assess remote memory:
   - Ask the client to describe a previous illness or surgery (e.g., 5 years ago) or a birthday or anniversary. Generally, remote memory will be intact until late in neurologic pathology and is least useful in assessing acute neurologic problems.

Attention Span and Calculation

8. Test the ability to concentrate or maintain *attention span* by asking the client to recite the alphabet or to count backward from 100. Test the ability to calculate by asking the client to subtract 7 or 3 progressively from 100, that is, 100, 93, 86, 79, or 100, 97, 94, 91 (referred to as *serial sevens* or *serial threes*). Normally, an adult can complete the serial sevens test in about 90 seconds with three or fewer errors. Because educational level, language, or cultural differences affect calculating ability, this test may be inappropriate for some people.

Level of Consciousness

9. Apply the Glasgow Coma Scale (Table 3–8, page 125): eye response, motor response, and verbal response. An assessment totaling 15 points indicates the client is alert and completely oriented. A client who is comatose scores 7 or less.

Cranial Nerves

10. For the specific functions and assessment methods of each cranial nerve, see Table 3–9 on page 126. Test each nerve not already evaluated in another component of the health

Continued on page 120

SKILL 3-17

Assessing the Neurologic System—*continued*

assessment. A quick way to remember which cranial nerves are assessed in the face is shown in ❶.

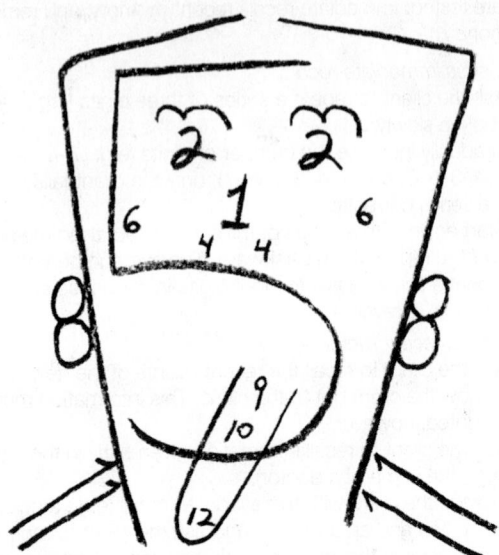

❶ Cranial nerves by the numbers: The next time you're trying to remember the locations and functions of the cranial nerves, picture this drawing. All 12 cranial nerves are represented, though some may be a little harder to spot than others. For example, the shoulders are formed by the number "11" because cranial nerve XI controls neck and shoulder movement. If you immediately recognize that the sides of the face and the top of the head are formed by the number "7," you're well on your way to using this memory device.

From "Strictly Clinical: Facing Cranial Nerve Assessment," by B. Bolek, 2006, *American Nurse Today, 1*(2), pp. 21–22.

Reflexes

11. Generalist nurses do not commonly assess each of the deep tendon reflexes except for the plantar (Babinski) reflex, indicative of possible spinal cord injury. Reflexes are reported using the following scale, comparing one side of the body with the other to evaluate the symmetry of response.

0 No reflex response
+1 Minimal activity (hypoactive)
+2 Normal response
+3 More active than normal
+4 Maximal activity (hyperactive)

Babinski Reflex

- Use a moderately sharp object, such as the handle of the percussion hammer, a key, or an applicator stick.
- Stroke the lateral border of the sole of the client's foot, starting at the heel, continuing to the ball of the foot, and then proceeding across the ball of the foot toward the big toe. ❷
- Observe the response. Normally, all five toes bend downward; this reaction is called a negative Babinski. In an abnormal (positive) Babinski response, the toes spread outward and the big toe moves upward.

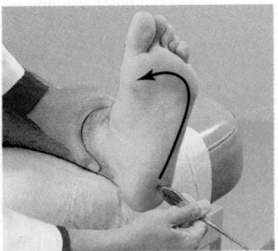

❷ Testing the plantar (Babinski) reflex.

MOTOR FUNCTION

Assessment	Normal Findings	Deviations from Normal
12. *Gross Motor and Balance Tests:* Generally, the Romberg test and one other gross motor function and balance tests are used.		
WALKING GAIT Ask the client to walk across the room and back, and assess the client's gait.	Has upright posture and steady gait with opposing arm swing; walks unaided, maintaining balance	Has poor posture and unsteady, irregular, staggering gait with wide stance; bends legs only from hips; has rigid or no arm movements
ROMBERG TEST Ask the client to stand with feet together and arms resting at the sides, first with eyes open, then closed. Stand close during this test. **Rationale:** *This prevents the client from falling.*	*Negative Romberg:* may sway slightly but is able to maintain upright posture and foot stance	*Positive Romberg:* cannot maintain foot stance; moves the feet apart to maintain stance If client cannot maintain balance with the eyes shut, client may have sensory ataxia (lack of coordination of the voluntary muscles) If balance cannot be maintained whether the eyes are open or shut, client may have cerebellar ataxia

Assessing the Neurologic System—*continued*

Assessment	Normal Findings	Deviations from Normal
STANDING ON ONE FOOT WITH EYES CLOSED		
Ask the client to close the eyes and stand on one foot. Repeat on the other foot. Stand close to the client during this test.	Maintains stance for at least 5 seconds	Cannot maintain stance for 5 seconds
HEEL–TOE WALKING		
Ask the client to walk a straight line, placing the heel of one foot directly in front of the toes of the other foot. ❸	Maintains heel–toe walking along a straight line	Assumes a wider foot gait to stay upright

❸ Heel–toe walking test.

TOE OR HEEL WALKING		
Ask the client to walk several steps on the toes and then on the heels.	Able to walk several steps on toes or heels	Cannot maintain balance on toes and heels
13. *Fine Motor Tests for the Upper Extremities:*		
FINGER TO NOSE		
Ask the client to abduct and extend the arms at shoulder height and then rapidly touch the nose alternately with one index finger and then the other. The client repeats the test with the eyes closed if the test is performed easily. ❹	Repeatedly and rhythmically touches the nose	Misses the nose or gives slow response

❹ Finger-to-nose test.

Continued on page 122

Assessing the Neurologic System—*continued*

SKILL 3–17

Assessment	Normal Findings	Deviations from Normal
ALTERNATING SUPINATION AND PRONATION OF HANDS ON KNEES Ask the client to pat both knees with the palms of both hands and then with the backs of the hands alternately at an ever-increasing rate. ❺	Can alternately supinate and pronate hands at rapid pace	Performs with slow, clumsy movements and irregular timing; has difficulty alternating from supination to pronation

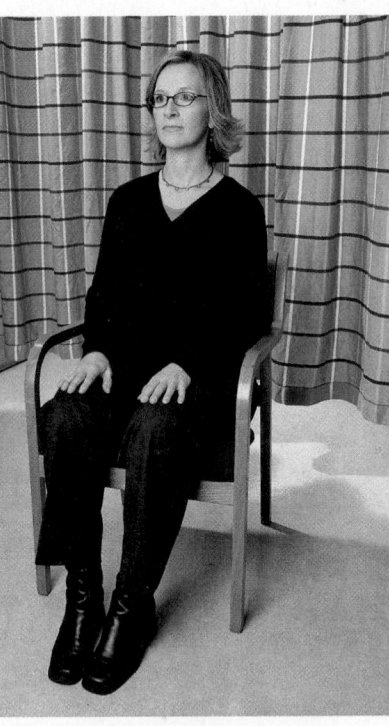 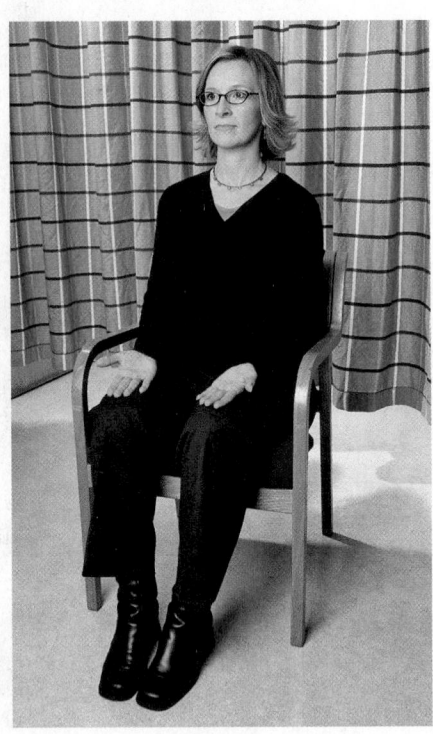

❺ Alternating supination and pronation of hands on knees test.

FINGER TO NOSE AND TO THE NURSE'S FINGER Ask the client to touch the nose and then your index finger, held at a distance of about 45 cm (18 in.), at a rapid and increasing rate. ❻	Performs with coordination and rapidity	Misses the finger and moves slowly

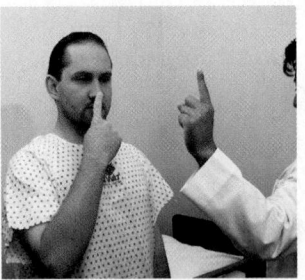 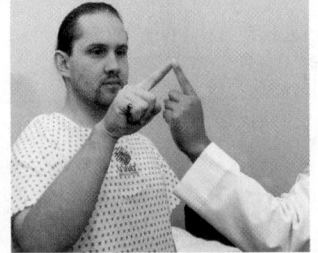

❻ Finger-to-nose and to the nurse's finger test.

FINGERS TO FINGERS Ask the client to spread the arms broadly at shoulder height and then bring the fingers together at the midline, first with the eyes open and then closed, first slowly and then rapidly. ❼	Performs with accuracy and rapidity	Moves slowly and is unable to touch fingers consistently

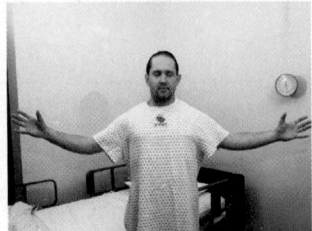 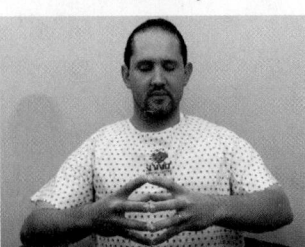

❼ Fingers-to-fingers test.

Assessing the Neurologic System—*continued*

Assessment	Normal Findings	Deviations from Normal

FINGERS TO THUMB (SAME HAND)

Ask the client to touch each finger of one hand to the thumb of the same hand as rapidly as possible. ❽

Rapidly touches each finger to thumb with each hand

Cannot coordinate this fine discrete movement with either one or both hands

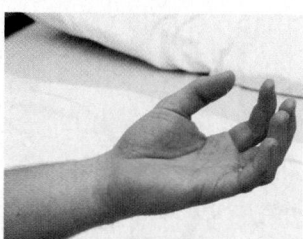

❽ Fingers-to-thumb (same hand) test.

14. *Fine Motor Tests for the Lower Extremities:* Ask the client to lie supine and to perform these tests.

HEEL DOWN OPPOSITE SHIN

Ask the client to place the heel of one foot just below the opposite knee and run the heel down the shin to the foot. Repeat with the other foot. The client may also use a sitting position for this test. ❾

Demonstrates bilateral equal coordination

Has tremors or is awkward; heel moves off shin

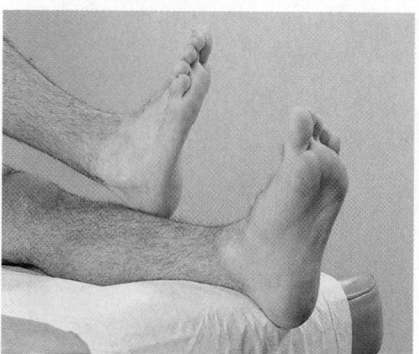

❾ Heel-down-opposite-shin test.

15. *Light-Touch Sensation:* Compare the light-touch sensation of symmetric areas of the body. **Rationale:** *Sensitivity to touch varies among different skin areas.*

- Ask the client to close the eyes and to respond by saying "yes" or "now" whenever the client feels the cotton wisp touching the skin.
- With a wisp of cotton, lightly touch one specific spot and then the same spot on the other side of the body. ❿
- Test areas on the forehead, cheek, hand, lower arm, abdomen, foot, and lower leg. Check a distal area of the limb first (i.e., the hand before the arm and the foot before the leg). **Rationale:** *The sensory nerve may be assumed to be intact if sensation is felt at its most distal part.*
- If areas of sensory dysfunction are found, determine the boundaries of sensation by testing responses about every 2.5 cm (1 in.) in the area. Make a sketch of the sensory loss area for recording purposes.

Light tickling or touch sensation

Loss of sensation (**anesthesia**); more than normal sensation (**hyperesthesia**); less than normal sensation (**hypoesthesia**); or an abnormal sensation such as burning, pain, or an electric shock (**paresthesia**)

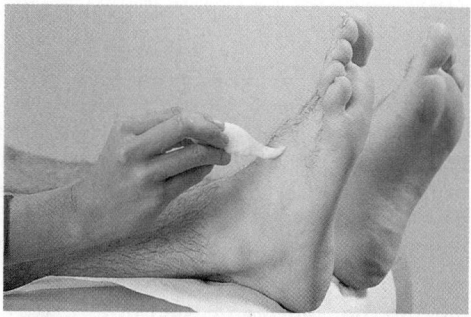

❿ Assessing light-touch sensation.

Continued on page 124

SKILL 3–17

Assessing the Neurologic System—*continued*

Assessment	Normal Findings	Deviations from Normal
16. *Pain Sensation:* Assess pain sensation as follows: • Ask the client to close the eyes and to say "sharp," "dull," or "don't know" when the sharp or dull end of a safety pin is felt. • Alternately, use the sharp and dull end to lightly prick designated anatomic areas at random (e.g., hand, forearm, foot, lower leg, abdomen). The face is not tested in this manner. • Allow at least 2 seconds between each test to prevent summation effects of stimuli, i.e., several successive stimuli perceived as one stimulus.	Able to discriminate "sharp" and "dull" sensations	Areas of reduced, heightened, or absent sensation (map them out for recording purposes)
17. *Position or Kinesthetic Sensation:* Commonly, the middle fingers and the large toes are tested for the kinesthetic sensation (sense of position). • To test the fingers, support the client's arm and hand with one hand. To test the toes, place the client's heels on the examining table. • Ask the client to close the eyes. • Grasp a middle finger or a big toe firmly between your thumb and index finger, and exert the same pressure on both sides of the finger or toe while moving it. ⑪ • Move the finger or toe until it is up, down, or straight out, and ask the client to identify the position. • Use a series of brisk, gentle up-and-down movements before bringing the finger or toe suddenly to rest in one of the three positions.	Can readily determine the position of fingers and toes	Unable to determine the position of one or more fingers or toes
18. Document findings in the client record using forms or checklists supplemented by narrative notes when appropriate. Describe any abnormal findings in objective terms, for example, "When asked to count backward by threes, client made seven errors and completed the task in four minutes."		

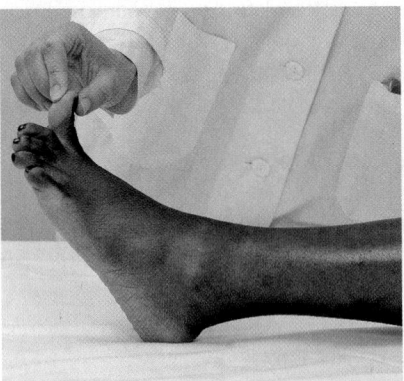

⑪ Position or kinesthetic sensation.

EVALUATION

• Relate findings to previous assessment data if available. Perform a detailed system-specific follow-up examination based on findings that deviated from those expected.

• Report deviations from expected findings to the primary care provider.

LIFESPAN CONSIDERATIONS   Assessing the Neurologic System

INFANTS

• Reflexes commonly tested in newborns include the following:
  • *Rooting:* Stroke the side of the face near the mouth; infant opens mouth and turns to the side that is stroked.
  • *Sucking:* Place nipple or finger 3 to 4 cm (1.2 to 1.6 in.) into mouth; infant sucks vigorously.

• *Tonic neck:* Place infant supine, turn head to one side; arm on side to which head is turned extends; on opposite side, arm curls up (fencer's pose).
• *Palmar grasp:* Place finger in infant's palm and press; infant curls fingers around.

LIFESPAN CONSIDERATIONS Assessing the Neurologic System—*continued*

- *Stepping:* Hold infant as if weight bearing on surface; infant steps along, one foot at a time.
  - *Moro:* Present loud noise or unexpected movement; infant spreads arms and legs, extends fingers, then flexes and brings hands together; may cry.
- Most of these reflexes disappear between 4 and 6 months of age.

CHILDREN
- Present the procedures as games whenever possible.
- Positive Babinski reflex is abnormal after the child ambulates or at age 2.
- For children under age 6, the Denver Developmental Screening Test II provides a comprehensive neurologic evaluation— particularly for motor function.
- Note the child's ability to understand and follow directions.
- Assess immediate recall or recent memory by using names of well-known media (e.g., movie or cartoon) characters. Normal recall in children is one less character than the age of the child in years. For example, normal recall for a 5-year-old would be four characters.
- Assess for signs of hyperactivity or abnormally short attention span.
- Children should be able to walk backward by age 2, balance on one foot for 5 seconds by age 4, heel–toe walk by age 5, and heel–toe walk backward by age 6.
- The Romberg test is appropriate over age 3.

OLDER ADULTS
- Because older adults tire more easily than younger clients, a total neurologic assessment is often done at a different time from the other parts of the physical assessment.
- A full neurologic assessment can be lengthy. Conduct in several sessions if indicated, and cease the tests if the client is noticeably fatigued.
- A decline in mental status is not a normal result of aging. Changes are more the result of physical or psychological

disorders (e.g., fever, fluid and electrolyte imbalances, medications). Acute, abrupt-onset mental status changes are usually caused by delirium. These changes are often reversible with treatment. Chronic subtle insidious mental health changes are usually caused by dementia and are usually irreversible.
- Intelligence and learning ability are unaltered with age. Many factors, however, inhibit learning (e.g., anxiety, illness, pain, cultural barrier).
- Short-term memory is often less efficient. Long-term memory is usually unaltered.
- Because old age is often associated with loss of support persons, depression can occur. Mood changes, weight loss, anorexia, constipation, and early morning awakening may be symptoms of depression.
- The stress of being in unfamiliar situations can cause confusion in older adults.
- As a person ages, reflex responses may become less intense.
- Although there is a progressive decrease in the number of functioning neurons in the central nervous system and in the sense organs, older adults usually function well because of the abundant reserves in the number of brain cells.
- Impulse transmission and reaction to stimuli are slower.
- Many older adults have some impairment of hearing, vision, smell, temperature and pain sensation, memory, or mental endurance.
- Coordination changes, including a reduced speed of fine finger movements. Standing balance remains intact, and Romberg's test remains negative.
- Reflex responses may slightly increase or decrease. Many show loss of Achilles reflex, and the plantar reflex may be difficult to elicit.
- When testing sensory function, the nurse needs to give older adults time to respond. Normally, older adults have unaltered perception of light touch and superficial pain, decreased perception of deep pain, and decreased perception of temperature stimuli. Many also reveal a decrease or absence of position sense in the large toes.

TABLE 3–8 Levels of Consciousness: Glasgow Coma Scale

Faculty Measured	Response	Score
Eye opening	Spontaneous	4
	To verbal command	3
	To pain	2
	No response	1
Motor response	To verbal command	6
	To localized pain	5
	Flexes and withdraws	4
	Flexes abnormally	3
	Extends abnormally	2
	No response	1
Verbal response	Oriented, converses	5
	Disoriented, converses	4
	Uses inappropriate words	3
	Makes incomprehensible sounds	2
	No response	1

TABLE 3–9   Cranial Nerve Functions and Assessment Methods

Cranial Nerve	Name	Type	Function	Assessment Method
I	Olfactory	Sensory	Smell	Ask client to close eyes and identify different mild aromas, such as coffee, vanilla, peanut butter, orange/lemon, chocolate.
II	Optic	Sensory	Vision and visual fields	Ask client to read Snellen-type chart; check visual fields by confrontation; and conduct an ophthalmoscopic examination (see Skill 3–6).
III	Oculomotor	Motor	Extraocular eye movement (EOM); movement of sphincter of pupil; movement of ciliary muscles of lens	Assess six ocular movements and pupil reaction (see Skill 3–6).
IV	Trochlear	Motor	EOM; specifically, moves eyeball downward and laterally	Assess six ocular movements (see Skill 3–6).
V	Trigeminal 　Ophthalmic branch	Sensory	Sensation of cornea, skin of face, and nasal mucosa	While client looks upward, lightly touch the lateral sclera of the eye with sterile gauze to elicit blink reflex. To test light sensation, have client close eyes, wipe a wisp of cotton over client's forehead and paranasal sinuses.
	Maxillary branch	Sensory	Sensation of skin of face and anterior oral cavity (tongue and teeth)	Assess skin sensation as for ophthalmic branch above.
	Mandibular branch	Motor and sensory	Muscles of mastication; sensation of skin of face	Ask client to clench teeth.
VI	Abducens	Motor	EOM; moves eyeball laterally	Assess directions of gaze.
VII	Facial	Motor and sensory	Facial expression; taste (anterior two thirds of tongue)	Ask client to smile, raise the eyebrows, frown, puff out cheeks, close eyes tightly. Ask client to identify various tastes placed on tip and sides of tongue: sugar (sweet), salt, lemon juice (sour), and quinine (bitter); identify areas of taste.
VIII	Auditory 　Vestibular branch 　Cochlear branch	Sensory Sensory	Equilibrium Hearing	Romberg test (see page 120). Assess client's ability to hear spoken word and vibrations of tuning fork.
IX	Glossopharyngeal	Motor and sensory	Swallowing ability, tongue movement, taste (posterior tongue)	Apply tastes on posterior tongue for identification. Ask client to move tongue from side to side and up and down.
X	Vagus	Motor and sensory	Sensation of pharynx and larynx; swallowing; vocal cord movement	Assessed with cranial nerve IX; assess client's speech for hoarseness.
XI	Accessory	Motor	Head movement; shrugging of shoulders	Ask client to shrug shoulders against resistance from your hands and turn head to side against resistance from your hand (repeat for other side).
XII	Hypoglossal	Motor	Protrusion of tongue; moves tongue up and down and side to side	Ask client to protrude tongue at midline, then move it side to side.

FEMALE GENITALS AND INGUINAL AREA

In generalist nursing practice, the assessment of the adult female genitals and reproductive tract includes examination of the inguinal lymph nodes and inspection of the external genitals. The extent of the assessment of the genitals and reproductive tract depends on the needs and problems of the individual client. Examination of the genitals usually creates uncertainty and apprehension in women and can cause embarrassment. The nurse must perform the examination in an objective and efficient manner.

Not all agencies permit male practitioners to examine the female genitals. Some agencies may require the presence of another female during the examination so that there is no question of unprofessional behavior. Most female clients accept examination by a male, especially if he is emotionally comfortable about performing the examination and does so in a matter-of-fact and competent manner. If the male nurse does not feel comfortable about this part of the examination or if the client is reluctant to be examined by a man, the nurse should refer this part of the examination to a female practitioner.

●○● NURSING PROCESS: ASSESSING THE FEMALE GENITALS AND INGUINAL AREA

Assessing the Female Genitals and Inguinal Area

SKILL 3-18

PLANNING
DELEGATION

Due to the substantial knowledge and skill required, assessment of the female genitals and inguinal lymph nodes is not delegated to UAP. However, individuals other than the nurse may record any aspect of the genital system that is observed during usual care. Abnormal findings must be validated and interpreted by the nurse.

INTERPROFESSIONAL PRACTICE

Assessing the female genitals and inguinal area is within the scope of practice of health care providers, specifically physician assistants conducting their own health assessment. Although these providers may verbally communicate their findings and plan to other health care team members, the nurse must also know where to locate their documentation in the client's medical record.

Equipment
- Clean gloves
- Drape
- Supplemental lighting, if needed

IMPLEMENTATION
Performance

1. Prior to conducting the examination, introduce self and verify the client's identity using agency protocol. Explain to the client what you are going to do, the reason for the examination, and how she can participate. Discuss how the findings will be used in planning further care or treatments.
2. Perform hand hygiene, apply gloves, and observe other appropriate infection control procedures.
3. Provide for client privacy. Request the presence of another woman if desired, required by agency policy, or requested by the client.

4. Inquire regarding the following: age of onset of menstruation, date of last menstrual period (LMP), regularity of cycle, duration, amount of daily flow, and whether menstruation is painful; incidence of pain during intercourse; vaginal discharge; number of pregnancies, number of live births, labor or delivery complications; urgency and frequency of urination at night; blood in urine, painful urination, incontinence; and history of sexually transmitted infection, past and present.
5. Cover the pelvic area with a sheet or drape at all times when not actually being examined. Position the client supine.

Assessment	Normal Findings	Deviations from Normal
6. Inspect the distribution, amount, and characteristics of pubic hair.	There are wide variations; generally kinky in the menstruating adult, thinner and straighter after menopause Distributed in the shape of an inverse triangle	Scant pubic hair (may indicate hormonal problem) Hair growth should not extend over the abdomen
7. Inspect the skin of the pubic area for parasites, inflammation, swelling, and lesions. To assess pubic skin adequately, separate the labia majora and labia minora.	Pubic skin intact, no lesions Skin of vulva area slightly darker than the rest of the body Minimal odor Labia round, full, and relatively symmetric in adult females	Lice, lesions, scars, fissures, swelling, erythema, excoriations, varicosities, or leukoplakia Malodorous discharge; thin, friable labia; protruding uterus
8. Palpate the inguinal lymph nodes. ❶ Use the pads of the fingers in a rotary motion, noting any enlargement or tenderness.	No enlargement or tenderness	Enlargement and tenderness

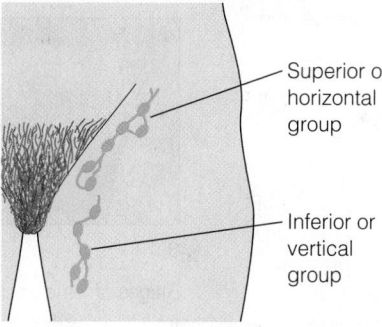

Superior or horizontal group

Inferior or vertical group

❶ Lymph nodes of the groin area.

Continued on page 128

Assessing the Female Genitals and Inguinal Area—*continued*

Assessment	Normal Findings	Deviations from Normal
9. Remove and discard gloves. • Perform hand hygiene. **10.** Document findings in the client record using forms or checklists supplemented by narrative notes when appropriate.		

EVALUATION

• Relate findings to previous assessment data if available. Perform a detailed system-specific follow-up examination based on findings that deviated from those expected.

• Significant deviations from normal indicate the need for an internal vaginal examination.

LIFESPAN CONSIDERATIONS | **Assessing the Female Genitals and Inguinal Lymph Nodes**

INFANTS

• Infants can be held in a supine position on the parent's lap with the knees supported in a flexed position and separated.
• In newborns, because of maternal estrogen, the labia and clitoris may be edematous and enlarged, and there may be a small amount of white or bloody vaginal discharge.
• Assess the mons and inguinal area for swelling or tenderness that may indicate presence of an inguinal hernia.

CHILDREN

• Ensure that you have the parent or guardian's approval to perform the examination and then explain to the child what you are going to do. Preschool children are taught not to allow others to touch their "private parts."
• Girls should be assessed for Tanner staging of pubertal development (see Box 3–8).
• Girls should be referred to a primary care provider for a Papanicolaou (Pap) test if sexually active, or by age 18 years.
• The clitoris is a common site for syphilitic chancres in younger females.

OLDER ADULTS

• Labia are atrophied and flattened.
• The clitoris is a potential site for cancerous lesions.
• The vulva atrophies as a result of a reduction in vascularity, elasticity, adipose tissue, and estrogen levels. Because the vulva is more fragile, it is more easily irritated.
• The vaginal environment becomes drier and more alkaline, resulting in an alteration of the type of flora present and a predisposition to vaginitis. Dyspareunia (difficult or painful intercourse) is also a common occurrence.
• The cervix and uterus decrease in size.
• The fallopian tubes and ovaries atrophy.
• Ovulation and estrogen production cease.
• Vaginal bleeding unrelated to estrogen therapy is abnormal in older women.
• Prolapse of the uterus can occur in older females, especially those who have had multiple pregnancies.

BOX 3–8 | **Five Stages of Pubic Hair Development in Females**

Stage 1: Preadolescence. No pubic hair except for fine body hair.
Stage 2: Usually occurs at ages 11 and 12. Sparse, long, slightly pigmented curly hair develops along the labia.
Stage 3: Usually occurs at ages 12 and 13. Hair becomes darker in color and curlier and develops over the pubic symphysis.
Stage 4: Usually occurs between ages 13 and 14. Hair assumes the texture and curl of the adult but is not as thick and does not appear on the thighs.
Stage 5: Sexual maturity. Hair assumes adult appearance and appears on the inner aspect of the upper thighs.

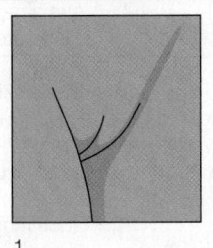 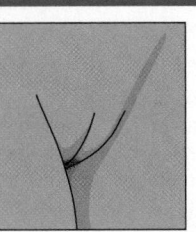
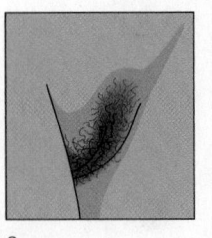 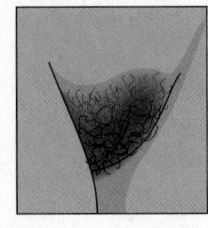 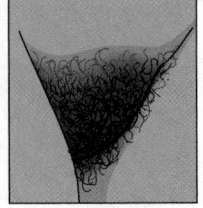

Stages of female pubic hair development.

MALE GENITALS AND INGUINAL AREA

In adult males, complete examination should include assessment of the external genitals, the inguinal area, and the prostate gland. As with females, generalist nurses routinely assess only the inguinal lymph nodes and external genitals. Examination of the male genitals by a female practitioner is becoming increasingly common, although not all agencies permit a female practitioner to examine the male genitals.

Some agencies may require the presence of another person during the examination so that there is no question of unprofessional behavior. Most male clients accept examination by a female, especially if she is emotionally comfortable about performing the examination and does so in a matter-of-fact and competent manner. If the female nurse does not feel comfortable about this part of the examination or if the client is reluctant to be examined by a woman, the nurse should refer this part of the examination to a male practitioner.

●○○● NURSING PROCESS: ASSESSING THE MALE GENITALS AND INGUINAL AREA

Assessing the Male Genitals and Inguinal Area

SKILL 3–19

PLANNING
DELEGATION

Due to the substantial knowledge and skill required, assessment of the male genitals and inguinal area is not delegated to UAP. However, individuals other than the nurse may record any aspect of the genital system that is observed during usual care. Abnormal findings must be validated and interpreted by the nurse.

INTERPROFESSIONAL PRACTICE

Assessing the male genitals and inguinal area is within the scope of practice of health care providers other than nurses, specifically physician assistants conducting their own health assessment. Although the providers may verbally communicate their findings and plan to other health care team members, the nurse must also know where to locate their documentation in the client's medical record.

Equipment
• Clean gloves

IMPLEMENTATION
Performance

1. Prior to conducting the examination, introduce self and verify the client's identity using agency protocol. Explain to the client what you are going to do, the reason for the examination, and how he can participate. Discuss how the findings will be used in planning further care or treatments.
2. Perform hand hygiene, apply gloves, and observe other appropriate infection control procedures.
3. Provide for client privacy. Request the presence of another person if desired, required by agency policy, or requested by the client.

4. Inquire regarding the following: usual voiding patterns and changes, bladder control, urinary incontinence, frequency, urgency, abdominal pain; symptoms of sexually transmitted infection; swellings that could indicate presence of hernia; and family history of nephritis, malignancy of the prostate, or malignancy of the kidney.
5. Cover the pelvic area with a sheet or drape at all times when not actually being examined.

Assessment	Normal Findings	Deviations from Normal
PUBIC HAIR		
6. Inspect the distribution, amount, and characteristics of pubic hair.	Triangular distribution, often spreading up the abdomen	Scant amount or absence of hair
PENIS		
7. Inspect the penile shaft and glans penis for lesions, nodules, swellings, and inflammation.	Penile skin intact Appears slightly wrinkled and varies in color as widely as other body skin Foreskin (if present) easily retractable from the glans penis Small amount of thick white smegma between the glans and foreskin	Presence of lesions, nodules, swellings, or inflammation Foreskin not retractable Large amount, discolored, or malodorous substance
8. Inspect the urethral meatus for swelling, inflammation, discharge, and position.	Pink and slitlike appearance Positioned at the tip of the penis	Inflammation; discharge Variation in meatal locations (e.g., hypospadias, on the underside of the penile shaft, and epispadias, on the upper side of the penile shaft)

Continued on page 130

SKILL 3–19

Assessing the Male Genitals and Inguinal Area—*continued*

Assessment	Normal Findings	Deviations from Normal
SCROTUM 9. Inspect the scrotum for appearance, general size, and symmetry. • Inspect all skin surfaces by spreading the rugated surface skin and lifting the scrotum as needed to observe posterior surfaces.	Scrotal skin is darker in color than that of the rest of the body and is loose Size varies with temperature changes (the dartos muscles contract when the area is cold and relax when the area is warm) Scrotum appears asymmetric (left testis is usually lower than right testis)	Discolorations; any tightening of skin (may indicate edema or mass) Marked asymmetry in size
INGUINAL AREA 10. Inspect both inguinal areas for bulges while the client is standing, if possible. • First, have the client remain at rest. • Next, have the client hold his breath and strain or bear down as though having a bowel movement. Bearing down may make the hernia more visible. 11. Remove and discard gloves. • Perform hand hygiene. 12. Document findings in the client record using forms or checklists supplemented by narrative notes when appropriate.	No swelling or bulges	Swelling or bulge (possible inguinal or femoral hernia)

EVALUATION
• Relate findings to previous assessment data if available. Perform a detailed system-specific follow-up examination based on findings that deviated from those expected.

• Report deviations from expected findings to the primary care provider.

LIFESPAN CONSIDERATIONS **Assessing the Male Genitals and Inguinal Area**

INFANTS
• The foreskin of the uncircumcised infant is normally tight at birth and should not be retracted. It will gradually loosen as the baby grows and is usually fully retractable by 2 to 3 years of age. Assess for cleanliness, redness, or irritation.
• Assess for placement of the urethral meatus.
• Palpate the scrotum to determine if the testes are descended; in the newborn and infant, the testes may retract into the inguinal canal, especially with stimulation of the cremasteric reflex.
• Assess the inguinal area for swelling or tenderness that may indicate the presence of an inguinal hernia.

CHILDREN
• Ensure that you have the parent or guardian's approval to perform the examination and then tell the child what you are going to do. Preschool children are taught not to allow others to touch their "private parts."

• In young boys, the cremasteric reflex can cause the testes to ascend into the inguinal canal. If possible have the boy sit cross-legged; this stretches the muscle and decreases the reflex.
• Table 3–10 shows the five Tanner stages of development of pubic hair, penis, and testes/scrotum.

OLDER ADULTS
• The penis decreases in size with age; the size and firmness of the testes decrease.
• Testosterone is produced in smaller amounts.
• More time and direct physical stimulation are required for an older man to achieve an erection, but he may experience premature ejaculation less often than he did at a younger age.
• Seminal fluid is reduced in amount and viscosity.
• Urinary frequency, nocturia, dribbling, and problems with beginning and ending the stream are usually the result of prostatic enlargement.

TABLE 3–10	Tanner Stages of Male Pubic Hair and External Genital Development (12 to 16 Years)			
Stage	**Pubic Hair**	**Penis**	**Testes/Scrotum**	
1	None, except for body hair like that on the abdomen	Size is relative to body size, as in childhood	Size is relative to body size, as in childhood	
2	Scant, long, slightly pigmented at base of penis	Slight enlargement occurs	Becomes reddened in color and enlarged	
3	Darker, begins to curl and becomes more coarse; extends over pubic symphysis	Elongation occurs	Continuing enlargement	
4	Continues to darken and thicken; extends on the sides, above and below	Increase in both breadth and length; glans develops	Continuing enlargement; color darkens	
5	Adult distribution that extends to inner thighs, umbilicus, and anus	Adult appearance	Adult appearance	

ANAL AREA

Examination of the anal area is part of every comprehensive physical examination. In many practice settings, the generalist nurse inspects but does not palpate the anal area.

●○● NURSING PROCESS: ASSESSING THE ANUS

Assessing the Anus

PLANNING
DELEGATION

Due to the substantial knowledge and skill required, assessment of the anus is not delegated to UAP. However, the condition of the anal area may be observed during usual care and may be recorded by individuals other than the nurse. Abnormal findings must be validated and interpreted by the nurse.

INTERPROFESSIONAL PRACTICE

Assessing the anus is within the scope of practice of health care providers, specifically physician assistants conducting their own health assessment. Although these providers may verbally communicate their findings and plan to other health care team members, the nurse must also know where to locate their documentation in the client's medical record.

Equipment
* Clean gloves

SKILL 3–20

Continued on page 132

Assessing the Anus—*continued*

IMPLEMENTATION
Performance

1. Prior to conducting the examination, introduce self and verify the client's identity using agency protocol. Explain to the client what you are going to do, the reason for the examination, and how he or she can participate. Discuss how the findings will be used in planning further care or treatments.
2. Perform hand hygiene, apply gloves, and observe other appropriate infection control procedures for all rectal examinations.
3. Provide for client privacy. Drape the client appropriately to prevent undue exposure of body parts.
4. Inquire if the client has any history of the following: bright blood in stools, tarry black stools, diarrhea, constipation, abdominal pain, excessive gas, hemorrhoids, or rectal pain; family history of colorectal cancer; when last stool specimen for occult blood was performed and the results; and for males, if not obtained during the genitourinary examination, signs or symptoms of prostate enlargement (e.g., slow urinary stream, hesitance, frequency, dribbling, and nocturia).
5. Position the client in a left lateral or Sims' position with the upper leg acutely flexed. A dorsal recumbent position with hips externally rotated and knees flexed may also be used. For males, a standing position while the client bends over the examining table may also be used.

Assessment	Normal Findings	Deviations from Normal
6. Inspect the anus and surrounding tissue for color, integrity, and skin lesions. Then, ask the client to bear down as though defecating. Bearing down creates slight pressure on the skin that may accentuate rectal fissures, rectal prolapse, polyps, or internal hemorrhoids. Describe the location of all abnormal findings in terms of a clock, with the 12 o'clock position toward the pubic symphysis. 7. Remove and discard gloves. • Perform hand hygiene. 8. Document findings in the client record using forms or checklists supplemented by narrative notes when appropriate.	Intact perianal skin; usually slightly more pigmented than the skin of the buttocks Anal skin is normally more pigmented, coarser, and moister than perianal skin and is usually hairless	Presence of fissures (cracks), ulcers, excoriations, inflammations, abscesses, protruding hemorrhoids (dilated veins seen as reddened protrusions of the skin), lumps or tumors, fistula openings, or rectal prolapse (varying degrees of protrusion of the rectal mucous membrane through the anus)

SAMPLE DOCUMENTATION

12/26/2015 1430 c/o itching and soreness around anal area. Anal skin clean, intact, slightly reddened. No signs of hemorrhoids or lesions. Encouraged to lie in lateral position more frequently. Reassess q shift. ———————————————————————— T. Nevel, RN

EVALUATION

• Relate findings to previous assessment data if available. Perform a detailed system-specific follow-up examination based on findings that deviated from those expected.

• Report deviations from expected findings to the primary care provider.

LIFESPAN CONSIDERATIONS   Assessing the Anus

INFANTS
• Lightly touching the anus should result in a brief anal contraction ("wink" reflex).

CHILDREN
• Erythema and scratch marks around the anus may indicate a pinworm parasite. Children with this condition may be disturbed by itching during sleep.

OLDER ADULTS
• Chronic constipation and straining at stool cause an increase in the frequency of hemorrhoids and rectal prolapse.

FLUID BALANCE

Physical assessment to evaluate a client's fluid balance includes aspects of assessment from many of the body systems including the skin, the oral cavity and mucous membranes, the eyes, the cardiovascular and respiratory systems, and neurologic and muscular status. Data from this physical assessment are used to expand and verify information obtained in the nursing history (Box 3–9). The focused physical assessment is summarized in Table 3–11.

BOX 3–9	Focused Health History Related to Fluid Balance

CURRENT AND PAST MEDICAL HISTORY
- Are you currently seeing a health care provider for treatment of any chronic diseases such as kidney disease, heart disease, high blood pressure, diabetes, or thyroid or parathyroid disorders?
- Have you experienced any acute conditions such as gastroenteritis, severe trauma, head injury, or surgery in the past 6 months? If so, describe them.

MEDICATIONS AND TREATMENTS
- Are you taking any medications on a regular basis such as diuretics, laxatives, steroids, hormones, or salt substitutes?
- Have you undergone any treatments such as dialysis, parenteral nutrition, or tube feedings in the past 6 months? If so, when and why?

FOOD AND FLUID INTAKE
- How much and what type of fluids do you drink each day?
- Do you restrict fluid intake in the evening in order to avoid the need to urinate during the night?
- Have there been any changes in your fluid intake in the past 6 months?
- Are you on any type of restricted diet?
- Has your fluid intake been affected by changes in appetite, nausea, or other factors such as pain or difficulty breathing?

FLUID OUTPUT
- Have you noticed any changes in the frequency or amount of urine output?
- Have you experienced any problems with vomiting, diarrhea, or constipation? If so, when and for how long?
- Have you noticed any other unusual fluid losses such as excessive sweating?

FLUID IMBALANCES
- Have you gained or lost weight in recent weeks? Was this gain or loss intentional?
- Have you recently experienced any symptoms such as excessive thirst, dry skin or mucous membranes, dark or concentrated urine, or low urine output?
- Do you have problems with swelling of your hands, feet, or ankles? Do you ever have difficulty breathing, especially when lying down or at night? How many pillows do you use to sleep?
- Have you experienced any of the following symptoms in the past 6 months: difficulty concentrating or confusion; dizziness or feeling faint; muscle weakness, twitching, cramping, or spasm; excessive fatigue; abnormal sensations such as numbness, tingling, burning, or prickling; abdominal cramping or distention; heart palpitations?

TABLE 3–11	Focused Physical Assessment for Fluid Balance

System	Assessment Focus	Technique	Possible Abnormal Findings
Skin	Color, temperature, moisture	Inspection, palpation	Flushed, warm, very dry Moist or diaphoretic Cool and pale
	Turgor	Gently grasp a fold of skin over sternum or inner aspect of thigh for adults; on the abdomen or medial thigh for children	Poor turgor: Skin remains tented for several seconds instead of immediately returning to normal position
	Edema	Inspect for visible swelling around eyes, in fingers, and in lower extremities	Skin around eyes is puffy, lids appear swollen; rings are tight; shoes leave impressions on feet
		Compress the skin over the dorsum of the foot, around the ankles, over the tibia, in the sacral area	Depression remains (pitting); see scale for describing edema in ❶ on page 68
Mucous membranes	Color, moisture	Inspection	Mucous membranes dry, dull in appearance; tongue dry and cracked
Eyes	Firmness	Gently palpate eyeball with lid closed	Eyeball feels soft to palpation
Cardiovascular system	Heart rate	Auscultation, cardiac monitor	Tachycardia, bradycardia; irregular; dysrhythmias
	Peripheral pulses	Palpation	Weak and thready; bounding
	Blood pressure	Auscultation of Korotkoff's sounds	Hypotension
		BP assessment lying and standing	Postural hypotension
	Capillary refill	Palpation	Slowed capillary refill
	Venous filling	Inspection of jugular veins and hand veins	Jugular venous distention; flat jugular veins, poor venous refill
Respiratory system	Respiratory rate and pattern	Inspection	Increased or decreased rate and depth of respirations
	Lung sounds	Auscultation	Crackles or moist rales
Neurologic system	LOC	Observation, stimulation	Decreased LOC, lethargy, stupor, or coma
	Orientation, cognition	Questioning	Disoriented, confused; difficulty concentrating

Three clinical measurements of fluid balance that the nurse can initiate independently are daily weights, vital signs, and fluid intake and output.

Daily Weights

Daily weight measurements provide an assessment of a client's fluid status. Significant changes in weight over a short time, such as more than 1 kg (2 lb) in a week, may be indicative of acute fluid changes. Each kilogram (2.2 lb) of weight is equivalent to 1 L of fluid. Rapid loss or gain of 5% to 8% of total body weight indicates moderate to severe fluid volume deficit or excess.

To obtain accurate weight measurements, the nurse should balance the scale before each use and weigh the client at the same time each day, wearing the same or similar clothing, and on the same scale. The type of scale (i.e., standing, bed, chair) should be documented.

Assessment of weight is important for clients in the community and extended care facilities who may be at risk for fluid imbalance. For these clients, measuring intake and output may be impractical. A program of regular weight measurement provides valuable information about this client's fluid volume status.

Vital Signs

Changes in a client's vital signs may indicate actual or impending fluid imbalances. For example, elevated body temperature may be a result of dehydration or a cause of increased body fluid losses.

Fluid Intake and Output

Measuring and recording of all fluid intake and output (I&O) during a 24-hour period provides important data about the client's fluid and electrolyte balance. Generally, I&O are measured for clients at risk for fluid imbalance due to their health problem or treatment.

The medical unit used to measure I&O is the milliliter (mL). In the community, fluid volumes may be measured in either metric (mL) or household (ounces, pints, quarts, gallons) units. Examples of common fluid volumes are given in Table 3–12.

TABLE 3–12	Fluid Containers and Their Common Volumes*	
Water glass	7 fluid ounces	210 mL
Juice glass	4 fluid ounces	120 mL
Cup	6 fluid ounces	180 mL
Soup bowl		
Adult	6 fluid ounces	180 mL
Child	3 fluid ounces	90 mL
Teapot	8 fluid ounces	240 mL
Creamer, small	1 fluid ounce	30 mL
Water pitcher	32 fluid ounces	960 mL
Jell-O, custard dish	3 fluid ounces	90 mL
Ice cream dish	4 fluid ounces	120 mL
Paper cup		
Large	7 fluid ounces	210 mL
Small	4 fluid ounces	120 mL

*The exact number of ounces per container varies by manufacturer and the degree to which it is filled. If an extremely accurate volume is needed, the nurse measures the fluid first and then pours it into the container.

●○○ NURSING PROCESS: ASSESSING FLUID BALANCE

Assessing Intake and Output

PLANNING

Assessing fluid intake and output is an ongoing process that requires the nurse to have measuring devices and methods of recording easily accessible. Most agencies have a form for recording incremental I&O. Usually there is a bedside record on which the nurse lists all items measured and the quantities per shift. These values are then transferred into the permanent chart record in the appropriate place (often on the vital signs record). ❶

DELEGATION

Measurement and recording of normal oral fluid intake or urinary and gastrointestinal output may be delegated to UAP. Measurement of parenteral fluid intake and output from wounds and tubes is generally not delegated to UAP.

INTERPROFESSIONAL PRACTICE

Assessing intake and output is within the scope of practice of many health care providers, although generally only nurses record this data in the client record. If the client requires measurement of intake or output and other providers are likely to supply fluid intake to the client or dispose of fluid output, it is essential that the nurse notify the provider of this requirement.

Equipment
- Graduated measuring containers
- I&O records
- Signs to post in room indicating that the client requires I&O recording

IMPLEMENTATION
Performance
1. Prior to conducting the assessment, introduce self and verify the client's identity using agency protocol. Explain to the client what you are going to do, the reason for the assessment, and how he or she can participate. Discuss how the findings will be used in planning further care or treatments.
2. Perform hand hygiene and observe other appropriate infection prevention procedures.

3. If necessary, record on the Kardex or nursing care plan that the client's I&O are to be measured, including when volumes should be totaled. In many cases, fluid balance is summed every shift and then totaled for the entire previous 24 hours. In extremely acute situations, the client's I&O may be evaluated hourly so that changes in treatment can be implemented immediately.

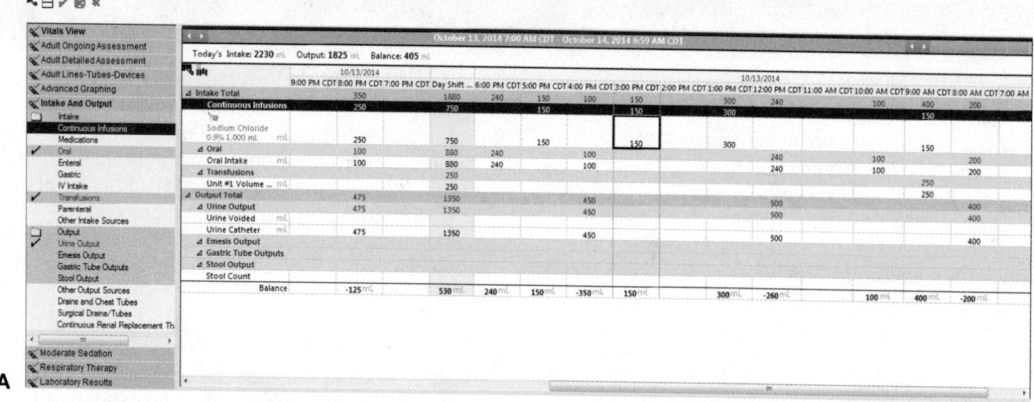

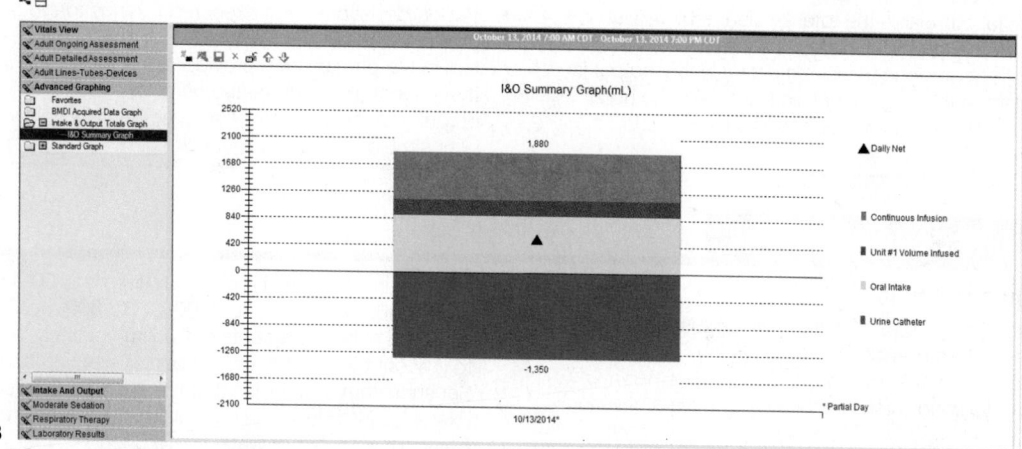

❶ *A*, A sample EHR fluid intake and output record; *B*, A sample 24 hour EHR summary graph.

4. Recording intake: Clients who wish to be involved in recording their own fluid intake measurements need to be taught how to compute the values and what to measure. Record each fluid item taken, specifying the time and type of fluid. All of the following fluids need to be recorded:

   - *Oral fluids.* Water, milk, juice, soft drinks, coffee, tea, cream, soup, and any other beverages. Include water taken with medications. To assess the amount of water taken from a water pitcher, measure what remains and subtract this amount from the volume of the full pitcher. Then refill the pitcher.

   - *Ice chips.* Record the fluid as approximately one half the volume of the ice chips. For example, if the ice chips fill a cup holding 200 mL and the client consumed all of the ice chips, the volume consumed would be recorded as 100 mL.

   - *Foods that are or tend to become liquid at room temperature.* These include ice cream, sherbet, custard, and gelatin. Do not measure foods that are pureed, because purees are simply solid foods prepared in a different form.

   - *Tube feedings.* Remember to include the amount of water flush following medication administration, at the end of intermittent feedings, or during continuous feedings.

   - *Parenteral fluids.* The exact amount of intravenous fluid administered is to be recorded. Blood transfusions and fluids used to flush medications are included.

   - *Intravenous medications.* Intravenous medications that are prepared with solutions such as normal saline (NS) and are administered as an intermittent or continuous infusion must also be included (e.g., ceftazidime 1 g in 50 mL of sterile water). Most intravenous medications are mixed in 50 to 100 mL of solution.

   - *Catheter or tube irrigants.* If the fluid used to irrigate urinary catheters, nasogastric tubes, and intestinal tubes or remaining after peritoneal dialysis (see Chapter 22 ∞) is not aspirated after instillation, the remaining fluid volume must be measured and recorded.

5. Recording output: Inform clients, family members, and all caregivers that accurate measurements of the client's fluid intake and output are required, explaining why and emphasizing the need to use a bedpan, urinal, commode, or in-toilet collection device (unless a urinary drainage system is in place). Instruct the client not to put toilet tissue into the container with urine. Clients who wish to be involved in recording their own fluid output measurements need to be taught how to handle the fluids and to compute the values. To measure fluid output, measure the following fluids (remember to observe appropriate infection prevention precautions):

   - *Urinary output.* Following each voiding, pour the urine into a measuring container, observe the amount, and record it and the time of voiding on the I&O form. For clients with retention catheters, empty the drainage bag into a measuring container at the end of the shift (or at prescribed times if output is to be measured more often). Sometimes, urine output is measured hourly. If the client is incontinent of urine, estimate and record these outputs. For example, for a client who is incontinent, the nurse might record "Incontinent × 3" or "Drawsheet soaked in 12-in. diameter." A more accurate estimate of the urine output of clients who are incontinent may be obtained by first weighing diapers or incontinent pads that are dry, and then subtracting this weight from the weight of the soiled items. Each gram of weight left after subtracting is equal to 1 mL of urine. If urine is frequently

Continued on page 136

SKILL 3-21

Assessing Intake and Output—*continued*

soiled with feces, the number of voidings may be recorded rather than the volume of urine.

- *Vomitus and liquid feces.* The amount, appearance, and type of fluid and the time of incident need to be specified.
- *Tube drainage, such as gastric or intestinal drainage.* The amount, appearance, and type of fluid and the time need to be specified.
- *Wound drainage and draining fistulas.* Wound drainage may be recorded by documenting the type and number of dressings or linen saturated with drainage or by measuring the exact amount of drainage collected in a vacuum drainage (e.g., Hemovac) or gravity drainage system.

6. Document in the client record using forms or checklists supplemented by narrative notes when appropriate. Fluid intake and output measurements are totaled at the end of each shift (every 8 to 12 hours), and the totals are recorded in the client's permanent record. Usually the staff on night shift totals the amounts of I&O recorded for each shift and records the 24-hour total. Check agency policy.

EVALUATION

- To determine whether the fluid output is proportional to fluid intake or whether there are any changes in the client's fluid status, the nurse (a) compares the total 24-hour fluid output measurement with the total fluid intake measurement and (b) compares both to previous measurements. Urinary output is normally equivalent to the amount of fluids ingested; the usual range is 1,500 to 2,000 mL in 24 hours, or 40 to 80 mL in 1 hour (0.5 mL/kg/hr).

- Relate findings to previous assessment data if available. Perform a detailed system-specific follow-up examination based on findings that deviated from those expected.
- Report deviations from expected findings to the primary care provider. The range of volumes that require immediate notification of the primary care provider will depend on many factors that cannot all be delineated here. One example is that urine output from an indwelling catheter that falls below 30 mL per hour should be reported. Check agency policy.

CLIENT TEACHING CONSIDERATIONS

Maintaining Fluid Balance

- Consume six to eight glasses of water daily unless told otherwise by the health care provider.
- Avoid excess amounts of fluids high in salt.
- Limit caffeine and alcohol intake because they have a diuretic effect.
- Increase fluid intake before, during, and after strenuous exercise, particularly when the environmental temperature is high, and replace lost electrolytes from excessive perspiration as needed with commercial electrolyte solutions.
- Learn about and monitor side effects of medications that affect fluid balance (e.g., diuretics) and ways to handle side effects.
- Recognize possible risk factors for fluid imbalance such as prolonged or repeated vomiting, frequent watery stools, or inability to consume fluids because of illness.
- Seek prompt professional health care for notable signs of fluid imbalance such as sudden weight gain or loss, decreased urine volume, swollen ankles, shortness of breath, dizziness, or confusion.

MONITORING FLUID INTAKE AND OUTPUT

- Teach and provide the rationale for monitoring fluid intake and output to the client and family as appropriate. Include how to use a commode or collection device ("hat") in the toilet, how to empty and measure urinary catheter drainage, and how to count or weigh diapers.
- Instruct and provide the rationale for regular weight monitoring to the client and family. Weigh at the same time of day, using the same scale and with the client wearing the same amount of clothing.
- Educate and provide the rationale to the client and family on when to contact a health care professional, such as in the cases of a significant change in urine output; any change of 2 kg (5 lb) or more in a 1- to 2-week period; prolonged episodes of vomiting, diarrhea, or inability to eat or drink; dry, sticky mucous membranes; extreme thirst; swollen fingers, feet, ankles, or legs; difficulty breathing, shortness of breath, or rapid heartbeat; and changes in behavior or mental status.

MAINTAINING FLUID INTAKE

- Establish a 24-hour plan for ingesting fluids. Generally, half of the desired total volume is given during the day, and the other half is divided between the evening and night, with most of that ingested during the evening. For example, if 2,500 mL is to be ingested in 24 hours, the plan may specify 0700–1500: 1,500 mL; 1500–2300: 700 mL; and 2300–0700: 300 mL. Try to avoid the ingestion of large amounts of fluid immediately before bedtime to prevent the need to urinate during sleeping hours.
- Set short-term outcomes that the client can realistically meet. Examples include ingesting a glass of fluid every hour while awake or a pitcher of water by 12 noon.
- If the client is on enteral or intravenous fluids and feeding at home, teach and provide the underlying rationale to caregivers about proper administration and care. Contact a home health or home intravenous service to provide services and teaching.
- Explain to the client the reason for the required intake and the specific amount needed.
- Identify fluids the client likes and make available a variety of those items, including fruit juices, soft drinks, and milk (if allowed). Remember that beverages such as coffee and tea have a diuretic effect, so their consumption should be limited.
- Help clients to select foods that tend to become liquid at room temperature (e.g., gelatin, ice cream, sherbet, custard), if these are allowed.
- Encourage clients when possible to participate in maintaining the fluid intake record. This assists them to evaluate the achievement of desired outcomes.
- Be alert to any cultural implications of food and fluids. Some cultures may restrict certain foods and fluids and view others as having healing properties.

HELPING CLIENTS INCREASE FLUID INTAKE

- Teach family members the rationale for the importance of offering fluids regularly to clients who are unable to meet their own needs because of age, impaired mobility or cognition, or other conditions such as impaired swallowing due to a stroke.
- For clients who are confined to bed, supply appropriate cups, glasses, and straws to facilitate appropriate fluid intake and keep the fluids within easy reach.
- Make sure fluids are served at the appropriate temperature: hot fluids heated and cold fluids chilled.

HELPING CLIENTS RESTRICT FLUID INTAKE

- Explain the reason for the restricted intake and how much and what types of fluids are permitted orally. Many clients need to be informed that ice chips, gelatin, and ice cream, for example, are considered fluid.

CLIENT TEACHING CONSIDERATIONS

- Help the client decide the amount of fluid to be taken with each meal, between meals, before bedtime, and with medications.
- Identify fluids or fluid-like substances the client likes and make sure that these are provided, unless contraindicated. A client who is allowed only 200 mL of fluid for breakfast, for example, should receive the type of fluid he or she favors.
- Set short-term goals that make the fluid restriction more tolerable. For example, schedule a specified amount of fluid at one or two hourly intervals between meals. Some clients may prefer fluids only between meals if the food provided at mealtime helps relieve thirst.
- Place allowed fluids in small containers such as a 4-ounce juice glass to allow the perception of a full container.
- Periodically offer the client ice chips as an alternative to water, because ice chips when melted are approximately half of the frozen volume.

- Provide frequent mouth care and rinses to reduce the thirst sensation.
- Instruct the client to avoid ingesting or chewing salty or sweet foods (hard candy or gum), because these foods tend to produce thirst. Sugarless gum may be an alternative for some clients.

REFERRALS

- Make appropriate referrals to home health or community social services for assistance with resources such as intravenous infusions and access, enteral feedings, and homemaker or home health aide services to help with ADLs.
- Provide a list of sources for supplies such as commodes, catheters and drainage bags, measuring devices, tube feeding formulas, and electrolyte replacement drinks.

Ambulatory and Community Settings **Assessing Intake and Output**   PATIENT-CENTERED CARE

Assess for the following:

CLIENT

- *Risk factors for imbalance:* the client's age, medications required such as diuretic therapy or corticosteroids, and presence of chronic diseases such as diabetes, heart disease, lung disease, or dementia
- *Self-care abilities for maintaining fluid intake:* mobility; ability to swallow, to access fluids and respond to thirst
- *Current level of knowledge* (as appropriate) about any fluid restrictions, actions and side effects of prescribed medications,

regular weight monitoring, gastric tube care and enteral feedings, and parenteral fluids and nutrition

FAMILY

- *Caregiver availability, skills, and responses:* availability and willingness to assume responsibility for care, knowledge and ability to provide assistance with maintaining adequate intake of fluids, knowledge of risk factors and early warning signs of problems
- *Family role changes and coping:* effect on financial status, parenting and spousal roles, social roles

---

Chapter 3 Review

FOCUSING ON CLINICAL THINKING

Consider This

1. What should you do if the client answers all history questions with simple one-word answers or gestures?
2. Your 78-year-old client has very thin skin with many bruises on her forearms and raised, pale, solid, soft lesions on her upper arms. What questions would you ask to help determine the cause of these lesions?
3. When speaking with a client during the nursing history, you note that one eye seems to be out of alignment with the other eye. What techniques would you use to determine that your observation is or is not valid?
4. You are performing the Rinne test on a client who has complained of difficulty hearing the television at home. The client states ability to hear the tuning fork when held next to the ear canal after ceasing to hear it while the tuning fork was held against the mastoid process. How would you interpret this result?
5. When auscultating a client's posterior thorax, you hear low-pitched sighing sounds at the left base and high-pitched squeaky sounds at the right base. Are these normal or abnormal findings? If not normal, what do the sounds indicate?

6. When auscultating the heart of an obese client, all sounds are extremely distant and difficult to hear. What might you do to enhance the auscultation?
7. When palpating a client's left breast, a thickened area about 1 cm (0.4 in.) wide and 2 cm (0.8 in.) long is noted in the upper outer quadrant. What actions should you take before ending this examination?
8. A client complains of constipation and vague abdominal discomfort. In listening for bowel sounds, you hear gurgling sounds about every 30 to 45 seconds. What action would you take next?
9. You are conducting a full assessment on an older client in a long-term care facility. What data would you gather from the medical record and from the usual caregivers prior to assessing the musculoskeletal system?
10. A client's spouse reports that the client has recently been irritable and forgetful. Which aspects of the neurologic examination would be most pertinent?

See Focusing on Clinical Thinking answers on student resource website.

TEST YOUR KNOWLEDGE

1. When percussing over the liver, the nurse hears a thudlike sound. Which type of percussion sound would the nurse document in the chart?
   1. Tympany
   2. Flatness
   3. Dullness
   4. Resonance

2. Which components should the nurse include under assessment of the client's history of present illness? Select all that apply.
   1. When the symptoms started
   2. How often the problem occurs
   3. How the problem will affect the client's future
   4. What treatments the client has tried
   5. Factors that aggravate or alleviate the problem

3. A nursing student is telling the instructor about the methods of examination. Which statement, if made by the nursing student, indicates the need for further teaching?
   1. "Four primary techniques are used in the physical examination: inspection, palpation, percussion, and auscultation."
   2. "Palpation is the examination of the body using the sense of touch."
   3. "Inspection is visual examination, which is assessing by using the sense of sight."
   4. "Auscultation is the process of listening to sounds produced by striking the body."

4. A nurse is preparing to perform an abdominal assessment on a client. Which of the following reflects the correct order for performing an abdominal assessment?
   1. Inspection, auscultation, palpation, and percussion
   2. Auscultation, palpation, inspection, and percussion
   3. Palpation, percussion, auscultation, and inspection
   4. Percussion, auscultation, palpation, and inspection

5. A 34-year-old woman is having a yearly checkup with her primary care provider. Which of the following is an appropriate breast health guideline for a woman this age?
   1. A screening mammogram every year
   2. A clinical breast exam by a health professional every 3 years
   3. A breast self-exam every 3 months
   4. A screening mammogram every 2 years

6. An adolescent male is noted to have dark curly pubic hair that is coarse and extends over the pubic symphysis. The penis is elongated and the scrotum is somewhat dark. Which Tanner stage of male pubic hair and external genital development does this client exhibit?
   1. Tanner stage 1
   2. Tanner stage 2
   3. Tanner stage 3
   4. Tanner stage 4

7. The nurse is performing a cardiac assessment on an older client. The nurse auscultates an S_4 heart sound during the assessment. Which action should the nurse do first?
   1. Notify the primary care provider immediately.
   2. Have another more experienced nurse assess the client.
   3. Document the findings in the progress note.
   4. Have the client sit in a high-Fowler's position to ease the cardiac workload.

8. Which statement demonstrates a good understanding of health assessment?
   1. "Independent clinical judgment drives the selection of which components of an assessment are indicated."
   2. "Commonly, the generalist nurse performs an in-depth screening assessment of all body systems."
   3. "An advanced practice nurse performs a brief screening of all systems prior to the generalist nurse's assessment."
   4. "An in-depth screening assessment is sometimes referred to as a head-to-toe assessment."

9. A nurse is assessing the nails of an older client. The nurse notes that the nails are thick and have white spots. What is the most likely reason for this finding?
   1. A calcium deficiency
   2. A zinc deficiency
   3. A protein deficiency
   4. An iron deficiency

10. At the change-of-shift report, the nurse is told that the client has rhonchi at the posterior bases on inspiration. At which of the lettered sites would the nurse expect to hear these sounds?
    1. A
    2. B
    3. C
    4. D
    5. E

See Answers to Test Your Knowledge in Appendix A.

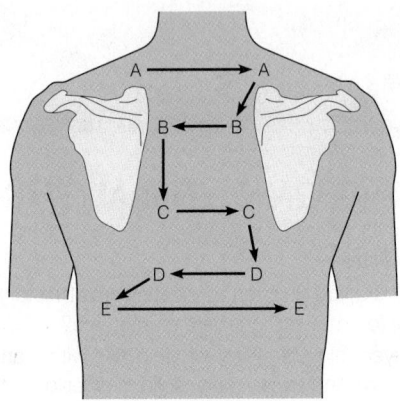

READINGS AND REFERENCES

References

Bolek, B. (2006). Strictly clinical: Facing cranial nerve assessment. *American Nurse Today,1*(2), 21–22.

Bowman, S., Eiserman, J., Beletsky, L., Stancliff, S., & Bruce, R. D. (2013). Reducing the health consequences of opioid addiction in primary care. *American Journal of Medicine, 126,* 565–571. doi:10.1016/j.amjmed.2012.11.031

D'Amico, D., & Barbarito, C. (2012). *Health and physical assessment in nursing* (2nd ed.). Upper Saddle River, NJ: Prentice Hall.

de Vries Feyens, C., & de Jager, C. P. (2011). Images in clinical medicine: Decreased skin turgor. *New England Journal of Medicine, 364*(4), e6. doi:10.1056/NEJMicm1005144

Smith, R. A., Manassaram-Baptiste, D., Brooks, D., Cokinides, V., Doroshenk, M., Saslow, D., . . . Brawley, O. W.

(2014). Cancer screening in the United States, 2014: A review of current American Cancer Society guidelines and current issues in cancer screening. *CA: A Cancer Journal for Clinicians, 64,* 30–51. doi:10.3322/caac.21212

U.S. Preventive Services Task Force. (2009). Screening for breast cancer: U.S. Preventive Services Task Force recommendation statement. *Annals of Internal Medicine, 151,* 716–726. doi:10.7326/0003-4819-151-10-200911170-00008

Weichbold, V., Holzer, A., Newesely, G., & Stephan, K. (2012). Results from high-frequency hearing screening in 14- to 15-year-old adolescents and their relation to self-reported exposure to loud music. *International Journal of Audiology, 51,* 650–654. doi:10.3109/14992027.201 2.679747

Selected Bibliography

Berman, A., & Snyder, S. (2016). *Kozier & Erb's fundamentals of nursing: Concepts, process, and practice* (10th ed.). Upper Saddle River, NJ: Pearson.

Bickley, L. S. (2012). *Bates' guide to physical examination and history taking* (12th ed.). Philadelphia, PA: Lippincott Williams & Wilkins.

Jarvis, C. (2011). *Physical examination & health assessment* (6th ed.). St. Louis, MO: Saunders.

Rhoads, J., & Petersen, S. W. (2011). *Advanced health assessment and diagnostic reasoning* (2nd ed.). Burlington, MA: Jones & Bartlett.

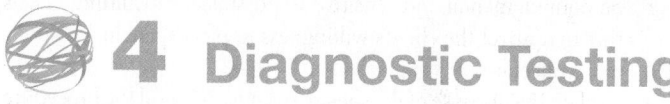

4 Diagnostic Testing

LEARNING OUTCOMES

At the completion of this chapter, the student will be able to:

1. Define the key terms used in the skills of diagnostic testing, aspiration/biopsy procedures, and care of clients receiving contrast media.
2. Describe the nursing responsibilities for specimen collection.
3. Explain the rationale for the collection of a:
   a. Capillary blood specimen.
   b. Stool specimen.
   c. Routine urine specimen.
   d. Timed urine specimen.
   e. Urine specimen for culture and sensitivity.
   f. Sputum specimen.
   g. Nose and throat specimen.
   h. Wound drainage specimen.
4. Recognize when it is appropriate to delegate specimen collection to unlicensed assistive personnel.

5. Verbalize the steps used in collecting a:
   a. Capillary blood specimen.
   b. Stool specimen.
   c. Routine urine specimen.
   d. Timed urine specimen.
   e. Urine specimen for culture and sensitivity.
   f. Sputum specimen.
   g. Nose and throat specimen.
   h. Wound drainage specimen.
6. Demonstrate appropriate documentation and reporting of specimen collection.
7. Describe the nurse's role in caring for clients undergoing aspiration or biopsy procedures.
8. Describe the nurse's role in caring for clients receiving contrast media.

SKILLS

Skill 4–1 Obtaining a Capillary Blood Specimen to Measure Blood Glucose
Skill 4–2 Obtaining and Testing a Stool Specimen
Skill 4–3 Collecting a Routine Urine Specimen
Skill 4–4 Collecting a Timed Urine Specimen
Skill 4–5 Collecting a Urine Specimen for Culture and Sensitivity by the Clean-Catch Method

Skill 4–6 Performing Urine Testing
Skill 4–7 Collecting a Sputum Specimen
Skill 4–8 Obtaining Nose and Throat Specimens
Skill 4–9 Obtaining a Wound Drainage Specimen

KEY TERMS

abdominal paracentesis, *161*
acid-fast bacillus (AFB), *154*
aerobic, *158*
anaerobic, *158*
angiogram, *164*
arteriogram, *164*
ascites, *161*
aspiration, *159*
biopsy, *159*
blood glucose meters, *140*
cannula, *161*
capillary blood glucose (CBG), *140*

cardiac catheterization, *164*
clean-catch urine specimen, *147*
contrast medium, *164*
dysuria, *151*
erythematous, *156*
exudate, *156*
guaiac test, *144*
hematuria, *151*
lancet, *141*
lancet injector, *141*
lumbar puncture (LP), *159*
manometer, *160*

midstream urine specimen, *147*
nasopharyngeal culture, *157*
nose culture, *156*
occult, *144*
ova and parasites, *144*
postural drainage, *154*
purosanguineous, *158*
purulent, *158*
pus, *159*
reagent, *140*
saliva, *154*
sanguineous, *158*

second-voided
    specimen, *153*
serosanguineous, *158*
serous, *158*
specimens, *140*
sputum, *154*
steatorrhea, *144*
thoracentesis, *161*
throat culture, *156*
trocar, *161*
venogram, *164*
void, *147*

Diagnostic tests are tools that provide information about the client. Frequently tests are used to help confirm a diagnosis, monitor an illness, and provide valuable information about the client's response to treatment. Nurses require knowledge of the most common diagnostic tests because one primary role of the nurse is to teach the client and family or significant other how to prepare for the test and the care that may be required following the test. Nurses must also know the implications of the test results in order to provide the most appropriate nursing care for the client.

DIAGNOSTIC TESTING PHASES

Diagnostic testing involves three phases: pretest, intratest, and post-test.

Pretest

The major focus of the pretest phase is client preparation. A thorough assessment and data collection (e.g., biologic, psychological, sociologic, cultural, and spiritual) assist the nurse in determining communication and teaching strategies. The nurse also needs to know what equipment and supplies are needed for the specific test. Common questions include the following: What type of sample will be needed and how will it be collected? Are medications given or withheld? How long is the test? Is a consent form required? Answers to these types of questions can help avoid costly mistakes and reduce inconvenience to all involved. Most facilities have information in the form of policy and procedure manuals about the tests available to the health care team. The laboratory at the facility can also act as a resource for information.

Intratest

This phase focuses on specimen collection and performing or assisting with certain diagnostic testing. The nurse uses standard precautions and sterile technique as appropriate. During the procedure the nurse provides emotional and physical support while monitoring the client as needed (e.g., vital signs, pulse oximetry, ECG). The nurse ensures correct labeling, storage, and transportation of the specimen to avoid invalid test results.

Post-Test

The focus of this phase is on nursing care of the client and follow-up activities and observations. As appropriate, the nurse compares the previous and current test results and modifies nursing interventions as needed. The nurse also reports the results to appropriate health team members. The National Patient Safety Goals identify the importance of reporting critical results of tests and diagnostic procedures.

SPECIMEN COLLECTION

The nurse contributes to the assessment of a client's health status by collecting **specimens** of body fluids. All hospitalized clients have at least one laboratory specimen collected during their stay at the health care facility. Laboratory examination of specimens such as urine, blood, stool, sputum, and wound drainage provides important information for diagnosing health problems as well as measuring a response to therapy.

Nurses often assume the responsibility for specimen collection. Thus, it is important that nurses know and implement Occupational Safety and Health Administration (OSHA) standards for all specimen collection. Depending on the type of specimen and skill required, the nurse may be able to delegate this task to unlicensed assistive personnel (UAP) under the supervision of the nurse.

Nursing responsibilities associated with specimen collection include the following:

- Provide client comfort, privacy, and safety. Clients may experience embarrassment or discomfort when providing a specimen. The nurse should provide the client with as much privacy as possible and handle the specimen discretely. The nurse needs to be nonjudgmental and sensitive to possible sociocultural beliefs that may affect the client's willingness to participate in the specimen collection.

- Explain the purpose of the specimen collection and the procedure for obtaining the specimen. Clients may experience anxiety about the procedure, especially if it is perceived as being intrusive or the client is afraid of an unknown test result. A clear explanation will help the client cooperate in the collection of the specimen. With proper instruction, many clients are able to collect their own specimens, which promotes independence and reduces or avoids embarrassment. Client participation may also ensure understanding of the importance for the diagnostic test and alleviate some anxiety over the test procedure.

- Use the correct procedure for obtaining a specimen, or ensure that the client or staff follows the correct procedure. Aseptic or sterile technique is used in specimen collection to prevent contamination and reduce transmission of microorganisms, which can cause inaccurate test results or infectious disease transmission. A nursing procedure or laboratory manual is often available if the nurse is unfamiliar with the procedure. If there is any question about the procedure, the nurse calls the laboratory for directions before collecting the specimen.

- Note relevant information on the laboratory requisition slip, for example, medications the client is taking that may affect the results.

- Transport the specimen to the laboratory promptly. Fresh specimens provide more accurate results. Ensure safety of other health care providers through implementation of safety measures when transporting all specimens.

- Report abnormal laboratory findings to the primary care provider in a timely manner consistent with the severity of the abnormal results.

CAPILLARY BLOOD GLUCOSE (CBG)

A **capillary blood glucose (CBG)** specimen is taken to measure the current blood glucose level when frequent tests are required or when a venipuncture cannot be performed. This technique is less painful than a venipuncture and easily performed. Hence, clients can perform this technique on themselves.

The development of home glucose test kits and **reagent** (substance used to produce a chemical reaction to detect or measure other substances) strips has simplified the testing of blood glucose and greatly facilitated the management of home care by clients with diabetes. A number of manufacturers have developed **blood glucose meters** (glucometers) (Figure 4–1 ■).

Advances in technology have resulted in clients having greater choices for a glucose meter that meets their needs. For example, a person with a visual impairment could choose a voice-activated glucose meter or a meter with a large visual display (Wahowiak, 2013). Some meters may be used for alternative site testing (AST). This is when the client obtains a blood sample from an area of the body other than the finger such as the palm of the hand, forearm, or thigh. It is important to instruct a client who is using one of these devices that AST may not be as accurate as fingertip testing. It is recommended that AST only be used by people with fairly stable diabetes and for testing before meals (Whitmore, 2012, p. 585). For high-tech clients, there are

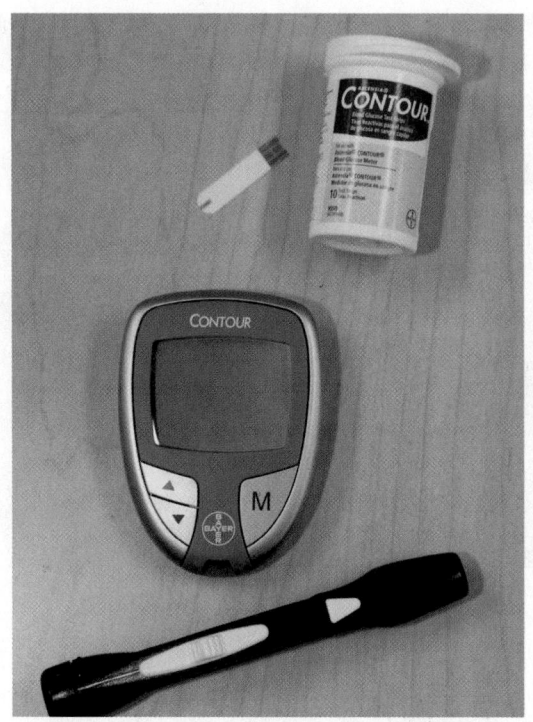

mini-meters available in different colors and meters that automatically analyze their trends in glucose control, medications, food, and exercise. This allows clients to see patterns and trends that can help them be successful in controlling their diabetes.

Blood glucose meters can vary in the following ways: amount of blood needed, code vs. noncode requirement, testing speed, size, ability to store results, cost of the meter, and test strips. It is important that clients who require glucose monitoring be comfortable and confident in the use of the meter. Once the client chooses a blood glucose meter, it is imperative for the nurse or client to review the manufacturer's operating guidelines. Being familiar with the proper use of the equipment helps ensure accurate readings. This will assist the client in controlling his or her diabetes. Clients who are comfortable taking their blood glucose readings and knowledgeable about interpreting the results will feel empowered to make changes, as needed, for optimal self-management.

Capillary blood specimens are commonly obtained from the lateral aspect or side of the finger in adults. This site avoids the nerve endings and calloused areas at the fingertip. The earlobe may be used if the client is in shock or if the fingers are edematous. Some newer monitors allow for obtaining specimens from less sensitive areas on the arms, legs, or abdomen (i.e., AST).

Figure 4–1 ■ Blood glucose meter, test strips, and lancet injector.

●○● NURSING PROCESS: MEASURING CAPILLARY BLOOD GLUCOSE

Obtaining a Capillary Blood Specimen to Measure Blood Glucose

ASSESSMENT
- Before obtaining a capillary blood specimen, determine:
  - The policies and procedures for the facility.
  - The frequency and type of testing.
  - The client's understanding of the procedure.
  - The client's response to previous testing.
- Assess the client's skin at the puncture site to determine if it is intact and the circulation is not compromised. Check color, warmth, and capillary refill.

- Review the client's record for medications that may prolong bleeding, such as anticoagulants, or medical problems that may increase the bleeding response.
- Assess the client's self-care abilities that may affect accuracy of test results, such as visual impairment and finger dexterity.

PLANNING
DELEGATION

Check the applicable nurse practice act and the facility policy and procedure manual to determine who can perform this skill. It is usually considered an invasive technique and one that requires problem solving and application of knowledge. It is the responsibility of the nurse to know the results of the test, and supervise ancillary personnel responsible for assisting the nurse.

Equipment
- Blood glucose meter (glucometer)
- Blood glucose reagent strip compatible with the meter
- 2×2 gauze
- Antiseptic swab
- Clean gloves
- Sterile **lancet** (a sharp device to puncture the skin)
- **Lancet injector** (a spring-loaded mechanism that holds the lancet)
- Warm cloth or other warming device (optional)

IMPLEMENTATION
Preparation
Review the type of meter and the manufacturer's instructions. Assemble the equipment at the bedside.

Performance
1. Prior to performing the procedure, introduce self and verify the client's identity using agency protocol. Explain to the client what

you are going to do, why it is necessary, and how he or she can participate. Discuss how the results will be used in planning further care or treatments.
2. Perform hand hygiene and observe other appropriate infection prevention procedures.
3. Provide for client privacy.

SKILL 4–1

Continued on page 142

Obtaining a Capillary Blood Specimen to Measure Blood Glucose—*continued*

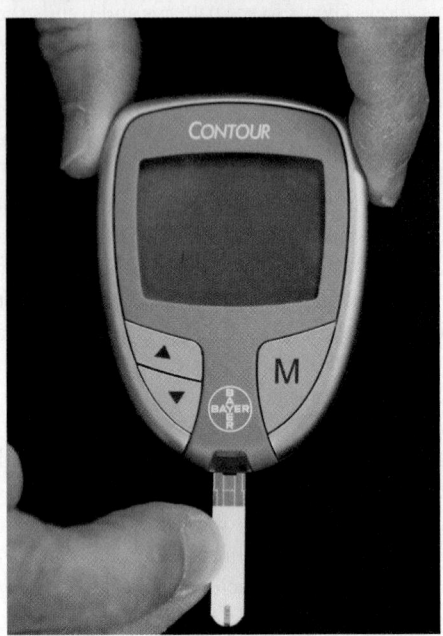

❶ Insert the test strip into the meter.

4. Prepare the equipment.
   * Some meters turn on by inserting the test strip into the meter. ❶
   * Calibrate the meter and run a control sample according to the manufacturer's instructions and/or confirm the code number. The newer no-code models do not require calibration. The technology is integrated into the test strips.
5. Select and prepare the vascular puncture site.
   * Choose a vascular puncture site (e.g., the side of an adult's finger). Avoid sites beside bone. Wrap the finger first in a warm cloth *or* hold a finger in a dependent (below heart level) position. If the earlobe is used, rub it gently with a small piece of gauze. **Rationale:** *These actions increase the blood flow to the area, ensure an adequate specimen, and reduce the need for a repeat puncture.*
   * Clean the site with the antiseptic swab or soap and water and allow it to dry completely. **Rationale:** *Alcohol can affect accuracy, and the site stings when punctured when wet with alcohol.*
6. Obtain the blood specimen.
   * Apply clean gloves.
   * Place the injector, if used, against the site, and release the needle, thus permitting it to pierce the skin. Make sure the lancet is perpendicular to the site. **Rationale:** *The lancet is designed to pierce the skin at a specific depth when it is in a perpendicular position relative to the skin.* ❷

   or

   * Prick the site with a lancet or needle, using a darting motion.
   * Gently squeeze (but do not touch) the puncture site until a drop of blood forms. The size of the drop of blood can vary depending on the meter. Some meters require as little as 0.3 mL of blood to accurately test blood sugar.
   * Hold the reagent strip under the puncture site until adequate blood covers the indicator square. ❸ The pad will absorb the blood and a chemical reaction will occur. Do not smear the blood. **Rationale:** *Smearing will cause an inaccurate*

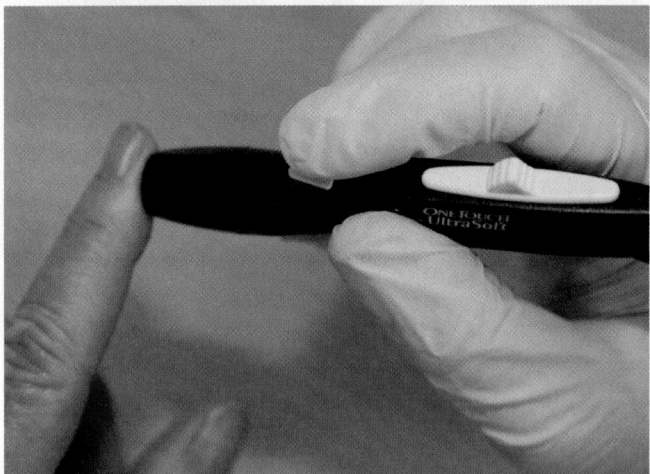

❷ Place the injector against the site.

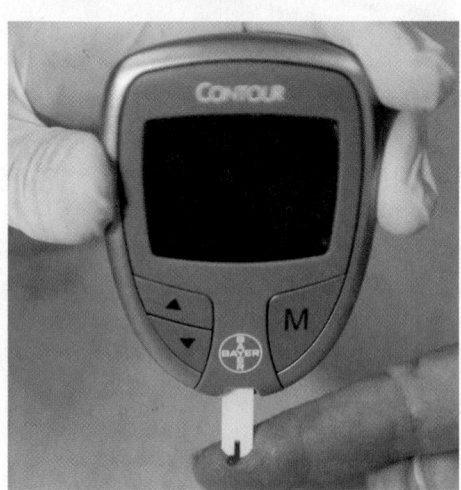

❸ Apply the blood to the test strip.

reading. Some meters wick the blood by just touching the puncture site with the strip.
   * Ask the client to apply pressure to the skin puncture site with a 2×2 gauze. **Rationale:** *Pressure will assist hemostasis.*
7. Expose the blood to the test strip for the period and the manner specified by the manufacturer. As soon as the blood is placed on the test strip:
   * Follow the manufacturer's recommendations on the glucose meter and monitor for the amount of time indicated by the manufacturer. **Rationale:** *The blood must remain in contact with the test strip for a prescribed time to obtain accurate results.*
   * Some glucometers have the test strip placed in the machine before the specimen is obtained.
8. Measure the blood glucose.
   * Place the strip into the meter according to the manufacturer's instructions. Refer to the specific manufacturer's recommendations for the specific procedure.

Obtaining a Capillary Blood Specimen to Measure Blood Glucose—*continued*

- After the designated time, most glucose meters will display the glucose reading automatically. Correct timing ensures accurate results. ④
- Turn off the meter and discard the test strip and 2×2 gauze in a biohazard container. Discard the lancet into a sharps container.
- Remove and discard gloves.
- Perform hand hygiene.

9. Document the method of testing and results on the client's record. If appropriate, record the client's understanding and ability to demonstrate the skill. The client's record may also include a flow sheet on which capillary blood glucose results and the amount, type, route, and time of insulin administration are recorded. Always check if a diabetic flow sheet is being used for the client.
10. Check for orders for sliding scale insulin based on capillary blood glucose results. Administer insulin as prescribed.

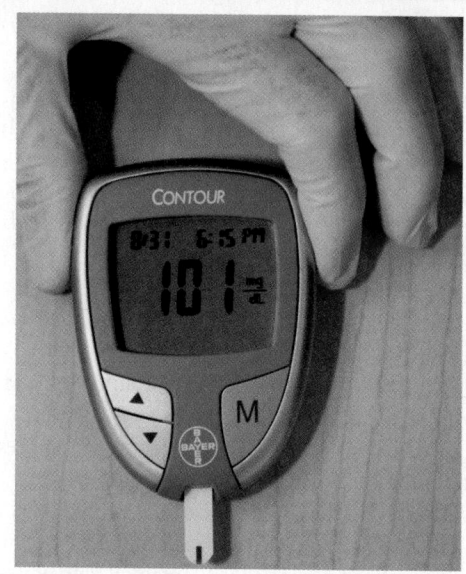

④ Read the results.

EVALUATION

- Compare the glucose meter reading with normal blood glucose level, status of puncture site, and motivation of the client to perform the test independently.
- Relate the blood glucose reading to previous readings and the client's current health status.
- Report abnormal results to the primary care provider. Some agencies may have a standing policy to obtain a venipuncture blood glucose if the capillary blood glucose exceeds a certain value.
- Conduct appropriate follow-up such as asking the client to explain the meaning of the results and/or demonstrating the procedure at the next scheduled test.
- Prepare the client for home glucose monitoring and review frequency, record keeping, and insulin administration if appropriate.

LIFESPAN CONSIDERATIONS   Capillary Blood Glucose

INFANTS

- The outer aspect of the heel is the most common site on neonates and infants for obtaining a capillary blood specimen. Placing a warm cloth on the infant's heel often increases the blood flow to the area.

CHILDREN

- Use the side of a fingertip for a young client older than age 2, unless contraindicated.
- When possible, allow the child to choose the puncture site.
- Praise the young client for cooperating and assure the child that the procedure is not a punishment.

OLDER ADULTS

- Older adults may have arthritic joint changes, poor vision, or hand tremors and may need assistance using the glucose meter or obtaining a meter that accommodates their limitations.
- The older adult may have difficulty obtaining diabetic supplies due to financial concerns or homebound status.
- Older adults often have poor circulation. Warming the hands by wrapping with a warm washcloth for 3 to 5 minutes or placing the hand dependent for a few moments may help in obtaining a blood sample.

Ambulatory and Community Settings   Capillary Blood Glucose

PATIENT-CENTERED CARE

- Assess the client or caregiver's ability and willingness to perform blood glucose monitoring at home.
- Teach the proper use of the lancet and glucose meter, and provide written guidelines. Allow time for a return demonstration. The client may need several visits to completely learn the procedure.
- Ensure the client's ability to obtain supplies and purchase reagent strips. The strips are relatively expensive and may not be covered by the client's insurance.
- Stress the importance of record keeping. Instruct the client on when to do glucose monitoring, how to record the blood glucose levels, and when to notify the primary care provider.
- Children with diabetes who need to perform finger-sticks should be taught about safe practices for cleaning blood from surfaces (household bleach is best) and about safe storage of equipment to prevent young children from having access to it. Identify a place in the school where the child can store glucose-monitoring equipment and perform the procedure in private.

STOOL SPECIMENS

Analysis of stool specimens can provide information about a client's health condition. Some of the reasons for testing feces include the following:

- *To analyze for dietary products and digestive secretions.* For example, an excessive amount of fat in the stool (**steatorrhea**) can indicate faulty absorption of fat from the small intestine. A decreased amount of bile can indicate obstruction of bile flow from the liver and gallbladder into the intestine. For these kinds of tests, the nurse needs to collect and send the total quantity of stool expelled at one time instead of a small sample.
- *To detect the presence of* **ova and parasites** *(intestinal organisms such as protozoa and worms and their eggs).* When collecting specimens for parasites, it is important that the sample be transported immediately to the lab while it is still warm. Usually, three stool specimens are evaluated to confirm the presence of and identify the organism so that appropriate treatment can be ordered. Always check agency policies and procedures for specimen collection. For example, a stool specimen for ova and parasites may be collected in specialized containers with preservatives.
- *To detect the presence of* **bacteria or viruses.** Only a small amount of feces is required for this test because the specimen will be cultured. Collection containers or tubes must be sterile, and aseptic technique must be used during collection. Stools need to be sent immediately to the laboratory. The nurse needs to note if the client is receiving any antibiotics on the lab requisition.

- *To determine the presence of* **occult** *(hidden) blood.* Bleeding can occur as a result of gastrointestinal ulcers, inflammatory disease, or tumors. The fecal occult blood test (FOBT) is the most frequently performed fecal analysis. There are two types of FOBTs: the traditional **guaiac test** (Hemoccult) and the fecal immunochemical test (FIT).

For the Hemoccult guaiac test, certain foods, medications, and vitamin C produce inaccurate test results. False-positive results can occur if the client has recently ingested (a) red meat (beef, lamb, liver, and processed meats); (b) raw vegetables or fruits, particularly radishes, turnips, horseradish, and melons; or (c) certain medications that irritate the gastric mucosa and cause bleeding, such as aspirin or other nonsteroidal anti-inflammatory drugs, steroids, iron preparations, and anticoagulants. False-negative results can occur if the client has taken more than 250 mg/day of vitamin C from all sources (dietary and supplemental) up to 3 days before the test—even if bleeding is present.

The other newer method used for FOBT is the FIT, which has a higher sensitivity and specificity for the detection of cancer than the guaiac test (Daly, 2012, p. 67). When comparing the two types of FOBT, the FIT has the following advantages: no dietary or medication restrictions, fewer false-positives, and only two samples are required as opposed to the three required for the guaiac test. There are two different types of FITs: a liquid-based method, which stores the stool sample in a liquid buffer, and a dry-slide method, which stores the sample on a collection card.

See Skill 4–2 for the traditional FOBT using the Hemoccult guaiac test.

●○● NURSING PROCESS: STOOL SPECIMENS AND TESTS

SKILL 4–2

Obtaining and Testing a Stool Specimen

ASSESSMENT

Assessment can include the following aspects:

- The client's need for assistance to defecate or use a bedpan
- Any abdominal discomfort before, during, or after defecation
- Status of perianal skin for any irritation, especially if the client defecates frequently and has liquid stools
- Any interventions related to the specimen collection (e.g., dietary or medication orders)

- Presence of hemorrhoids that may bleed (particularly important for clients who are constipated, because constipated stool can aggravate existing hemorrhoids and any bleeding can affect test results)
- Any interventions (e.g., medication) ordered to follow a defecation.

PLANNING

Before obtaining a specimen, determine the reason for collecting the stool specimen and the correct method of obtaining and handling it (i.e., how much stool to obtain, whether a preservative needs to be added to the stool, and whether it needs to be sent immediately to the laboratory). It may be necessary to confirm this information by checking with the agency laboratory. In many situations, only a single specimen is required; in others, timed specimens are necessary, and every stool passed is collected within a designated time period. Check whether the client needs to be placed on a diet free of red meat and whether to discontinue oral iron preparations before an occult blood test.

DELEGATION

UAP may obtain and collect stool specimen(s). The nurse, however, needs to consider the collection process before delegating this task. For example, a random stool specimen collected in a specimen container may be delegated, but the nurse should do a stool culture requiring a sterile swab in a test tube. Use of an incorrect collection technique can cause inaccurate test results.

The task of obtaining and testing a stool specimen for occult blood may be performed by UAP. It is important that the nurse instruct the UAP to tell the nurse if blood is detected and/or if the test is positive. In addition, the stool specimen should be saved to allow the nurse to repeat the test.

Equipment
Collecting a Stool Specimen
- Clean bedpan or bedside commode
- Clean gloves
- Cardboard or plastic specimen container (labeled) with a lid or, for stool culture, a sterile swab in a test tube, as policy dictates
- Two tongue blades
- Paper towel
- Completed laboratory requisition

Testing the Stool for Occult Blood
- Clean bedpan or bedside commode
- Clean gloves
- Two tongue blades
- Paper towel
- Test product

Obtaining and Testing a Stool Specimen—*continued*

IMPLEMENTATION

Preparation

Assemble the needed equipment. Post a sign in the client's bathroom if a timed specimen is required (e.g., "Save All Stools").

Performance

1. Prior to performing the procedure, introduce self and verify the client's identity using agency protocol. Explain to the client what you are going to do, why it is necessary, and how he or she can participate. Discuss how the results will be used in planning further care or treatments. Give ambulatory clients the following information and instructions:
   - The purpose of the stool specimen and how the client can assist in collecting it
   - To defecate in a clean bedpan or bedside commode
   - Not to contaminate the specimen, if possible, with urine or menstrual discharge
   - To void before the specimen collection
   - Not to place toilet tissue in the bedpan after defecation, because contents of the paper can affect the laboratory analysis
   - To notify the nurse as soon as possible after defecation, particularly for specimens that need to be sent to the laboratory immediately after collection.
2. Perform hand hygiene and observe other appropriate infection prevention procedures.
   - When obtaining stool samples—that is, when handling the client's bedpan, when transferring the stool sample to a specimen container, and when disposing of the bedpan contents—the nurse follows medical aseptic technique meticulously.
3. Provide for client privacy.
4. Assist clients who need help.
   - Assist the client to a bedside commode or a bedpan placed on a bedside chair or under the toilet seat in the bathroom.
   - Apply gloves to prevent hand contamination, and clean the client as required. Inspect the skin around the anus for any irritation, especially if the client defecates frequently and has liquid stools.
5. Transfer the required amount of stool to the stool specimen container.
   - Use one or two tongue blades to transfer some or all of the stool to the specimen container, taking care not to contaminate the outside of the container. The amount of stool to be sent depends on the purpose for which the specimen is collected. Usually, 2.5 cm (1 in.) of formed stool or 15 to 30 mL of liquid stool is adequate. For some timed specimens, however, the entire stool passed may need to be sent. Visible pus, mucus, or blood should be included in the sample.
   - For a culture, dip a sterile swab into the specimen, preferably where purulent fecal matter is present in the feces. Place the swab in a sterile test tube using sterile technique.
   - For an FOBT using the traditional Hemoccult test, see step 7.
   - Wrap the used tongue blades in a paper towel before disposing of them in a waste container. **Rationale:** *These measures help prevent the spread of microorganisms by contact with other articles.*
   - Place the lid on the container as soon as the specimen is in the container. **Rationale:** *Putting the lid on immediately prevents the spread of microorganisms.*
6. Ensure client comfort.
   - Empty and clean the bedpan or commode, and return it to its place.
   - Remove and discard the gloves.
   - Perform hand hygiene.

7. Label and send the specimen to the laboratory.
   - Ensure that the specimen label and the laboratory requisition have the correct information on them and are securely attached on the specimen container. **Rationale:** *Inappropriate identification of the specimen can lead to errors of diagnosis or therapy for the client.*
   - Ensure that specimens are placed in appropriate biohazard containers or specimen bags.
   - Arrange for the specimen to be taken to the laboratory. Specimens to be cultured or tested for parasites need to be sent immediately. If this is not possible, follow the directions on the specimen container. In some instances, refrigeration is indicated because bacteriologic changes take place in stool specimens left at room temperature. Never place a stool specimen in a refrigerator that contains food or medication. **Rationale:** *This prevents contamination of "clean" items with "dirty" items. It also follows OSHA standards for biohazard materials.*

FOBT Using the Hemoccult Test:
- Apply clean gloves.
- Follow the manufacturer's directions. For example:
  - For a Hemoccult slide, smear a thin layer of feces over the circle inside the envelope, and drop reagent solution onto the smear ❶, *A* and *B*.

A

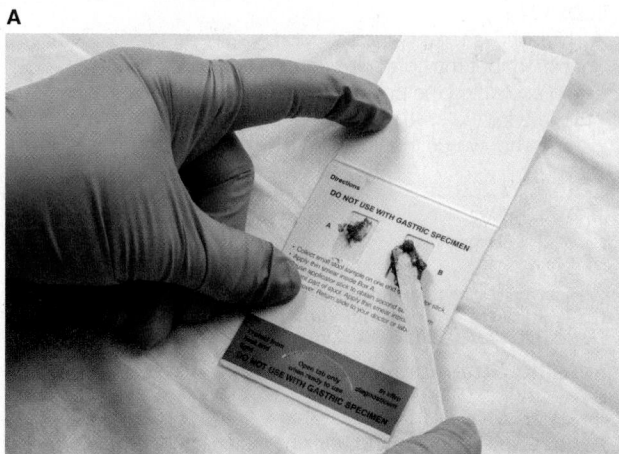

B

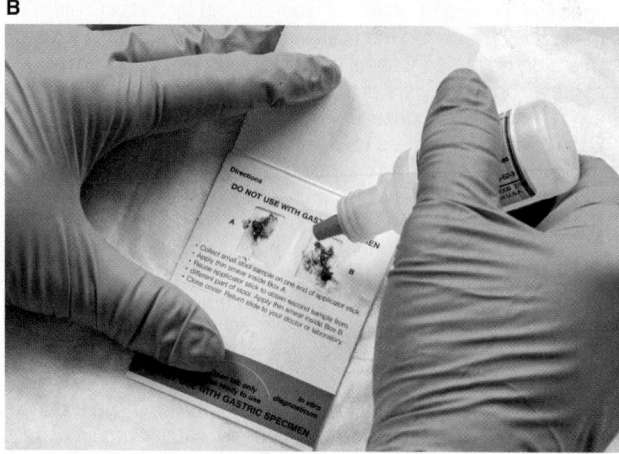

❶ *A,* Opening the front cover of a Hemoccult slide and applying a thin smear of feces on the slide. *B,* Opening the flap on the back of the slide and applying two drops of developing fluid over each smear.

Continued on page 146

SKILL 4–2

Obtaining and Testing a Stool Specimen—*continued*

- Note the reaction. For all tests, a blue color indicates a positive result, that is, the presence of occult blood. Because the results are color based, a nurse who is color blind should not be responsible for reading the results.
- Remove and discard gloves.
- Perform hand hygiene.

8. Document all relevant information.
- Record the collection of the specimen on the client's chart. Include the date and time of the collection and all nursing

assessments (e.g., color, odor, consistency, and amount of feces); presence of abnormal constituents, such as blood or mucus; results of test for occult blood if obtained; discomfort during or after defecation; status of perianal skin; and any bleeding from the anus after defecation.
- For an FOBT, record the type of test product used and the reaction.

EVALUATION

- Report positive test results for occult blood to the primary care provider.

- Conduct appropriate follow-up after stool specimen tests are completed, such as discussing with the primary care provider any changes in the client's health care plan or need for additional testing as a result of the tests.

LIFESPAN CONSIDERATIONS   Stool Specimen

INFANTS
- To collect a stool specimen for an infant, the stool is scraped from the diaper, being careful not to contaminate the stool with urine.

CHILDREN
- A child who is toilet trained should be able to provide a fecal specimen, but may prefer being assisted by a parent.
- When explaining the procedure to the child, use words appropriate for the child's age rather than medical terms. Ask the parent what words the family normally uses to describe a bowel movement.

- A specimen for pinworms is collected by the parent early in the morning, after sleep and before the child has a bowel movement. Scotch tape is attached to a tongue blade, and the sticky side is laid flat against the perineum and anus to pick up any eggs or small worms. The tongue blade is then examined under a microscope.

OLDER ADULTS
- Older adults may need assistance if serial stool specimens are required.

CLIENT TEACHING CONSIDERATIONS

Assessing Stool for Occult Blood

USING A HEMOCCULT TEST
- Avoid restricted foods, medications, and vitamin C for the period recommended by the manufacturer and during the test. Usually specified foods and vitamin C are restricted for 3 days before the test and specified medications for 7 days before the test.
- Use a ballpoint pen to label the specimens with your name, address, age, and date of specimen. Usually three specimens are collected from consecutive and different bowel movements. Each specimen must be dated accurately.
- Avoid collecting specimens during your menstrual period and for 3 days afterward, and while you have bleeding hemorrhoids or blood in your urine.
- Remove toilet bowl cleaners from the toilet bowl. Flush the toilet twice before proceeding with the test.
- Avoid contaminating the specimen with urine or toilet tissue. Empty your bladder before the test. To facilitate specimen collection, transfer the stool to a clean, dry container. Wear clean gloves.
- Use the tongue blade provided to transfer the specimen to the test folder or tape. Only a small amount of stool is required. Take the sample from the center of a formed stool to ensure a uniform sample.
- Wrap the tongue blade in a paper towel and dispose of it in the waste receptacle. Do not flush the stick.

- Follow the manufacturer's directions explicitly for the test product being used. Test products vary. For example, for the Hemoccult test, a thin layer of feces is smeared over the boxes inside the envelope, and a drop of developing solution is applied on the opposite side of the specimen paper. For the Hematest, a thin layer of feces is smeared onto guaiac filter paper, a tablet is placed in the middle of the specimen, and two or three drops of water are added to the tablet. If there is space for two specimens in the test folder, take the sample from two different areas of the stool specimen.
- Consult your primary care provider if there is any problem understanding the instructions.
- Return completed specimens to your primary care provider or laboratory as instructed.

USING A FIT
- The sampling procedure varies depending on the specific test. For the liquid FIT, a test strip inside the sampling tube is exposed to the stool sample and the resulting change in color indicates a positive or negative result (Daly, 2012, p. 68). For the dry-slide method, the sample is collected using a long-handled brush to stroke the surface of the stool while in the toilet bowl. The brush bristles are then dabbed on the test card. After the card is dried, the sample is sent to the laboratory for testing (Kessenich & Cronin, 2013, p. 7).

- Ask the client or caregiver to call when the stool specimen is obtained. If a laboratory test is needed, the home health nurse can pick up the specimen or a family member may take it to the laboratory.

- Place the stool specimen inside a plastic biohazard bag. Carry the bag in a sealed container marked "Biohazard" and take it to the laboratory promptly. Do not expose the specimen to extreme temperatures in the car.

URINE SPECIMENS

The nurse is responsible for collecting urine specimens for a number of tests: clean voided specimens for routine urinalysis, timed urine specimens for a variety of tests that depend on the client's specific health problem, and clean-catch or midstream urine specimens for urine culture.

Routine Urine Specimen

A clean voided specimen is usually adequate for routine examination. Many clients are able to collect a clean voided specimen and provide the specimen independently with minimal instructions. Male clients generally are able to **void** (urinate) directly into the specimen container, and female clients usually sit or squat over the toilet, holding the container between their legs during voiding.

At least 10 mL of urine is generally sufficient for a routine urinalysis. Clients who are seriously ill, physically incapacitated, or disoriented may need to use a bedpan or urinal in bed; others may require supervision or assistance in the bathroom. Skill 4–3 describes how to collect a routine urine specimen.

Timed Urine Specimen

Some urine examinations require collection of all urine produced and voided over a specific period of time, ranging from 1 to 2 hours to 24 hours. Timed specimens generally either are refrigerated or contain a preservative to prevent bacterial growth or decomposition of urine components. Each voiding of urine is collected in a small, clean container and then emptied immediately into the large refrigerated bottle or carton. See Skill 4–4 for a detailed description. Some of the reasons timed urine specimens are tested include the following:

- To assess the ability of the kidney to concentrate and dilute urine.
- To determine disorders of glucose metabolism (e.g., diabetes mellitus).
- To determine levels of specific constituents (e.g., albumin, amylase, creatinine, urobilinogen, certain hormones such as estriol or corticosteroids) in the urine.

Clean-Catch or Midstream Urine Specimen

Clean-catch or **midstream urine specimens** are collected when a urine culture is ordered to identify microorganisms causing urinary tract infection. Care is taken to ensure that the specimen is as free as possible from contamination by microorganisms around the urinary meatus. Clean-catch specimens are collected in a sterile specimen container with a lid. Disposable clean-catch kits are available (Figure 4–2 ■). Skill 4–5 explains how to collect a clean-catch urine specimen for culture.

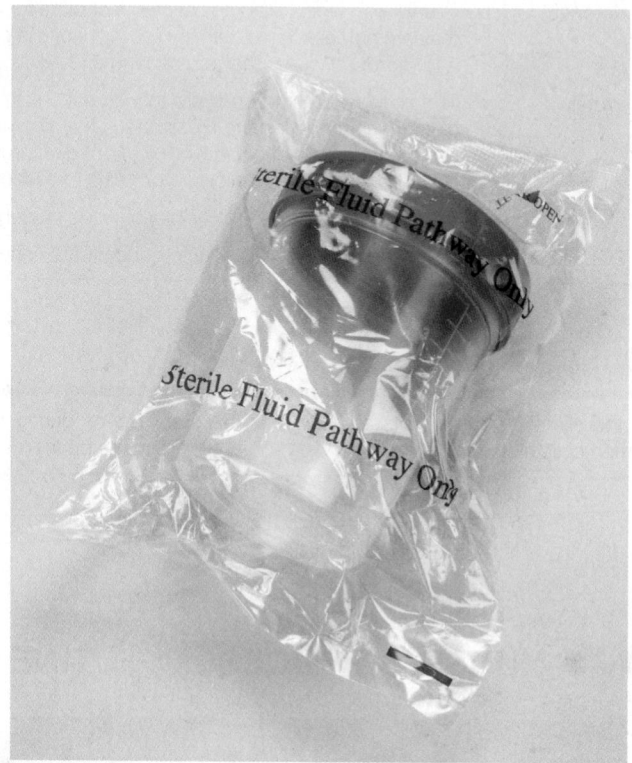

Figure 4–2 ■ Disposable clean-catch specimen equipment.

Urine Tests

Several simple urine tests are often done by nurses on the nursing units. These include tests for specific gravity, pH, and the presence of abnormal constituents such as glucose, ketones, protein, and occult blood (Table 4–1).

Nurses in a health care facility or clients in the home setting can use commercially prepared kits to test abnormal constituents in the urine. These kits contain the required equipment and an appropriate reagent. Reagents may be in the form of a tablet, fluid, or paper test strips or dipsticks. When the urine contacts the reagent, a chemical reaction occurs, causing a color change that is then compared with a chart to interpret the significance of the color. Specific directions for the amount of urine needed, the time required for the chemical reaction, and the meaning of the colors produced vary among manufacturers. Thus, it is essential that nurses and clients read and follow directions supplied by each manufacturer. In addition, testing materials need to be checked to ascertain that they are not outdated. Some facilities may require a color testing assessment prior to the urine testing. This ensures accurate interpretation of colors to determine abnormal constituents in the urine.

TABLE 4–1 Simple Urine Tests Done by Nurses on the Unit or by Clients in the Home

Test	Purpose	Normal	Equipment Used for Testing
Urinary pH	To measure the relative acidity or alkalinity of urine and to assess the client's acid–base status.	Slightly acidic with an average pH of 6	Litmus paper or a test strip
Glucose	To screen clients for diabetes mellitus and to assess clients during pregnancy for abnormal glucose tolerance.	Negative	Reagent tablets or a test strip
Ketones	Clients with type 1 diabetes should test urine for ketones when they are not feeling well, when blood glucose is consistently over 240 mg/dL, or when they are running a fever.	Negative	Reagent tablets or a test strip
Protein	Protein molecules normally are too large to escape from glomerular capillaries into the filtrate. If the glomerular membrane has been damaged, however (e.g., from glomerulonephritis), it can become "leaky," allowing proteins to escape.	Negative	Reagent test strip
Occult blood	To determine if occult (not visible) blood is present.	Negative	Reagent test strip
Specific gravity	To measure a kidney's ability to concentrate urine.	1.010–1.025	Reagent test strip

CLINICAL ALERT!

If the client or staff forgets and discards the client's urine during a timed collection, the procedure must be restarted from the beginning.

Skill 4–6 describes the tests that use a reagent: specific gravity, pH, glucose, ketones, and occult blood.

Collecting a Routine Urine Specimen

Routine urine examination is usually done on the first voided specimen in the morning because it tends to have a higher, more uniform concentration and a more acidic pH than specimens later in the day.

●○● NURSING PROCESS: ROUTINE URINE SPECIMEN

SKILL 4–3

Collecting a Routine Urine Specimen

ASSESSMENT

Before collecting the specimen, the nurse determines:
- Whether the client can assist with the procedure or may require supervision or assistance.
- If any of the client's medications may discolor the urine or affect the test results.
- If the client is able to provide the specimen independently. At least 10 mL of urine is generally sufficient for a routine urinalysis.

PLANNING
DELEGATION

UAP may be assigned to collect a routine urine specimen. Provide the UAP with clear directions on how to instruct the client to collect his or her own urine specimen or how to correctly collect the specimen for the client who may need to use a bedpan or urinal.

Equipment
- Clean gloves as needed
- Clean bedpan, urinal, or commode for clients who are unable to void directly into the specimen container
- Wide-mouthed specimen container
- Completed laboratory requisition
- Completed specimen identification label

IMPLEMENTATION
Preparation

Obtain needed equipment. Determine if the client requires supervision or assistance in the bathroom. Clients who are seriously ill, physically incapacitated, or disoriented may need to use a bedpan or urinal in bed. A fracture bedpan may be needed for a client with a hip fracture.

Performance

1. Prior to performing the procedure, introduce self and verify the client's identity using agency protocol. Explain to the client what you are going to do, why it is necessary, and how he or she can participate. Discuss how the results will be used in planning further care or treatments. Give ambulatory clients the following information and instructions:
   - Explain the purpose of the urine specimen and how the client can assist.
   - Explain that all specimens must be free of fecal contamination, so voiding needs to occur at a different time from defecation.
   - Instruct clients to discard the toilet tissue in the toilet or in a waste bag rather than in the bedpan. **Rationale:** *Tissue in the specimen makes laboratory analysis more difficult.*
   - Give the client the specimen container, and direct the client to the bathroom to void into it.

Collecting a Routine Urine Specimen—*continued*

2. Perform hand hygiene and observe other appropriate infection prevention procedures.
3. Provide for client privacy.
4. Assist clients who are seriously ill, physically incapacitated, or disoriented. Provide required assistance in the bathroom or help the client to use a bedpan or urinal in bed.
5. Ensure that the specimen is sealed and the container is clean.
   - Put the lid tightly on the container. **Rationale:** *This prevents spillage of the urine and contamination of other objects.*
   - If the outside of the container has been contaminated by urine, apply clean gloves and clean it with soap and water. **Rationale:** *This prevents the spread of microorganisms.*
   - Remove and discard gloves.
   - Perform hand hygiene.

6. Label and transport the specimen to the laboratory, using appropriate biohazard specimen bags or containers.
   - Ensure that the specimen label and the laboratory requisition have the correct information on them. Attach them securely to the specimen container. **Rationale:** *Inappropriate identification of the specimen can lead to errors of diagnosis or therapy for the client.*
   - Arrange for the specimen to be taken immediately to the laboratory or placed in a refrigerator. **Rationale:** *Urine deteriorates relatively rapidly from bacterial contamination when left at room temperature; specimens should be analyzed immediately after collection. If the urine specimen is delayed from reaching the lab by more than 1 hour, a new specimen may be needed.*
7. Document the collection of the specimen on the client's chart. Include the date and time of collection and the appearance and odor of the urine.

EVALUATION
Conduct appropriate follow-up such as checking the test results and informing the primary care provider as needed.

LIFESPAN CONSIDERATIONS | Urine Specimen

INFANTS
- The process for cleaning the perineal area and the urethral opening is similar to the process for an adult. A specimen bag, however, is used to collect the urine specimen. The specimen bag has an adhesive backing that attaches to the skin. After the infant has voided a desired amount, gently remove the bag from the skin.
- If you are having trouble obtaining a bagged urine specimen from an infant, try cutting a hole in the diaper (front for a boy and middle for a girl) and pulling part of the bag through. You can see when urine is collected without having to untape the diaper.

CHILDREN
- When collecting a routine urine specimen, explain the procedure in simple, nonmedical terms to the child and ask the child to void using a potty chair or a bedpan placed inside the toilet.

- Give the child a clean specimen container to play with.
- Allow a parent to assist the child, if possible. The child may feel more comfortable with a parent.

OLDER ADULTS
- For a clean-catch urine specimen, an older adult may have difficulty controlling the stream of urine.
- An older female adult with arthritis may have difficulty holding the labia apart during the collection of a clean-catch urine specimen.

Ambulatory and Community Settings | Urine Specimen | PATIENT-CENTERED CARE

- Assess the client's ability and willingness to collect a timed urine specimen. If poor eyesight or hand tremors are a problem, suggest using a clean funnel to pour the urine into the container.
- Always wash hands well with warm, soapy water before and after collecting urine samples.
- Always wear gloves if handling another person's urine.

- The home should have a refrigerator or other method for cooling the urine samples. Tell the client to keep the specimen container in a plastic or paper bag in the refrigerator, separate from other refrigerator contents. The client may also use a cooler with ice.

Collecting a Timed Urine Specimen

For timed urine specimens, appropriate specimen containers with or without preservative in accordance with the specific test are generally obtained from the laboratory and placed in the client's bathroom or in the "dirty" utility room. Signs to remind staff and client of the test in progress are placed in the client's room. Specimen identification labels need to indicate the date and time of each voiding in addition to the usual identification information. They may also be numbered sequentially (e.g., first specimen, second specimen, third specimen).

●○● NURSING PROCESS: TIMED URINE SPECIMEN

Collecting a Timed Urine Specimen

ASSESSMENT

- Determine the client's ability to understand instructions and to provide urine samples independently. Are there any fluid or dietary requirements associated with the test?
- Are there any medication restrictions or requirements for the test?

PLANNING
DELEGATION

UAP may be assigned to assist in the collection of a timed urine specimen. Provide clear directions about the collection procedure, proper storage of the specimen container, and the importance of saving all of the client's urine to avoid the need to restart the collection process.

- Completed laboratory requisition
- Bedpan or urinal
- Sign on or near the bed indicating the specific times for urine collection
- Clean gloves, as needed
- Ice-filled container if a refrigerator is not available

Equipment

- Appropriate specimen containers with or without preservative in accordance with the specific test
- Completed specimen identification labels

IMPLEMENTATION
Preparation

Obtain a specimen container with preservative (if indicated) from the laboratory. Label the container with identifying information for the client, the test to be performed, time started, and time of completion. Provide a clean receptacle to collect urine (bedpan, commode, or toilet collection device). Post signs in the client's chart, Kardex, room, and bathroom alerting personnel to save all urine during the specified time.

Performance

1. Prior to performing the procedure, introduce self and verify the client's identity using agency protocol. Explain to the client what you are going to do, why it is necessary, and how he or she can participate. Discuss how the results will be used in planning further care or treatments. Give the client the following information and instructions:
   - The purpose of the test and how the client can assist
   - When the specimen collection will begin and end (For example, a 24-hour urine test commonly begins at 0700 hours and ends at the same hour the next day.)
   - That all urine must be saved and placed in the specimen containers once the test starts
   - That the urine must be free of fecal contamination and toilet tissue
   - That each specimen must be given to the nursing staff immediately so that it can be placed in the appropriate specimen bottle.
2. Perform hand hygiene and observe other appropriate infection prevention procedures.
3. Provide for client privacy.
4. Start the collection period.
   - Ask the client to void in the toilet or bedpan or urinal. *Discard* this urine (check agency procedure), and document the time the test starts with this discarded specimen. Collect all subsequent urine specimens, including the one specimen collected at the end of the period.
   - Ask the client to ingest the required amount of liquid for certain tests or to restrict fluid intake. Follow the test directions.
   - Intake and output should be implemented and documented.

- Instruct the client to void all subsequent urine into the bedpan or urinal and to notify the nursing staff when each specimen is provided. Some tests require voiding at specified times.
- Number the specimen containers sequentially (e.g., first specimen, second specimen, third specimen) if separate specimens are required.
5. Collect all of the required specimens.
   - Place each specimen into the appropriately labeled container. For some tests, each specimen is not kept separately but is poured into a large bottle. Note: *All* urine specimens must be collected for timed collections. If one voiding is missed, the timed urine collection may need to be restarted.
   - If the outside of the specimen container is contaminated with urine, apply gloves and clean it with soap and water. **Rationale:** *Cleaning prevents the transfer of microorganisms to others.*
   - Ensure that each specimen is refrigerated throughout the timed collection period. If not refrigerated, specimens are often kept on ice. **Rationale:** *Refrigeration or another form of cooling prevents bacterial decomposition of the urine.*
   - Measure the amount of each urine specimen if required.
   - Ask the client to provide the last specimen 5 to 10 minutes before the end of the collection period.
   - Inform the client that the test is completed.
   - Remove the signs and the specimen equipment from the client's unit and bathroom.
   - Remove and discard gloves.
   - Perform hand hygiene.
6. Document all relevant information.
   - Record the starting time of the test, the name of the test, and completion of the specimen collection on the client's chart. Include the date and specific time. In addition, if indicated for the specific test, note the time each urine specimen was collected, the volume of each specimen, the appearance of the urine, and other relevant data such as fluid intake or restrictions.

EVALUATION

- Conduct follow-up such as checking the test results and informing the primary care provider as needed.
- Discuss abnormal test results with the primary care provider to facilitate nursing interventions if appropriate.

Collecting a Urine Specimen for Culture and Sensitivity by Clean Catch

A clean-catch or midstream voided specimen is collected when a urine culture is ordered by the primary care provider. The purpose of the specimen is to determine the presence of microorganisms, the type of organism(s), and the antibiotics to which the organisms are sensitive.

●○● NURSING PROCESS: URINE SPECIMEN FOR CULTURE AND SENSITIVITY

Collecting a Urine Specimen for Culture and Sensitivity by the Clean-Catch Method

ASSESSMENT
- Determine the ability of the client to provide the specimen.
- Assess the color, odor, and consistency of the urine and the presence of clinical signs of urinary tract infection, for example, frequency, urgency, **dysuria** (painful or difficult urination), **hematuria** (blood in the urine), flank pain, or cloudy urine with foul odor.

PLANNING
DELEGATION

UAP may perform the collection of a clean-catch or midstream urine specimen. It is important, however, that the nurse inform the UAP how to instruct the client in the correct process for obtaining the specimen. Proper cleansing of the urethra should be emphasized to avoid contaminating the urine specimen.

Equipment
Equipment used varies from agency to agency. Some agencies use commercially prepared disposable clean-catch kits. Others use agency-prepared sterile trays. Both prepared trays and kits generally contain the following items:
- Clean gloves
- Antiseptic towelettes
- Sterile specimen container
- Specimen identification label

In addition, the nurse needs to obtain the following:
- Completed laboratory requisition form
- Urine receptacle, if the client is not ambulatory
- Basin of warm water, soap, washcloth, and towel for the nonambulatory client

IMPLEMENTATION
Preparation
Collect the necessary equipment needed for the collection of the specimen. Use visual aids, if available, to assist the client to understand the midstream collection technique.

Performance
1. Prior to performing the procedure, introduce self and verify the client's identity using agency protocol. Explain to the client that a urine specimen is required, give the reason, and explain the method to be used to collect it. Discuss how the results will be used in planning further care or treatments.
2. Perform hand hygiene and observe other appropriate infection prevention procedures.
3. Provide for client privacy.
4. For an ambulatory client who is able to follow directions, instruct the client on how to collect the specimen.
   - Direct or assist the client to the bathroom.
   - Ask the client to wash and dry the genitals and perineal area with soap and water. **Rationale:** *Washing the perineal area reduces the number of skin and transient bacteria, decreasing the risk of contaminating the urine specimen.*
   - Ask the client if he or she is sensitive to any antiseptic or cleansing agents. **Rationale:** *This will avoid unnecessary irritation of the genitals or perineum.*
   - Instruct the client on how to clean the urinary meatus with antiseptic towelettes. **Rationale:** *The antiseptic further reduces bacterial contamination of the urinary meatus and the risk of contaminating the specimen.*

For Female Clients
- Use each towelette only once. Clean the perineal area from front to back and discard the towelette. ❶ Use all towelettes provided (usually two or three). **Rationale:** *Cleaning from front to back cleans the area of least contamination to the area of greatest contamination.*

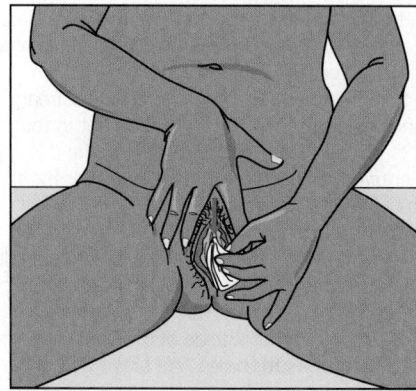

❶ Cleansing the female urinary meatus. Spread the labia minora with one hand and with the other hand, cleanse the perineal area from front to back.

For Male Clients
- If uncircumcised, retract the foreskin slightly to expose the urinary meatus.
- Using a circular motion, clean the urinary meatus and the distal portion of the penis. ❷ Use each towelette only once, then discard. Clean several inches down the shaft of the penis. **Rationale:** *This cleans from the area of least contamination to the area of greatest contamination.*
5. For a client who requires assistance, prepare the client and equipment.
   - Apply clean gloves.
   - Wash the perineal area with soap and water, rinse, and dry.
   - Assist the client onto a clean commode or bedpan. If using a bedpan or urinal, position the client as upright as allowed or tolerated. **Rationale:** *Assuming a normal anatomic position for voiding facilitates urination.*

Continued on page 152

Collecting a Urine Specimen for Culture and Sensitivity—*continued*

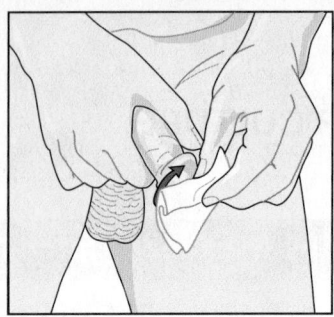

❷ Cleansing the male urinary meatus. Retract the foreskin if needed. Using a towelette, cleanse the urinary meatus by moving in a circular motion from the center of the urethral opening around the glans and down the distal portion of the shaft of the penis.

- Remove and discard gloves.
- Perform hand hygiene.
- Open the clean-catch kit, taking care not to contaminate the inside of the specimen container or lid. Place the lid in the upright position. **Rationale:** *It is important to maintain sterility of the specimen container to prevent contamination of the specimen.*
- Apply clean gloves.
- Clean the urinary meatus and perineal area as described in step 4.

6. Collect the specimen from a nonambulatory client or instruct an ambulatory client on how to collect it.
   - Instruct the client to start voiding. **Rationale:** *Bacteria in the distal urethra and at the urinary meatus are cleared by the first few milliliters of urine expelled.*
   - Place the specimen container into the midstream of urine and collect the specimen, taking care not to touch the container to the perineum or penis. **Rationale:** *It is important to avoid contaminating the interior of the specimen container and the specimen itself.*
   - Collect urine in the container.
   - Cap the container tightly, touching only the outside of the container and the cap. **Rationale:** *This prevents contamination or spilling of the specimen.*
   - If necessary, clean the outside of the specimen container with disinfectant. **Rationale:** *This prevents transfer of microorganisms to others.*
   - Remove and discard gloves.
   - Perform hand hygiene.

7. Label the specimen and transport it to the laboratory.
   - Ensure that the specimen label is attached to the specimen cup, not the lid, and the laboratory requisition provides the correct information. Place the specimen in a plastic bag that has a biohazard label on it. Attach the requisition securely to the bag. **Rationale:** *Inaccurate identification or information on the specimen container can result in errors of diagnosis or therapy.*
   - Arrange for the specimen to be sent to the laboratory immediately. **Rationale:** *Bacterial cultures must be started immediately before any contaminating organisms can grow, multiply, and produce false results.*

8. Document pertinent data.
   - Record collection of the specimen; any pertinent observations of the urine such as color, odor, or consistency; and any difficulty in voiding that the client experienced.
   - Indicate on the lab slip if the client is taking any current antibiotic therapy or if the client is menstruating.

SAMPLE DOCUMENTATION

6/15/2015 0800 Informed of MD order for clean-catch urine for C&S. Instructed how to perform. Stated she understood. Urine specimen cloudy. States she continues to have burning on urination. Urine specimen sent to lab. Antibiotic started per MD orders.
———————————————————————— T. Sanchez, RN

Variation: Obtaining a Urine Specimen from a Closed Drainage System

Sterile urine specimens can be obtained from closed drainage systems by inserting a sterile needle attached to a syringe through a drainage port in the tubing. Aspiration of urine from catheters can be done only with self-sealing rubber catheters—not plastic, silicone, or Silastic catheters. When self-sealing rubber catheters are used, the needle is inserted just above the location where the catheter is attached to the drainage tubing. The area from which to obtain urine may be marked by a patch on the catheter. Closed drainage urinary systems now have needleless ports, which avoids use of a needle to obtain a sample. ❸ This protects the nurse from a needlestick injury and maintains the integrity and sterility of the catheter system by eliminating the need to puncture the tubing. The needleless port accepts a Luer-Lok syringe. Position the syringe perpendicular to the center of the port and insert, twist, and lock into the port. When the specimen is obtained and the syringe removed, the port seals itself.

To collect a specimen from a Foley (retention) catheter or a drainage tube, follow these steps:

- Apply clean gloves.
- If there is no urine in the catheter, clamp the drainage tubing at least 8 cm (3 in.) below the sampling port for about 30 minutes. **Rationale:** *This allows fresh urine to collect in the catheter.*
- Wipe the area where the needle or Luer-Lok syringe will be inserted with a disinfectant swab. The site should be distal to the tube leading to the balloon to avoid puncturing this tube. **Rationale:** *Disinfecting the needle insertion site removes any microorganisms on the surface of the catheter, thereby avoiding contamination of the needle and the entrance of microorganisms into the catheter.*
- Insert the needle at a 30° to 45° angle. This angle of entrance facilitates self-sealing of the rubber. Insert the Luer-Lok syringe at a 90° angle for the needleless port.
- Withdraw the required amount of urine, for example, 3 mL for a urine culture or 10 mL for a routine urinalysis.
- Unclamp the catheter.

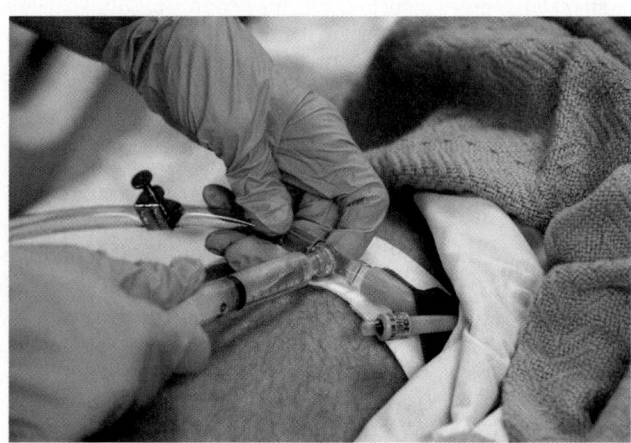

❸ Obtaining a urine specimen from a retention catheter using a needleless port.

Collecting a Urine Specimen for Culture and Sensitivity—*continued*

- Transfer the urine to the specimen container. If a sterile culture tube is used, make sure the needle or syringe (depending on the system) does not touch the outside of the container.
- Discard the syringe and needle or syringe (depending on the system) in an appropriate sharps container.
- Cap the container.

- Remove and discard gloves.
- Perform hand hygiene.
- Label the container, and send the urine to the laboratory immediately for analysis or refrigeration.
- Record collection of the specimen and any pertinent observations of the urine on the appropriate records.

EVALUATION

- Report lab results to the primary care provider.
- Discuss findings of the laboratory test with the primary care provider.

- Conduct appropriate follow-up nursing interventions as needed, such as administering *ordered* medications and client teaching.

●○○● NURSING PROCESS: URINE TESTING

Performing Urine Testing

ASSESSMENT

- Determine the rationale for the test for each individual client, for example, to determine hydration status, acidity or alkalinity of the client's urine, the presence of glucose and ketone bodies in the urine, or the presence of occult blood in the urine.
- Testing urine for glucose is not a measure of current blood glucose level and is considered an inadequate measurement. Testing urine for glucose is *only* for people who *cannot* or *will not*

test their blood glucose levels (American Diabetes Association [ADA], n.d.).
- Urine testing for ketone level is advised for clients with type 1 diabetes who are at home and not feeling well, running a fever, or have a blood glucose level that is consistently over 240 mg/dL (ADA, n.d.).

PLANNING
DELEGATION

Urine testing may be performed by UAP. It is important for the UAP to understand the specific specimen collection procedure and report the results of the test to the nurse. Inform the UAP to save the urine sample to allow the nurse to repeat the test if necessary.

Equipment
For All Tests

- Clean gloves

For Specific Gravity

- Multiple-test dipstick that has a separate reagent area for specific gravity

For Urine pH

- Dipstick or litmus paper (red or blue)

For Glucose

- Reagent tablet or reagent test strip
- Appropriate color chart
- Clean test tube and a dropper, if a tablet is used

For Ketone Bodies

- Reagent tablet or dipstick

For Occult Blood

- Reagent strip

IMPLEMENTATION
Preparation

- Use a fresh urine sample.
- Determine the appropriate equipment and testing product for the client.
- Follow the manufacturer's instructions.

Performance

1. Prior to performing the procedure, introduce self and verify the client's identity using agency protocol. Explain to the client what you are going to do, why it is necessary, and how he or she can participate. Discuss how the results will be used in planning further care or treatments.
2. Perform hand hygiene and observe other appropriate infection prevention procedures.
3. Provide for client privacy.
4. To measure specific gravity:
   - Apply clean gloves and place a dipstick into the urine specimen.
   - Observe the color and compare it to a standardized color chart on the bottle.

5. To measure pH:
   - Apply a glove and dip a strip of either red or blue litmus paper into the urine specimen.
   - Observe the color of the litmus paper and compare it to a standardized color chart on the bottle. The blue litmus paper, more commonly used, remains blue if the urine is alkaline and turns red if it is acidic. The red litmus paper remains red in the presence of acidic urine and turns blue if the urine is alkaline. Whichever litmus strip is used, red always indicates acidic urine and blue always indicates alkaline urine.
6. To test for glucose:
   - Obtain a freshly voided specimen. Most agencies require a **second-voided specimen**: Ask the client to void, and in 30 minutes to void again, providing a specimen for the test this time. **Rationale:** *A second-voided specimen more accurately reflects the present condition of the body. Urine that has accumulated in the bladder (e.g., overnight) reflects the condition of the body at the time the urine was produced (e.g., 0300 hours).*

Continued on page 154

Performing Urine Testing—*continued*

- To carry out the test, apply gloves and follow the directions specified by the manufacturer. If Clinitest tablets are used, be careful not to touch the bottom of the test tube because it becomes extremely hot when the tablet boils in the presence of urine and water.

7. To test for ketone bodies:
- Apply a glove and place one or two drops of urine on a reagent tablet (e.g., an Acetest tablet) or dip a reagent test strip (e.g., Ketostix) into the urine.
- Observe and compare the results with the appropriate color chart to determine the quantity of ketones present. ❶

8. To test for occult blood:
- Apply a glove, and dip the reagent strip (e.g., Hemastix) into a sample of urine.
- Compare the color change with a color chart in the same manner as with other reagent strips.

9. For all tests:
- Discard the urine following the tests. Clean the equipment with soap and water.
- Remove and discard gloves.
- Perform hand hygiene.

10. Document the results in accordance with the product used and agency practice.

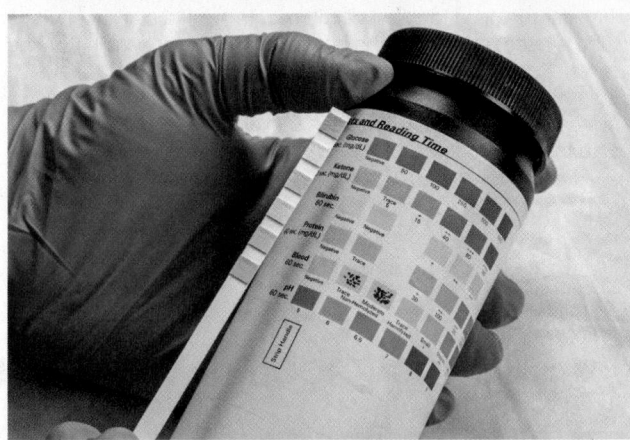

❶ After dipping the reagent strip (dipstick) into fresh urine, wait the stated time period and compare the results to the color chart.

EVALUATION
- Relate test results to the client's health status and nursing assessments.
- Compare test results to prior results. Is a pattern developing? Is the pattern reflective of a positive or negative outcome for the client?

- Report abnormal results to the primary care provider.

SPUTUM, NOSE, AND THROAT SPECIMENS

Sputum is the mucous secretion from the lungs, bronchi, and trachea. It is important to differentiate it from **saliva**, the clear liquid secreted by the salivary glands in the mouth, sometimes referred to as "spit." Healthy individuals do not produce sputum.

Sputum specimens are ordered for culture and sensitivity to identify a specific microorganism and its drug sensitivities. Cytology studies of the respiratory system often require serial collection of three early-morning specimens, which are tested to identify cancer in the lung and its specific cell type. Tests to determine the presence of **acid-fast bacillus (AFB)** also require serial collection of sputum specimens, often for 3 consecutive days, to identify the presence of

tuberculosis (TB). Some agencies use a special glass container when the presence of AFB is suspected.

Clients need to cough to bring sputum up from the lungs, bronchi, and trachea into the mouth and expectorate it into a collecting container. Sputum specimens are often collected in the morning. On awakening, the client can cough up the secretions that have accumulated during the night. Skill 4–7 describes how to collect a sputum specimen. Sometimes, specimens are collected following an aerosolized respiratory treatment or during **postural drainage** (the client is positioned to allow gravity to facilitate drainage of secretions from the lung) when the client can usually produce sputum. When a client cannot cough, the nurse must sometimes use pharyngeal suctioning (see Chapter 26 ∞) to obtain a specimen.

●○○● NURSING PROCESS: SPUTUM SPECIMEN

Collecting a Sputum Specimen

ASSESSMENT
- Determine the client's ability to cough and expectorate secretions. What type of assistance is required to produce the specimen, for example, the need to splint an abdominal incision, the need to be placed in postural drainage position

beforehand, or the need to perform deep-breathing exercises beforehand?
- Assess baseline data such as skin color and rate, depth, and pattern of respiration.

PLANNING

Before collecting a sputum specimen, identify the purpose for which it is to be obtained. This often determines the number of specimens to obtain and the time of day to obtain them.

DELEGATION

UAP can obtain a sputum specimen that is expectorated by a client. It is important to instruct the UAP about when to collect the specimen, how to position the client, and how to correctly collect the specimen. If a sputum specimen is to be obtained by use of pharyngeal suctioning, however, the nurse should perform the procedure because it is an invasive, sterile process and requires knowledge application and problem solving.

Equipment

- Sterile specimen container with a cover
- Clean gloves (if assisting the client)
- Disinfectant and swabs, or liquid soap and water
- Paper towels
- Completed label
- Completed laboratory requisition
- Mouthwash

IMPLEMENTATION

Preparation

Determine the method of collection and gather the appropriate equipment.

Performance

1. Prior to performing the procedure, introduce self and verify the client's identity using agency protocol. Explain to the client what you are going to do, why it is necessary, and how he or she can participate. Discuss how the results will be used in planning further care or treatments. Give the client the following information and instructions:
   - The purpose of the test, the difference between sputum and saliva, and how to provide the sputum specimen
   - Not to touch the inside of the sputum container
   - To expectorate the sputum directly into the sputum container
   - To keep the outside of the container free of sputum, if possible
   - How to hold a pillow firmly against an abdominal incision if the client finds it painful to cough
   - The amount of sputum required (usually, 1 to 2 tsp [4 to 10 mL] of sputum is sufficient for analysis).
2. Perform hand hygiene and observe other appropriate infection prevention procedures.
3. Provide for client privacy.
4. Provide necessary assistance to collect the specimen.
   - Assist the client to a standing or a sitting position (e.g., high- or semi-Fowler's position or on the edge of a bed or in a chair). **Rationale:** *These positions allow maximum lung ventilation and expansion.*
   - Ask the client to hold the sputum cup on the outside, or, for a client who is not able to do so, apply gloves and hold the cup for the client. ❶
   - Ask the client to breathe deeply and then cough up secretions. **Rationale:** *A deep inhalation provides sufficient air to force secretions out of the airways and into the pharynx.*
   - Hold the sputum cup so that the client can expectorate into it, making sure that the sputum does not come in contact with the outside of the container. **Rationale:** *Containing the sputum within the cup restricts the spread of microorganisms to others.*
   - Assist the client to repeat coughing until a sufficient amount of sputum has been collected.
   - Cover the container with the lid immediately after the sputum is in the container. **Rationale:** *Covering the container prevents the inadvertent spread of microorganisms to others.*
   - If spillage occurs on the outside of the container, clean the outer surface with a disinfectant. Some agencies recommend washing the outside of all containers with liquid soap and water and then drying with a paper towel.

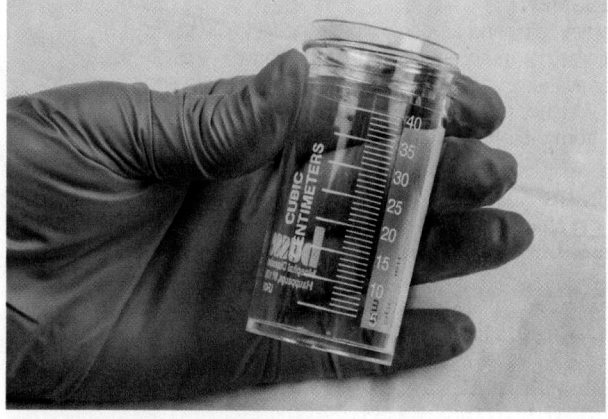

❶ Sputum specimen container.

   - Remove and discard the gloves.
   - Perform hand hygiene.
5. Ensure client comfort and safety.
   - Assess the client for respiratory difficulty and provide oxygen per the primary care provider's orders.
   - Assist the client to rinse his or her mouth with a mouthwash as needed.
   - Assist the client to a position of comfort that allows maximum lung expansion as required.
6. Label and transport the specimen to the laboratory.
   - Ensure that the specimen label and the laboratory requisition contain the correct information. Attach the label and requisition securely to the specimen. **Rationale:** *Inaccurate identification or information on the specimen container can lead to errors of diagnosis or therapy.*
   - Arrange for the specimen to be sent to the laboratory immediately or refrigerated. **Rationale:** *Bacterial cultures must be started immediately before any contaminating organisms can grow, multiply, and produce false results.*
7. Document all relevant information.
   - Document the collection of the sputum specimen on the client's chart. Include the amount, color, consistency (e.g., thick, tenacious, watery), presence of hemoptysis (blood in the sputum), odor of the sputum, any measures needed to obtain the specimen (e.g., postural drainage), the general amount of sputum produced, any discomfort experienced by the client, and any interventions implemented to ensure adequate air exchange postprocedure (such as O_2 saturation monitoring or administration of O_2).

EVALUATION

- In addition to assessing the client's sputum, relate respiration rate and any abnormalities or difficulty breathing after the specimen collection to your baseline data. For example, assess the color of the client's skin and mucous membranes, especially any cyanosis, which can indicate impaired blood oxygenation. Monitor vital signs and pulse oximetry if appropriate.
- Report the lab results of the sputum specimen(s) to the primary care provider.

LIFESPAN CONSIDERATIONS | Sputum Specimens

OLDER ADULTS
- Older adults may need encouragement to cough because a decreased cough reflex occurs with aging.
- Allow time for the older adult to rest and recover between coughs when obtaining a sputum specimen.

Nose and Throat Specimens

A **throat culture** sample is collected from the mucosa of the oropharynx and tonsillar regions using a culture swab. The sample is then cultured and examined for the presence of disease-producing microorganisms. A **nose culture** sample is collected from the mucosa of the nasal passages using a culture swab. Skill 4–8 describes how to obtain nose and throat specimens.

●○● NURSING PROCESS: NOSE AND THROAT SPECIMENS

Obtaining Nose and Throat Specimens

ASSESSMENT
- Before collecting a nose or throat specimen, determine (a) whether the client is suspected of having a contagious disease (e.g., diphtheria) that requires special precautions and (b) whether a specimen is required from the nasal cavity as well as from the pharynx and/or the tonsils.

- Assess the nasal mucosa and throat, noting in particular areas of inflammation and purulent drainage.
- Ask if the client has any complaints of soreness or tenderness.
- Determine the presence of clinical signs of infection (e.g., fever, chills, fatigue).

PLANNING
DELEGATION

Obtaining nose and throat cultures is an invasive skill that requires the application of scientific knowledge and potential problem solving to ensure client safety. Therefore, the nurse needs to perform this skill and does not delegate it to UAP.

Equipment
- Clean gloves
- Two sterile, cotton-tipped swabs in sterile culture tubes with transport medium
- Penlight
- Tongue blade (optional)
- Otoscope with a nasal speculum (optional)
- Container for the used nasal speculum
- Completed labels for each specimen container
- Completed laboratory requisition

IMPLEMENTATION
Preparation
Prepare the client and the equipment:
- Assist the client to a sitting position. **Rationale:** *This is the most comfortable position for many people and the one in which the pharynx is most readily visible.*
- Apply gloves if the client's mucosa will be touched.
- Open the culture tube and place it on the sterile wrapper. **Rationale:** *This prevents microorganisms from entering the tube.*
- Remove one sterile applicator and hold it carefully by the stick end, keeping the remainder sterile. The swab end is kept from touching any objects that could contaminate it.

Performance
1. Prior to performing the procedure, introduce self and verify the client's identity using agency protocol. Explain to the client what you are going to do, why it is necessary, and how he or she can participate. Discuss how the results will be used in planning further care or treatments. Inform the client that he or she may gag while swabbing the throat or feel like sneezing during the swabbing of the nose; however, the procedure will take less than 1 minute.
2. Perform hand hygiene and observe other appropriate infection prevention procedures.
3. Provide for client privacy.
4. Collect the specimen.

For a Throat Specimen
- Ask the client to tilt the head back, open the mouth, extend the tongue, and say "ah." **Rationale:** *When the tongue is extended, the pharynx is exposed. Saying "ah" relaxes the throat muscles and helps minimize contraction of the constriction muscle of the pharynx (the gag reflex).*

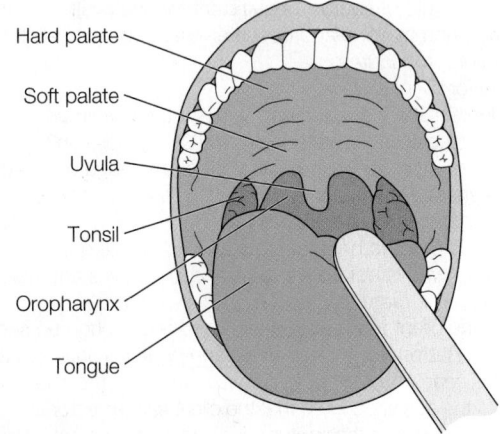

❶ Depressing the tongue to view the pharynx.

- Use the penlight to illuminate the posterior pharynx while depressing the tongue with a tongue blade. Depress the anterior third of the tongue firmly without touching the throat. ❶ **Rationale:** *Touching the throat stimulates the gag reflex. Check for inflamed areas.*
- Insert a swab into the mouth without touching any part of the mouth or tongue. **Rationale:** *The swab should not pick up microorganisms in the mouth.*
- Gently and quickly, swab along the tonsils, making sure to contact any areas on the pharynx that are particularly **erythematous** (reddened) or that contain **exudate** (purulent drainage). **Rationale:** *By moving the swab quickly, you can avoid initiating the gag reflex or causing discomfort. Erythematous areas and areas with exudate will likely have*

Obtaining Nose and Throat Specimens—*continued*

the most microorganisms. Rotating the swab where exudate is present may maximize the amount of specimen collected.

- Remove the swab without touching the mouth or lips. **Rationale:** *This prevents the swab from transmitting microorganisms to the mouth.*
- Insert the swab into the sterile tube without allowing it to touch the outside of the container. Push the tip of the swab into the liquid medium. Make sure the swab is placed in the correctly labeled tube. **Rationale:** *Touching the outside of the tube could transmit microorganisms to it and then to others.*
- Crush the ampule of culture medium at the bottom of the tube.
- Place the top securely on the tube, taking care not to touch the inside of the cap. **Rationale:** *Touching the inside of the cap could transmit additional microorganisms into the tube.*
- Repeat the above steps with the second swab.
- Discard the tongue blade in the waste container.
- Remove and discard gloves.
- Perform hand hygiene.

For a Nasal Specimen

- Ask the client to blow the nose to clear the nasal passages. Check nostrils with a penlight to check for patency.
- If using a nasal speculum, gently insert the lighted nasal speculum up one nostril.
- Insert the sterile swab carefully through the speculum, without touching the edges. **Rationale:** *This prevents the swab*

from picking up microorganisms from the speculum. When working without a speculum, pass the swab along the septum and the floor of the nose.

- When the area of mucosa that is reddened or contains exudate is reached, rotate the swab quickly.
- Remove the swab without touching the speculum.
- Remove the nasal speculum if used.
- Insert the swab into the culture tube. Crush the ampule at the bottom of the tube and push the tip of the swab into the liquid medium.
- Repeat the above steps for the other nostril.

5. Label and transport the specimens to the laboratory.
   - See Skill 4–7, step 6.
6. Document all relevant information.
   - Record the collection of the nose and/or throat specimens on the client's chart. Include the assessments of the nasal mucosa and pharynx, and any discomfort the client experienced.

Variation: Obtaining a Nasopharyngeal Culture

A **nasopharyngeal culture** uses the same steps as a nasal culture with the following exceptions: A special cotton-tipped swab on a flexible wire is used. While this swab is still in the package, bend the sterile swab in a curve and then open the package without contaminating the swab. Gently pass the swab through the more patent nostril about 8 to 10 cm (3 to 4 in.) into the nasopharynx.

EVALUATION

- While taking the specimen, assess the pharynx, tonsils, and nares for appearance, color, and amount and consistency of any exudate. Compare this information to future assessment data.

- Report lab results to the primary care provider.

LIFESPAN CONSIDERATIONS | **Throat Specimens**

INFANTS
- When taking a throat swab, avoid occluding an infant's nose because infants normally breathe only through the nose.

CHILDREN
- Have a parent stand the young child between the parent's legs with the child's back to the parent and the parent's arms gently

but firmly around the child. As the parent tips the child's head back, ask the child to open wide and stick the tongue out. Assure the child that the procedure will be over quickly and may "tickle" but should not hurt.

WOUND DRAINAGE SPECIMEN

Wounds are assessed to determine the progress of healing. One complication of wound healing is infection. A wound can be infected with microorganisms at the time of injury, during surgery, or postoperatively. Wounds that occur as a result of injury (e.g., bullet and knife wounds) are most likely to be contaminated at the time of injury. Surgery involving the intestines can also result in infection from the microorganisms inside the intestine. Surgical infection is most likely to become apparent 2 to 11 days postoperatively.

Kinds of Wound Drainage

Fluid containing cells that have escaped from blood vessels during the inflammatory phase of wound healing and is deposited

in tissue or on tissue surfaces is called *exudate*. The nature and amount of exudates vary according to the tissue involved, the intensity and duration of the inflammation, and the presence of microorganisms. There are three major types of exudates: serous, purulent, and sanguineous. Descriptions of these exudates are provided in Table 4–2.

Wound cultures can either confirm or rule out the presence of infection. Sensitivity studies are helpful in the selection of appropriate antibiotic therapy. The nurse obtains a wound culture whenever an infection is suspected. Skill 4–9 describes how to obtain a specimen of wound drainage.

TABLE 4–2   **Kinds of Wound Drainage**

Type of Exudate	Description	Constituents
Serous	Watery, clear.	Serum, few cells
Purulent	Thicker because of the presence of pus; varies in color (e.g., tinges of blue, green, or yellow). The color may depend on the causative organism.	Leukocytes, liquefied dead tissue debris, and dead and living bacteria
Sanguineous (hemorrhagic)	Dark or bright red. A bright sanguineous exudate indicates fresh bleeding, whereas dark sanguineous exudate means older bleeding.	Red blood cells
Serosanguineous	Clear and blood-tinged drainage. Commonly seen in surgical incisions.	Serum and red blood cells
Purosanguineous	Pus and blood. Often seen in a wound that is infected.	Leukocytes, liquefied dead tissue debris, bacteria, and red blood cells

●○● NURSING PROCESS: WOUND DRAINAGE SPECIMEN

Obtaining a Wound Drainage Specimen

SKILL 4–9

ASSESSMENT
- Assess the appearance of the wound and surrounding tissue. Check the character and amount of wound drainage. Is the client complaining of pain at the wound site?
- Assess for signs of infection such as fever, chills, or elevated white blood cell (WBC) count.

PLANNING
Before obtaining a specimen of wound drainage, determine (a) whether the wound should be cleaned before taking the specimen and (b) whether the site from which to take the specimen has been specified.

Equipment
- Clean gloves
- Protective eyewear, if appropriate
- Sterile gloves
- Moisture-resistant bag
- Sterile dressing set
- Normal saline and irrigating syringe
- Culture tube with swab and culture medium (aerobic and anaerobic tubes are available) or sterile syringe with needle for anaerobic culture
- Completed labels for each container
- Completed requisition to accompany the specimens to the laboratory

DELEGATION

Obtaining a wound culture is an invasive procedure that requires the application of sterile technique, knowledge of wound healing, and potential problem solving to ensure client safety. Therefore, the nurse needs to perform this skill and does not delegate it to UAP.

IMPLEMENTATION
Preparation
Check the medical orders to determine if the specimen is to be collected for an **aerobic** (growing only in the presence of oxygen) or **anaerobic** (growing only in the absence of oxygen) culture. Aerobic organisms are generally found on the surface of the wound, whereas anaerobic organisms would be found in deep wounds, tunnels, and cavities. Administer an analgesic 30 minutes before the procedure if the client is complaining of pain at the wound site to prevent unnecessary discomfort during the procedure.

Performance
1. Prior to performing the procedure, introduce self and verify the client's identity using agency protocol. Explain to the client what you are going to do, why it is necessary, and how he or she can participate. Discuss how the results will be used in planning further care or treatments.
2. Perform hand hygiene and observe other appropriate infection prevention procedures.
3. Provide for client privacy.
4. Remove any moist outer dressings that cover the wound.
   - Apply clean gloves.
   - Remove the outer dressing, and observe any drainage on the dressing. Hold the dressing so that the client does not

see the drainage. **Rationale:** *The appearance of the drainage could upset the client.*
   - Determine the amount, color, consistency, and odor of the drainage. For example, "one 4×4 gauze saturated with yellow-greenish, thick, malodorous drainage."
   - Discard the dressing in the moisture-resistant bag. Handle it carefully so that the dressing does not touch the outside of the bag. **Rationale:** *Touching the outside of the bag will contaminate it.*
   - Remove and discard gloves.
   - Perform hand hygiene.
5. Open the sterile dressing set using sterile technique.
   - See Skill 7–1 on page 214.
6. Assess the wound.
   - Apply sterile gloves.
   - Assess the appearance of the tissues in and around the wound and the drainage. Infection can cause reddened tissues with a thick discharge, which may be foul-smelling, whitish, or colored.
7. Cleanse the wound.
   - Using gauze swabs or irrigation, cleanse the wound with normal saline until all visible exudates have been removed. See Skill 31–5 on page 677.

Obtaining a Wound Drainage Specimen—*continued*

- After cleansing, apply a sterile gauze pad to the wound. **Rationale:** *This absorbs excess saline.*
- If a topical antimicrobial ointment or cream is being used to treat the wound, use a swab to remove it. **Rationale:** *Residual antiseptic must be removed prior to culture.*
- Remove and discard sterile gloves.
8. Obtain the aerobic culture.
   - Apply clean gloves.
   - Open a specimen tube and place the cap upside down on a firm, dry surface so that the inside will not become contaminated, or if the swab is attached to the lid, twist the cap to loosen the swab. Hold the tube in one hand and take out the swab in the other.
   - Rotate the swab back and forth over clean areas of granulation tissue from the sides or base of the wound. **Rationale:** *Microorganisms most likely to be responsible for a wound infection reside in viable tissue.*
   - Do not collect **pus** or pooled exudates to culture. **Rationale:** *These secretions contain a mixture of contaminants that are not the same as those causing the infection.*
   - Avoid touching the swab to intact skin at the wound edges. **Rationale:** *This prevents the introduction of superficial skin organisms into the culture.*
   - Return the swab to the culture tube, taking care not to touch the top or the outside of the tube. **Rationale:** *The outside of the container must remain free of pathogenic microorganisms to prevent their spread to others.*
   - Crush the inner ampule containing the medium for organism growth at the bottom of the tube. **Rationale:** *This ensures that the swab with the specimen is surrounded by culture medium.*
   - Twist the cap to secure.
   - If a specimen is required from another site, repeat the steps. Specify the exact site (e.g., inferior drain site or lower aspect of incision) on the label of each container. Be sure to put each swab in the appropriately labeled tube.
9. Dress the wound.
   - Apply any ordered medication to the wound.

- Cover the wound with a sterile moist transparent wound dressing. See Skill 31–3 on page 675.
- Remove and discard gloves.
- Perform hand hygiene.
10. Arrange for the specimen to be transported to the laboratory immediately. Be sure to include the completed requisition.
11. Document all relevant information.
    - Record on the client's chart the taking of the specimen and source.
    - Include the date and time; the appearance of the wound; the color, consistency, amount, and odor of any drainage; the type of culture collected; and any discomfort experienced by the client.

SAMPLE DOCUMENTATION

5/27/2015 1000 Obtained specimen from (R) hip for anaerobic culture. Pressure ulcer 3 × 3 cm, 6 mm deep, minimal amt. thick, yellow drainage. No odor. Skin around wound reddened. Rates pain at 1 on 0–10 scale. —————————————— N. Jamaghani, RN

Variation: Obtaining a Specimen for Anaerobic Culture Using a Sterile Syringe and Needle

- Apply clean gloves.
- Insert a sterile 10-mL syringe (without needle) into the wound, and aspirate 1 to 5 mL of drainage into the syringe.
- Attach the needle to the syringe, and expel all air from the syringe and needle.
- Immediately inject the drainage into the anaerobic culture tube.

or

Use an anaerobic culture swab system in which the swab is immediately placed into a tube filled with an oxygen-free gas or gel environment.
- Label the tube appropriately.
- Remove and discard gloves.
- Perform hand hygiene.
- Send the tube of drainage to the laboratory immediately. Do not refrigerate the specimen.

EVALUATION

- Compare findings of wound assessment and drainage to previous assessments to determine any changes.
- Report the culture results to the primary care provider.

- Conduct appropriate follow-up such as administering antibiotics or modifying wound treatment as ordered.

ASPIRATION AND BIOPSY PROCEDURES

Aspiration is the withdrawal of fluid that has abnormally collected (e.g., pleural cavity, abdominal cavity) or to obtain a specimen (e.g., cerebrospinal fluid). A **biopsy** is the removal and examination of tissue. Usually the biopsy is performed to determine a diagnosis or to detect malignancy. Both aspiration and biopsy are invasive procedures and require strict sterile technique.

CLINICAL ALERT!

Determine if the facility requires a signed, informed consent form for aspiration/biopsy procedures.

Lumbar Puncture

In a **lumbar puncture (LP)**, or spinal tap, cerebrospinal fluid (CSF) is withdrawn through a needle (Figure 4–3 ■) inserted into the

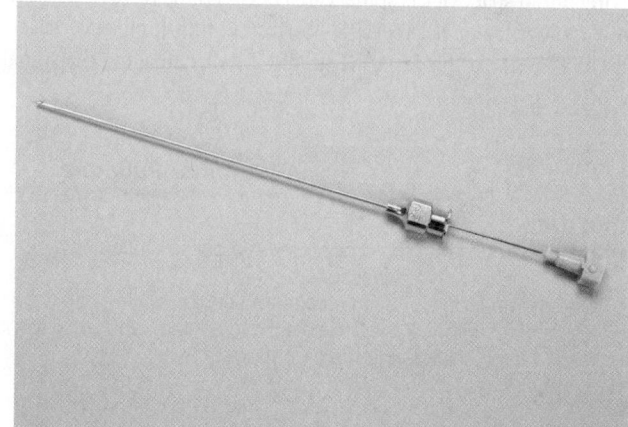

Figure 4–3 ■ A spinal needle with the stylet protruding from the hub.

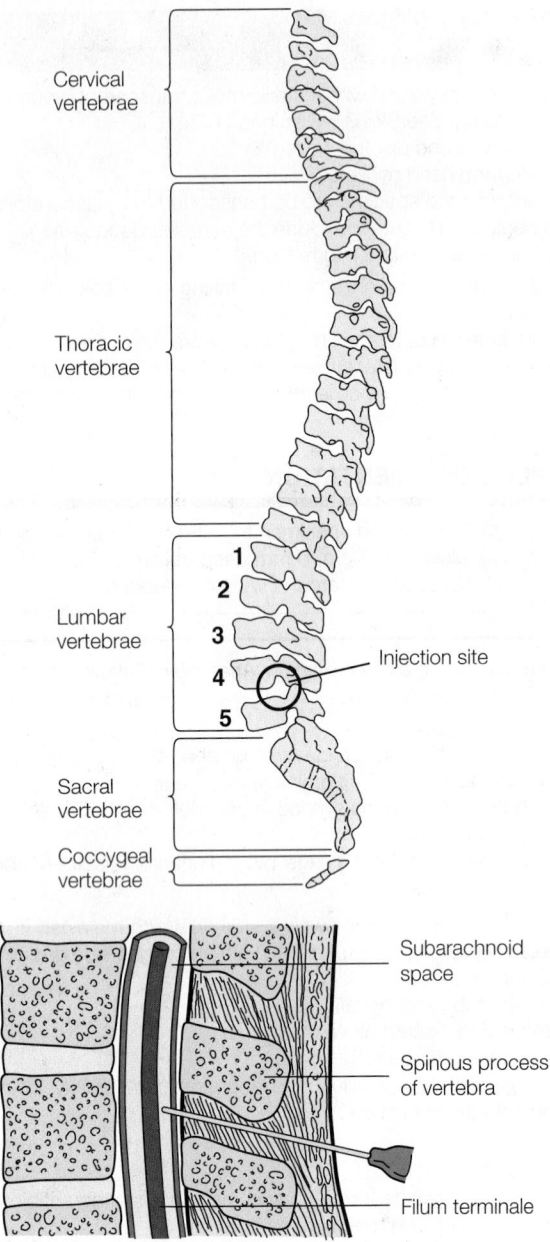

Figure 4–4 ■ A diagram of the vertebral column, indicating a site for insertion of the lumbar puncture needle into the subarachnoid space of the spinal canal.

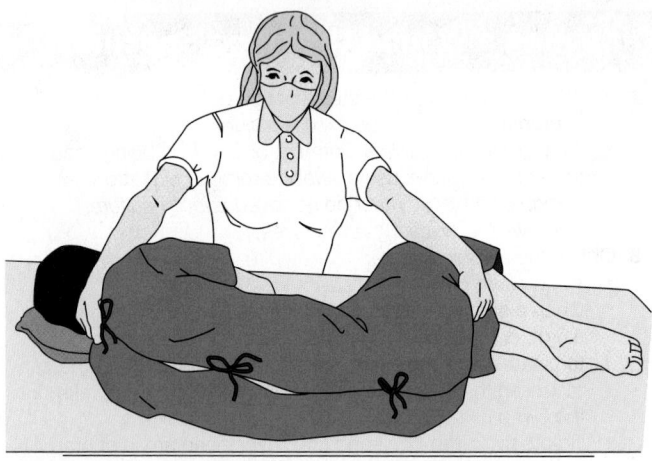

Figure 4–5 ■ Supporting the client for a lumbar puncture.

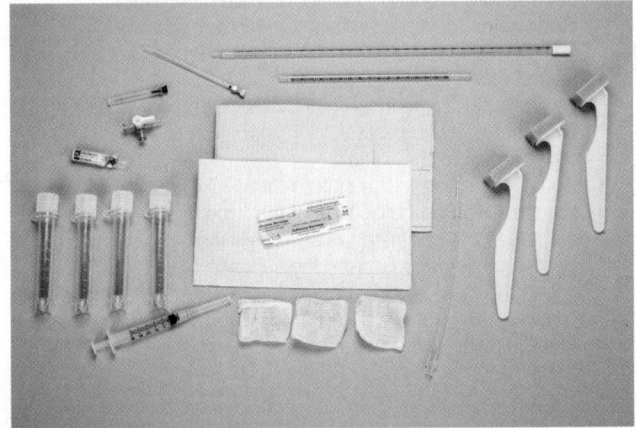

Figure 4–6 ■ A preassembled lumbar puncture set. Note the manometer at the top of the set.

subarachnoid space of the spinal canal between the third and fourth lumbar vertebrae or between the fourth and fifth lumbar vertebrae (Figure 4–4 ■). At this level the needle avoids damaging the spinal cord and major nerve roots. The client is positioned laterally with the head bent toward the chest, the knees flexed onto the abdomen, and the back at the edge of the bed or examining table (Figure 4–5 ■). In this position the back is arched, increasing the spaces between the vertebrae so that the spinal needle can be inserted readily. The nurse helps the client maintain this position to help prevent accidental needle displacement. During a lumbar puncture, the primary care provider frequently takes CSF pressure readings using a **manometer**, a glass or plastic tube calibrated in millimeters (Figure 4–6 ■). The primary care provider collects samples of CSF. After the procedure, apply a small sterile dressing over the puncture site.

LIFESPAN CONSIDERATIONS | **Lumbar Puncture**

CHILDREN
- Briefly demonstrate the procedure on a doll or stuffed animal. Allow time to answer questions.
- One member of the health care team should stay in close physical contact with the child, maintain eye contact, and talk to and reassure the child during the procedure.

OLDER ADULTS
- Some clients need help maintaining the flexed position due to arthritis, weakness, or tremors.
- Provide an extra blanket to keep the client warm during the procedure. Older adults have a decreased metabolism and less subcutaneous fat.
- If the client has a hearing loss, speak slowly, distinctly, and loud enough, especially when unable to make eye contact.

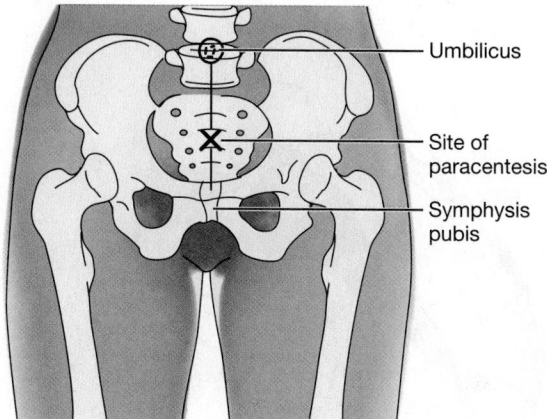

Figure 4–7 ■ A common site for an abdominal paracentesis.

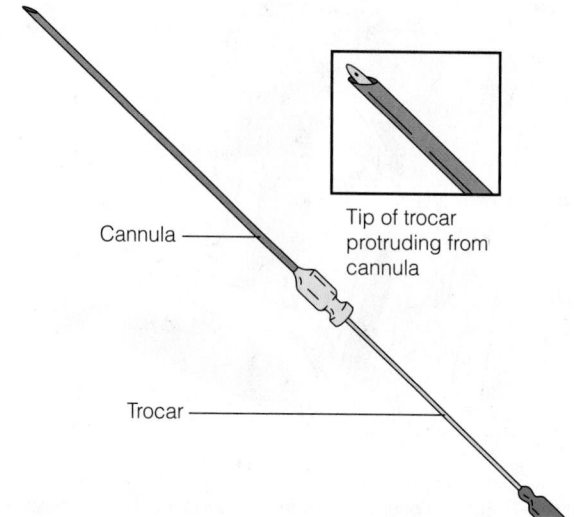

Figure 4–8 ■ A trocar and cannula may be used for an abdominal paracentesis.

Abdominal Paracentesis

Normally the body creates just enough peritoneal fluid for lubrication. The fluid is continuously formed and absorbed into the lymphatic system. However, in some disease processes, a large amount of fluid accumulates in the abdominal cavity; this condition is called **ascites**. Normal ascitic fluid is serous, clear, and light yellow in color. An **abdominal paracentesis** is carried out to obtain a fluid specimen for laboratory study and to relieve pressure on the abdominal organs due to the presence of excess fluid.

A primary care provider performs the procedure with the assistance of a nurse. Strict sterile technique is followed. A common site for abdominal paracentesis is midway between the umbilicus and the symphysis pubis on the midline (Figure 4–7 ■). The primary care provider makes a small incision with a scalpel, inserts the **trocar** (a sharp, pointed instrument) and **cannula** (tube), and then withdraws the trocar, which is inside the cannula (Figure 4–8 ■). Tubing is attached to the cannula, and the fluid flows through the tubing into a receptacle. If the purpose of the paracentesis is to obtain a specimen, the primary care provider may use a long aspirating needle attached to a syringe rather than making an incision and using a trocar and cannula. Normally about 1,500 mL is the maximum amount of fluid drained at one time to avoid hypovolemic shock. The fluid is drained very slowly for the same reason. Some fluid is placed in the specimen container before the cannula is withdrawn. The small incision may or may not be sutured; in either case, it is covered with a small sterile bandage.

Thoracentesis

Normally, only sufficient fluid to lubricate the pleura is present in the pleural cavity. However, excessive fluid can accumulate as a result of injury, infection, or other pathology. In such a case or in the case of pneumothorax, a primary care provider may perform a **thoracentesis** to remove the excess fluid or air to ease breathing. Thoracentesis is also performed to introduce chemotherapeutic drugs intrapleurally.

The nurse assists the client to assume a position that allows easy access to the intercostal spaces. This is usually a sitting position with the arms above the head, which spreads the ribs and enlarges the intercostal space. Two positions commonly used are one in which the arm is elevated and stretched forward (Figure 4–9A ■) and one in which the client leans forward over a pillow (Figure 4–9B). To ensure that the needle is inserted below the fluid level when fluid is to be removed (or above any fluid if air is to be removed), the primary care provider will palpate and percuss the chest and select the exact site for insertion of the needle. A site on the lower posterior chest is often used to remove fluid (Figure 4–10 ■), and a site on the upper anterior chest is used to remove air. A chest x-ray prior to the procedure will help pinpoint the best insertion site.

The primary care provider and the assisting nurse follow strict sterile technique. The primary care provider attaches a syringe and/or stopcock to the aspirating needle. The stopcock must be in the closed position so that no air will enter the pleural space. The primary

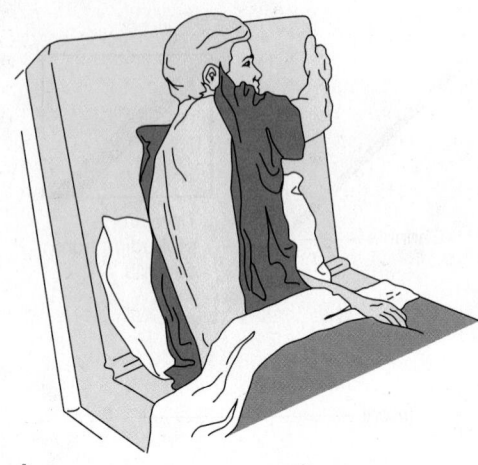

A

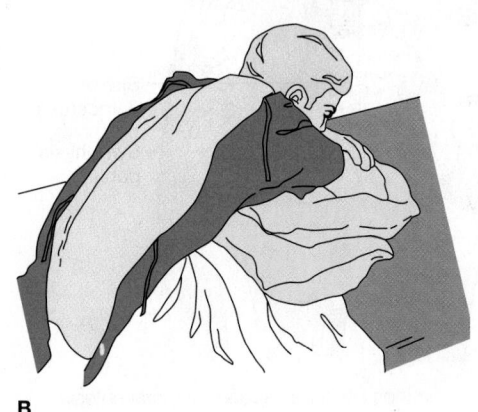

B

Figure 4–9 ■ Two positions commonly used for a thoracentesis: *A,* sitting on one side with arm held to the front and up; *B,* sitting and leaning forward over a pillow.

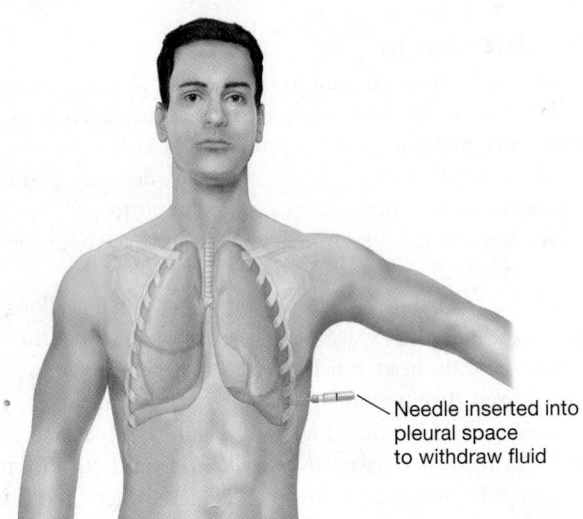

Needle inserted into
pleural space
to withdraw fluid

Figure 4–10 ■ Needle is inserted into the pleural space on the lower posterior chest to withdraw fluid.
Source: From *Medical Terminology: A Living Language,* 5th ed. (p. 241), by B. Fremgen and S. Frucht, 2013, Upper Saddle River, NJ: Prentice Hall.

care provider inserts the needle through the intercostal space to the pleural cavity. In some instances, the primary care provider threads a small plastic tube through the needle and then withdraws the needle. (The tubing is less likely to puncture the pleura.)

If a syringe is used to collect the fluid, the plunger is pulled out to withdraw the pleural fluid as the stopcock is opened. If a large container is used to receive the fluid, the tubing is attached from the stopcock to the adapter on the receiving bottle. When the adapter and stopcock are opened, gravity allows fluid to drain from the pleural cavity into the container, which should be kept below the level of the client's lungs. After the fluid has been withdrawn, the primary care provider removes the needle or plastic tubing. A small sterile dressing is applied over the puncture site.

LIFESPAN CONSIDERATIONS **Thoracentesis**

OLDER ADULTS
• Some older adults will need help maintaining the proper position due to arthritis, tremors, or weakness.
• Provide support with pillows during the procedure.
• Absence of body fat in older adults can help the primary care provider locate the intercostal spaces.
• Provide an extra blanket to keep your client warm during the procedure. Older adults have a decreased metabolism and less subcutaneous fat.

Bone Marrow Biopsy

Another type of diagnostic study is the *biopsy.* A biopsy is a procedure whereby tissue is obtained for examination. Biopsies are performed on many different types of tissues, for example, bone marrow, liver, breast, lymph nodes, and lung.

A bone marrow biopsy is the removal of a specimen of bone marrow for laboratory study. The biopsy is used to detect specific diseases of the blood, such as pernicious anemia and leukemia. The bones of the body commonly used for a bone marrow biopsy are the sternum, iliac crests, anterior or posterior iliac spines, and proximal tibia in children. The *posterior superior iliac crest* is the preferred site with the client placed prone or on the side (Figure 4–11 ■).

After injecting a local anesthetic, a small incision may be made with a scalpel to avoid tearing the skin or pushing skin into the bone marrow with a needle. The primary care provider then introduces a bone marrow needle with stylet into the red marrow of the spongy bone (Figure 4–12 ■).

Once the needle is in the marrow space, the stylet is removed and a 10-mL syringe is attached to the needle. The plunger is withdrawn until 1 to 2 mL of marrow has been obtained. The primary care provider replaces the stylet in the needle, withdraws the needle, and places the specimen in test tubes and/or on glass slides. The nurse places a small sterile dressing over the puncture site.

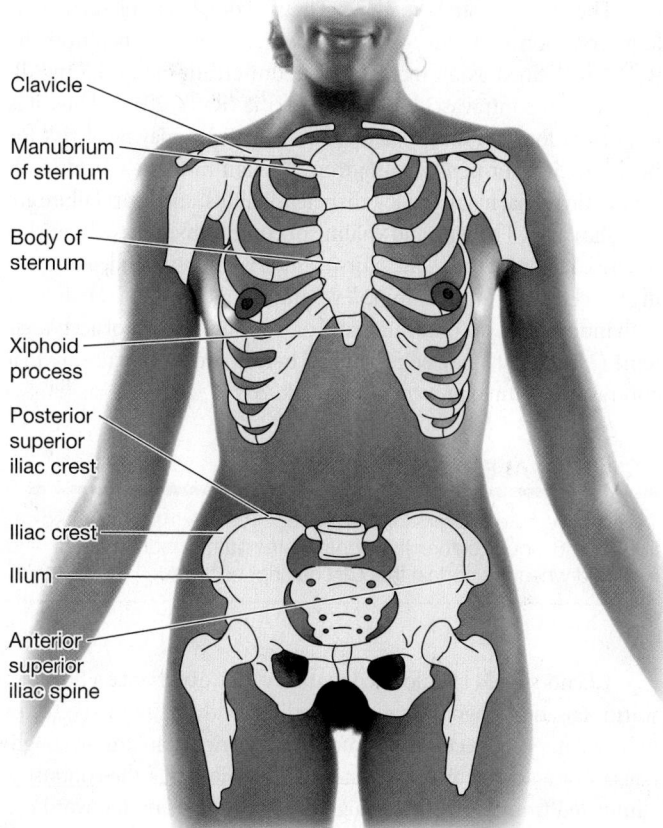

Figure 4–11 ■ The sternum and the iliac crests are common sites for a bone marrow biopsy.

Liver Biopsy

A liver biopsy is a short procedure, generally performed at the client's bedside, in which a sample of liver tissue is aspirated. A primary care provider inserts a needle in the intercostal space between two of the right lower ribs and into the liver (Figure 4–13 ■) or through the abdomen below the right rib cage (subcostally).

The client exhales and stops breathing while the primary care provider inserts the biopsy needle, injects a small amount of sterile normal saline to clear the needle of blood or particles of tissue picked up during insertion, and aspirates liver tissue by drawing back on the plunger of the syringe. After the needle is withdrawn, the nurse applies pressure to the site to prevent bleeding, often by positioning the client on the biopsy site (Figure 4–14 ■). The site is covered with a sterile dressing.

Because many clients with liver disease have blood clotting defects and are prone to bleeding, prothrombin time and platelet count are normally taken well in advance of the test. If the test results are abnormal, the biopsy may be contraindicated. Table 4–3 describes the nurse's role before, during, and after the aspiration/biopsy procedures discussed here.

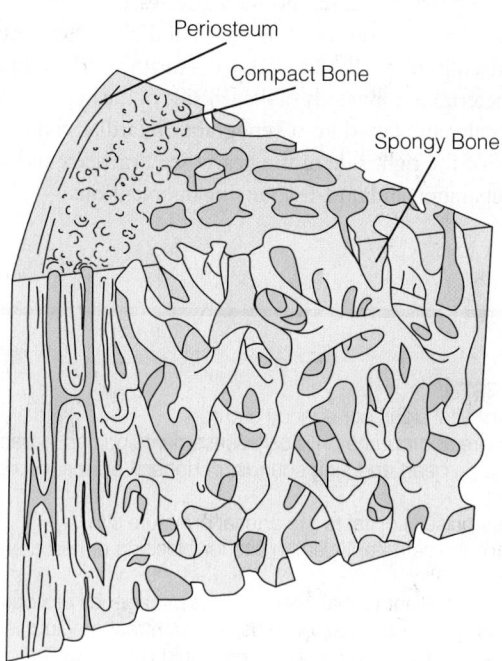

Figure 4–12 ■ A cross section of a bone.

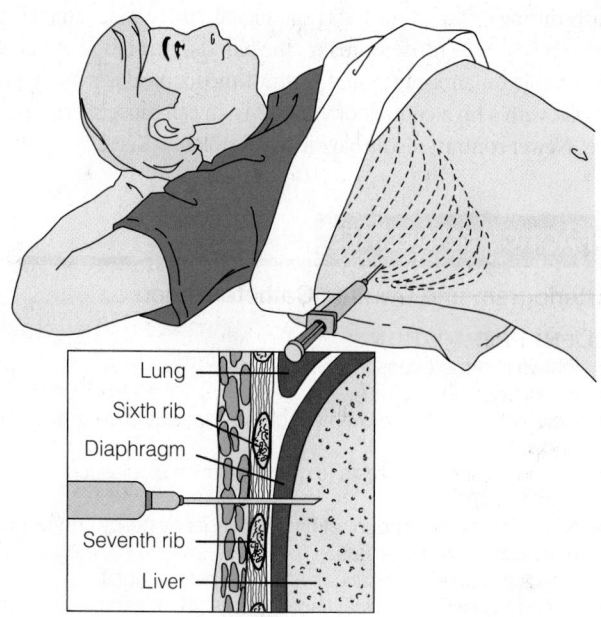

Figure 4–13 ■ A common site for a liver biopsy.

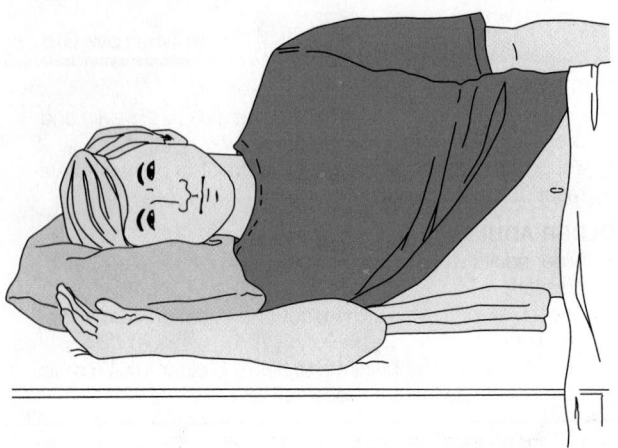

Figure 4–14 ■ The position used to provide pressure on a liver biopsy site.

LIFESPAN CONSIDERATIONS **Liver Biopsy**

OLDER ADULTS
- Observe for skin irritation from tape applied to the sterile dressing. Older adults often have fragile skin.
- Ask the client to empty the bladder before the procedure. The older adult may need to void more often and in smaller amounts.

CLINICAL ALERT!

Ask clients if they are allergic to iodine or shellfish. An allergy to shellfish may be caused by an allergy to iodine.

CARE OF CLIENTS RECEIVING CONTRAST MEDIA

A **contrast medium** or dye is a solution that is injected intravenously during certain x-ray tests (e.g., angiogram, cardiac catheterization). The contrast medium makes the blood in the blood vessels or heart visible on an x-ray. Many contrast media products are hyperosmolar with a high content of iodine, which can cause allergic reactions. Newer contrast media have a low osmolality (Kee, 2013, p. 405).

The use of contrast media can cause complications such as allergic reaction or kidney damage. Contrast-induced nephropathy (CIN) is defined as an increase in serum creatinine of 0.5 mg/dL after receiving intravascular contrast media (Rank, 2013). Thus, it is important for the nurse to assess for clients who may be at risk for nephrotoxicity or nephropathy from the contrast dye. Clients with preexisting renal insufficiency, diabetes mellitus, and heart failure are at highest risk. The type and volume of contrast media used can also be a risk factor for the client. Nursing interventions include monitoring the client's serum creatinine level and hydration status. Hydration with intravenous isotonic fluids and oral administration of acetylcysteine (Mucomyst) may be prescribed before and after exposure to a contrast medium to prevent CIN (Rank, 2013).

CLINICAL ALERT!

Clients who take metformin (Glucophage) usually have the medication held 6 hours before the contrast medium is administered and resumed when it is certain that CIN has not occurred.

Clients should be informed that they may experience a flushing, warm sensation when the contrast medium or dye is injected intravenously. After the injection, they may also experience an urge to cough, nausea, or a salty or metallic taste. Tell the client that the contrast is eliminated from the body through the kidneys. Using the word *dye* may lead some clients to believe that the injection may cause their body color to change. The nurse needs to clarify that this is not true.

Common x-ray tests that use contrast media include angiograms and cardiac catheterization studies. An **angiogram** is an imaging test that allows visualization of blood vessels in many parts of the body, including the brain, heart, kidney, abdomen, and legs. An **arteriogram** specifically visualizes arteries, and a **venogram** studies the veins. A **cardiac catheterization** is performed to visualize heart structure, coronary arteries, and blood flow.

The most common site of insertion of the catheter for the contrast media injection is the femoral artery for an arteriogram and cardiac catheterization for study of the left side of the heart. In contrast, the femoral vein is used for a venogram or cardiac catheterization for study of the right side of the heart. See Practice Guidelines for client preparation and post-test nursing interventions.

PRACTICE GUIDELINES

Arteriogram and Cardiac Catheterization

CLIENT PREPARATION
- Obtain informed consent.
- Check allergies.
- Review the procedure with the client. Assess the client's level of understanding.
- Obtain results of lab tests (e.g., coagulation studies, creatinine, hematocrit).
- NPO. Check the amount of time with agency policy and/or primary care provider orders.
- Check if routine medications are to be held or not.
- Perform baseline physical assessments. Mark peripheral pulses for cardiac catheterization and appropriate arteriograms. This provides locations for comparison after the procedure.
- Ask the client to void prior to the procedure.

POST-TEST
- Monitor vital signs per agency protocol.
- Compare appropriate physical assessment findings to baseline data (e.g., heart and lung sounds, peripheral pulses, neurologic status).
- Assess pulse(s) distal to the arterial puncture site.
- Monitor the catheter insertion site for bleeding or hematoma formation.
- Instruct the client to maintain bed rest per agency protocol.
- Provide adequate intake of fluids. The contrast medium is a hypertonic solution and can produce a fluid volume deficit.
- Assess for discomfort. The client may experience pain in the back because of positioning during the procedure. Discomfort at the puncture site is usually relieved by a mild analgesic.

TABLE 4–3   Assisting with Aspiration and Biopsy Procedures

Procedure	Before the Procedure	During the Procedure	After the Procedure
Lumbar puncture	Prepare the client: • Explain the procedure to the client and support people. The primary care provider will be taking a small sample of spinal fluid from the lower spine. A local anesthetic will be given to minimize discomfort. Explain when and where the procedure will occur (e.g., the bedside or in a treatment room) and who will be present (e.g., the primary care provider and the nurse). Explain that it will be necessary to lie in a certain position without moving for about 15 min. A slight pinprick will be felt when the local anesthetic is injected, and a sensation of pressure will be felt as the spinal needle is inserted. • Have the client empty the bladder and bowels prior to the procedure to prevent unnecessary discomfort. • Position and drape the client. • Open the lumbar puncture set.	Support and monitor the client throughout: • Stand in front of the client and support the back of the neck and knees if the client needs help remaining still. • Reassure the client throughout the procedure by explaining what is happening. Encourage normal breathing and relaxation. • Observe the client's color, respirations, and pulse during the procedure. Ask the client to report headache or persistent pain at the insertion site. Handle specimen tubes appropriately: • Wear gloves when handling test tubes. • Label the specimen tubes in sequence. • Send the CSF specimens to the lab immediately. Place a small sterile dressing over the puncture site.	Ensure the client's comfort and safety: • Assist the client to a dorsal recumbent position with only one head pillow. The client may remain in this position for a pre-scribed time period. It has been thought that lying flat prevents a post–lumbar puncture headache but this has not been supported by research. • Determine whether analgesics are ordered and can be given for headaches. • Offer oral fluids frequently, unless contraindicated, to help restore the volume of CSF. Monitor the client: • Observe for swelling or bleeding at the puncture site. • Monitor changes in neurologic status. • Determine whether the client is experiencing any numbness, tingling, or pain radiating down the legs. Document the procedure on the client's chart: • Include date and time performed; the primary care provider's name; the color, character (e.g., clear, cloudy, bloody), and amount of CSF; and the number of specimens obtained. Also document nursing assessments and interventions.
Abdominal paracentesis	Prepare the client: • Explain the procedure: obtaining the specimen usually takes about 15 min. Emphasize the importance of re-maining still during the procedure. Tell the client when and where the procedure will occur and who will be present. • Have the client void just before the paracentesis to reduce the possibility of puncturing the urinary bladder. • Help the client assume a sitting position in bed, in a chair, or on the edge of the bed supported by pillows. • Maintain the client's privacy and pro-vide blankets for warmth.	Assist and monitor the client: • Support the client verbally and describe the steps of the pro-cedure as needed. • Observe the client closely for signs of distress (e.g., abnor-mal pulse rate, skin color, and blood pressure). • Observe for signs of hypovo-lemic shock induced by the loss of fluid: pallor, dyspnea, diaphoresis, drop in BP, and restlessness or increased anxiety. • Place a small sterile dressing over the site of the incision after the cannula or aspirating needle is withdrawn.	Monitor the client closely: • Observe for hypovolemic shock. • Observe for scrotal edema with male clients. • Monitor vital signs, urine output, and drainage from the puncture site every 15 min for at least 2 h and every hour for 4 h or as the client's condition indicates. • Measure the abdominal girth at the level of the umbilicus. Document all relevant information: • Include date and time performed; the primary care provider's name; abdominal girth before and after; the color, clarity, and amount of drained fluid; and the nurse's assess-ments and interventions. Transport the correctly labeled specimens to the laboratory.

Continued on page 166

TABLE 4–3   **Assisting with Aspiration and Biopsy Procedures—*continued***

Procedure	Before the Procedure	During the Procedure	After the Procedure
Thoracentesis	Prepare the client: • Explain the procedure to the client. Normally, the client may experience some discomfort and a feeling of pressure when the needle is inserted. The procedure may bring considerable relief if breathing has been difficult. The procedure takes only a few minutes, depending primarily on the time it takes for the fluid to drain from the pleural cavity. To avoid puncturing the lungs, it is important for the client not to cough while the needle is inserted. Explain when and where the procedure will occur and who will be present. • Help position the client and cover the client as needed with a bath blanket.	Support and monitor the client throughout: • Support the client verbally and describe the steps of the procedure as needed. • Observe the client for signs of distress, such as dyspnea, pallor, and coughing. Collect drainage and laboratory specimens. Place a small sterile dressing over the site of the puncture.	Monitor the client: • Assess pulse rate and respiratory rate and skin color. • Do not remove more than 1,000 mL of fluid from the pleural cavity within the first 30 min. • Observe changes in the client's cough, sputum, respiratory depth, and breath sounds; note complaints of chest pain. Position the client appropriately: • Some agency protocols recommend that the client lie on the unaffected side with the head of the bed elevated 30° for at least 30 min because this position facilitates expansion of the affected lung and eases respirations. Document all relevant information: • Include date and time performed; the primary care provider's name; the amount, color, and clarity of fluid drained; if any specimens were obtained; and nursing assessments and interventions provided. Transport the specimens to the laboratory.
Bone marrow biopsy	Prepare the client: • Explain the procedure. The client may experience pain when the marrow is aspirated and hear a crunching sound as the needle is pushed through the cortex of the bone. The procedure usually takes 15–30 min. Explain when and where the procedure will occur, who will be present, and which site will be used. • Help the client assume a supine position (with one pillow if desired) for a biopsy of the sternum (sternal puncture) or a prone position for a biopsy of either iliac crest. Fold the bedclothes back or drape the client to expose the area. • Administer a sedative as ordered.	Monitor and support the client throughout: • Describe the steps of the procedure as needed and provide verbal support. • Observe the client for pallor, diaphoresis, and faintness due to bleeding or pain. • Place a small sterile dressing over the site of the puncture after the needle is withdrawn. • Some agency protocols recommend direct pressure over the site for 5–10 min to prevent bleeding. Assist with preparing specimens as needed.	Monitor the client: • Assess for discomfort and bleeding from the site. The client may experience some tenderness in the area. Bleeding and hematoma formation need to be assessed for several days. Report bleeding or pain to the nurse in charge. • Provide an analgesic as needed and ordered. Document all relevant information: • Include date and time of the procedure; the primary care provider's name; and any nursing assessments and interventions. Document any specimens obtained. Transport the specimens to the laboratory.

TABLE 4–3	**Assisting with Aspiration and Biopsy Procedures**—*continued*		
Procedure	**Before the Procedure**	**During the Procedure**	**After the Procedure**
Liver biopsy	Prepare the client: • Give preprocedural medications as ordered. Vitamin K may be given for several days before the biopsy to reduce the risk of hemorrhage. • Explain the procedure and tell the client that the primary care provider will take a small sample of liver tissue by putting a needle into the client's side or abdomen. Explain that a sedative and local anesthetic will be given, so the client will feel no pain. Explain when and where the procedure will occur, who will be present, the time required, and what to expect as the procedure is being performed (e.g., the client may experience mild discomfort when the local anesthetic is injected and slight pressure when the biopsy needle is inserted). • Ensure that the client fasts for at least 2 h before the procedure. • Administer the appropriate sedative about 30 min beforehand or at the specified time. • Help the client assume a supine position with the upper right quadrant of the abdomen exposed. Cover the client with the bedclothes so that only the abdominal area is exposed.	Monitor and support the client throughout: • Support the client in a supine position. • Instruct the client to take a few deep inhalations and exhalations and to hold the breath after the final exhalation for up to 10 seconds as the needle is inserted, the biopsy obtained, and the needle withdrawn. Holding the breath after exhalation immobilizes the chest wall and liver and keeps the diaphragm in its highest position, avoiding injury to the lung and laceration of the liver. • Instruct the client to resume breathing when the needle is withdrawn. • Apply pressure to the site of the puncture to help stop any bleeding. Apply a small dressing to the site of the puncture.	Position the client appropriately: • Assist the client to a right side-lying position with a small pillow or folded towel under the biopsy site. Instruct the client to remain in this position for several hours. Monitor the client: • Assess the client's vital signs every 15 min for the first hour following the test or until the signs are stable. Then monitor vital signs every hour for 24 h or as needed. • Determine whether the client is experiencing abdominal pain. Severe abdominal pain may indicate bile peritonitis. • Check the biopsy site for localized bleeding. Pressure dressings may be required if bleeding does occur. Document all relevant information: • Include date and time performed; the primary care provider's name; and all nursing assessments and interventions. Transport the specimens to the laboratory.

Chapter 4 Review

FOCUSING ON CLINICAL THINKING

Consider This

1. What if, when measuring CBG, you do not obtain enough blood to cover the indicator square on the reagent strip?
2. What should you do if the stool becomes contaminated with urine or toilet paper when collecting a stool specimen?

3. What should you do if the client or staff forgot and discarded the client's urine during the collection of a timed 24-hour urine specimen?
4. What if your assessments clearly indicate a wound infection but the culture results return indicating no growth?

See Focusing on Clinical Thinking answers on student resource website.

TEST YOUR KNOWLEDGE

1. A client submitted a stool specimen. The primary care provider tells the client that the test reveals the presence of occult blood and steatorrhea. The nurse explains to the client that the results of the test indicate which of the following?
   1. Ova and parasites are present in the stool.
   2. The large intestine is not functioning properly.
   3. The stool contains blood and an excessive amount of fat.
   4. The pancreas is not functioning properly.

2. A nurse is caring for a client who needs a 24-hour urine specimen. Which nursing actions are appropriate for this client? Select all that apply.
   1. Place a sign in the client's room to remind staff of the test in progress.
   2. Provide clear instructions to the unlicensed assistive personnel (UAP) assisting with the specimen collection.
   3. Ensure that the urine is free of fecal contamination and toilet tissue.
   4. Discard the first sample and document the time the test starts with this discarded specimen.
   5. Collect all subsequent urine specimens, including the one specimen collected at the end of the period.

3. A nurse tests a urine specimen. The test strip indicates the client is positive for the presence of protein in the urine. The nurse knows that this finding can indicate which of the following?
   1. The acid–base status of the urine
   2. Damage to the glomerular membrane
   3. Hidden blood in the urine
   4. Abnormal glucose tolerance

4. The nurse is caring for a client with a Foley catheter. The primary care provider orders a urine test for culture and sensitivity. Which actions indicate correct performance by the nurse? Select all that apply.
   1. Wearing sterile gloves during the collection process
   2. Clamping the drainage tubing 3 inches below the sampling plot
   3. Wiping the area where the needle or Luer-Lok syringe will be inserted with a disinfectant swab
   4. Withdrawing 10 mL from the Foley bag and transferring it to the specimen container
   5. Sending the specimen immediately to the lab

5. A nurse collected a sputum specimen from a client. The specimen was blood tinged, foul smelling, thick, and a very large quantity. Which documentation recording is most accurate for this client?
   1. Copious amount of blood-tinged, foul-smelling, thick sputum specimen sent to lab.
   2. Sputum specimen noted to be minimal, tenacious, foul smelling, and negative for hemoptysis.
   3. Sputum specimen was copious, odorous, watery, and positive for hemoptysis. Sent to lab.
   4. Sputum specimen minimal, thick, foul smelling, and negative for hemoptysis.

6. The nurse is caring for a client scheduled for a lumbar puncture. Which actions by the nurse are appropriate? Select all that apply.
   1. Encourage normal breathing and relaxation with the client.
   2. Reassure the client throughout the procedure by explaining what is happening.
   3. Have the client empty the bladder and bowels prior to the procedure.
   4. Withdraw a small sample of spinal fluid from the lower spine.
   5. Apply a small sterile dressing over the puncture site.

7. A nurse is caring for a client who is scheduled for an angiogram. The client has a history of renal insufficiency related to diabetes. The nurse expects which orders from the primary care provider? Select all that apply.
   1. Obtain daily serum creatinine level.
   2. Administer metformin (Glucophage) PO.
   3. Administer acetylcysteine (Mucomyst) PO.
   4. Restrict fluids to 1,000 mL/24 h.
   5. Check for iodine allergy.

8. The nurse is working in a long-term care facility and planning to delegate the collection of a specimen to unlicensed assistive personnel. Which could the nurse delegate appropriately?
   1. Assist the primary care provider with obtaining a cerebrospinal fluid collection.
   2. Collect a wound specimen for culture and sensitivity.
   3. Collect a venous blood specimen.
   4. Collect a routine urine specimen.

9. The nurse is preparing to collect a wound drainage specimen for culture and sensitivity from a postoperative wound. What action would the nurse take before collecting the specimen?
   1. Apply clean gloves.
   2. Apply sterile gloves.
   3. No need to wear gloves as long as the wound is not touched.
   4. Apply sterile gown and gloves.

10. The nurse is preparing to collect a routine urine specimen from a female client. Place the steps involved in the procedure in the correct order.
    1. Label the container.
    2. Instruct the client on how to collect the specimen.
    3. Obtain the necessary equipment.
    4. Perform hand hygiene.
    5. Explain the need and purpose of collection of the urine specimen to the client.

See Answers to Test Your Knowledge in Appendix A.

READINGS AND REFERENCES

References

American Diabetes Association. (n.d.). *Living with diabetes: Checking your blood glucose*. Retrieved from http://www.diabetes.org/living-with-diabetes/treatment-and-care/blood-glucose-control/checking-your-blood-glucose.html

Daly, J. (2012). Fecal immunochemical tests for colorectal cancer screening. *American Journal of Nursing, 112*(10), 67–69. doi:10.1097/01.NAJ.0000421031.02199.65

Fremgen, B., & Frucht, S. (2013). *Medical terminology: A living language* (5th ed.). Upper Saddle River, NJ: Prentice Hall.

Kee, J. (2013). *Pearson handbook of laboratory and diagnostic tests with nursing implications* (7th ed.). Upper Saddle River, NJ: Pearson.

Kessenich, C. R., & Cronin, K. (2013). Fecal occult blood testing in older adult patients with anemia. *Nurse Practitioner, 38*(1), 6–8. doi:10.1097/01.NPR.0000423386.26198.d4

Rank, W. (2013). Preventing contrast media-induced nephrotoxicity. *Nursing, 43*(4), 48–51. doi:10.1097/01.NURSE.0000427100.98269.76.

Wahowiak, L. (2013). Blood glucose meters. What to look for—and what to know. *Diabetes Forecast, 66*(1), 38–47.

Whitmore, C. (2012). Blood glucose monitoring: An overview. *British Journal of Nursing, 21*(10), 583–587.

Selected Bibliography

Ayanian, J., & Carethers, J. (2012). Bridging behavior and biology to reduce socioeconomic disparities in colorectal cancer risk. *Journal of the National Cancer Institute, 104*(18), 1343–1344. doi:10.1093/jnci/djs356

Berman, A., Snyder, S., & Frandsen, G. (2016). *Kozier & Erb's fundamentals of nursing: Concepts, process, and practice* (10th ed.). Upper Saddle River, NJ: Pearson.

Davis, T. C., Rademaker, A., Bailey, S. C., Platt, D., Esparza, J., Wolf, M. S., & Arnold, C. L. (2013). Contrasts in rural and urban barriers to colorectal cancer screening. *American Journal of Health Behavior, 37*(3), 289–298. doi:10.5993/AJHB.37.3.1

Diabetes Forecast. (2013, January). Blood glucose meters 2013. Retrieved from http://www.forecast.diabetes.org/meters-jan2013

Fisher, W. A., Cornman, D. H., Kohut, T., Schachner, H., & Stenger, P. (2013). What primary care providers can do to address barriers to self-monitoring of blood glucose. *Clinical Diabetes, 31*(1), 34–42. doi:10.2337/diaclin.31.1.34

Jean-Jacques, M., Kaleba, E., Gatta, J., Gracia, G., Ryan, E., & Choucair, B. (2012). Program to improve colorectal cancer screening in a low-income, racially diverse population: A randomized controlled trial. *Annals of Family Medicine, 10*, 412–417. doi:10.1370/afm.1381

Seggelke, S. A., & Everhart, B. (2012). Managing glucose levels in hospital patients. *American Nurse Today, 7*(9), 27–31.

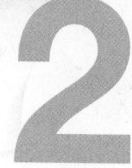

2 Applying the Nursing Process

This unit looks at skills essential for gathering data including vital signs, health assessment, and diagnostic testing. A comprehensive and effective plan of care can only be developed when accurate data are collected during the nursing assessment. The nursing assessment provides the information needed for analysis, diagnosis, and planning. The nurse is always assessing, whether meeting a client for the first time or caring for a client at the end of the shift, in order to determine client needs or client responses to care or to recognize new problems.

CLIENT: Hazel   AGE: 84 Years   CURRENT MEDICAL DIAGNOSIS: Congestive Heart Failure

Medical History: Hazel was treated for myocardial infarctions at ages 55, 63, and again at age 70. The damage to her heart muscle resulted in congestive heart failure and chronic renal failure. She was admitted to the acute care facility today, secondary to a 2-day weight gain of 8 pounds, peripheral edema, and shortness of breath secondary to pulmonary edema. Her vital signs are temperature 36.9°C (98.4°F) axillary, pulse 108 beats/min irregular and thready, respirations 28/min, and blood pressure 152/94 mmHg in her left arm.

Personal and Social History: Hazel lives with her 85-year-old husband who has been diagnosed with dementia. In addition to caring for her husband, she also cares for her three great-grandchildren while her granddaughter works. She lives in the same home she and her husband bought 53 years ago, and says she plans to die in her home. The home has bedrooms on the second floor and a laundry room in the basement, resulting in her walking down two flights of stairs when she wants to do the family's laundry. Her daughter and son live out of state, and her 24-year-old granddaughter and three great-grandchildren live approximately 2 miles away.

Questions

Assessment

1. When obtaining Hazel's vital signs, why did the nurse measure the client's temperature using the axillary site?
2. What data will the nurse collect in order to assess Hazel's oxygenation status?
3. How will the nurse best position Hazel during the assessment? Why is this the best position for this client?

Analysis

4. List two possible nursing diagnoses that can be identified from the medical/personal history and assessment data above.

Planning

5. Based on the assessment data and nursing diagnoses, identify one desired outcome.

Implementation

6. Prior to beginning Hazel's physical assessment, what teaching will the nurse provide?
7. The provider has ordered a 24-hour urine collection. What teaching will the nurse provide for Hazel?

Evaluation

8. How will the nurse know if the expected outcome has been achieved?

See *Applying the Nursing Process* suggested answers on student resource website.

Assisting with Client Hygiene and Comfort

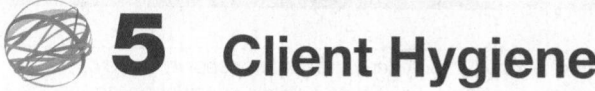

5 Client Hygiene

LEARNING OUTCOMES

At the completion of this chapter, the student will be able to:

1. Define the key terms used in the skills of hygienic care.
2. Describe the kinds of hygienic care nurses provide to clients.
3. Identify factors that influence personal hygiene.
4. Describe various types of baths.
5. Describe guidelines for bathing individuals with dementia.
6. Recognize when it is appropriate to delegate hygienic care to unlicensed assistive personnel.

7. Verbalize the steps used in:
   a. Bathing an adult or pediatric client.
   b. Providing perineal-genital care.
   c. Brushing and flossing the teeth.
   d. Providing special oral care.
   e. Providing hair care.
   f. Providing foot care.
   g. Removing, cleaning, and inserting a hearing aid.
8. Demonstrate appropriate documentation and reporting of hygienic care.

SKILLS

Skill 5–1 Bathing an Adult Client
Skill 5–2 Providing Perineal-Genital Care
Skill 5–3 Brushing and Flossing the Teeth
Skill 5–4 Providing Special Oral Care for an Unconscious or Debilitated Client

Skill 5–5 Providing Hair Care
Skill 5–6 Providing Foot Care
Skill 5–7 Removing, Cleaning, and Inserting a Hearing Aid

KEY TERMS

abbreviated bath, *172*
alopecia, *187*
as-needed (prn) care, *171*
bag bath, *172*
cerumen, *192*
cleaning baths, *172*
complete bed bath, *172*
dandruff, *187*
dentifrice, *182*

early morning care, *171*
earmold, *192*
gingivitis, *181*
hearing aid, *192*
hirsutism, *187*
hour of sleep care, *171*
morning care, *171*
partial bath, *172*
pediculosis (lice), *187*

pericare, *179*
perineal care, *179*
personal hygiene, *171*
plaque, *181*
pyorrhea, *181*
scabies, *187*
self-help bed bath, *172*
shower, *173*
sitz bath, *173*

sulcular technique, *182*
tartar, *181*
therapeutic baths, *173*
towel bath, *173*
tub bath, *173*
xerostomia, *182*

Personal hygiene is the self-care by which people attend to such functions as bathing, toileting, general body hygiene, and grooming. Hygiene is a highly personal matter determined by various factors, including individual and cultural values and practices. It involves care of the skin, hair, nails, teeth, oral and nasal cavities, eyes, ears, and perineal-genital areas.

It is important for nurses to know exactly how much assistance a client needs for hygienic care. Clients may require help after urinating or defecating, after vomiting, and whenever they become soiled, for example, from wound drainage or from profuse perspiration. In addition, culture-specific beliefs and practices influence hygienic care. Table 5–1 lists factors that influence hygienic practices.

Nurses commonly use the following terms to describe the various types of hygienic care:

- **Early morning care** is provided to clients as they awaken in the morning. This care consists of providing a urinal or bedpan to the

client confined to bed, washing the face and hands, and giving oral care.

- **Morning care** is often provided after clients have breakfast, although it may be provided before breakfast. It usually includes providing for elimination needs, a bath or shower, perineal care, and oral, nail, and hair care. Making the client's bed is part of morning care.
- **Hour of sleep care**, or *PM care*, is provided to clients before they go to sleep for the night. It usually involves providing for elimination needs, washing face and hands, giving oral care, and possibly giving a back massage. Some clients prefer bathing in the evening. If possible, the nurse needs to accommodate the client's routine schedule for personal hygiene.
- **As-needed (prn) care** is provided as required by the client. For example, a client who is diaphoretic (sweating profusely) may need bathing and a change of clothes and linen frequently.

TABLE 5–1   Factors That Influence Individual Hygienic Practices

Factor	Variables
Culture	North American culture places a high value on cleanliness. Many North Americans bathe or shower once or twice a day, whereas people from some other cultures bathe once a week. Some cultures consider privacy essential for bathing, whereas others practice communal bathing. Body odor is offensive in some cultures and accepted as normal in others.
Religion	Ceremonial washings are practiced by some religions.
Environment	Finances may affect the availability of facilities for bathing. For example, homeless people may not have warm water available; soap, shampoo, shaving lotion, and deodorants may be too expensive for people who have limited resources.
Developmental level	Children learn hygiene in the home. Practices vary according to the individual's age; for example, preschoolers can carry out most tasks independently with encouragement.
Health and energy	Ill people may not have the motivation or energy to attend to hygiene. Some clients who have neuromuscular impairments may be unable to perform hygienic care.
Personal preferences	Some people prefer a shower to a tub bath. People have different preferences regarding the time of bathing (e.g., morning versus evening).

BATHING AND SKIN CARE

Bathing removes accumulated oil, perspiration, dead skin cells, and some bacteria. The nurse can appreciate the quantity of oil and dead skin cells produced by the body when observing the client's skin after the removal of a cast that has been on for 6 weeks. The skin is crusty, flaky, and dry underneath the cast. Applications of oil over several days are usually necessary to remove the debris. Excessive bathing, however, can interfere with the intended lubricating effect of the sebum, causing dryness of the skin. This is an important consideration of older clients who produce limited sebum (fatty secretions of the sebaceous glands).

In addition to cleaning the skin, bathing also stimulates circulation. A warm or hot bath dilates superficial arterioles, bringing more blood and nourishment to the skin. Vigorous rubbing has the same effect. Rubbing with long smooth strokes from the distal to proximal parts of extremities (from the point farthest from the body to the point closest) is particularly effective in facilitating venous blood flow unless there is some underlying condition (e.g., blood clot) that would contraindicate this action. Vigorous rubbing is avoided in older clients with little subcutaneous tissue and those on medications that thin skin or cause easy bruising such as steroids or anticoagulants. Bathing also produces a sense of well-being. It is refreshing and relaxing and frequently improves spirit, appearance, and self-concept. Some people take a morning shower for its refreshing, stimulating effect. Others prefer an evening bath because it is relaxing. These effects are more evident when a person is ill. For example, it is not uncommon for clients who have had a restless or sleepless night to feel relaxed, comfortable, and sleepy after a morning bath.

Bathing offers an excellent opportunity for the nurse to assess clients who are ill, and opens the door to establishing trust. The nurse can observe the condition of the client's skin and physical conditions such as reddened pressure areas over bony prominences. While assisting a client with a bath, the nurse can also assess the client's psychosocial needs (e.g., orientation to time and ability to cope with the illness) and physical ability to implement self-care. The nurse can also assess a client's learning needs during a bath, such as a client with diabetes needing to learn foot care.

Planning to assist a client with personal hygiene includes consideration of the client's personal preferences, health, and limitations; the best time to give the care; and the equipment, facilities, and personnel available. A client's personal preferences—about when and how to bathe, for example—should be followed as long as they are compatible with the client's health and the equipment available. Another consideration for the nurse is to assess the client's comfort level with the gender of the caregiver. Hygienic care, particularly bathing, can be embarrassing and stressful to modest individuals, regardless of gender. Women in some cultures (e.g., Hindu, Iranian, Arab, and Navajo Indian) are generally modest. Nurses must respect a client's modesty, whether male or female, and provide adequate privacy and sensitivity. If possible, try to provide a caregiver of the same gender (Purnell, 2014). Nurses need to provide whatever assistance the client requires, either directly or by delegating this task to other nursing personnel, or including a family caregiver in the task if the client prefers.

Categories of Baths

Two categories of baths are given to clients: cleaning and therapeutic. **Cleaning baths** are given chiefly for hygienic purposes and include these types:

- **Complete bed bath**. The nurse washes the entire body of a dependent client in bed.
- **Self-help bed bath**. Clients confined to bed are able to bathe themselves with help from the nurse for washing the back and perhaps the feet.
- **Partial bath (abbreviated bath)**. Only parts of the client's body that might cause discomfort or odor, if neglected, are washed: the face, hands, axillae, perineal area, and back. Omitted are the arms, chest, abdomen, legs, and feet. The nurse provides this care for dependent clients and assists self-sufficient clients confined to bed by washing their backs. Some ambulatory clients prefer to take a partial bath at the sink. The nurse can assist them by washing their backs.
- **Bag bath**. This bath is a commercially prepared, disposable product that contains 10 to 12 presoaked disposable washcloths that contain no-rinse cleanser solution (Figure 5–1 ■). The package is warmed in a microwave. The warming time is about 1 minute, but the nurse needs to determine how long it takes to attain a desirable and evenly distributed temperature. Each area of the body is cleaned with a different cloth and then air-dried. Because the body is not rubbed dry, the emollient in the solution remains on

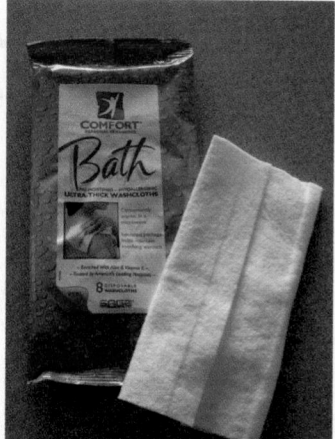

Figure 5–1 ■ A commercial bag bath product.

the skin. The disposable bag bath is often a desirable form for bathing clients in critical care and long-term care settings.

- **Towel bath**. This bath is similar to a bag bath but uses regular towels. It is useful for clients who are confined to bed and clients with dementia. The client is covered and kept warm throughout the bathing process by a bath blanket. The nurse gradually replaces the bath blanket with a large towel that has been soaked with warm water and no-rinse soap. The client is then gently massaged with the warm, wet, soapy towel. The wet towel is replaced with a large dry towel for drying the client's skin.

- **Tub bath**. Tub baths are preferred to bed baths because it is easier to wash and rinse in a tub. Tubs are also used for therapeutic baths. The amount of assistance the nurse offers depends on the abilities of the client. Specially designed tubs are available for dependent clients. These tubs greatly reduce the work of the nurse in lifting clients in and out of the tub and offer greater benefits than a sponge bath in bed. Safety precautions must be implemented per agency protocol.

- **Shower**. Many ambulatory clients are able to use shower facilities and require only minimal assistance from the nurse. Clients in long-term care settings are often given showers and may need to use a shower chair. The wheels on a shower chair allow clients to be transported from their room to the shower. The shower chair also has a commode seat to facilitate cleansing of the client's perineal area during the shower process (Figure 5–2 ■).

Therapeutic baths are given for physical effects such as to soothe irritated skin or to promote healing of an area (e.g., the perineum). Two common types are the sitz bath and the medicated bath. For the **sitz bath**, the client sits in warm water to help soothe and heal the perineum. For example, mothers after childbirth or clients who have had rectal surgery may find a sitz bath soothing. Some clients may also use a sitz bath to help alleviate discomfort from hemorrhoids. A tub can be used for a sitz bath, or a disposable plastic sitz bath unit that sits over a toilet bowl can be used.

The medicated therapeutic bath is generally taken in a tub one-third or one-half full with water at a comfortable temperature. Medications may be placed in the water (e.g., sodium bicarbonate, Aveeno oatmeal products, bath oils). The baths are useful for soothing irritated or itchy skin (e.g., from sunburn, hives, skin diseases). The client usually remains in the bath for no longer than 20 to 30 minutes. If the client's back, chest, and arms are to be treated, these areas need to be immersed in the solution. For safety reasons, advise the client

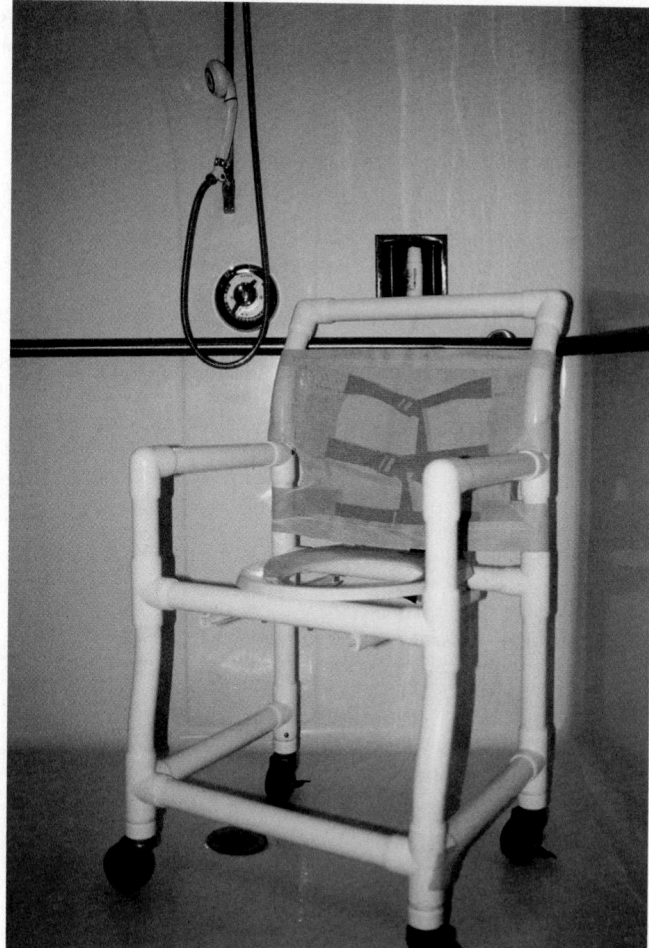

Figure 5–2 ■ A shower chair.

to use a bath mat, especially if the product added to the water will make the surface of the tub slippery. Skill 5–1 provides guidelines for bathing clients.

Long-Term Care Setting

From a historical perspective, the bath has always been a part of nursing care and is considered a component of the "art" of nursing. In today's nursing world, however, the bath is seen as a necessary, routine task and is often delegated to nonprofessionals.

In spite of the previously listed beneficial values associated with bathing, the choice of bathing procedure often depends on the amount of time available to the nurse or unlicensed assistive personnel (UAP) and the client's self-care ability. The bath routine (e.g., day, time, and number/week) for clients in health care settings is often determined by agency policy, which often results in the bath becoming routine and depersonalized versus therapeutic, satisfying, and person centered. New models and a culture change process are emerging in long-term care and residential care settings. That is, these settings are trying to become less about tasks and more about people and the relationships between people. This person-centered approach to bathing is especially important for the older person in a long-term care setting. Bathing needs to focus on the experience for the client rather than the outcome (i.e., getting a bath or shower).

A nurse who provides person-centered care asks questions such as these: What is the client's usual method of maintaining cleanliness?

BOX 5–1 **General Guidelines for Bathing Individuals with Dementia**

- Focus on the person rather than the task.
  - Evaluate to determine if the person needs pain control before the bath.
  - Time the bath to fit the person's history, preferences, and mood.
  - Cover! Keep the person covered as much as possible to keep him or her warm.
  - Move slowly and let the person know when you are going to move or touch him or her.
  - Use a gentle touch. Use soft cloths. Pat dry rather than rubbing.
- Be flexible. Adapt your approach to meet the needs of the person.
  - Consider adapting your methods (e.g., distracting the person with singing while bathing), the environment (e.g., correct size of shower chair, reducing noise, playing music), and the procedure (e.g., consistently assigning same caregiver, inviting family to help).
  - Encourage flexibility in scheduling of the bath based on the person's preference.
- Use persuasion, not coercion.
  - Give choices and respond to individual requests.

- Help the person feel in control.
  - Use a supportive, calm approach and praise the person often.
- Be prepared.
  - Gather everything that you will need for the bath (e.g., towels, washcloths, clothes) before approaching the person.
- Stop when a person becomes distressed. It is *not* normal to have cries, screams, or protests from the person.
  - Stop what you are doing and assess for causes of the distress.
  - Adjust your approach.
  - Shorten or stop the bath.
  - Try to end on a positive note.
  - Reapproach later to wash critical areas if necessary.
- Ask for help.
  - Talk with others, including the family, about different ways to help make the bath more comfortable for the person.

From "Dementia-Friendly Bathing," by S. Hoban, 2012, *Long-Term Living*, *61*(10), pp. 41–42; "Practical Care: Creative Strategies for Bathing," by R. H. Johnson, 2011, *Nursing & Residential Care*, *13*(8), pp. 392–394; and "Nursing Home Bathing Transformed," by E. F. Barbera, 2011, *Long-Term Living*, *60*(10), pp. 41–43

Are there any past negative experiences related to bathing? Are factors such as pain or fatigue increasing the client's difficulty with the demands and stimuli associated with bathing or showering? A client's resistance to the bathing experience can be a cue to the nurse to consider other methods of maintaining cleanliness. For example, if the shower causes distress, is there another form of bathing (such as the bag or towel bath) that may be more therapeutic and comforting?

An individualized approach focusing on therapeutic and comforting outcomes of bathing is especially important for clients with dementia. Alzheimer's disease is the most common cause of dementia among people ages 65 and older. As the incidence of dementia increases, so does the need to preserve the dignity of people with dementia. Preserving dignity is especially a priority in the residential care environment where more than two thirds of residents have some form of dementia (Gaspard & Cox, 2012, p. 43). This statistic has implications for nursing care. For example, people with dementia become agitated as soon as they are told it is time to bathe and many are afraid of the noise of running water and of water on the face (Hoban, 2012). See Box 5–1 for strategies that can reduce the stress of the bathing experience for both the person with dementia and the caregiver.

Providing personal hygiene to clients with dementia is often an ongoing challenge. Being sensitive to the rhythm of their behavior and looking for cues can often offset problems related to this. Clients with dementia, whether they are at home or in a health care facility, often have certain times of the day when they are more agitated—these are times to avoid doing things that will increase their fear and agitation. If a client is agitated, it is sometimes helpful to wait (e.g., half an hour or so) before trying to give the bath, because the client may forget his or her protesting and be willing to participate.

In addition, collaboration between the nurse and UAP is a critical element to implementing the individualized person-focused approach for clients with cognitive impairments who exhibit aggressive behavior during bathing. The nurse, after observing a difficult bathing situation, should discuss with the UAP possible alternative strategies or methods that might be implemented for the client. More than one intervention may be required (e.g., reassurance, simple explanations, moving slowly). It is important for the nurse to subsequently evaluate the client's response to the new intervention(s). The nurse has a role in educating UAP about dementia and collaboratively problem solving bathing challenges (Gaspard & Cox, 2012).

●○● NURSING PROCESS: BATHING AND SKIN CARE

Bathing an Adult Client

SKILL 5-1

ASSESSMENT
Assess:
- Physical or emotional factors (e.g., fatigue, sensitivity to cold, need for control, anxiety, or fear).
- Condition of the skin (color, texture and turgor, presence of pigmented spots, temperature, lesions, excoriations, abrasions, and bruises). Areas of erythema (redness) on the sacrum, bony prominences, and heels should be assessed for possible pressure sores.

- Presence of pain and need for adjunctive measures (e.g., an analgesic) before the bath.
- Range of motion of the joints.
- Any other aspect of health that may affect the client's bathing process (e.g., mobility, strength, cognition).
- Need for use of clean gloves during the bath

Bathing an Adult Client—*continued*

PLANNING
DELEGATION

The nurse often delegates the skill of bathing to UAP. However, the nurse remains responsible for assessment and client care. The nurse needs to do the following:

- Inform the UAP of the type of bath appropriate for the client and precautions, if any, specific to the needs of the client.
- Remind the UAP to notify the nurse of any concerns or changes (e.g., redness, skin breakdown, rash) so the nurse can assess, intervene if needed, and document.
- Instruct the UAP to encourage the client to perform as much self-care as appropriate in order to promote independence and self-esteem.
- Obtain a complete report about the bathing experience from the UAP.

Equipment

- Basin or sink with warm water (between 43°C and 46°C [110°F and 115°F])
- Soap and soap dish
- Linens: bath blanket, two bath towels, washcloth, clean gown or pajamas or clothes as needed, additional bed linen and towels, if required
- Clean gloves, if appropriate (e.g., presence of body fluids or open lesions)
- Personal hygiene articles (e.g., deodorant, powder, lotions)
- Shaving equipment
- Table for bathing equipment
- Laundry bag

IMPLEMENTATION
Preparation

Before bathing a client, determine (a) the purpose and type of bath the client needs; (b) self-care ability of the client; (c) any movement or positioning precautions specific to the client; (d) other care the client may be receiving, such as physical therapy or x-rays, in order to co-ordinate all aspects of health care and prevent unnecessary fatigue; (e) the client's comfort level with being bathed by someone else; and (f) necessary bath equipment and linens.

Caution is needed when bathing clients who are receiving intravenous (IV) therapy. Easy-to-remove gowns that have Velcro or snap fasteners along the sleeves may be used. If a special gown is not available, the nurse needs to pay special attention when changing the client's gown after the bath (or whenever the gown becomes soiled). In addition, special attention is needed to reassess the IV site for security of IV connections and appropriate taping around the IV site.

The nurse should use universal precautions when bathing a client, particularly when performing perineal care. It is not always necessary, however, to wear gloves while providing a bath. The nurse should use clinical judgment when deciding to wear gloves and offer an explanation to the client.

Performance

1. Prior to performing the procedure, introduce self and verify the client's identity using agency protocol. Explain to the client what you are going to do, why it is necessary, and how he or she can participate. Discuss the client's preferences for bathing and explain any unfamiliar procedures to the client.
2. Perform hand hygiene and observe other appropriate infection prevention procedures.
3. Provide for client privacy by drawing the curtains around the bed or closing the door to the room. Some agencies provide signs indicating the need for privacy. **Rationale:** *Hygiene is a personal matter.*
4. Prepare the client and the environment.
   - Invite a family member or significant other to participate if desired or requested by the client.
   - Close windows and doors to ensure the room is a comfortable temperature. **Rationale:** *Air currents increase loss of heat from the body by convection.*
   - Offer the client a bedpan or urinal or ask whether the client wishes to use the toilet or commode. **Rationale:** *Warm water and activity can stimulate the need to void. The client will be more comfortable after voiding, and voiding before cleaning the perineum is advisable.*
   - Encourage the client to perform as much personal self-care as possible. **Rationale:** *This promotes independence, exercise, and self-esteem.*
   - During the bath, assess each area of the skin carefully.

For a Bed Bath

5. Prepare the bed and position the client appropriately.
   - Position the bed at a comfortable working height. Lower the side rail on the side close to you. Keep the other side rail *up*. Assist the client to move near you. **Rationale:** *This avoids undue reaching and straining, promotes good body mechanics, and allows the nurse to wash both sides of the client's body without moving around the bed. It also ensures client safety.*
   - Place a bath blanket over the top sheet. Remove the top sheet from under the bath blanket by starting at the client's shoulders and moving linen down toward the client's feet. ❶ Ask the client to grasp and hold the top of the bath blanket while pulling linen to the foot of the bed. **Rationale:** *The bath blanket provides comfort, warmth, and privacy.* Note: If the bed linen is to be reused, place it over the bedside chair. If it is to be changed, place it in the linen hamper, not on the floor. **Rationale:** *Placing used linens in the linen hamper, rather than on the floor, prevents the spread of microorganisms.*
   - Remove the client's gown while keeping the client covered with the bath blanket. Place the gown in the linen hamper.
6. Make a bath mitt with the washcloth. **Rationale:** *A bath mitt retains water and heat better than a cloth loosely held and prevents the ends of the washcloth from dragging across the skin.* See ❷ for the triangular method and ❸ for the rectangular method of making a bath mitt.

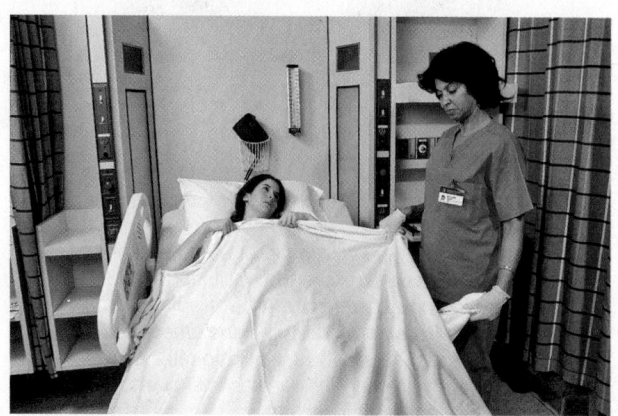

❶ Remove the top sheet from under the bath blanket.

Continued on page 176

SKILL 5–1

Bathing an Adult Client—*continued*

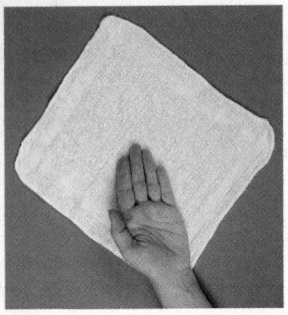 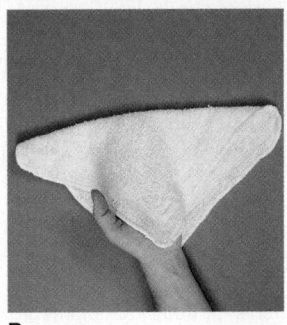 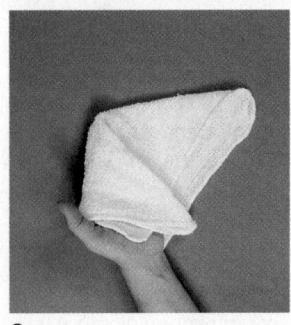 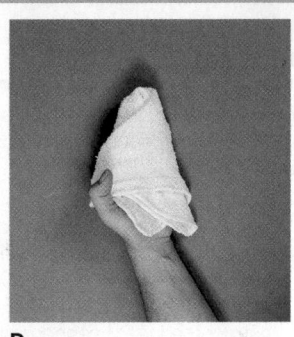

A   **B**   **C**   **D**

❷ Making a bath mitt, triangular method. *A,* Lay your hand on the washcloth; *B,* fold the top corner over your hand; *C,* fold the side corners over your hand; *D,* tuck the second corner under the cloth on the palm side to secure the mitt.

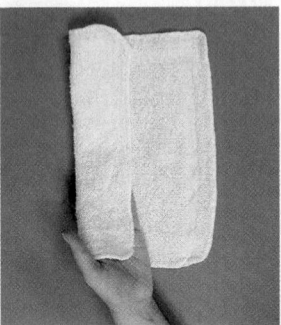 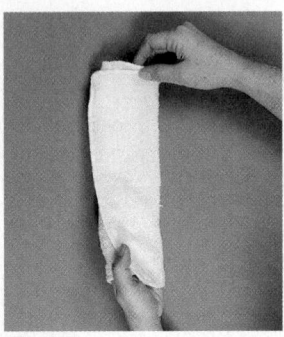 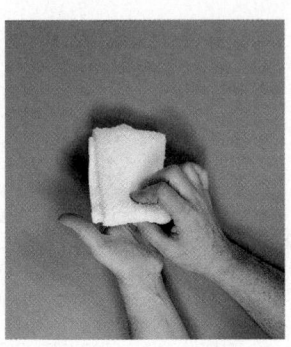

A   **B**   **C**

❸ Making a bath mitt, rectangular method. *A,* Lay your hand on the washcloth and fold one side over your hand; *B,* fold the second side over your hand; *C,* fold the top of the cloth down and tuck it under the folded side against your palm to secure the mitt.

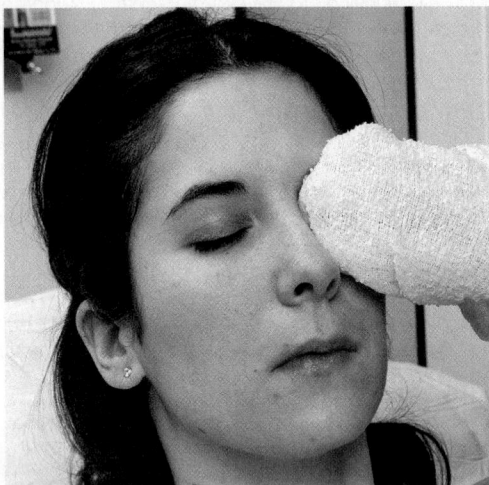

❹ Using a separate corner of the washcloth for each eye, wipe from the inner to the outer canthus.

7. Wash the face. **Rationale:** *Begin the bath at the cleanest area and work downward toward the feet.*
   • Place a towel under the client's head.
   • Wash the client's eyes with water only and dry them well. Use a separate corner of the washcloth for each eye. **Rationale:** *Using separate corners prevents transmission of microorganisms from one eye to the other.* Wipe from the inner to the outer canthus. ❹ **Rationale:** *This prevents secretions from entering the nasolacrimal ducts.*

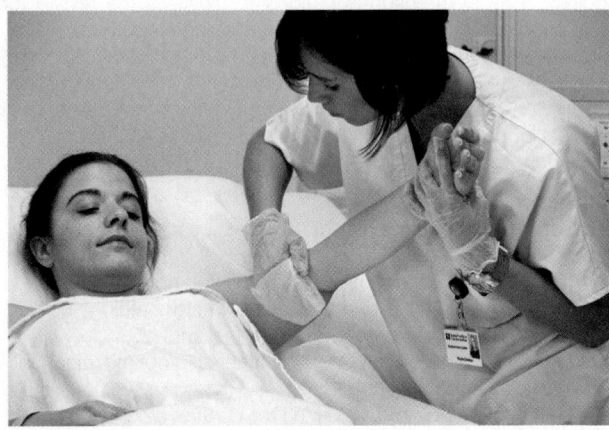

❺ Washing the arm using long, firm strokes from wrist to shoulder area.

   • Ask whether the client wants soap used on the face. **Rationale:** *Soap has a drying effect, and the face, which is exposed to the air more than other body parts, tends to be drier.*
   • Wash, rinse, and dry the client's face, ears, and neck.
   • Remove the towel from under the client's head.
8. Wash the arms and hands. (Omit the arms for a partial bath.)
   • Place a towel lengthwise under the arm away from you. **Rationale:** *It protects the bed from becoming wet.*
   • Wash, rinse, and dry the arm by elevating the client's arm and supporting the client's wrist and elbow. Use long, firm strokes from wrist to shoulder, including the axillary area. ❺

Bathing an Adult Client—*continued*

Rationale: *Firm strokes from distal to proximal areas promote circulation by increasing venous blood return.*

- Apply deodorant or powder if desired. Special caution is needed for clients with respiratory alterations. **Rationale:** *Powder is not recommended for these clients due to potential adverse respiratory effects.*
- *Optional:* Place a towel on the bed and put a washbasin on it. Place the client's hands in the basin. **Rationale:** *Many clients enjoy immersing their hands in the basin and washing themselves. Soaking loosens dirt under the nails.* Assist the client as needed to wash, rinse, and dry the hands, paying particular attention to the spaces between the fingers.
- Repeat for the hand and arm nearest you. Exercise caution if an intravenous infusion is present, and check its flow after moving the arm. Avoid submersing the IV site.

9. Wash the chest and abdomen. (Omit the chest and abdomen for a partial bath. However, the areas under a woman's breasts may require bathing if this area is irritated or if the client has significant perspiration under the breasts.)
   - Place the bath towel lengthwise over the chest. Fold the bath blanket down to the client's pubic area. **Rationale:** *This keeps the client warm while preventing unnecessary exposure of the chest.*
   - Lift the bath towel off the chest, and bathe the chest and abdomen with your mitted hand using long, firm strokes. ❻ Give special attention to the skin under the breasts and any other skinfolds, particularly if the client is overweight. Rinse and dry well.
   - Replace the bath blanket when the areas have been dried.

10. Wash the legs and feet. (Omit legs and feet for a partial bath.)
    - Expose the leg farthest from you by folding the bath blanket toward the other leg, being careful to keep the perineum covered. **Rationale:** *Covering the perineum promotes privacy and maintains the client's dignity.*
    - Lift the leg and place the bath towel lengthwise under the leg. Wash, rinse, and dry the leg using long, smooth, firm strokes from the ankle to the knee to the thigh. ❼ **Rationale:** *Washing from the distal to proximal areas promotes circulation by stimulating venous blood flow.*
    - Reverse the coverings and repeat for the other leg.
    - Wash the feet by placing them in a basin of water.
    - Dry each foot. Pay particular attention to the spaces between the toes. If preferred, wash one foot after that leg before washing the other leg.

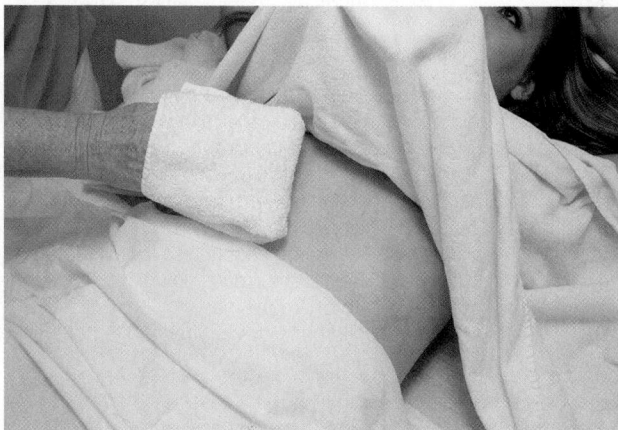

❻ Washing the chest and abdomen.

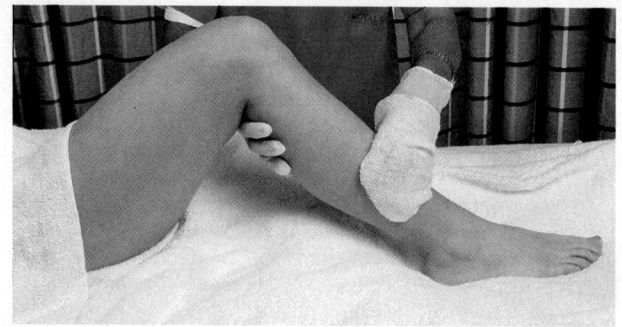

❼ Washing the far leg.

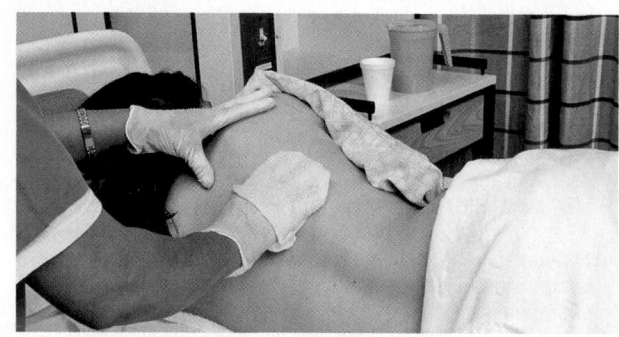

❽ Washing the back.

- Obtain fresh, warm bathwater now or when necessary. **Rationale:** *Water may become dirty or cold.* Because surface skin cells are removed with washing, the bathwater from dark-skinned clients may be dark; however, this does not mean the client is dirty. Lower the bed and raise the side rails when refilling the basin. **Rationale:** *This ensures the safety of the client.*

11. Wash the back and then the perineum.
    - Assist the client into a prone or side-lying position facing away from you. Place the bath towel lengthwise alongside the back and buttocks while keeping the client covered with the bath blanket as much as possible. **Rationale:** *This provides warmth and prevents undue exposure.*
    - Wash and dry the client's back, moving from the shoulders to the buttocks, and upper thighs, paying attention to the gluteal folds. ❽ **Rationale:** *Wash from the area of least contamination (the back) to that of greatest (gluteal folds).*
    - Remove and discard gloves if used.
    - Perform a back massage now or after completion of the bath (see Skill 9–4 in Chapter 9 ∞).
    - Assist the client to the supine position and determine whether the client can wash the perineal area independently. If the client cannot do so, drape the client as shown in Skill 5–2 ❶, apply gloves, and wash the area.

12. Assist the client with grooming aids such as powder, lotion, or deodorant.
    - Use powder sparingly. Release as little as possible into the atmosphere. **Rationale:** *This will avoid irritation of the respiratory tract by powder inhalation. Excessive powder can cause caking, which leads to skin irritation.*
    - Help the client put on a clean gown or pajamas.
    - Assist the client to care for hair, mouth, and nails. Some clients prefer or need mouth care prior to their bath.

Continued on page 178

SKILL 5–1

Bathing an Adult Client—*continued*

For a Tub Bath or Shower

13. Prepare the client and the tub.
  - Fill the tub about one-third to one-half full of water at 43°C to 46°C (110°F to 115°F). **Rationale:** *Sufficient water is needed to cover the perineal area.*
  - Cover all intravenous catheters or wound dressings with plastic coverings, and instruct the client to prevent wetting these areas if possible.
  - Put a rubber bath mat or towel on the floor of the tub if safety strips are not on the tub floor. **Rationale:** *These prevent slippage of the client during the bath or shower.*

14. Assist the client into the shower or tub.
  - Assist the client taking a standing shower with the initial adjustment of the water temperature and water flow pressure, as needed. Some clients need a chair to sit on in the shower because of weakness. Hot water can cause older clients to feel faint due to vasodilation and decreased blood pressure from positional changes.
  - If the client requires considerable assistance with a tub bath, a hydraulic bathtub chair may be required (see the *Variation* section later in this skill).
  - Explain how the client can signal for help, leave the client for 2 to 5 minutes, and place an "Occupied" sign on the door. For safety reasons, do not leave a client with decreased cognition or clients who may be at risk (e.g., history of seizures, syncope).

15. Assist the client with washing and getting out of the tub.
  - Wash the client's back, lower legs, and feet, if necessary.
  - Assist the client out of the tub. If the client is unsteady, place a bath towel over the client's shoulders and drain the tub of water before the client attempts to get out of it. **Rationale:** *Draining the water first lessens the likelihood of a fall. The towel prevents chilling.*

16. Dry the client, and assist with follow-up care.
  - Follow step 12.
  - Assist the client back to his or her bed.
  - Clean the tub or shower in accordance with agency practice, discard the used linen in the laundry hamper, and place the "Unoccupied" sign on the door.

17. Document the following:
  - Type of bath given (i.e., complete, partial, or self-help). This is usually recorded on a flow sheet.
  - Skin assessment, such as excoriation, erythema, exudates, rashes, drainage, or skin breakdown.
  - Nursing interventions related to skin integrity.
  - Ability of the client to assist or cooperate with bathing.
  - Client response to bathing. Also, document the need for reassessment of vital signs if appropriate.
  - Educational needs regarding hygiene.
  - Information or teaching shared with the client or the family.

Variation: Bathing Using a Hydraulic Bathtub Chair

A hydraulic lift, often used in long-term care or rehabilitation settings, can facilitate the transfer of a client who is unable to ambulate to a tub. The lift also helps eliminate strain on the nurse's back.

- Bring the client to the tub room in a wheelchair or shower chair.
- Fill the tub and check the water temperature with a bath thermometer. **Rationale:** *This avoids thermal injury to the client.*
- Lower the hydraulic chair lift to its lowest point, outside the tub.
- Transfer the client to the chair lift and secure the seat belt.
- Raise the chair lift above the tub.
- Support the client's legs as the chair is moved over the tub. **Rationale:** *This avoids injury to the legs.*
- Position the client's legs down into the water and slowly lower the chair lift into the tub.
- Assist in bathing the client, if appropriate.
- Reverse the procedure when taking the client out of the tub.
- Dry the client and transport him or her to the room.

EVALUATION

- Note the client's tolerance of the procedure (e.g., respiratory rate and effort, pulse rate, behaviors of acceptance or resistance, statements regarding comfort).
- Conduct appropriate assessment follow-up, such as determining and documenting:
  - Condition and integrity of skin (dryness, turgor, redness, and lesions).
- Client strength. Note range of motion and circulation, movement, and sensation for all extremities.
- Percentage of bath done without assistance.
- Relate to prior assessment data, if available.

LIFESPAN CONSIDERATIONS   Bathing

INFANTS
- Sponge baths are suggested for the newborn because daily tub baths are not considered necessary. After the bath, the infant should be immediately dried and wrapped. Parents need to be advised that the infant's ability to regulate body temperature has not yet fully developed and newborns' bodies lose heat readily.

CHILDREN
- Encourage a child's participation as appropriate for developmental level.
- Closely supervise children in the bathtub. Do not leave them unattended.

ADOLESCENTS
- Assist adolescents as needed to choose deodorants and antiperspirants. Secretions from newly active sweat glands react with bacteria on the skin, causing a pungent odor.

OLDER ADULTS
- Changes of aging can decrease the protective function of the skin in older adults. These changes include fragile skin, less oil and moisture, and a decrease in elasticity.
- To minimize skin dryness in older adults, avoid use of soap. The ideal time to moisturize the skin is immediately after bathing.
- Avoid excessive powder because it causes moisture loss and is a hazardous inhalant. Cornstarch should also be avoided because in the presence of moisture it breaks down into glucose and can facilitate the growth of organisms.
- Protect older adults and children from injury related to hot water burns.

CLIENT TEACHING CONSIDERATIONS

Skin Problems and Care

DRY SKIN

- Use cleansing creams to clean the skin rather than soap or detergent, which cause drying and, in some cases, allergic reactions.
- Thoroughly rinse soap or detergent, if used, from the skin.
- Bathe less frequently when environmental temperature and humidity are low.
- Increase fluid intake.
- Humidify the air with a humidifier or by keeping a tub or sink full of water.
- Use moisturizing or emollient creams that contain lanolin, petroleum jelly, or cocoa butter to retain skin moisture.
- Moisturizers should be applied in the direction of hair growth, after bathing, immediately after the client has patted self dry so there is still moisture in the skin.
- Daily use of a moisturizer is recommended.

SKIN RASHES

- Keep the area clean by washing it with a mild soap. Rinse the skin well, and pat it dry.
- To relieve itching, try a tepid bath or soak. Some over-the-counter preparations, such as Caladryl lotion, may help but should be used with full knowledge of the product.
- Avoid scratching the rash to prevent inflammation, infection, and further skin lesions.
- Choose clothing carefully. Wearing too much clothing can cause perspiration and aggravate a rash.

ACNE

Gently wash the face no more than twice daily using a cleanser or mild soap made specifically for people with acne.
- Avoid using oily creams, which aggravate the condition.
- Avoid using cosmetics that block the ducts of the sebaceous glands and the hair follicles.
- Never squeeze or pick at the lesions. This increases the potential for infection and scarring.

Ambulatory and Community Settings | Safety

Hygiene

- Focus on promoting function, independence, and autonomy during the bathing process. This will help clients avoid dependence on caretakers in the long-term care setting.
- The type of bath chosen depends on assessment of the home, caregiver, availability of running water, and condition of bathing facilities.

Suggestions for bathing in the home setting include the following:
- Consider purchasing a bath seat that fits in the tub or shower.
- Install a hand shower for use with a bath seat and shampooing.
- Use a nonskid surface on the tub or shower.
- Install hand bars on both sides of the tub or shower to facilitate transfers in and out of the tub or shower.
- Carefully monitor the temperature of the bathwater.
- Apply lotion and oil after a bath, not during, because these solutions can make a tub surface slippery.

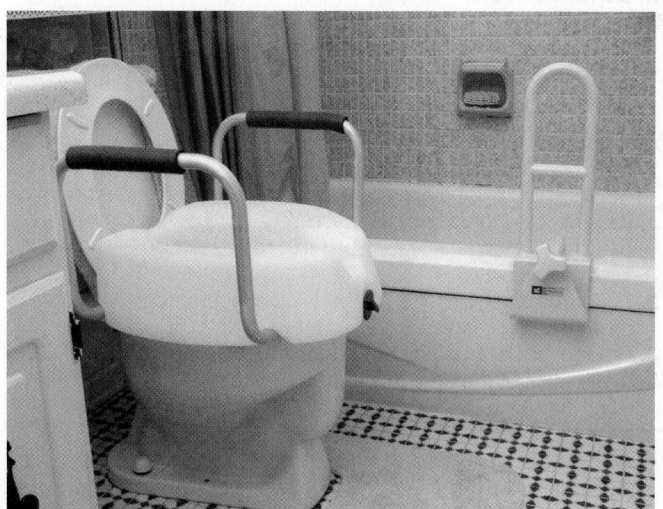

Tub/shower seat in the home.
Steven Barnes/Medical/Alamy

Raised toilet seat and hand bar on the side of the bathtub.
Scimat/Photo Researchers, Inc.

PERINEAL-GENITAL CARE

Perineal-genital care is also referred to as **perineal care** or **peri-care**. Perineal care as part of the bed bath is embarrassing for many clients. Nurses also may find it embarrassing initially, particularly with clients of the opposite sex. Many clients who require a bed bath from the nurse are able to clean their own perineal area with minimal

assistance. The nurse may need to hand a moistened washcloth and soap to the client, rinse the washcloth, and provide a towel.

Because some clients are unfamiliar with terminology for the genitals and perineum, it may be difficult for nurses to explain what is expected. Most clients, however, understand what is meant if the nurse simply says, "I'll give you a washcloth to finish your bath." Older clients may be familiar with the term *private parts*. Whatever expression the nurse uses, it needs to be one that the client understands and one that is comfortable for the nurse to use.

The nurse needs to provide perineal care efficiently and matter-of-factly. Nurses should wear gloves while providing this care for the comfort of the client and to protect themselves from infection. Skill 5–2 explains how to provide perineal-genital care.

CLINICAL ALERT!

Always wash or wipe from "clean to dirty." For a female client, cleanse the perineal area from front to back. For a male client, cleanse the urinary meatus by moving in a circular motion from the center of the urethral opening around the glans.

●○● NURSING PROCESS: PROVIDING PERINEAL-GENITAL CARE

Providing Perineal-Genital Care

SKILL 5-2

ASSESSMENT
Assess for the presence of:
- Irritation, excoriation, inflammation, or swelling.
- Excessive discharge.
- Odor; pain or discomfort.
- Urinary or fecal incontinence.
- Recent rectal or perineal surgery.
- Indwelling catheter.

Determine:
- Perineal-genital hygiene practices.
- Self-care abilities.

PLANNING
DELEGATION

Perineal-genital care can be delegated to UAP; however, if the client has recently had perineal, rectal, or genital surgery, the nurse needs to assess if it is appropriate for the UAP to perform perineal-genital care.

Equipment
Perineal-Genital Care Provided in Conjunction with the Bed Bath
- Bath towel
- Bath blanket
- Clean gloves

- Bath basin with warm water at 43°C to 46°C (110°F to 115°F)
- Soap
- Washcloth

Special Perineal-Genital Care
- Bath towel
- Bath blanket
- Clean gloves
- Solution bottle, pitcher, or container filled with warm water or a prescribed solution
- Bedpan to receive rinse water
- Perineal pad

IMPLEMENTATION
Preparation
- Determine whether the client is experiencing any discomfort in the perineal-genital area.
- Obtain and prepare the necessary equipment and supplies.

Performance
1. Prior to performing the procedure, introduce self and verify the client's identity using agency protocol. Explain to the client what you are going to do, why it is necessary, and how he or she can participate, being particularly sensitive to any embarrassment felt by the client.
2. Perform hand hygiene and observe other appropriate infection prevention procedures.
3. Provide for client privacy by drawing the curtains around the bed or closing the door to the room. Some agencies provide signs indicating the need for privacy. **Rationale:** *Hygiene is a personal matter.*
4. Prepare the client:
   - Fold the top bed linen to the foot of the bed and fold the gown up to expose the genital area.
   - Place a bath towel under the client's hips. **Rationale:** *The bath towel prevents the bed from becoming soiled.*
5. Position and drape the client and clean the upper inner thighs.
   - Cover the body and legs with the bath blanket positioned so a corner is at the head, the opposite corner at the feet, and the other two on the sides. Drape the legs by tucking the bottom corners of the bath blanket under and then over the inner sides of the legs. ① **Rationale:** *Minimum exposure lessens embarrassment and helps to provide warmth.* Bring the middle portion of the base of the blanket up and then over the pubic area.

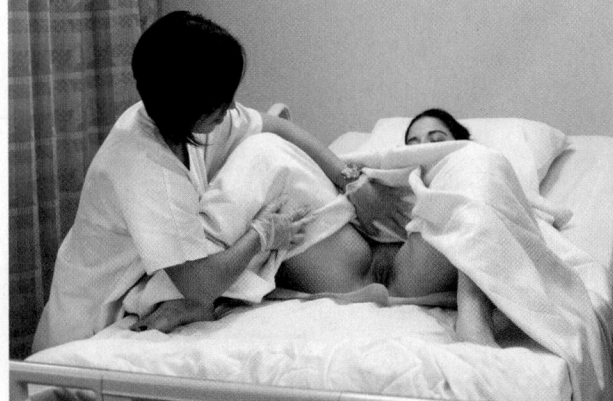

① Draping the client for perineal-genital care.

   - Position the female in a back-lying position with the knees flexed and spread well apart.
   - Position the male client in a supine position with knees slightly flexed and hips slightly externally rotated.
   - Apply gloves. Wash and dry the upper inner thighs.
6. Inspect the perineal area.
   - Note particular areas of inflammation, excoriation, or swelling, especially between the labia in females and the scrotal folds in males.
   - Also note excessive discharge or secretions from the orifices and the presence of odors.
7. Wash and dry the perineal-genital area.

Providing Perineal-Genital Care—*continued*

For Female Clients

- Clean the labia majora. Then spread the labia to wash the folds between the labia majora and the labia minora. ❷ **Rationale:** *Secretions that tend to collect around the labia minora facilitate bacterial growth.*
- Use separate quarters of the washcloth for each stroke, and wipe from the pubis to the rectum. For menstruating women and clients with indwelling catheters, use clean wipes. Use a clean wipe for each stroke. **Rationale:** *Using separate quarters of the washcloth or new wipes prevents the transmission of microorganisms from one area to the other. Wipe from the area of least contamination (the pubis) to that of greatest (the rectum).*
- Rinse the area well. You may place the client on a bedpan and use a Peri-Wash or a solution bottle to pour warm water over the area. Dry the perineum thoroughly, paying particular attention to the folds between the labia. **Rationale:** *Moisture supports the growth of many microorganisms.*

For Male Clients

- Wash and dry the penis, using firm strokes.
- If the client is uncircumcised, retract the prepuce (foreskin) to expose the glans penis (the tip of the penis) for cleaning. Replace the foreskin after cleaning and drying the glans penis. ❸

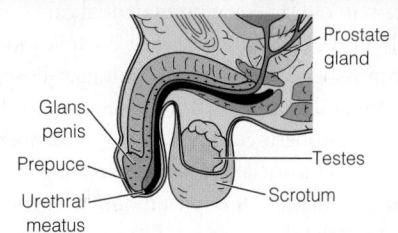

❸ Male genitals.

Rationale: *Retracting the foreskin is necessary to remove the smegma (thick, cheesy secretion) that collects under the foreskin and facilitates bacterial growth. Replacing the foreskin prevents constriction of the penis, which may cause edema.*

- Wash and dry the scrotum. The posterior folds of the scrotum may need to be cleaned when the buttocks are cleaned (see step 9). **Rationale:** *The scrotum tends to be more soiled than the penis because of its proximity to the rectum; thus it is usually cleaned after the penis.*

8. Inspect perineal orifices for intactness.
   - Inspect particularly around the urethra in clients with indwelling catheters. **Rationale:** *A catheter may cause excoriation around the urethra.*
9. Clean the natal cleft (between the gluteal folds) and the entire buttocks.
   - Assist the client to turn onto the side facing away from you.
   - Pay particular attention to the anal area and posterior folds of the scrotum in males. Clean the anus with toilet tissue before washing it, if necessary.
   - Dry the area well.
   - For postdelivery or menstruating females, apply a perineal pad as needed from front to back. **Rationale:** *This prevents contamination of the vagina and urethra from the anal area.*
10. Remove and discard gloves.
    - Perform hand hygiene.
11. Document any unusual findings such as redness, excoriation, skin breakdown, discharge or drainage, and any localized areas of tenderness.

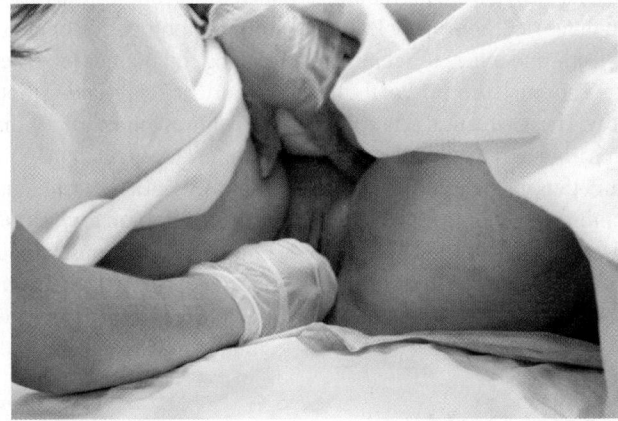

❷ Cleaning the labia.

EVALUATION

- Relate current assessments to previous assessments.
- Conduct appropriate follow-up such as prescribed ointment for excoriation.
- Report any deviation from normal to the primary care provider.

ORAL HYGIENE

Good oral hygiene includes daily stimulation of the gums, mechanical brushing and flossing of the teeth, flushing of the mouth, and regular checkups by a dentist. The nurse is often in a position to help clients maintain oral hygiene by helping or teaching them to clean their teeth and oral cavity, by inspecting whether clients (especially children) have done so, or by actually providing mouth care to clients who are ill or incapacitated. The nurse can also be instrumental in identifying problems that require the intervention of a dentist or oral surgeon and arranging a referral.

Clients at Risk

Dental caries (cavities) and periodontal disease are the two problems that most frequently affect the teeth. Both problems are commonly associated with plaque and tartar deposits. **Plaque** is an invisible soft film that adheres to the enamel surface of teeth; it consists of bacteria, molecules of saliva, and remnants of epithelial cells and leukocytes. When plaque is unchecked, tartar (dental calculus) is formed. **Tartar** is a visible, hard deposit of plaque and dead bacteria that forms at the gum lines. Tartar buildup can alter the fibers that attach the teeth to the gum and eventually disrupt bone tissue. Periodontal disease is characterized by **gingivitis** (red, swollen gingiva), bleeding, receding gum lines, and the formation of pockets between the teeth and gums. In advanced periodontal disease (**pyorrhea**), the teeth are loose and pus is evident when the gums are pressed.

Certain clients are prone to oral problems because of an inability to maintain oral hygiene. Among these are older clients and those who are seriously ill, confused, comatose, depressed, or dehydrated. Effective oral hygiene relies on fine motor skills, adequate vision, and motivation. It can be a problem for an older adult who has cognitive, visual, or physical impairments (Bissett & Preshaw, 2011). Oral problems are common in older people in residential care homes (Burns, 2012). Critically ill clients can experience complications that may lead to ventilator-associated pneumonia, a longer hospital stay, increased cost of care, and even death if oral assessment and care are not properly performed (Roberts & Moule, 2011). A number of research studies have shown an association between pathogenic oral bacteria and the incidence of aspiration pneumonia in clients following a stroke. Furthermore, the studies showed strong evidence that the intervention of improved oral hygiene significantly decreased the risk of pneumonia (Dickinson, 2012). In addition, people with nasogastric tubes or who are receiving oxygen are likely to develop dry oral mucous membranes, especially if they breathe through their mouths. Clients who have had oral or jaw surgery must have meticulous oral hygiene care to prevent the development of infections.

CLINICAL ALERT!

Clients in long-term care settings are at high risk for oral health problems. The nurse must assess the client's oral health and teach the UAP about the importance of and methods to promote oral hygiene.

Healthy-appearing individuals, too, may be at risk. High-risk variables such as lack of knowledge, inadequate nutrition, lack of money and/or insurance for dental care, excessive intake of refined sugars, and family history of periodontal disease also need to be identified. Some older adults may also be at risk, for example, those who choose salty and enamel-eroding sugary foods because of a decline in their number of taste buds. The decreased saliva production in older adults, which produces a dry mouth and thinning of the oral mucosa, is another factor.

A dry mouth can be aggravated by poor fluid intake, heavy smoking, alcohol use, high salt intake, anxiety, and many medications. Medications that can cause dryness of the mouth include diuretics; laxatives, if used excessively; and tranquilizers, such as chlorpromazine (Thorazine) and diazepam (Valium). Some chemotherapeutic agents used to treat cancer also cause oral dryness and mucositis (inflammation of mucous membranes). A common side effect of the anticonvulsant drug phenytoin (Dilantin) is gingival hyperplasia. Optimal oral hygiene (e.g., brushing with a soft toothbrush and flossing) is needed.

Clients who are receiving or have received radiation treatments to the head and neck may have permanent damage to salivary glands. This results in a very dry mouth and can often be treated by providing a thick liquid called *artificial saliva*. Some clients prefer to just sip on liquids to moisten the mouth. Radiation can also cause damage to teeth and jaw structure, with actual damage occurring years after the radiation.

The rate of edentulism (without teeth) among older adults continues to decline (Burns, 2012). As a result, older adults are at risk for dental cavities and periodontal disease. Older adults who have self-care deficits are at an increased risk because they cannot maintain their oral hygiene practices and/or may not be able to visit the dentist on a routine basis. Furthermore, those who suffer the worst oral health and hygiene include older adults residing in nursing homes and older adults with dementia. Poor oral hygiene among frail and dependent nursing home residents can place them at risk for serious illness such as pneumonia. Furthermore, along with the increasing evidence that poor oral health is a serious problem among older adults is the lack of effective oral care by health caregivers. Examples of interventions that can improve the oral health of residents in long-term care settings include consistent oral assessment by the nurses, instruction of UAP on how to deliver effective oral care, providing sufficient oral hygiene supplies, and expectations of the administration that oral care should receive the same priority as other kinds of care. Nurses have an important role in promoting and implementing optimal geriatric oral health care.

Some people have artificial teeth in the form of a plate—a complete set of teeth for one jaw. A person may have a lower plate or an upper plate or both. When only a few artificial teeth are needed, the individual may have a bridge rather than a plate. A bridge may be fixed or removable. Artificial teeth are fitted to the individual and usually will not fit another person. People who wear dentures or other types of oral prostheses should be encouraged to use them. Ill-fitting dentures or other oral prostheses can cause discomfort and chewing difficulties. They may also contribute to oral problems as well as poor nutrition and lack of enjoyment of food. Those who do not wear their prostheses are prone to shrinkage of the gums, which results in further tooth loss.

Like natural teeth, artificial dentures collect microorganisms and food. They need to be cleaned regularly, at least once a day. They can be removed from the mouth, scrubbed with a toothbrush, rinsed, and reinserted. Some people use a **dentifrice** (toothpaste) for cleaning teeth, and others use commercial cleaning compounds for plates.

Thorough brushing of the teeth is important in preventing tooth decay. The mechanical action of brushing removes food particles that can harbor and incubate bacteria. It also stimulates circulation in the gums, thus maintaining their healthy firmness. One of the techniques recommended for brushing teeth is called the **sulcular technique**, which removes plaque and cleans under the gingival margins. Various types of toothpastes are available. Fluoride toothpaste is often recommended because of its antibacterial protections. Skill 5–3 describes brushing the teeth using the sulcular technique and flossing the teeth.

Special Oral Hygiene

For the client who is debilitated or unconscious or who has excessive dryness, sores, or irritations of the mouth, it may be necessary to clean the oral mucosa and tongue in addition to the teeth. Agency practices differ with regard to special mouth care and the frequency with which it is provided. Depending on the health of the client's mouth, special care may be needed every 2 to 8 hours.

Mouth care for clients who are unconscious or debilitated is important because their mouths tend to become dry and consequently predisposed to tooth decay and infections. Saliva has antiviral, antibacterial, and antifungal effects. Dry mouth—called **xerostomia**—occurs when the supply of saliva is reduced. This condition can be caused by side effects of certain medications (e.g., antihistamines, antidepressants, antihypertensives). The drying irritates the soft tissues in the mouth, which can cause inflammation and susceptibility to infection (American Dental Association, 2013). Other reasons for a client to experience xerostomia include oxygen therapy, tachypnea, and NPO status where the client cannot take fluids by mouth.

For clients with special oral hygiene needs, the nurse focuses on removal of plaque and microorganisms as well as client comfort. If possible, a soft-bristled toothbrush should be used because it provides the best means of plaque removal. A sodium bicarbonate toothpaste or diluted sodium bicarbonate (i.e., one part sodium bicarbonate to three parts water) will help dissolve and remove viscous oral debris (Chan, Lee, Poh, Ng, & Prabhakaran, 2011, p. 177). If the client cannot tolerate the use of a toothbrush, the nurse can use an oral swab or a gauze wrapped around a gloved finger and soaked with saline to swab the teeth, tongue, and oral mucosa. A foam swab (Figure 5–3 ■) can be used to provide oral hygiene to dependent clients. Lemon-glycerin swabs are not recommended because they irritate and dry the oral mucosa and can decalcify teeth. Mouthwashes containing alcohol can irritate the oral mucosa and cause dryness. Mineral oil is contraindicated as a moisturizer for the lips or inside the mouth because aspiration of it can initiate an infection (lipid pneumonia). A water-soluble moisturizer, absorbed by the skin and tissue, provides important hydration. Saliva substitutes can also help moisturize the oral cavity. Skill 5–4 focuses on oral care for the unconscious client but may be adapted for conscious clients who are seriously ill or have mouth problems.

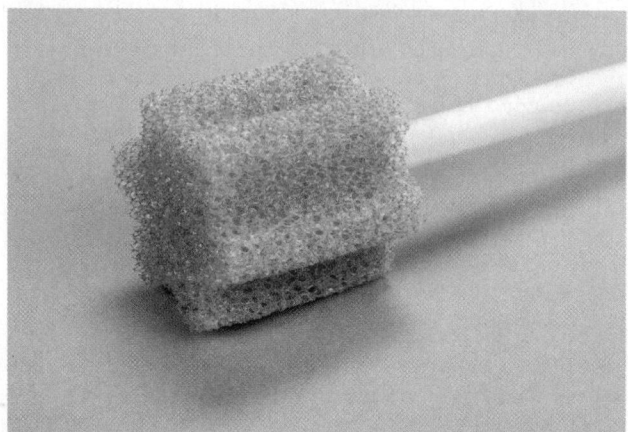

Figure 5–3 ■ Example of a foam swab used to clean the mouth of a dependent client.

●○● NURSING PROCESS: ORAL HYGIENE

Brushing and Flossing the Teeth

SKILL 5-3

ASSESSMENT
- Determine the extent of the client's self-care abilities.
- Assess the client's usual mouth care practices.
- Inspect lips, gums, oral mucosa, and tongue for deviations from normal.
- Identify presence of oral problems such as tooth caries, halitosis, gingivitis, and loose or broken teeth.
- Check if the client has bridgework or wears dentures. If the client has dentures, ask if any tenderness or soreness is present and, if so, the location of the area(s) for ongoing assessment.

PLANNING
DELEGATION

Oral care, brushing and flossing of teeth, and denture care can be delegated to the UAP. After performing the above assessment, the nurse should instruct the UAP as to the type of oral care and amount of assistance needed by the client. Remind the UAP to report changes in the client's oral mucosa.

Equipment
Brushing and Flossing
- Towel
- Clean gloves
- Curved basin (emesis basin)
- Toothbrush (soft bristle)
- Cup of tepid water

- Dentifrice (toothpaste)
- Mouthwash
- Dental floss, at least two pieces 20 cm (8 in.) in length
- Floss holder (optional)

For Cleaning Artificial Dentures
- Clean gloves
- Tissue or piece of gauze
- Denture container
- Clean washcloth
- Toothbrush or stiff-bristled brush
- Dentifrice or denture cleaner
- Tepid water
- Container of mouthwash
- Curved basin (emesis basin)
- Towel

IMPLEMENTATION
Preparation
Assemble all necessary equipment.

Performance
1. Prior to performing the procedure, introduce self and verify the client's identity using agency protocol. Explain to the client what you are going to do, why it is necessary, and how he or she can participate.
2. Perform hand hygiene and observe other appropriate infection prevention procedures.
3. Provide for client privacy by drawing the curtains around the bed or closing the door to the room. Some agencies provide signs indicating the need for privacy. **Rationale:** *Hygiene is a personal matter.*

4. Prepare the client.
   - Assist the client to a sitting position in bed, if health permits. If not, assist the client to a side-lying position with the head turned. **Rationale:** *This position prevents liquids from draining down the client's throat.*
5. Prepare the equipment.
   - Place the towel under the client's chin.
   - Apply clean gloves.
   - Use a soft toothbrush (a small one for a child) and the client's choice of dentifrice.
   - Moisten the bristles of the toothbrush with tepid water and apply the dentifrice to the toothbrush.
   - For the client who must remain in bed, place or hold the curved basin under the client's chin, fitting the small curve around the chin or neck.
   - Inspect the mouth and teeth.

Continued on page 184

6. Brush the teeth.

- Hand the toothbrush to the client, or brush the client's teeth as follows:

  a. Hold the brush against the teeth with the bristles at a 45° angle. The tips of the outer bristles should rest against and penetrate under the gingival sulcus. ❶ The brush will clean under the sulcus of two or three teeth at one time. **Rationale:** *This sulcular technique removes plaque and cleans under the gingival margins.*

  b. Move the bristles up and down gently in short strokes from the sulcus to the crowns of the teeth. ❷

  c. Repeat until all outer and inner surfaces of the teeth and sulci of the gums are cleaned.

  d. Clean the biting surfaces by moving the brush back and forth over them in short strokes. ❸

  e. Brush the tongue gently with the toothbrush. **Rationale:** *Brushing removes bacteria and freshens breath. A coated tongue may be caused by poor oral hygiene, low fluid intake, and side effects of medications. Brushing gently and carefully helps prevent gagging or vomiting.*

- Hand the client the water cup or mouthwash to rinse the mouth vigorously. Then ask the client to spit the water and excess dentifrice into the basin. Some agencies supply a standard mouthwash. Alternatively, a mouth rinse of normal saline can be an effective cleaner and moisturizer. **Rationale:** *Vigorous rinsing loosens food particles and washes out already loosened particles.*

- Repeat the preceding step until the mouth is free of dentifrice and food particles.

- Remove the curved basin and help the client wipe the mouth.

7. Floss the teeth.

- Assist the client to floss independently, or floss the teeth of an alert and cooperative client as follows. Waxed floss is less likely to fray than unwaxed floss; particles between the teeth attach more readily to unwaxed floss than to waxed floss.

  a. Wrap one end of the floss around the third finger of each hand. ❹

  b. To floss the upper teeth, use your thumb and index finger to stretch the floss. Move the floss up and down between the teeth. When the floss reaches the gum line, gently slide the floss into the space between the gum and the tooth. Gently move the floss away from the gum with up and down motions. Start at the back on the right side and work around to the back of the left side, or work from the center teeth to the back of the jaw on either side.

  c. To floss the lower teeth, use your index fingers to stretch the floss. ❺

- Give the client tepid water or mouthwash to rinse the mouth and a curved basin in which to spit the water.

- Assist the client in wiping the mouth.

8. Remove and dispose of equipment appropriately.

- Remove and clean the curved basin.
- Remove and discard gloves.
- Perform hand hygiene.

9. Document assessment of the teeth, tongue, gums, and oral mucosa. Include any problems such as sores or inflammation, bleeding, and swelling of the gums. Brushing and flossing teeth are not usually recorded.

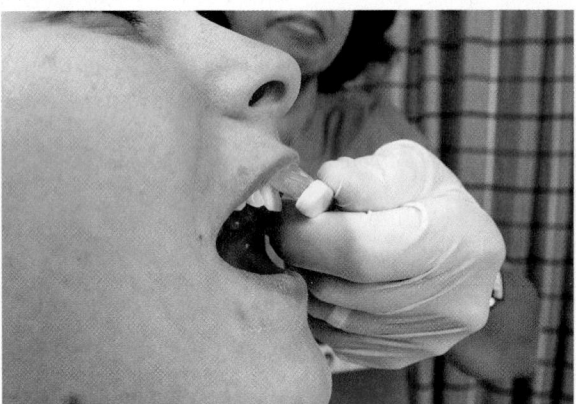

❶ The sulcular technique: Place the bristles at a 45° angle with the tips of the outer bristles under the gingival margins.

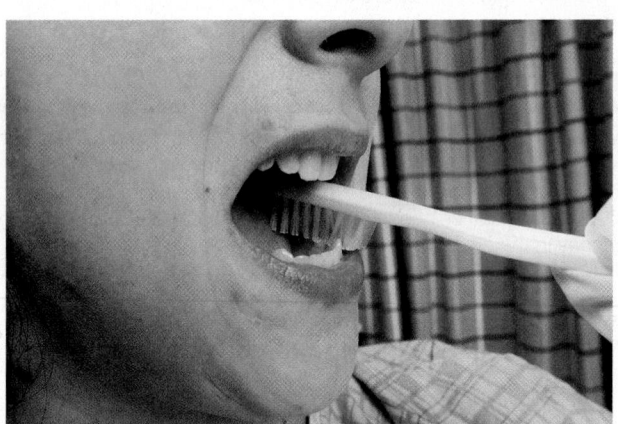

❸ Brushing the biting surfaces.

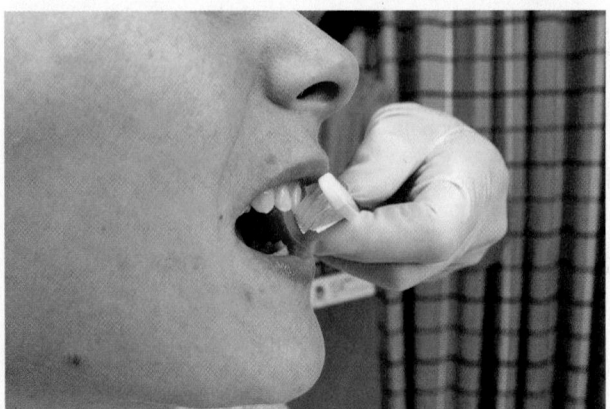

❷ Brushing from the sulcus to the crowns of the teeth.

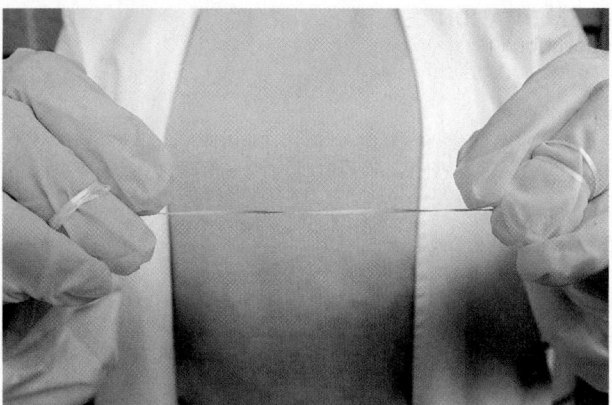

❹ Stretching the floss between the third finger of each hand.

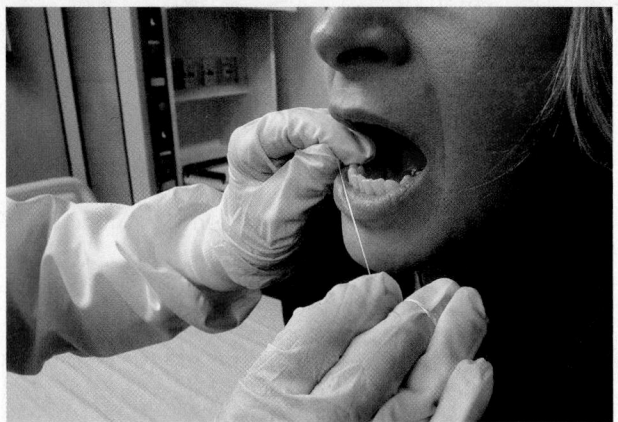

⑤ Flossing the lower teeth by using the index fingers to stretch the floss.

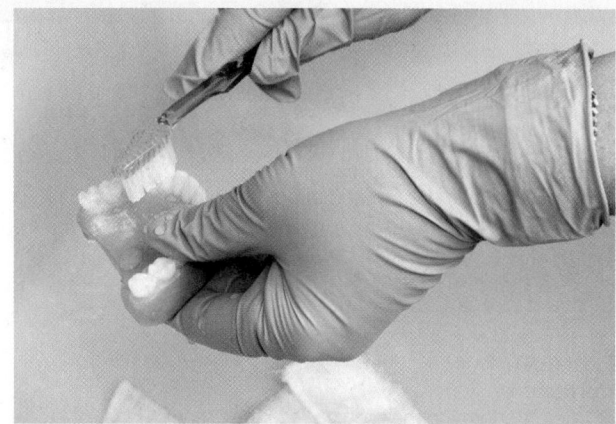

⑦ A washcloth prevents damage if the dentures are dropped.

Variation: Cleaning Artificial Dentures

1. Remove the dentures.
- Apply gloves. **Rationale:** *Wearing gloves decreases the likelihood of spreading infection.*
- If the client cannot remove the dentures, using a tissue or gauze, grasp the upper plate at the front teeth with your thumb and second finger, and move the denture up and down slightly. ⑥ **Rationale:** *The slight movement breaks the suction that holds the plate on the roof of the mouth.*
- Lower the upper plate, move it out of the mouth, and place it in the denture container.
- Lift the lower plate, turning it so that the left side, for example, is slightly lower than the right, to remove the plate from the mouth without stretching the lips. Place the lower plate in the denture container.
- Remove a partial denture by exerting equal pressure on the border of each side of the denture, not on the clasps, which can bend or break.

2. Clean the dentures.
- Take the denture container to a sink. Take care not to drop the dentures. Place a washcloth in the bowl of the sink. ⑦ **Rationale:** *A washcloth prevents damage if the dentures are dropped.*
- Using a toothbrush or special stiff-bristled brush, scrub the dentures with the cleaning agent and tepid water.
- Rinse the dentures with tepid running water. **Rationale:** *Rinsing removes the cleaning agent and food particles.* If the dentures are stained, soak them in a commercial cleaner. Be sure to follow the manufacturer's directions. To prevent corrosion, dentures with metal parts should not be soaked overnight.

3. Inspect the dentures and the mouth.
- Observe the dentures for any rough, sharp, or worn areas that could irritate the tongue or mucous membranes of the mouth, lips, and gums.
- Inspect the mouth for any redness, irritated areas, or indications of infection.
- Assess the fit of the dentures. People who have them should see a dentist at least once a year to check the fit and the presence of any irritation to the soft tissues of the mouth. Clients who need repairs to their dentures or new dentures may need a referral for financial assistance.

4. Return the dentures to the mouth.
- Offer some mouthwash and a curved basin to rinse the mouth. If the client cannot insert the dentures independently, insert the plates one at a time. Hold each plate at a slight angle while inserting it, to avoid injuring the lips. ⑧
- *Note:* If clients perform self-cleaning of dentures, ensure that dentures are placed in the appropriate container. **Rationale:** *Many older clients leave dentures on food trays and risk losing them when food trays are removed. Replacement dentures may not be covered by Medicare.*

5. Assist the client as needed.
- Wipe the client's hands and mouth with the towel.
- If the client does not want to or cannot wear the dentures, store them in a denture container with water. Label the container with the client's name and identification number. (Do not place the container on the food tray.)

6. Remove and discard gloves.
- Perform hand hygiene.

7. Document all assessments and include any problems such as an irritated area on the mucous membrane.

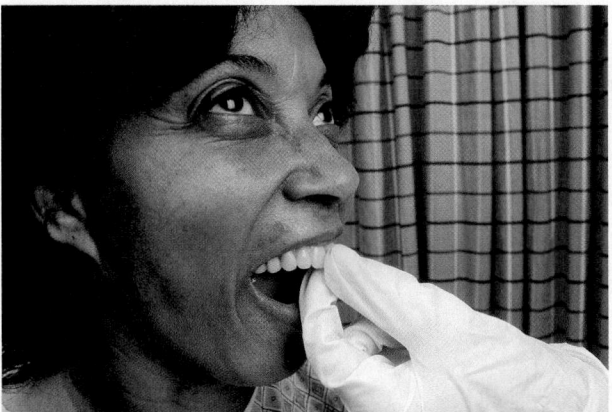

⑥ Removing the top dentures by first breaking the suction.

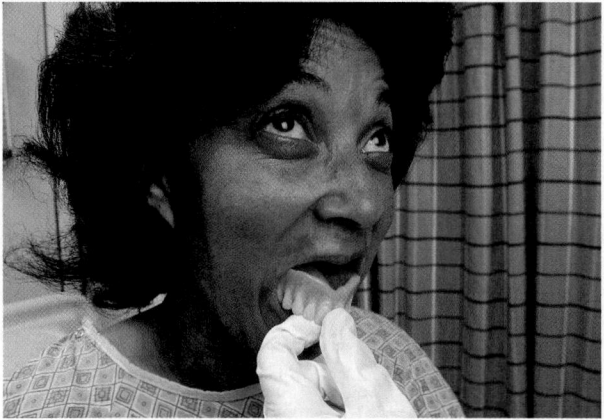

⑧ Inserting the dentures at a slight angle.

SKILL 5-4

Providing Special Oral Care for an Unconscious or Debilitated Client

Equipment
- Towel
- Clean gloves
- Curved basin (emesis basin)
- Bite-block to hold the mouth open and teeth apart (optional)
- Toothbrush
- Cup of tepid water
- Dentifrice or denture cleaner
- Tissue or piece of gauze to remove dentures (optional)
- Denture container as needed
- Mouthwash
- Rubber-tipped bulb syringe
- Suction catheter with suction apparatus when aspiration is a concern
- Foam swabs and cleaning solution for cleaning the mucous membranes
- Water-soluble lip moisturizer

IMPLEMENTATION
Performance
1. Prior to performing the procedure, if the client is conscious, introduce self and verify the client's identity using agency protocol. Explain to the client and the family what you are going to do and why it is necessary.
2. Perform hand hygiene and observe other appropriate infection prevention procedures.
3. Provide for client privacy by drawing the curtains around the bed or closing the door to the room. Some agencies provide signs indicating the need for privacy. **Rationale:** *Hygiene is a personal matter.*
4. Prepare the client.
   - Position the unconscious client in a side-lying position, with the head of the bed lowered. **Rationale:** *In this position, the saliva automatically runs out by gravity rather than being aspirated into the lung and allows for suctioning, if needed. This position is chosen for the unconscious client receiving mouth care.* If the client's head cannot be lowered, turn it to one side. **Rationale:** *The fluid will readily run out of the mouth or pool in the side of the mouth, where it can be suctioned.*
   - Place the towel under the client's chin.
   - Place the curved basin against the client's chin and lower cheek to receive the fluid from the mouth. ❶
   - Apply gloves.
5. Clean the teeth and rinse the mouth.
   - If the client has natural teeth, brush the teeth as described in Skill 5–3. Brush gently and carefully to avoid injuring the gums. If the client has artificial teeth, clean them as described in the *Variation* component of Skill 5–3.
   - Rinse the client's mouth by drawing about 10 mL of water or alcohol-free mouthwash into the syringe and injecting it gently into each side of the mouth. **Rationale:** *If the solution is injected with force, some of it may flow down the client's throat and be aspirated into the lungs.*
   - Watch carefully to make sure that all of the rinsing solution has run out of the mouth into the basin. If not, suction the fluid from the mouth. **Rationale:** *Fluid remaining in the mouth may be aspirated into the lungs.*
   - Repeat rinsing until the mouth is free of dentifrice, if used.
6. Inspect and clean the oral tissues.
   - If the tissues appear dry or unclean, clean them with the foam swabs or gauze and cleaning solution following agency policy.

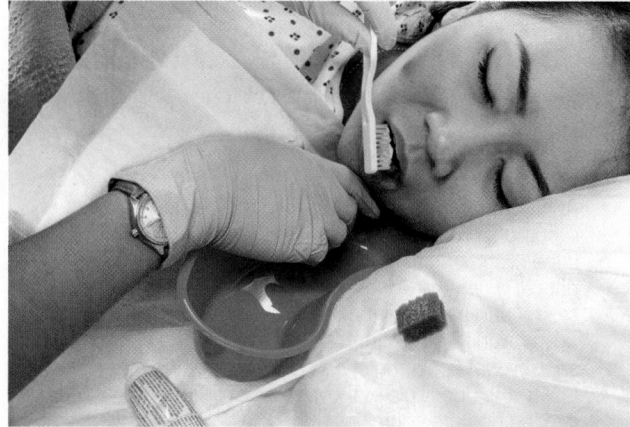

❶ Position of client and placement of curved basin when providing special mouth care.

   - Picking up a moistened foam swab, wipe the mucous membrane of one cheek. Discard the swab in a waste container; use a fresh one to clean the next area. **Rationale:** *Using separate applicators for each area of the mouth prevents the transfer of microorganisms from one area to another.*
   - Clean all mouth tissues in an orderly progression, using separate applicators: the cheeks, roof of the mouth, base of the mouth, and tongue.
   - Observe the oral tissues closely for inflammation, dryness, or lesions.
   - Rinse the client's mouth as described in step 5.
7. Ensure client comfort.
   - Remove the basin, and dry around the client's mouth with the towel. Replace artificial dentures, if indicated.
   - Lubricate the client's lips with water-soluble moisturizer. **Rationale:** *Lubrication prevents cracking and subsequent infection.*
   - Remove and discard gloves.
   - Perform hand hygiene.
8. Document assessment of the teeth, tongue, gums, and oral mucosa. Include any problems such as sores or inflammation and swelling of the gums.

EVALUATION
- Consider the client's medical diagnosis and treatment (e.g., chemotherapy, oxygen) and the necessary nursing interventions related to oral hygiene.
- Conduct an ongoing assessment, if appropriate, of the oral mucosa, gums, tongue, and lips. Report deviations from normal to the primary care provider.
- Conduct appropriate follow-up such as a referral to a dentist for dental caries.

INFANTS
- Most dentists recommend that dental hygiene should begin when the first tooth erupts and be practiced after each feeding. Cleaning can be accomplished by using a wet washcloth or small gauze moistened with water.

CHILDREN
- Beginning at about 18 months of age, brush the child's teeth with a soft toothbrush. Use only a toothbrush moistened with water. Introduce toothpaste later and use one that contains fluoride.
- Frequent snacking on products containing sugar increases the child's risk for developing cavities.

OLDER ADULTS
- Oral care is often difficult for certain older adults to perform due to problems with dexterity or cognitive problems with dementia.
- Most long-term health care facilities have dentists that come on a regular basis to see clients with special needs.
- Dryness of the oral mucosa is a common finding in older adults. Because this can lead to tooth decay, advise clients to discuss it with their dentist or primary care provider.
- Decay of the tooth root is common among older adults. When the gums recede, the tooth root is more vulnerable to decay.
- Promoting good oral hygiene can have a positive effect on older adults' ability to eat.

CLIENT TEACHING CONSIDERATIONS

Measures to Prevent Tooth Decay

- Brush the teeth thoroughly after meals and at bedtime. Assist children or inspect their mouths to be sure the teeth are clean. If the teeth cannot be brushed after meals, vigorous rinsing of the mouth with water is recommended.
- Floss the teeth daily.
- Ensure an adequate intake of nutrients, particularly calcium; phosphorus; vitamins A, C, and D; and fluoride.

- Avoid sweet foods and drinks between meals. Take them in moderation at meals.
- Eat coarse, fibrous foods (cleansing foods), such as fresh fruits and raw vegetables.
- Have topical fluoride applications as prescribed by the dentist.
- Have a checkup by a dentist every 6 months.

Ambulatory and Community Settings | Oral Hygiene

- Assess the oral hygiene practices and attitude toward oral hygiene of family members and the client.
- Remind adults to replace their toothbrush every 3 to 4 months and a child's toothbrush more frequently.

PATIENT-CENTERED CARE

- The client with a nasogastric tube or who is receiving oxygen is likely to develop dry oral mucous membranes, especially if the client breathes through the mouth. More frequent oral hygiene will be needed.

HAIR CARE

The appearance of the hair often reflects a person's feelings of self-concept and sociocultural well-being. Becoming familiar with hair care needs and practices that may be different from our own is an important aspect of providing competent nursing care to all clients. People who feel ill may not groom their hair as before. A dirty scalp and hair are itchy and uncomfortable, and can have an odor. The hair may also reflect state of health (e.g., excessive coarseness and dryness may be associated with endocrine disorders such as hypothyroidism). Box 5–2 lists common hair problems. Each person has particular ways of caring for hair. Many dark-skinned people need to oil their hair daily because it tends to be dry. Oil prevents the hair from breaking and the scalp from drying. A wide-toothed comb is usually used because finer combs pull and break the hair. Some people brush their hair vigorously before going to bed; others comb their hair frequently.

Brushing and Combing Hair

To be healthy, hair needs to be brushed daily. Brushing has three major functions: It stimulates the circulation of blood in the scalp, it distributes the oil along the hair shaft, and it helps to arrange the hair.

Long hair may present a problem for clients confined to bed because it may become matted. Combing and brushing the hair, at least

BOX 5–2 | Common Hair Problems

- **Alopecia** (hair loss)—can be caused by chemotherapeutic agents and radiation of the head.
- **Dandruff**—a diffuse scaling of the scalp, often accompanied by itching. Can usually be treated effectively with a commercial shampoo.
- **Pediculosis (lice)**—there are three common kinds:
  - *Head lice* (*Pediculus capitis*): Found on the scalp and tend to stay hidden in the hairs.
  - *Body lice* (*Pediculus corporis*): Tend to cling to clothing so that when a client undresses, the lice may not be in evidence on the body. These lice suck blood from the person and lay their eggs on the clothing.
  - *Crab lice* (*Pediculus pubis*): Stay hidden in pubic hair.
- **Scabies**—a contagious skin infestation by the itch mite. The mites cause intense itching that is more pronounced at night.
- **Hirsutism**—the growth of excessive body hair. The cause of excessive body hair is not always known.

once a day, will prevent matting. A brush with stiff bristles provides the best stimulation to blood circulation in the scalp. The bristles should not be so sharp, however, that they injure the client's scalp. A comb with dull, even teeth is advisable. A comb with sharp teeth might injure the scalp; combs that are too fine can pull and break the hair.

Some clients are pleased to have their hair tied neatly in the back or braided until other assistance is available or until they feel better and can look after it themselves. Braiding also prevents tangling and matting for clients confined to bed.

CLINICAL ALERT!

Excessively matted or tangled hair may be infested with lice.

Dark-skinned people often have thicker, drier, curlier hair than light-skinned people. Very curly hair may stand out from the scalp. Although the shafts of curly or kinky hair look strong and wiry, they have less strength than straight hair shafts and can break easily. Many African American people have hair that is naturally curly, and it can easily become matted and tangled in a short period of time. African Americans generally wash their hair less often than other ethnic groups because the hair is drier. Frequent shampooing could damage their hair.

Some African Americans have their hair straightened. Even if straightened, the hair tends to tangle and mat easily, especially at the back and the sides if the client is confined to bed. Other African Americans style their hair in braids (Figure 5–4 ■). These braids do not have to be unbraided for shampooing and washing. If, however, unbraiding becomes necessary, the nurse should obtain the client's permission to do so. Some African American clients may use oil by applying it between the braids and massaging it into the scalp. The oil prevents the hair strands from breaking and the scalp from becoming too dry. Not all African American individuals have curly or kinky hair. Some have naturally straight hair. Keeping the scalp and hair clean and oiled remains important and necessary. Skill 5–5 describes how to provide hair care for clients.

Shampooing the Hair

Hair should be washed as often as needed to keep it clean. There are several ways to shampoo clients' hair, depending on their health, strength, and age. The client who is well enough to take a shower can shampoo while in the shower. The client who is unable to shower

Figure 5–4 ■ An African American's hair styled with braids.
Cavan Images/Getty Images

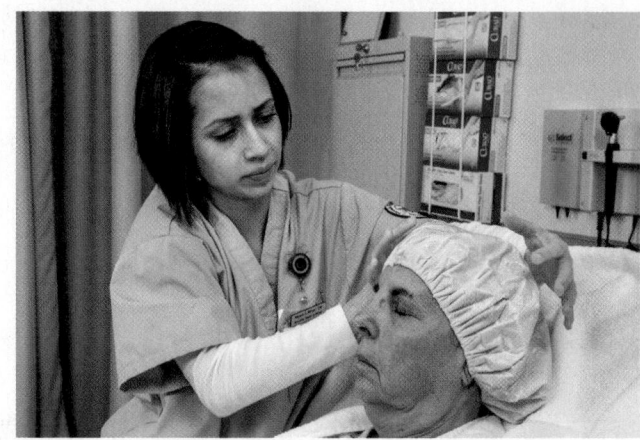

Figure 5–5 ■ Using a rinse-free shampoo cap.

may be given a shampoo while sitting on a chair in front of a sink. The back-lying client who can move to a stretcher can be given a shampoo on a stretcher wheeled to a sink. The client who must remain in bed can be given a shampoo with water brought to the bedside. A commercial product, similar to the bag bath, called a *head bath*, is another approach. It consists of a specially designed cap (looks like a shower cap) placed over the hair. The cap contains rinse-free shampoo and conditioner, and gently massaging the cap cleans the hair and scalp (Figure 5–5 ■). In some agencies, volunteer beauticians with portable shampoo chairs may be available to assist with hair care.

Water used for the shampoo should be 40.5°C (105°F) for an adult or child to be comfortable and not injure the scalp. Usually the client will supply a liquid or cream shampoo. If the shampoo is being given to destroy lice, a medicated shampoo should be used. Dry shampoos are also available that can remove some of the dirt, odor, and oil. Their main disadvantage is that they dry the hair and scalp.

How often a person needs a shampoo is highly individual, depending largely on the person's activities and the amount of sebum secreted by the scalp. Oily hair tends to look stringy and dirty, and it feels unclean to the person.

Beard and Mustache Care

Beards and mustaches also require daily care. The most important aspect of the care is to keep them clean. Food particles tend to collect in beards and mustaches, and they need washing and combing periodically. Clients may desire a beard or mustache trim to maintain a well-groomed appearance.

CLINICAL ALERT!

A beard or mustache should not be shaved off without the client's consent.

Male clients often shave or are shaved after a bath. Frequently clients supply their own electric or safety razors. See Box 5–3 for the steps involved in shaving facial hair with a safety razor. If a client is taking an anticoagulant (e.g., warfarin [Coumadin], heparin), an electric shaver should be used.

BOX 5–3 **Using a Safety Razor to Shave Facial Hair**

- Wear gloves in case facial nicks occur and you come in contact with blood.
- Apply shaving cream or soap and water to soften the bristles and make the skin more pliable.
- Hold the skin taut, particularly around creases, to prevent cutting the skin.
- Hold the razor so that the blade is at a 45° angle to the skin, and shave in short, firm strokes in the direction of hair growth.

- After shaving the entire area, wipe the client's face with a wet washcloth to remove any remaining shaving cream and hair.
- Dry the face well, then apply aftershave lotion or powder as the client prefers.
- To prevent irritating the skin, pat on the lotion with the fingers and avoid rubbing the face.

Note: Check agency policy as some do not allow safety razors because of the risk of impaired skin integrity from cutting the skin.

●○● NURSING PROCESS: PROVIDING HAIR CARE

Providing Hair Care

SKILL 5-5

ASSESSMENT
Determine:

- History of the following conditions or therapies: recent chemotherapy, hypothyroidism, radiation of the head, unexplained hair loss, and growth of excessive body hair.
- Usual hair care practices and routinely used hair care products (e.g., hair spray, shampoo, conditioners, hair oil preparation, hair dye, curling or straightening preparations).
- Whether wetting the hair will make it difficult to comb. Kinky hair is easier to comb when wet and is very difficult to comb when it dries.

Assess:

- Condition of the hair and scalp. Is the hair straight, curly, or kinky? Is the hair matted or tangled? Is the scalp dry?
- Evenness of hair growth over the scalp, in particular, any patchy loss of hair; hair texture, oiliness, thickness, or thinness; presence of lesions, infections, or infestations on the scalp; presence of hirsutism.
- Self-care abilities (e.g., any problems managing hair care).

PLANNING
DELEGATION

Brushing and combing hair, shampooing hair, and shaving facial hair can be delegated to UAP unless the client has a condition in which the procedure would be contraindicated (e.g., cervical spinal injury or trauma). The nurse needs to assess the UAP's knowledge and experience of hair care for clients of other cultures, if appropriate.

Equipment

- Clean brush and comb (A wide-toothed comb is usually used for many dark-skinned people because finer combs pull the hair into knots and may also break the hair.)
- Towel
- Hair oil preparation, if appropriate

IMPLEMENTATION
Performance

1. Prior to performing the procedure, introduce self and verify the client's identity using agency protocol. Explain to the client what you are going to do, why it is necessary, and how he or she can participate.
2. Perform hand hygiene and observe other appropriate infection prevention procedures.
3. Provide for client privacy by drawing the curtains around the bed or closing the door to the room. Some agencies provide signs indicating the need for privacy. **Rationale:** *Hygiene is a personal matter.*
4. Position and prepare the client appropriately.
   - Assist the client who can sit to move to a chair. **Rationale:** *Hair is more easily brushed and combed when the client is in a sitting position.* If health permits, assist a client confined to a bed to a sitting position by raising the head of the bed. Otherwise, assist the client to alternate side-lying positions, and do one side of the head at a time.
   - If the client remains in bed, place a clean towel over the pillow and the client's shoulders. Place it over the sitting client's shoulders. **Rationale:** *The towel collects any removed hair, dirt, and scaly material.*
   - Remove any pins or ribbons in the hair.

5. Remove any mats or tangles gradually.
   - Mats can usually be pulled apart with fingers or worked out with repeated brushings.
   - If the hair is very tangled, rub alcohol or an oil, such as mineral oil, on the strands to help loosen the tangles.
   - Comb out tangles in a small section of hair toward the ends. Stabilize the hair with one hand and comb toward the ends of the hair with the other hand. **Rationale:** *This avoids scalp trauma.*
6. Brush and comb the hair.
   - For short hair, brush and comb one side at a time. Divide long hair into two sections by parting it down the middle from the front to the back. If the hair is very thick, divide each section into front and back subsections or into several layers.
7. Arrange the hair as neatly and attractively as possible, according to the individual's desires.
   - Braiding long hair helps prevent tangles.
8. Document assessments and special nursing interventions. Daily combing and brushing of the hair are not normally recorded.

Continued on page 190

SKILL 5-5

Providing Hair Care—*continued*

Variation: Providing Hair Care for African American Clients
- Position and prepare the client.
- Separate the hair into four sections, proceeding from one section to the next.
- Untangle the hair first, if appropriate. Use fingers to reduce hair breakage and discomfort. Move fingers in a circular motion starting at the roots and gently moving up to the tip of the hair.
- Comb the hair. Dampen the hair with water or a leave-in conditioner. **Rationale:** *This will help loosen any tangles.*

- Apply hair oil preparation as the client indicates. Using a large and open-toothed comb, grasp a small section of hair and, holding the hair at the tip, start untangling at the tip and work down toward the scalp.
- Ask the client if he or she would like the hair braided. **Rationale:** *Braiding will decrease tangling; however, the choice is the client's.*

EVALUATION
- Conduct ongoing assessments for problems such as dandruff, alopecia (hair loss), pediculosis, scalp lesions, or excessive dryness or matting.

- Evaluate effectiveness of medication (e.g., for treating pediculosis), if appropriate.

LIFESPAN CONSIDERATIONS **Hair Care**

INFANTS
- Some newborns have hair on their scalp, and others are free of hair at birth but grow hair over the scalp during the first year of life.

CHILDREN
- In adolescence, the sebaceous glands increase in activity as a result of increased hormone levels. As a result, hair follicle openings enlarge to accommodate the increased amount of sebum, which can make the adolescent's hair more oily.

OLDER ADULTS
- The older adult's hair tends to be drier than normal. With age, axillary and pubic hair becomes finer and scanter, in contrast to the eyebrows, which become bristly and coarse. Many women develop hair on their face, which may be a concern to them.

FOOT CARE

Foot hygiene is particularly important for clients who have an infection or abrasion. Because of reduced peripheral circulation to the feet, clients with diabetes or peripheral vascular disease are particularly prone to infection if skin breakage occurs. Many foot problems can be prevented by teaching the client simple foot care guidelines.

CLINICAL ALERT!

Clients with diabetes are at high risk for lower extremity amputations (LEAs). Routine foot assessment and client education in proper foot care can significantly reduce the risk for LEA.

Foot and nail care (Box 5–4) is often provided during the client's bath but may be provided at any time during the day to accommodate the client's preference or schedule. The frequency of foot care is determined by the nurse and the client and is based on objective assessment data and the client's specific problems. Skill 5–6 describes how to provide foot care.

CLINICAL ALERT!

Clients with diabetes often have extremely dry skin. Tell them to use a nonperfumed lotion and to avoid putting lotion between the toes. Advise to not soak their feet in water because it is drying to the skin.

BOX 5–4 **Nail Care**

- Check the agency's policy regarding nail care. Often, podiatrists must be consulted for clients with diabetes.
- To provide nail care, the nurse needs a nail cutter or sharp scissors, a nail file, an orange stick to push back the cuticle, hand lotion or mineral oil to lubricate any dry tissue around the nails, and a basin of water to soak the nails if they are particularly thick or hard.
- One hand or foot is soaked, if needed, and dried. Then, the nail is cut or filed straight across beyond the end of the finger or toe. Avoid trimming or digging into nails at the lateral corners. **Rationale:** *Trimming toes at the corners predisposes the client to ingrown toenails.*
- Clients who have diabetes or circulatory problems should have their nails filed rather than cut. Inadvertent injury to tissues can occur if scissors are used.
- After the initial cut or filing, the nail is filed to round the corners and the nurse cleans under the nail.
- Gently push back the cuticle, taking care not to injure it.

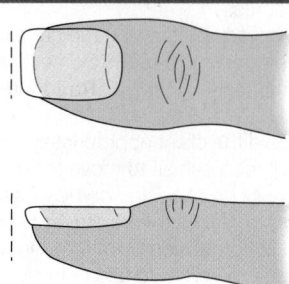

Fingernails are trimmed straight across.

- The next finger or toe is cared for in the same manner.
- Any abnormalities, such as an infected cuticle or inflammation of the tissue around the nail, are recorded and reported.

●○● NURSING PROCESS: PROVIDING FOOT CARE

Providing Foot Care

ASSESSMENT

Determine:

- History of any problems with foot discomfort, foot odor, foot mobility, circulatory problems (e.g., swelling, changes in skin color and/or temperature, and pain), or structural problems (e.g., bunion, hammer toe, or overlapping digits).
- Usual foot care practices (e.g., frequency of washing feet and cutting nails, foot hygiene products used, how often socks are changed, whether the client ever goes barefoot, whether the client sees a podiatrist).

Assess:

- Skin surfaces for cleanliness, odor, dryness, and intactness.
- Each foot and toe for shape, size, presence of lesions (e.g., corn, callus, wart, or rash), areas of tenderness, and ankle edema.
- Heels for erythema, blisters, or breaks in skin integrity.
- Skin temperatures of both feet to assess circulatory status.
- Pedal pulses: dorsalis pedis and posterior tibialis.
- Feet of bedbound clients for foot drop.
- Self-care abilities (e.g., any problems managing foot care).

PLANNING
DELEGATION

Foot care for the client who does *not* have diabetes can be delegated to UAP. Remind the UAP to notify the nurse of anything that looks out of the ordinary. Review with the UAP the agency policy about cutting or trimming nails.

- Moisture-resistant disposable pad
- Towels
- Soap
- Washcloth
- Toenail cleaning and trimming equipment, if agency policy permits
- Lotion or foot powder

Equipment

- Wash basin containing warm water
- Pillow

IMPLEMENTATION
Preparation

Assemble all of the necessary equipment and supplies if nails need trimming and agency policy permits.

Performance

1. Prior to performing the procedure, introduce self and verify the client's identity using agency protocol. Explain to the client what you are going to do, why it is necessary, and how he or she can participate.
2. Perform hand hygiene and observe other appropriate infection prevention procedures.
3. Provide for client privacy by drawing the curtains around the bed or closing the door to the room. Some agencies provide signs indicating the need for privacy. **Rationale:** *Hygiene is a personal matter.*
4. Prepare the equipment and the client.
   - Fill the washbasin with warm water at about 40°C to 43°C (105°F to 110°F). **Rationale:** *Warm water promotes circulation, comforts, and refreshes.*
   - Assist the ambulatory client to a sitting position in a chair, or the bed client to a supine or semi-Fowler's position.
   - Place a pillow under the bed client's knees, if not contra-indicated. **Rationale:** *This provides support and prevents muscle fatigue.*
   - Place the washbasin on the moisture-resistant pad at the foot of the bed for a bed client or on the floor in front of the chair for an ambulatory client.
   - For a bed client, pad the rim of the washbasin with a towel. **Rationale:** *The towel prevents undue pressure on the skin.*
5. Wash the foot and soak it.
   - Place one of the client's feet in the basin and wash it with soap, paying particular attention to the interdigital areas. Prolonged soaking is generally not recommended for clients with diabetes or individuals with peripheral vascular disease. **Rationale:** *Prolonged soaking may remove natural skin*

oils, thus drying the skin and making it more susceptible to cracking and injury.
   - Rinse the foot well to remove soap. **Rationale:** *Soap irritates the skin if not completely removed.*
   - Rub calloused areas of the foot with the washcloth. **Rationale:** *This helps remove dead skin layers.*
   - If the nails are brittle or thick and require trimming, replace the water and allow the foot to soak for 10 to 20 minutes. **Rationale:** *Soaking softens the nails and loosens debris under them.*
   - Clean the nails as required with an orange stick. **Rationale:** *This removes excess debris that harbors microorganisms.*
   - Remove the foot from the basin and place it on the towel.
6. Dry the foot thoroughly and apply lotion or foot powder.
   - Blot the foot gently with the towel to dry it thoroughly, particularly between the toes. **Rationale:** *Harsh rubbing can damage the skin. Thorough drying reduces the risk of infection.*
   - Apply lotion or lanolin cream to the foot but not between the toes. **Rationale:** *This lubricates dry skin and keeps the area between the toes dry.*

   or

   - Apply a foot powder containing a nonirritating deodorant if the feet tend to perspire excessively. **Rationale:** *Foot powders have greater absorbent properties than regular bath powders; some also contain menthol, which makes the feet feel cool.*
7. If agency policy permits, trim the nails of the first foot while the second foot is soaking.
   - See the discussion on nails in Box 5–4 for the appropriate method to trim nails. Note that in many agencies, toenail trimming requires a primary care provider's order or is con-traindicated for clients with diabetes mellitus, toe infections, and peripheral vascular disease, unless performed by a

Continued on page 192

Providing Foot Care—*continued*

podiatrist, general practice physician, or advanced practice provider such as a nurse practitioner.

8. Document any foot problems observed.

- Foot care is not generally recorded unless problems are noted.

- Record any signs of inflammation, infection, breaks in the skin, corns, troublesome calluses, bunions, and pressure areas. This is of particular importance for clients with peripheral vascular disease and diabetes.

EVALUATION
- Inspect nails and skin after the soak.
- Compare to prior assessment data.
- Report any abnormalities to the primary care provider.

CLIENT TEACHING CONSIDERATIONS

Foot Care

WASH THE FEET DAILY, AND DRY THEM WELL, ESPECIALLY BETWEEN THE TOES

- When washing, inspect the skin of the feet for breaks or red or swollen areas. Use a mirror if needed to visualize all areas.
- To prevent burns, check the water temperature before immersing the feet.
- Cover the feet, except between the toes, with creams or lotions to moisten the skin. Lotion will also soften calluses. A lotion that reduces dryness effectively is a mixture of lanolin and mineral oil.
- To prevent or control an unpleasant odor due to excessive foot perspiration, wash the feet frequently and change socks and shoes at least daily. Special deodorant sprays or absorbent foot powders are also helpful.
- File the toenails rather than cutting them to avoid skin injury. File the nails straight across the ends of the toes. If the nails are too thick or misshapen to file, consult a podiatrist.
- Wear clean stockings or socks daily. Avoid socks with holes or darns that can cause pressure areas.
- Wear comfortable, well-fitting shoes that neither restrict the foot nor rub on any area; rubbing can cause corns and calluses. Check worn shoes for rough spots in the lining. Break

in new shoes gradually by increasing the wearing time 30 to 60 minutes each day.
- Avoid walking barefoot, because injury and infection may result. Wear slippers in public showers and in change areas to avoid contracting athlete's foot or other infections.
- Several times each day, exercise the feet to promote circulation. Point the feet upward, point them downward, and move them in circles.
- Avoid wearing constricting garments such as knee-high elastic stockings, and avoid sitting with the legs crossed at the knees, which may decrease circulation.
- When the feet are cold, use extra blankets and wear warm socks rather than using heating pads or hot water bottles, which may cause burns. Test bathwater before stepping into it.
- Wash any cut on the foot thoroughly, apply a mild antiseptic, and notify the primary care provider.
- Avoid self-treatment for corns or calluses. Pumice stones and some callus and corn applications are injurious to the skin. Do not cut calluses or corns. Consult a podiatrist or primary care provider first.
- Notify the primary care provider if you notice abnormal sores or drainage, pain, or changes in temperature, color, and sensation of the foot.

EARS

Normal ears require minimal hygiene. Clients who have excessive **cerumen** (earwax) and dependent clients who have hearing aids may require assistance from the nurse.

Cleaning the Ears

The auricles of the ear are cleaned during the bed bath. The nurse or client must remove excessive cerumen that is visible or that causes discomfort or hearing difficulty. Visible cerumen may be loosened and removed by retracting the auricle up and back. If this measure is ineffective, the use of a cerumenolytic (wax-softening agent used to soften the cerumen) or irrigation may be necessary. Irrigation, however, may cause complications including pain, tinnitus, and external otitis media (Holcomb, 2009; Stevenson, 2010). Because ear irrigations have the potential to cause discomfort or even injury, the nurse must have competence in aural irrigation prior to performing the procedure.

Clients with hearing aids are at greater risk for cerumen impaction for two reasons. The hearing aid (a foreign body) causes excessive cerumen production, and the presence of the hearing aid prevents the body's normal mechanism for removal of cerumen.

It is important for nurses to advise clients to never use bobby pins, toothpicks, or cotton-tipped applicators to remove cerumen. Bobby pins and toothpicks can injure the ear canal and rupture the tympanic membrane. Cotton-tipped applicators can cause wax to become impacted within the canal and have also been shown to enhance cerumen production (Holcomb, 2009).

Care of Hearing Aids

A **hearing aid** is a battery-powered, sound-amplifying device used by people with hearing impairments. It consists of a microphone that picks up sound and converts it to electric energy, an amplifier that magnifies the electric energy electronically, a receiver that converts the amplified energy back to sound energy, and an **earmold** that directs the sound into the ear. See Box 5–5 for a description of several types of hearing aids.

For correct functioning, hearing aids require appropriate handling during insertion and removal, regular cleaning of the earmold, and replacement of dead batteries. With proper care, hearing aids generally last 5 to 10 years. Earmolds generally need readjustment every 2 to 3 years.

Skill 5–7 describes how to remove, clean, and insert a hearing aid.

BOX 5–5 **Types of Hearing Aids**

- *Behind-the-ear (BTE) with earmold:* This is widely used because it fits snugly behind the ear. The hearing aid case, which holds the microphone, amplifier, and receiver, is attached to the earmold by a plastic tube.

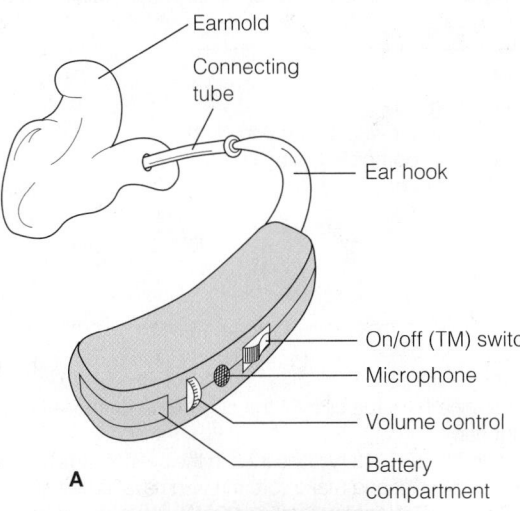

Earmold

Connecting tube

Ear hook

On/off (TM) switch

Microphone

Volume control

Battery compartment

A

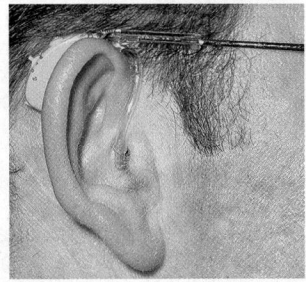

B

A, A behind-the-ear (BTE) hearing aid with earmold; *B,* a BTE hearing aid attached to glasses.
Jane Schemilt/Science Photo Library, Photo Researchers, Inc.

- *In-the-ear (ITE):* This one-piece aid has all its components housed in the earmold. It is more visible but has more room for features such as volume control.

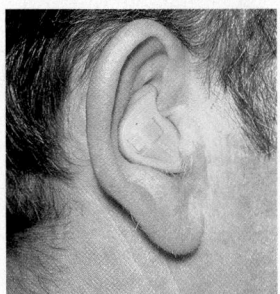

An in-the-ear (ITE) hearing aid.
Jane Schemilt/Science Photo Library, Photo Researchers, Inc.

- *Completely-in-the-canal (CIC):* Almost invisible to an observer. Has to be custom designed to fit the individual's ear.
- *Eyeglasses aid:* This is similar to the behind-the-ear aid, but the components are housed in the temple of the eyeglasses. A hearing aid can be in one or both temples of the glasses.
- *Body hearing aid:* This pocket-sized aid, used for more severe hearing losses, clips onto an undergarment, shirt pocket, or harness carrier supplied by the manufacturer. The case, containing the microphone and amplifier, is connected by a cord to the receiver, which snaps into the earpiece.

- *Behind-the-ear (BTE) open fit:* The newest in hearing aid technology. No earmold. Barely visible with a clear tube that runs down into the ear canal. Does not occlude the ear canal.

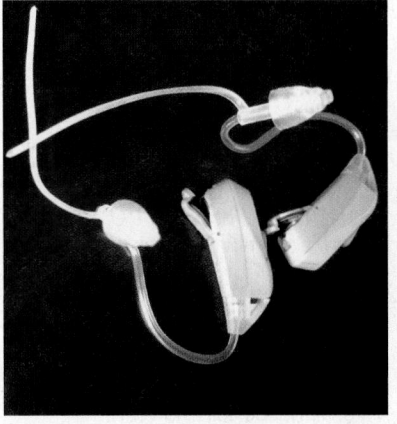

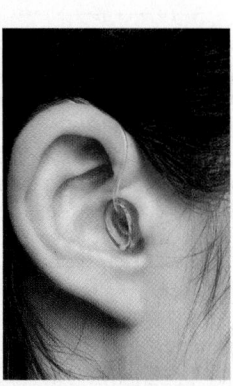

A   B

A, A behind-the-ear (BTE) open fit hearing aid; *B,* a BTE open fit hearing aid in place.
A, David Gunn/Getty; B, Diane MacDonald/Getty Images.

- *In-the-canal (ITC):* Compact and barely visible, fitting inside the ear canal. In addition to having cosmetic appeal, the ITC does not interfere with telephone use or the wearing of eyeglasses. However, it is not suitable for clients with progressive hearing loss; it requires adequate ear canal diameter and length for a good fit; and it tends to plug with cerumen more than other aids.

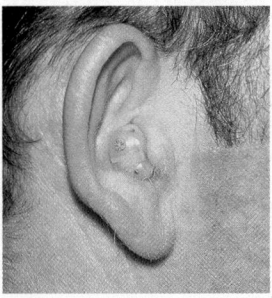

An in-the-canal (ITC) hearing aid.
Jane Schemilt/Science Photo Library, Photo Researchers, Inc.

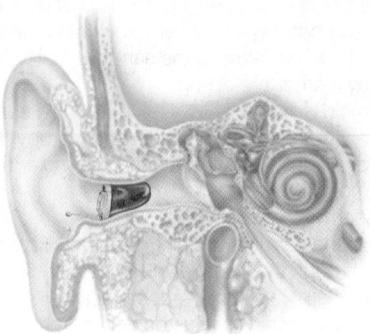

A completely-in-the-canal (CIC) hearing aid in place.

SKILL 5-7

●○● NURSING PROCESS: EARS

Removing, Cleaning, and Inserting a Hearing Aid

ASSESSMENT

Determine if the client has experienced any problems with the hearing aid and hearing aid practices. Assess for the presence of inflammation, excessive wax, drainage, or discomfort in the external ear.

PLANNING
DELEGATION

A nurse can delegate the task of caring for a hearing aid to the UAP. It is important, however, for the nurse to first determine that the UAP knows the correct way to care for a hearing aid. Instruct the UAP to report the presence of ear inflammation, discomfort, excess wax, or drainage to the RN.

Equipment
- Client's hearing aid
- Soap, water, and towels or a damp cloth
- Pipe cleaner or toothpick (optional)
- New battery (if needed)

IMPLEMENTATION
Performance

1. Prior to performing the procedure, introduce self and verify the client's identity using agency protocol. Explain to the client what you are going to do, why it is necessary, and how he or she can participate.
2. Perform hand hygiene and observe other appropriate infection prevention procedures.
3. Provide for client privacy by drawing the curtains around the bed or closing the door to the room. Some agencies provide signs indicating the need for privacy. **Rationale:** *Hygiene is a personal matter.*
4. Remove the in-the-ear (ITE) hearing aid.
   - Turn the hearing aid off and lower the volume. The on/off switch may be labeled "O" (off), "M" (microphone), "T" (telephone), or "TM" (telephone/microphone). **Rationale:** *The batteries continue to run if the hearing aid is not turned off.*
   - Remove the earmold by rotating it slightly forward and pulling it outward.
   - If the hearing aid is not to be used for several days, remove the battery. **Rationale:** *Removal prevents corrosion of the hearing aid from battery leakage.*
   - Store the hearing aid in a safe place and label with the client's name. Avoid exposure to heat and moisture. **Rationale:** *Proper storage prevents loss or damage.*
5. Clean the earmold.
   - Detach the earmold if possible. **Rationale:** *Removal facilitates cleaning and prevents inadvertent damage to the other parts.* Disconnect the earmold from the receiver of a body hearing aid or from the hearing aid case of behind-the-ear and eyeglass hearing aids where the tubing meets the hook of the case. Do not remove the earmold if it is glued or secured by a small metal ring.
   - If the earmold is detachable, soak it in a mild soapy solution. Rinse and dry it well. Do not use isopropyl alcohol. **Rationale:** *Alcohol can damage the hearing aid.*
   - If the earmold is not detachable or is for an in-the-ear aid, wipe the earmold with a damp cloth.
   - Check that the earmold opening is patent. Blow any excess moisture through the opening or remove debris (e.g., earwax) with a pipe cleaner or toothpick.
   - Reattach the earmold if it was detached from the rest of the hearing aid.

6. Insert the hearing aid.
   - Determine from the client if the earmold is for the left or the right ear.
   - Check that the battery is inserted in the hearing aid. Turn off the hearing aid, and make sure the volume is turned all the way down. **Rationale:** *A volume that is too loud is distressing.*
   - Inspect the earmold to identify the ear canal portion. Some earmolds are fitted for only the ear canal and concha; others are fitted for all the contours of the ear. The canal portion, common to all, can be used as a guide for correct insertion.
   - Line up the parts of the earmold with the corresponding parts of the client's ear.
   - Rotate the earmold slightly forward, and insert the ear canal portion.
   - Gently press the earmold into the ear while rotating it backward.
   - Check that the earmold fits snugly by asking the client if it feels secure and comfortable.
   - Adjust the other components of a behind-the-ear or body hearing aid.
   - Turn the hearing aid on, and adjust the volume according to the client's needs.
7. Correct problems associated with improper functioning.
   - If the sound is weak or there is no sound:
     a. Ensure that the volume is turned high enough.
     b. Ensure that the earmold opening is not clogged.
     c. Check the battery by turning the hearing aid on, turning up the volume, cupping your hand over the earmold, and listening. A constant whistling sound indicates the battery is functioning. If necessary, replace the battery. Be sure that the negative (–) and positive (+) signs on the battery match those where indicated on the hearing aid.
     d. Ensure that the ear canal is not blocked with wax, which can obstruct sound waves.
   - If the client reports a whistling sound or squeal after insertion:
     e. Turn the volume down.
     f. Ensure that the earmold is properly attached to the receiver.
     g. Reinsert the earmold.
8. Document pertinent data.
   - The removal and the insertion of a hearing aid are not normally recorded.
   - Report and record any problems the client has with the hearing aid.

EVALUATION

- Speak to the client in a normal conversational tone and observe client behaviors.
- Compare the client's hearing ability to previous assessments.
- Report to the primary care provider any deviations from normal for the client.

Ambulatory and Community Settings **Hearing Aids**

- People who need a hearing aid may not wear one because they view the hearing aid as a stigma of old age.
- It is important for the client who has just purchased a hearing aid to know that it often takes weeks or even months to adjust to the hearing aid. At first, the sounds will seem shrill as they start hearing high-frequency sounds that had been forgotten. Remind them that it is a hearing aid, not a hearing cure. Encourage them to not give up.

- The client needs to adjust to the hearing aid gradually by increasing the amount of time each day until the aid can be worn for a full day.
- Encourage clients to purchase their hearing aids from a company that has a minimum warranty of a 30-day return policy.
- Emphasize the importance of maintaining the hearing aid, that is, having it cleaned and checked regularly.

Chapter 5 Review

FOCUSING ON CLINICAL THINKING

Consider This

1. An unlicensed assistive personnel (UAP) comes to you and informs you that a client "refuses her bath." The UAP tells you that the client has an unpleasant body odor and her hair is oily and matted. What should you do?

2. A client complains of not being able to hear after the cleaning of his hearing aid. What should you do?

See Focusing on Clinical Thinking answers on student resource website.

TEST YOUR KNOWLEDGE

1. The nurse asks the nursing student to give a client early morning care before breakfast. What would the nursing student do for this client?
   1. Provide for elimination needs, a bath or shower, and oral care.
   2. Provide for elimination needs, wash face and hands, and give a back massage.
   3. Provide care only as needed by this client.
   4. Provide a urinal or bedpan, wash the face and hands, and give oral care.

2. Which factors may influence a person's personal hygiene practices? Select all that apply.
   1. Culture
   2. Religion
   3. Health and energy
   4. Personal preferences
   5. Development level

3. Medication is to be placed in the client's bathwater, and the client is to remain in the tub for 20 to 30 minutes. Which type of bath will the nurse provide to this client?
   1. A partial bath
   2. A therapeutic bath
   3. A cleaning bath
   4. A bag bath

4. An unlicensed assistive personnel (UAP) is caring for an older client with dementia. Which action by the UAP would require intervention by the nurse?
   1. Performing morning care as quickly as possible to limit client disruption
   2. Using a supportive, calm approach and praising the client often
   3. Stopping the bath when the client becomes distressed
   4. Using a gentle touch with the client

5. The nurse is teaching the unlicensed assistive personnel (UAP) about using a safety razor to shave facial hair. Which action by the UAP indicates successful teaching by the nurse?
   1. Shaves the client using no cream or water to reduce friction
   2. Holds the razor blade at a 90° angle to the skin
   3. Holds the skin taut to prevent cutting the skin
   4. After shaving, rubs the client's face dry

6. A home care nurse is instructing a client with diabetes and peripheral vascular disease about foot care. Which statement made by the client demonstrates understanding of the material?
   1. "I will first dip my toes in the water to check the water temperature."
   2. "I will wash my feet every 2 days if I notice excessive sweating."
   3. "I will cut my toenails to an appropriate length."
   4. "When my feet are cold, I will use extra blankets and wear warm socks."

7. Which of the following would be appropriate for the nurse to delegate to unlicensed assistive personnel?
   1. Bathing a client diagnosed with hemophilia (a bleeding disorder)
   2. Bathing a client diagnosed with osteogenesis imperfecta (a disorder with abnormal bone fragility)
   3. Bathing an anxious client who is scheduled for surgery this morning
   4. Bathing a client diagnosed with chronic atrial fibrillation (irregular heart rate)

8. The nurse is preparing to bathe an 18-month-old child and begins by washing which part of the child's body first?
   1. Abdomen
   2. Diaper area
   3. Face
   4. Extremities

9. The nurse is bathing an 85-year-old woman recently admitted to the hospital with a fractured right humerus. While performing the bath the nurse notices several bruises on the woman's back in various stages of healing, a 1-inch-wide abrasion that starts at the shoulder and ends at the lumbar spine area, and a bump on the back of her head. What would be the nurse's priority action?
   1. Accurately document the assessment findings and call the primary care provider immediately to report them.

2. Document the bruises and abrasion in the client's chart and mention the findings the next time the primary care provider arrives.
3. Report the abuse of the client to the authorities immediately.
4. Document the assessment findings in the client's medical record.

10. While providing hygienic care to the client, the nurse notes a large amount of a yellow waxy substance in the client's ear canal. The nurse documents which of the following as cleaned from the client's ear canal?
    1. Yellow waxy substance
    2. Cerumen
    3. Earwax
    4. Purulent material

See Answers to Test Your Knowledge in Appendix A.

READINGS AND REFERENCES

References

American Dental Association. (2013). *Dry mouth*. Retrieved from http://www.mouthhealthy.org/en/az-topics/d/dry-mouth.aspx

Barbera, E. F. (2011). Nursing home bathing transformed. *Long-Term Living, 60*(10), 41–43.

Bissett, S., & Preshaw, P. (2011). Guide to providing mouth care for older people. *Nursing Older People, 23*(10), 14–21.

Burns, B. (2012). Oral care for older people in residential care. *Nursing & Residential Care, 14*, 26–31.

Chan, E., Lee, Y., Poh, T., Ng, L., & Prabhakaran, L. (2011). Translating evidence into nursing practice: Oral hygiene for care dependent adults. *International Journal of Evidence-Based Healthcare, 9*, 172–183. doi:10.1111/j.1744-1609.2011.00214.x

Dickinson, H. (2012). Maintaining oral health after stroke. *Nursing Standard, 26*(49), 35–39. doi:10.7748/ns2012.08.26.49.35.c9233

Gaspard, G., & Cox, L. (2012). Bathing people with dementia. When education is not enough. *Journal of Gerontological Nursing, 38*(9), 43–51. doi:10.3928/00989134-20120807-05

Hoban, S. (2012). Dementia-friendly bathing. *Long-Term Living, 61*(10), 41–42.

Holcomb, S. S. (2009). Get an earful of the new cerumen impaction guidelines. *Nurse Practitioner, 34*(4), 14–19. doi:10.1097/01.NPR.0000348316.45989.0e

Johnson, R. H. (2011). Practical care: Creative strategies for bathing. *Nursing & Residential Care, 13*, 392–394.

Purnell, L. D. (2014). *Transcultural health care: A culturally competent approach* (4th ed.). Philadelphia, PA: F. A. Davis.

Roberts, N., & Moule, P. (2011). Chlorhexidine and toothbrushing as prevention strategies in reducing ventilator-associated pneumonia rates. *Nursing in Critical Care, 16*(6), 295–302. doi:10.1111/j.1478-5153.2011.00465.x

Stevenson, J. (2010). Dealing with stubborn earwax. *Practice Nurse, 39*(8), 17–18.

Selected Bibliography

Berman, A., Snyder, S., & Frandsen, G. (2016). *Kozier & Erb's fundamentals of nursing: Concepts, process, and practice* (10th ed.). Upper Saddle River, NJ: Pearson.

Conley, P., McKinsey, D., Graff, J., & Ramsey, A. R. (2013). Does an oral care protocol reduce VAP in patients with a tracheostomy? *Nursing, 43*(7), 18–23. doi:10.1097/01.NURSE.0000428709.81378.7c

Eisenhower, C., & Farrington, E. A. (2012). Advancements in the treatment of head lice in pediatrics. *Journal of Pediatric Healthcare, 26*, 451–461. doi:10.1016/j.pedhc.2012.05.004

Gallagher, M., & Hall, G. R. (2014). Evidence-based practice guideline. Bathing persons with Alzheimer's disease and related dementias. *Journal of Gerontological Nursing, 49*(2), 14–20. doi:10.3928/00989134-20131220-01

Gunning, K., Pippitt, K., Kiraly, B., & Sayler, M. (2012). Pediculosis and scabies: Treatment update. *American Family Physician, 86*, 535–541.

Heavey, E. (2014). Open wide: Oral health in primary care. *Nursing, 44*(3), 59–62. doi:10.1097/01.NURSE.0000441882.95371.8c

Hersh, S. P. (2010). Cerumen: Insights and management. *Annals of Long Term Care, 18*(7), 39–42.

Kassakian, S. Z., Mermel, L. A., Jefferson, J. A., Parenteau, S. L., & Machan, J. T. (2011). Impact of chlorhexidine bathing on hospital-acquired infections among general medical patients. *Infection Control and Hospital Epidemiology, 32*, 238–243. doi:10.1086/658334

Keefe, S. (2010). Bath safety & dementia. *Advance for Long-Term Care Management, 15*(6), 9–10.

Kleinpell, R. M. (2012). *Is chlorhexidine bathing really better than soap and water?* Retrieved from http://www.medscape.com/viewarticle/773904

Legg, T. L. (2012). Oral care in older adults with dementia: Challenges and approaches. *Journal of Gerontological Nursing, 38*(8), 10–13. doi:10.3928/00989134-20120703-01

Morton, J. A. (2013). Notes on noise. *Nursing, 43*(5), 37–40. doi:10.1097/01.NURSE.0000428697.87216.a8

Quinn, B., Baker, D. L., Cohen, S., Stewart, J. L., Lima, C. A., & Parise, C. (2014). Basic nursing care to prevent nonventilator hospital-acquired pneumonia. *Journal of Nursing Scholarship, 46*, 11–19. doi:10.1111/jnu.12050

Ray, K. D., & Fitzsimmons, S. (2014). Music–assisted bathing. Making shower time easier for people with dementia. *Journal of Gerontological Nursing, 49*(2), 9–13. doi:10.3928/00989134-20131220-09

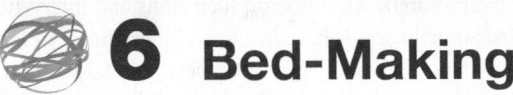

6 Bed-Making

LEARNING OUTCOMES

At the completion of this chapter, the student will be able to:

1. Define the key terms used in the skill of bed-making.
2. Describe the elements to consider when providing clients with a hygienic and comfortable environment.
3. Identify indications for common bed positions.
4. Recognize when it is appropriate to delegate bed-making to unlicensed assistive personnel.

5. Verbalize the steps used in making:
   a. A closed and open unoccupied bed.
   b. A surgical bed.
   c. An occupied bed.

SKILLS

KEY TERMS

Because people are usually confined to bed when ill, often for long periods, the bed becomes an important element in the client's life. A place that is clean, safe, and comfortable contributes to the client's ability to rest and sleep and to a sense of well-being. From a holistic perspective, bed-making can be viewed as the preparation of a healing space.

Basic furniture in a health care facility includes the bed, bedside cabinet, overbed table, one or more chairs, and a storage space for clothing. Most bed units also have a call light, light fixtures, electric outlets, and hygienic equipment in the bedside cabinet. Three types of equipment often installed in an acute care facility are a suction outlet for several kinds of suction, an oxygen outlet for most oxygen equipment, and a sphygmomanometer to measure the client's blood pressure (BP). Some long-term care agencies also permit clients to have personal furniture, such as a television, a chair, and lamps, at the bedside. In the home, a client often has personal and medical equipment near the bed.

SUPPORTING A HYGIENIC AND COMFORTABLE ENVIRONMENT

In Florence Nightingale's book, *Notes on Nursing*, she discussed many concepts including ventilation and warming, light, cleanliness of rooms, noise, and beds and bedding. These concepts are just as important today, and the nurse is often an influencing factor (e.g., dimming lights, controlling noise, providing a clean bed). When providing a hygienic and comfortable environment, it is important to consider the client's age, severity of illness, and level of activity.

Room Temperature

A room temperature between 20°C and 23°C (68°F and 74°F) is comfortable for most clients. Clients who are very young, very old, or acutely ill may need a warmer room temperature. The nurse should be able to facilitate control of the temperature of the client's room. This may require the nurse to communicate with another department in the facility.

Ventilation

Effective ventilation is important to remove unpleasant odors and stale air. Odors caused by urine, draining wounds, feces, or vomitus, for example, can be offensive to people. Room deodorizers can help eliminate odors; however, they may be contraindicated for clients with respiratory alterations. Most hospitals are smoke-free and prohibit smoking in client rooms and throughout the entire hospital.

Noise

Hospital environments can be quite noisy, and special care needs to be taken to reduce noise in the hallways and nursing care units. Distractions such as environmental noises and staff communication noise are particularly troublesome for hospitalized clients. For example, increased noise has been linked to stress reaction, sleep disturbance, and increased perception of pain, and also has been demonstrated to delay wound healing (Mazer, 2012). Environmental noises include the sound of paging systems, telephones, and call lights; doors closing; elevator chimes; industrial floor cleaners; and carts being wheeled through corridors.

In acute care settings, a multitude of medical device alarms create a noisy environment for both client and nurse. This situation has produced the term *alarm fatigue*. Device alarms are intended to alert nurses to a potential problem; however, medical devices create many false alarms. For example, one study revealed that only 3.6% of cardiac alarm conditions indicated critical events (Mazer, 2012, p. 351). As a result, apathy and desensitization occur and the alarms are less likely to be acted on or are even disabled (Cvach, 2012). Alarm hazards are receiving national attention. The ECRI Institute, a federal patient safety organization, raised alarm hazards to number one on its 2012 list of "Top 10 Health Technology Hazards" (Ferenc, 2012). In addition, the U.S. Food and Drug Administration (FDA) and The Joint Commission are investigating alarm fatigue because "of high noise levels that can hinder the performance of the healthcare staff" (FDA, 2012). Cvach (2012) reported that organizations committed to finding solutions have formed interdisciplinary alarm management committees to conduct an alarm risk assessment and explore strategies for alarm reduction (p. 273).

Staff communication is a major source of noise, particularly at staff change of shift in the morning when staff conversations and many of the environmental noises occur simultaneously. It is important for nurses to raise their awareness of noise on their units and intervene to find solutions. Some hospitals have instituted "quiet times" in the afternoon on nursing units; "quiet" signs are placed around the unit, the lights are lowered, and activity and noise purposefully decreased so clients can rest or nap. The "quiet times" are in the afternoon because many of the required activities for client care take place in the morning.

Hospital Beds

The frame of a hospital bed is divided into three sections. This permits the head and the foot to be elevated separately. Most hospital beds have electric motors to operate the movable joints. The motor is usually activated by pressing a button, located either at the side of the bed or on a small panel separate from the bed but attached to it by a cable, which the client can readily use. Table 6–1 shows common bed positions.

Hospital beds are usually 66 cm (26 in.) high and 0.9 m (3 ft) wide, narrower than the usual bed, so that the nurse can reach the client from either side of the bed without undue stretching. The length is usually 1.9 m (6.5 ft). Some beds can be extended in length to accommodate very tall clients. Long-term care facilities for ambulatory

TABLE 6–1   Commonly Used Bed Positions

Position	Description	Uses
Flat Flat Foot of bed · Head of bed	Mattress is completely horizontal.	Client sleeping in a variety of bed positions, such as back-lying, side-lying, and prone (face down) To maintain spinal alignment for clients with spinal injuries To assist clients to move and turn in bed Bed-making by nurse
Fowler's position 	Semi-sitting position in which head of bed is raised to an angle between 45° and 60°, typically at 45°. Knees may be flexed or horizontal.	Convenient for eating, reading, visiting, watching TV Relief from lying positions To promote lung expansion for client with respiratory problem To assist a client to a sitting position on the edge of the bed
Semi-Fowler's position 	Head of bed is raised between 15° and 45°, typically at a 30° angle.	Relief from lying position To promote lung expansion
Trendelenburg's position 	Head of bed is lowered and the foot is raised in a straight incline.	To promote venous circulation in certain clients To provide postural drainage of lung lobes
Reverse Trendelenburg's position 	Head of bed is raised and the foot is lowered. Straight tilt in direction opposite to Trendelenburg's position.	To promote stomach emptying and prevent esophageal reflux in clients with hiatal hernia

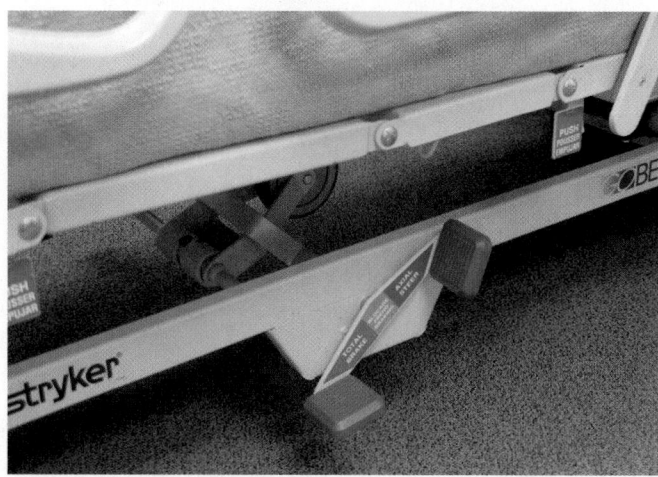

Figure 6–1 ■ Lock for bed wheels.

clients usually have low beds to facilitate movement in and out of bed. Most hospital beds have high and low positions that can be adjusted either mechanically or electrically by a button or lever. The high position permits the nurse to reach the client without undue stretching or stooping. The low position allows the client to step easily to the floor. It is important for the nurse to place the bed in the low position before leaving the bedside.

It is important for the nurse to check that the wheels on the bed are locked when the bed is stationary. The locks may be located on the wheels or at the middle of the bed frame (Figure 6–1 ■). Locking the wheels prevents accidental movement of the bed when the client independently gets out of bed or when a nurse is helping a client to transfer from the bed to a chair, thus ensuring client safety.

Mattresses

Mattresses are usually covered with a water-repellent material that resists soiling and can be cleaned easily. Most mattresses have handles on the sides called lugs by which the mattress can be moved.

Many special mattresses are also used in hospitals to relieve pressure on the body's bony prominences, such as the heels. They are particularly helpful for clients confined to bed for a long time. See Chapter 10 ∞ for more information on specialized beds.

Side Rails

Side rails, also referred to as bed rails, are used on both hospital beds and stretchers. They are of various shapes and sizes and are usually made of metal. A bed can have two full-length side rails or four half- or quarter-length side rails (also called split rails). Some side rails have two positions: up and down. Others have three: high, intermediate, and low. Devices to raise and lower side rails differ. Often one or two knobs are pulled to release the side and permit it to be moved. When side rails are being used, it is important that the nurse never leave the bedside while the rail is lowered.

For decades, the use of side rails has been routine practice with the rationale that the side rails serve as a safe and effective means of preventing clients from falling out of bed. Research, however, has not validated this assumption. In fact, studies have shown that raised side rails do not deter clients from getting out of bed unassisted and have led to more serious falls, injuries, and even death (Minnick, Mion, Johnson, Catrambone, & Leipzig, 2008). If all of the bed's side rails are up and restrict the client's freedom to leave the bed, and the client did not voluntarily request all rails to be up, they are considered a restraint by the Centers for Medicare and Medicaid Services (CMS). If, however, one side rail is up to assist the client to get in and out of the bed, it is not a restraint.

In addition to falls because of raised side rails, side rail entrapment can occur. The FDA has received reports of over 400 deaths as a direct result of side rail entrapment from a variety of health care settings, including hospitals (Minnick et al., 2008, p. 36). Entrapment occurs when a client gets caught or entangled in the openings or gaps around the hospital bed. This usually involves a side rail. There are seven areas or zones where clients are most often entrapped (Figure 6–2 ■). Clients at highest risk for entrapment include older or frail adults and clients who are agitated, delirious,

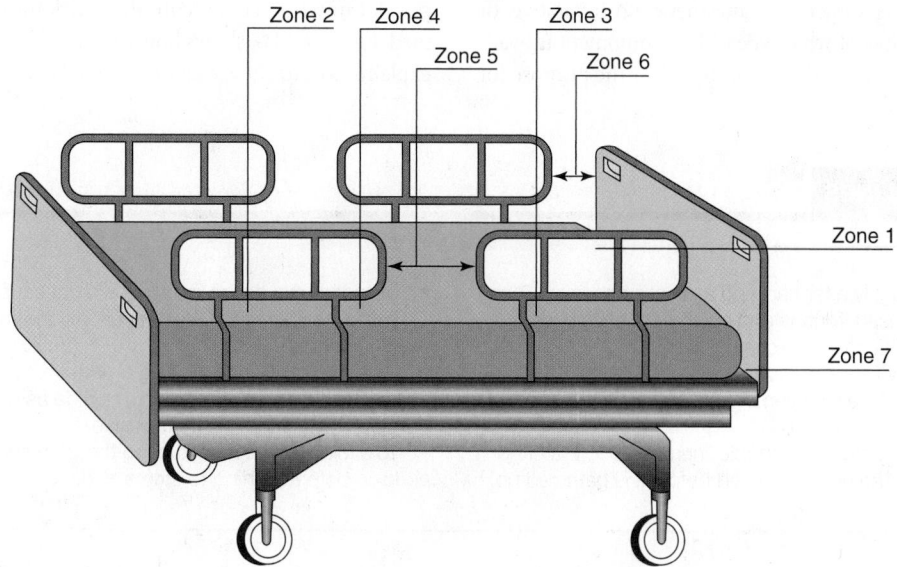

Figure 6–2 ■ Potential entrapment zones: Zone 1—within the rail; Zone 2—under the rail, between the rail supports, or next to a single rail support; Zone 3—between the rail and the mattress; Zone 4—under the rail, at the ends of the rail; Zone 5—between split bed rails; Zone 6—between the end of the rail and the side edge of the headboard or footboard; Zone 7—between the headboard or footboard and the mattress end.

confused, and hypoxic. The risk of entrapment increases when there are large gaps or openings in the bed because these openings can entrap a client's head, neck, or chest.

The CMS mandates that nurses in both acute care and long-term care decrease the routine use of side rails. Alternatives to side rails do exist and can include low-height beds, mats placed at the side of the bed, motion sensors, and bed alarms.

SAFETY ALERT! | SAFETY

Side rail entrapment, injuries, and deaths do occur. When side rails are used, the nurse must assess the client's physical and mental status and closely monitor high-risk (frail, older, or confused) clients.

Footboards

Footboards are used to support the immobilized client's foot in a normal right angle to the legs to prevent plantar flexion contractures, sometimes called "foot drop." The footboard is usually a solid support placed on the bed where the soles of the feet touch. It is secured to the mattress or bed frame. Placing high-top sneakers on the client's feet can also help maintain proper alignment of the feet.

Intravenous Rods

Intravenous (IV) rods (poles, stands, standards), usually made of metal, support IV infusion containers while fluid is being administered to a client. These rods were traditionally free standing on the floor beside the bed. Now, they are often attached to the hospital beds. Some hospital units have overhead hanging rods on a track for IVs.

MAKING BEDS

Nurses need to be able to prepare hospital beds in different ways for specific purposes. In most instances, beds are made after the client receives certain care and when beds are unoccupied. At times, however, nurses need to make an **occupied bed** or prepare a bed for a client who is having surgery (an anesthetic, postoperative, or **surgical bed**). Regardless of what type of bed equipment is available, whether the bed is occupied or unoccupied, or the purpose for

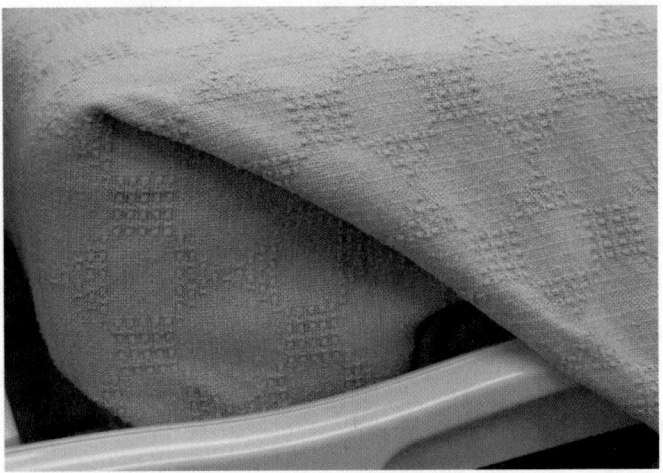

Figure 6–3 ■ Mitered corners help keep bed linens secure.

which the bed is being prepared, certain practice guidelines pertain to all bed-making.

Unoccupied Bed

An **unoccupied bed** (one not occupied by a client) can be either closed or open. Generally the top covers of an **open bed** are folded down toward the bottom of the bed (thus the term *open bed*) to make it easier for a client to get in the bed. Open and closed beds are made the same way, except that for the **closed bed** the top sheet, blanket, and bedspread are drawn up to the top of the bed (covering the bed) and under the pillows. The closed bed is often used in long-term care settings where the resident is up and about for most of the day.

Beds are often changed after bed baths. The linen (e.g., sheets, drawsheets, pillowcases, bedspread) can be collected before the bath. The linen is not usually changed unless it is soiled. Check the policy at each clinical agency. Unfitted or flat sheets, blankets, and bedspreads are mitered at the corners of the bed. A miter is made by placing the linen at the corner of the bed at an angle (Figure 6–3 ■). The purpose of mitering is to secure the bedclothes while the bed is occupied. Figure 6–4 ■ shows how to miter the corner of a bed. Skill 6–1 explains how to change an unoccupied bed.

PRACTICE GUIDELINES

Bed-Making

- Wash hands thoroughly after handling a client's bed linen. Clean gloves need to be used if linens and equipment have been soiled with secretions and/or excretions.
- Hold soiled linen away from uniform.
- Linen for one client is never (even momentarily) placed on another client's bed or on the floor.
- Place soiled linen directly in a portable linen hamper or tucked into a pillowcase at the end of the bed before it is gathered up for disposal.

- Do not shake soiled linen in the air because shaking can disseminate secretions and excretions and the microorganisms they contain.
- When stripping and making a bed, conserve time and energy by stripping and making up one side as much as possible before working on the other side.
- To avoid unnecessary trips to the linen supply area, gather all linen before starting to strip a bed.

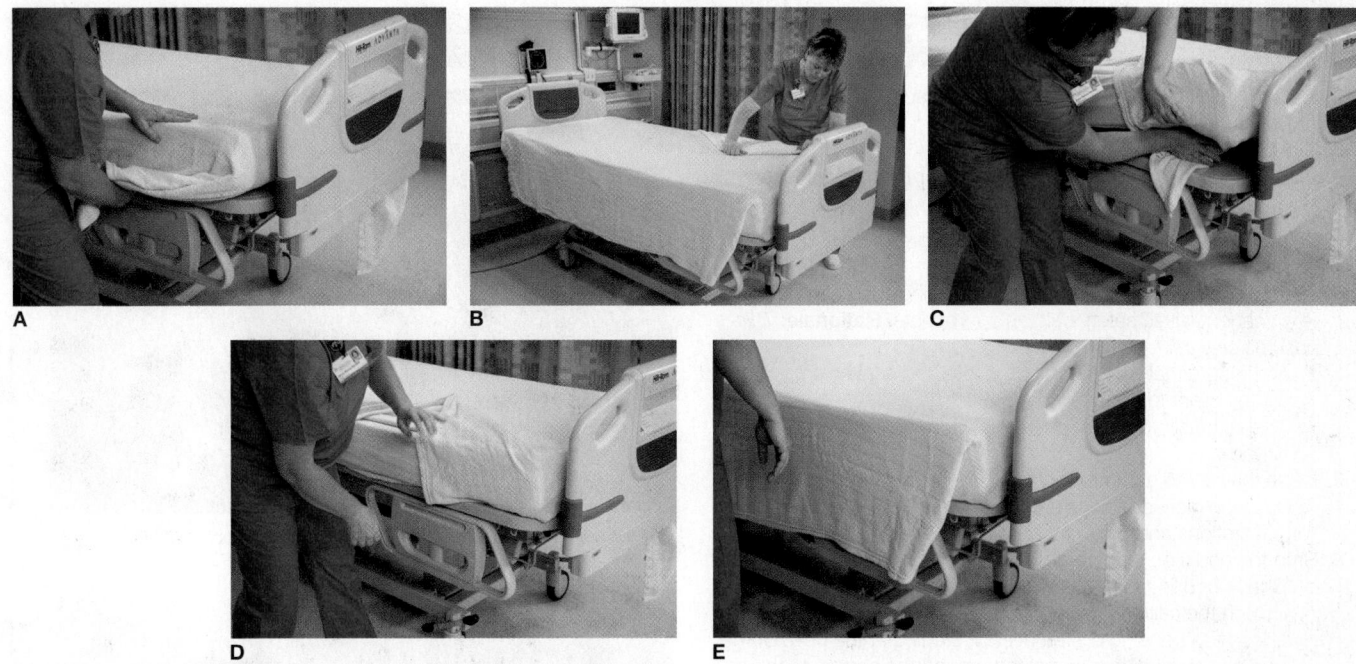

Figure 6–4 ■ Mitering the corner of a bed. *A,* Tuck in the bedcover (sheet, blanket, and/or spread) firmly under the mattress at the bottom or top of the bed. *B,* Lift the bedcover so that it forms a triangle with the side edge of the bed and the edge of the bedcover is parallel to the end of the bed. *C,* Tuck the part of the cover that hangs below the mattress under the mattress while holding the triangle up or against the bed. *D,* Bring the tip of the triangle down toward the floor while the other hand holds the fold of the cover against the side of the mattress. *E,* Remove the hand and tuck the remainder of the cover under the mattress, if appropriate. The sides of the top sheet, blanket, and bedspread may be left hanging freely rather than tucked in, if desired.

●○○● NURSING PROCESS: MAKING BEDS

Changing an Unoccupied Bed

ASSESSMENT
Assess:
- Client's health status to determine that the client can safely get out of bed.
- Client's BP, pulse, and respirations if indicated. **Rationale:** *The client may experience postural hypotension when moved from a lying position to sitting or standing, particularly if it is the first time out of bed for awhile.*
- Client's mobility status. **Rationale:** *This may influence the need for additional assistance with transferring the client from the bed to a chair.*
- Tubes and equipment connected to the client. **Rationale:** *This may influence the need for additional linens or waterproof pads.*

PLANNING
DELEGATION

Bed-making is often delegated to unlicensed assistive personnel (UAP). If appropriate, inform the UAP of the proper disposal method for linens that contain drainage. Ask the UAP to inform you immediately if any tubes or dressings become dislodged or removed. Stress the importance of the call light being readily available while the client is out of bed.

Equipment
- Clean gloves, if needed
- Two flat sheets or one fitted and one flat sheet
- Cloth drawsheet (optional)
- One blanket
- One bedspread
- Incontinent pads (optional)
- Pillowcase(s) for the head pillow(s)
- Plastic laundry bag or portable linen hamper, if available

IMPLEMENTATION
Preparation
Determine what linens the client may already have in the room. **Rationale:** *This avoids stockpiling of unnecessary extra linens.*

Performance
1. If the client is in bed, prior to performing the procedure, introduce self and verify the client's identity using agency protocol. Explain to the client what you are going to do, why it is necessary, and how he or she can participate.

Continued on page 202

SKILL 6-1

Changing an Unoccupied Bed—*continued*

2. Perform hand hygiene and observe other appropriate infection prevention procedures.
3. Provide for client privacy.
4. Place the fresh linen on the client's chair or overbed table; do not use another client's bed. **Rationale:** *This prevents* **cross contamination** *(the movement of microorganisms from one client to another) via soiled linen.*
5. Assess and assist the client out of bed using assistive devices (e.g., cane, walker, safety belt) as appropriate. **Rationale:** *This ensures client safety.*
   - Make sure that this is an appropriate and convenient time for the client to be out of bed.
   - Assist the client to a comfortable chair; provide warmth and privacy.
6. Raise the bed to a comfortable working height.
7. Apply clean gloves if linens and equipment have been soiled with secretions and/or excretions.
8. Strip the bed (i.e., remove bed linens).
   - Check bed linens for any items belonging to the client, and detach the call bell or any drainage tubes from the bed linen.
   - Loosen all bedding systematically, starting at the head of the bed on the far side and moving around the bed up to the head of the bed on the near side. **Rationale:** *Moving around the bed systematically prevents stretching and reaching and possible muscle strain.*
   - Remove the pillowcases, if soiled, and place the pillows on the bedside chair near the foot of the bed.
   - Fold reusable linens, such as the bedspread and top sheet on the bed, into fourths. First, fold the linen in half by bringing the top edge even with the bottom edge, and then grasp it at the center of the middle fold and bottom edges. ❶ **Rationale:** *Folding linens saves time and energy when reapplying the linens on the bed and keeps them clean.*
   - Remove the incontinent pad and discard it if soiled.
   - Roll all soiled linen inside the bottom sheet, hold it away from your uniform, and place it directly into the linen hamper, not on the floor. ❷ **Rationale:** *These actions are essential to prevent the transmission of microorganisms to the nurse and others.*
   - Wipe the mattress with disinfectant if soiled.
   - Grasp the mattress securely, using the lugs if present, and move the mattress up to the head of the bed.
   - Remove and discard gloves if used.
   - Perform hand hygiene.
9. Apply the bottom sheet and drawsheet (optional).
   - If using a flat sheet, place the folded bottom sheet with its center fold on the center of the bed. Make sure the sheet is

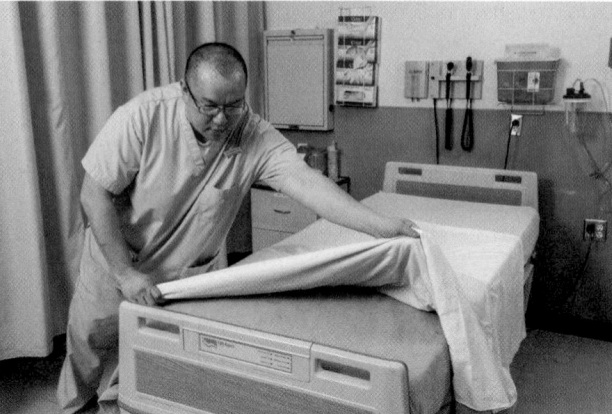

❶ Fold reusable linens into fourths when removing them from the bed.

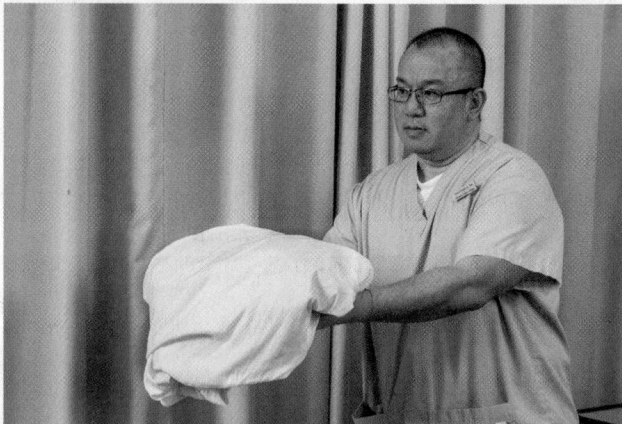

❷ Roll soiled linen inside the bottom sheet and hold away from the body.

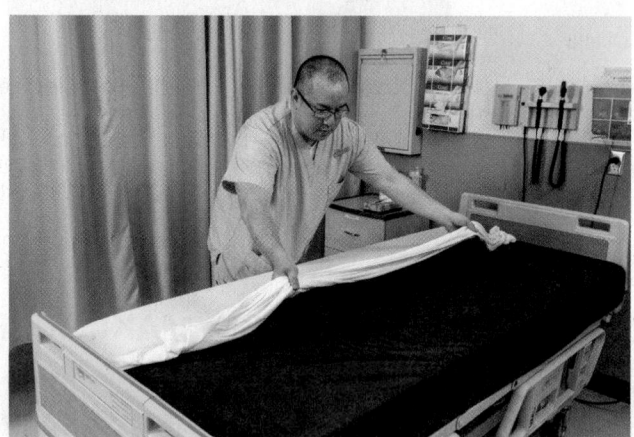

❸ Placing the bottom sheet on the bed.

hem side down for a smooth foundation. Spread the sheet out over the mattress, and allow a sufficient amount of sheet at the top to tuck under the mattress. **Rationale:** *The top of the sheet needs to be well tucked under to remain securely in place, especially when the head of the bed is elevated.* If using a fitted sheet, pull sheet over ends of mattress. ❸ Place the flat sheet along the edge of the mattress at the foot of the bed and do not tuck it in (unless it is a contour or fitted sheet).
   - Miter the sheet at the top corner on the near side (see Figure 6–4) and tuck the sheet under the mattress using the palms of the hands faced down, working from the head of the bed to the foot. **Rationale:** *This prevents the sheet from dragging out from under the mattress as the hands are being removed.*
   - If a drawsheet is used, place it over the bottom sheet so that the center fold is at the centerline of the bed, and the top and bottom edges extend from the middle of where the client's back would be on the bed to the area where the mid-thigh or knee would be. Fanfold the uppermost half of the folded drawsheet at the center or far edge of the bed and tuck in the near edge.
   - *Optional:* Before moving to the other side of the bed, place the top linens on the bed hem side up, unfold them, tuck them in, and miter the bottom corners. **Rationale:** *Completing one entire side of the bed at a time saves time and energy.*

Changing an Unoccupied Bed—*continued*

10. Move to the other side and secure the bottom linens.
- Tuck in the bottom sheet under the head of the mattress, pull the sheet firmly, and miter the corner of the sheet.
- Pull the remainder of the sheet firmly so that there are no wrinkles. **Rationale:** *Wrinkles can cause discomfort for the client and breakdown of skin. Tuck the sheet in at the side.*
- Tuck in the drawsheet, if appropriate.

11. Apply or complete the top sheet, blanket, and spread.
- Place the top sheet, hem side up, on the bed so that its center fold is at the center of the bed and the top edge is even with the top edge of the mattress.
- Unfold the sheet over the bed.
- **Optional:** Make a vertical or a horizontal toe pleat in the sheet. A toe pleat provides additional room for the client's feet and helps prevent foot drop.
- **Vertical toe pleat:** Make a fold in the sheet 5 to 10 cm (2 to 4 in.) perpendicular to the foot of the bed. ❹
- **Horizontal toe pleat:** Make a fold in the sheet 5 to 10 cm (2 to 4 in.) across the bed near the foot. ❺
- Loosening the top covers around the feet after the client is in bed is another way to provide additional space.
- Follow the same procedure for the blanket and the spread, but place the top edges about 15 cm (6 in.) from the head of the bed to allow a cuff of sheet to be folded over them.
- Tuck in the sheet, blanket, and spread at the foot of the bed, and miter the corner, using all three layers of linen. Leave the sides of the top sheet, blanket, and spread hanging freely unless toe pleats were provided.
- Fold the top of the top sheet down over the spread, providing a cuff. ❻ **Rationale:** *The cuff of sheet makes it easier for the client to pull the covers up.*
- Move to the other side of the bed and secure the top bedding in the same manner.

12. Put clean pillowcases on the pillows as required.
- Grasp the closed end of the pillowcase at the center with one hand.

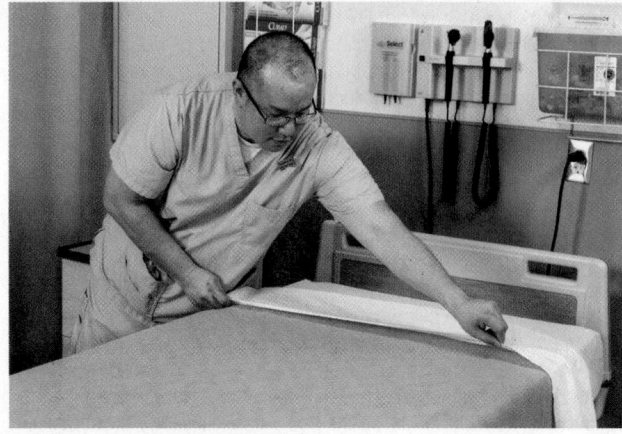
❻ Making a cuff of the top linens.

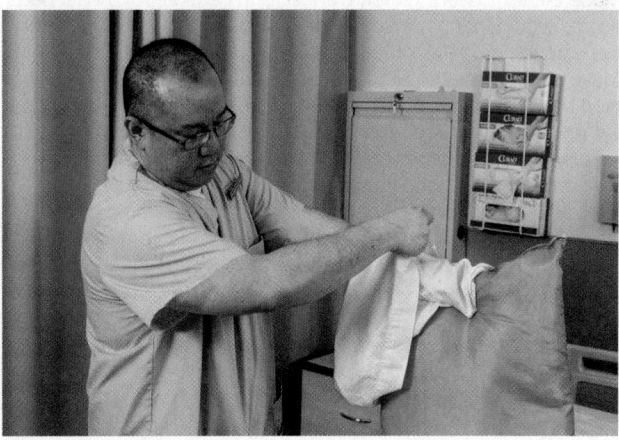
❼ Method for putting a clean pillowcase on a pillow.

- Gather up the sides of the pillowcase and place them over the hand grasping the case. Then grasp the center of one short side of the pillow through the pillowcase. ❼
- With the free hand, pull the pillowcase over the pillow.
- Adjust the pillowcase so that the pillow fits into the corners of the case and the seams are straight. **Rationale:** *A smoothly fitting pillowcase is more comfortable than a wrinkled one.*
- Place the pillows appropriately at the head of the bed.

13. Provide for client comfort and safety.
- Attach the call light so that the client can conveniently reach it. Some call lights have clamps that attach to the sheet or pillowcase. Others are attached by a safety pin. Most beds now have a call light button on the side rail.
- If the bed is currently being used by a client, either fold back the top covers at one side or fanfold them down to the end of the bed. **Rationale:** *This makes it easier for the client to get into the bed.*
- Place the bedside cabinet and the overbed table so that they are available to the client.
- Leave the bed in the high position if the client is returning by stretcher, or place in the low position if the client is returning to bed after being up ambulating or sitting in a chair.
- Perform hand hygiene.

14. Document and report pertinent data.
- Many agencies use a checklist that indicates if bed linens were changed.
- Record any nursing assessments, such as the client's physical status and pulse and respiratory rates before and after being out of bed, as indicated.

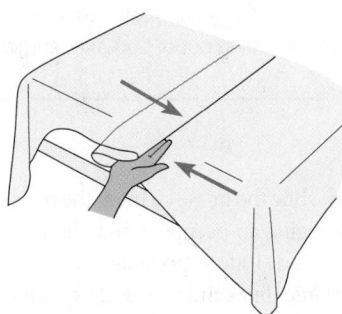
❹ A vertical toe pleat.

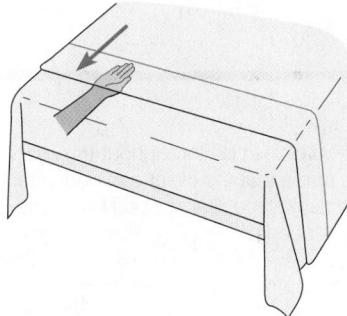
❺ A horizontal toe pleat.

Continued on page 204

Changing an Unoccupied Bed—*continued*

Variation: Making a Surgical Bed

A surgical bed is used for the client who is having surgery and will return to bed for the postoperative phase. When making a surgical bed, the linens are horizontally fanfolded to facilitate transfer of the client into the bed. In some agencies, the client is brought back to the unit on a stretcher and transferred to the bed in the room. In other agencies, the client's bed is brought to the surgery suite and the client is transferred there. In the latter situation, the bed needs to be made with clean linens as soon as the client goes to surgery so that it can be taken to the operating room when needed.

• Strip the bed.
• Place and leave the pillows on the bedside chair. **Rationale:** *Pillows are left on a chair to facilitate transferring the client into the bed.*
• Apply the bottom linens as for an unoccupied bed. Place a bath blanket on the foundation of the bed if this is agency practice. **Rationale:** *A flannel bath blanket provides additional warmth.*
• Place the top covers (sheet, blanket, and bedspread) on the bed as you would for an unoccupied bed. Do not tuck them in, miter the corners, or make a toe pleat.
• Make a cuff at the top of the bed as you would for an unoccupied bed. Fold the top linens up from the bottom.
• On the side of the bed where the client will be transferred, fold up the two outer corners of the top linens so they meet in the middle of the bed, forming a triangle. **❽**
• Pick up the apex or point of the triangle and fanfold the top linens lengthwise to the side of the bed opposite from where the client will enter the bed. **Rationale:** *This facilitates the client's transfer into the bed.*
• Leave the bed in high position with the side rails down. **❾** **Rationale:** *The high position facilitates the transfer of the client.*
• Lock the wheels of the bed if the bed is not to be moved. **Rationale:** *Locking the wheels keeps the bed from rolling when the client is transferred from the stretcher to the bed.*

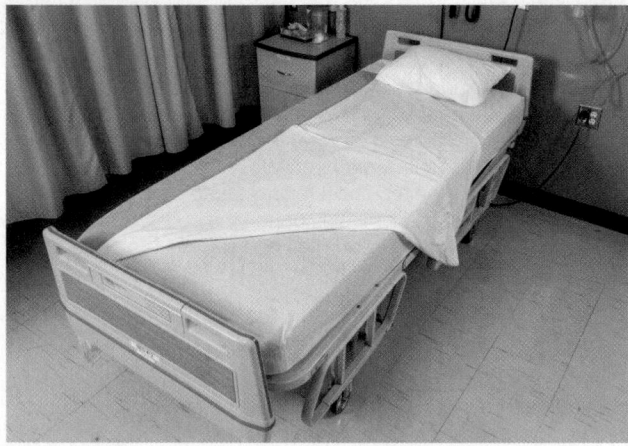

❽ Fold up the two outer corners of the top linens, forming a triangle.

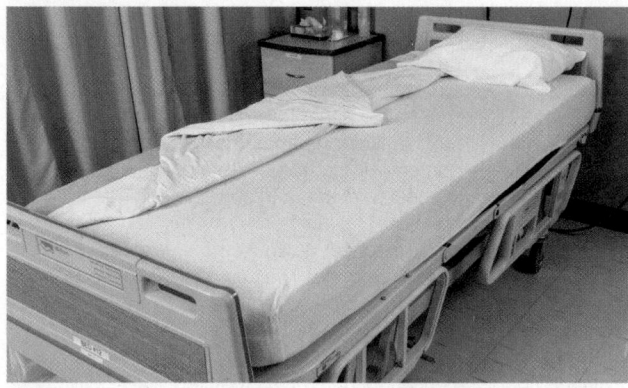

❾ Surgical bed. The linens are horizontally fanfolded to one side of the bed to facilitate transfer of the client into the bed.

EVALUATION

• Make sure the call light is accessible to the client.
• Relate client parameters of activity (e.g., BP, pulse, and respirations) to previous assessment data, particularly if the client has been on bed rest for an extended period of time or if it is the first time that the client is getting out of bed after surgery.

OCCUPIED BED

Some clients may be too weak to get out of bed. Either the nature of their illness may contraindicate their getting out of bed, or they may be restricted in bed by the presence of traction or other therapies. Thus, the nurse needs to be able to make an occupied bed. The client remains in the bed while the nurse changes the bed linens and makes the bed. When changing an occupied bed, the nurse works quickly and disturbs the client as little as possible to conserve the client's energy. The Practice Guidelines and Skill 6–2 explain how to change an occupied bed.

PRACTICE GUIDELINES

Changing an Occupied Bed

• Maintain the client in good body alignment. Never move or position a client in a manner that is contraindicated by the client's health. Obtain help if necessary to ensure safety.
• Move the client gently and smoothly. Rough handling can cause the client discomfort and abrade the skin.

• Explain what you plan to do throughout the procedure before you do it. Use terms that the client can understand.
• Use the bed-making time, like the bed bath time, to assess and meet the client's needs.

●○● NURSING PROCESS: OCCUPIED BEDS

Changing an Occupied Bed

ASSESSMENT

- Assess skin condition and need for a special mattress (e.g., an egg-crate mattress), footboard, bed cradle, or heel protectors.
- Assess the client's ability to reposition self. **Rationale:** *This will determine if additional assistance is needed.*

- Determine the presence of incontinence or excessive drainage from other sources indicating the need for protective waterproof pads.
- Note specific orders or precautions for moving and positioning the client.

PLANNING
DELEGATION

Bed-making is often delegated to UAP. Inform the UAP to what extent the client can assist or if another person will be needed to assist the UAP. Instruct the UAP about the handling of any dressings and/or tubes of the client and also the need for special equipment (e.g., footboard, heel protectors), if appropriate.

Equipment

- Two flat sheets or one fitted and one flat sheet
- Cloth drawsheet (optional)
- One blanket
- One bedspread
- Incontinent pads (optional)
- Pillowcase(s) for the head pillow(s)
- Plastic laundry bag or portable linen hamper, if available

IMPLEMENTATION
Preparation

Determine what linens the client may already have in the room. **Rationale:** *This avoids stockpiling of unnecessary extra linens.*

Performance

1. Explain to the client what you are going to do, why it is necessary, and how he or she can participate. Prior to performing the procedure, introduce self and verify the client's identity using agency protocol.
2. Perform hand hygiene and observe other appropriate infection prevention procedures. Apply clean gloves if linen is soiled with body fluids.
3. Provide for client privacy.
4. Remove the top bedding.
   - Remove any equipment attached to the bed linen, such as a signal light.
   - Loosen all top linen at the foot of the bed, and remove the spread and the blanket.
   - Leave the top sheet over the client (the top sheet can remain over the client if it is being changed and if it will provide sufficient warmth), or replace it with a bath blanket as follows:
      a. Spread the bath blanket over the top sheet.
      b. Ask the client to hold the top edge of the blanket.
      c. Reaching under the blanket from the side, grasp the top edge of the sheet and draw it down to the foot of the bed, leaving the blanket in place. ❶
      d. Remove the sheet from the bed and place it in the soiled linen hamper.

5. Change the bottom sheet and drawsheet.
   - Raise the side rail that the client will turn toward. **Rationale:** *This protects clients from falling and allows them to support themselves in the side-lying position.* If there is no side rail, have another nurse support the client at the edge of the bed.
   - Assist the client to turn on the side away from the nurse and toward the raised side rail.
   - Loosen the bottom linens on the side of the bed near the nurse.
   - Fanfold the dirty linen (i.e., drawsheet and the bottom sheet) toward the center of the bed ❷ as close to and under the client as possible. **Rationale:** *Doing this leaves the near half of the bed free to be changed.*
   - Place the new bottom sheet on the bed, and vertically fanfold the half to be used on the far side of the bed as close to the client as possible. ❸ Tuck the sheet under the near half of the bed and miter the corner if a contour sheet is not being used.
   - Place the clean drawsheet on the bed with the center fold at the center of the bed. Fanfold the uppermost half vertically at the center of the bed and tuck the near side edge under the side of the mattress. ❹
   - Assist the client to roll over toward you, over the fanfolded bed linens at the center of the bed, onto the clean side of the bed.
   - Move the pillows to the clean side for the client's use. Raise the side rail before leaving the side of the bed.
   - Move to the other side of the bed and lower the side rail.
   - Remove the used linen and place it in the portable hamper.
   - Unfold the fanfolded bottom sheet from the center of the bed.

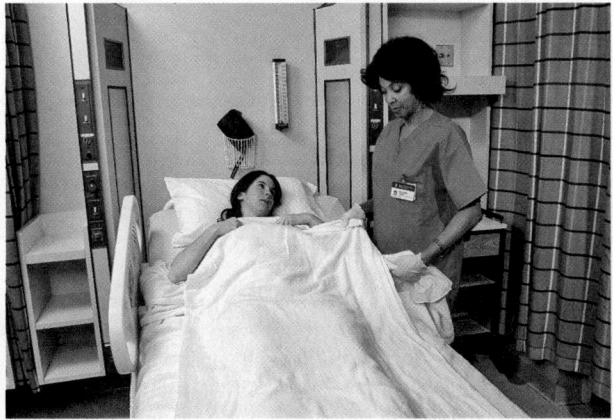

❶ Removing top linens under a bath blanket.

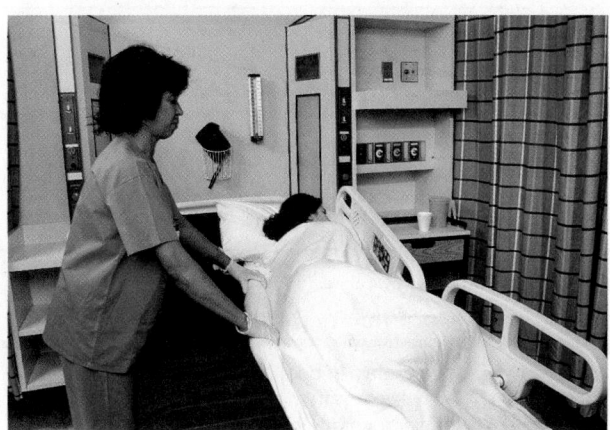

❷ Moving soiled linen as close to the client as possible.

SKILL 6-2

Changing an Occupied Bed—*continued*

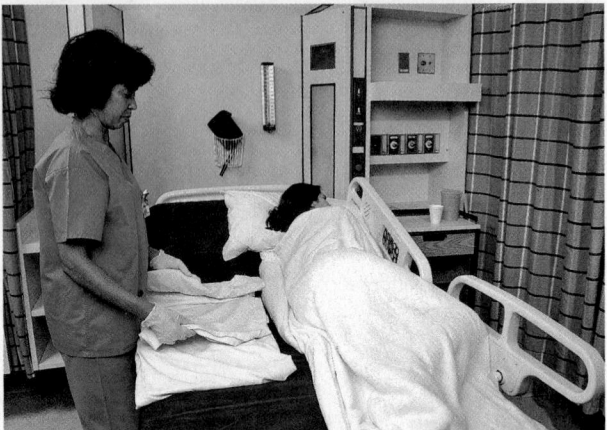

❸ Placing a new bottom sheet on half of the bed.

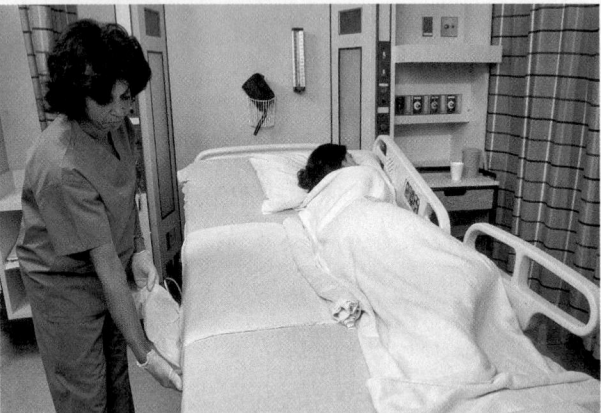

❹ Placing a clean drawsheet on the bed.

- Facing the side of the bed, use both hands to pull the bottom sheet so that it is smooth and tuck the excess under the side of the mattress.
- Unfold the drawsheet fanfolded at the center of the bed and pull it tightly with both hands. Pull the sheet in three

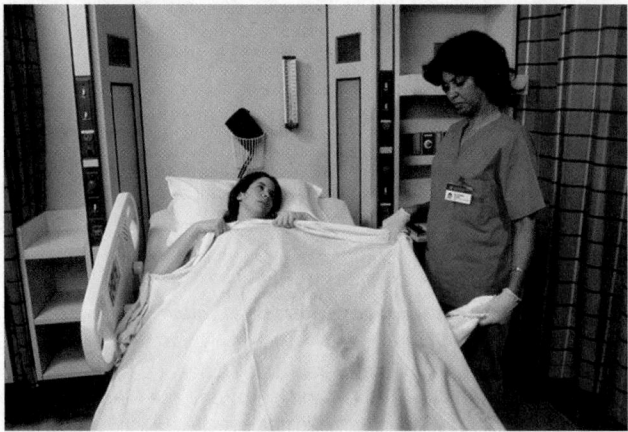

❺ Client holds the top edge of sheet while the nurse removes the bath blanket.

divisions: (a) Face the side of the bed to pull the middle division, (b) face the far top corner to pull the bottom division, and (c) face the far bottom corner to pull the top division.
- Tuck the excess drawsheet under the side of the mattress.
6. Reposition the client in the center of the bed.
   - Reposition the pillows at the center of the bed.
   - Assist the client to the center of the bed. Determine what position the client requires or prefers and assist the client to that position.
7. Apply or complete the top bedding.
   - Spread the top sheet over the client and either ask the client to hold the top edge of the sheet or tuck it under the shoulders. The sheet should remain over the client when the bath blanket or used sheet is removed. ❺
   - Complete the top of the bed.
8. Ensure continued safety of the client.
   - Raise the side rails. Place the bed in the low position before leaving the bedside.
   - Attach the call light to the bed linen within the client's reach.
   - Put items used by the client within easy reach.
   - Perform hand hygiene.
9. Document. Many agencies use a checklist that indicates if bed linens were changed.

Evaluation
- Conduct appropriate follow-up, such as determining the client's comfort and safety, patency of all drainage tubes, and the client's access to the call light to summon help when needed.

- Reassess all tubing, oxygen apparatus, IV pumps, and so forth. **Rationale:** *This prevents errors in supportive devices resulting from the procedure.*

LIFESPAN CONSIDERATIONS   Bed-Making

CHILDREN
- Check if the child has a favorite blanket and if it was brought from home. If so, make sure you replace it on the bed after changing the bed linens.

OLDER ADULTS
- Because of the older adult's thin, tender, and fragile skin, be sure to check that the linens are dry and free of wrinkles and be especially careful when pulling linens underneath the older client.

Ambulatory and Community Settings   Bed-Making

- If the client needs to remain in bed, determine the caregiver's knowledge and experience with making an occupied bed. The nurse may need to demonstrate how to change the linen. Emphasize safety for the client and use of correct body mechanics for the caregiver.

PATIENT-CENTERED CARE

- Assess and discuss with the caregiver the following: need for linens (e.g., incontinence, drainage), available linen supply, and laundry accommodations.

Chapter 6 Review

FOCUSING ON CLINICAL THINKING

Consider This

1. What should you do if the UAP complains of back discomfort during or after making a bed?

See Focusing on Clinical Thinking answers on student resource website.

TEST YOUR KNOWLEDGE

1. The nurse wants the unlicensed assistive personnel (UAP) to make an unoccupied open bed. How would the nurse describe this to the UAP?
   1. Make the bed while the client is in the bed and with the top covers folded back.
   2. Make the bed while the client is out of bed and with the top covers folded back.
   3. Make the bed while the client is in the bed with the top covers drawn to the top of the bed.
   4. Make the bed while the client is out of the bed with the top covers drawn to the top of the bed.

2. To allow for more room for the client's feet, the nurse made a fold in the sheet 5 to 10 cm across the bed near the foot. Which term correctly describes the nurse's action?
   1. A miter of the sheet
   2. A vertical toe pleat
   3. A fanfold of the sheet
   4. A horizontal toe pleat

3. The nurse enters a client's room to perform an assessment. The client is complaining of syncope and the blood pressure reads 64/36 mmHg. The nurse places the client in Trendelenburg's position. How is the client placed in bed?
   1. Positioned completely horizontal
   2. Sitting in bed with the head of the bed raised 30°
   3. Positioned with the head of the bed raised and the foot lowered
   4. Positioned with the head of the bed lowered and the foot raised

4. A client has his left pleural chest tube removed. Within minutes of the chest tube removal, the client develops difficulty breathing. In which position should the nurse place this client?
   1. Fowler's
   2. Trendelenburg's
   3. Semi-Fowler's
   4. Reverse Trendelenburg's

5. A student nurse is learning how to make a surgical bed. Which statement made by the student nurse indicates the need for further teaching?
   1. "A flannel bath blanket provides additional warmth for the client."
   2. "I will place top covers on the bed as I would for an unoccupied bed."
   3. "I will tuck the sheets in and miter the corners of the sheets."
   4. "Pillows are left on a chair to facilitate transferring the client into the bed."

6. Which practice guidelines need to be implemented during bed-making? Select all that apply.
   1. Hold soiled linen close to the uniform.
   2. Linen for one client can be placed on another client's bed.
   3. Place soiled linen directly in a portable linen hamper.
   4. Gather all linen before starting to strip a bed.
   5. Do not shake soiled linen in the air.

7. The nurse plans to delegate bed-making to the UAP. Which of the following clients' beds could the nurse safely delegate? Select all that apply.
   1. The postoperative client who had a lumbar laminectomy performed yesterday
   2. The client in traction following surgery for an internal fixation of the femur this morning
   3. The client on complete bed rest secondary to improving symptoms of Guillain-Barré syndrome (a neurologic disorder)
   4. The older adult client who has been chronically confined to bed
   5. The client in traction following a fractured cervical vertebra

8. A client is complaining of not being able to sleep while in the hospital. Which of the following interventions by the nurse is appropriate? Select all that apply.
   1. Keep the door to the room open.
   2. Post a "Do Not Disturb" sign on the client door.
   3. Lower lights.
   4. Lower room temperature below 20°C (68°F).
   5. Decrease the noise level at change of shift.

9. The nurse is caring for a client who has recently suffered a cerebrovascular accident (stroke) and has orders for bathroom privileges only. When changing this client's bed, the nurse would make a/an
   1. Occupied bed.
   2. Unoccupied bed.
   3. Surgical bed.
   4. Closed bed.

10. Which of the following would the nurse consider appropriate for an alert adult client? Select all that apply.
    1. The 6'6" client has an extended-length bed.
    2. All of the side rails are up.
    3. The bed is in the low position.
    4. The wheels on the bed are in the "lock" position.
    5. The two upper (top) quarter-length side rails are up.

See Answers to Test Your Knowledge in Appendix A.

READINGS AND REFERENCES

References

Cvach, M. (2012). Monitor alarm fatigue: An integrative review. *Biomedical Instrumentation & Technology, 46*, 268–277. doi:10.2345/0899-8205-46.4.268

Ferenc, I. (2012). Alarm fatigue to get heightened attention. *Hospitals & Health Networks, 86*(5), 18.

Mazer, S. E. (2012). Creating a culture of safety. Reducing hospital noise. *Biomedical Instrumentation & Technology, 46*, 350–355. doi:10.2345/0899-8205-46.5.350

Minnick, A. F., Mion, L. C., Johnson, M. E., Catrambone, C., & Leipzig, R. (2008). The who and why's of side rail use.

Nursing Management, 39(5), 36–44. doi:10.1097/01 .NUMA.0000318064.41092.f2

U. S. Food and Drug Administration. (2012). The Joint Commission aim to reduce alarm fatigue. *AACN Bold Voices, 4*(8), 9.

Selected Bibliography

Berman, A., Snyder, S., & Frandsen, G. (2016). *Kozier & Erb's fundamentals of nursing: Concepts, process, and practice* (10th ed.). Upper Saddle River, NJ: Pearson.

Eggertson, L. (2012). Hospital noise. *Canadian Nurse, 108*(4), 29–31.

Morton, J. A. (2013). Notes on noise. *Nursing, 43*(5), 37–40. doi:10.1097/01.NURSE.0000428697.87216.a8

Sendelbach, S. (2012). Alarm fatigue. *Nursing Clinics of North America, 47*, 375–382. doi:10.1016/j.cnur.2012.05.009

Stokowski, L. A. (2014). Time to battle alarm fatigue: Better monitoring and management. Retrieved from http://www .medscape.com/viewarticle/820738_print

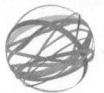

7 Infection Prevention

LEARNING OUTCOMES

At the completion of this chapter, the student will be able to:

1. Define the key terms used in infection control and prevention.
2. Describe six links in the chain of infection.
3. Recognize when it is appropriate to delegate infection control and prevention skills to unlicensed assistive personnel.
4. Verbalize the steps used in:
   a. Establishing and maintaining a sterile field.
   b. Applying and removing sterile gloves.
   c. Implementing transmission-based precautions including bagging articles and managing equipment used for clients who are in isolation.
5. Compare and contrast standard precautions and transmission-based isolation precaution systems.
6. Demonstrate appropriate documentation and reporting of infection control and prevention skills.

SKILLS

Skill 7–1 Establishing and Maintaining a Sterile Field
Skill 7–2 Applying and Removing Sterile Gloves (Open Method)
Skill 7–3 Implementing Transmission-Based Precautions

KEY TERMS

airborne precautions, 220
antiseptics, 211
asepsis, 211
contact precautions, 220

disinfectants, 211
droplet nuclei, 211
droplet precautions, 220
medical asepsis, 211

sepsis, 220
standard precautions, 220
sterile field, 213
surgical asepsis, 211

transmission-based
  precautions, 220
vector-borne transmission, 210
vehicle-borne transmission, 210

This chapter presents the chain of infection and ways of protecting clients and caregivers at each link in the chain. Foundational to the skills presented in this chapter is the concept of host susceptibility and the ways in which each client's immunodefense mechanisms can be bolstered and amplified. Many of the skills nurses offer clients stimulate innate immune function, which boosts resistance to infectious disease. By facilitating regular positional changes (Chapter 10 ∞), bed exercises, early ambulation (Chapter 11 ∞), and deep-breathing exercises (Chapter 24 ∞), nurses stimulate circulation of lymph and healthy immune functioning in clients. By teaching nutritional principles (Chapter 19 ∞) and offering suggestions for stress management and the cultivation of healthy relationships, nurses encourage lifestyle choices that tap into the mind–body connection and enhance immune function.

Chapter 1 ∞ of this text presented the concepts of hand hygiene, standard precautions, and use of personal protective equipment (PPE). Those skills are used with all clients. The Centers for Disease Control and Prevention (CDC) published *Guidelines for Isolation Precautions: Preventing Transmission of Infectious Agents in Healthcare Settings 2007* (Siegel, Rhinehart, Jackson, Chiarello, & the Healthcare Infection Control Practices Advisory Committee, 2007) expands those skills by adding recommendations for respiratory hygiene/cough etiquette and placing increased emphasis on needle safety. When standard precautions cannot adequately block the transmission of pathogenic microorganisms, more advanced infection prevention practices are used.

CHAIN OF INFECTION

Six links make up the chain of infection: the etiologic agent, or microorganism; the place where the organism naturally resides (reservoir); a portal of exit from the reservoir; a method (mode) of transmission; a portal of entry into a host; and the susceptibility of the host (Figure 7–1 ■). The goal of infection control and prevention measures is to break the chain whenever and wherever possible so that disease is not transmitted from one person to another.

SAFETY ALERT!   SAFETY

A person does not need to have an identified infection in order to pass potentially infective microorganisms to another person. Even normal microorganisms for one person can infect another person.

Method of Transmission

After a microorganism leaves its source or reservoir (Table 7–1), it requires a means of transmission to reach another person or host through a receptive portal of entry. Three mechanisms are available for doing so:

1. *Direct contact transmission.* Direct contact transmission involves immediate and direct transfer of microorganisms from person to person through touching, biting, kissing, or sexual intercourse. Transfer of contaminated blood or tissue from one individual to another is also direct transmission. Droplet spread

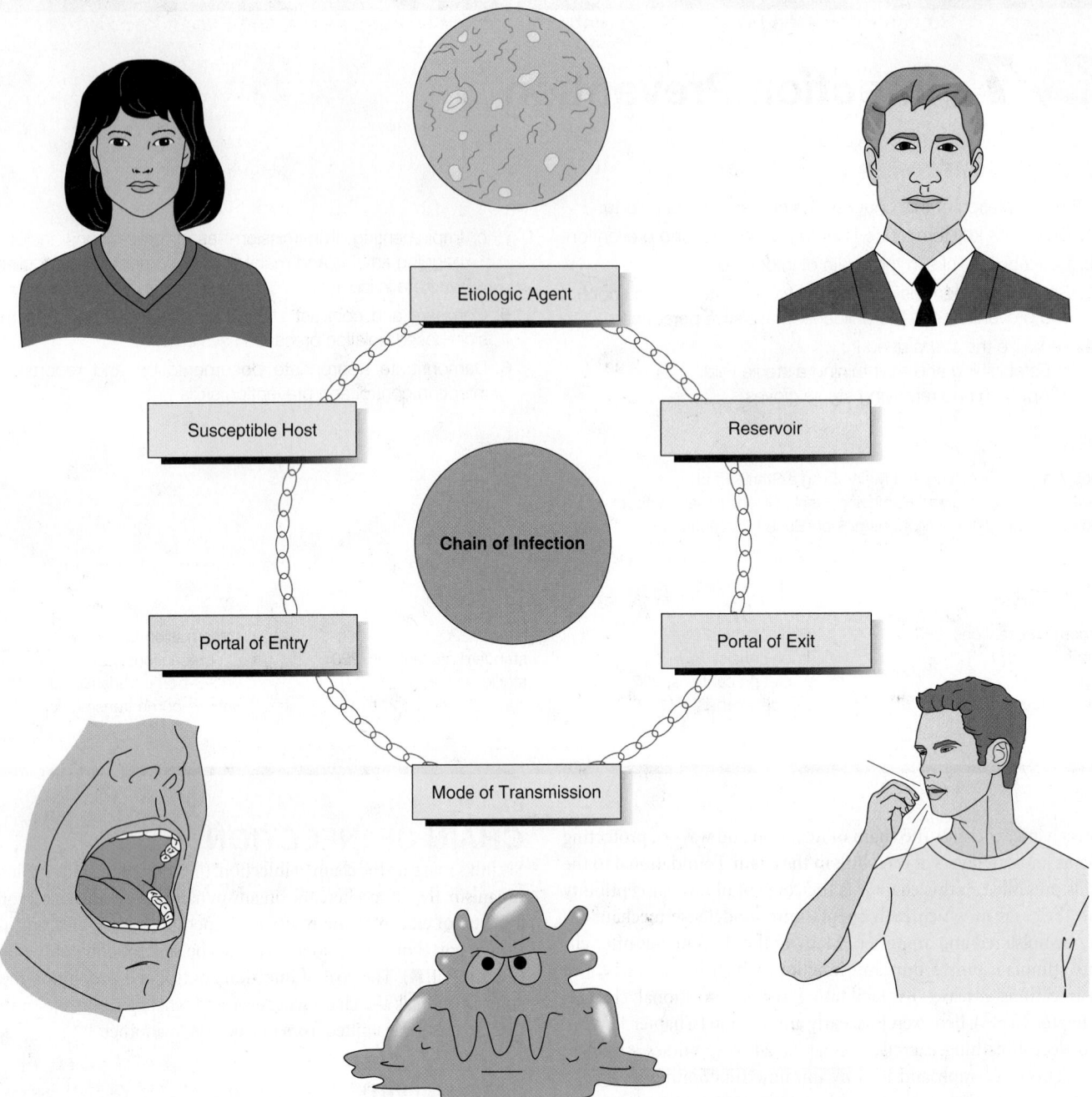

Figure 7-1 ■ The chain of infection.

is a form of direct transmission but can occur only if the source and the host are within 1m (3 ft) of each other. Sneezing, coughing, spitting, singing, or talking can project droplet spray into the conjunctiva or onto the mucous membranes of the eye, nose, or mouth of another person.

2. *Indirect contact transmission.* Indirect contact transmission may be either vehicle-borne or vector-borne.

   a. Vehicle-borne transmission. A vehicle is any substance that serves as an intermediate means to transport and introduce an infectious agent into a susceptible host through a suitable portal of entry. Fomites (inanimate materials or objects), such as handkerchiefs, toys, soiled clothes, cooking or eating utensils, surgical instruments, needles, thermometers,

or dressings, can act as vehicles. Water and food are other vehicles. For example, food or water may become contaminated by a food handler who carries the hepatitis A virus. The food is then ingested by a susceptible host.

   Health care workers' hands are also vehicles for transmission of infectious agents. This occurs when the worker touches an infected or colonized client and then touches another client without using effective hand hygiene between the two clients.

   b. Vector-borne transmission. A vector is an animal or flying or crawling insect that serves as an intermediate means of transporting the infectious agent. Transmission may occur when the vector injects salivary fluid during biting or when

TABLE 7–1 Human Body Area Reservoirs, Common Infectious Microorganisms, and Portals of Exit

Body Area Reservoir	Common Infectious Organisms	Portals of Exit
Respiratory tract	Parainfluenza virus *Mycobacterium tuberculosis* *Staphylococcus aureus*	Nose or mouth through sneezing, coughing, breathing, or talking
Gastrointestinal tract	Hepatitis A virus *Salmonella* species *Clostridium difficile*	Mouth: saliva, vomitus; Anus: feces; Ostomies: feces
Urinary tract	*Escherichia coli* enterococci *Pseudomonas aeruginosa*	Urethral meatus and urinary diversion
Reproductive tract	*Neisseria gonorrhoeae* *Treponema pallidum* Herpes simplex virus type 2 Hepatitis B virus (HBV)	Vagina: vaginal discharge; Urinary meatus: semen, urine
Blood	HBV Human immunodeficiency virus (HIV) *Staphylococcus aureus* *Staphylococcus epidermidis*	Open wound, needle puncture site, any disruption of intact skin or mucous membrane surfaces
Tissue	*Staphylococcus aureus* *Escherichia coli* *Proteus* species *Streptococcus* beta-hemolytic A or B	Drainage from cut or wound

it deposits feces or other materials on the skin through a bite wound or a traumatized skin area.

3. ***Airborne transmission.*** Airborne transmission may involve droplets or dust. **Droplet nuclei**, the residue of evaporated droplets emitted by an infected host such as someone with tuberculosis (TB), can remain in the air for long periods. Dust particles containing infectious agent spores from the soil can also become airborne. The material is transmitted by air currents to a suitable portal of entry, usually the respiratory tract, of another person.

Breaking the Chain of Infection

Various practices break the chain of infection or interrupt the infectious disease process (Table 7–2). For example, the etiologic agent is interrupted by the use of **antiseptics** (agents that inhibit the growth of some microorganisms) and **disinfectants** (agents that destroy microorganisms other than spores) and by sterilization. The aim of most hospital precautions is breaking the chain during the mode of transmission phase of the cycle.

Reducing Risks for Infection

Planned nursing strategies to reduce the risk of transmission of organisms from one person to another include the use of meticulous asepsis. **Asepsis** is the freedom from infection or infectious material. The two basic types of asepsis are medical and surgical. **Medical asepsis** includes all practices intended to confine a specific microorganism to a specific area, limiting the number, growth, and spread of microorganisms. **Surgical asepsis**, or sterile technique, refers to those practices that keep an area or objects free of all microorganisms. It includes practices that destroy all microorganisms and *spores* (microscopic dormant structures formed by some pathogens that are very hardy and often survive common cleaning techniques).

SAFETY ALERT! `SAFETY`

2014 The Joint Commission National Patient Safety Goals (2013)

GOAL 7: REDUCE THE RISK OF HEALTH CARE–ASSOCIATED INFECTIONS.

- Comply with either the current CDC hand hygiene guidelines or the current World Health Organization (WHO) hand hygiene guidelines.
  Rationale: Following the best practices identified in these guidelines helps ensure standardized, proven approaches to hand hygiene.
- Implement evidence-based practices to prevent health care–associated infections due to multidrug-resistant organisms (MDROs) in acute care hospitals.
  Rationale: *Each health care agency needs to determine which practices are most appropriate for its unique client population and circumstances that lead to the prevalence of particular MDROs.*
- Implement evidence-based practices to prevent central line–associated bloodstream infections. *Note:* This requirement covers short- and long-term central venous catheters and peripherally inserted central catheter (PICC) lines.
- Implement evidence-based practices for preventing surgical site infections.

MAINTAINING SURGICAL ASEPSIS

An object is sterile only when it is free of all microorganisms. It is well known that surgical asepsis is practiced in operating rooms and special diagnostic areas. Surgical asepsis is also employed for many procedures in general care areas, such as when changing wound dressings, performing urinary catheterizations, and administering intravenous (IV) therapy. In these situations, all of the principles of surgical asepsis are applied as in the operating room; however, not all of the sterile techniques that follow are always required. For example,

TABLE 7–2   Nursing Interventions That Break the Chain of Infection

Link	Interventions	Rationales
Etiologic agent (microorganism)	Ensure that articles are correctly cleaned and disinfected or sterilized before use.	Correct cleaning, disinfecting, and sterilizing reduce or eliminate microorganisms.
	Educate clients and support people about appropriate methods to clean, disinfect, and sterilize articles.	Knowledge of ways to reduce or eliminate microorganisms reduces the numbers of microorganisms present and the likelihood of transmission.
Reservoir (source)	Change dressings and bandages when they are soiled or wet.	Moist dressings are ideal environments for microorganisms to grow and multiply.
	Assist clients to carry out appropriate skin and oral hygiene.	Hygienic measures reduce the numbers of resident and transient microorganisms and the likelihood of infection.
	Dispose of damp, soiled linens appropriately.	Damp, soiled linens harbor more microorganisms than dry linens.
	Dispose of feces and urine in appropriate receptacles.	Urine and feces in particular contain many microorganisms.
	Ensure that all fluid containers, such as bedside water jugs and suction and drainage bottles, are covered or capped.	Prolonged exposure increases the risk of contamination and promotes microbial growth.
	Empty suction and drainage bottles at the end of each shift or before they become full, or according to agency policy.	Drainage harbors microorganisms that, if left for long periods, proliferate and can be transmitted to others.
Portal of exit from the reservoir	Avoid talking, coughing, or sneezing over open wounds or sterile fields, and cover the mouth and nose when coughing and sneezing.	These measures limit the number of microorganisms that escape from the respiratory tract.
Method of transmission	Cleanse hands between client contacts, after touching body substances, and before performing invasive procedures or touching open wounds.	Hand hygiene is an important means of controlling and preventing the transmission of microorganisms.
	Instruct clients and support people to cleanse hands before handling food or eating, after eliminating, and after touching infectious material.	Hand hygiene helps prevent transfer of microorganisms from one person to another.
	Wear gloves when handling secretions and excretions.	Gloves prevent soiling of the hands.
	Wear gowns if there is danger of soiling clothing with body substances.	Gowns prevent soiling of the clothing.
	Place discarded soiled materials in moisture-proof refuse bags.	Moisture-proof bags prevent the spread of microorganisms to others.
	Hold used bedpans steadily to prevent spillage, and dispose of urine and feces in appropriate receptacles.	Feces in particular contain many microorganisms.
	Initiate and implement infection prevention strategies for all clients.	All clients may harbor potentially infectious microorganisms that can be transmitted to others.
	Wear masks and eye protection when in close contact with clients who have infections transmitted by droplets from the respiratory tract.	Masks and eyewear reduce the spread of droplet-transmitted microorganisms.
	Wear masks and eye protection when sprays of body fluid are possible (e.g., during irrigation procedures).	Masks and eye protection provide protection from microorganisms in clients' body substances.
Portal of entry to the susceptible host	Use aseptic technique for invasive procedures (e.g., injections, catheterizations).	Invasive procedures penetrate the body's natural protective barriers to microorganisms.
	Use sterile technique when exposing open wounds or handling dressings.	Open wounds are vulnerable to microbial infection.
	Place used disposable needles and syringes in puncture-resistant containers for disposal.	Injuries from needles contaminated by blood or body fluids from an infected client or carrier are a primary cause of HBV and HIV transmission to health care workers.
	Provide all clients with their own personal care items.	People have less resistance to another person's microorganisms than to their own.
Susceptible host	Maintain the integrity of the client's skin and mucous membranes.	Intact skin and mucous membranes protect against invasion by microorganisms.
	Ensure that the client receives a balanced diet and proper hydration.	A balanced diet supplies proteins and vitamins necessary to build or maintain body tissues and healthy immune function.
	Educate the public about the importance of immunizations.	Certain immunizations may protect people against virulent infectious diseases.
	Encourage deep, slow, full breathing, ambulation, and movement.	These actions enhance ventilation and circulation throughout the body.
	Offer stress management strategies and encourage healthy relationships.	Tap into the mind–body connection to enhance healing.

before an operating room procedure, the nurse generally puts on a mask and cap, performs a surgical hand scrub, and then applies a sterile gown and gloves. In a general care area, the nurse may only perform hand hygiene and use sterile gloves. The nine basic principles of surgical asepsis and practices that relate to each principle appear in Table 7–3.

Sterile Field

A **sterile field** is a microorganism-free area. Nurses often establish a sterile field by using the innermost side of a sterile wrapper or by using a sterile drape. When the field is established, sterile supplies and sterile solutions can be placed on it. Sterile forceps are used in many instances to handle and transfer the sterile supplies.

So that sterility can be maintained, equipment is wrapped in a variety of materials. Commercially prepared items are frequently wrapped in plastic, paper, or glass. Commercially prepared sterile liquids for both internal and external use are often supplied in plastic or glass containers. Sterile liquids (e.g., sterile water for irrigations) are preferably packaged in amounts adequate for one use only because once a container has been opened, there can be no assurance that it will remain sterile. Open bottles of sterile liquids are never used longer than 24 hours.

TABLE 7–3	Principles and Practices of Surgical Asepsis
Principles	**Practices**
All objects used in a sterile field must be sterile.	All articles are sterilized appropriately by dry or moist heat, chemicals, or radiation before use. Always check a package containing a sterile object for intactness, dryness, and expiration date. Sterile articles can be stored for only a prescribed time; after that, they are considered unsterile. Any package that appears already open, torn, punctured, or wet is considered unsterile. Storage areas should be clean, dry, off the floor, and away from sinks. Always check chemical indicators of sterilization before using a package. The indicator is often a tape used to fasten the package or contained inside the package. The indicator changes color during sterilization, indicating that the contents have undergone a sterilization procedure. If the color change is not evident, the package is considered unsterile. Commercially prepared sterile packages may not have indicators but are marked with the word *sterile*.
Sterile objects become unsterile when touched by unsterile objects.	Handle sterile objects that will touch open wounds or enter body cavities only with sterile forceps or sterile gloved hands. Discard or resterilize objects that come into contact with unsterile objects. Whenever the sterility of an object is questionable, assume the article is unsterile.
Sterile items that are out of sight or below the waist or table level are considered unsterile.	Once left unattended, a sterile field is considered unsterile. Sterile objects are always kept in view. Nurses do not turn their backs on a sterile field. Only the front part of a sterile gown, from shoulder to waist (or table height, whichever is higher), and the cuff of the sleeves to 2 inches above the elbows are considered sterile. Always keep sterile gloved hands in sight and above waist/table level; touch only objects that are sterile. Sterile draped tables in the operating room or elsewhere are considered sterile only at surface level.
Sterile objects can become unsterile by prolonged exposure to airborne microorganisms.	Keep doors closed and traffic to a minimum in areas where sterile procedures are performed, because moving air can carry dust and microorganisms. Keep areas in which sterile procedures are carried out as clean as possible by frequent damp cleaning with detergent germicides to minimize contaminants in the area. Keep hair clean and short or secure it to prevent hair from falling on sterile objects. Microorganisms on the hair can make a sterile field unsterile. Wear surgical caps in operating rooms, delivery rooms, and burn units. Refrain from sneezing or coughing over a sterile field. This can make it unsterile because droplets containing microorganisms from the respiratory tract can travel 1 m (3 ft). Some agencies recommend that masks covering the mouth and the nose should be worn by anyone working over a sterile field or an open wound. When working over a sterile field, keep talking to a minimum. To prevent microorganisms from falling over a sterile field, refrain from reaching over a sterile field unless sterile gloves are worn and refrain from moving unsterile objects over a sterile field.
Fluids flow in the direction of gravity.	Unless gloves are worn, always hold wet forceps so that the tips are positioned below the handles. When the tips are held higher than the handles, fluid can flow onto the handle and become contaminated by the hands. When the forceps are again pointed downward, the contaminated fluid flows back down and contaminates the tips. During a surgical hand wash, hold the hands higher than the elbows to prevent contaminants from the forearms from reaching the hands.

(continued)

TABLE 7–3 | **Principles and Practices of Surgical Asepsis—*continued***

Principles	Practices
Moisture that passes through a sterile object draws microorganisms from unsterile surfaces above or below to the sterile surface by capillary action.	Sterile moisture-proof barriers are used beneath sterile objects. Liquids are frequently poured into containers on a sterile field. If they are spilled onto the sterile field, the barrier keeps the liquid from seeping beneath it. Keep the sterile covers on sterile equipment dry. Damp surfaces can attract microorganisms in the air. Replace sterile drapes that do not have a sterile barrier underneath when they become moist.
The edges of a sterile field are considered unsterile.	A 2.5-cm (1-in.) margin at each edge of an opened drape is considered unsterile because the edges are in contact with unsterile surfaces. Place all sterile objects more than 2.5 cm (1 in.) inside the edges of a sterile field. Any article that falls outside the edges of a sterile field is considered unsterile.
The skin cannot be sterilized and is unsterile.	Use sterile gloves or sterile forceps to handle sterile items. Prior to a surgical aseptic procedure, cleanse the hands to reduce the number of microorganisms on them.
Conscientiousness, alertness, and honesty are essential qualities in maintaining surgical asepsis.	When a sterile object becomes unsterile, it does not necessarily change in appearance. The person who sees a sterile object become contaminated must correct or report the situation. Do not set up a sterile field ahead of time for future use.

●○● NURSING PROCESS: ESTABLISHING AND MAINTAINING A STERILE FIELD

SKILL 7–1

Establishing and Maintaining a Sterile Field

ASSESSMENT
Review the client's record or discuss with the client exactly what procedure will be performed that requires a sterile field. Assess the client for the presence of or excessive risk for infection and the client's ability to participate in the procedure.

PLANNING
Determine, if possible, what supplies and techniques have been used in the past to perform the sterile procedure for this client. Also attempt to determine if the procedure will be performed again in the future so that you can conduct appropriate client teaching and ensure that adequate supplies will be available.

Schedule the procedure that requires a sterile field at a time consistent with the primary care provider's order, the need for the procedure, and the client's other activities.

DELEGATION

Sterile procedures are not delegated to unlicensed assistive personnel (UAP).

INTERPROFESSIONAL PRACTICE

Sterile fields and procedures may be within the scope of practice for many health care providers. These providers may perform the procedure independently or with a nurse or other provider. Although these providers may verbally communicate about the procedure to the health care team members, the nurse must also know where to locate their documentation in the client's medical record.

Equipment
- Package containing a sterile drape
- Sterile equipment as needed (e.g., wrapped sterile gauze, wrapped sterile bowl, antiseptic solution, sterile forceps)

IMPLEMENTATION
Preparation
- Ensure that the package is clean and dry; if moisture is noted on the inside of a plastic-wrapped package or the outside of a cloth-wrapped package, it is considered contaminated and must be discarded.
- Check the sterilization expiration dates on the package, and look for any indications that it has been previously opened. Spots or stains on cloth or paper-wrapped objects may indicate contamination, and these objects should not be used.
- Follow agency practice for disposal of possibly contaminated packages.

Performance
1. Prior to establishing the sterile field, introduce self and verify the client's identity using agency protocol. Explain to the client what you are going to do, why it is necessary, and how he or she can participate. Discuss how the results will be used in planning further care or treatments.
2. Perform hand hygiene and observe other appropriate infection prevention procedures (see Skills 1–1, 1–2, 1–3, and 7–3).
3. Provide for client privacy if appropriate.
4. Open the package. If the package is inside a plastic cover, remove the cover.

To Open a Wrapped Package on a Surface
- Place the package in the work area so that the top flap of the wrapper opens away from you.
- Reaching around the package (not over it), pinch the top flap on the outside of the wrapper between the thumb and index finger.❶ **Rationale:** *Touching only the outside of the wrapper maintains the sterility of the inside of the wrapper. Pull the flap open, laying it flat on the far surface.*

Establishing and Maintaining a Sterile Field—*continued*

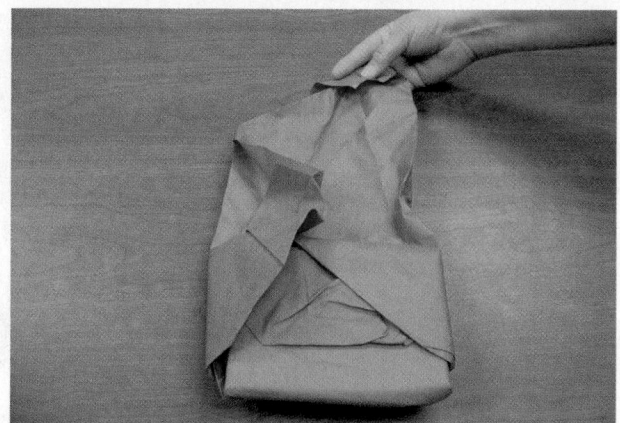

1 Opening the first flap of a sterile wrapped package.

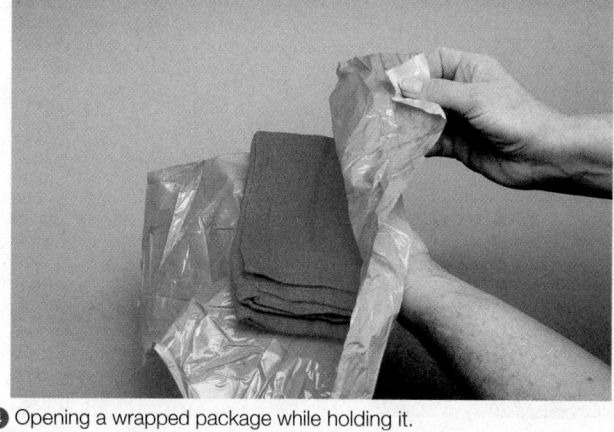

4 Opening a wrapped package while holding it.

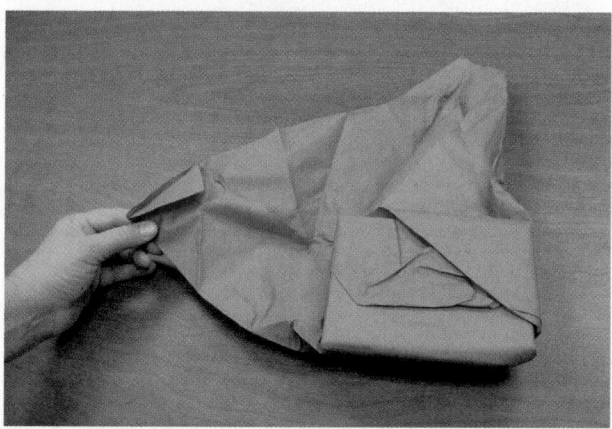

2 Opening the second flap to the side.

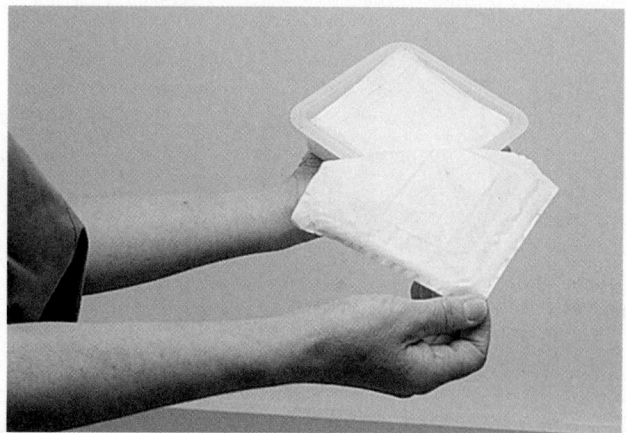

5 Opening a sterile package that has an unsealed corner.

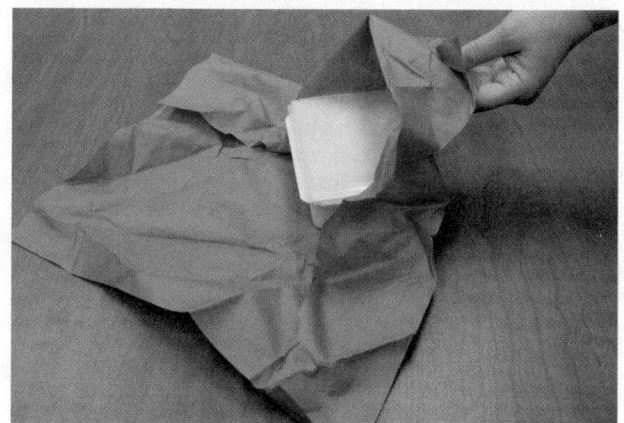

3 Pulling the last flap toward oneself by grasping the corner.

- Repeat for the side flaps. Use the right hand for the right flap, and the left hand for the left flap. **2** **Rationale:** *By using both hands, you avoid reaching over the sterile contents.*
- Pull the fourth flap toward you by grasping the corner that is turned down. **3**

Variation: Opening a Wrapped Package While Holding It
- Hold the package in one hand with the top flap opening away from you.

- Using the other hand, open the package as described above, pulling the corners of the flaps well back. **4** Tuck each of the corners into the hand holding the package so that they do not flutter and contaminate sterile objects. The hands are considered contaminated, and at no time should they touch the contents of the package.

Variation: Opening Commercially Prepared Packages
- If the flap of the package has an unsealed corner, hold the container in one hand, and pull back on the flap with the other hand. **5**
- If the package has a partially sealed edge, grasp both sides of the edge, one with each hand, and pull apart gently. **6**

5. Establish a sterile field by using a drape.
- Open the package containing the drape as described above.
- With one hand, pluck the corner of the drape that is folded back on the top touching only one side of the drape.
- Lift the drape out of the cover, and allow it to open freely without touching any objects. **7** **Rationale:** *If the drape touches the outside of the package or any unsterile surface, it is considered contaminated.*
- With the other hand, carefully pick up another corner of the drape, holding it well away from you and, again, touching only the same side of the drape as the first hand.
- Lay the drape on a clean and dry surface, placing the bottom (i.e., the freely hanging side) farthest from you. **8**

Continued on page 216

Establishing and Maintaining a Sterile Field—*continued*

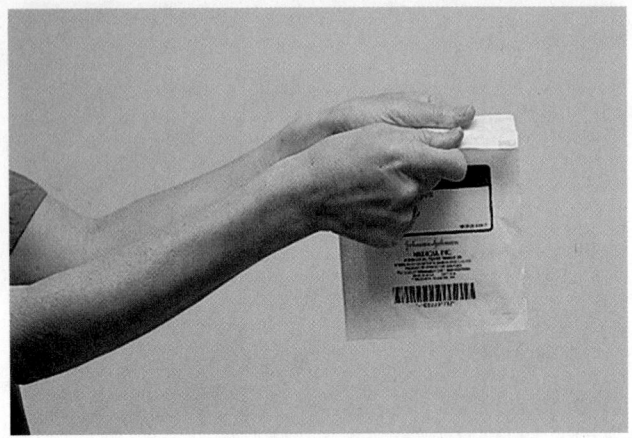

6 Opening a sterile package that has a partially sealed edge.

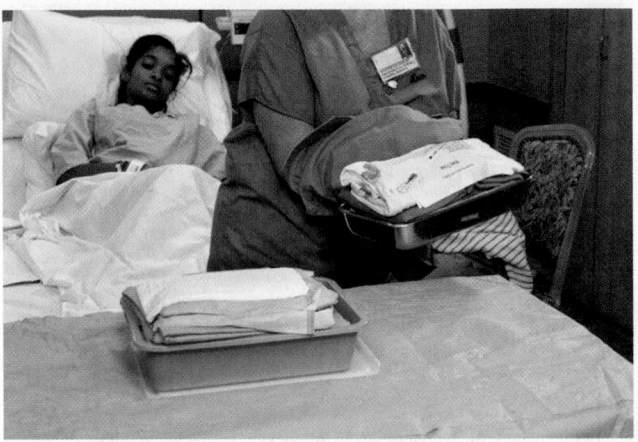

9 Adding wrapped sterile supplies to a sterile field.

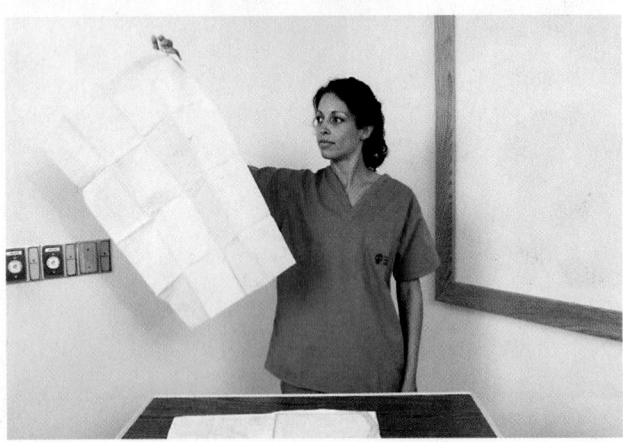

7 Allowing a drape to open freely without touching any objects.

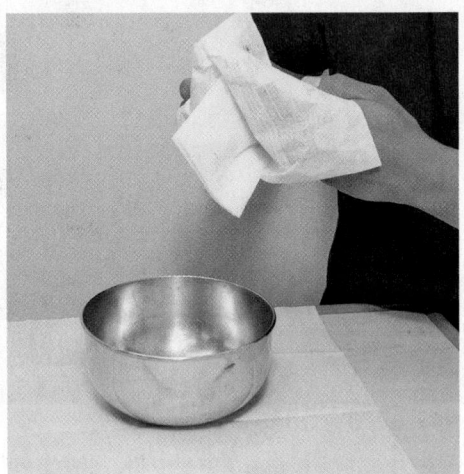

10 Adding commercially packaged gauze to a sterile field.

* With the free hand, grasp the corners of the wrapper, and hold them against the wrist of the other hand. **9 Rationale:** *The sterile wrapper now covers the unsterile hand.*
* Place the sterile bowl, drape, or other supply on the sterile field by approaching from an angle rather than holding the arm over the field.
* Discard the wrapper.

Variation: Adding Commercially Packaged Supplies to a Sterile Field

* Open each package as previously described.
* Hold the package 15 cm (6 in.) above the field, and allow the contents to drop on the field. **10** Keep in mind that 2.5 cm (1 in.) around the edge of the field is considered contaminated. **Rationale:** *At a height of 15 cm (6 in.), the outside of the package is not likely to touch and contaminate the sterile field.*

Adding Solution to a Sterile Bowl
Liquids may need to be poured into containers within a sterile field. Unwrapped bottles that contain sterile solution are considered sterile on the inside and contaminated on the outside because the bottle may have been handled. Bottles used in an operating room may be sterilized on the outside as well as the inside, however, and these are handled with sterile gloves.

* Obtain the exact amount of solution, if possible. **Rationale:** *Once a sterile bottle has been opened, its sterility cannot*

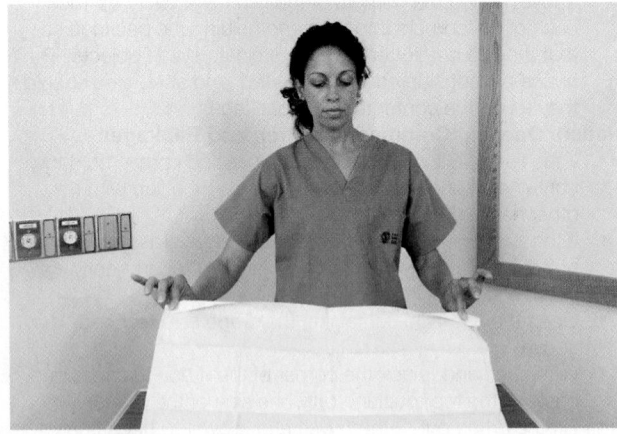

8 Placing a drape on a surface.

    Rationale: By placing the lowermost side farthest away, you avoid leaning over the sterile field and contaminating it.
6. Add necessary sterile supplies, being careful not to touch the drape with the hands.

Adding Wrapped Supplies to a Sterile Field
* Open each wrapped package as described in the preceding steps.

Establishing and Maintaining a Sterile Field—*continued*

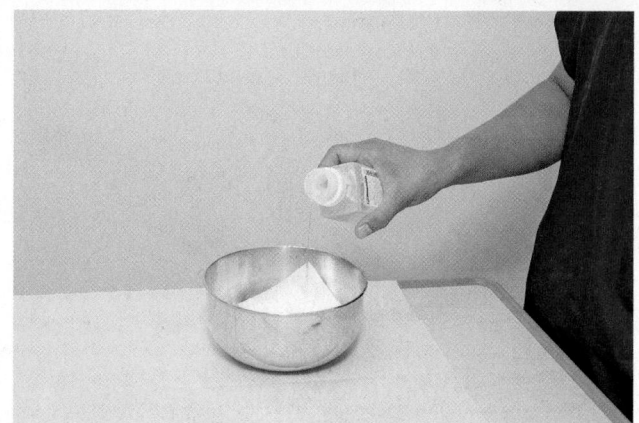

⑪ Adding a liquid to a sterile bowl.

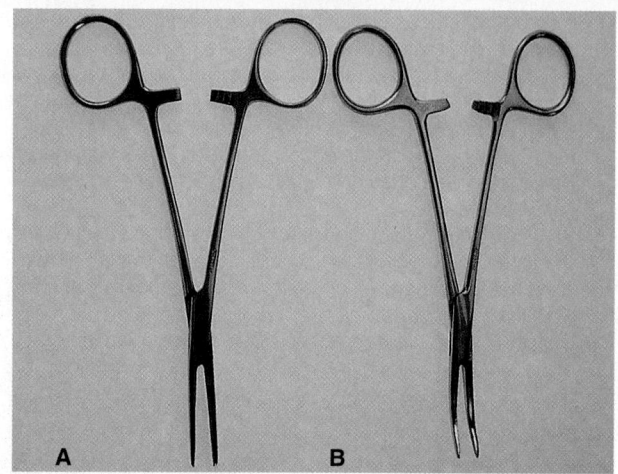

⑫ Hemostats: *A*, straight; *B*, curved.

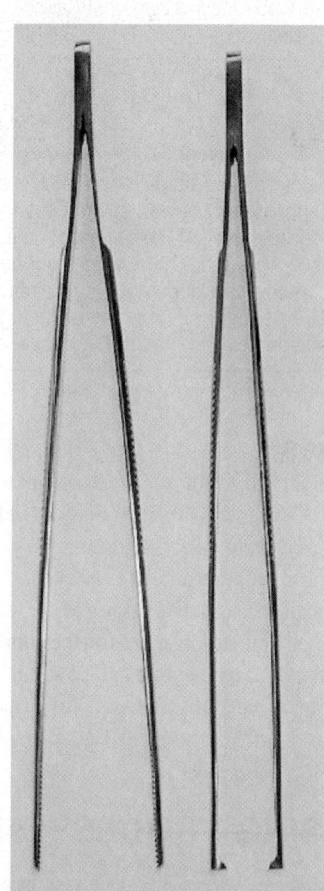

⑬ Tissue forceps: *A*, plain; *B*, toothed.

be ensured for future use. Follow agency policy for reuse of opened sterile solution bottles.

- Before pouring any liquid, read the label three times to make sure you have the correct solution and concentration (strength). Wipe the outside of the bottle with a damp towel to remove any large particles that could fall into the bowl or field.
- Remove the lid or cap from the bottle and invert the lid before placing it on a surface that is not sterile. **Rationale:** *Inverting the lid maintains the sterility of the inside surface because it is not allowed to touch an unsterile surface.*
- Hold the bottle at a slight angle so that the label is upper-most. ⑪ **Rationale:** *Any solution that flows down the outside of the bottle during pouring will not damage or obliterate the label.*
- Hold the bottle of fluid at a height of 10 to 15 cm (4 to 6 in.) over the bowl and to the side of the sterile field so that as little of the bottle as possible is over the field. **Rationale:** *At this height, there is less likelihood of contaminating the sterile field by touching the field or by reaching an arm over it.*
- Pour the solution gently to avoid splashing the liquid. **Rationale:** *If a barrier drape (one that has a water-resistant layer) is not used and the drape is on an unsterile surface, moisture will contaminate the field by wicking microorganisms through the drape.*
- Tilt the neck of the bottle back to vertical quickly when done pouring so that none of the liquid flows down the outside of the bottle. **Rationale:** *Such drips would contaminate the sterile field if the outside of the bottle is not sterile.*
- If the bottle will be used again, replace the lid securely and write on the label the date and time of opening. **Rationale:** *Replacing the lid immediately maintains the sterility of the inner aspect of the lid and the solution. Depending on agency policy, a sterile container of solution that is opened may be used only once and is then discarded (such as in the operating room). In other settings, policy may permit recapped bottles to be reused within 24 hours.*

7. Use sterile forceps to handle sterile supplies. Forceps are usu-ally used to move a sterile article from one place to another, for example, when transferring sterile gauze from its package to a sterile dressing tray. Forceps may be disposable or resterilized after use. Commonly used forceps include hemostats ⑫ and tissue forceps. ⑬

- If forceps tips are wet, keep the tips lower than the wrist at all times, unless you are wearing sterile gloves. ⑭

Rationale: *Gravity prevents liquids on the tips of the forceps from flowing to the unsterile handles and later back to the tips.*

- Hold sterile forceps above waist or table level, whichever is higher. **Rationale:** *Items held below waist or table level are considered contaminated.*

Continued on page 218

Establishing and Maintaining a Sterile Field—*continued*

- Hold sterile forceps within sight. **Rationale:** *While out of sight, forceps may, unknown to the user, become unsterile. Any forceps that go out of sight should be considered unsterile.*
- When using forceps to lift sterile supplies, be sure that the forceps do not touch the edges or outside of the wrapper. **Rationale:** *The edges and outside of the sterile field are considered unsterile.*
- When placing forceps whose handles were in contact with the bare hand, position the handles outside the sterile area. **Rationale:** *The handles of these forceps harbor microorganisms from the bare hand.*
- Deposit a sterile item on a sterile field without permitting moist forceps to touch the sterile field when the surface under the absorbent sterile field is unsterile and a barrier drape is not used.

8. Document that sterile skill was used in the performance of the procedure.

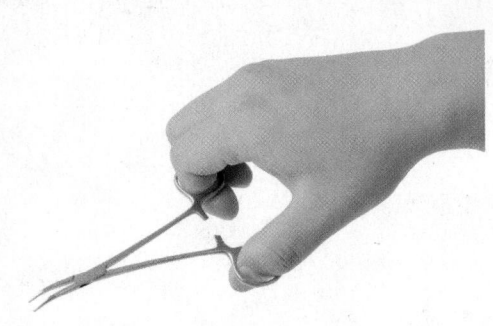

⑭ Holding forceps with an ungloved hand, keeping the tips lower than the wrist.

EVALUATION

Conduct any follow-up indicated during your care of the client. Ensure that adequate numbers and types of sterile supplies are available for the next health care provider.

Ambulatory and Community Settings **Establishing and Maintaining a Sterile Field** | **PATIENT-CENTERED CARE**

- Clean and wipe dry a flat surface for the sterile field.
- Keep pets and noninvolved small children out of the area when setting up for and performing sterile procedures.
- Dispose of all soiled materials in a waterproof bag. Check with the agency as to how to dispose of medical refuse.
- Remove all instruments from the home or other setting where others might accidentally find them. **Rationale:** *New or used*

instruments can be sharp or capable of causing injury. Used instruments may transmit infection. Check with the agency for instructions on cleansing of reusable supplies and disposal of single-use instruments.
- If appropriate, teach the client and family members the principles and rationale underlying the use of a sterile field.

Sterile Gloves

Sterile gloves may be applied by the open method or the closed method. The open method is most frequently used outside the operating room, since the closed method requires that the nurse wear a sterile gown. Sterile gloves are worn during many procedures to enable the nurse to handle sterile objects freely and to prevent clients at risk (e.g., those with open wounds) from becoming infected by microorganisms on the nurse's hands.

Sterile gloves are packaged with a cuff of about 5 cm (2 in.) and with the palms facing upward when the package is opened. The package usually indicates the size of the glove (e.g., size 6 or 7 1/2, or small, medium, large).

Sterile gloves protect the nurse from contact with blood and body fluids. Latex gloves are not recommended due to possible allergies (see Chapter 1 ∞). Nitrile gloves are more flexible than vinyl, mold to the wearer's hands, and allow freedom of movement. Wear nitrile gloves when performing tasks that (a) demand flexibility, (b) place stress on the material (e.g., turning stopcocks [valves for regulating the flow of a fluid] or handling sharp instruments or tape), and (c) involve a high risk of exposure to pathogens. Vinyl gloves should be chosen for tasks that are unlikely to stress the glove material, those requiring minimal precision, and those that present minimal risk of exposure to pathogens.

●○● NURSING PROCESS: APPLYING AND REMOVING STERILE GLOVES

Applying and Removing Sterile Gloves (Open Method)

ASSESSMENT

Review the client's record and orders to determine exactly what procedure will be performed that requires sterile gloves. Check the client record and ask about latex allergies. Use nonlatex gloves whenever possible.

PLANNING

Think through the procedure that requires sterile gloves, planning which steps need to be completed before the gloves can be applied. Determine what additional supplies are needed to perform the procedure for this client. Always have an extra pair of sterile gloves available.

DELEGATION

Sterile procedures are not delegated to UAP.

Applying and Removing Sterile Gloves (Open Method)—*continued*

INTERPROFESSIONAL PRACTICE

Sterile gloves are used by many health care providers. All providers should be comfortable pointing out to each other when any break in sterile technique is detected.

IMPLEMENTATION

Preparation

Ensure the sterility of the package of gloves.

Performance

1. Prior to performing the procedure that requires sterile gloves, introduce self and verify the client's identity using agency protocol. Explain to the client what you are going to do, why it is necessary, and how he or she can participate. Discuss how the results will be used in planning further care or treatments.

2. Perform hand hygiene and observe other appropriate infection prevention procedures (see Skills 1–1, 1–2, 1–3, and 7–3).

3. Provide for client privacy if appropriate.

4. Open the package of sterile gloves.
   - Place the package of gloves on a clean, dry surface. **Rationale:** *Any moisture on the surface could contaminate the gloves.*
   - Some gloves are packed in an inner as well as an outer package. Open the outer package without contaminating the gloves. See Skill 7–1.
   - Remove the inner package from the outer package.
   - Open the inner package as in step 4 of Skill 7–1 or according to the manufacturer's directions. Some manufacturers provide a numbered sequence for opening the flaps and folded tabs to grasp. If no tabs are provided, pluck the flap so that the fingers do not touch the inner surfaces. **Rationale:** *The inner surfaces, which are next to the sterile gloves, will remain sterile.*

5. Put the first glove on the dominant hand.
   - If the gloves are packaged so that they lie side by side, grasp the glove for the dominant hand by its folded cuff edge (on the palmar side) with the thumb and first finger of the nondominant hand. Touch only the inside of the cuff. ❶ **Rationale:** *The hands are not sterile. By touching only the inside of the glove, the nurse avoids contaminating the outside.*

or

   - If the gloves are packaged one on top of the other, grasp the cuff of the top glove, using the opposite hand.
   - Insert the dominant hand into the glove and pull the glove on. Keep the thumb of the inserted hand against the palm of the hand during insertion. ❷ **Rationale:** *If the thumb is kept against the palm, it is less likely to contaminate the outside of the glove.*
   - Leave the cuff in place once the unsterile hand releases the glove. **Rationale:** *Attempting to further unfold the cuff is likely to contaminate the glove.*

6. Put the second glove on the nondominant hand.
   - Pick up the other glove with the sterile gloved hand, inserting the gloved fingers under the cuff and holding the gloved thumb close to the gloved palm. ❸
   - Pull on the second glove carefully. Hold the thumb of the gloved first hand as far as possible from the palm. ❹ **Rationale:** *In this position, the thumb is less likely to touch the arm and become contaminated.*

Equipment

- Packages of sterile gloves

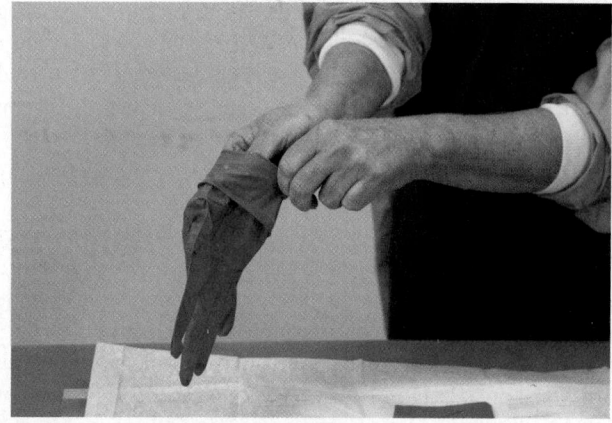

❷ Putting on the first sterile glove.

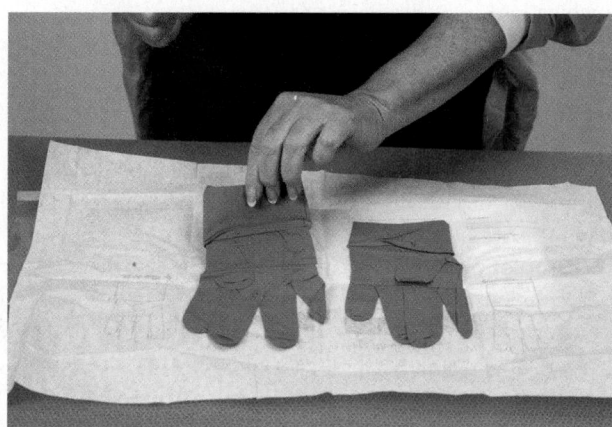

❶ Picking up the first sterile glove.

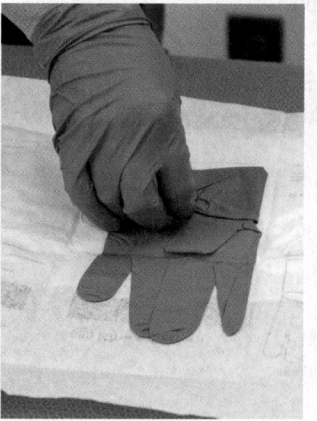

❸ Picking up the second sterile glove.

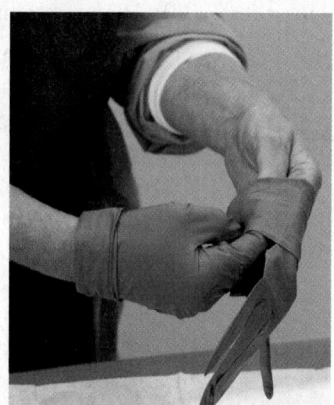

Continued on page 220

SKILL 7-2

Applying and Removing Sterile Gloves (Open Method)—*continued*

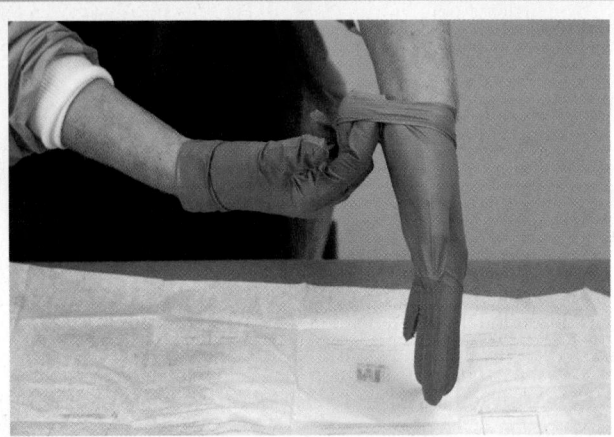

④ Putting on the second sterile glove.

- Adjust each glove so that it fits smoothly, and carefully pull the cuffs up by sliding the fingers under the cuffs.
7. Remove and dispose of used gloves.
   - The technique for removing sterile gloves is the same as that for removing unsterile gloves. If they are soiled with secretions, remove them by turning them inside out. See removal of gloves in Skill 1–3 on page 10.
   - Perform hand hygiene.
8. Document that sterile technique was used in the performance of the procedure.

EVALUATION

Conduct any follow-up indicated during your care of the client. Ensure that adequate numbers and types of sterile supplies are available for the next health care provider.

CARING FOR CLIENTS WITH KNOWN OR SUSPECTED INFECTIONS

As discussed in Chapter 1 ∞, nurses care for all clients using **standard precautions**(see Skill 1–1). That is, the risk of caregiver exposure to client body tissues and fluids rather than the suspected presence or absence of infectious organisms determines the use of clean gloves, gowns, masks, and eye protection. Isolation refers to measures designed to prevent the spread of infection or potentially infectious material.

Sepsis is the condition in which acute organ dysfunction occurs secondary to infection. This organ dysfunction presents as a number of indicators including altered vital signs, elevated white blood count, hypotension, renal impairment, and elevated blood lactate. Due to the prevalence of and mortality rates from sepsis, several international organizations have worked to create best practices for responding to the presence of sepsis. These guidelines, or bundles of interventions, were published by the Surviving Sepsis Campaign (Dellinger et al., 2013). The key recommendations are as follows:

- Measure serum lactate.
- Obtain blood cultures before beginning antibiotic therapy.
- Perform imaging studies promptly to confirm potential source of infection.
- Administer broad-spectrum antibiotic therapy within 1 hour of diagnosis of severe sepsis.
- Administer IV fluid resuscitation to restore blood pressure.
- Provide medication therapy when cardiac output remains low despite fluid resuscitation.
- Use mechanical ventilation as indicated (see Chapter 28 ∞).
- Provide prophylaxis for complications of immobility and other treatments.

Nurses play a key role in the early identification of signs of sepsis and in implementing the recommended interventions. Depending on the causative agent of the infection, isolation precautions may be required. In 2007, the CDC published updated recommendations for isolation precautions in hospitals (Siegel et al., 2007).

Standard Precautions (see Chapter 1 ∞)

The updated guidelines reinforced the need for effective hand hygiene, PPE, and environmental controls. They also added respiratory hygiene/cough etiquette that calls for covering the mouth and nose when sneezing or coughing, proper disposal of tissues, and separating potentially infected individuals from others by at least 1 m (3 ft) or having them wear a surgical mask.

Transmission-Based Precautions (see Skill 7–3)

Transmission-based precautions are used in addition to standard precautions when those precautions do not completely block the chain of infection and the infections are spread in one of three ways: by airborne transmission, by droplet transmission, or by contact. Transmission-based precautions may be used singly or in combination.

Airborne precautions are used for clients known to have or suspected of having serious illnesses transmitted by airborne droplet nuclei smaller than 5 microns. Examples of such illnesses include measles (rubeola), varicella (including disseminated zoster), and TB. The CDC has also prepared special guidelines for preventing the transmission of TB. The most current information may be found on the CDC Division of Tuberculosis Elimination website.

Droplet precautions are used for clients known or suspected to have serious illnesses transmitted by particle droplets larger than 5 microns. Examples of such illnesses are diphtheria (pharyngeal); mycoplasma pneumonia; pertussis; mumps; rubella; streptococcal pharyngitis, pneumonia, or scarlet fever in infants and young children; and pneumonic plague.

Contact precautions are used for clients known or suspected to have serious illnesses easily transmitted by direct client contact or by contact with items in the client's environment. According to the

CDC (Siegel et al., 2007), such illnesses include gastrointestinal, respiratory, skin, or wound infections or colonization with multidrug-resistant bacteria; specific enteric infections such as *C. difficile* and enterohemorrhagic *E. coli* O157:H7, *Shigella*, and hepatitis A and noroviruses for diapered or incontinent clients; respiratory syncytial virus, parainfluenza virus, or enteroviral infections in infants and young children; and highly contagious skin infections such as herpes simplex virus, impetigo, pediculosis, and scabies.

Another organism requiring contact precautions is methicillin-resistant *S. aureus* (MRSA). Approximately half of all MRSA infections are acquired in the hospital, one fourth are associated with having received health care but onset is in the community; the remainder are considered community acquired (Jarvis, Jarvis, & Chinn, 2012). Due to aggressive health care emphasis on prevention of MRSA transmission using standard and contact precautions, rates have decreased but are still unacceptably high. More Americans die each year from MRSA than die from AIDS (MRSA Research Center, 2013).

In addition to the preceding conditions, special contact precautions are used for vancomycin-resistant enterococci (VRE) infections.

The CDC recommends use of an antimicrobial soap for hand hygiene and no sharing of equipment among clients with and without VRE. The client should have a private room (or a room with other clients who have VRE), and such isolation should continue until at least three cultures taken 1 week apart are negative (Siegel et al., 2007).

Some diseases require a combination of transmission-based precautions. For clients infected with the coronavirus that causes severe acute respiratory syndrome (SARS-CoV), standard (including eye protection), contact, and airborne precautions are indicated (Siegel et al., 2007).

When certain conditions exist, transmission-based precautions are indicated until the presence or absence of the suspected agent has been confirmed. For example, for a generalized petechial rash with fever and a history of travel in an area known to have viral hemorrhagic fever, droplet and contact precautions are used until viruses such as Ebola or Lassa have been ruled out. In contrast, airborne precautions should be initiated if a maculopapular rash with fever, cough, and nasal congestion are present and rubeola has not been eliminated as a possible cause.

●○● NURSING PROCESS: CARING FOR CLIENTS WITH KNOWN OR SUSPECTED INFECTIONS

Implementing Transmission-Based Precautions

Assessment
If precautions have not already been ordered or specified, determine needed precautions based on the client's history and current signs and symptoms. Consult with appropriate infection prevention personnel as needed. In most cases, the strictest precautions indicated should always be used until a definitive diagnosis has been made.

Planning
Notify all agency departments as specified by policy. These may include placing biohazard or isolation labels on equipment, rooms, or charts and notifying the dietary, housekeeping, laboratory, and other relevant departments of the precautions being implemented.

Explain to the client and the client's family the necessity of precautions. Keep in mind the feelings of strangeness, alienation, or even shame that clients may experience as they look at masked faces and only receive touch from gloved hands. Using the skill of therapeutic presence will convey compassion as nursing care is provided under these circumstances.

DELEGATION
Care of clients requiring transmission-based precautions may be delegated to UAP. However, the nurse is responsible for ensuring that all personnel are aware of the specific isolation procedures required for the individual client and can implement them.

INTERPROFESSIONAL PRACTICE
Transmission-based precautions are required for all health care providers. All providers should be comfortable pointing out to each other when any break in technique is detected.

Equipment
As indicated by the specific precautions:
- Clean gloves
- Isolation (water-resistant) gown
- Surgical or N95 (particulate) respirator mask
- Protective eyewear
- A private room or specialized isolation room that has an anteroom with control airflow where individuals can perform hand hygiene and apply and remove PPE
- Dedicated (preferably disposable) equipment such as blood pressure cuff, thermometer, and stethoscope

IMPLEMENTATION
Performance
1. Prior to performing the procedure, introduce self and verify the client's identity using agency protocol. Explain to the client what you are going to do, why it is necessary, and how he or she can participate. It is extremely important for clients and family members to understand the rationale for use of barriers to infection transmission. They must be given the opportunity to ask questions and express feelings. Hospitalized clients are already socially isolated from others, and the use of additional barriers can initiate negative feelings such as depression and withdrawal.

SKILL 7-3

Continued on page 222

Implementing Transmission-Based Precautions—*continued*

2. Use standard precautions (see Skill 1–1). Perform hand hygiene using soap and water if hands are visibly soiled. Otherwise, use alcohol-based hand rub.

3. Implement indicated precautions.
   - Place used disposable sharps (e.g., needles and syringes, scalpels, lancets) from all clients directly into designated sharps containers. Do not disassemble or recap sharps. **Rationale:** *Manipulating open sharps increases the chances of sustaining a puncture injury.*

Airborne Precautions
- Place the client in an airborne infection isolation room (AIIR). An AIIR is a private room that has negative air pressure, 6 to 12 air changes per hour, and either discharge of air to the outside or a filtration system for the room air. Keep the room door closed.
- If a private room is not available, place the client with another client who is infected with the same organism.
- Wear an N95 respirator mask when entering the room. Steps for applying and removing N95 masks are shown in the Practice Guidelines on page 224.
- Susceptible individuals should not enter the room of a client who has rubeola (measles) or varicella (chickenpox). If they must enter, they should wear a respirator mask.
- Limit movement of the client outside the room to essential purposes. Place a surgical mask on the client while outside the room.

Droplet Precautions
- Place the client in a private room.
- If a private room is not available, place the client with another client who is infected with the same organism.
- Wear a mask when entering the room if you will be working within 1 m (3 ft) of the client.
- Limit movement of the client outside the room to essential purposes. Place a surgical mask on the client while outside the room.

Contact Precautions
- Place the client in a private room.
- If a private room is not available, place the client with another client who is infected with the same organism.
- Perform hand hygiene. Use soap and water for clients with *C. difficile* or *Bacillus anthracis* because alcohol and other cleansing agents are not effective against spores (Siegel et al., 2007).
- Apply clean gloves. Remove gloves and perform hand hygiene after contact with infectious material. Apply a new set of clean gloves as indicated.
- Wear a gown (see standard precautions) when entering a room if there will be any client contact or contact with potentially contaminated areas.
- Bag contaminated articles.
  a. Identify and separate items that are disposable from those that are reusable.
  b. Place garbage and disposable items such as dressings or single-use equipment in the plastic bags that line

the wastebasket and tie the bag. If the bag is sturdy and impermeable to microorganisms (waterproof or solid enough to prevent organisms from moving through it even when wet), a single bag is adequate. If not, place the first bag inside another impermeable bag. Some agencies have a particular location where such garbage is to be placed, and some use bags of a particular color (e.g., red) to indicate potentially infective waste.

   c. Place contaminated reusable items in an impermeable bag and send to the proper area for decontamination. In some agencies, glass and metal are separated from plastic and rubber equipment because they require different methods of decontamination.

   d. Always holding linen away from the uniform, place soiled linen directly in the linen hamper bag. Close the bag and send to the laundry as specified by policy. In some agencies, a bag that dissolves in hot water (melt-away) is used as the first bag and then the entire bundle is placed in a cloth or plastic bag. **Rationale:** *In this way, laundry workers need never actually touch soiled linens. In other agencies, all contaminated linen is double-bagged.*

   e. Specimens to be sent to the laboratory must be placed in an impermeable labeled container with a secure lid. If the outside of the container is contaminated, place the container in a sealable plastic bag. In some agencies, all specimen containers are placed in a sealed plastic bag.

   f. Food dishes and silverware require no special handling. Some agencies use disposable dishes for convenience.

- Remove PPE at the doorway before leaving the room or in the anteroom, in the proper sequence, and dispose of it properly. Perform hand hygiene.
  a. Remove gloves without touching hands to the outside of the gloves.
  b. Remove goggles or face shield.
  c. Remove gown without touching hands to the outside of the gown.
  d. Make sure the uniform does not contact possible contaminated surfaces.
  e. Remove the mask, grasping only the ties or elastic.
  f. Cleanse hands immediately.

- Variations may be required for care of clients with multidrug-resistant organisms (MDROs). For example, in some cases, cohorting (grouping) of clients with the same MDRO onto a single nursing unit may decrease transmission (Siegel et al., 2007).

4. Document observance of infection prevention procedures in the client record using forms or checklists supplemented by narrative notes when appropriate.

EVALUATION
Report any concerns regarding breaks in isolation technique to the appropriate persons (often the infection prevention nurse). An infection prevention committee monitors unusual occurrences of infections.

CHILDREN

Infections are an expected part of childhood. The majority of these infections are caused by viruses. In some cases, severe, even life-threatening infections occur. Considerations related to children include the following:

- Newborns may not be able to respond to infections due to an underdeveloped immune system. As a result, in the first few months of life, infections may not be associated with typical signs and symptoms (e.g., an infant with an infection may not have a fever).
- Newborns are born with some naturally acquired immunity transferred from the mother across the placenta.
- Breast-fed infants enjoy higher levels of immunity against infections than formula-fed infants.
- Children who are immune compromised (e.g., leukemia, HIV) or have a chronic health condition (e.g., cystic fibrosis, sickle cell disease, congenital heart disease) need extra precautions to prevent exposure to infectious agents.

OLDER ADULTS

Normal aging may predispose older adults to increased risk of infection and delayed healing. Anatomic and physiological agents that are protective when a person is younger often change in structure and function with increasing age and then provide a decrease in their protective ability. Changes take place in the skin, respiratory tract, gastrointestinal system, kidneys, and immune system. Special considerations for older adults include the following:

- Nutrition may be poor in older adults. Certain components, especially adequate protein, are necessary to build up and maintain the immune system.
- Diabetes mellitus, which occurs more frequently in older adults, increases the risk of infection and delayed healing by causing an alteration in nutrition and impaired peripheral circulation, which decrease the oxygen transport to the tissues.
- The normal inflammatory response is delayed. This often causes atypical responses to infections with unusual presentations. Instead of displaying the redness, swelling, and fever usually associated with infections, atypical symptoms such as confusion and disorientation, agitation, incontinence, falls, lethargy, and general fatigue are often seen first.

Recognizing these changes in older adults is important in the early detection and treatment of the related potential for infections and delayed healing. Nursing interventions to promote prevention include the following:

- Provide and teach ways to improve nutritional status.
- Use strict aseptic technique (especially in health care facilities).
- Encourage older adults to have regular immunizations for flu and pneumonia.
- Be alert to subtle atypical signs of infection and act quickly to diagnose and treat.

Infection Prevention

Describe ways to manipulate the bed, the room, and other household facilities to prevent injury or to contain possible cross contamination.

- Instruct to clean obviously soiled linen separately from other laundry. Wash in hot water if possible, adding a cup of bleach or phenol-based disinfectant such as Lysol concentrate to the wash, and rinse in cold water.
- Based on assessment of client and family knowledge, teach proper hand hygiene (e.g., before handling foods, before eating, after toileting, before and after any required home care treatment, and after touching any body substances such as wound drainage) and related hygienic measures to all family members.
- Promote nail care. Keep fingernails short, clean, and well manicured to eliminate rough edges or hangnails, which can harbor microorganisms.
- Instruct not to share personal care items such as toothbrushes or used washcloths and towels. Describe how infections can be transmitted from shared personal items.
- Discuss antimicrobial soaps and effective disinfectants.
- Discuss the relationship between hygiene, rest, activity, and nutrition in the chain of infection.
- Instruct about cleaning reusable equipment and supplies. Use soap and water, and disinfect with a chlorine bleach solution.
- Teach the client and family members the signs and symptoms of infection, and when to contact a health care provider. Determine by verbal questions the level of understanding of the topic after each teaching session.
- Teach the client and family members how to avoid infections.
- Suggest techniques for safe food preservation and preparation (e.g., wash raw fruits and vegetables before eating them, refrigerate all opened and unpackaged foods).
- Remind to avoid coughing, sneezing, or breathing directly on others. Cover the mouth and nose to prevent the transmission of airborne microorganisms.
- Inform of the importance of maintaining sufficient fluid intake to promote urine production and output. This helps flush the bladder and urethra of microorganisms.
- Emphasize the need for proper immunizations of all family members.

PRACTICE GUIDELINES

Using an N95 Respirator Mask

- Before handling the respirator, wash hands thoroughly with soap and water.
- If you have used a respirator before that fit you, you should use the same make, model, and size.
- Inspect the respirator for damages. If your respirator has been damaged, DO NOT USE IT. Get a new one.
- Anything that comes between the respirator and your face will make the respirator less effective. Do not allow facial hair, hair, jewelry, glasses, or clothing to come between your face and the respirator, or interfere with the placement of the respirator on the face.

If respirators are used for people performing work-related duties, employers must comply with the Occupational Safety and Health Administration's Respiratory Protection Standard, 29 CFR 1910.134. Consult www.OSHA.gov for more information.

Application

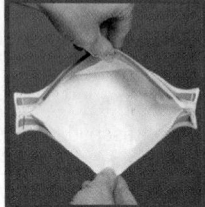

1 Remove the respirator from its packaging and hold with straps facing upward. Place the bottom strap under the center flaps next to the "ATTENTION" statement.

2 Fully open the top and bottom panels, bending the nosepiece around your thumb at center of the foam. Straps should separate when panels are opened. Make certain the bottom panel is unfolded and completely opened.

3 Place the respirator on your face so that the foam rests on your nose and the bottom panel is securely under your chin.

4 Pull the top strap over your head and position it high on the back of the head. Then, pull the bottom strap over your head and position it around your neck and below your ears.

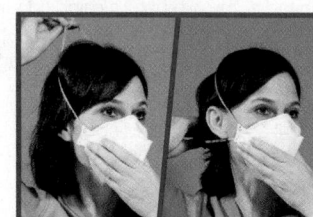

5 Adjust for a comfortable fit by pulling the top panel toward the bridge of your nose and the bottom panel under your chin.

Make certain hair, facial hair, jewelry and clothing are not between your face and the respirator as they will interfere with fit.

6 Place your fingertips from both hands at the top of the metal nosepiece. Using two hands, mold the nose area to the shape of your nose by pushing inward while moving your fingertips down both sides of the nosepiece.

Note: Always use two hands when molding the nosepiece. Pinching the nosepiece with one hand may result in improper fit and less effective respirator performance.

7 Place one or both hands completely over the middle panel. Inhale and exhale sharply. Be careful not to disturb the position of the respirator. If air leaks around your nose, re-adjust the nosepiece as described in Step 6. If air leaks around respirator edges, adjust panels and position of straps and make certain respirator edges fit snugly against the face. **If you cannot achieve a proper seal, do not enter the contaminated area. See your supervisor.**

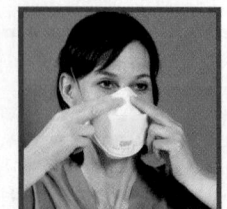

Perform a User Seal Check
Check the seal of your respirator each time you use the respirator.

Removal
Can be performed using one or both hands

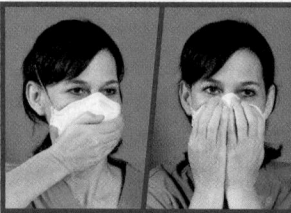

One hand　Two hand　One hand　Two hand

1 Without touching the respirator facepiece, slowly lift the bottom strap from around your neck up over your head.

2 Lift off the top strap. Do not touch the respirator.

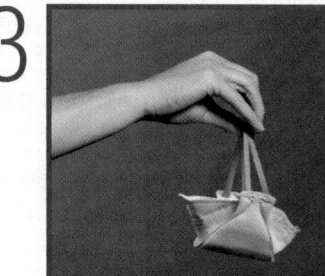

3 Store or discard according to your facility's infection control policy.

| **PATIENT-CENTERED CARE** |

- Assist with injury-proofing the home to prevent the possibility of tissue injury (e.g., use of padding, handrails, removal of hazards).
- Explore ways to control the environmental temperature and airflow (especially if the client has an airborne pathogen).

- Determine the advisability of visitors and family members in proximity to an infected client.
- Ensure access to and proper use of hand-cleansing supplies, gloves, and other barriers as indicated by the type of infection or risk.

Chapter 7 Review

FOCUSING ON CLINICAL THINKING

Consider This
- While the nurse is dropping commercially packaged sterile gauze onto an already established sterile field, the gauze lands with one corner almost off the edge of the field. Does this present any concerns regarding its sterility? If so, how would you handle the situation?
- After establishing a sterile field and applying sterile gloves, you realize that you have forgotten to open the bottle of saline that needs to be poured into a bowl on the field. The bottle is not sterile on the outside. What are two ways you could solve this dilemma?

- A client is being admitted to the hospital with a diagnosis of severe diarrhea, unknown origin. What infection prevention precautions would be appropriate at this time?
- You are assigned to care for a client who has a disseminated herpes zoster infection (shingles). In reviewing the agency infection prevention manual, you learn that individuals who have not had chickenpox should not enter this client's room. Individuals who have had chickenpox or a blood titer indicating immunity to chickenpox may interact with the client. Explain why this is the case.

See Focusing on Clinical Thinking answers on student resource website.

TEST YOUR KNOWLEDGE

1. The nurse knows that any substance can serve as an intermediate means to transport and introduce an infectious agent into a susceptible host through a suitable portal of entry. Which term best describes this type of transmission?
   1. Direct transmission
   2. Vehicle-borne transmission
   3. Airborne transmission
   4. Vector-borne transmission

2. Which statement, if made by a nurse, indicates the need for further teaching about the six links in the chain of infection?
   1. "The goal of infection prevention measures is to break the chain whenever and wherever possible so that disease is not transmitted from one person to another."
   2. "Direct transmission can occur through touching, biting, kissing, or sexual intercourse."
   3. "Airborne transmission may involve droplets or dust."
   4. "Direct transmission can be either vehicle-borne or vector-borne."

3. A nurse is preparing to establish a sterile field. Which technique, if done by the nurse, could compromise the maintenance of the sterile field?
   1. Use of a package that has condensation in it
   2. Placement of the package so that the top flap of the wrapper opens away from the nurse
   3. Dropping sterile items on the field so that they land more than 2.5 cm (1 in.) from the border of the field
   4. Reaching around rather than over the field

4. Which technique of applying sterile gloves indicates a good understanding of this technique? Select all that apply.
   1. Place the package of gloves on a clean, dry surface.
   2. Open the outer package without contaminating the gloves or the inner package.
   3. Put the first glove on the nondominant hand.
   4. Pick up the other glove with the sterile gloved hand, inserting the gloved fingers under the cuff and holding the gloved thumb close to the gloved palm.
   5. Once both gloves are on, unroll any portion of the cuff that had been caught during application.

5. A nurse is caring for a client with tuberculosis. The transmission-based precautions used are in addition to standard precautions. Which of the following would the nurse use and be consistent with infection prevention guidelines? Select all that apply.
   1. A surgical mask at all times while in the client's room
   2. An N95 respirator mask when within 1 m (3 ft) of the client
   3. Gloves for all contact with the client
   4. Hand hygiene before applying and after removing gloves
   5. A gown when performing a physical examination of the client

6. A nurse is assigned to care for a client on contact precautions. Which action by the nurse would require immediate intervention on the part of the supervisor?
   1. The nurse changes gloves after contact with infectious material.
   2. The nurse places used disposable sharps directly into designated sharps containers.
   3. The nurse removes the used gown outside the client's room.
   4. The nurse sends a specimen to the laboratory in a plastic container with a secure lid, and in a plastic bag.

7. In delegating to unlicensed assistive personnel, which task would need to be completed only by the registered nurse?
   1. Caring for a client on standard precautions
   2. Collecting a urine specimen from a client who is infectious
   3. Performing a sterile procedure on a client on contact precautions
   4. Caring for a client on airborne precautions

8. The nurse caring for a client on droplet precautions is preparing to document care of that client. Which aspects of care should the nurse document in the narrative notes?
   1. Characteristics of a productive cough
   2. Which aspects of care were delegated to UAP
   3. Treatments provided by the respiratory therapist
   4. Oral and skin hygiene

9. A client is HIV positive, taking antiviral medications as ordered, and has no HIV-related problems. The client is being admitted for an appendectomy. What type of precautions would be required when caring for this client?
   1. Droplet precautions
   2. Contact precautions
   3. Airborne precautions
   4. Standard precautions

10. The nurse is caring for several clients requiring transmission-based precautions. Which of the following skills could the nurse safely delegate to the unlicensed assistive personnel? Select all that apply.
    1. Explaining isolation requirements to a client in airborne isolation
    2. Teaching the parents of a child in isolation how to follow the necessary precautions
    3. Obtaining vital signs from a client in airborne isolation
    4. Transporting a client requiring standard precautions to radiology
    5. Instructing a client who has been on airborne precautions for discharge

See Answers to Test Your Knowledge in Appendix A.

READINGS AND REFERENCES

References

Dellinger, R. P., Levy, M. M., Rhodes, A., Annane, D., Gerlach, H., Opal, S. M., . . . Surviving Sepsis Campaign Guidelines Committee including the Pediatric Subgroup. (2013). Surviving Sepsis Campaign: International guidelines for management of severe sepsis and septic shock: 2012. *Critical Care Medicine, 41*, 580–637. doi:10.1097//CCM.0b013e31827e83af

Jarvis, W. R., Jarvis, A. A., & Chinn, R. Y. (2012). National prevalence of methicillin-resistant *Staphylococcus aureus* in inpatients at United States health care facilities, 2010. *American Journal of Infection Control, 40*, 194–200. doi:10.1016/j.ajic.2012.02.001

The Joint Commission. (2013). *National Patient Safety Goals effective January 1, 2014. Hospital accreditation program.* Retrieved from http://www.jointcommission.org/assets/1/6/HAP_NPSG_Chapter_2014.pdf

MRSA Research Center. (2013). *What disease kills more Americans a year than AIDS?* Retrieved from http://mrsa-research-center.bsd.uchicago.edu/index.html

Siegel, J. D., Rhinehart, E., Jackson, M., Chiarello, L., & Healthcare Infection Control Practices Advisory Committee. (2007). *2007 guidelines for isolation precautions: Preventing transmission of infectious agents in healthcare settings.* Atlanta, GA: Centers for Disease Control and Prevention. Retrieved from http://www.cdc.gov/hicpac/pdf/isolation/Isolation2007.pdf

Selected Bibliography

Aitken, L., Williams, G., Harvey, M., Blot, S., Kleinpell, R., Labeau, S., . . . Ahrens, T. (2011). Nursing considerations to complement the Surviving Sepsis Campaign guidelines. *Critical Care Medicine, 39*, 1800–1818. doi:10.1097/CCM.0b013e31821867cc

Berman, A., Snyder, S., & Frandsen, G. (2016). *Kozier & Erb's fundamentals of nursing: Concepts, process, and practice* (10th ed.). Upper Saddle River, NJ: Pearson.

Casanova, L. M., Rutala, W. A., Weber, D. J., & Sobsey, M. D. (2012). Effect of single- versus double-gloving on virus transfer to health care workers' skin and clothing during removal of personal protective equipment. *American Journal of Infection Control, 40*, 369–374. doi:10.1016/j.ajic.2011.04.324

Centers for Disease Control and Prevention. (2010). *Self-study modules on tuberculosis.* Retrieved from http://www.cdc.gov/tb/publications/slidesets/selfstudymodules/default.htm

Fayerberg, E., Bouchard, J., & Kellie, S. M. (2013). Knowledge, attitudes and practice regarding *Clostridium difficile*: A survey of physicians in an academic medical center. *American Journal of Infection Control, 41*, 266–269. doi:10.1016/j.ajic.2012.03.013

Harding, A. D., Almquist, L. J., & Hashemi, S. (2011). The use and need for standard precautions and transmission-based precautions in the emergency department. *Journal of Emergency Nursing, 37*, 367–373. doi:10.1016/j.jen.2010.11.017

Miller, B. A., Chen, L. F., Sexton, D. J., & Anderson, D. J. (2010). *The impact of hospital-onset healthcare facility associated (HO-HCFA)* Clostridium difficile *infection (CDI) in community hospitals: Surpassing methicillin-resistant* Staphylococcus aureus *(MRSA) as the new superbug.* Abstract presented at the Fifth Decennial International Conference on Healthcare-Associated Infections. Retrieved from http://shea.confex.com/shea/2010/webprogram/Paper2801.html

Neo, F., Edward, K., & Mills, C. (2012). Current evidence regarding non-compliance with personal protective equipment: An integrative review to illuminate implications for nursing practice. *ACORN: Journal of Perioperative Nursing in Australia, 25*(4), 22–30.

Pastagia, M., Kleinman, L., Cruz, E., & Jenkins, S. (2012). Predicting risk for death from MRSA bacteremia. *Emerging Infectious Diseases, 18*, 1072–1080. doi:10.3201/eid1807.101371

Spence, M. R., & McQuaid, M. (2011). The interrelationship of isolation precautions and adverse events in an acute care facility. *American Journal of Infection Control, 39*, 154–155. doi:10.1016/j.ajic.2010.04.213

8 Heat and Cold Measures

LEARNING OUTCOMES

At the completion of this chapter, the student will be able to:

1. Define the key terms used in the skills of heat and cold measures.
2. Identify essential guidelines for applying heat and cold.
3. Identify indications and contraindications for heat and cold measures.
4. Recognize when it is appropriate to delegate application of heat and cold measures to unlicensed assistive personnel.
5. Verbalize the steps used in:
   a. Applying dry heat.
   b. Applying dry cold.
   c. Applying compresses and moist packs.
6. Demonstrate appropriate documentation and reporting of application of heat and cold measures.

SKILLS

Skill 8–1 Applying Dry Heat Measures: Hot Water Bottle, Electric Heating Pad, Aquathermia Pad, Disposable Hot Pack

Skill 8–2 Applying Dry Cold Measures: Ice Bag, Ice Collar, Ice Glove, Disposable Cold Pack

Skill 8–3 Applying Compresses and Moist Packs

KEY TERMS

aquathermia pad, 227
compress, 227

rebound phenomenon, 228

vasoconstriction, 227

vasodilation, 227

Heat and cold are applied to the body to promote comfort and the repair and healing of tissues. The form of thermal application depends on its purpose. Cold applied to a body part draws heat from the area; heat, of course, warms the area. Applying heat or cold produces physiological changes in the temperature of the tissues, size of the blood vessels, capillary blood pressure, capillary surface area for exchange of fluids and electrolytes, and tissue metabolism. The duration of the application also affects the response. See Table 8–1 for a summary of the physiological effects of heat and cold. These explain, for example, why cold is used on a recent musculoskeletal injury (e.g., 24 to 72 hours old) while heat is more appropriate for an injury that has passed its acute phase.

Heat and cold can be applied to the body in both dry and moist forms. Dry heat is applied locally by means of a hot water bottle, electric pad, **aquathermia pad** (an electric device that circulates warm water through a flat case), or disposable heat pack. Moist heat can be provided by a **compress** (a damp dressing applied with pressure), hot pack, soak, or bath. Heat causes **vasodilation** (an increase in the diameter of blood vessels), which allows more blood to reach an area. The increased blood flow simultaneously brings white blood cells and other healing elements to the site and removes waste products.

Dry cold is administered for local effect by an ice bag, ice collar, ice glove, or disposable cold pack. In addition, continuous cold therapy (cryotherapy) following joint surgery or injury can be delivered by a cooling unit similar to the aquathermia pad (Su et al., 2012). Moist cold can be provided by a compress or a cooling sponge bath.

Cold is often applied to the body to decrease bleeding or inflammation by constricting blood vessels (**vasoconstriction**) and to decrease pain by slowing nerve conduction rate, producing numbness, and acting as a counterirritant. Selected indications for the use of heat and cold are found in Table 8–2.

GUIDELINES FOR APPLYING HEAT AND COLD

An understanding of the adaptive response of thermal receptors, the rebound phenomenon, systemic effects, tolerance to heat and cold, contraindications, and the mind-body connection is essential when administering hot and cold applications.

Adaptation of Thermal Receptors

Temperature (thermal) receptors in body tissues adapt to temperature changes. When a cold receptor is subjected to an abrupt fall in temperature or when a heat receptor is subjected to an abrupt rise in temperature, the receptor is strongly stimulated initially. This strong stimulation declines rapidly during the first few seconds and then more slowly during the next half hour or more as the receptor adapts to the new temperature.

Nurses and clients need to understand this adaptive response when applying heat and cold. Clients may be tempted to modify the temperature of a thermal application because of the change in sensation following adaptation. Increasing the temperature of a hot application after adaptation has occurred can cause serious burns.

TABLE 8–1	Physiological Effects of Heat and Cold

Heat	Cold
Vasodilation	Vasoconstriction
Increases capillary permeability	Decreases capillary permeability
Increases cellular metabolism	Decreases cellular metabolism
Increases inflammation	Slows bacterial growth, decreases inflammation
Sedative effect	Local anesthetic effect

TABLE 8–3	Temperatures for Hot and Cold Applications

Description	Temperature	Application
Very cold	Below 15°C (59°F)	Ice bags
Cold	15°C–18°C (59°F–65°F)	Cold pack
Cool	18°C–27°C (65°F–80°F)	Cold compresses
Tepid	27°C–37°C (80°F–98°F)	Alcohol sponge bath
Warm	37°C–40°C (98°F–104°F)	Warm bath, aquathermia pads
Hot	40°C–46°C (104°F–115°F)	Hot soak, irrigations, hot compresses*
Very hot	Above 46°C (above 115°F)	Hot water bags for adults*

Note: The temperature of the water used to create the hot soak or compress, or to fill a hot water bottle exceeds the surface temperature of 43°C (110°F) that is safe to apply to skin.

Decreasing the temperature of a cold application can cause pain and serious impairment of circulation to the body part. See Table 8–3 for recommended temperatures of hot and cold applications.

Rebound Phenomenon

The **rebound phenomenon** occurs at the time the maximum therapeutic effect of the hot or cold application is achieved and the opposite effect begins. For example, heat produces maximum vasodilation in 20 to 30 minutes; continuation of the application beyond 30 minutes brings tissue congestion, and the blood vessels then *constrict*. If the heat application is continued further, the client is at risk for burns, because the constricted blood vessels cannot dissipate the heat adequately via the blood circulation.

With cold applications, maximum vasoconstriction occurs when the involved skin reaches a temperature of 15°C (60°F). The ruddiness of the skin of a person who has been walking in cold weather is caused by oxygenated red blood cells trapped in the skin when vasoconstriction occurs. Below 15°C, vasodilation begins. This

mechanism is protective: It helps to prevent freezing of body tissues normally exposed to cold, such as the nose and ears. Continued cold causes alternating vasodilation and vasoconstriction (called the Lewis Hunting effect).

Systemic Effects

Heat applied to a localized body area, particularly a large body area, may decrease cardiac output and pulmonary ventilation. These increases result from excessive peripheral vasodilation, which diverts large supplies of blood from the internal organs and produces a drop in blood pressure. A significant drop in blood pressure can cause fainting. Clients who have cardiac or pulmonary disease and who have circulatory disturbances such as arteriosclerosis are more prone to this effect than healthy individuals.

TABLE 8–2	Selected Indications for the Use of Heat and Cold

Indication	Effect of Heat	Effect of Cold
Muscle spasm	Relaxes muscles and increases their contractility.	Relaxes muscles and decreases muscle contractility.
Inflammation	Increases blood flow, softens exudates.	Vasoconstriction decreases capillary permeability, decreases blood flow, slows cellular metabolism.
Pain	Relieves pain, possibly by promoting muscle relaxation, increasing circulation, and promoting psychological relaxation and a feeling of comfort; acts as a counterirritant.	Decreases pain by slowing nerve conduction rate and blocking nerve impulses; produces numbness, acts as a counterirritant, increases pain threshold.
Joint contracture	Reduces contracture and increases joint range of motion by allowing greater distention of muscles and connective tissue.	
Joint stiffness	Reduces joint stiffness by decreasing viscosity of synovial fluid and increasing tissue distensibility.	
Traumatic injury		Decreases bleeding by constricting blood vessels; decreases edema by reducing capillary permeability.

Evidence-Based Practice Rebound Phenomenon

EVIDENCE-BASED PRACTICE

An understanding of the rebound phenomenon is essential for the nurse and client. Thermal applications must be halted *before* the rebound phenomenon begins.

Evidence-Based Practice Shivering   **EVIDENCE-BASED PRACTICE**

If the nurse's interventions to reduce a fever cause the client to shiver, the client's temperature will actually rise instead of fall. Shivering also increases oxygen consumption. Various medications and alternative cooling methods can be used to reduce shivering if rapid temperature reduction is critical (Gessner, Dugan, & Janusek, 2012).

With extensive cold applications (such as when a client is placed on a cooling blanket) and vasoconstriction, a client's blood pressure can increase, because blood is shunted from the cutaneous circulation to the internal blood vessels. This shunting of blood, a normal protective response to prolonged cold, is the body's attempt to maintain its core temperature. Shivering, another generalized effect of prolonged cold, is a normal response as the body attempts to warm itself.

Tolerance and Contraindications

Various parts of the body have different tolerances to heat and cold. The physiological tolerance of individuals also varies (Box 8–1).

Specific conditions contraindicate the use of hot or cold applications. In addition, certain conditions call for precautions when administering heat and cold therapy (Box 8–2).

The Mind–Body Connection

Thermal interventions afford nurses opportunities to help clients tap into the mind–body connection to amplify healing effects. Thoughts change physiological function, and physiological processes affect our mental function. For example, by using the power of imagination, clients can be guided to visualize their pain or injury as a particular color. Then, they can imagine the color of the area or tissue if it were healed or pain free. During the hot or cold application, they can imagine that the thermal intervention is causing color change in the affected area in the direction of healing. These kinds of exercises are powerful because of the effectiveness of imagery on physiological function. In addition, using them can increase clients' feelings of control as they learn to use their own mind–body potential to help themselves.

BOX 8–1 Variables Affecting Physiological Tolerance to Heat and Cold

- *Body part.* The back of the hand and foot are not very temperature sensitive. In contrast, the inner aspect of the wrist and forearm, the neck, and the perineal area are temperature sensitive.
- *Size of the exposed body part.* The larger the area exposed to heat and cold, the lower the tolerance.
- *Individual tolerance.* The very young and the very old generally have the lowest tolerance. Individuals who have neurosensory impairments may have a high tolerance, but the risk of injury is greater.
- *Length of exposure.* People feel hot and cold applications most while the temperature is changing. After a period of time, tolerance increases.
- *Intactness of skin.* Injured skin areas are more sensitive to temperature variations.

BOX 8–2 Contraindications to the Use of Heat and Cold Therapies

Determine the presence of any conditions indicating the need for special precautions during heat and cold therapy:

- *Neurosensory impairment.* Individuals with sensory impairments are unable to perceive that heat is damaging the tissues and are at risk for burns, or they are unable to perceive discomfort from cold and cannot prevent tissue injury.
- *Impaired mental status.* Individuals who are confused or have an altered level of consciousness need monitoring and supervision during applications to ensure safe therapy.
- *Impaired circulation.* Individuals with peripheral vascular disease, diabetes, or congestive heart failure lack the normal ability to dissipate heat via the blood circulation, which puts them at risk for tissue damage with heat applications. Cold applications are contraindicated for these individuals.
- *Open wounds.* Tissues around an open wound are more sensitive to heat and cold.

Determine the presence of any conditions contraindicating the use of heat:

- *First 24 hours after traumatic injury.* Heat increases bleeding and swelling.
- *Active hemorrhage.* Heat causes vasodilation and increases bleeding.
- *Noninflammatory edema.* Heat increases capillary permeability and edema.
- *Skin disorder that causes redness or blisters.* Heat can burn or cause further damage to the skin.

Determine the presence of any conditions contraindicating the use of cold:

- *Open wounds.* Cold can increase tissue damage by decreasing blood flow to an open wound.
- *Impaired circulation.* Cold can further impair nourishment of the tissues and cause tissue damage. In clients with Raynaud's disease, cold increases arterial spasm.
- *Allergy or hypersensitivity to cold.* Some clients have an allergy to cold that may be manifested by an inflammatory response, for example, erythema, hives, swelling, joint pain, and occasional muscle spasm. Some react with a sudden increase in blood pressure, which can be hazardous if the person is hypertensive.

SKILL 8–1

●○● NURSING PROCESS: APPLYING HEAT OR COLD

Applying Dry Heat Measures: Hot Water Bottle, Electric Heating Pad, Aquathermia Pad, Disposable Hot Pack

ASSESSMENT
Assess:
- The capacity of the client to recognize when the heat is injurious. **Rationale:** *This establishes whether the client is aware of heat and can discern a temperature that is too hot for the tissues.*
- The client's general physical condition. **Rationale:** *Clients who are very young, very old, or debilitated do not tolerate heat well.*
- The area to be treated for:
  - Alterations in skin integrity, such as the presence of edema, bruises, redness, open lesions, discharge, and bleeding.

- Circulatory status (color, temperature, and sensation). **Rationale:** *Tissues that feel cold, have a pale or bluish hue, and lack sensation or feel numb indicate circulatory impairment.*
- Level of discomfort and range of motion if muscle spasm or pain is being treated.
- Pulse, respirations, and blood pressure. **Rationale:** *Assessing these factors is particularly important before heat is applied to large areas of the body.* See Table 8–1 and Box 8–2 for the effects of heat on vital signs.

PLANNING
Before applying heat, determine:
- Type of heat to be used, the temperature, and the duration and frequency of the application (check the order if necessary).
- Agency protocol about the type of equipment used to deliver the heat, the temperature recommended, and the length of applications.
- At what time the heat treatment should be applied.

DELEGATION

Application of certain heat measures (e.g., baths) may be delegated to unlicensed assistive personnel (UAP) if they meet the general criteria for delegation (see Chapter 1∞). However, in all cases, assessment of the client and the determination that the measure is safe to employ are the responsibility of the nurse. UAP may observe the area being treated during usual care and must report abnormal findings to the nurse. Abnormal findings must be validated and interpreted by the nurse.

INTERPROFESSIONAL PRACTICE

Applying heat may be within the scope of practice for several health care providers. For example, in addition to nurses, both physical therapists and occupational therapists use thermal modalities. Although the therapists may verbally communicate their findings and plan to the health care team members, the nurse must also know where to locate their documentation in the client's medical record.

Equipment
Hot Water Bottle (Bag)
- Hot water bottle with a stopper
- Cover
- Hot water and a thermometer

Electric Heating Pad
- Electric pad and control
- Cover (waterproof if there will be moisture under the pad when it is applied)
- Gauze ties (optional)

Aquathermia Pad
- Pad
- Distilled water
- Control unit
- Cover
- Gauze ties or tape (optional)

Disposable Hot Pack
- One or two commercially prepared disposable hot packs

IMPLEMENTATION
Preparation
Test all equipment for proper functioning and integrity (lack of leaks) before taking it to the client.

Performance
1. Prior to performing the procedure, introduce self and verify the client's identity using agency protocol. Explain to the client what you are going to do, why it is necessary, and how he or she can participate. Discuss how the results will be used in planning further care or treatments.
2. Perform hand hygiene and observe other appropriate infection prevention procedures.
3. Provide for client privacy.
   - Expose only the area to be treated.
4. Apply the heat.

Variation: Hot Water Bottle (Most commonly used in the home setting)
- Measure the temperature of the water. Follow agency practice for the appropriate temperature. The following temperatures are commonly used:
  a. 46°C to 52°C (115°F to 125°F) for a healthy adult

  b. 40°C to 46°C (104°F to 115°F) for a debilitated or unconscious adult.
- Fill the hot water bottle about two-thirds full.
- Expel the air from the bottle. **Rationale:** *Air remaining in the bottle prevents it from molding to the body part being treated.*
- Secure the stopper tightly.
- Hold the bottle upside down, and check for leaks.
- Dry the bottle.
- Wrap the bottle in a towel or hot water bottle cover. ❶
- Apply the bottle to the body part using pillows to support it if necessary.

Variation: Electric Heating Pad (Most commonly used in the home setting)
- Ensure that the body area is dry. **Rationale:** *Electricity in the presence of moisture can conduct a shock.*
- Check that the electric pad is functioning properly. The cord should be free from cracks, wires should be intact, heating components should not be exposed, and temperature distribution over the pad should be even.
- Place the cover on the pad. Some models have waterproof covers to be used when the pad is placed over a moist dressing.

Applying Dry Heat Measures—*continued*

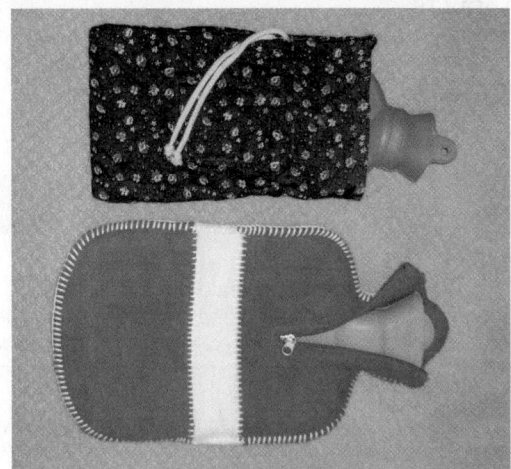

❶ Hot water bottles with cloth covers.

Rationale: *Moisture could cause the pad to short-circuit and burn or shock the client.*
- Plug the pad into the electric socket.
- Set the control dial for the correct temperature.
- After the pad has heated, place the pad over the body part to which heat is being applied.
- Use gauze ties instead of safety pins to hold the pad in place, if needed. **Rationale:** *A pin might strike a wire, damaging the pad and giving an electric shock to the client.*

Variation: Aquathermia Pad (Also called a K-Pad) ❷
- Fill the unit with water as specified by the manufacturer. The unit will warm the water, which circulates through the pad.
- Secure the lid.
- Regulate the temperature if it has not been preset. Normal temperature is 40°C to 46°C (104°F to 115°F). Check the manufacturer's instructions.
- Cover the pad with a towel or pillowcase.

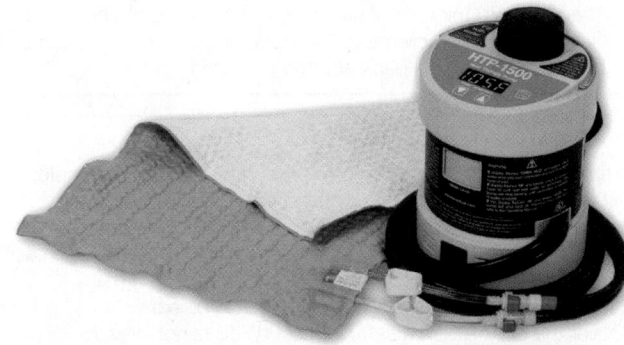

❷ An aquathermia heating unit and pad.
Courtesy Adroit Medical Systems, Inc

❸ Commercially prepared disposable hot packs.

- Plug in the unit.
- Check for any leak or malfunctions of the pad before use.
- Use tape or gauze ties to hold the pad in place. Never use safety pins. They can cause leakage.
- If unusual redness or pain occurs, discontinue the treatment, and report the client's reaction.

Variation: Disposable Hot Pack ❸
- Microwave, strike, squeeze, or knead the pack according to the manufacturer's directions.
- Note the manufacturer's instructions about the length of time that heat is produced.
- Depending on the type of pack, wrap in a towel or enclose in a cover prior to application.

5. Give the client the following instructions for all types of dry heat:
   - Do not insert any sharp, pointed object (e.g., a pin) into the bottle, pack, or pad.
   - Do not lie directly on the bottle or pad. **Rationale:** *The surface below the object promotes heat absorption instead of normal heat dissipation.*
   - To prevent injury, avoid adjusting the heat higher than specified. **Rationale:** *The degree of heat felt shortly after application will decrease, because the body's temperature receptors quickly adapt to the temperature. This adaptive mechanism can lead to tissue injury if the temperature is adjusted higher.*
   - Call the nurse if any discomfort is felt.
6. Leave the heat in place for only the designated time to avoid the rebound phenomenon, usually 30 minutes. Check the application and skin area after 5 to 10 minutes to be sure the skin is intact.
7. Document the application of the heat and the client's response in the client record, using forms or checklists supplemented by narrative notes when appropriate.

EVALUATION
- Perform a follow-up examination of the client to determine the effectiveness of the heat therapy and assess for any complications. Relate findings to previous assessment data if available.
- Report significant deviations from normal to the primary care provider.

INFANT/CHILD
- The temperature of water in a hot water bottle should be 40.5°C to 46°C (105°F to 115°F) for a child under 2 years of age.

OLDER ADULTS
- Use special care when assessing the area to be treated and when evaluating the effects of the treatment because older adults have many of the conditions predisposing to injury with heat measures.

Applying Dry Cold Measures: Ice Bag, Ice Collar, Ice Glove, Disposable Cold Pack

SKILL 8-2

ASSESSMENT
Assess:
- The capacity of the client to recognize when the cold is injurious. **Rationale:** *This establishes whether the client is aware of cold and can discern a temperature that is too cold for the tissues.*
- The client's general physical condition. **Rationale:** *Clients who are very young, very old, or debilitated do not tolerate cold well.*
- The area to be treated for:
  - Alterations in skin integrity, such as the presence of edema, bruises, redness, open lesions, discharge, and bleeding.

- Circulatory status (color, temperature, and sensation). **Rationale:** *Tissues that feel cold, have a pale or bluish hue, and lack sensation or feel numb indicate circulatory impairment.*
- Level of discomfort and range of motion if muscle spasm or pain is being treated.
- Pulse, respirations, and blood pressure. **Rationale:** *Assessing these factors is particularly important before cold is applied to large body areas.* See Table 8–1 and Box 8–2 for the effects of cold.

PLANNING
Before applying cold, determine:
- Type of cold to be used, the temperature, and the duration and frequency of the application (check the order if necessary).
- Agency protocol about the type of equipment used to deliver the cold, the temperature recommended, and the length of applications.
- At what time the treatment should be applied.

DELEGATION

Application of certain cold measures (e.g., cooling baths) may be delegated to UAP if they meet the general criteria for delegation (see Chapter 1 ∞). However, in all cases, assessment of the client and the determination that the measure is safe to employ are the responsibility of the nurse. UAP may observe the area being treated during usual care and must report abnormal findings to the nurse. Abnormal findings must be validated and interpreted by the nurse.

INTERPROFESSIONAL PRACTICE

Applying cold may be within the scope of practice for several health care providers. For example, in addition to nurses, both physical therapists and occupational therapists use thermal modalities. Although the therapists may verbally communicate their findings and plan to the health care team members, the nurse must also know where to locate their documentation in the client's medical record.

Equipment
- Ice bag, collar, glove, or cold pack
- Ice chips
- Protective covering
- Roller gauze, a binder or a towel, and tape

CLINICAL ALERT!

In the home, a bag of frozen peas or corn can substitute for an ice bag. After 15 to 20 minutes of use, they can be refrozen and reused as an ice bag. Caution clients not to cook and eat vegetables that have been used as an ice pack and then refrozen.

IMPLEMENTATION
Preparation
- Test all equipment for proper functioning and integrity (lack of leaks) before taking it to the client.

Performance
1. Prior to performing the procedure, introduce self and verify the client's identity using agency protocol. Explain to the client what you are going to do, why it is necessary, and how he or she can participate. Discuss how the results will be used in planning further care or treatments.
2. Perform hand hygiene and observe other appropriate infection prevention procedures.
3. Provide for client privacy.
   - Expose only the area to be treated, and provide warmth to avoid chilling.
4. Prepare the client.
   - Assist the client to a comfortable position, and support the body part requiring the application.
5. Apply the cold measure.

Variation: Ice Bag, Collar, or Glove ❶
- Fill the device one-half to two-thirds full of crushed ice. **Rationale:** *Partial filling makes the device more pliable so that it can be molded to a body part.*

- Remove excess air by bending or twisting the device. **Rationale:** *Air inflates the device so that it cannot be molded to the body part.*
- Insert the stopper securely into an ice bag or collar, or tie a knot at the open end of a glove. **Rationale:** *This prevents leakage of fluid when the ice melts.*
- Hold the device upside down, and check it for leaks.
- Cover the device with a soft cloth cover, if it is not already equipped with one. **Rationale:** *The cover absorbs moisture that condenses on the outside of the device. It is also more comfortable for the client.*
- Hold the device in place with roller gauze, ties, a binder, or a towel. Secure with tape as necessary.

Variation: Disposable Cold Pack ❷
- Strike, squeeze, or knead the cold pack according to the manufacturer's instructions. **Rationale:** *The action activates the chemical reaction that produces the cold.*
- Cover with a soft cloth cover if the pack does not have a cover. Most commercially prepared cold packs have soft outer coverings to permit application directly to the body part.

6. Instruct the client as follows for all types of dry cold:
   - Remain in position for the duration of the treatment.
   - Call the nurse if discomfort is felt.

SKILL 8-2

Applying Dry Cold Measures—*continued*

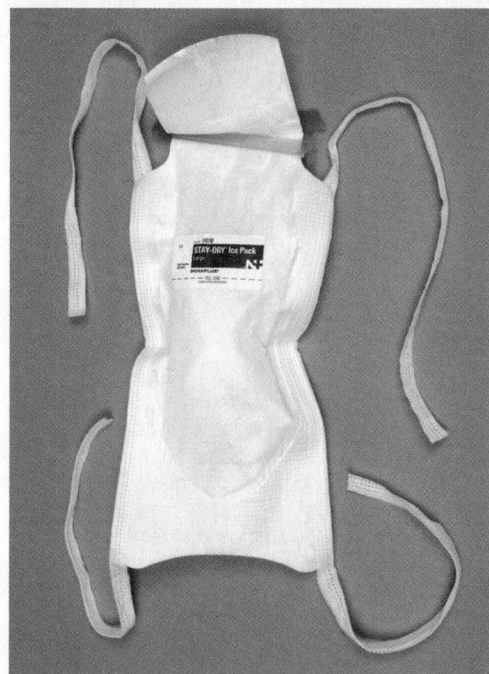

❶ Disposable ice bag.

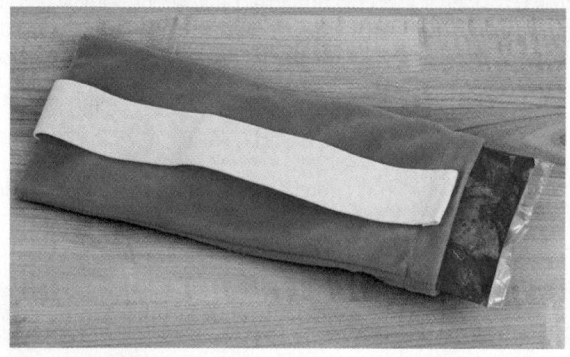

❷ A commercial chemical cold pack.
Sasimoto/Shutterstock.

7. Monitor the client during the application.
- Assess the client in terms of comfort and skin reaction (e.g., pallor, mottled appearance) as frequently as necessary for the client's safety (e.g., every 5 to 10 minutes). Check more often if the client has had previous negative responses to applications or if the client has difficulty reporting problems.
- Report untoward reactions and remove the application.

8. Leave the cold in place for only the designated time. **Rationale:** *Avoid the rebound phenomenon and the harmful effects of prolonged cold.*
9. Document the application of the cold and the client's response in the client record using forms or checklists supplemented by narrative notes when appropriate.

CLINICAL ALERT!

Ice packs used to reduce fever should be applied to the neck, groin, and axillae.

SAMPLE DOCUMENTATION

3/30/2015 2245 Rt foot and ankle remain swollen from toes to lower calf. Reports pain is 7/10. Full ROM of toes and ankle, pedal pulses present. Skin warm, no bruising or wounds noted. Padded ice pack applied × 10 minutes. Reports pain 5/10. ————— P. Wilder, RN

EVALUATION

- Perform a follow-up examination of the client to determine the effectiveness of the cold therapy and assess for any complications. Relate findings to previous assessment data if available.

- Report significant deviations from normal to the primary care provider.

Compresses and Moist Packs

Compresses and moist packs can be either warm or cold. A compress may be applied to a wound (see Chapter 31∞) or injury. When there is a break in the skin or when the body part (e.g., an eye) is vulnerable to microbial invasion, sterile technique is necessary; therefore, sterile gloves or sterile forceps are needed to apply the compress, and all materials (solution, container, thermometer, towels, gauze squares, and petroleum jelly) must be sterile (see Skills 7–1 and 7–2). When warm compresses are ordered, the solution is heated to the temperature indicated by the primary care provider, for example, 40.5°C (105°F).

A moist pack is a hot or cold moist cloth applied to an area of the body (Figure 8–1 ■). Moist packs are usually not sterile; after application, they are covered with a water-resistant material (e.g., plastic wrap) to contain the temperature and moisture and prevent the transfer of airborne microorganisms to the area.

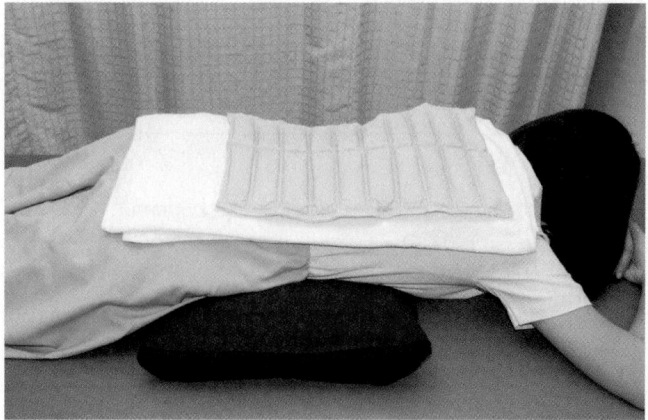

Figure 8–1 ■ A hot pack is often used to treat back pain.
123RF Images.

SKILL 8-3

Culturally Responsive Care   **Perspectives on Heat and Cold** | PATIENT-CENTERED CARE |

- The use of heat and cold therapies varies considerably across cultures. In many cultures, the mother who has just delivered a baby is offered warm or hot foods and kept warm with blankets because childbirth is seen as a "cold" condition.
- To reduce a person's fever, conventional scientific thought recommends cooling the body. The primary care provider may order cool liquids for the client to drink and cool compresses to be applied to the client's forehead, axillae, or groin. In contrast, many cultures believe that the best way to treat a fever is to increase elimination of toxins through sweat baths. Clients from these cultures may want to cover up with several blankets, take hot baths, and drink hot beverages.
- The nurse must consider cultural beliefs and preferences when planning and implementing heat and cold measures to ensure they are culturally acceptable.

Applying Compresses and Moist Packs

ASSESSMENT

Assess:

- The capacity of the client to recognize when the temperature of the compress or pack is injurious. **Rationale:** *This establishes whether the client is aware of potentially harmful temperature variations.*
- The client's level of consciousness and general physical condition.
- The area to be treated for:
  - Alterations in skin integrity, such as the presence of edema, bruises, redness, open lesions, discharge, and bleeding.
- Circulatory status (color, temperature, and sensation). **Rationale:** *Tissues that feel cold, have a pale or bluish hue, and lack sensation or feel numb indicate circulatory impairment.*
- Level of discomfort and range of motion if muscle spasm or pain is being treated.
- Pulse, respirations, and blood pressure. **Rationale:** *Assessing these factors is particularly important before heat or cold is applied to large body areas.* See Table 8–1 and Box 8–2 for the effects of heat and cold on vital signs.

PLANNING

Before applying, determine:

- The type of compress or pack to be used, the temperature, and the duration and frequency of the application (check the order if necessary).
- At what time the treatment should be applied.

DELEGATION

Application of unsterile compresses or packs may be delegated to UAP if they meet the general criteria for delegation (see Chapter 1 ∞). However, in all cases, assessment of the client and the determination that the measure is safe to employ are the responsibility of the nurse. UAP may observe the area being treated during usual care and must report abnormal findings to the nurse. Abnormal findings must be validated and interpreted by the nurse.

INTERPROFESSIONAL PRACTICE

Applying compresses and moist packs is within the scope of practice for several health care providers. For example, in addition to nurses, both physical therapists and occupational therapists may apply them. Although the therapists may verbally communicate their plan to the health care team members, the nurse must also know where to locate their documentation in the client's medical record.

Equipment

Use sterile equipment and supplies for an open wound.

Compress

- Clean gloves or sterile gloves (for an open wound)
- Container for the solution
- Solution at the strength and temperature specified by the primary care provider or the agency
- Gauze squares
- Cotton applicator sticks
- Petroleum jelly
- Insulating towel
- Plastic wrap
- Ties (e.g., roller gauze or masking tape)
- Hot water bottle or aquathermia pad (optional)
  or
- Ice bag (optional)
- Sterile dressing, if required

Moist Pack

- Clean gloves
- Flannel pieces or towel packs
- Hot-pack machine for heating the packs
  or
- Basin of water with some ice chips for cooling the packs
- Cotton applicator sticks
- Petroleum jelly
- Insulating material (e.g., flannel or towels)
- Plastic wrap
- Hot water bottle (optional)
  or
- Ice bag (optional)
- Sterile dressing, if required

IMPLEMENTATION

Preparation

If possible, perform care so that the application of the compress or pack will not need to be interrupted for other activities such as toileting.

Performance

1. Prior to performing the procedure, introduce self and verify the client's identity using agency protocol. Explain to the client what you are going to do, why it is necessary, and how he or she can participate. Discuss how the results will be used in planning further care or treatments.
2. Perform hand hygiene and observe other appropriate infection prevention procedures.
3. Provide for client privacy.
   - Expose only the area to be treated.

Applying Compresses and Moist Packs—*continued*

4. Prepare the client.
   - Assist the client to a comfortable position.
   - Expose the area for the compress or pack.
   - Provide support for the body part requiring the compress or pack.
   - If indicated, apply clean gloves, and remove the wound dressing. Remove and discard gloves.
   - Perform hand hygiene.
5. Moisten the compress or the pack.
   - Place the gauze in the solution.

   or

   - Heat the flannel or towel in a towel warmer cabinet or chill it in the basin of water and ice chips.
6. Protect the surrounding skin as indicated.
   - If a wound is exposed, apply petroleum jelly to the skin surrounding the wound, not on the wound or open areas of the skin, using a cotton applicator stick. **Rationale:** *Jelly protects the skin from possible burns, maceration, and the irritating effects of some solutions.*
7. Apply the moist compress or pack.
   - Wring out the gauze compress so that the solution does not drip from it. For a sterile compress, use sterile forceps or sterile gloves to wring out the gauze.
   - Apply the gauze lightly and gradually to the designated area and, if tolerated by the client, mold the compress close to the body. **Rationale:** *Air is a poor conductor of cold or heat, and molding excludes air.*

   or

   - Wring out the flannel (for a sterile pack, use sterile gloves).
   - Apply the flannel to the body area, molding it closely to the body part.
8. Immediately insulate and secure the application. ❶
   - Cover the gauze or flannel quickly with a dry towel and a piece of plastic wrap. **Rationale:** *This step helps maintain the temperature of the application and thus its effectiveness.*
   - Secure the compress or pack in place with gauze ties or tape.

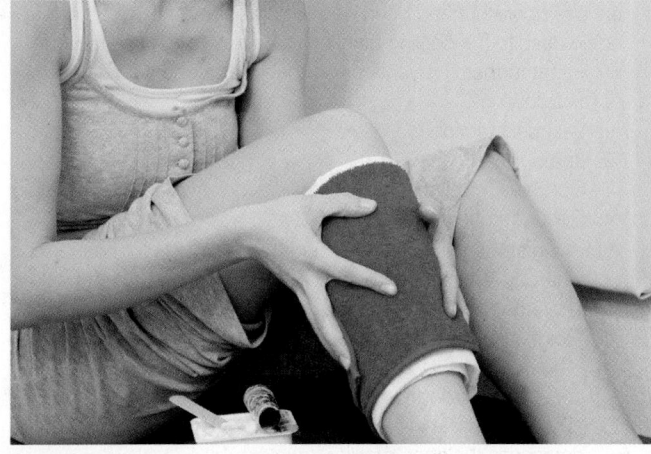

❶ A towel is wrapped around a cold compress.
Allesalltag/Alamy.

   - *Optional:* Apply a hot water bottle, aquathermia pad, or ice bag over the plastic wrap to maintain the heat or cold.
9. Monitor the client.
   - Assess the client for discomfort at 5- to 10-minute intervals. If the client feels any discomfort, assess the area for erythema, numbness, maceration, or blistering.
   - For applications to large areas of the body, note any change in the pulse, respirations, and blood pressure.
   - In the event of unexpected reactions, terminate the treatment and report to the nurse in charge.
10. Remove the compress or pack at the specified time.
    - Compresses and packs with an external heat or cold source on top may remain in place. Without external heat or cold, they need to be changed every few minutes.
    - Apply a sterile dressing if one is required.
11. Document the application of the compress or pack and the client's response in the client record using forms or checklists supplemented by narrative notes when appropriate.

EVALUATION

- Perform a follow-up examination of the client to determine the effectiveness of the therapy and assess for any complications. Relate findings to previous assessment data if available.

- Report significant deviations from expected to the primary care provider.

Chapter **8** Review

FOCUSING ON CLINICAL THINKING

Consider This

1. The client reports using a heating pad at home for low back pain. The client says it used to help but now, even on the highest setting, it doesn't feel very warm. What are three possible explanations for this experience?

2. Your friend has an injured ankle and asks you whether ice or heat should be applied. Based on your understanding of the effects of heat and cold on various tissues, how would you respond?

3. The primary care provider has ordered cooling baths for a client whose temperature is greater than 40°C (104°F). You observe the nursing assistant using cool tap water and rubbing the client's legs. The client is shivering. Which of these observations require you to intervene?

See Focusing on Clinical Thinking answers on student resource website.

TEST YOUR KNOWLEDGE

1. A client has been on a cooling blanket for some time. The client's temperature had been decreasing but it is now creeping up again despite the cooling blanket treatment. The nurse recognizes that further interventions are needed to counteract which of the following?
   1. Vasoconstriction
   2. Immobility
   3. Compression
   4. Rebound phenomenon

2. A nursing student is learning about the indications for heat and cold therapy. Which statement, if made by the nursing student, indicates the need for further teaching?
   1. "Joint stiffness is decreased by the application of heat."
   2. "The use of cold in traumatic injury decreases bleeding by constricting blood vessels."
   3. "The use of heat in muscle spasms relaxes muscles, but decreases their contractility."
   4. "Pain is decreased due to the slowed nerve conduction effect of cold."

3. A nurse is determining which tasks to delegate to unlicensed assistive personnel (UAP). Which task, if performed by UAP, would require immediate intervention by the nurse?
   1. Administration of a warm bath
   2. Application of an ice pack
   3. Determination to use ice bags to treat fever
   4. Safety check of a heating pad

4. A nurse is applying a heating pad to a client. Which action could cause potential harm to the client?
   1. Apply moisture to the site that requires the heating pad.
   2. Place a cover on the heating pad.
   3. Reassess the site after 15 minutes.
   4. Use gauze ties instead of safety pins to hold the pad in place.

5. A nurse is preparing to administer an ice bag to a client who is having knee pain. Which nursing intervention is correct for this procedure?
   1. Fill the device completely with ice.
   2. Remove excess air by bending or twisting the device.
   3. Hold the device upright and check for leaks.
   4. Leave the device uncovered for optimal temperature.

6. For which of the following clients would the nurse question use of heat? Select all that apply.
   1. A client who presents with an active hemorrhage
   2. A client with a localized malignant tumor
   3. A client who has just sustained a traumatic injury
   4. A client who presents with a skin disorder
   5. A client with a nonbleeding open wound

7. The nurse applies cold treatment to a client. Which interventions are important to include in the nurse's documentation? Select all that apply.
   1. Circulatory status
   2. Comfort level
   3. Application method
   4. Skin reaction
   5. Temperature of the cold device

8. A nurse is preparing an aquathermia pad for a client. At which temperature should the nurse prepare this for the client?
   1. 27°C to 37°C (80°F to 98°F)
   2. 37°C to 40°C (98°F to 104°F)
   3. 40°C to 46°C (104°F to 115°F)
   4. Above 46°C (above 115°F)

9. The nurse is caring for a client requiring a hot compress. After applying the moist compress, the nurse applies an electric heating appliance to keep the compress warm. The client calls the nurse a few minutes later to say the compress has become cold. The nurse checks the compress and finds it is still as warm as when it was first applied. What would be the nurse's best response?
   1. "I will turn up the temperature on the heater to make it warmer."
   2. "The compress feels cooler because your body has adjusted to the warmth."
   3. "No, the compress is still warm."
   4. "Your body has adjusted to the warmth but if I turn up the temperature it could cause a burn."

10. The nurse applied a hot pack to a client's leg 20 minutes ago. When the nurse returns to assess the site, the leg is red and blistered. What would be the nurse's priority action?
    1. Notify the primary care provider.
    2. Apply an ice pack.
    3. Remove the hot pack.
    4. Apologize to the client.

See Answers to Test Your Knowledge in Appendix A.

READINGS AND REFERENCES

References

Gessner, P., Dugan, G., & Janusek, L. (2012). Target temperature within 3 hours: Community hospital's experience with therapeutic hypothermia. *AACN Advanced Critical Care, 23*, 246–257. doi:10.1097/NCI.0b013e31824c6489

Su, E. P., Perna, M., Boettner, F., Mayman, D. J., Gerlinger, T., Barsoum, W., . . . Lee, G. (2012). A prospective, multicenter, randomised trial to evaluate the efficacy of a cryopneumatic device on total knee arthroplasty recovery. *Journal of Bone and Joint Surgery, 94* (11, Suppl. A), 153–156. doi:10.1302/0301-620X.94B11.30832

Selected Bibliography

Berman, A., & Snyder, S. (2016). *Kozier & Erb's fundamentals of nursing: Concepts, process, and practice* (10th ed.). Upper Saddle River, NJ: Pearson.

Bucher, L., Buruschkin, R., Kenyon, D. M., Stenton, K., & Treseder, S. (2013). Improving outcomes with therapeutic hypothermia. *Nursing, 43*(1), 30–37. doi:10.1097/01.NURSE.0000423953.77012.d5

Garcia, E. G. (2013). *Pain: Thermotherapy* (Joanna Briggs Institute Evidence Summary). Retrieved from http://www.joannabriggs.edu.au

Oliveira, S., Silva, F., Riesco, M., Rosario, D., & Nobre, M. (2012). Comparison of application times for ice packs used

to relieve perineal pain after normal birth: A randomised clinical trial. *Journal of Clinical Nursing, 21*, 3382–3391. doi:10.1111/j.1365-2702.2012.04195.x

Park, S., Mangat, H., Berger, K., & Rosengart, A. (2012). Efficacy spectrum of antishivering medications: Meta-analysis of randomized controlled trials. *Critical Care Medicine, 40*, 3070–3082. doi:10.1097/CCM.0b013e31825b931e

Presciutti, M., Bader, M., & Hepburn, M. (2012). Shivering management during therapeutic temperature modulation: Nurses' perspective. *Critical Care Nurse, 32*(1), 33–42. doi:10.4037/ccn2012189

Wessinger, L., Marotta, R., & Kelechi, T. J. (2011). Hot or cold? Treating cellulitis. *Nursing, 41*(3), 46–48. doi:10.1097/01.NURSE.0000394067.76673.0b

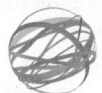

9 Pain Management

LEARNING OUTCOMES

At the completion of this chapter, the student will be able to:

1. Define key terms used in the skills of pain management.
2. Describe the various types of pain.
3. Describe factors that affect the pain experience.
4. List barriers to pain management.
5. Identify key factors in pain management.
6. Describe the two major components of pain assessment.
7. Identify data to collect and analyze when obtaining a comprehensive pain history.
8. Describe pharmacologic pain management, including classifications of medications and routes for opioid delivery.
9. Describe nonpharmacologic pain management interventions.

10. Recognize when it is appropriate to delegate pain management skills to unlicensed assistive personnel.
11. Verbalize the steps used in:
    a. Assessing the client in pain.
    b. Managing pain with a patient-controlled analgesia pump.
    c. Managing a transcutaneous electrical nerve stimulation unit.
    d. Providing a back massage.
    e. Teaching progressive muscle relaxation.
    f. Assisting with guided imagery.
12. Demonstrate appropriate documentation and reporting of pain assessment and interventions.

SKILLS

KEY TERMS

Pain is an unpleasant and highly personal experience that may be imperceptible to others, while consuming all parts of an individual's life. The best definition of pain comes from Margo McCaffery, an internationally known nurse expert on pain. Her often-quoted definition of pain says "pain is whatever the person says it is, and exists whenever he says it does" (Pasero & McCaffery, 2011, p. 21). This definition certainly portrays how subjective pain is. Another widely agreed-on definition of pain is "an unpleasant sensory and emotional experience associated with actual or potential tissue damage, or described in terms of such damage" (International Association for the Study of Pain, 2012). Three aspects of this definition have important implications for nurses. First, pain is a physical *and* emotional experience, not all in the body or all in the mind. Second, it is in response to actual *or* potential tissue damage, so there may

not be abnormal lab or radiographic reports despite real pain. Finally, pain is described in terms of such damage (e.g., neuropathic pain). Given that some clients are reluctant to disclose the presence of pain unless asked, nurses will not know of the client's pain until they assess for it. Additionally, it is clear that even clients who are nonverbal (e.g., preverbal children, intubated clients, clients with cognitive impairments, and those who are unconscious) experience pain that demands nursing assessment and treatment even if clients are unable to "describe in terms" the nature of their discomfort. Pain interferes with functional abilities and quality of life. Severe or persistent pain affects all body systems, causing potentially serious health problems while increasing the risk of complications, delays in healing, and an accelerated progression of fatal illnesses (Arnstein, 2010).

Pain management is the alleviation of pain or a reduction in pain to a level of comfort (palliation) that is acceptable to the client. To **palliate** pain means to ease, reduce, or allay without curing, and this is often the most realistic goal for those with chronic pain. Even if the original cause of the pain heals, the changes in the nervous system resulting from suboptimal pain management can result in the development of persistent or chronic pain. Persistent pain also contributes to insomnia, weight gain or loss, constipation, hypertension, deconditioning, chronic stress, and depression. These effects interfere with work, recreation, domestic activities, and personal care activities to the point that leads many people experiencing pain to question whether life is worth living. Effective pain management is an important aspect of nursing care to promote healing, prevent complications, reduce suffering, and prevent the development of incurable pain states. To be a true client advocate, nurses must realize their role is truly to be an advocate for pain relief.

Pain is more than a symptom of a problem; it is a high-priority problem in itself. Pain presents both physiological and psychological dangers to health and recovery. Severe pain is viewed as an emergency situation deserving attention and prompt professional treatment.

THE NATURE OF PAIN

Although pain is a universal experience, the nature of the experience is unique to the individual based, in part, on the type of pain experienced, the psychosocial context or meaning, and the response needed. Adding to the complexity, pain may be a physiological warning system alerting the nurse to a problem or unmet need demanding attention; or it may be a diseased, malfunctioning segment of the nervous system. Advances in the understanding of physiological mechanisms may someday replace the currently used categories of acute pain or chronic (persistent) pain. In addition to the underlying mechanisms, nurses need to consider a holistic view of care and how these physiological signals affect the mind, body, spirit, and social interactions.

TYPES OF PAIN

Pain may be described in terms of location, duration, intensity, and etiology.

Location

Classifications of pain based on where it is in the body (e.g., headache, backache, chest pain) may be problematic. For example, the International Headache Society (n.d.) recognizes approximately 80 different types of headaches. Many have similar clinical presentations but different clinical needs. Nevertheless, location of pain is an important consideration. For example, if after knee surgery, a client reports moderately severe chest pain, the nurse must act immediately to further evaluate and treat this discomfort. The ability to discriminate between cardiac and noncardiac chest pain challenges even expert clinicians, but the fact that chest pain is evaluated and treated differently than knee pain in this client is understandable. Complicating the categorization of pain by location is the fact that some pains **radiate** (spread or extend) to other areas (e.g., low back to legs). Pain may also be **referred** (appear to arise in different areas) to other parts of the body. For example, cardiac pain may be felt in the shoulder or left arm, with or without chest pain. **Visceral pain** (pain arising from organs) is often perceived in an area remote from the organ causing the pain (Figure 9–1 ■).

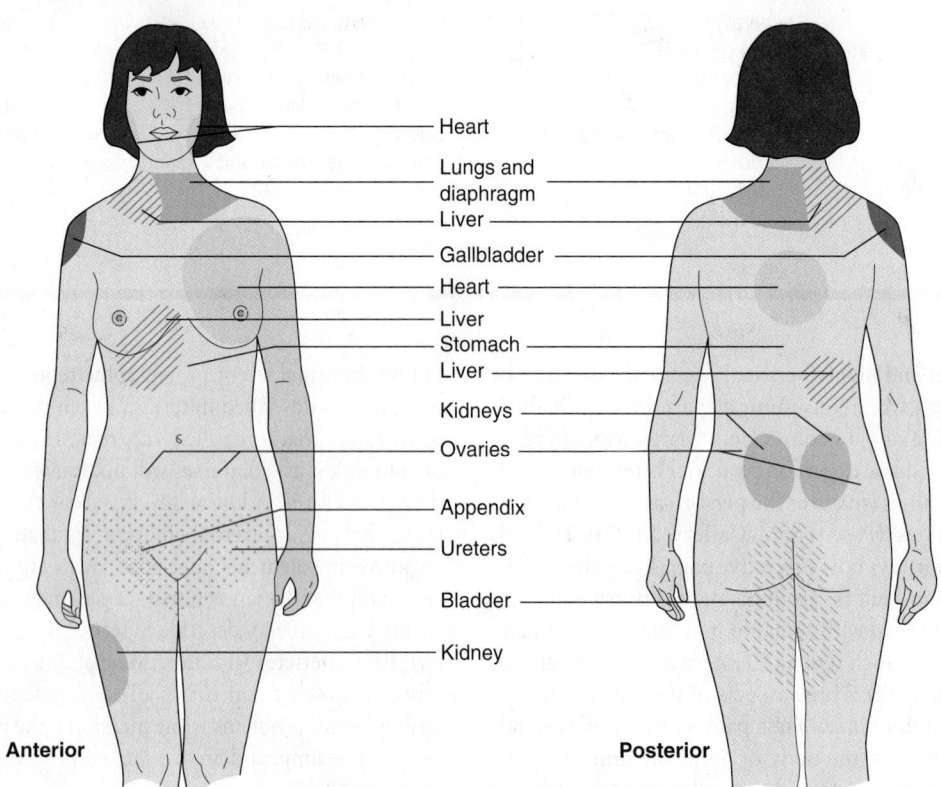

Figure 9–1 ■ Common sites of referred pain from various body organs.

Anterior

Posterior

Heart
Lungs and diaphragm
Liver
Gallbladder
Heart
Liver
Stomach
Liver
Kidneys
Ovaries
Appendix
Ureters
Bladder
Kidney

Duration

When pain lasts only through the expected recovery period, it is described as **acute pain**, whether it has a sudden or slow onset and regardless of the intensity. **Chronic pain**, also known as persistent pain, is prolonged, usually recurring or persisting over 3 months or longer, and interferes with functioning. Acute and chronic pain cause different physiological and behavioral responses, as shown in Table 9–1. Although experts may disagree on whether the cutoff point for chronic pain should be 3 or 6 months after onset or after expected healing time, NANDA International (Herdman & Kamitsuru, 2014) specifies the accepted nursing diagnosis of *Chronic Pain* to be mild to severe, constant or recurring, without an anticipated or predictable end, and a duration of greater than three (>3) months (p. 442).

Cancer pain may result from the direct effects of the disease and its treatment, or it may be unrelated. Over time, other diagnoses have been included in the "malignant pain" category, such as HIV/AIDS or burn pain, which tend to be treated more aggressively than "noncancer pain."

Intensity

Most practitioners classify intensity of pain by using a standard scale: 0 (no pain) to 10 (worst possible pain). Linking the rating to health and functioning scores, pain in the 1 to 3 range is considered mild pain, a rating of 4 to 6 is moderate pain, and pain reaching 7 to 10 is ranked severe pain and is associated with the worst outcomes.

Etiology

Designating types of pain by etiology can be done under the broad categories of nociceptive pain and neuropathic pain. **Nociceptive pain** is experienced when an intact, properly functioning nervous system sends signals that tissues are damaged, requiring attention and proper care. For example, the pain experienced following a cut or broken bone alerts the person to avoid further damage until it is properly healed. Once stabilized or healed, the pain goes away; thus, this pain is transient. There may also be persistent forms of nociceptive pain. For example, a person who has lost the protective cartilage

in joints will have pain when those joints are stressed, because the bone-to-bone contact damages tissues. This common form of arthritis produces pain in millions of individuals, some of whom have intermittent pain, whereas others have constant pain for years.

Subcategories of nociceptive pain include somatic or visceral. **Somatic pain** originates in the skin, muscles, bone, or connective tissue. The sharp sensation of a paper cut or aching of a sprained ankle are common examples of somatic pain. Visceral pain results from activation of pain receptors in the organs and/or hollow viscera. Visceral pain tends to be characterized by cramping, throbbing, pressing, or an aching quality. Often visceral pain is associated with feeling sick (e.g., sweating, nausea, or vomiting) as in the examples of labor pain, angina pectoris, or irritable bowel.

Neuropathic pain is associated with damaged or malfunctioning nerves due to illness (e.g., post-herpetic neuralgia, diabetic peripheral neuropathy), injury (e.g., phantom limb pain, spinal cord injury pain), or undetermined reasons. Neuropathic pain is typically chronic; it is described as burning, "electric shock," and/or tingling, dull, and aching. Episodes of sharp, shooting pain can also be experienced. Neuropathic pain tends to be difficult to treat.

The two subtypes of neuropathic pain are based on the part of the nervous system believed to be damaged. **Peripheral neuropathic pain** (e.g., phantom pain, post-herpetic neuralgia, carpal tunnel syndrome) follows damage and/or sensitization of peripheral nerves. **Central neuropathic pain** (e.g., spinal cord injury pain, post-stroke pain, multiple sclerosis pain) results from malfunctioning nerves in the central nervous system (CNS). **Sympathetically maintained pain** occurs occasionally when abnormal connections between pain fibers and the sympathetic nervous system perpetuate problems with both the pain and sympathetically controlled functions (e.g., edema, temperature, and blood flow regulation). Common pain syndromes are briefly described in Clinical Manifestations.

CONCEPTS ASSOCIATED WITH PAIN

It is useful for nurses to differentiate pain threshold from pain tolerance. **Pain threshold** is the least amount of stimuli that is needed for a person to label a sensation as pain. Threshold studies are typically conducted in a laboratory with many controls and measured amounts of stimuli (typically electrically generated). Pain threshold may vary slightly from person to person, and may be related to age, gender, or race, but it changes little in the same individual over time. **Pain tolerance** is the maximum amount of painful stimuli that a person is willing to withstand without seeking avoidance of the pain or relief. Pain tolerance varies considerably from person to person, even within the same person at different times and in different circumstances. For example, a woman may tolerate a considerable amount of labor pain because she does not want to alter her level of alertness or the vitality of her baby. She likely would not tolerate a fraction of that pain during a routine dental procedure before requesting appropriate medicine.

Hyperalgesia, hyperpathia, allodynia, and dysesthesia are conditions of abnormal pain processing that may signal the development of neuropathic processes. If recognized early these may be reversed; if ignored, however, they may lead to the development of incurable pain syndromes. The terms **hyperalgesia** and *hyperpathia* may be used interchangeably to denote heightened responses to a painful stimuli (e.g., severe pain response to a paper cut). This is differentiated from **allodynia**, in which nonpainful stimuli (e.g., contact with

TABLE 9–1	Comparisons of Acute and Chronic Pain	
Acute Pain	**Chronic Pain**
Mild to severe	Mild to severe
Sympathetic nervous system responses:	Parasympathetic nervous system responses:
• Increased pulse rate	• Vital signs normal
• Increased respiratory rate	
• Elevated blood pressure	
• Diaphoresis	• Dry, warm skin
• Dilated pupils	• Pupils normal or dilated
Related to tissue injury; resolves with healing	Continues beyond healing
Client appears restless and anxious	Client appears depressed and withdrawn
Client reports pain	Client often does not mention pain unless asked
Client exhibits behavior indicative of pain: crying, rubbing area, holding area	Pain behavior often absent

CLINICAL MANIFESTATIONS

Common Chronic Pain Syndromes

- *Post-herpetic neuralgia.* This pain, which currently affects 2 million Americans, occurs when a case of herpes zoster (shingles) typically erupts decades after a primary infection (chickenpox) during a period of stress or compromised immune functioning. After the painful unilateral vesicular rash fades, burning or electric-shock pain in the area may persist for months or years. Advancing age is a risk factor for persistent post-herpetic neuralgia. A vaccine has been approved and is recommended for all people over the age of 60 to prevent shingles, and the possibility of post-herpetic neuralgia.
- *Phantom pain.* Phantom sensations, the feeling that a lost body part is present, occur in most people after amputation. For many, this sensation is painful. It may occur spontaneously, or it may be evoked (e.g., using a poor-fitting prosthesis). When the amputation involves a limb, it is termed *phantom limb pain,* whereas following breast surgery, it is called *postmastectomy pain*. If the limb was painful or mangled before the amputation, that is commonly the sensation that is experienced (unless the discomfort is completely relieved prior to surgery). It is important for the nurse to explain the reasons for phantom limb pain, because clients may have difficulty understanding why they have pain when the limb is gone. They may start to question their sanity.
- *Trigeminal neuralgia.* This is an intense stablike pain that is distributed by one or more branches of the trigeminal nerve (fifth cranial). The pain is usually experienced on parts of the face and head. It is so severe that it produces facial muscle spasms.
- *Headache.* An estimated 40% of the worldwide population suffers at least one severe, disabling headache per year. This commonly occurring painful condition can be caused by either intracranial or extracranial problems, serious or benign conditions. To establish a plan to prevent or treat headache, the nurse needs to assess the quality, location, onset, duration, and frequency of the pain, as well as any signs and symptoms that precede the headache. There are many types of headaches, but the three most common are migraine, tension-type, and cluster. Migraine and tension-type headaches are three times more common in women than in men, whereas cluster headaches occur primarily in men.
- *Low back pain.* Nearly everyone has low back pain at some time during their life. Most occurrences of low back pain go away within a few days. Chronic back pain persists for more than 3 months. It is often progressive and the cause can be difficult to determine.
- *Fibromyalgia.* An estimated 5 million Americans have fibromyalgia, a chronic disorder characterized by widespread musculoskeletal pain, fatigue, and multiple tender points. This disease is poorly understood and primarily occurs in women. The term *tender points* refers to tenderness that occurs in precise, localized areas, particularly in the neck, spine, shoulders, and hips. People with this syndrome may also experience sleep disturbances, morning stiffness, irritable bowel syndrome, anxiety, and other symptoms. Although the symptoms present as muscle pain, stiffness, and weakness, it is considered by many to be a problem of abnormal CNS functioning, particularly as it relates to the way nerves process pain.

linen, water, or wind) produce pain, and from **dysesthesia**, which is an unpleasant abnormal sensation. Dysesthesia mimics or imitates the pathology of a central neuropathic pain disorder, such as the pain that follows a stroke or spinal cord injury. See Box 9–1 for a review of concepts associated with pain.

FACTORS AFFECTING THE PAIN EXPERIENCE

Numerous factors can affect a person's perception of and reaction to pain. These include the person's ethnic and cultural values, developmental stage, environment and support people, previous pain experiences, the meaning of the pain, and emotional responses to pain.

Ethnic and Cultural Values

Ethnic background and cultural heritage have long been recognized as factors that influence both a person's reaction to pain and the expression of that pain. Behavior related to pain is a part of the socialization process. For example, individuals in one culture may have learned to be expressive about pain, whereas individuals from another culture may have learned to keep those feelings to themselves and not bother others.

BOX 9–1	Concepts Associated with Pain

Acute pain: Pain that is directly related to tissue injury and resolves when tissue heals.

Cancer pain: Pain associated with the disease, treatment, or some other factor in individuals with cancer.

Chronic or persistent pain: Pain that persists beyond 3 to 6 months secondary to chronic disorders or nerve malfunctions that produce ongoing pain after healing is complete.

Intractable pain: A pain state (generally severe) for which there is no cure possible after accepted medical evaluation and treatments have been implemented. The focus of treatment turns from cure to pain reduction, functional improvement, and the enhancement of quality of life.

Neuropathic pain: Pain that is related to damaged or malfunctioning nervous tissue in the peripheral and/or central nervous system.

Nociceptive pain: Pain that is directly related to tissue damage. May be somatic (e.g., damage to skin, muscle, bone) or visceral (e.g., damage to organs).

Pain threshold: The least amount of stimuli that is needed for a person to label a sensation as pain.

Pain tolerance: The most pain an individual is willing or able to tolerate before taking evasive actions.

The following states indicate abnormal nerve functioning, and the associated cause needs to be identified/treated (as soon as possible) before irreversible damage occurs:

Allodynia: Sensation of pain from a stimulus that normally does not produce pain (e.g., light touch).

Dysesthesia: An unpleasant abnormal sensation that can be either spontaneous or evoked.

Hyperalgesia: Increased sensation of pain in response to a normally painful stimulus.

The following concepts are important reasons to prevent pain or treat it as soon as possible to prevent the amplification, spread, and persistence of pain:

Sensitization: An increased sensitivity of a receptor after repeated activation by noxious stimuli.

Windup: Progressive increase in excitability and sensitivity of spinal cord neurons, leading to persistent, increased pain.

Culturally Responsive Care

Transcultural Differences in Responses to Pain

Expressions of pain vary from culture to culture and may vary from person to person within a culture. Treat each client as an individual and provide the type of pain relief that is the best fit for the client.

AFRICAN AMERICANS

- Some believe pain and suffering is a part of life and is to be endured.
- Some may deny or avoid dealing with pain until it becomes unbearable.
- Some believe that prayer and laying on of hands will free a person from suffering and pain.

HISPANIC/LATINO

- Mexican Americans may tend to view pain as a part of life and as an indicator of the seriousness of an illness.
- Some believe that enduring pain is a sign of strength.
- Puerto Ricans may tend to be loud and outspoken in their expressions of pain. This is a socially learned way to cope, and it is important for the nurse to not judge or disapprove.

ASIAN AMERICANS

- Chinese culture values silence. As a result, some clients may be quiet when in pain because they do not want to cause dishonor to themselves and their family. Therefore, offer pain medications frequently because they generally agree to the use of pain medications; they may be afraid to ask for them.
- Japanese may have a stoic (minimal verbal and nonverbal expressions) response to pain. They may even refuse pain

medication. Bearing pain is considered a virtue and a matter of family honor.
- Filipino clients may believe that pain is "God's will" and therefore to be endured, not expressed. Some older Filipino clients may refuse pain medication.
- If the client is a Buddhist, remaining calm when in pain is viewed as bringing oneself to a higher state of being.

NATIVE AMERICANS

- In general, Native Americans are quiet, are less expressive verbally and nonverbally, and may tolerate a high level of pain. They tend to not request pain medication and may tolerate pain until they are physically disabled.

ARAB AMERICANS

- Pain is regarded as unpleasant and they anticipate immediate relief from their symptoms. Expressive emotional and vocal responses to pain are reserved for immediate family, not for health professionals. As a result, this may lead to conflicting perceptions among the family members and the nurse regarding the effectiveness of a client's pain relief. For example, the nurse may believe the client has adequate pain management, whereas the family is requesting additional pain medication for their family member.

From *Transcultural Health Care: A Culturally Competent Approach*, 4th ed. (pp. 109, 173, 193, 246, 387, 423), by L. D. Purnell, 2013, Philadelphia, PA: F.A. Davis; and *Pocket Guide to Culturally Sensitive Health Care* (pp. 12, 27, 123, 136, 157) by B. Stuart, C. Cherry, & J. Stuart, 2011, Philadelphia, PA: F.A. Davis.

Although there appears to be little variation in pain threshold, cultural background can affect the level of pain that an individual is willing to tolerate. In some Middle Eastern and African cultures, self-infliction of pain is a sign of mourning or grief. In other groups, pain may be anticipated as part of ritualistic practices, in which tolerance of pain signifies strength and endurance. Additionally, there are significant variations in the expression of pain. Studies have shown that individuals of northern European descent tend to be more stoic and less expressive of their pain than individuals from southern European backgrounds. See Culturally Responsive Care for transcultural differences in responses to pain.

Nurses must realize their own attitudes and expectations about pain. For example, in a large study of clients with pain ($n = 374,891$) admitted to an emergency department with similar pain reports, Pasero and McCaffery (2011) report that Caucasian clients were more likely to receive opioids than African American, Hispanic, Asian, and other clients (p. 160). This may be because of a hidden bias that nurses are not aware of at a conscious level. Nurses who deny or downplay the pain they observe in others may be culturally incompetent (unaware and emotionally apathetic toward others' viewpoints). To become culturally responsive, nurses must become knowledgeable about differences in the meaning of and appropriate responses to pain. They must be sympathetic to concerns and develop the skills needed to address pain in a culturally sensitive way.

Developmental Stage

The age and developmental stage of a client is an important variable that will influence both the reaction to and the expression of pain. Age variations and related nursing interventions are presented in Table 9–2.

The field of pain management for infants and children has grown significantly. It is now accepted that anatomic, physiological,

and biochemical elements necessary for pain transmission are present in newborns, regardless of their gestational age. For far too many years, the myth of infants and children not "feeling" pain has prevailed. Now, it is universally accepted that environmental, non-pharmacologic, *and* pharmacologic interventions should be used to prevent, reduce, or eliminate pain in neonates. Physiological indicators may vary in infants, so behavioral observation is recommended for pain assessment. Children may be less able than an adult to articulate their experience or needs related to pain, which may result in their pain being undertreated. Children, however, as young as 3 years can accurately report the location and intensity of their pain if evaluated properly.

With puberty comes the emergence of some pain syndromes, particularly for women. Unfortunately, women are overrepresented in a large number of painful disorders, including headaches, fibromyalgia, lupus, and menstrual-related disorders. Men are more vulnerable to pain related to their occupational or risk-taking patterns, including burn pain, post-trauma pain, and pain related to HIV/AIDS. A needless disparity continues that the very young, the very old, women, and ethnic minorities are undertreated for their pain more frequently than their adult male counterparts. Studies report that racial disparities in pain and health exist (Narayan, 2010).

Studies have shown that 57% of older adults living in the United States often experience pain, with 35% to 48% of community-dwelling older adults experiencing daily pain (Tabloski & Connell, 2014, p. 211). With the number of older individuals in our society increasing dramatically, by 2030, nurses will be caring for older adults in all settings of care in greater numbers.

Older adults constitute the largest group of individuals seeking health care services. The prevalence of pain in the older population is generally higher due to both acute and chronic disease conditions.

TABLE 9–2 Variations in the Pain Experience

Age Group	Pain Perception and Behavior	Selected Nursing Interventions
Infant	Perceives pain. Responds to pain with increased sensitivity. Older infant tries to avoid pain; for example, turns away and physically resists.	Give a glucose pacifier. Use tactile stimulation. Play music or tapes of a heartbeat.
Toddler or preschooler	Develops the ability to describe pain and its intensity and location. Often responds with crying and anger because child perceives pain as a threat to security. Reasoning with child at this stage is not always successful. May consider pain a punishment. Feels sad. May learn there are gender differences in pain expression. Tends to hold someone accountable for the pain.	Distract the child with toys, books, pictures. Involve the child in blowing bubbles as a way of "blowing away the pain." Appeal to the child's belief in magic by using a "magic" blanket or glove to take away pain. Hold the child to provide comfort. Explore misconceptions about pain.
School-age child	Tries to be brave when facing pain. Rationalizes in an attempt to explain the pain. Responsive to explanations. Can usually identify the location and describe the pain. With persistent pain, may regress to an earlier stage of development.	Use imagery to turn off "pain switches." Provide a behavioral rehearsal of what to expect and how it will look and feel. Provide support and nurturing.
Adolescent	May be slow to acknowledge pain. Recognizing pain or "giving in" may be considered weakness. Wants to appear brave in front of peers and not report pain.	Provide opportunities to discuss pain. Provide privacy. Present choices for dealing with pain. Encourage music or TV for distraction.
Adult	Behaviors exhibited when experiencing pain may be gender-based behaviors learned as a child. May ignore pain because to admit it is perceived as a sign of weakness or failure. Fear of what pain means may prevent some adults from taking action.	Deal with any misconceptions about pain. Focus on the client's control in dealing with the pain. Allay fears and anxiety when possible.
Older Adults	May have multiple conditions presenting with vague symptoms. May perceive pain as part of the aging process. May have decreased sensations or perceptions of the pain. Lethargy, anorexia, and fatigue may be indicators of pain. May withhold complaints of pain because of fear of the treatment, of any lifestyle changes that may be involved, or of becoming dependent. May describe pain differently, that is, as "ache," "hurt," or "discomfort." May consider it unacceptable to admit or show pain.	Thorough history and assessment are essential. Spend time with the client and listen carefully. Clarify misconceptions. Encourage independence whenever possible.

The pain threshold does not appear to change with aging, although the effect of analgesics may increase due to physiological changes related to drug metabolism and excretion (Arnstein, 2010).

Environment and Support People

A strange environment such as a hospital, with its noises, lights, and activity, can compound pain. In addition, the lonely person who is without a support network may perceive pain as severe, whereas the person who has supportive people around may perceive less pain. Some people prefer to withdraw when they are in pain, whereas others prefer the distraction of people and activity around them. Family caregivers can be a significant support for a person in pain. With the trend toward increased outpatient and home care, families are assuming more responsibility for the management of pain. Education related to the assessment and management of pain can positively affect the perceived quality of life for both clients and their caregivers.

Expectations of significant others can affect a person's perceptions of and responses to pain. In some situations, girls may be permitted to express pain more openly than boys. Family role can also affect how a person perceives or responds to pain. For instance, a single mother supporting three children may ignore pain because of her need to stay on the job. The presence of support people often changes a client's reaction to pain. For example, toddlers often tolerate pain more readily when supportive parents or nurses are nearby.

Previous Pain Experiences

Previous pain experiences alter a client's sensitivity to pain. People who have personally experienced pain or who have been exposed to the suffering of someone close are often more threatened by anticipated pain than people without a pain experience. In addition, the success or lack of success of pain relief measures influences a person's expectations for relief and future response to interventions. For example, a person who has tried several nondrug pain relief measures without success may have little hope about the helpfulness of nursing interventions and may demand medication as the only thing that helps the pain.

Meaning of Pain

Some clients may accept pain more readily than others, depending on the circumstances and the client's interpretation of its significance. A client who associates the pain with a positive outcome may withstand the pain amazingly well. For example, a woman giving birth to a child or an athlete undergoing knee surgery to prolong his career may tolerate pain better because of the benefit associated with it. These clients may view the pain as a temporary inconvenience rather than a potential threat or disruption to daily life.

By contrast, clients with unrelenting chronic pain may suffer more intensely. Chronic pain affects the body, mind, spirit, and social relationships in an undesirable way. Physically, the pain limits functioning and contributes to the disuse or deconditioning alluded to previously. For many, the change in activities of daily living (ADLs) (e.g., eating, sleeping, toileting) also takes a toll. The side effects of the many medications used to try to control the pain also place a heavy burden on the body.

Mentally, individuals with chronic pain change their outlook, becoming more pessimistic, often to the point of helplessness and hopelessness. Mood often becomes impaired when pain persists, because the sadness of being unable to do important or enjoyable activities combines with self-doubts and learned helplessness to produce depression. Anxiety, worry, and uncertainty about coping with the pain may escalate emotionally, to the point of panic. Spiritually, pain may be viewed in a variety of ways. It may be perceived as a punishment for wrongdoing, a betrayal by the higher power, a test of fortitude, or a threat to the essence of who the person is. Pain may be a source of spiritual distress, or it may be a source of strength and enlightenment. Socially, pain often strains valued relationships, in part because of the impaired ability to fulfill role expectations.

Emotional Responses to Pain

Anxiety often accompanies pain. Prolonged anxiety associated with pain can lead to other emotional disturbances, such as depression or difficulty coping. Fear of the unknown and the inability to control the pain or the events surrounding it often augment the pain perception. When clients are experiencing pain, they often become fatigued. Fatigue reduces a person's ability to cope, thereby increasing pain perception. With anxiety, depression, and fatigue, sleep disturbances can occur. When pain interferes with sleep, fatigue and muscle tension often result and increase the pain; thus, a cycle of pain, fatigue, and increased pain develops. Assessing clients with chronic pain for the presence of insomnia, major depression, and suicide potential is vitally important. People in pain who believe that they have control of their pain have decreased fear and anxiety that decreases their pain perception. A perception of lacking control or a sense of helplessness tends to increase pain perception.

BARRIERS TO PAIN MANAGEMENT

Misconceptions and biases about pain management involve attitudes of the nurse or the client as well as knowledge deficiencies. Clients respond to pain experiences based on their culture, personal experiences, and the meaning the pain has for them. For many people, pain is expected and accepted as a normal aspect of illness. Clients and families may lack knowledge of the adverse effects of pain and may have been provided incorrect information regarding the use of analgesics. Clients may not report pain because they expect nothing can be done, they think it is not severe enough, or they feel it would distract or prejudice the health care provider. Other common misconceptions are shown in Table 9–3.

Another barrier to effective pain management is the exaggerated fear of becoming addicted, especially when long-term opioid use is prescribed. Both nurses and clients often hold this fear. It is important for all individuals to know the difference between tolerance, physical dependence, and addiction.

Tolerance occurs when the client's opioid dose, over time, leads to a decreased sensitivity of the drug's analgesic effect. In other words, increasing doses of the opioid are needed to provide the same level of pain relief (Pasero & McCaffery, 2011, p. 295). **Physical dependence** is an expected physical response when a client, who

---

TABLE 9–3 **Misconceptions About Pain**

Misconception	Correction
Clients experience severe pain only when they have had major surgery.	Even after minor surgery, clients can experience intense pain.
The nurse or other health care professionals are the authorities about a client's pain.	The person who experiences the pain is the only authority about its existence and nature.
Administering analgesics regularly for pain will lead to addiction.	Clients are unlikely to become addicted to an analgesic provided to treat pain.
The amount of tissue damage is directly related to the amount of pain.	Pain is a subjective experience, and the intensity and duration of pain vary considerably among individuals.
Visible physiological or behavioral signs accompany pain and can be used to verify its existence.	Even with severe pain, periods of physiological and behavioral adaptation can occur.

is on long-term opioid therapy, has the opioid significantly reduced or withdrawn. The client experiences withdrawal symptoms such as nausea, vomiting, diarrhea, chills, and changes in vital signs (Oliver et al., 2012; Dunn, 2012). Pasero and McCaffery (2011) state, "physical dependence is one of the most frequently misunderstood terms and is often confused with addiction or 'dependence'" (p. 298). They maintain that the term *dependence* should be avoided because it is used in addiction medicine as another term for addiction. Physical dependence is associated with *physiological* dependence (potential ability for withdrawal), while addiction is associated with a *psychological* dependence to the drug. **Addiction** is a chronic, relapsing, treatable disease influenced by genetic, psychosocial, and environmental factors (Pasero & McCaffery, 2011; Oliver et al., 2012). Dunn (2012) describes how addiction is characterized by four Cs: a) craving for the substance, b) lack of control over the substance, c) compulsive use, and d) continued use despite harm (p. 66). Pasero and McCaffery (2011) remind us that it is important for the nurse to remember the following: 1) tolerance, physical dependence, and addiction are separate conditions with each requiring different treatment (p. 33), and 2) "taking opioids for pain relief is not addiction, no matter how long an individual takes opioids or at what doses. Individuals taking opioid drugs for relief of pain are using them therapeutically" (p. 299).

Pseudoaddiction is a condition that results from the undertreatment of pain in which the client may become so focused on obtaining medications for pain relief that he or she becomes angry and demanding, may "clock watch," and may otherwise seem inappropriately "drug seeking." Nurses can differentiate between pseudoaddiction and addiction if the client's negative behaviors resolve when the pain is treated effectively (Arnstein, 2010; Liberto & Fornili, 2013).

Nurses will provide care for clients who have substance abuse problems or addiction. Thus, a client could come to the acute care setting for an elective surgery, through the emergency department, or have cancer and the nurse will be caring for a client who has two separate problems: pain and addiction. Unfortunately, clients with a present or past history of substance abuse may suffer a great deal of pain needlessly. This is likely due to nurses' fear of addiction when administering opioid medications. Because addiction is a disease, clients must be cared for appropriately. The American Society for Pain Management Nursing (ASPMN) and the International Nurses Society on Addictions (IntNSA) hold the position that "patients with substance use disorders and pain have the right to be treated with dignity, respect, and the same quality of pain assessment and management as all other patients" (Oliver et al., 2012, p. 169).

It is important to first treat the pain. A myth held by nurses is that if they treat the pain, they are contributing to the addiction, but this is not true. In fact, undertreating the pain may cause the client with an addictive disorder to increase the drug use. Often, clients who are addicted require more pain medication, often more than the nurse is comfortable giving. Pain and addiction are two separate problems. To best help the client, if possible, nurses should consult with a pain management expert and an addiction specialist.

Cultural differences can also become a barrier to providing effective pain management. In providing culturally responsive care to those in pain, all of the usual considerations apply. This includes addressing linguistic issues and using certified interpreters whenever needed, respecting social and intimate space issues, and considering the client's comfort with the gender of the caregiver. The meaning of the pain experience, and the acceptability of and preference for various pain management approaches, must also be explored with the client. The best approach is to ask questions, and never make assumptions. Great variability exists within cultural groups, and it is always best to clarify the individual client's needs whenever possible.

KEY STRATEGIES IN PAIN MANAGEMENT

Key strategies to reduce pain include acknowledging and accepting the client's pain, assisting support people, reducing misconceptions about pain, reducing fear and anxiety, and preventing pain.

Acknowledging and Accepting the Client's Pain

According to the professional standards of conduct, nurses have a duty to ask clients about their pain and to believe their reports of discomfort. Challenging the client's report of discomfort undermines the environment of trust that is an essential component in the therapeutic relationship. Consider these four ways of communicating this belief:

1. Acknowledge the possibility of the pain: "Many people with your condition are bothered by leg pain. Are you experiencing any leg discomfort? What does it feel like? How concerned/upset are you about it?"
2. Listen attentively to what the client says about the pain, restating your understanding of the reported discomfort. Adding an empathetic statement like "I'm sorry you are hurting, it must be very upsetting. I want to help you feel better" lets the client know you believe the pain is real and intend to help.
3. Convey that you need to ask about the pain because, despite some similarities, everybody's experience is unique, for example: "Many people with your condition report having some discomfort. Do you have any pain or other discomfort now?"
4. Attend to the client's needs promptly. It is unconscionable to believe the client's report of pain and then do nothing. After determining the client has pain, discuss options and plan actions for providing relief.

Culturally Responsive Care | **PATIENT-CENTERED CARE**

Clients in Pain

To provide culturally sensitive pain management, nurses must first be aware of their own personal beliefs, values, and behaviors about pain; and subsequently, be open to the cultural effects of how clients perceive and react to pain. It is important, therefore, to develop an effective and caring relationship with the client.

- Respect each client:
  - Believe the client's statement of pain.
  - Recognize that clients hold different beliefs about pain.
  - Ask about the client's beliefs and how they cope with pain.
- Respect each client's response to pain:
  - Recognize that clients have the right to respond to pain in the way they learned is appropriate.
  - Recognize that expressions of pain vary widely and no expression is good or bad, just different.
- Avoid stereotyping. Expressions of pain vary between and within cultures.

From: "Culture's Effects on Pain Assessment and Management," by M. C. Narayan, 2010, *American Journal of Nursing, 110*(4), 38–47, doi:10.1097/01.NAJ.0000370157.33223.6d; "*Clinical Coach for Effective Pain Management*" by P. Arnstein, 2010, Philadelphia, PA: F. A. Davis; and "*Compact Clinical Guide to Acute Pain Management: An Evidence-Based Approach for Nurses*" by Y. D'Arcy, 2011, New York, NY: Springer.

Perception is reality. The client's self-report of pain is what must be used to determine pain intensity. The nurse is obligated to record the pain intensity as reported by the client. By challenging the believability of the client's report, the nurse is undermining the therapeutic relationship and preventing the fulfillment of advocacy and helping people with pain, which is called for in the American Nurses Association's Standards of Professional Performance for Pain Management Nursing.

Assisting Support People

Support people often need assistance to respond in a helpful manner to the person experiencing pain. Nurses can help by giving accurate information about the pain and providing opportunities for caregivers to discuss their emotional reactions, which may include anger, fear, frustration, and feelings of inadequacy. Teaching the support people about the disease and medications (including warning signs to report) and nondrug pain-relieving techniques they can help with (e.g., massage, application of ice, coached relaxation techniques) may diminish their feelings of helplessness and strengthen their relationship. Support people also may need the nurse's understanding, reassurance, and perhaps access to resources that will help them cope as they add the caregiver role to an already stressful life circumstance.

Reducing Misconceptions About Pain

Reducing a client's misconceptions about pain and its treatment will remove one of the barriers to optimal pain relief. The nurse should explain to the client that pain is a highly individual experience and that the client is the only one who really experiences the pain, although others can understand and empathize. Misconceptions are also dealt with when the nurse and client discuss the context of pain control as part of the healing process. For example, clients may refuse pain medicine out of concern for addiction, explaining that the pain is more tolerable as long as they remain totally still. This misconception overstates the risk of addiction (estimated at less than 5% of clients without a history of substance abuse when treated for acute pain), while underestimating the risks associated with immobility (atelectasis, muscle atrophy, decubitus ulcers, infections, etc.).

Reducing Fear and Anxiety

It is important to help relieve strong emotions capable of amplifying pain (e.g., anxiety, anger, and fear). When clients have no opportunity to talk about their pain and associated fears, their perceptions and reactions to the pain can be intensified. Often, these emotions are related to uncertainty about the future, feeling mistreated in the past, or having unmet expectations. By providing accurate information, the nurse can also reduce many of the client's fears or anxiety; and clarifying expectations can minimize frustration and anger. Specifically, client education about the range of pain that is considered normal for the condition as well as the types of discomforts that signal a potential for problems will help alleviate this fear and uncertainty.

Preventing Pain

A preventive approach to pain management involves the provision of measures to treat the pain before it occurs or before it becomes severe. **Preemptive analgesia** is the administration of analgesics *before* surgery to decrease or relieve pain *after* surgery. An example would be treating clients preoperatively with local infiltration of an anesthetic or an oral or parenteral administration of an opioid to reduce postoperative pain. This concept is controversial with little evidence-based research to support the practice (D'Arcy, 2011, p. 200).

Nurses, however, can use a preemptive approach by providing an analgesic around the clock (ATC) and supplementing with as-needed (prn) doses after surgery or prior to painful procedures (e.g., dressing changes, physical therapy). This strategy prevents the windup and sensitization described earlier that spreads, intensifies, and prolongs pain.

PAIN ASSESSMENT

Accurate pain assessment is essential for effective pain management. Many health facilities make pain assessment the **fifth vital sign**. This strategy of linking pain assessment to routine vital sign assessment and documentation represents a push to make pain assessment a routine aspect of care for all clients. Given the highly subjective and individually unique nature of pain, a comprehensive assessment of the pain experience (physiological, psychological, behavioral, emotional, and sociocultural) provides the necessary foundation for optimal pain control.

The extent and frequency of the pain assessment varies according to the situation and organizational policy. For clients experiencing acute or severe pain, the nurse may focus only on location, quality, severity, and early intervention. Clients with less severe or chronic pain can usually provide a more detailed description of the

---

PRACTICE GUIDELINES

Strategies for Colleague Accountability in Pain Management

What do we do if the health care team does not respond positively to a client's report of pain?

- Speak up! Inappropriate professional behavior will persist if not challenged. If necessary, file an "incident" or "variance" report for persistent patterns or egregious violations of standards of care. These types of behaviors (ignoring reports of pain, failing to treat or mistreating people with pain) are not only unethical, but legally indefensible because a standard of care is not being met.
- Clarify that the sensation of pain is subjective and that professionals have a duty to believe clients' reports of their symptoms.

- Cite recommendations from evidence-based clinical practice guidelines (e.g., American Pain Society, Agency for Health Care Policy and Research), The Joint Commission standards, organization-specific documents (e.g., mission statement, patient bill of rights, practice standards), or relevant research/quality reports. As necessary, distribute or post with key passages highlighted.
- Involve key committees, managers, and administrators in studying and addressing the problem from a cost, quality, competency, and credentialing perspective.

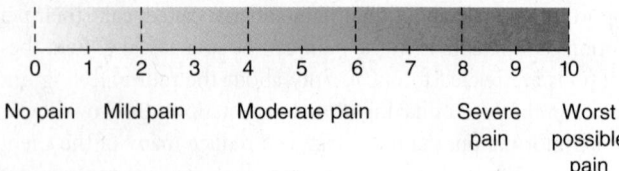

Figure 9–2 ■ An 11-point (0–10) pain intensity scale with word modifiers.

experience. As the fifth vital sign, pain status should be assessed and documented every time vital signs are taken. A simple question such as "Are you experiencing any discomfort right now?" and having the client rate discomfort on an 11-point (0–10) scale is usually sufficient (Figure 9–2 ■). Frequency of pain assessment may vary depending on the pain control measures being used and the clinical circumstances. For example, in the initial postoperative period, pain is assessed as often as every 15 minutes and then extended to every 2 to 4 hours as the interval between vital sign assessment lengthens.

CLINICAL ALERT!

Remember: Pain is the fifth vital sign. Pain assessment should be done (in a brief fashion) every time vital signs are taken, and should include a subjective self-report component whenever possible.

Major barriers to better pain control for both nurses and clients relate to failure to assess pain, underestimation of pain, failure to accept the client's report of pain, failure to act on the client's report of pain, and concerns about addiction (Pasero & McCaffery, 2011). Given that many clients will not voice their pain unless asked about it, the nurse *must* initiate pain assessments. Some of the many reasons clients may be reluctant to report pain are listed in Box 9–2. Because the words *pain* or *complain* may have emotional or sociocultural

BOX 9–2	Why Clients May Be Reluctant to Report Pain

- Unwillingness to trouble staff who are perceived as busy
- Do not want to be labeled as a "complainer" or "bad"
- Fear of the injectable route of analgesic administration—especially children
- Belief that unrelieved pain is to be expected as part of the recovery process or aging
- Difficulty communicating or unable to communicate discomfort
- Concern about risks associated with opioid drugs (e.g., addiction)
- Concern about unwanted side effects, especially of opioid drugs
- Concern that use of drugs now will render the drug inefficient later in life
- Fear about the cause of pain or that reporting pain will lead to further tests and expenses
- Belief that nothing can be done to control pain
- Belief that enduring pain and suffering may lead to spiritual enlightenment
- Culture affects behavioral responses to pain and treatment preferences (e.g., some cultures are comfortable expressing pain, whereas others are stoic and are not comfortable expressing or reporting pain)

meaning attached, it is better to ask, "Do you have any discomforts to report?" rather than "Do you have any complaints of pain?" It is also essential that nurses listen to and believe the client's statements of pain. Believing the client's statement is crucial in establishing the sense of trust needed to develop a therapeutic relationship.

Pain assessments consist of two major components: (1) a pain history to obtain facts from the client and (2) direct observation of behavioral and physiological responses of the client. The goal of assessment is to gain an objective understanding of a subjective experience.

Pain History

While taking a pain history, the nurse must provide opportunity for clients to express in their own words how they view the pain and the situation. This will help the nurse understand what the pain means to the client and how the client is coping with it. Remember that each person's pain experience is unique and that the client is the best interpreter of the pain experience. This history should be geared to the specific client. For example, questions asked of a motor vehicle crash victim would be different from those asked of a postoperative client or someone experiencing chronic pain. The initial pain assessment for someone in severe acute pain may consist of only a few questions before intervention occurs. In contrast, for the person with chronic pain, the nurse may ask more questions focusing on the client's coping mechanisms, effectiveness of current pain management, and ways in which the pain has affected the client's body, thoughts and feelings, activities, and relationships.

Data that should be obtained in a comprehensive pain history include pain location, intensity, quality, patterns, precipitating factors, alleviating factors, associated symptoms, effect on ADLs, coping resources, and affective responses. Two other types of data that are important to a pain history are past pain experiences and meaning of the pain to the person, both of which were discussed earlier in the chapter.

LOCATION

To ascertain the specific location of the pain, ask the client to point to the site of the discomfort. A chart consisting of drawings of the body can assist in identifying pain locations. The client marks the location of pain on the chart. This tool can be especially effective with clients who have more than one source of pain. A client who has multiple pains of different character can use symbols to draw the distribution of different pain types (e.g., circle aching areas, mark areas where shock-like pain is felt with an X).

When assessing the location of a child's pain, the nurse needs to understand the child's vocabulary. For example, "tummy" might refer either to the abdomen or to part of the chest. Asking the child to point to the pain helps clarify the child's word usage to identify location. The use of figure drawings can assist in identifying pain locations. Parents can also be helpful in interpreting the meaning of a child's words.

When documenting pain location, the nurse may use various body landmarks. Further clarification is possible with the use of terms such as *proximal, distal, medial, lateral,* and *diffuse.*

PAIN INTENSITY OR RATING SCALES

The single most important indicator of the existence and intensity of pain is the client's report of pain. In practice, however, nurses

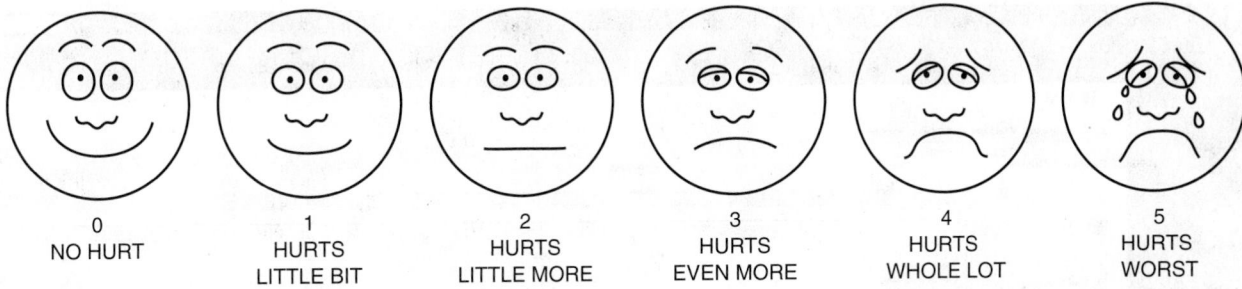

0	1	2	3	4	5
NO HURT	HURTS LITTLE BIT	HURTS LITTLE MORE	HURTS EVEN MORE	HURTS WHOLE LOT	HURTS WORST

Explain to the person that each face is for a person who feels happy because he has no pain (hurt) or sad because he has some or a lot of pain. Face 0 is very happy because he doesn't hurt at all. Face 1 hurts just a little bit. Face 2 hurts a little more. Face 3 hurts even more. Face 4 hurts a whole lot. Face 5 hurts as much as you can imagine, although you don't have to be crying to feel this bad. Ask the person to choose the face that best describes how he is feeling.

Rating scale is recommended for persons age 3 years and older.

Brief word instructions: Point to each face using the words to describe the pain intensity. Ask the child to choose the face that best describes own pain and record the appropriate number.

Figure 9–3 ■ The FACES rating scale.
Copyright 1983, Wong-Baker FACES® Foundation. www.WongBakerFACES.org. Used by permission of The WongBaker FACES® Foundation. Originally published in Whaley & Wong's Nursing Care of Infants and Children, ©Elsevier Inc.

tend to use less reliable measures for assessing pain such as changes in vital signs and observing for client behaviors they interpret as drug seeking (D'Arcy, 2011). Pain assessment that is inaccurate or incomplete leads to undertreatment of pain. The use of pain intensity scales is an easy and reliable method of determining the client's pain intensity. Such scales provide consistency for nurses to communicate with the client (adults and children over the age of 7) and other health care providers. To avoid confusion, numerical rating scales (NRS) should use a 0 to 10 range with 0 indicating "no pain" and the highest number indicating the "worst pain possible" for that individual. An 11-point (0–10) rating scale was shown earlier in Figure 9–2. The inclusion of word modifiers on the scale can assist some clients who find it difficult to apply a number level to their pain. For example, after ruling out "0" and "10" (neither no pain nor the worst possible pain), a nurse can ask the client if it is mild (ratings in the 1–3 range), moderate (ratings in the 4–6 range), or severe (ratings in the 7–10 range).

Another way to evaluate the intensity of pain for clients who are unable to use the numeric rating scales is to determine the extent of pain awareness and degree of interference with functioning. For example, 0 = no pain; 2 = awareness of pain only when paying attention to it; 4 = can ignore pain and do things; 6 = cannot ignore pain, interferes with functioning; 8 = impairs ability to function or concentrate; and 10 = intense incapacitating pain. It is believed that the degree that pain interferes with functioning is a good marker for the severity of pain, especially for those with chronic pain.

CLINICAL ALERT!

Emphasize to the client that, at times, treatment may need to balance the demands of providing pain reduction with functional improvement. Too much pain medicine might impair alertness or gait; too much pain impairs alertness and ability to move. Thus, a client may have to tolerate mild pain in order to do what is necessary to maximize functioning and recovery (e.g., cough, deep breathe, and walk).

When noting pain intensity it is important to determine any related factors that may be affecting the pain. When the intensity changes, the nurse needs to consider the possible cause. For example, the abrupt cessation of acute abdominal pain may indicate a ruptured appendix. Several factors affect the perception of intensity: (a) the amount of distraction, or the client's concentration on another event; (b) the client's state of consciousness; (c) the level of activity; and (d) the client's expectations.

Not all clients understand or relate to numerical pain intensity scales. These include preverbal children, older adults with impairments in cognition or communication, and people who do not speak English. For these clients the Wong-Baker FACES Rating Scale (Figure 9–3 ■) may be easier to use. The FACES scale includes a number scale along with an illustrated facial expression so that the pain intensity can be documented. When using the FACES rating scale, it is important to remember that the client's facial expression does not need to match the picture. The client points to the picture that represents how much pain the client is experiencing.

When clients are unable to verbalize their pain for reasons of age, mental capacity, medical interventions, or other reasons, nurses need to accurately assess the intensity of each client's pain and the effectiveness of the pain management interventions. For these clients, patience and time are required, and the nurse must rely on observation of behavior.

Several validated behavioral pain rating scales are useful in specific populations. The FLACC scale has been validated in children 2 months to 7 years old and rates pain behaviors manifested in Facial expressions, Leg movement, Activity, Cry, and Consolability measures that yield a 0 to 10 score. A scale specifically designed for older adults with advanced dementia is PAINAD. This scale looks at five specific indicators: breathing, vocalization, facial expression, body language, and consolability (D'Arcy, 2011; Pasero & McCaffery, 2011). Given the diversity of pain and behaviors among clients spanning a broad range of age and physical and mental

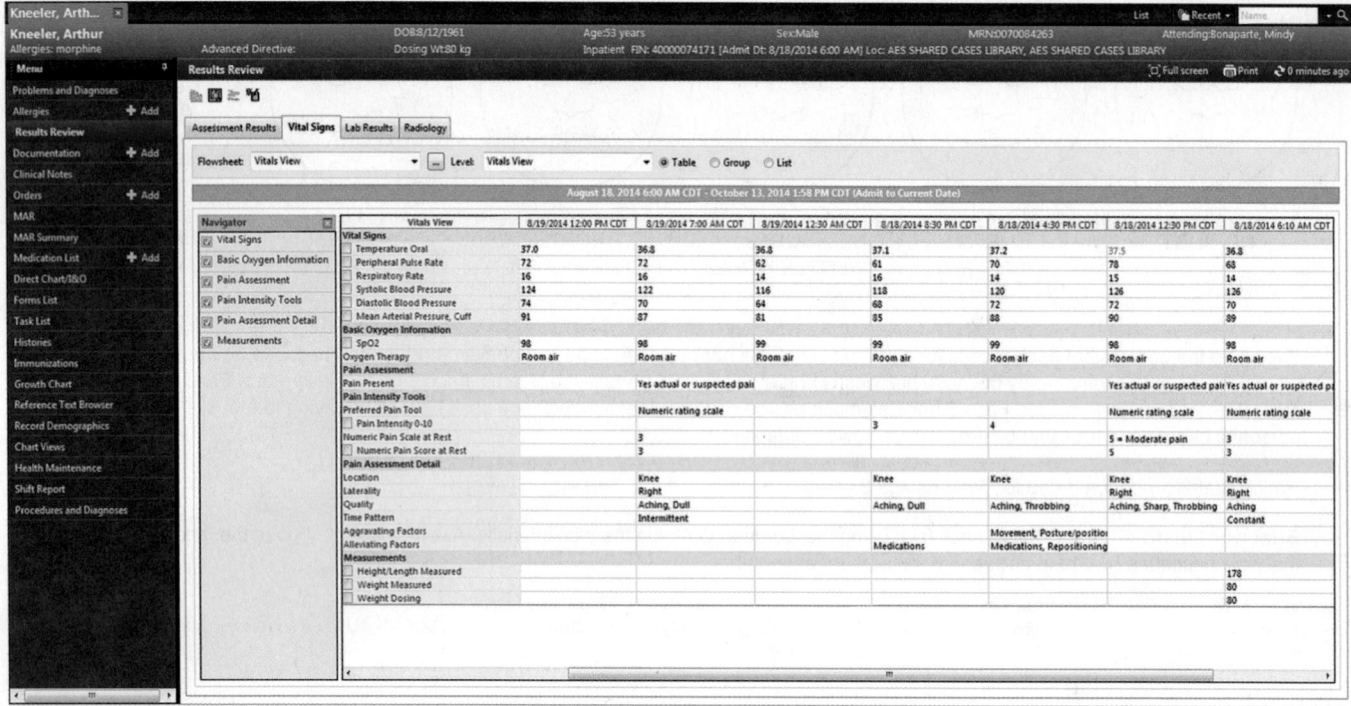

Figure 9–4 ■ Pain management flow sheet in an electronic health record.
"Pain Management Flow Sheet" from Cerner Electronic Health Record. Copyright © by Cerner Corporation. Used by permission of Cerner Corporation.

capabilities, it is unrealistic to believe a single pain assessment tool can be applied across all populations. The pain scale needs to fit the client being assessed.

For effective use of pain rating scales, clients need not only to understand the use of the scale but also to be educated about how the information will be used to determine changes in their condition and the effectiveness of pain management interventions. Clients should also be asked to indicate what level of comfort is acceptable so that they can perform specific activities. To align the client's goals and expectations with reality, it is important to note that acute pain can typically be cut by 50% and chronic pain can be cut by 25%. To ensure that optimal pain management is achieved, the client works together with professionals toward established goals of pain reduction and functional improvement.

The use of a pain numerical rating scale together with a FACES pain flow sheet has been shown to be effective in improving pain management (Pasero & McCaffery, 2011). Documentation can be completed by the nurse, the client, or a caregiver and can be used in acute, outpatient, and home care settings. See Figure 9–4 ■ for an example of a pain documentation form in an electronic health record (EHR).

PAIN QUALITY

Descriptive adjectives help people communicate the quality of pain. A headache may be described as "unbearable" or an abdominal pain as "piercing like a knife." The astute clinician can collect subtle clinical clues from the quality of the pain described; thus, it is important to record the description verbatim. Some of the commonly used pain descriptors are listed in Table 9–4. Note that the term *unbearable* is listed as an affective term and *piercing* is a sensory term. Both pains are real physical conditions signaling an underlying condition, but the affective description "unbearable" suggests that there is a coexisting emotional distress that needs to be addressed as well. Pain described as

TABLE 9–4	Commonly Used Pain Descriptors	
Term	**Sensory Words**	**Affective Words**
Pain	Searing	Unbearable
	Scalding	Killing
	Sharp	Intense
	Piercing	Torturing
	Drilling	Agonizing
	Wrenching	Terrifying
	Shooting	Exhausting
	Burning	Suffocating
	Crushing	Frightful
	Penetrating	Punishing
		Miserable
Hurt	Hurting	Heavy
	Pricking	
	Pressing	Throbbing
	Tender	
Ache	Numb	Annoying
	Cold	Nagging
	Flickering	Tiring
	Radiating	Troublesome
	Dull	Gnawing
	Sore	Uncomfortable
	Aching	Sickening
	Cramping	Tender

burning or shock-like tends to be neuropathic in origin and may be responsive to anticonvulsants (e.g., gabapentin or pregabalin), with or without an opioid (e.g., morphine, fentanyl, hydromorphone).

PATTERN

The pattern of pain includes time of onset, duration, and recurrence or intervals without pain. The nurse therefore determines when the pain began; how long the pain lasts; whether it recurs and, if so, the length of the interval without pain; and when the pain last occurred. Attention to the pattern of pain helps the nurse anticipate and meet the needs of the client, as well as recognize patterns of grave concern (e.g., chest pain only on exertion).

PRECIPITATING FACTORS

Certain activities sometimes precede pain. For example, physical exertion may precede chest pain, or abdominal pain may occur after eating. These observations can help prevent pain and determine its cause. Environmental factors such as extreme cold or heat and extremes of humidity can affect some types of pain. For example, people with rheumatic conditions have worse pain on cold, damp days or just before a large storm. Physical and emotional stressors can also precipitate pain. Strong emotions can trigger a migraine headache or an episode of chest pain. Extreme physical exertion can trigger muscle spasms in the neck, shoulders, or back.

ALLEVIATING FACTORS

Nurses must ask clients to describe anything that they have done to alleviate the pain (e.g., home remedies such as herbal teas, medications, rest, applications of heat or cold, prayer, or distractions like TV, reading, and games). It is important to explore the effect any of these measures had on the pain, whether relief was obtained, or whether the pain became worse. It is helpful to recommend a diary be kept to gather this information.

ASSOCIATED SYMPTOMS

Also included in the clinical appraisal of pain are associated symptoms such as nausea, vomiting, dizziness, and diarrhea. These symptoms may relate to the onset of the pain or they may result from the presence of the pain.

EFFECT ON ACTIVITIES OF DAILY LIVING

Knowing how ADLs are affected by pain helps the nurse understand the client's perspective on the pain's severity. The nurse asks the client to describe how the pain has affected the following aspects of life:

- Sleep
- Appetite
- Concentration
- Work/school
- Interpersonal relationships
- Marital relations/sex
- Home activities
- Driving/walking
- Leisure activities
- Emotional status (mood, irritability, depression, anxiety)

A rating scale of none, a little, or a great deal, or another range can be used to determine the degree of alteration.

COPING RESOURCES

Each individual will exhibit personal ways of coping with pain. Strategies may relate to earlier pain experiences or the specific meaning of the pain; some may reflect religious or cultural influences. Nurses can encourage and support the client's use of methods known to have helped in modifying pain, unless they are specifically contraindicated. Strategies may include seeking quiet and solitude, learning

about the condition, pursuing interesting or exciting activities (for distraction), saying prayers (or other meaningful rituals), or getting social support (from family, friends, or support groups).

AFFECTIVE RESPONSES

Affective responses vary according to the situation, the degree and duration of pain, the interpretation of it, and many other factors. The nurse needs to explore the client's feelings of anxiety, fear, exhaustion, depression, or a sense of failure. Because many people with chronic pain become depressed and potentially suicidal, it may also be necessary to assess the client's suicide risk. In such situations, the nurse needs to ask the client, "Do you ever feel so bad that you want to die? Have you considered harming yourself or others recently?" The vast majority of people experiencing chronic pain are not actively suicidal and do not have a specific, lethal plan. For those who express suicidal intent, nurses need to be familiar with state regulations, organizational policies, and resources available to guide practice in this area.

Observation of Behavioral and Physiological Responses

The client's self-report is the gold standard for pain assessment. Not all clients, however, are able to self-report. This group, referred to as "nonverbal" clients, include clients who are very young, cognitively impaired, critically ill, or comatose and some individuals at the end of life. These clients are definitely a challenge as the nurse provides effective pain management.

There are wide variations in nonverbal responses to pain. For clients who are very young, aphasic, confused, or disoriented, nonverbal expressions may be the only means of communicating pain. Facial expression is often the first indication of pain, and it may be the only one. Clenched teeth, tightly shut eyes, open somber eyes, biting of the lower lip, and other facial grimaces may be indicative of pain. Vocalizations such as moaning and groaning or crying and screaming are sometimes associated with pain (Box 9–3).

Immobilization of the body or a part of the body may also indicate pain. The client with chest pain often holds the left arm across the chest. A person with abdominal pain may assume the position of greatest comfort, often with the knees and hips flexed, and moves reluctantly.

Purposeless body movements can indicate pain—for example, tossing and turning in bed or flinging the arms about. Involuntary movements such as a reflexive jerking away from a needle inserted through the skin indicate pain. An adult may be able to control this reflex; however, a child may be unable or unwilling to do so.

BOX 9–3   Behavioral Responses to Pain

- Clenched teeth, tightly shut eyes, biting of lower lip, facial grimaces, open somber eyes
- Moaning, groaning, whimpering, crying, screaming
- Rubbing a part of the body, rocking, assuming a fetal position
- Immobilization or holding, supporting, or guarding of a part of the body
- Hostility and/or aggression (often seen in older adult clients)
- Confusion, restlessness (frequently seen in older adult clients)
- Purposeless or rhythmic body movements (often seen in children)

| **BOX 9–4** | **Hierarchy of Importance of Pain Measures: A Framework for Determining Presence of Pain in "Nonverbal" Clients to Develop a Treatment Plan** |

1. Attempt to obtain a self-report.
- Do not assume a client is unable to self-report until you have attempted to use a reliable and valid self-report tool. If unable to provide a self-report, proceed with the following steps.

2. Consider potential causes of pain (e.g., acute pain, chronic pain, procedures known to cause pain).
- When pain is assumed to be present, provide appropriate treatment.
- Some institutions use the abbreviation "APP" (assume pain present).

3. Observe client behaviors.
- For example, observe facial expressions and watch for restlessness, crying, changes in activity.
- Behavioral pain assessment tools may be helpful. It is important to remember that a behavioral pain score is not considered equivalent to a self-report of pain intensity (e.g., a behavior pain score of 4/10 does not equal a self-report of pain intensity of 4/10).

4. Obtain information from family members and caregivers who know the client well.
- These proxy assessments should be combined with other evidence when possible.

5. Attempt an analgesic trial and observe changes in the client's behavior.
- Provide a low dose of an analgesic if pain is suspected.
- Observe for behavioral changes.
- A low dose of analgesic may not be high enough. If that dose was tolerated and if there is no change in behavior, the dose should be increased or another analgesic added and observe for change in behavior.
- If behaviors improve, assume pain was the cause, continue the analgesic and add appropriate nonpharmacologic interventions.

From "Pain Assessment in the Patient Unable to Self-Report: Position Statement with Clinical Practice Recommendations," by K. Herr, P. J. Coyne, M. McCaffery, R. Manworren, & S. Merkel, 2011, *Pain Management Nursing*, 12(4), pp. 230–250; "Pain Assessment in Nonverbal Older Adults with Advanced Dementia," by S. M. Miller, 2011, *Journal for Nurse Practitioners*, 7(9), pp. 781–782; and *Pain Assessment and Pharmacologic Management*, by C. Pasero and M. McCaffery, 2011, p. 123, St. Louis, MO: Mosby Elsevier.

Behavioral changes such as confusion and restlessness may be indicators of pain in both cognitively intact and cognitively impaired older adult clients (Chapman, 2010; D'Arcy, 2011). Older adults with chronic pain may become hostile or aggressive.

Rhythmic body movements or rubbing may indicate pain. An adult or child may assume a fetal position and rock back and forth when experiencing abdominal pain. During labor a woman may massage her abdomen rhythmically with her hands.

It is important to note that because behavioral responses are controllable, they may not be very revealing. When pain is chronic, behavioral responses are rarely overt because the individual develops personal coping styles for dealing with pain, discomfort, or suffering.

Physiological responses vary with the origin and duration of the pain. Early in the onset of acute pain, the sympathetic nervous system is stimulated, resulting in increased blood pressure, pulse rate, respiratory rate, pallor, diaphoresis, and pupil dilation. The body does not sustain the increased sympathetic function over a prolonged period and, therefore, the sympathetic nervous system adapts, making the physiological responses less evident or even absent. Physiological responses are most likely to be absent in people with chronic pain because of autonomic nervous system adaptation. Thus, measures of physiological responses (e.g., pulse, blood pressure) are poor indicators of the presence, absence, or severity of pain and should not be used.

When clients are unable to self-report pain, an alternative approach based on the Hierarchy of Importance of Pain Measures is recommended as a framework for pain assessment (Pasero & McCaffery, 2011). See Box 9–4.

Daily Pain Diary

For clients who experience chronic pain, a daily diary may help the client and nurse identify pain patterns and factors that exacerbate or mediate the pain experience. In home care the family or other caregiver can be taught to complete the diary if the family member is unable to do it alone. The record can include the following:

- Time of onset of pain
- Activity or situation
- Physical pain character (quality) and intensity level (0–10)
- Emotions experienced and intensity level (0–10)
- Use of analgesics or other relief measures
- Pain rating after intervention taken
- Comments.

Pain diaries have been shown to improve pain management. They avoid "recall bias" where the client tries to remember or recall pain levels. A pain diary allows the client to understand and express the pain experience and possibly determine patterns that can help providers suggest better interventions. The diary may also increase the client's sense of control by helping the client use medication more effectively. For example, a pain diary may show the client that waiting too long to take an analgesic means that it takes longer to control the pain.

The recorded data in the diary provides the basis for developing or modifying the plan for care. For this tool to be effective, it is important for the nurse to educate the client and family about the value and use of the diary in achieving effective pain control. Review the diary at each visit, asking questions, sharing observations, and providing hints. Determining the client's abilities to use the diary is essential.

●○● NURSING PROCESS: ASSESSING THE CLIENT IN PAIN

Assessing the Client in Pain

PLANNING

Nurses must be prepared to assess pain for all clients, no matter what their age, communication abilities, or level of awareness and understanding. Having several methods for assessment, and being familiar with each method, will ensure that all clients are given opportunities to experience relief from suffering.

DELEGATION

The nurse is responsible for the initial and regular reassessment of pain. As the fifth vital sign, it may be that unlicensed assistive personnel (UAP) most frequently assess clients for pain if they are responsible for vital signs. After the assessment and in collaboration with the client, the nurse can discuss and delegate the performance of appropriate comfort measures to UAP. For example, the UAP may reposition the client at regular intervals, give the client a back massage, or provide rest periods. Emphasize to the UAP the importance of reporting any changes in the client's pain to the nurse.

Equipment

- Pain assessment flow sheet
- Pain rating scale

IMPLEMENTATION

Preparation

Identify those factors that may cause the client to be in pain. For example, does the client have a prior history of low back pain or diabetic neuropathy? Has the client had a major surgical procedure? Has the client experienced recent trauma? Note the client's baseline vital signs.

Performance

1. Prior to performing the procedure, introduce self and verify the client's identity using agency protocol. Explain to the client what you are going to do, why it is necessary, and how he or she can participate. Discuss how the results will be used in planning further care or treatments.
2. Perform hand hygiene and observe other appropriate infection prevention procedures.
3. Provide for client privacy.
4. Assess the client's perception of pain. For clients experiencing acute or severe pain, the nurse may focus on the first three aspects of the assessment—determining location, intensity, and quality—and quickly follow with an intervention. Clients with less severe or chronic pain can usually provide a more detailed description and the nurse can obtain a comprehensive pain assessment.
   - *Location.* Ask the client to place a mark on the figure on the pain assessment flow sheet or form with a figure, if appropriate. If there is more than one area of pain, use letters (e.g., A, B, C) to differentiate between the various sites. If the client is unable or unwilling to mark the figure, ask the client to tell you where the pain is located. Follow up by asking the client to point to the painful site with one finger. **Rationale:** *This will help verify if the verbal description and the location are the same.*
   - *Intensity.* Ask the client to rate the pain using the appropriate scale per agency policy.
   - *Quality.* Ask the client, "What words would you use to describe your pain?" **Rationale:** *Although this question may be difficult for the client to answer, the assessment is most accurate when the client provides the description.*
   - *Onset, duration, and recurrence.* This assessment can include such questions as "How long have you been having pain?" "Have you noticed any activity (e.g., swallowing, eating, stress, urinating, exertion) that increases or decreases the pain?" "How long does the pain last?" "How often does the pain occur?" "Is the pain better or worse at certain times of the day or night?"
   - *Manner of expressing pain.* Observe for behavioral cues such as grimacing, crying, or a change in body posture. **Rationale:** *Learning how a client expresses pain is particularly important for the client who cannot communicate or is very young, very old, or unable to hear.*
   - *Precipitating factors.* Ask what causes or increases the pain. **Rationale:** *Knowledge of those activities can both help prevent the pain from occurring and, sometimes, help determine the cause.*
   - *Alleviating factors.* Ask questions such as "What makes the pain go away or lessen?" "What methods of relief have you tried?" "How long did you use them?" "How effective were they?" **Rationale:** *Asking these questions can assist the nurse and the client to determine if some of the methods (such as listening to music or relaxation) can continue to be used while at the health care facility.*
   - *Associated symptoms.* Ask if there are any other symptoms (e.g., nausea, vomiting, dizziness) that occur prior to, with, or after the pain. **Rationale:** *These symptoms may relate to the onset of the pain or may result from the presence of the pain.*

Continued on page 252

Assessing the Client in Pain—*continued*

- *Effects of pain.* Explore the client's feelings and the effect the pain has on the client's life. This is particularly important for the client with chronic pain. **Rationale:** *Assessing the areas of sleep, appetite, physical activity, relationships, emotions, and concentration provides the nurse with information about the level of the client's functioning on a daily basis.*
- *Other comments.* Ask if there is any other information that would be helpful for the primary care providers and nurses to know. Emphasize that you want to work with the client and family to get the best control of the pain.

5. Assess physiological response to pain. Note blood pressure, pulse rate, respiratory rate, skin color, and presence of diaphoresis. **Rationale:** *Signs of sympathetic nervous system stimulation (fight or flight) may be present with acute pain; however, clients with chronic pain may not have physical signs because of CNS adaptation.*

6. Assess the affected body part, if appropriate. **Rationale:** *Additional assessment may provide additional information about the pain and possible intervention.*

7. Document findings of the pain assessment and include the intervention(s) and the client's response to the interventions. **Rationale:** *Thorough assessment and documentation assists the nurse to gain insights into the nature and pattern of the client's pain and ensures continuity of care.* Maintaining a pain management flow sheet (see Figure 9–4) will clarify and communicate each client's pain experience to enhance effective pain relief efforts.

In settings where a pain management flow sheet is not used, data can be documented in the client record as follows:

SAMPLE DOCUMENTATION

7/22/2015 0900 Admitted for elective foot surgery. Reports dull, throbbing, continuous pain in right cheek and jaw area radiating to right shoulder. Rates pain at 6/10. States pain began 6 months ago. Holding jaw throughout interview, became teary when describing negative effects on sleep, mood, and daily functioning. Associates onset with stress at work, and states she has been clenching her teeth throughout the day and grinding her teeth during sleep. States pain seems worse today with anxiety about surgery. Reports that Advil and heating pad relieve pain temporarily. Given moist heat pack to use now and relaxation breathing demonstrated with client participation. ———————————————— M. Blaszko, RN
7/22/2015 0930 Rates pain at 2/10. Referrals to TMJ specialist and counseling made. Discussed maintaining a daily pain diary to identify patterns and to share with primary care provider. ———————————————— M. Blaszko, RN

Variation: Daily Pain Diary

For clients who experience chronic pain, a daily diary may illuminate pain patterns and factors that exacerbate or mediate the pain experience. In home care, the family or other caregiver can be taught to complete the diary. The record can include:

- Time or onset of pain and activity or situation preceding pain
- Relevant data (e.g., weather conditions the client deems significant)
- Physical pain character (quality) and intensity level (0–10)
- Emotions experienced and intensity level (0–10)
- Use of analgesics or other relief measures
- Duration of pain
- Time spent in relief activities and effectiveness of these activities.

EVALUATION

- Conduct appropriate follow-up assessments to determine the effectiveness of the pain management intervention. Include the client's response, the changes in the pain, and the client's perceptions of the effectiveness of the therapy.
- Relate findings to previous assessment data if available.
- Report significant deviations from normal to the primary care provider.

Ambulatory and Community Settings   **Pain Assessment**   PATIENT-CENTERED CARE

Assess the following:

CLIENT
- *Level of knowledge:* pharmacologic and nonpharmacologic pain relief measures selected; adverse effects and measures to counteract these effects; warning signs to report to the primary care provider
- *Self-care abilities for analgesic administration:* ability to use analgesics appropriately; physical dexterity to take pills or to administer intravenous medications and to store medications safely; ability to obtain prescriptions or over-the-counter medications at the pharmacy

FAMILY
- *Caregiver availability, skills, and willingness:* primary and secondary individuals able and willing to assist with pain management; shopping if the client has restricted activity; ability to comprehend selected therapies (e.g., infusion pumps, imagery, massage, positioning, and relaxation techniques) and perform them or assist the client with them as needed
- *Family role changes and coping:* effect on financial status, parenting and spousal roles, sexuality, social roles

COMMUNITY
- *Resources:* availability of and familiarity with resources such as supplies, home health aide, or financial assistance

---

PAIN MANAGEMENT

Pain management includes two basic types of nursing interventions: pharmacologic and nonpharmacologic. Nursing management of pain consists of both independent and collaborative nursing actions. In general, noninvasive measures may be performed as an independent nursing function, but administration of analgesic medications requires a medical order from a primary care provider. However, because many analgesics are ordered to be administered on an as-needed (prn) basis that includes range orders, the decision to administer the prescribed medication is frequently the nurse's, requiring judgment as to the dose and the time of administration. Range orders are defined as "medication orders in which the selected dose varies

BOX 9–5	The Use of "As-Needed" Range Orders for Opioid Analgesics

To promote safety, it is vital that primary care providers, nurses, and pharmacists understand and agree how to properly write, interpret, and carry out prn range orders. Therefore, each institution should develop its own policies and procedures for the use of range orders.

RECOMMENDATIONS:
Prescriber:
- The order should provide clear direction to the nurse administering the analgesic.
- The order should include a dosage range with a fixed time interval. (The past practice of ordering one to two tablets every 3–4 hours is no longer acceptable . . . there should be only one time interval.)
- There should be no duplication of different opioids by the same route (e.g., IV morphine and IV hydromorphone).
- It is unsafe to order more than one analgesic by different routes *unless* the orders provide clear guidelines for use. For example, prn IV hydromorphone for severe pain, PO hydrocodone for moderate pain, and PO ibuprofen for mild pain.
- Written orders for the same opioid but different routes should provide clear direction for use (e.g., use oral route unless client is NPO or nauseous/vomiting).

Nurses:
- Implementation of the range orders should be based on a thorough pain assessment and knowledge of the medication.
- It is important to consider the pharmacokinetics of the opioid, especially for very young or very old clients.
- Do not administer partial doses at frequent intervals (i.e., giving oxycodone 10 mg every 2 hours when the order is for oxycodone 10 to 20 mg every 3 hours). This frequent, ineffective dose of the analgesic within the range leads to an ineffective underdose of analgesic for the client.
- Always evaluate the client's response to the dose and interval.
- If the partial dose in the range is ineffective, avoid making the client wait the full interval. Wait until the peak effect of the first dose has been reached before giving another dose.
- Make sure that the client's response to the dose and the dosing interval is documented.

From "The Use of 'As-Needed' Range Orders for Opioid Analgesics in the Management of Pain: A Consensus Statement of the American Society of Pain Management Nurses and the American Pain Society," by D. Drew et al., 2014, *Pain Management Nursing*, 15(2), pp. 551–554; and "Controlling Pain: Facing Up to the Challenge of Range Orders," by P. K. Rosier, 2012, *Nursing*, 42(12), pp. 64–65.

over a prescribed range according to the patient's situation and status" (Rosier, 2012, p. 64). For example, a prn range order for "morphine 2 to 6 mg IV every 2 h prn for pain" or "oxycodone 5–10 mg PO every 4 h prn for pain" provides flexibility in dosing to meet individual client's analgesic needs. In the past, there was an inconsistent understanding of how to interpret and carry out prn range orders. As a result, the American Society of Pain Management Nurses and the American Pain Society recently published a position statement on the use of "as-needed" range orders for opioid analgesics. The Joint Commission approves of the use of range orders as long as appropriate policies and procedures are in place and nurses are knowledgeable about their implementation (Rosier, 2012). These recent changes to the

way prn range orders are written provide a little more structure than in the past; however, professional nursing judgment remains a key factor in relieving pain by determining which medication in what dosage would best meet the client's comfort needs. See Box 9–5 for additional information from the position statement on prn range orders.

Client and family teaching is essential, because pain must be monitored in the home setting as well. Pain can go undertreated in home environments because caregivers may fear addiction and side effects. Caregivers may also have concerns that pain indicates disease progression, and may not want to fully acknowledge their loved one's pain. Guidelines for monitoring pain in ambulatory and home care settings are included in Client Teaching Considerations.

CLIENT TEACHING CONSIDERATIONS

Monitoring Pain

- Teach the client to keep a pain diary to monitor pain onset, activity before pain, pain intensity, use of analgesics or other relief measures, and so on.
- Instruct the client to contact a health care professional if planned pain control measures are ineffective.

PAIN CONTROL
- Teach the use of preferred and selected nonpharmacologic techniques such as relaxation, guided imagery, distraction, music therapy, massage, and so on.
- Discuss the actions, side effects, dosages, and frequency of administration of prescribed analgesics.
- Suggest ways to handle side effects of medications.
- Provide accurate information about tolerance, physical dependence, and addiction if opioid analgesics are prescribed and these topics are of concern.
- Instruct the client to use pain control measures before the pain becomes severe.
- Inform the client of the effects of untreated pain.
- Instruct clients with breakthrough (sudden, brief onset) pain regarding potential interactions with other medications and risk of overdosages. It is wise for a client to use only one pharmacy

to allow for tracking of pain medications. A client who has more than four episodes of breakthrough pain a day needs further evaluation by a pain specialist.
- Demonstrate and have the client or caregiver return demonstrate appropriate skills to administer analgesics (e.g., skin patches, injections, infusion pumps, or patient-controlled analgesia). If a home infusion pump is being used, caregivers need to be able to:
  a. Demonstrate stopping and starting the pump.
  b. Change the medication cartridge and tubing.
  c. Adjust the delivery dose.
  d. Demonstrate site care.
  e. Identify signs indicating the need to change an injection site.
  f. Describe care of the pump and insertion site when the client is ambulatory, bathing, sleeping, or traveling.
  g. Perform problem solving for pumps when alarms are activated.
  h. Change the battery.

RESOURCES
- Provide appropriate information about how to access community resources, home care agencies, and associations that offer self-help groups and educational materials.

Because pain is a multifaceted experience involving a client's body, mind, and spirit, a combination of strategies that will address the body, mind, and spirit is best for the client in pain. These strategies include pharmacologic and nonpharmacologic interventions. Research supports the use of multimodal strategies to effectively address pain. Exercise, relaxation, and challenging negative thoughts enhance the effectiveness of medications in reducing pain, depression, and anxiety, and improving physical ability and functional status. Teaching positive coping and self-management skills early in the chronic pain process greatly improve outcomes.

The simple act of altering the rate and depth of respiration by breathing slowly and deeply changes the amounts and types of pain and stress-reducing neuropeptides (such as endorphins) released into the body. Childbirth breathing is routinely taught to pregnant women to help them manage the pain of delivery. Available research indicates that a positive correlation exists between preoperative anxiety and postoperative pain. It makes sense that relaxation measures offered prior to surgery would have positive effects on postoperative pain. Control of breathing is built into many of the nonpharmacologic skills for pain management presented in this chapter (e.g., progressive muscle relaxation, guided imagery, and massage). Encouraging clients to breathe more deeply into the abdomen and to slow and quiet their breathing can enhance the effects of pain medications, as well. Usually a combination of pharmacologic and nonpharmacologic strategies must be adjusted to maximize the client's pain relief.

Pharmacologic Pain Management

Pharmacologic pain management involves the use of **opioids** (narcotics), nonopioids such as **nonsteroidal anti-inflammatory drugs (NSAIDs)**, and coanalgesic drugs (Box 9–6). The World Health Organization (WHO), in 1986, published guidelines regarding the use of analgesics with its logical three-step approach, also known as an analgesic ladder, to treat cancer pain. The WHO analgesic ladder was translated into 22 languages and became one of the adopted standards for general pain therapy for the last 28 years. The three-step ladder focuses on aligning the proper analgesic with the intensity of pain.

WORLD HEALTH ORGANIZATION THREE-STEP ANALGESIC LADDER

For clients with mild pain (1 to 3 on a 0 to 10 scale), step 1 of the analgesic ladder, nonopioid analgesics (with or without a coanalgesic), is the appropriate starting point. If the client has mild pain that persists or increases despite using full doses of step 1 medications, or if the pain is moderate (4 to 6 on a 0 to 10 scale), then a step 2 routine is appropriate. At the second step, an opioid for moderate pain (e.g., codeine, tramadol) or a combination of opioid and nonopioid medicine (e.g., oxycodone with acetaminophen, hydrocodone with ibuprofen) is provided with or without coanalgesic medications. If the client has moderate pain that persists or increases despite using full doses of step 2 medications, or if the pain is severe (7 to 10 on a 0 to 10 scale), then a step 3 schedule is medically indicated. At the third step, an opioid for severe pain (e.g., morphine, hydromorphone, fentanyl) is administered and titrated in ATC scheduled doses until the pain is relieved.

CLINICAL ALERT!

Combining opioid and nonopioid analgesics to treat pain is frequently overlooked. Each has different mechanisms of action, side effects, and toxicity profiles. Alternating the two or giving them at the same time creates no danger and often produces a synergistic rather than merely additive effect. By combining nonopioids and opioids, pain management can be enhanced, reducing doses of analgesics and decreasing the risks of side effects for both. This practice is sometimes referred to as multimodal therapy.

The WHO analgesic ladder has been the cornerstone of pain management for over two decades. Current literature, however, is questioning if it is still a valid tool (Leung, 2012; Vargas-Schaffer, 2010; Zeppetella, 2011). Some suggest a two-step ladder; others call for a four- or five-step ladder. A common theme is that the WHO analgesic ladder focuses on pharmacotherapy and ignores the emotional and cognitive aspects of pain management. Leung (2012) proposes that pain management should not be a linear approach of going up or down the narrow rungs of an analgesic ladder, but instead the rungs should be broadened horizontally to become platforms. These platforms would include the analgesics *and* other therapies to

---

BOX 9–6	Categories and Examples of Analgesics

NONOPIOID ANALGESICS/NSAIDs
- Acetaminophen (Tylenol, Datril)
- Acetylsalicylic acid (aspirin)
- Choline magnesium trisalicylate (Trilisate)
- Ibuprofen (Motrin, Advil)
- Indomethacin sodium trihydrate (Indocin)
- Naproxen (Naprosyn), naproxen sodium (Anaprox)
- Ketorolac (Toradol)
- Piroxicam (Feldene)
- Meloxicam (Mobic)
- Celecoxib (Celebrex) COX-2 NSAID

OPIOID ANALGESICS FOR MODERATE PAIN
- Hydrocodone (Lortab, Vicodin)
- Codeine (Tylenol No. 3)

- Tramadol (Ultram, Ultracet)
- Pentazocine (Talwin)

OPIOID ANALGESICS FOR SEVERE PAIN
- Fentanyl citrate (Sublimaze, transdermal patches, Actiq lozenges)
- Hydromorphone hydrochloride (Dilaudid)
- Oxycodone (OxyContin)
- Morphine sulfate (morphine)
- Oxymorphone (Opana)
- Methadone (Dolophine)

COANALGESICS
- Tricyclic antidepressants (nortriptyline, amitriptyline)
- Anticonvulsants (gabapentin, pregabalin)
- Topical local anesthetic (Lidoderm)

alleviate pain (e.g., physical therapy, counseling, support group, yoga, meditation, hypnosis, relaxation therapy, and other complementary and alternative medicine (CAM) options). The use of multidrug strategies coupled with multimodal therapies may permit opioid dose reduction and improve client outcomes.

NONOPIOIDS/NSAIDs

Nonopioids include acetaminophen and NSAIDs such as ibuprofen or aspirin. All are useful for the management of acute and chronic pain.

Aspirin is the most common NSAID and is available over the counter (OTC). Because it can prolong bleeding time, clients should stop taking it 1 week prior to any surgical procedure. Aspirin should never be given to children under 12 years of age due to the possibility of Reye's syndrome. The nurse must also be aware that aspirin can cause excessive anticoagulation if a client is taking the anticoagulant warfarin.

Acetaminophen (Tylenol) does not affect platelet function and rarely causes gastrointestinal (GI) distress. It does, however, have serious side effects such as hepatotoxicity and possible renal toxicity, especially with high doses or with long-term use. Studies show that even with recommended doses up to 4 grams per day, some clients may be at an increased risk for liver toxicity (Pasero & McCaffery, 2011). The U.S. Food and Drug Administration (FDA) currently requires warnings against taking alcohol with acetaminophen. It is recommended that young and healthy people limit their acetaminophen consumption to less than 3 grams per day, with susceptible individuals (e.g., older adults, those with a history of alcoholism, dehydration, or liver disease) limiting their consumption to less than 2 grams per day (Arnstein, 2010; D'Arcy, 2011). Given that acetaminophen is so well tolerated, it is often a hidden ingredient in OTC remedies (e.g., pain, fever, allergy, cough and cold preparations), so clients must be instructed to read the ingredient list of all OTC medicines they take. Box 9–7 lists common prescription pain medications that contain acetaminophen.

NSAIDs have anti-inflammatory, analgesic, and antipyretic effects, whereas acetaminophen has only analgesic and antipyretic effects. All NSAIDs relieve pain by inhibiting the enzyme cyclooxygenase (COX) that is activated by damaged tissue, which results in decreased synthesis of prostaglandins. The COX-1 specific isoforms are found in platelets, the GI tract, kidneys, and most other tissue, and are believed to be the cause of the well-known side effects of NSAIDs (GI bleeding, diminished renal blood flow, inhibited clotting, etc.).

In the 1990s a second isoform (COX-2) was found and believed to be specific only for pain and inflammation. The resulting new "safer" (COX-2 selective) NSAIDs were tested, approved, and widely used. These drugs demonstrated significantly less GI bleeding, but uncommon cardiovascular events and rare skin problems occurred in susceptible individuals. The only COX-2 currently available in the United States is celecoxib (Celebrex). Although the COX-2 NSAIDs have fewer GI side effects, they are no safer on renal function than the COX-1 NSAIDs. All prescription NSAIDs now must carry the strong "black box" warning of the risks of using these drugs. Even nonprescription NSAIDs (e.g., aspirin, ibuprofen, naproxen) must be labeled to warn consumers of the potential dangers of using those products.

Individual drugs in this category vary little in their analgesic potency, but do vary in their anti-inflammatory properties, metabolism, excretion, and side effects. These drugs have a ceiling effect and a narrow therapeutic index. The term *ceiling effect* means that once the maximum analgesic benefit is achieved, additional amounts of the drug will not produce more analgesia; however, more toxicity may occur. The *narrow therapeutic index* indicates that there is not much margin for safety between the dose that produces a desired effect and the dose that may produce a toxic, even lethal effect. The most common side effect of nonopioid analgesics is gastrointestinal, such as heartburn or indigestion. These effects can become toxic or lethal when silent GI bleeding occurs. Given the interference with platelet aggregation, a small stomach ulcer can bleed a lot, making it a potentially life-threatening condition. Clients should be taught to take NSAIDs with food and a full glass of water, and be routinely monitored by a health professional if they take these preparations daily for more than a couple of weeks.

Table 9–5 lists common misconceptions about nonopioids.

CLINICAL ALERT!

Many health care professionals underestimate the effectiveness of ordinary aspirin and acetaminophen. An ordinary dose of aspirin or acetaminophen relieves as much pain as 1.5 mg of parenteral morphine, whereas standard doses of mixed analgesics (e.g., Tylenol No. 3 or Percocet) are approximately equivalent to 2.5 to 5 mg of morphine.

OPIOIDS

There are three primary types of opioids:

1. *Full agonists.* A full **agonist analgesic** is morphine, the gold standard opioid. Other full agonists include oxycodone (e.g., Percocet, OxyContin), hydromorphone (e.g., Dilaudid), and fentanyl (Duragesic, Actiq). There is no ceiling on the level of analgesia from these drugs; their dose can be steadily increased to relieve pain. There is also no maximum daily dose limit unless they are in compound with a nonopioid analgesic drug.

BOX 9–7	Common Prescription Pain Medications That Contain Acetaminophen

Medication	
• Tylenol No. 3	(325 mg acetaminophen/ 30 mg codeine)
• Percocet	(325 mg acetaminophen/ 5 mg oxycodone)
• Lortab	(500 mg acetaminophen/ 5, 7.5, or 10 mg hydrocodone)
• Vicodin	(500 mg acetaminophen/ 5 mg hydrocodone)
• Vicodin ES (750 mg)	(750 mg acetaminophen/ 7.5 mg hydrocodone)
• Tylox	(500 mg acetaminophen/ 5 mg oxycodone)
• Darvocet-N 100	(650 mg acetaminophen/ 100 mg propoxyphene)

TABLE 9–5   Misconceptions About Nonopioids

Misconception	Correction
Regular daily use of NSAIDs is much safer than taking opioids.	Side effects from long-term use of NSAIDs are considerably more severe and life threatening than the side effects from daily doses of oral morphine or other opioids. The most common side effect from long-term use of opioids is constipation, whereas NSAIDs can cause gastric ulcers, increased bleeding time, and renal insufficiency. Acetaminophen can cause hepatotoxicity.
A nonopioid should not be given at the same time as an opioid.	It is safe to administer a nonopioid and opioid at the same time. Giving a dose of nonopioid at the same time as a dose of opioid poses no more danger than giving the doses at different times. In fact, many opioids are compounded with a nonopioid (e.g., Percocet [oxycodone and acetaminophen]).
Administering antacids with NSAIDs is an effective method of reducing gastric distress.	Administering antacids with NSAIDs can lessen distress but may be counterproductive. Antacids reduce the absorption and therefore the effectiveness of the NSAID by releasing the drug in the stomach rather than in the small intestine where absorption occurs.
Nonopioids are not useful analgesics for severe pain.	Nonopioids alone are rarely sufficient to relieve severe pain, but they are an important part in the total analgesic plan. One of the basic principles of analgesic therapy is this: Whenever pain is severe enough to require an opioid, adding a nonopioid should be considered.
Gastric distress (e.g., abdominal pain) is indicative of NSAID-induced gastric ulceration.	Most clients with gastric lesions have no symptoms until bleeding or perforation occurs.

From *Pain Assessment and Pharmacologic Management*, by C. Pasero and M. McCaffery, 2011, St. Louis, MO: Mosby Elsevier. Reprinted with permission from Elsevier.

2. *Mixed agonists–antagonists.* **Agonist–antagonist analgesic** drugs can act like opioids and relieve pain when given to a client who has not taken any pure opioids. However, they can block or inactivate other opioid analgesics when given to a client who has been taking pure opioids. These drugs include dezocine (Dalgan), pentazocine hydrochloride (Talwin), butorphanol tartrate (Stadol), and nalbuphine hydrochloride (Nubain). If a client has been receiving a full agonist (e.g., morphine, Percocet, or Vicodin for pain) daily for more than a couple of weeks, the administration of a mixed agonist–antagonist may result in an immediate and severe withdrawal reaction. These drugs also have a ceiling effect that limits the dose. They are not recommended for use with clients who are terminally ill. In the opioid-naïve client (one who has not taken opioids for a week or longer) with acute pain (e.g., migraine headache), these agents have a favorable effect and low side effect burden.

3. *Partial agonists.* Partial agonists have a ceiling effect in contrast to a full agonist. One example is buprenorphine (Buprenex). This drug has good analgesic potency and is emerging as an alternative to methadone for opioid maintenance/narcotic treatment programs. The safety and favorable side effect profile make it an increasingly popular choice.

OPIOID ANALGESICS FOR MODERATE PAIN   These include drugs such as codeine, hydrocodone, and tramadol. Most of these drugs are combinations of a nonopioid with an opioid. These medicines are generally two to four times more potent than nonopioids alone, and have some of the risks of both drug classes. These drugs are controlled substances and must be ordered by a physician or nurse practitioner, adhering to applicable federal and state laws. They also have a ceiling effect due to the nonopioid

and a maximum daily dose limit. There are advantages to giving combination drugs, such as lowering the amount of any one medicine needed in a 24-hour period, thus reducing the potential for side effects or toxicity; however, nurses need to be familiar with each medication and be aware of daily dose limits of the ingredients as well as the potential to receive duplicate medications for different clinical indications (e.g., Tylenol in the mixed drug, Tylenol for fever, and Tylenol in the headache preparation).

These opioids have a narrow therapeutic index. Codeine at doses of 30 to 60 mg produces dose-limiting GI distress in many people. A specific enzyme in the body (CYP450) is required to make codeine active in order for analgesia to be effected. About 10% of the population lack this enzyme and are "poor metabolizers," meaning they may not get any pain relief at all from codeine (D'Arcy, 2011).

OPIOID ANALGESICS FOR SEVERE PAIN   Pure agonist opioid analgesics include opium derivatives, such as morphine, hydromorphone, oxycodone, fentanyl, and methadone. *Opioid* is the pharmacologic class of pain relievers and is the correct medical term, rather than the term *narcotics*. Many opioids are "scheduled" as a controlled substance (narcotic) due to the potential for misuse. In addition to pain reduction, changes in mood may make the person feel more comfortable even though the pain persists. As the most potent class of pain relievers, these drugs are indicated for severe pain, or when other medications have failed to control moderately severe or worse pain. Among this class, meperidine (Demerol) has received a lot of attention in recent years as a medication to avoid because of its short half-life, toxic metabolite, and potential to induce tremors and seizures with repeated doses. It should not be used with infants and children, older adults, and clients with cancer pain or sickle cell disease (Pasero & McCaffery,

2011). Most acute care settings have taken it off their formularies for pain control.

Methadone is a synthetic opioid used for severe pain. The nurse needs to be aware of the potential for serious problems when a client is on methadone. Due to its long half-life (15 to 60 hours), there is an increased risk of sedation and respiratory depression, especially in older adults.

OPIOID SIDE EFFECTS   When administering any analgesic, the nurse must review side effects. Side effects of the opioids typically include respiratory depression, sedation, nausea/vomiting, urinary retention, blurred vision, sexual dysfunction, and constipation. The adverse effect of most concern is respiratory depression (e.g., 8 breaths per minute or less), which usually occurs early in therapy among opioid-naïve clients, with dose escalation, or in clients with drug–drug or drug–disease interactions. Clinically, the client will appear overly sedated, and respirations will be slow and deep with periods of apnea. The nurse needs to assess a client's level of alertness and respiratory rate for baseline data before administering narcotics. Clients will often manifest an increase in sedation *before* they manifest a decrease in respiratory rate and depth. The use of a scale to assess sedation during opioid pain management is common in hospitals in the United States. A number of sedation scales are available; thus, it is important for nurses to know how to use their facility's choice of sedation scale. A commonly used scale is the Pasero Opioid-Induced Sedation Scale (POSS), which uses a scale ranging from 1 (alert and awake) to

---

BOX 9–8	**Pasero Opioid-Induced Sedation Scale**

S = Sleep, easy to arouse
1 = Awake and alert
2 = Slightly drowsy, easily aroused
3 = Frequently drowsy, arousable, drifts off to sleep during conversation
4 = Somnolent, minimal, or no response to physical stimulation

From *Pain Assessment and Pharmacologic Management* (p. 510), by C. Pasero and M. McCaffery, Copyright 2011, St. Louis, MO: Mosby Elsevier. Reprinted with permission from Elsevier.

---

4 (minimal or no response to verbal and physical stimulation). See the sedation rating scale in Box 9–8. Pasero and McCaffery (2011) suggest an easy way for the nurse to assess sedation is to ask the client a simple question, such as "What did you have for breakfast today?" and observe the client's ability to stay awake and answer the question (p. 509). If the client is excessively sedated, he or she will fall asleep in the middle of answering the question. This behavior is unacceptable and requires close monitoring of respiratory rate and sedation level. Early recognition of an increasing level of sedation or respiratory depression will enable the nurse to implement appropriate measures promptly (e.g., pulse oximetry monitoring, obtaining an order to decrease the opioid dosage).

Box 9–9 provides suggested measures to prevent and treat side effects of opioid analgesics. Tolerance to all opioid side effects usually

---

BOX 9–9	**Common Opioid Side Effects and Preventive and Treatment Measures**

CONSTIPATION
- Increase fluid intake (e.g., 6 to 8 glasses daily).
- Increase fiber and bulk-forming agents to the diet (e.g., fresh fruits and vegetables). Increasing exercise is often ineffective in controlling this type of constipation.
- Administer daily stool softeners combined with a mild laxative (e.g., Senokot-S) as a first line of prevention against constipation (as ordered) for clients on opioid maintenance therapy.
- Stimulants (bisacodyl), osmotic laxatives (lactulose, sorbitol, and polyethylene glycol), enemas (tap water and sodium phosphate), and even prokinetic agents (metoclopramide) may be ordered for refractory cases of constipation.
- A new medication was recently approved for opioid-induced constipation in end-of-life care, methylnaltrexone bromide (Relistor). It is to be given subcutaneously, when other methods prove ineffective (D'Arcy, 2011).

NAUSEA AND VOMITING
- Inform the client that tolerance to this emetic effect generally develops after several days of opioid therapy.
- Provide an antiemetic: 5HT antagonist ondansetron (Zofran), phenothiazines (Compazine, Phenergan), or the GI stimulant metoclopramide (Reglan).
- Obtain primary care provider orders to change the dose or analgesic agent as indicated.

SEDATION
- Inform the client that tolerance usually develops over 3 to 5 days.
- Consider requesting a primary care provider's order for a stimulant in the morning (e.g., caffeine, Dexedrine, or Ritalin for adult clients) or an alternative route of administration (e.g., epidural) for clients with persistent pain and sedation.

- Observe the client for evidence of respiratory depression that may occur with sedation.

RESPIRATORY DEPRESSION
- Per primary care provider order, administer an opioid antagonist, such as naloxone hydrochloride (Narcan), cautiously by diluting 1 ampule in 10 mL of saline and then administering 1 mL per minute until the respirations are equal to or more than 10/min. Make provisions for repeat administration, continuous infusion, or a longer-acting version of a reversal agent because the half-life of naloxone is considerably shorter than that of most opioids being reversed.
- Be aware of the CNS depression risks of other medications such as hypnotics, benzodiazepines, and sedatives, especially in the opioid-naïve client.
- Remember to titrate naloxone to prevent seizures, arrhythmias, and returning pain.
- Attempt to stimulate the client to take deep breaths every 15 to 30 minutes. Stop, change, or slow the administration of opioids until respirations are restored.

PRURITUS
- Apply cool packs, lotion, and diversional activity.
- Administer an antihistamine (e.g., diphenhydramine hydrochloride [Benadryl]).
- Inform the client that tolerance also develops to pruritus within a few days; otherwise, as with other unresolved side effects, switching to another opioid may prove beneficial.

URINARY RETENTION
- May need to catheterize client, or change or lower the analgesic dose.

occurs within a few days, except for constipation. Because of this, the nurse must initiate and continue measures to prevent constipation during the entire time the client is on opioids.

Older clients are particularly sensitive to the analgesic properties of opioids and may require less medication, or medication administered at less frequent intervals than younger clients. This sensitivity may be related to reduced or delayed excretion of the drug in older clients. As such, the clinical pearl of "start low (25% to 50% dose reduction) and go (titrate) slow" is often followed in the older population.

CLINICAL ALERT!

Constipation is an almost universal adverse effect of opioid use. All clients should receive prophylactic stimulant laxative therapy, unless contraindicated. Stool softeners are not useful alone, but are a good choice when combined with a stimulant laxative (e.g., Senokot-S). If those products are ineffective, a regimen of cathartic laxatives (e.g., bisacodyl), followed by more aggressive forms of treatment (e.g., osmotic laxatives, enema, manual disimpaction), may be necessary.

SAFETY ALERT!   SAFETY

Assessing for sedation and respiratory status is critical during the first 12 to 24 hours after starting opioid therapy. The most critical period is during the peak effect of the first dose (15 minutes if administered IV; first hour after IM, oral, or rectal route). An exception is with opioids administered via the spinal route. Respiratory depression may increase over time with epidural infusions and with intrathecal analgesia; respiratory depression may manifest 24 hours after the spinal injection even after the analgesic effect has worn off. In general, the longer the client receives opioids, the wider the safety margin as the client develops a tolerance to the sedative and respiratory depressive effects of the drug.

SAFETY ALERT!   SAFETY

As a precaution, have naloxone (Narcan), sodium chloride 0.9% diluent, and injection equipment on hand for each client receiving an opioid-containing epidural infusion.

EQUIANALGESIC DOSING The term **equianalgesia** refers to the relative potency of various opioid analgesics compared to a standard dose of parenteral morphine (gold standard opioid). This tool helps professionals individualize the analgesic regimen by guiding the adjustment of medication, dose, time interval, and route of administration. An equianalgesic table can be used to help provide doses of approximately equal ability to relieve pain.

COANALGESICS A **coanalgesic** agent (formerly known as an adjuvant) is a medication that is not classified as a pain medication. However, coanalgesics have properties that may reduce pain alone or in combination with other analgesics, relieve other discomforts, potentiate the effect of pain medications, or reduce the pain medication's side effects. Examples of coanalgesics that relieve pain are antidepressants (increase pain relief, improve mood, and improve sleep); anticonvulsants (stabilize nerve membranes, reducing excitability and spontaneous firing); and local anesthetics (block the transmission of pain signals). Anxiolytics, sedatives, and antispasmodics are examples of medicines that relieve other discomforts; however, they do not alleviate pain and thus should be used in addition to rather than instead of analgesics. Examples of medications used to reduce the side effects of analgesics include stimulants, laxatives, and antiemetics.

Coanalgesics appear to be particularly beneficial for the management of neuropathic pain. Tricyclic antidepressant drugs seem to be particularly useful for central neuropathic pain, which often manifests as pain with a burning, unusual, or stinging quality. Anticonvulsant drugs, such as gabapentin (Neurontin) or pregabalin (Lyrica), seem particularly useful for peripheral neuropathic conditions that often present with a stabbing, shooting, or electrical-shock quality. Local anesthetics such as the Lidoderm patch also alleviate neuropathic as well as other types of pain, and are particularly useful for clients with the skin sensitivity known as allodynia. There is a growing scientific and clinical basis for the use of these medications in relieving pain, especially persistent pain that is not relieved by the analgesic classes of medication alone.

Administration of Placebos

A **placebo** is "any sham medication or procedure designed to be void of any known therapeutic value" (Arnstein, Broglio, Wuhrman, & Kean, 2011, p. 226). An example would be a sugar pill or an injection of saline. In contrast, the *placebo effect* is "the positive response some patients/participants experience after receiving a placebo" (Arnstein et al., 2011, p. 226). Some professionals try to justify the use of placebos to elicit the desirable placebo effect or in a misguided attempt to determine if the client's pain is "real." The use of placebos outside the context of an approved research study is deceptive and represents fraudulent and unethical treatment. Many professional and pain management organizations (e.g., ANA Code of Ethics for Nurses, American Society for Pain Management Nursing, American Pain Society, Oncology Nursing Society) have published position papers that adamantly oppose the use of placebos without consent.

Routes for Opioid Delivery

Opioids can be given in the following routes: oral, transnasal, transdermal, transmucosal, topical, rectal, subcutaneous, intramuscular, IV (bolus and continuous), intraspinal (epidural and intrathecal), and continuous local anesthetics. Box 9–10 describes some of these administration routes.

ORAL

Oral administration of opioids remains the preferred route of delivery because of ease of administration. Given that the duration of action of most opioids is approximately 4 hours, people with chronic pain have had to awaken during the night to medicate themselves for pain. To avoid this problem, long-acting or sustained-release forms of morphine with a duration of 8 or more hours have been developed. Examples of long-acting morphine are MS Contin, a controlled-release tablet; and Avinza, a morphine sulfate extended-release capsule. Clients receiving long-acting morphine may also need prn "rescue" doses of immediate-release analgesics such as the short-acting oral transmucosal fentanyl citrate (Actiq) for acute breakthrough pain. Another method of oral opioid delivery is high-concentration liquid morphine. This formulation enables clients who can swallow only small amounts to continue taking the drug orally.

BOX 9–10	Routes for Opioid Delivery

- *Oral:* Preferred because of ease of administration. Duration of action is approximately 4 hours. Long-acting forms with durations of 8 or more hours are also available. Another method of oral opioid delivery is high-concentration liquid morphine that allows clients who can swallow only small amounts to continue taking the drug orally.
- *Transnasal:* Has the advantage of rapid action of the medication because of direct absorption through the vascular nasal mucosa.
- *Transdermal:* Delivers a relatively stable plasma drug level and is noninvasive. Can provide drug delivery for up to 72 hours.
- *Rectal:* This route is useful for clients who have difficulty swallowing or nausea and vomiting.
- *Subcutaneous:* A traditional route.
- *Intramuscular:* The least desirable route because of variable absorption, pain involved with administration, and the need to repeat administration every 3 to 4 hours.
- *Intravenous:* Provides rapid and effective pain relief with few side effects. Can be administered by IV bolus or by continuous infusion controlled by the client using a patient-controlled analgesia machine at the bedside (see Skill 9–2).
- *Intraspinal:* Infusion of opioids into the epidural or intrathecal (subarachnoid) space (see page 260).

TRANSNASAL

Transnasal administration has the advantage of rapid action of the medication because of direct absorption through the vascular nasal mucosa. A commonly used agent is a mixed agonist–antagonist butorphanol (Stadol) for acute migraine headaches. Treating migraine headaches via the nasal route of administration is particularly beneficial because of the nausea, vomiting, and gastroparesis that occur with that condition, making oral medications relatively contraindicated.

TRANSDERMAL

Transdermal drug therapy is advantageous in that it delivers a relatively stable plasma drug level and is noninvasive. Fentanyl (Duragesic) is a lipophilic synthetic opioid (i.e., binds to subcutaneous fat) and is currently available as a skin patch with various dosages (12 to 100 mcg). The nurse must remember that fentanyl is 100 times more potent than morphine and is ordered in micrograms (mcg) not milligrams (mg). It provides drug delivery for up to 72 hours. The transdermal route is distinguished from the topical route, in that the effects of the medications are systemic after the medication is absorbed. Nurses must teach clients not to use heat with the fentanyl patch (e.g., hot tubs, heating pads) because increased absorption may occur. A client with a fever may absorb the medication faster because of the vasodilation from the increased skin temperature. Used patches should be disposed of in a tamper-proof container. This is especially true in the home setting because the used patch can contain enough residual medication to harm a small child or animal if ingested (Mayo Clinic, 2012).

TRANSMUCOSAL

Many clients with cancer-related pain experience breakthrough pain even though they are on a fixed schedule for pain control. The transmucosal route is helpful for breakthrough pain because the oral mucosa is well vascularized, which facilitates rapid absorption. Two forms of fentanyl are available for transmucosal delivery: oral transmucosal fentanyl citrate (OTFC; Actiq) and fentanyl buccal tablet (FBT; Fentora).

TOPICAL

The topical route is when medications work directly at the point they are placed on the body. They are useful for painful procedures (lumbar punctures or bone marrow biopsies) or injections. These products can also offer effective pain relief for chronic pain syndromes such as peripheral neuropathy and/or low back pain. OTC examples include Aspercreme and LMX4 (4% lidocaine).

Prescription topical medications include EMLA cream (lidocaine and prilocaine), Synera (lidocaine and tetracaine), and Zingo (lidocaine hydrochloride powder). Lidoderm is a topical patch approved for post-herpetic neuralgia. It has been found to be useful in other types of neuropathic pain. It must be applied on intact skin and left in place for 12 hours and then off for 12 hours.

A new form of the NSAID diclofenac (Voltaren) is now available, by prescription, for acute short-term pain due to minor strains, sprains, and contusions (bruises). It is called the Flector patch.

RECTAL

Several nonopioid and opioid medicines are now available in suppository form. The rectal route is particularly useful for clients who have dysphagia (difficulty swallowing) or nausea and vomiting. It is best to use commercially available rectal preparations, or have them compounded by a licensed compound pharmacist.

SUBCUTANEOUS

Although the subcutaneous route has been used extensively to deliver opioids, another technique uses subcutaneous catheters and infusion pumps to provide continuous subcutaneous infusion (CSCI) of narcotics. CSCI is particularly helpful for clients (a) whose pain is poorly controlled by oral medications, (b) who are experiencing dysphagia or GI obstruction, or (c) who have a need for prolonged use of parenteral narcotics. CSCI involves the use of a small, light, battery-operated pump that administers the drug through a #23- or #25-gauge butterfly needle. The needle can be inserted into the anterior chest, the subclavicular region, the abdominal wall, the outer aspects of the upper arms, or the thighs. Client mobility is maintained with the application of a shoulder bag or holster to hold the pump. The frequency of site change ranges from 3 to 7 days. The maximum fluid volume should be less than 3 mL/h for continuous infusion (Pasero & McCaffery, 2011).

Because family caregivers must operate the pump and also change and care for the injection site, the nurse needs to provide appropriate instruction. Caregivers need to be able to:

- Describe the basic parts and symbols of the system.
- Identify ways to determine whether the pump is working.
- Change the battery.
- Change the medication.
- Demonstrate stopping and starting the pump.
- Demonstrate tubing care, site care, and changing of the injection site.
- Identify signs indicating the need to change an injection site.

- Describe general care of the pump when the client is ambulatory, bathing, sleeping, or traveling.
- Identify actions to take to solve problems when the alarm signals.

INTRAMUSCULAR

The intramuscular (IM) route should be abandoned for administration of analgesics (Pasero & McCaffery, 2011). Disadvantages include variable absorption, unpredictable onset of action and peak effect, as well as the tissue damage that may result, even if properly administered. Regardless of precautions taken, there is pain involved with administration.

INTRAVENOUS

The IV route provides rapid and effective pain relief with few side effects. However, just as the onset of pain relief occurs in 5 to 10 minutes, so can adverse effects, such as respiratory depression. The analgesic can be administered by IV bolus or by slow continuous infusion. Caution is needed to prevent the introduction of air or bacteria into the tubing, and to prevent introducing medications that are incompatible with other medications dissolved in the IV solution.

INTRASPINAL

An increasingly popular method of delivery is the infusion of opioids into the **epidural** or intrathecal (subarachnoid) space (Figure 9–5 ■). Analgesics administered via the intraspinal route are delivered adjacent to the opioid receptors in the dorsal horn of the spinal cord. Two commonly used medications are morphine sulfate and fentanyl. All medicines administered via the intraspinal route need to be sterile and preservative free (preservatives are neurotoxic). The major benefit of intraspinal drug therapy is that superior analgesia is achieved with less medication. The epidural space is most commonly used because the dura mater acts as a protective barrier against infection, including meningitis, and there is less risk of developing a "spinal headache." Intraspinal catheters are not in constant contact with blood, and thus an

infusion can be stopped and restarted later without concern that the catheter has become clotted.

Intrathecal administration delivers medication directly into the cerebrospinal fluid (CSF) that bathes and nourishes the spinal cord. Medicines quickly and efficiently bind to the opioid receptor sites in the dorsal horn when administered in this way, speeding the onset and peak effect, while prolonging the duration of action of the analgesic. An example of how the route of administration affects the relative potency of opioids is as follows: A client who needs 300 mg of oral morphine per day to control pain will need 100 mg of parenteral morphine, 10 mg of epidural morphine, and only 1 mg of intrathecal morphine in a 24-hour period. Very little drug is absorbed by blood vessels into the systemic circulation. In fact, the drug must circulate through the CSF to be excreted. As a result, there may be a delayed onset (24 hours after administration) of respiratory depression, because medication that has left the spinal opioid sites travels through the brain to be eliminated.

In contrast, the epidural space is separated from the spinal cord by the dura mater, which acts as a barrier to drug diffusion. In addition, it is filled with fatty tissue and an extensive venous system. With this diffusion delay, some medications (especially fat-soluble medications like fentanyl) from the epidural space enter the systemic circulation via the venous plexus. Thus, a higher dose of opioid is required to create the desired effect, which can produce side effects of itching, urinary retention, and/or respiratory depression. Often, an opioid (e.g., fentanyl) and a local anesthetic (e.g., bupivacaine) are combined to lower the dose of opioid needed. As a result, some clients may develop muscular weakness in their legs or orthostatic hypotension in response to the local anesthetic, resulting in an increased risk of falls.

Intraspinal analgesia can be administered by three modes of operation:

1. **Bolus.** A single or repeated bolus dose(s) may be provided. When clients have spinal anesthesia (e.g., during a cesarean section), a bolus of 1 mg intrathecal preservative-free morphine

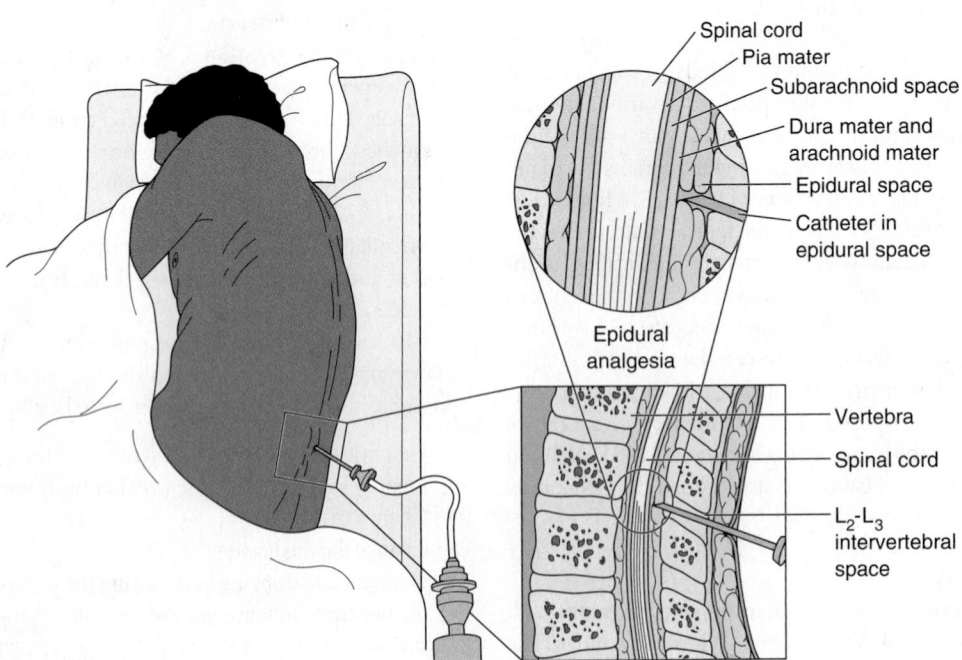

Figure 9–5 ■ Placement of intraspinal catheter in the epidural space.

can provide significant pain control for up to 24 hours. A newer formulation of morphine called DepoDur provides up to 48 hours of analgesia. For shorter acting medications, an epidural catheter may be intact and accessed by a qualified health professional (e.g., anesthesiologist or nurse anesthetist) to administer bolus doses on an as-needed basis. Check your state regulations and agency policy regarding who can provide these bolus doses, how they are documented, and the postbolus monitoring procedures.

2. *Continuous infusion administered by pump.* The pump may be external (for acute or chronic pain) or surgically implanted (for chronic pain) to provide a continuous infusion of pain relievers into the epidural or intrathecal space.

3. *Continuous plus intermittent bolus.* With this mode of operation, the client receives a continuous infusion with bolus "rescue" doses administered for breakthrough pain. Often a pump with *patient-controlled epidural analgesia (PCEA)* capabilities is used for this mode of operation. This is similar to patient-controlled analgesia (detailed later) in which a basal rate may or may not be used to meet the client's anticipated analgesic need, and the client has the ability to request an incremental dose at set intervals by pressing a button. PCEA is often used to manage acute postoperative pain, chronic pain, and intractable cancer pain. The "walking epidurals" used for women in labor are typically PCEA devices that are programmed in the bolus mode without a continuous infusion (basal rate) set.

The anesthesiologist or nurse anesthetist inserts a needle into the intrathecal or epidural space (typically in the lumbar region) and threads a catheter through the needle to the desired level. The catheter is connected to tubing that is then positioned along the spine and over the client's shoulder for the nurse to access. The entire catheter and tubing are taped securely to prevent dislodgment. Often an occlusive, transparent dressing is placed over the insertion site for easy identification of catheter displacement or local inflammation. Temporary catheters, used for short-term acute pain management, are usually placed at the lumbar or thoracic vertebral level and often removed after 2 to 4 days. Permanent catheters, for clients with chronic pain, may be tunneled subcutaneously through the skin and exit at the client's side or be connected to a pump implanted in the abdomen. Tunneling of the catheter reduces the risk of infection and displacement of the catheter. After the catheter is inserted, the nurse is responsible for monitoring the infusion and assessing the client per institutional policy. Nursing care of clients with intraspinal infusions is summarized in Table 9–6.

Misconceptions about spinal analgesia do exist. They often involve either overstating or ignoring the risks of spinal analgesia. This is due in part to the importance of the technique of the professional inserting the catheter, which varies considerably. In general, clients receiving epidural analgesia do not need to be monitored in an intensive care setting, but they do need vigilant assessment of their pain, neurologic and respiratory status, and the insertion site frequently during the course of therapy (Pasero & McCaffery, 2011).

CONTINUOUS LOCAL ANESTHETICS

Continuous subcutaneous administration of long-acting local anesthetics into or near the surgical site is a technique being used to provide postoperative pain control. This technique has been used for a variety of surgical procedures, including knee arthroplasty, abdominal hysterectomy, hernia repair, and mastectomy. Nursing interventions for the client with infusion of a continuous local anesthetic include the following:

- Conduct pain assessment and documentation every 2 to 4 hours while the client is awake.
- Check the dressing every shift to ensure it is intact. The dressing is not usually changed in order to avoid dislodging the catheter. Contact the primary care provider if the dressing becomes loose.
- Check the site of the catheter. It should be clean and dry.

TABLE 9–6	Nursing Interventions for Clients Receiving Analgesics Through an Epidural Catheter	
Nursing Goals	**Interventions**
Maintain client safety.	Label the tubing, the infusion bag, and the front of the pump with tape marked EPIDURAL to prevent confusion with similar-looking IV lines (most epidural tubing is yellow for this reason). Post a sign above the client's bed indicating an epidural is in place. Secure all connections with tape. If there is no continuous infusion, apply tape over all injection ports on the epidural line to avoid the injection of substances intended for IV administration into the epidural catheter. Do not use alcohol in any care of the catheter or insertion site because it can be neurotoxic. Ensure that any solution injected or infused intraspinally is sterile, preservative free, and safe for intraspinal administration.
Maintain catheter placement.	Secure temporary catheters with tape. When bolus doses are used, gently aspirate prior to medication administration to determine that the catheter has not migrated into the subarachnoid space. (Expect less than 1 mL of fluid return in syringe.) Assist the client in repositioning or moving out of bed. Teach the client to avoid tugging on the catheter. Assess the insertion site for leakage with each bolus dose or at least every 8–12 h.
Prevent infection.	Use strict aseptic techniques with all epidural-related procedures. Maintain sterile occlusive dressing over the insertion site. Assess the insertion site for signs of infection.
Maintain urinary and bowel function.	Monitor intake and output. Assess for bowel and bladder distention.
Prevent respiratory depression.	Assess sedation level and respiratory status q1h for the first 24 h and thereafter q4h. Do not administer other opioids or CNS depressants unless ordered. Keep an ampule of naloxone hydrochloride (0.4 mg) at the bedside. Notify the clinician in charge if the respiratory rate falls below 8 per minute or if the client is difficult to rouse.

- Assess the client for signs of local anesthetic toxicity (e.g., cardiac arrhythmias; dizziness; ringing in the ears; a metallic taste; tingling or numbness of the lips, gums, or tongue) or neurologic deficit distal to the catheter insertion site.
- Notify the primary care provider of signs of local anesthetic toxicity or neurologic deficit. If detected early, prompt treatment can be initiated and serious complications avoided.

Patient-Controlled Analgesia

Patient-controlled analgesia (PCA) is an interactive method of pain management that permits clients to treat their pain by self-administering doses of analgesics. The IV route is the most common in an acute care setting. Its use for postoperative pain has been well documented. It is also helpful when oral pain management is not possible. The PCA mode of therapy minimizes the roller-coaster effect of peaks of sedation and valleys of pain that occur with the traditional method of prn dosing. With the parenteral routes, the client administers a predetermined dose of an opioid by an electronic infusion pump. This allows the client to maintain a more constant level of relief yet requires less medication for pain relief. PCA can be effectively used for clients with acute pain related to a surgical incision, traumatic injury, or labor and delivery, and for chronic pain as with cancer.

The prescriber orders the analgesic, dose, demand (bolus) dose interval, and lockout interval. Standardized medications and order sets are recommended. The most commonly used opioids for PCA are morphine, hydromorphone (Dilaudid), and fentanyl. Meperidine (Demerol) is no longer recommended for PCA use because of toxic CNS effects (e.g., seizures) when administered by continuous infusion (D'Arcy, 2011; Pasero & McCaffery, 2011). Whether in an acute hospital setting, an ambulatory clinic, or with home care, the nurse is responsible for the initial instruction regarding use of the PCA. To avoid incorrect pump programming, two registered nurses should double-check the initial settings and for any changes in dose or medication and both should document this on the medical record (Pasero & McCaffery, 2011). The nurse also is responsible for ongoing monitoring of the therapy (i.e., checking at least once every 2 to 4 hours). The client's pain level, respiratory rate, sedation level, ability to understand, and use of the device must be assessed at regular intervals. Postoperative clients may also have oxygen levels or carbon dioxide levels monitored. Some PCA pumps have an in-line capnography system that monitors carbon dioxide levels while the PCA is being used (D'Arcy, 2011). Analgesic use is documented in the client's record. The most significant adverse effects are respiratory depression and hypotension; however, they occur rarely.

Although PCA pumps vary in design, they all have similar protective features. The line of the PCA pump, a syringe-type pump, is usually introduced into the injection port of a primary IV fluid line (Figure 9–6 ■). The primary care provider determines the drug concentration (amount of drug per milliliter of solution), the PCA bolus dose (amount of medication the client will receive when a bolus is self-administered), and the lockout, which is also called the delay interval (the amount of time that must pass between PCA doses). When clients need a dose of analgesic, they can push a button attached to the infusion pump and the preset dose (bolus) is delivered. The lockout interval is usually set at 6 or 8 minutes for postoperative clients. This means that clients can give themselves a dose of medication every 6 or 8 minutes. Even if the client pushes the button more frequently,

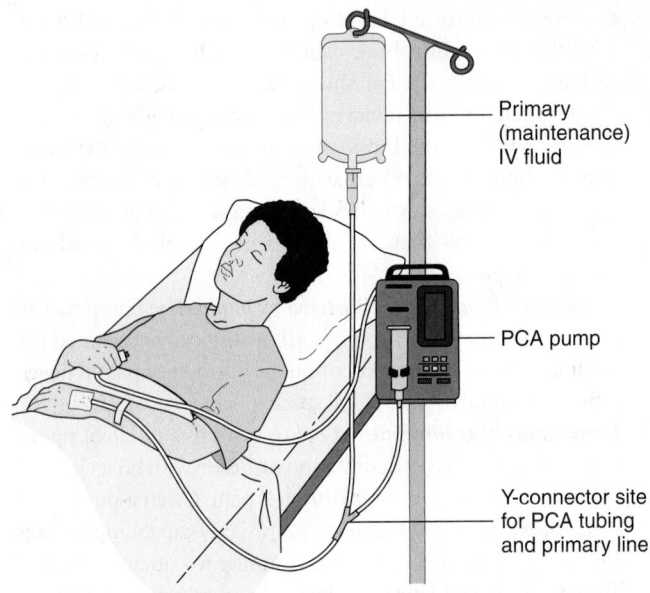

Figure 9–6 ■ PCA line introduced into the injection port of a primary IV line.

he or she will receive only one bolus during the lockout interval. The hour interval is set at either 1 or 4 hours (depending on agency policy). The primary care provider can also prescribe an hour interval, which is the maximum amount of opioid a client can receive in an hour-limit time period. Most PCA pumps can be programmed for a 1- or 4-hour limit. The 1-hour limit is preferable because it allows for closer PCA monitoring by the nurse; that is, the nurse is alerted earlier if the client is not receiving adequate analgesia and requires an increase in opioid dose (Pasero & McCaffery, 2011). Many pumps are capable of delivering a basal rate (continuous infusion), with or without additional PCA doses administered by the client. This practice, however, is no longer recommended for opioid-naïve clients because of the risk of oversedation. It is more appropriate, if not necessary, for the postoperative client who is an opioid-tolerant client with chronic pain. This client, when NPO, may need to have his or her usual daily opioid oral medication dose changed to PCA delivery postoperatively (D'Arcy, 2011, p. 213).

As PCA use has increased, so have errors and other problems, such as adverse (untoward, undesirable, and usually unanticipated) events. Problems that reduce PCA safety include improper client selection, pump problems, programming errors, and PCA by proxy.

Clients who use PCA must be able to understand how to use PCA and be able to physically push the button independently. Clients who are not good candidates for PCA include infants and young children, older clients who are confused, individuals who are obese or have asthma or sleep apnea, and clients taking other drugs that potentiate opioids, such as muscle relaxants.

Improperly programming the PCA pump is the most common human error (Pasero & McCaffery, 2011). Examples of such errors include confusing milliliters and milligrams, making decimal point errors (i.e., order is for 0.5 mg and the pump is programmed for 5 mg), using the loading dose for the bolus dose, and setting the lockout function incorrectly. To increase safety upon PCA initiation, many institutions now require that two nurses independently check client ID, drug and concentration, and PCA pump settings.

PCA by proxy is a term that describes activation of the PCA pump by *anyone other than the client* (Cooney et al., 2013). For example, a well-intentioned family member pushes the button when the client is sleeping or already sedated and causes oversedation. A natural safety feature of PCA is that clients who are sleeping or sedated will not push the button and overmedicate themselves. That is why it is important for the client to be the only one who pushes the button. To counteract this, some institutions put signs on the PCA pump stating "Only the client to push PCA button."

The ASPMN differentiates between PCA by proxy (unauthorized activation of the pump) and authorized agent-controlled analgesia (AACA). AACA is a method of pain control in which a consistently available and competent individual is authorized by a prescriber and properly educated to push the PCA button when the client is unable, and in response to the client's pain (Cooney et al., 2013, p. 178). *Nurse-controlled analgesia (NCA)* is the term used when the authorized person is the nurse responsible for the client. The term is *caregiver-controlled analgesia (CCA)* when a nonprofessional individual (e.g., parent, significant other) is the authorized person. AACA is not appropriate if the client is determined to be able to use PCA.

●○● NURSING PROCESS: PATIENT-CONTROLLED ANALGESIA PUMP

Managing Pain with a PCA Pump

SKILL 9-2

ASSESSMENT
Assess
- Pain (intensity, location, presence of radiation, associated factors, precipitating factors, and alleviating factors).
- Client's allergies.
- Baseline vital signs.
- Client's understanding of the purpose and function of the PCA pump.

- Inspect and palpate the IV insertion site for signs of infection, infiltration, or a dislocated catheter.
- Inspect the surrounding skin for redness, pallor, or swelling.
- Palpate the surrounding tissues for coldness and the presence of edema, which could indicate leakage of the IV fluid into the tissues.

PLANNING
Adequate time for client teaching must be allowed. A planned approach for teaching this skill is essential.

DELEGATION

Initiating and maintaining a PCA pump requires application of nursing knowledge, aseptic technique, critical thinking, and administration of a controlled substance and, therefore, is not delegated to UAP. The nurse can inform UAP of the intended therapeutic effects and specific side effects of the medication and direct UAP to report specific client observations (e.g., unrelieved pain) to the nurse for follow-up. UAP must not administer a dose (push the button) for the client.

Equipment
- PCA pump and appropriate tubing
- Operational manual for specific pump to be used
- Alcohol swab

IMPLEMENTATION
Preparation
- Before initiating PCA therapy, determine factors that may contra-indicate use (e.g., impaired mental status, impaired respiratory status), the amount of narcotic specified by the order, bolus and continuous infusion dosage parameters, and type of primary fluid. Calculate:
  - The initial bolus dose based on the number of milligrams of drug per milliliter of fluid.
  - The dose per intermittent bolus delivery.
  - The 1- or 4-hour lockout drug limit.
- Check the medication administration record (MAR).
  - Check the label on the medication carefully against the MAR to make sure that the correct medication is being prepared.
- Organize the equipment.

Performance
1. Prior to performing the procedure, introduce self and verify the client's identity using agency protocol. Explain the purpose and operation of the PCA.
2. Perform hand hygiene and observe other appropriate infection prevention procedures.

3. Provide for client privacy.
4. Prepare the client.
   - If not previously assessed, take the baseline vital signs. If any of the findings are above or below the predetermined parameters, consult the primary care provider before administering the medication.
5. Set up the PCA infusion line according to the manufacturer's instructions.
   - Attach a needleless adapter to the end of the PCA tubing.
   - Prime the PCA tubing.
   - Clamp the tubing. **Rationale:** *This prevents accidental bolusing and flushing of the primary line with the opioid.*
   - Place the medication syringe in the PCA machine according to the operational instructions.
6. Connect the PCA infusion line to the primary fluid line.
   - Cleanse the injection port of the primary IV with an alcohol swab.
   - Connect the PCA tubing to the primary fluid line at the injection port closest to the client.

Continued on page 264

SKILL 9-2

Managing Pain with a PCA Pump—*continued*

7. Deliver the loading dose, as prescribed.
   • Set the pump for a lockout time of zero minutes.
   • Set the volume to be delivered based on calculated dosage volume for the loading dose.
   • Inject the loading dose by pressing the loading dose control button.
8. Set the safety parameters for the infusion on the PCA pump according to the manufacturer's instructions. For example:
   • *Dose volume limits.* **Rationale:** *This will limit the amount of drug that the client can receive when the client pushes the control button.*
   • *Lockout interval between each dose.* The lockout interval is generally between 5 and 15 minutes. **Rationale:** *This sets the minimum time that must elapse before the client can receive another dose of the drug. Lockout time is based on the usual onset of the IV narcotic and the assessment of the client.*
   • *Dosage limit.* Set the dosage limit (usually 1 or 4 hours) as specified on the orders. **Rationale:** *This is an additional safety feature to limit the amount of medication delivered.*

9. Lock the machine.
   • Close the door on the pump.
   • Look for any digital cues or alarms that may indicate the machine is not set, and make corrections as needed.
   • Lock the machine with the key.
10. Begin the infusion.
    • Place the client control button within reach.
11. Monitor the client.
    • Monitor the status of the client every 2 hours during the first 24 to 36 hours of infusion and regularly thereafter, depending on the client's health and agency protocol.
12. Monitor the infusion.
    • Observe the IV site for signs of infiltration and phlebitis.
    • Inspect the tubing for kinks that may occlude the line.
    • Note the total number of doses and milligrams received.
13. Document all relevant information.
    • Record the initiation of PCA, the dose setting, the doses received, pain intensity, and all assessments. See agency protocol for specific guidelines.

EVALUATION
• Conduct appropriate follow-up:
  • Pain status
  • Respiratory rate and character
  • Amount of medication used
  • Frequency of use
• Relate to previous findings, if available.
• Report significant deviations from normal to the primary care provider.

LIFESPAN CONSIDERATIONS PCA Pump

CHILDREN
• Include the parents in teaching.
• Assess the child's ability to understand and use the client control button. Pasero and McCaffery (2011) report that "PCA has been used effectively and safely in developmentally normal children as young as 4 years old" (p. 314).
• Use distraction techniques to avoid dislodging or disconnection by the child.
• Use pediatric elbow immobilizers (no-nos, Snuggle Wraps) if distraction is not effective in keeping the child from playing with tubing and ports.

OLDER ADULTS
• Carefully monitor for drug side effects.
• Use cautiously for individuals with impaired pulmonary or renal function.
• Assess the client's cognitive and physical ability to use the client control button.

CLIENT TEACHING CONSIDERATIONS

Client Self-Management of Pain

Choose a time to teach the client about pain management when the pain is controlled so that the client is able to focus on the teaching. Teaching the client about self-management of pain can include the following:

• Demonstrate the operation of the PCA pump and explain that the client can safely push the button without fear of overmedicating. Sometimes it helps clients who are reluctant to repeatedly push the button to know that they must dose themselves (i.e., push the button) 5 to 10 times to receive the same amount of medication (10 mg morphine equivalent) they would receive in a standard "shot."
• Describe the use of the pain scale and encourage the client to respond in order to demonstrate understanding.
• Explore a variety of nonpharmacologic pain relief techniques that the client is willing to learn and use to promote pain relief and optimize functioning.
• Explain to the client the need to notify staff when ambulation is desired (e.g., for bathroom use) if applicable.

Ambulatory and Community Settings Safety

PCA Pump
• Monitor for signs and symptoms of oversedation such as excessive drowsiness, slowed respiratory rate, or change in mental state.

• Do not adjust settings without consulting with the appropriate primary care provider.
• Tape to the back of the pump the following emergency contact numbers: emergency medical services, primary care provider, home care agency, and pump manufacturer.

Nonpharmacologic Pain Management

Nonpharmacologic pain management consists of a variety of physical, cognitive–behavioral, and lifestyle pain management strategies that target the body, mind, spirit, and social interactions (Table 9–7).

TABLE 9–7	Nonpharmacologic Interventions for Pain Control

Target Domain of Pain Control	Intervention
Body	Reducing pain triggers, promoting comfort Deep, slow breathing Massage Applying heat or ice Electric stimulation (TENS) Positioning, bracing (selective immobilization) Acupressure Diet, nutritional supplements Exercise, pacing activities Invasive interventions (e.g., blocks) Sleep hygiene
Mind	Relaxation, imagery Self-hypnosis Pain diary, journal writing Distracting attention Repatterning thinking Attitude adjustment Reducing fear, anxiety, stress Reducing sadness, helplessness Information about pain
Spirit	Music therapy Prayer, meditation Self-reflection regarding life and pain Meaningful rituals Energy work (e.g., therapeutic touch, Reiki) Spiritual healing
Social interactions	Functional restoration Improved communication Family therapy Pet therapy Problem solving Vocational training Volunteering Support groups

Physical modalities include cutaneous stimulation, ice or heat, immobilization or therapeutic exercises, transcutaneous electrical nerve stimulation, and acupuncture. Mind–body (cognitive–behavioral) interventions include distracting activities, relaxation techniques and imagery (see Skills 9–5 and 9–6), meditation, biofeedback, hypnosis, cognitive reframing, emotional counseling, prayer and spiritual activities, and energy-directed approaches such as therapeutic touch or Reiki. Lifestyle management approaches include symptom monitoring, stress management, exercise, nutrition, disability management, counseling, and attention to quality of relationships, to name a few. All of these approaches are necessary for clients with chronic pain, and can significantly improve perception of pain and quality of life.

PHYSICAL INTERVENTIONS

The goals of physical intervention include providing comfort, altering physiological responses to reduce pain perception, and optimizing functioning. **Cutaneous stimulation** can provide effective temporary pain relief. It distracts the client by focusing attention on tactile stimuli and away from the painful sensations, thus reducing pain perception. Selected cutaneous stimulation techniques include:

1. *Massage.* Varying styles and degrees of pressure are used, including lymphatic, Swedish (see Skill 9–4), Thai, craniosacral, deep tissue, ice massage, and hot stones.
2. *Application of heat and cold.* Includes warm baths, heating pads, ice bags, hot or cold compresses, and warm or cold sitz baths (see Chapter 8 ∞).
3. **Acupressure.** Based on the ancient Chinese system of acupuncture, this technique uses the fingers to apply pressure to specific points along meridians throughout the body.
4. *Contralateral stimulation.* This technique is the application of any of the above cutaneous modalities to the exact location on the opposite side of the body.

Additional physical approaches to pain management include immobilizing a painful body part through bracing with splints and supportive devices, and **transcutaneous electrical nerve stimulation (TENS)**. See Table 9–8 for additional information regarding nonpharmacologic physical interventions. Skill 9–3 describes how to manage a TENS unit.

TABLE 9–8	Nonpharmacologic Physical Interventions

Physical Intervention	Comments
Cutaneous stimulation techniques:	Can provide effective temporary pain relief. They distract the client and focus attention on the tactile stimuli, away from the painful sensations, thus reducing pain perception.
• Massage	A comfort measure that can aid relaxation, decrease muscle tension, and possibly ease anxiety.
• Heat and cold applications	A warm bath, heating pads, ice bags, ice massage, hot or cold compresses, and warm or cold sitz baths in general relieve pain and promote healing of injured tissues.
• Acupressure	A form of healing in which the therapist exerts finger pressure on specific sites. According to the theory underlying acupressure, 657 designated points can be massaged. These points are similar to those used in acupuncture and shiatsu massage.
• Contralateral stimulation	Stimulating the skin in an area opposite to the painful area (e.g., stimulating the left knee if the pain is in the right knee). The contralateral area may be scratched for itching, massaged for cramps, or treated with cold packs or analgesic ointments. This method is useful when the painful area cannot be touched because it is hypersensitive, when the painful area is inaccessible because of the presence of a cast or bandages, or when the pain is felt in a missing part (phantom pain).
• Immobilization	Immobilizing or restricting the movement of a painful body part may help to manage episodes of acute pain. Splints or supportive devices should hold joints in the position of optimal function and should be removed regularly to provide range-of-motion exercises.

TRANSCUTANEOUS ELECTRICAL NERVE STIMULATION

TENS is a method of applying low-voltage electrical stimulation directly over identified pain areas, at an acupressure point, along peripheral nerve areas that innervate the pain area, or along the spinal column. The TENS unit consists of a portable, battery-operated device with lead wires and electrode pads that are applied to the chosen area of skin (Figure 9–7 ■). The purposes of a TENS unit are to (1) reduce chronic and acute pain, (2) decrease opioid requirements and reduce the chances of depressed respiratory function from opioid usage, and (3) facilitate client involvement in managing pain control. The use of TENS is contraindicated for clients with pacemakers or arrhythmias, or in areas of skin breakdown. It is generally not used on the head or over the chest.

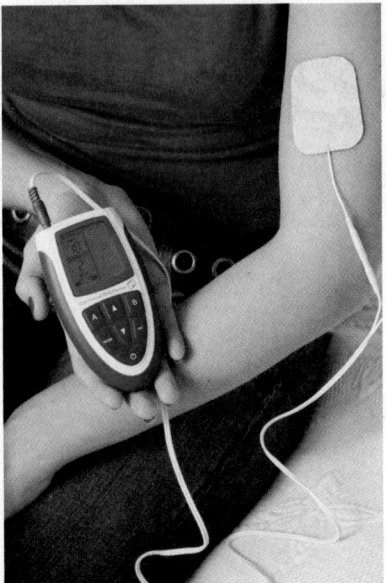

Figure 9–7 ■ A transcutaneous electrical nerve stimulator (TENS).
Hilary Morgan/Alamy

●○● NURSING PROCESS: TRANSCUTANEOUS ELECTRICAL NERVE STIMULATION

Managing a TENS Unit

SKILL 9-3

ASSESSMENT
Assess:
- Client's mental status and ability to follow instructions in using the TENS unit.
- Intactness of skin and absence of signs of infection and irritation.
- Appearance of incisional area of postoperative client.
- Characteristics of pain (intensity, location, associated factors, precipitating factors, and alleviating factors).
- Amount of pain medication required before and during treatment.

PLANNING
Before applying a TENS unit, determine the presence of factors contraindicating usage, such as the presence of a cardiac pacemaker, history of dysrhythmias, myocardial ischemia, myocardial infarction, first-trimester pregnancy, confusion, or history of peripheral vascular problems altering neurosensory perception.

DELEGATION

The assessment for and application of a TENS unit requires specialized knowledge and problem solving. It is important that the nurse understand how this method of pain management works. In an acute care health setting, the nurse would not delegate the skill of managing a TENS unit to UAP. A TENS unit is often ordered for home use, and the nurse is responsible for teaching the client or caregiver how to safely and effectively use the device.

Equipment
- TENS unit
- Bath basin with warm water
- Soap
- Washcloth
- Towel
- Conduction cream, gel, or water (see manufacturer's instructions)
- Hypoallergenic tape

IMPLEMENTATION
Performance
1. Prior to performing the procedure, introduce self and verify the client's identity using agency protocol. Explain to the client what you are going to do, why it is necessary, and how he or she can participate. The TENS unit may not completely eliminate pain but should reduce pain to a level that allows the client to rest more comfortably and/or carry out everyday activities.
2. Perform hand hygiene and observe other appropriate infection prevention procedures.
3. Provide for client privacy.
4. Prepare the equipment.
   - Insert the battery into the TENS unit to test its functioning.
   - With the TENS unit off, plug the lead wires into the battery-operated unit at one end, leaving the electrodes at the other end.

Managing a TENS Unit—*continued*

5. Clean the application area.
   * Wash, rinse, and dry the designated area with soap and water. **Rationale:** *This reduces skin irritation and facilitates adhesion of the electrodes to the skin for a longer period of time.*
6. Apply the electrodes to the client.
   * If the electrodes are not pre-gelled, moisten them with a small amount of water or apply conducting gel. (Consult the manufacturer's instructions.) **Rationale:** *This facilitates electrical conduction.*
   * Place the electrodes on a clean, unbroken skin area. Choose the area according to the location, nature, and origin of the pain.
   * Ensure that the electrodes make full surface contact with the skin. Tape all sides evenly with hypoallergenic tape. **Rationale:** *This prevents an inadvertent burn.*
7. Turn the unit on.
   * Ascertain that the amplitude control is set at level 0.
   * Slowly increase the intensity of the stimulus (amplitude) until the client notes a slight increase in discomfort.
   * When the client notes discomfort, slowly decrease the amplitude until the client notes a pleasant sensation. Once this has been achieved, keep the TENS unit set at this level to maintain blockage of the pain sensation. Most clients select frequencies between 60 and 100 Hz.
8. Monitor the client.
   * If the client complains of itching, pricking, or burning, explore the following options:
     a. Turn the pulse-width dial down.
     b. Check that the entire electrode surface is in contact with the skin.
     c. Increase the distance between the electrodes.
     d. Select another type of electrode suitable for the model of TENS unit in use.
     e. Discontinue the TENS and consider the possibility of another brand of TENS.
   * If the sensation of the stimulus is unpleasant, too intense, or distracting, turn down both the amplitude and the pulse-width dial.
   * If the client complains of headache or nausea during application or use, turn down both the amplitude and the

pulse-width dial. Repositioning of the electrodes may also be helpful.
   * If further troubleshooting is not effective, discontinue the use of the TENS unit and notify the primary care provider.
9. After the treatment:
   * Turn off the controls and unplug the lead wires from the control box.
   * Clean the electrodes according to the manufacturer's instructions. Clean the client's skin with soap and water.
   * Replace the used battery pack with a charged battery. Begin recharging the used battery.
   * If continuous therapy is used, remove the electrode patches and inspect the skin at least once daily.
10. Provide client teaching.
   * Review instructions for use with the client and verify that the client understands.
   * Have the client demonstrate the use of the TENS unit and verbalize ways to troubleshoot if headache, nausea, or unpleasant sensations occur.
   * Instruct the client not to submerge the unit in water but instead to remove and reapply it after bathing.
11. Document all relevant information.
   * Record the date and time TENS therapy was initiated, the location of electrode placement and status of skin in that area, the character and quality of the pain, settings of TENS unit used, and side effects experienced and the client's response.

SAMPLE DOCUMENTATION

7/30/2015 1100 Reports sharp pain in right hip that radiates down back of right leg. Rates pain at 3/10, and achieves some relief with positional changes that take weight off hip. TENS applied over lateral aspect of right hip at 70 Hertz. —————— M. Johnstone, RN

7/30/2015 1110 Reports nausea. Frequency reduced to 60 Hertz; states nausea resolved. —————— M. Johnstone, RN

7/30/2015 1140 TENS discontinued. Rates pain at 0–1/10. No report of nausea. Skin intact. —————— M. Johnstone, RN

EVALUATION

* Perform a follow-up assessment of the client to determine pain relief or side effects experienced.
* Relate findings to previous assessment data if available.
* Report significant deviations from normal to the primary care provider.

Ambulatory and Community Settings **TENS Unit**

PATIENT-CENTERED CARE

TENS units are frequently ordered for home use to relieve chronic pain. Instruct the client or caregiver on:
* How to use and care for the TENS equipment.
* How to troubleshoot if side effects or problems occur and who to call if the equipment malfunctions.
* Where and how to obtain supplies needed for the TENS unit.
* How to remove the electrodes daily and check for skin breakdown at the electrode sites.

MASSAGE

Massage is a comfort measure that can aid relaxation, promote circulation of blood and lymph, decrease muscle tension, and may ease anxiety because the physical contact communicates caring. By increasing superficial circulation as well as neurologic distraction, pain intensity can be directly reduced as a result of massage. The use of creams, oils, aromatherapy, or liniments may amplify therapeutic potential. Massage is contraindicated in areas of skin breakdown, suspected clots, or infections.

Ironically, nurses in acute care settings seldom use this basic nursing skill. The intensity of the acute care environment and the time demands of high-technology nursing may be contributing factors leading to the disappearance of the back massage. Nurses, however, need to reconsider this simple, effective, traditional skill when research indicates the positive client outcomes. Skill 9–4 provides guidelines for giving a back massage.

Providing a Back Massage

ASSESSMENT

- Assess behaviors indicating potential need for a back massage, such as a complaint of stiffness, muscle tension in the back or shoulders, or difficulty sleeping related to tenseness or anxiety.
- Determine if the client is willing to have a massage, because some individuals may not enjoy a massage.

- Assess for contraindications to back massage (e.g., coagulation issues, clots, impaired skin integrity, back surgery, vertebral issues, risk of fracture).

PLANNING

Ensure that you have the full amount of time available for the massage. Although the actual skill may require only about 5 minutes, the entire process should be conducted in a calm and unhurried manner.

Equipment

- Lotion
- Towel for excess lotion

DELEGATION

The nurse can delegate this skill to UAP; however, the nurse should first assess for UAP's comfort and ability, any contraindications, and client willingness to participate.

IMPLEMENTATION

Preparation

Determine (a) previous assessments of the skin, (b) special lotions to be used, and (c) positions contraindicated for the client. Arrange for a quiet environment with no interruptions to promote maximum effect of the back massage.

Performance

1. Prior to performing the procedure, introduce self and verify the client's identity using agency protocol. Explain to the client what you are going to do, why it is necessary, and how he or she can participate. Encourage the client to give you feedback as to the amount of pressure you are using during the back rub.
2. Perform hand hygiene and observe other appropriate infection prevention procedures.
3. Provide for client privacy.
4. Prepare the client.
   - Assist the client to move to the near side of the bed within your reach and adjust the bed to a comfortable working height. **Rationale:** *This prevents back strain.*
   - Establish which position the client prefers. The prone position is recommended for a back rub. The side-lying position can be used if a client cannot assume the prone position.
   - Expose the back from the shoulders to the inferior sacral area. Cover the remainder of the body. **Rationale:** *This prevents chilling and minimizes exposure.*
5. Massage the back.
   - Pour a small amount of lotion onto the palms of your hands and hold it for a minute. The lotion bottle can also be placed in a bath basin filled with warm water. **Rationale:** *Back rub preparations tend to feel uncomfortably cold to people. Warming the solution facilitates client comfort.*
   - Using your palm, begin in the sacral area using smooth, circular strokes.
   - Move your hands up the center of the back and then over both scapulae.
   - Massage in a circular motion over the scapulae.
   - Move your hands down the sides of the back.
   - Massage the areas over the right and left iliac crests. Massage the back in an orderly pattern using a variety of strokes and appropriate pressure. ❶

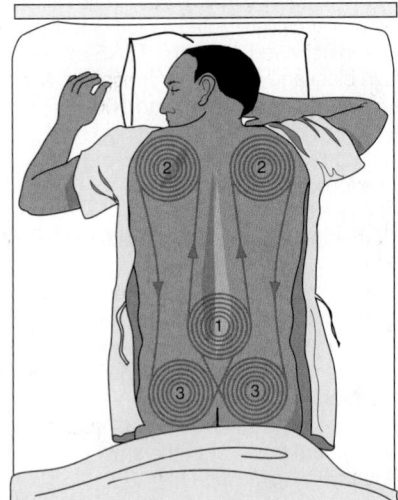

❶ One suggested pattern for a back massage.

   - Apply firm, continuous pressure without breaking contact with the client's skin.
   - Repeat above for 3 to 5 minutes, obtaining more lotion as necessary.
   - While massaging the back, assess for skin redness and areas of decreased circulation.
   - Pat dry any excess lotion with a towel.
6. Document that a back massage was performed and the client's response. Record any unusual findings.

SAMPLE DOCUMENTATION

6/22/2015 1400 Reports aching, intermittent back pain. Wincing and grimacing when attempting to move in bed. Rates pain at 4–5 on 0–10 scale. States uses massage to help relieve pain when at home. Back massaged. Stated the massage helped him "to relax." Lights dimmed and door to room closed. ———————— M. Black, RN
1430 Rates pain at 1–2/10. States feels "much more comfortable." Moving in bed with ease. ———————— M. Black, RN

EVALUATION

Compare the client's current response to his or her previous response. Is there a positive client outcome such as increased relaxation and decrease in pain and anxiety as a result of the back massage?

COGNITIVE–BEHAVIORAL PAIN MANAGEMENT STRATEGIES

Mind–body (cognitive–behavioral) interventions include distraction activities, relaxation techniques, imagery, meditation, biofeedback, hypnosis, counseling, peer support groups, and therapeutic touch. Incorporating these as part of a comprehensive approach to pain management is essential and can give those who experience pain a sense of control and involvement in their own care.

Whereas pharmacologic interventions aim at the pain itself, cognitive–behavioral modalities aim at reducing the resistance to pain, thus reducing suffering. The goals of cognitive–behavioral interventions include providing comfort, altering psychological responses to reduce pain perception, and optimizing functioning. Selected cognitive–behavioral interventions include distraction, eliciting the relaxation response, repatterning unhelpful thinking, facilitating coping with emotions, and spiritual interventions.

DISTRACTION   Distraction draws the person's attention away from the pain and lessens the perception of pain. In some instances, distraction can make a client completely unaware of pain. Distraction makes the person unaware of the pain only for the amount of time and to the extent that the distracting activity holds his or her "undivided" attention. For example, a client recovering from surgery may feel no pain while watching a football game on television, yet feel pain again during commercials or when the game is over. Different types of distraction are shown in Box 9–11. Using multiple forms of distraction simultaneously adds value to the activity. For example, listening to music can be distracting; however, value can be added by tapping to the music, singing along, or playing along on a musical instrument. Play therapy can be a distraction for children.

ELICITING THE RELAXATION RESPONSE   Stress increases pain, in part by increasing muscle tension, activating the sympathetic nervous system, and putting the client at risk for stress-related types of pain (e.g., tension headaches). The relaxation response decreases and counteracts the harmful effects of stress, including the effect it has on physical, cognitive, and emotional functioning. Producing this response requires more than simply helping a client relax; rather it involves a structured technique designed to focus the mind and relax muscle groups. Basic techniques with helpful scripts are available for common techniques including progressive relaxation, breath-focus relaxation, and meditation. The nurse can coach the client, urge self-directed meditation, or provide an audiotaped guide to help elicit the relaxation response. Many clients can achieve the desired state after a few attempts, but mastery of this skill requires daily practice over a few weeks. In general, relaxation techniques by themselves do not have remarkable pain-relieving properties; however, they can reduce pain that may have been exacerbated by stress. Some clients may become more consciously aware of their pain while practicing relaxation techniques before they have learned mastery of controlling "mind chatter" and remaining mentally focused.

Once the client has mastered the basic skills for eliciting the relaxation response, techniques of imagery or self-hypnosis can be used. Both imagery and hypnosis begin with attaining a deep state of relaxation and are capable of altering the experience of pain; for example, having the client replace the pain with a feeling of pleasant numbness. Additional post-hypnotic suggestions can then be made, linking these pleasant numb sensations to coping efforts used during

---

BOX 9–11   Types of Distraction

VISUAL DISTRACTION
- Reading or watching TV
- Video and computer games (also tactile)
- Blowing bubbles (also tactile)
- Watching a baseball game
- Guided imagery

AUDITORY DISTRACTION
- Humor
- Music

TACTILE DISTRACTION
- Slow, rhythmic breathing
- Massage
- Needlework such as knitting, embroidery, cross-stitch (also intellectual)
- Holding or stroking a pet or toy

INTELLECTUAL DISTRACTION
- Crossword puzzles, Sudoku number puzzles
- Card games
- Hobbies

---

the day (e.g., "every time you stop to take a slow, deep, diaphragmatic breath, you will feel this pleasant numbness instead of pain").

Music therapy can also be useful for providing relaxation and distraction from pain (D'Arcy, 2011). With iPods and portable CD players, clients can listen to their favorite tunes as a helpful distraction.

REPATTERNING UNHELPFUL THINKING   Some people harbor strong self-doubts, unrealistic expectations (e.g., "I just want someone to make the pain go away"), rumination (e.g., "I keep thinking about my pain and the person who did this to me"), helplessness (e.g., "I can't do anything"), and magnification (e.g., "My life is ruined, I'll never be a good parent because of my pain"). These cognitive patterns have been identified as important contributors to treatment failures, the intensification of pain, disability, and depression. Nurses can help by challenging the truthfulness and helpfulness of these thoughts, and replacing them with realistic and confidence-building ones that are particularly powerful predictors of more effective coping, better clinical outcomes, and improved quality of life.

FACILITATING COPING   Nurses can help by intervening with clients who are anxious, are sad, or express overly pessimistic or helpless points of view. Awareness of the client's misperceptions or unrealistic expectations also helps the professional avoid a common cause of therapeutic failure. Therapeutic communication with an emphasis on listening, providing encouragement, teaching self-management skills, sharing vicarious experiences, and persuading clients to act on their own behalf are strategies that enhance coping. Helping clients to better communicate with the professional staff, family members, and friends can also promote coping. Counseling from trained professionals may be indicated for those clients with severe emotional distress, but must be offered to them in a sensitive way that does not convey the notion that the pain is "in their head." Chronic pain support groups have been effective for many clients.

SELECTED SPIRITUAL INTERVENTIONS   The spiritual dimension encompasses a person's innermost concerns and values, including the ascribed purpose, meaning, and driving force in the person's life. It may include rituals that help the individual become part of a community or feel a bond with the universe that is not necessarily religious in nature. For those who express their spirituality in a religious context, it is appropriate to offer prayer, intercessory prayer (being prayed for by others), or access to meaningful rituals. Scriptural readings may provide strength and comfort to clients in pain, and should be offered only when desired by the client. For some clients, a caring presence, attentive listening, and facilitating the process of acceptance can help reduce spiritual distress, whereas other clients benefit from manipulation of energy patterns (e.g., therapeutic touch).

Some clients may view pain as a punishment from God, as illustrated in the Mexican American cultural concept of *castigo* (punishment). For these clients, it could be helpful to provide opportunities to discuss their situation with a culturally aware resource person well versed in theology (e.g., a clergyperson). To hold such beliefs inside without attempting to increase understanding can contribute to pain and suffering.

When using imagery techniques with clients, multisensory input relating to spiritual and religious experiences can be powerfully healing. Seek understanding of the client's needs, preferences, and fears in this area. For some, imagining themselves being held in the loving arms/presence of healing light, God, the mother Mary, Buddha, or some other figure can be very comforting.

When using relaxation breathing techniques with clients, the breath can be viewed as a direct connection with God, and life energy. The word *inspiration* means "to take in the spirit." The image of breathing in the healing spirit, and breathing out the pain, can be calming and empowering. To say to oneself while breathing in, "I am breathing in the healing power of God," and out, "I am releasing my pain as I breathe out," can serve as powerful, faith-based affirmations for cognitive restructuring.

Through improved spiritual insights, individuals with pain can find meaning in what seems incomprehensible and learn to cope with the intolerable. This process often begins by making peace with their past, being spiritually aware in the present, and making a commitment to go forward with life despite the pain (Arnstein, 2010). By shifting awareness from within to external sources of power, pain sufferers can transcend the limits of their pain to find new energy and a renewed sense of purpose.

Skill 9–5, *Teaching Progressive Muscle Relaxation*, and Skill 9–6, *Assisting with Guided Imagery*, provide examples of mind–body interventions. These interventions are relatively easy to use and make use of the powerful relaxation effects of diaphragmatic breathing. They can empower clients and facilitate feelings of hope and creativity in the midst of chronic pain. In general, the more clients and their loved ones know about self-management of their pain, the better they will do.

LIFESPAN CONSIDERATIONS **Pain Management**

INFANT
- Giving an infant, particularly a very-low-birth-weight infant, a water and sucrose solution administered through a pacifier provides some pain reduction during procedures that may be painful, but should not replace anesthetic or analgesic medications when indicated.

CHILD
- Distract the child with toys, books, or pictures.
- Hold the child to console and promote comfort.
- Explore misconceptions about pain and correct in understandable "concrete" terms. Be aware of how your explanations may be misunderstood. For example, telling a child that surgery will not hurt because the child will be "put to sleep" will be very upsetting to a child who knows of an animal that was "put to sleep."
- Children can use their imagination during guided imagery. To use the "pain switch," ask the child to imagine a pain switch

(even give it a color) and tell the child to visualize turning the switch off in the area where there is pain. A "magic glove" or "magic blanket" is an imaginary object that the child applies on areas of the body (e.g., hand, thigh, back, hip) to lessen discomfort.

OLDER ADULTS
- Promote the client's use of pain control measures that have worked in the past for the client.
- Spend time with the client and listen carefully.
- Clarify misconceptions. Encourage independence whenever possible.
- Carefully review the treatment plan to avoid drug–drug, food–drug, or disease–drug interactions.
- Physicians and nurse practitioners with advanced certification in hospice and palliative medicine (HPM) are often members of the interdisciplinary team that work with the client and family to provide the best possible hospice care.

Ambulatory and Community Settings **Pain Management** **PATIENT-CENTERED CARE**

- Teach the client to keep a pain diary to monitor pain onset, activity before pain, pain intensity, use of analgesics or other relief measures, and so on.
- Instruct the client to contact a health care professional if planned pain control measures are ineffective.
- Teach the use of preferred and selected nonpharmacologic techniques such as relaxation, guided imagery, distraction, music therapy, massage, and so on.

- Instruct the client to use pain control measures before the pain becomes severe.
- Inform the client of the effects of untreated pain.
- Provide appropriate information about how to access community resources, home care agencies, and associations that offer self-help groups and educational materials.

●○● NURSING PROCESS: COGNITIVE–BEHAVIORAL PAIN MANAGEMENT STRATEGIES

Teaching Progressive Muscle Relaxation

ASSESSMENT
- Assess the client's willingness to participate in relaxation or imagery exercises. Note the nature and location of any pain.
- Check the client's vital signs, if appropriate.
- Note any signs of stress being exhibited by the client.

PLANNING
Cognitive–behavioral strategies require an uninterrupted period of time, at least 15 minutes. A degree of quiet and privacy is also necessary, because these strategies require the client to concentrate and relax.

DELEGATION
Noninvasive pain management techniques can be delegated to UAP if they have experience using the technique and are comfortable doing so. The nurse is responsible for assessing the client's willingness to participate in the relaxation or imagery exercise. The nurse instructs UAP to report the client's response to the nurse.

Equipment
- A printed relaxation script that an individual can read until the client learns the technique. Many are available online and through stress management resource books and tapes.
- CD player or iPod (optional). The CD or iPod could be used to provide the script for the exercise or for the playing of background music.

IMPLEMENTATION
Preparation
Allow 10 to 15 minutes of uninterrupted time for the session. Ensure that the environment is private, quiet, and at a temperature that suits the client. The client should have an empty bladder. **Rationale:** *Interruptions or distractions interfere with the client's ability to achieve full relaxation. Once clients learn how to use this technique, they will be able to do it in less than 5 minutes as part of self-care and ongoing stress management.*

Performance
1. Prior to performing the procedure, introduce self and verify the client's identity using agency protocol. Explain to the client what you are going to do, why it is necessary, and how he or she can participate.
2. Perform hand hygiene and observe other appropriate infection prevention procedures.
3. Provide for client privacy.
4. Prepare the client:
   - Tell the client how progressive muscle relaxation works.
   - Provide a rationale for the procedure. **Rationale:** *It has been noted that muscular tension accompanies most stress states. By aiming to reduce muscle tension, the negative effects of stress on the mind–body can be lessened.*
   - Ask the client to identify the stressors operating in the client's life and the reactions to these stressors. **Rationale:** *Awareness is important as the client learns how to cope effectively.*
   - Demonstrate the method of tensing and relaxing groups of muscles and have the client do it with you. It is easy to start with making fists—tensing the muscles with 100% effort the first time, and then with only 50% effort the second time. **Rationale:** *Demonstration and initial practice enable the client to understand the progression of muscle relaxation more clearly.*
   - Assist the client to a comfortable position.
5. If music is to be used, select music that is instrumental, calming, neutral, and unfamiliar to the client. **Rationale:** *Music should not be recognizable and should not intentionally elicit memories or emotion. In this way, the music will enhance relaxation. Classical music can sometimes be too "busy" and may evoke memories and emotion that could be distracting for the client.*
   - Ensure that all body parts are supported and the joints slightly flexed with no strain or pull on the muscles (e.g., arms and legs should not be crossed). **Rationale:** *Assuming a position of comfort facilitates relaxation.*
6. Encourage the client to begin slow, deep diaphragmatic or abdominal breathing to rest the mind and begin relaxing the body. Inhaling through the nose and exhaling through the mouth (pursed lips are best) slows down the breath and enhances relaxation.
7. Instruct the client to tense and then relax each group of muscles starting from the head and moving down the body. Use a tone of voice throughout the exercise that invites participation rather than directs.
   - The following script suggestions are just one way of doing the technique:
     a. Take in a deep breath, and close your eyes tightly shut, furrowing your brows and wrinkling your forehead. Hold this contraction with the most effort you can, and then release as you exhale slowly. Again, take a breath and contract these same muscles with half the effort you used last time. Hold, hold, and now release with your breath, feeling the tension leave your body as a soothing wave of relaxation flows over your head and face. . . . You could keep your eyes softly closed throughout this exercise. . . .
     b. You might want to clench your jaw as you breathe in, feeling the muscles in your cheeks and throat and base of your tongue tightening as you hold, hold, and then release. You could repeat this contraction as you inhale, and hold with less tension this time, and then release as you exhale, allowing all of these muscles to soften, allowing your teeth to rest just slightly apart.
     c. Next, pull your shoulders up toward your ears as you take a full and gentle breath in and hold as tightly as you can. Now relax and release your shoulders with your breath, allowing a soothing wave of relaxation to flow into your neck and shoulder area. This time hunch your shoulders up with only half the effort you used last time . . . hold it . . . and release, allowing any tension to run down your arms and through your hands and out the tips of your fingers. . . .
     d. Next, you could inhale and make tight fists of both hands and hold these fists as strongly as you can. Release your fists and your breath. Take another breath in and make fists again, this time with less effort . . . hold . . . and release, allowing tension to leave your hands, being replaced with softness.

Continued on page 272

Teaching Progressive Muscle Relaxation—*continued*

e. Now we can focus on the arms. As you breathe in, think about contracting the muscles of the arms, perhaps making fists again, and feeling the entire length of your arms tightening and flexing. Hold, hold, and release, feeling the tension leaving your arms and flowing out through your hands and fingertips. This time breathe in and tighten your arms with less effort, and then release with your breath, feeling a sense of comfort and peace as the tension leaves you now.

f. You could focus on your abdominal muscles, and pull them in tightly as if to button your navel onto the front of your spine. You may even notice tension in your back muscles, and hold this as tightly as you can. Exhale and release all of these muscles, feeling as if a band of tightness around your midsection is being released. Breathe in and tense this abdominal and low back band of muscles again. Hold more gently this time and then release, exhaling slowly. Enjoy the feelings as your muscles become relaxed and loose.

g. You could inhale deeply and flex your hip and buttock muscles, feeling yourself lift as the muscles contract. Hold, and then release as you exhale. This time, flex these muscles a bit more gently, aware of the peace that is flowing throughout your body as you continue to relax.

h. You could inhale and flex your heels away from your body as you pull your toes hard, hard toward your face. Hold this, feeling your calf and thigh muscles flexing as well, and then release as you exhale. Inhale again and this time press your toes away from your face and feel the tension throughout the entire length of your leg once again. You can repeat this with less effort, and feel the whole body relax and release.

- Encourage the client to breathe slowly and deeply during the entire procedure. **Rationale:** *Quiet, full, slow breathing with an emphasis on prolonged exhalation elicits a parasympathetic response that is the opposite of the fight-or-flight response.*
- Speak in a calm voice that encourages relaxation, and coach the client to mentally focus on each muscle group being addressed. **Rationale:** *By suggesting rather than directing throughout the process, you avoid triggering any underlying control issues in the client.*

8. Ask the client to state whether any tension remains after all muscle groups have been tensed and relaxed.
   - Repeat the procedure for muscle groups that are not relaxed.
9. Terminate the relaxation exercise slowly by counting from 1 to 3, suggesting that the client will feel calm and alert.
   - Ask the client to move the body slowly: first the hands and feet, then arms and legs, and finally the head and neck.
10. Remind the client that this technique can be used any time the client needs to release tension or wants to feel more relaxed.
11. Document the client's response to the exercise.

SAMPLE DOCUMENTATION

7/20/2015 2300 Reports "mild" headache, 1–2/10 on pain scale. Also expressing anxiety about recent diagnosis, and having difficulty falling asleep. Progressive muscle relaxation taught using relaxation music as a background. Participated fully, stated "headache is gone." Asleep when nurse returned with sleep med. Sleep med held. ———————————————— B. Montgomery, RN

EVALUATION

A subjective report of pain (on a scale of 0 to 10) can be used before and after the progressive muscle relaxation session to demonstrate whether the strategy has been helpful in reducing pain. In addition, assessing for associated fear, anxiety, and perceptions of relaxation is also important. Reduction in fear and anxiety levels is desirable, even if the pain experience itself is still the same. Relaxation reduces the resistance to pain, and the degree of suffering is therefore reduced.

Assisting with Guided Imagery

IMPLEMENTATION
Preparation
Allow 10 to 15 minutes for this process. Provide a private, comfortable, quiet environment free of distractions. Ensure thermal comfort and make sure the client has an empty bladder. **Rationale:** *Comfort and freedom from distractions are necessary for the client to relax and focus on the exercise.*

Performance
1. Prior to performing the procedure, introduce self to the client and verify the client's identity using agency protocol. Explain the rationale and benefits of imagery. Ask the client about the goals for the session. Imagery can provide relaxation and feelings of empowerment, lead to creative problem solving, and facilitate healing. The content used will vary depending on the client's goals. Many books, tapes, and CDs are available for those who want to learn more about this powerful technique. **Rationale:** *The client is an active participant in an imagery exercise and can offer direction for the session.*
2. Perform hand hygiene and observe other appropriate infection prevention procedures.

3. Provide for client privacy.
4. Assist the client to a comfortable position.
   - Assist the client to a reclining position and ask the client to close the eyes. **Rationale:** *A position of comfort can enhance the client's focus during the imagery exercise.*
5. Implement actions to induce relaxation.
   - Speak clearly in a calming and neutral tone of voice. **Rationale:** *Positive voice coaching can enhance the effect of imagery. A shrill or loud voice can distract the client from the image.*
   - Ask the client to take slow, full diaphragmatic/abdominal breaths and to relax all muscles. Use progressive muscle relaxation exercises as needed to assist the client to achieve total relaxation (see Skill 9–5).
   - Guide the client through relaxation breathing and then through muscle relaxation. Then begin to guide the client toward a most beautiful or peaceful place. The client may have been to this place before or may be imagining this place. Do not impose your own suggestions as to where they might be. Clients know where they want and need to

SKILL 9-6

Assisting with Guided Imagery—*continued*

go! Slowly guide them to approach and then finally enter the place. Prompt them to use all of their senses as they look around the place, listen to the sounds of the place, feel the air, feel what's underfoot, and smell the fragrances of the place. Have them find and move toward a safe spot where they can rest awhile.

- While clients are in their safe spot, you can assist them to do some work. For example, if they need stress management or pain relief, they can picture themselves (from the safety of this, their very safe spot) in a potentially tense situation. Then have them inhale and exhale slowly three times, saying to themselves "relax, relax, relax" with each exhalation. For internal healing work, encourage the client to focus on a meaningful image of power and to use it to control the specific problem. Or, the client can be educated beforehand to use anatomic and physiological imagery for self-healing. These kinds of goals are facilitated with some prior preparation on the part of the nurse and client, and many resources exist to prepare people for this work. Ask the client to use all the senses when practicing imagery. **Rationale:** *Using all the senses enhances the client's benefit from imagery.* Clients may be asked to assign a color to their pain, and then identify a color signifying "no pain." Then, they can use imagery to change the color of their pain to the "no-pain color."

6. Take the client out of the image by suggesting that it is time for the client to leave this most beautiful and safe place. Suggest that the client can return at any time desired and that breathing will lead the way.
   - Slowly count from 1 to 3, suggesting that the client should come back into the here and now. Tell the client to open the eyes on 3 and that he or she will feel rested and refreshed.
   - Remain until the client is alert. If the client remains in a trancelike state, simply repeat that he or she will wake up on the number 3, and count to 3 again. No harm will occur if you allow the client to remain "asleep," or you can gently touch the client to facilitate awakening.
7. Following the experience, ask the client to describe the physical and emotional feelings elicited by the imagery session. The meanings images have for the individual client can be very helpful in the therapeutic process. Direct the client to explore the response to images because this enables the client to modify the imagery for future sessions.
8. Encourage the client to practice the imagery technique.
   - Imagery is a technique that can be done independently by the client once the client knows how.
9. Document the client's response to the exercise, noting signs of increased relaxation and reduced anxiety.

EVALUATION
- Conduct a follow-up assessment of the client for signs of relaxation and/or decreased pain (e.g., decreased muscle tension; slow, restful breathing; and peaceful affect).

- Determine the client's feelings regarding success or problems with the relaxation skill or the effectiveness of the image selected.
- Relate findings to previous assessment data if available.

Chapter **9** Review

FOCUSING ON CLINICAL THINKING

Consider This
1. You are caring for two clients, both with the diagnosis of low back pain. One client's low back pain resulted from an on-the-job injury yesterday. He lifted a heavy object without using proper body mechanics. The other client's pain has been bothering him for over 12 months, and there is no known cause despite many medical tests. Describe the differences in your nursing assessment, goals, and nursing interventions.
2. You are a home health nurse visiting a client recently diagnosed with cancer. The client has had a great deal of pain lately. You notice that he yawns a lot during your visit and also that his wife is listless and doesn't follow the conversation that you are having with her husband. What assessments would you include for this family?

3. Describe how you would assess pain intensity for each of the following clients who are experiencing pain:
   a. A 4-year-old child
   b. A teenager
   c. A 30-year-old
   d. An 82-year-old with impaired hearing
4. Some clients grew up hearing the slogan, "Just Say No to Drugs." What are the implications, if any, of this statement on effective pain management?

See Focusing on Clinical Thinking answers on student resource website.

TEST YOUR KNOWLEDGE

1. The nurse enters the client's room and sees the client visiting with family members, laughing with them, and watching television. The client informs the nurse that he is in a great deal of pain and believes it is time for his pain medication. How would the nurse document this interaction?
   1. "Client says he is in pain but he is laughing with his visitors and watching TV."
   2. "Client reports pain but he is laughing and watching TV with visitors."
   3. "Client reports pain and requests medication. Client and visitors watching TV and laughing."
   4. "Client reports pain but does not appear to be in any distress. Laughing and watching TV with visitors."

2. The nurse is preparing to administer a full agonist analgesic and recognizes which of the following characteristics for this type of analgesic? Select all that apply.
   1. It should not be administered to clients who are terminally ill.
   2. Its dose can be steadily increased as needed to relieve pain.
   3. There is no maximum daily dose limit.
   4. There is no ceiling on level of analgesia from this drug.
   5. An example of this type of analgesic would include morphine, oxycodone, or hydromorphone.

3. An 86-year-old client is restless and moaning. His daughter states the client did not sleep well during the night and he seems to be confused at times. What is the nurse's first action?
   1. Administer the client's prn analgesic.
   2. Ask the client if he wants a sleeping pill.
   3. Ask the daughter to stay and watch her father in case he becomes more confused.
   4. Determine whether the client can provide a self-report of pain.

4. A client with a history of chronic low back pain has not been able to obtain effective pain management. Which does the nurse see as a barrier to pain management?
   1. The client refuses to take any drug that has the potential to be addictive.
   2. The client has no allergies to medications.
   3. The client has been actively participating in physical therapy.
   4. The client visits the doctor every 3 months.

5. The nurse is caring for a postoperative client who is complaining of pain and requests a nonnarcotic pain reliever. The nurse suggests a narcotic analgesic would be more effective. The client responds by saying she doesn't want to be "doped up" when her family comes to visit and will take the narcotic after the last family member leaves for the day. Which would be the nurse's best action?
   1. Administer the narcotic analgesic anyway because the nurse knows that would be the best thing for the client.
   2. Administer the nonnarcotic analgesic as requested and meet the family member visiting in the hall to suggest a short visit so the narcotic analgesic can be given sooner.
   3. Administer the nonnarcotic analgesic as requested, instruct the client to call if the pain becomes unmanageable, and reassess the client within 30 minutes.
   4. Explain to the client why she should take the narcotic analgesic and that family visits will be suspended for the day if she insists on the nonnarcotic analgesic.

6. The nurse enters the postoperative client's room to assess the client and finds vital signs are normal, the wound dressing is dry and intact, and the client did not complain of pain. What did this nurse forget? The nurse should have:
   1. Changed the client's bed linen.
   2. Administered an analgesic prophylactically to prevent unmanageable pain.
   3. Gotten the client out of bed and into a chair.
   4. Asked if the client was experiencing any discomfort.

7. The nurse is obtaining a pain history on two clients, one with chronic pain and another with acute pain. Which question is not as significant to ask of the client with acute pain?
   1. "Where is the pain located?"
   2. "On a scale of 1 to 10 with 10 being the worst pain you have ever experienced in your life, how would you rate your current pain?"
   3. "Has the pain kept you from performing any of the things you normally do every day?"
   4. "When did the pain begin?"

8. The nurse is preparing to administer an analgesic to a client with terminal cancer who is experiencing severe pain. Which medication would be the best analgesic for this client?
   1. Morphine
   2. Demerol
   3. Percocet with acetaminophen
   4. Aspirin

9. The nurse is providing preoperative teaching to the client about the use of patient-controlled analgesia (PCA). Which statement by the client informs the nurse that the teaching has been effective?
   1. "I have to be careful not to push the button too often or I will overdose myself."
   2. "Using a PCA will allow me to use more medication and relieve my pain better."
   3. "Using a PCA will allow me to have a more constant level of pain control and I will need less medication."
   4. "When I am asleep my wife can push the button to keep me comfortable."

10. When assessing a client's pain following a motor vehicle crash, the nurse learns that the client has some discomfort but would prefer not to take medication prior to her child's visit. Which would be an appropriate nursing action to increase the client's comfort level?
    1. Assist the client to get out of bed and into the bedside chair.
    2. Assist the client to control her breathing.
    3. Administer morphine sulfate IV push.
    4. Cancel visiting hours so the client may practice guided imagery.

See Answers to Test Your Knowledge in Appendix A.

READINGS AND REFERENCES

References

Arnstein, P. (2010). *Clinical coach for effective pain management.* Philadelphia, PA: F.A. Davis.

Arnstein, P., Broglio, K., Wuhrman, E., & Kean, M. B. (2011). Use of placebos in pain management. *Pain Management Nursing, 12,* 225–229. doi:10.1016/j.pmn.2010.10.033

Chapman, S. (2010). Managing pain in the older person. *Nursing Standard, 25*(11), 35–39. doi:10.7748/ns2010 .11.25.11.35.c8103

Cooney, M. F., Czarnecki, M., Dunwoody, C., Eksterowixz, N., Merkel, S., Oakes, L., & Wuhrman, E. (2013). American Society for Pain Management nursing position statement with clinical practice guidelines: Authorized agent controlled analgesia. *Pain Management Nursing, 14,* 176–181. doi:10.1016/j.pmn.2013.07.003

D'Arcy, Y. (2011). *Compact clinical guide to acute pain management: An evidence-based approach for nurses.* New York, NY: Springer.

Drew, D., Gordon, D., Renner, L., Morgan, B., Swensen, H., & Manworren, R. (2014). The use of "as-needed" range orders for opioid analgesics in the management of pain: A consensus statement of the American Society of Pain Management Nurses and the American Pain Society. *Pain Management Nursing, 15*(2), 551–554. doi:10.1016/ j.pmn.2014.03.001

Dunn, D. (2012). Controlling pain: How substance abuse impacts pain management in acute care. *Nursing, 42*(8), 66–68. doi:10.1097/01.NURSE.0000414643.35700.1b

Herdman, T. H., & Kamitsuru, S. (Eds.). (2014). *NANDA International Nursing Diagnoses: Definitions & Classification, 2015–2017.* Oxford, United Kingdom: Wiley-Blackwell.

Herr, K., Coyne, P. J., McCaffery, M., Manworren, R., & Merkel, S. (2011). Pain assessment in the patient unable to self-report: Position statement with clinical practice recommendations. *Pain Management Nursing, 12,* 230–250. doi:10.1016/j.pmn.2011.10.002

International Association for the Study of Pain. (2012). *IASP taxonomy.* Retrieved from http://www.iasp-pain.org/ Education/Content.aspx?ItemNumber=1698

International Headache Society. (n.d.). *IHS classification ICHD-II.* Retrieved from http://ihs-classification.org/en

Leung, L. (2012). From ladder to platform: A new concept for pain management. *Journal of Primary Health Care, 4*(3), 254–258.

Liberto, L. A., & Fornili, K. S. (2013). Managing pain in opioid-dependent patients in general hospital settings. *MEDSURG Nursing, 22*(1), 33–37.

Mayo Clinic. (2012). *Fentanyl (transdermal route).* Retrieved from http://www.mayoclinic.com/health/drug-information/ DR601815/DSECTION=proper-use

Miller, S. M. (2011). Pain assessment in nonverbal older adults with advanced dementia. *Journal of Nurse Practitioners, 7*(9), 781–782. doi:10.1016/j.nurpra.2011.08.014

Narayan, M. C. (2010). Culture's effects on pain assessment and management. *American Journal of Nursing, 110*(4), 38–47. doi:10.1097/01.NAJ.0000370157.33223.6d

Oliver, J., Coggins, C., Compton, P., Hagan, S., Matteliano, D., Stanton, M., . . . Turner, H. N. (2012). American Society for Pain Management nursing position statement: Pain management in patients with substance use disorders. *Pain Management Nursing, 13,* 169–183. doi:10.1016/ j.pmn.2012.07.001

Pasero, C., & McCaffery, M. (2011). *Pain assessment and pharmacologic management.* St. Louis, MO: Mosby Elsevier.

Purnell, L. D. (2013). *Transcultural health care: A culturally competent approach* (4th ed.). Philadelphia, PA: F.A. Davis.

Rosier, P. K. (2012). Controlling pain: Facing up to the challenge of range orders. *Nursing, 42*(12), 64–65.

Stuart, B., Cherry, C., & Stuart, J. (2011). *Pocket guide to culturally sensitive health care.* Philadelphia, PA: F.A. Davis.

Tabloski, P. A. & Connell, W. F. (2014). *Gerontological nursing* (3rd ed.). Upper Saddle River, NJ: Pearson.

Vargas-Schaffer, G. (2010). Is the WHO analgesic ladder still valid? *Canadian Family Physician, 56*(6), 514–517.

Wong-Baker FACES® Foundation. (1983). *Wong-Baker FACES® pain rating scale.* www.WongBakerFACES.org.

Zeppetella, G. (2011). The WHO analgesic ladder: 25 years on. *British Journal of Nursing, 20*(17), S4–S6.

Selected Bibliography

Arnstein, P., & Herr, K. (2013). Risk evaluation and mitigation strategies for older adults with persistent pain. *Journal of Gerontological Nursing, 39*(4), 56–65. doi:10.3928/00989134-20130221-01

Berman, A., Snyder, S., & Frandsen, G. (2016). *Kozier & Erb's fundamentals of nursing. Concepts, process, and practice* (10th ed.). Upper Saddle River, NJ: Pearson.

D'Arcy, Y. (2010). Managing chronic pain in acute care: Getting it right. *Nursing, 40*(4), 49–51.

Duke, G., Haas, B. K., Yarbrough, S., & Northam, S. (2013). Pain management knowledge and attitudes of baccalaureate nursing students and faculty. *Pain Management Nursing, 14,* 11–19. doi:10.1016/j.pmn.2010.03.006

Jarzyna, D., Jungquist, C. R., Pasero, C., Willens, J. S., Nisbet, A., Oakes, L., . . . Polomano, R. C. (2011). American Society for Pain Management nursing guidelines on monitoring for opioid-induced sedation and respiratory depression. *Pain Management Nursing, 12,* 118–145. doi:10.1016/j.pmn.2011.06.008

Marchand, S. (2012). *The phenomenon of pain.* Seattle, WA: International Association for the Study of Pain.

Reynolds, J., Drew, D., & Dunwoody, C. (2013). American Society for Pain Management nursing position statement: Pain management at the end of life. *Pain Management Nursing, 14,* 172–175. doi:10.1016/j.pmn.2013.07.002

Rose, L., Haslam, L., Dale, C., Knechtel, L., & McGillion, M. (2013). Behavioral pain assessment tool for critically ill adults unable to self-report pain. *American Journal of Critical Care, 22,* 246–254. doi:10.4037/ajcc2013200

Schatman, M. E. (2011). The role of the health insurance industry in perpetuating suboptimal pain management. *Pain Medicine, 12,* 415–426. doi:10.1111/j.1526-4637 .2011.01061.x

Willens, J. S., Jungquist, C. R., Cohen, A., & Polomano, R. (2013). ASPMN survey—Nurses' practice patterns related to monitoring and preventing respiratory depression. *Pain Management Nursing, 14,* 60–65. doi:10.1016/ j.pmn.2013.01.002

3

Applying the Nursing Process

This unit looks at comfort and hygiene skills including bathing, bed-making, infection control, heat and cold applications, and pain management. Comfort and hygiene needs are highly personal, and the nurse must consider the client's wishes, culture, and unique requirements when planning and providing care. The client should be involved as much as possible in both decision making and care delivery to increase his or her well-being and autonomy.

CLIENT: Juan   AGE: 42 Years   Current Medical Diagnosis: Fractured Left Femur and Left Ulna

Medical History: Juan fell asleep while driving home from his night shift job and was involved in a collision with another vehicle. He fractured his left femur, requiring placement of pins and traction. He also fractured his left ulna which was casted with a synthetic cast following closed reduction surgery. He has multiple abrasions and lacerations. A laceration above his left ear required sutures and has become infected with a methicillin-resistant *Staphylococcus aureus* (MRSA) infection. He was placed on contact precautions. Juan has an infusing IV with a patient-controlled analgesia (PCA) pump for pain management in his right arm via a percutaneous intravenous central catheter (PICC).

Personal and Social History: Juan lives with his wife in a three-story townhouse in the suburbs of a major city. He works the night shift in a department store. His wife is a high school chemistry teacher. She is 18 weeks pregnant with their first child. The parents and siblings of both Juan and his wife live within a 30-mile radius of their home. As a result, Juan has many visitors including family, friends, and coworkers.

Questions

Assessment

1. The nurse is assessing Juan for pain, which he ranks as a 6 on a 0–10 scale. What other information will the nurse assess?
2. The nurse offers Juan a back rub to help him relax as a nonpharmacologic pain management technique. What assessments will the nurse perform while providing the back rub?

Analysis

3. List two possible nursing diagnoses that can be identified from the medical/personal history and assessment data above.

Planning

4. The nurse plans care for Juan to include applications of ice to his fractured left arm to manage pain and edema. What expected outcomes would the nurse include in the plan of care related to this intervention?

5. Juan tells the nurse he usually showers every day and washes his hair in the shower. The nurse, developing his plan of care, includes interventions to shampoo his hair three times a week. For what outcomes would the nurse have associated this intervention?

Implementation

6. The nurse initiates contact isolation for Juan to reduce the risk of spreading MRSA. Describe the components of contact isolation to be used for this client.
7. What type of client hygiene interventions would the nurse include in Juan's plan of care?

Evaluation

8. Describe the steps to take if the outcomes have not been met or have been only partially met.

See Applying the Nursing Process suggested answers on student resource website.

Mobility and Safety

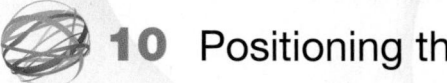
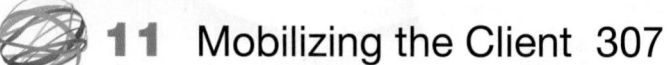
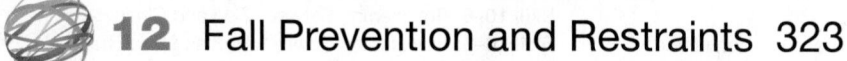
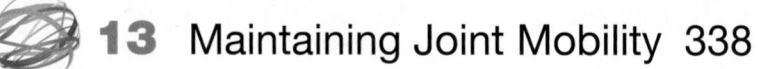

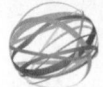 # 10 Positioning the Client

LEARNING OUTCOMES

At the completion of this chapter, the student will be able to:

1. Define the key terms used in body mechanics and the skills of positioning clients.
2. Identify essential guidelines for safe and efficient body movements.
3. Describe the limits of body mechanics regarding nurse and client safety.
4. Demonstrate how to effectively support and maintain proper alignment of clients for the described bed positions included in this chapter.
5. Recognize when it is appropriate to delegate positioning of clients to unlicensed assistive personnel.
6. Verbalize the steps used in:
   a. Supporting the client's position in bed.
   b. Moving a client up in bed.
   c. Turning a client to the lateral or prone position in bed.
   d. Logrolling a client.
   e. Assisting the client to sit on the side of the bed.
   f. Transferring between bed and chair.
   g. Transferring between bed and stretcher.
   h. Using a mobile floor-based hydraulic lift.
7. List indications and contraindications for assistive devices when lifting and transferring clients.
8. Demonstrate appropriate documentation and reporting of positioning skills.

SKILLS

KEY TERMS

In this chapter, readers will be given essential guidelines for safe and efficient strategies for assisting clients to move and change positions. The use of assistive equipment, adequate numbers of staff, and proper body alignment of nurse and client are discussed. Skills for assisting clients into various positions, turning clients in bed, and transferring clients from a bed to a chair or stretcher are included. During all positional changes, the comfort and dignity of clients must be protected. Ensure modesty by preventing improper exposure throughout the positional change. Protect dignity by giving careful and complete instructions, not rushing, encouraging clients to help themselves as much as possible, and using a caring tone of voice and eye contact.

BODY MECHANICS

Body mechanics is the term used to describe the efficient, coordinated, and safe use of the body to move objects and carry out the activities of daily living. Until recently, nurses believed that "correct"

body mechanics would facilitate the safe and efficient use of appropriate muscle groups to maintain balance, reduce the energy required, reduce fatigue, and decrease the risk of injury for both nurses and clients, especially during transferring, lifting, and repositioning. In reality, more than 30 years of evidence indicate the following:

- Educating nurses in body mechanics alone will not prevent job-related injuries.
- Back belts have not been shown to be effective in reducing back injury.
- Nurses who are physically fit are at no less risk of injury. Research has shown that physical fitness may *increase* the risk of injury because of being asked to help others four times more often (American Nurses Association [ANA], n.d.).
- The widely accepted National Institute for Occupational Safety and Health (NIOSH) "lifting equation," which recommended that workers observe a limit of 51 pounds of lifting, *cannot* be safely applied to nursing practice.

- The long-term benefits of using the proper equipment (e.g., mechanical lifts) far outweigh the costs related to injuries.
- Staff will use equipment when they have participated in the decision-making process for purchasing the equipment

In the field of nursing, work-related musculoskeletal disorders (MSDs), such as back and shoulder injuries, persist as the leading and most costly U.S. occupational health problem. In fact, during 2011, workers in the health care/social assistance workplace suffered a higher rate of MSDs than construction, mining, or manufacturing workers (Bureau of Labor Statistics, 2013). Moreover, 62% of 4,614 nurses who responded to a 2011 ANA health and safety survey reported that one of their top concerns was disabling musculoskeletal injury. Eight out of 10 said that musculoskeletal pain was a frequent occurrence and that they continued to work despite the pain (ANA, 2011). Manually moving and lifting clients often cause MSDs. Increasingly, health care facilities are focusing on "no lift" policies for their employees, and 35 pounds of client weight should be the maximum a nurse should attempt. This limit should be further reduced if the health care worker is lifting in a restricted space, sitting or kneeling, twisting, one-handed, or with arms extended; if working longer than 8 hours; or if the client is combative, cannot follow direction, or has physical or medical conditions that impact his or her being lifted or moved (ANA, 2013, p.13). If the weight to be lifted exceeds 35 pounds or the other conditions exist, assistive devices should be used. These devices include floor-based and ceiling-mounted lifts, slings, sit-to-stand devices, sliding boards, friction-reducing devices, transfer sheets or power-assist air-cushioned mattresses, and lateral transfer and transport chairs.

The ANA has been involved in the effort to protect nurses from MSDs for many years and has taken the official position of supporting actions and policies that result in the elimination of manual handling of clients in order to establish a safe environment for nurses and clients. Safe patient handling and mobility (SPHM) programs can greatly reduce health care worker injuries. Prompted by ANA's Handle with Care Campaign that started in 2003, 11 states have enacted "safe patient handling" laws related to the implementation of SPHM programs. However, there is no consistency among these 11 states. For example, one state requires replacing manual lifting with lifting devices and another state requires health care facilities to develop a comprehensive safe patient handling plan (ANA, n.d.).

Recently, the Centers for Medicare and Medicaid Services (CMS), the Institute of Medicine (IOM), the World Health Organization (WHO), the National Quality Foundation (NQF), and ANA supported the concepts of universal standards and an interdisciplinary approach to SPHM (ANA, 2013). As a result, a workgroup of national subject-matter experts from multiple health care disciplines was formed. Two years later in 2013, this workgroup published *Safe Patient Handling and Mobility Interprofessional National Standards Across the Care Continuum*. The workgroup focused on ensuring that the standards would be helpful and realistic for health care workers in all health care settings and focused on evidence-based outcomes without being prescriptive (ANA, 2013).

These standards are voluntary performance standards to help health care facilities establish policies and procedures. It is the hope, however, that similar to the requirement of universal precautions, the SPHM standards will become required instead of optional ("Safe

lifting," 2013). To this end, ANA is working with congressional bill sponsors in support of national legislation.

Until all work settings provide safe environments in which nurses have the equipment they need, content pertaining to body mechanics will be included here. Readers are encouraged to support "no manual lift" and "no solo lift" policies in their workplaces, and to become involved in legislation and equipment purchase initiatives. Nurses must participate in this shift in safety awareness, and are encouraged to support the SPHM standards of the ANA and to keep abreast of congressional action on bills to enforce safer client handling.

SAFETY ALERT! | SAFETY

Because safe manual client lifting applies only to weights of less than 35 pounds, many children should be lifted using technology. This is an issue in hospitals, in pediatric home care, and also in school nursing. Many children with special needs attend public schools and may need to be moved and lifted during the school day to meet their medical requirements.

Elements of Body Movement

Body movement requires coordinated muscle activity and neurologic integration. It involves the basic elements of body alignment (posture), balance, and coordinated movement.

BODY ALIGNMENT AND POSTURE

Proper body **alignment** and posture bring body parts into position in a manner that promotes optimal balance and maximal body function whether the client is standing, sitting, or lying down. Good body alignment and good **posture** are synonymous terms. When the body is well aligned, strain on the joints, muscles, tendons, or ligaments is minimized and internal structures and organs are supported.

BALANCE

Balance is a state of equilibrium in which opposing forces counteract each other. Good body alignment is essential to body balance. It is difficult to differentiate balance from body alignment, although, as mentioned above, balance is the result of proper alignment. A person maintains balance as long as the **line of gravity** (an imaginary vertical line drawn through an object's center of gravity) passes through the **center of gravity** (the point at which all of the mass of an object is centered) and the **base of support** (the foundation on which an object rests).

The usual line of gravity begins at the top of the head and falls between the shoulders, through the trunk, slightly anterior to the sacrum, and between the weight-bearing joints and base of support (Figure 10–1 ■).

In a well-aligned standing person, the center of gravity remains fairly stable. When a person moves, however, the center of gravity shifts continuously in the direction of the moving body parts. Balance depends on the interrelationship of the center of gravity, the line of gravity, and the base of support. When a person moves, the closer the line of gravity is to the center of the base of support, the greater the person's stability (Figure 10–2 A ■).

Conversely, the closer the line of gravity is to the edge of the base of support, the more precarious the balance (Figure 10–2 B). If

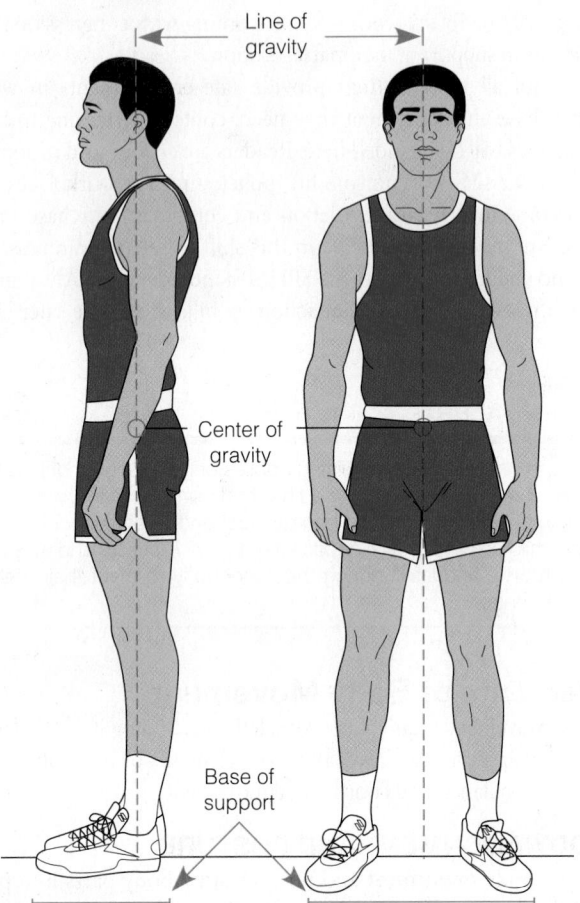

Figure 10–1 ■ The center of gravity and the line of gravity influence standing alignment.

therefore, can be greatly enhanced by (a) widening the base of support and (b) lowering the center of gravity, bringing it closer to the base of support. The base of support is easily widened by spreading the feet farther apart. The center of gravity is readily lowered by flexing the hips and knees until a squatting position is achieved. The importance of these alterations cannot be overemphasized for nurses.

COORDINATED BODY MOVEMENT

Body mechanics involves the integrated functioning of the musculoskeletal and nervous systems. Muscle tone, joint mobility, the neuromuscular reflexes, and the coordinated movements of opposing voluntary muscle groups play important roles in producing balanced, smooth, purposeful movement.

Principles of Body Mechanics

Elements of body mechanics as they apply to lifting, pulling, pushing, and pivoting are important for nurses to know. However, body mechanics alone is not enough to protect the nurse from the heavy weight, awkward postures, and repetition involved in manual handling. Safe client handling and movement requires use of assistive devices and equipment.

LIFTING

It is important to remember that nurses should *not* lift more than 35 pounds without assistance from proper equipment and/or other individuals. Types of assistive equipment include mobile powered or mechanical lifts, ceiling-mounted lifts, sit-to-stand powered lifts, friction-reducing devices, and transfer chairs. See Figures 10–3 ■ through 10–8 ■.

PULLING AND PUSHING

When pulling or pushing an object, a person maintains balance with least effort when the base of support is increased in the direction in

the line of gravity falls outside the base of support, the person falls (Figure 10–2 *C*).

The broader the base of support and the lower the center of gravity, the greater the stability and balance. Body balance,

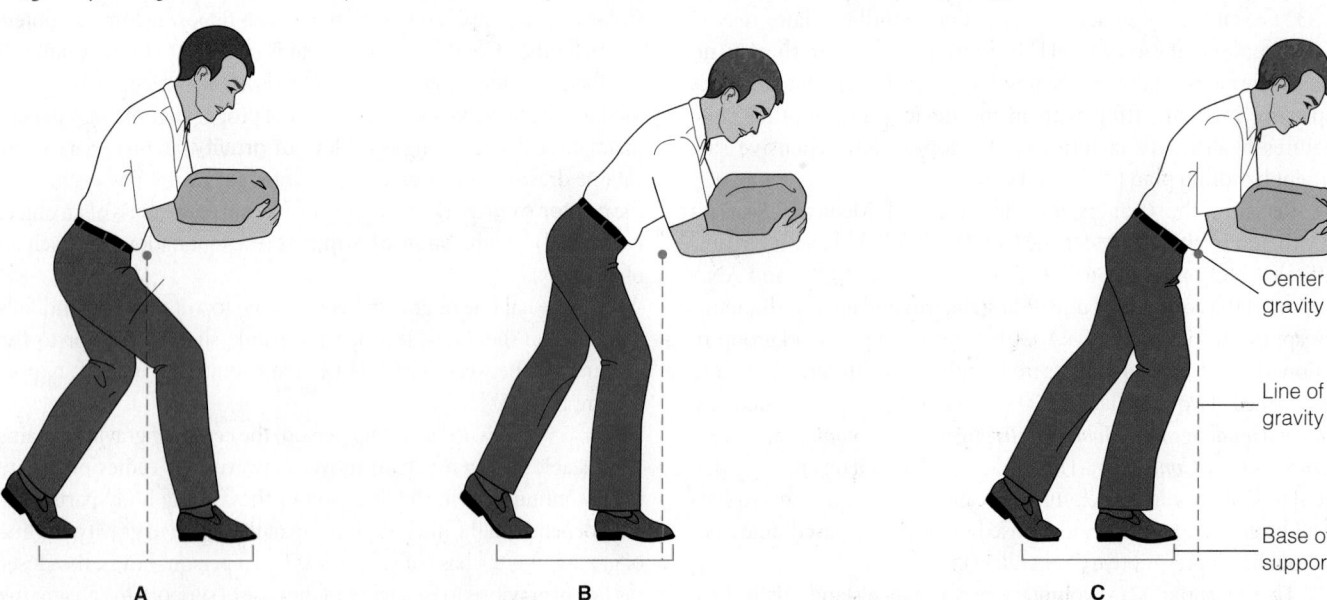

Figure 10–2 ■ *A,* Balance is maintained when the line of gravity falls close to the base of support. *B,* Balance is precarious when the line of gravity falls at the edge of the base of support. *C,* Balance cannot be maintained when the line of gravity falls outside the base of support.

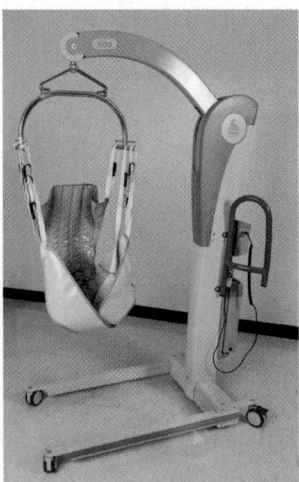

Figure 10–3 ■ A mobile electric lift moves clients from bed, chair, toilet, and floor.

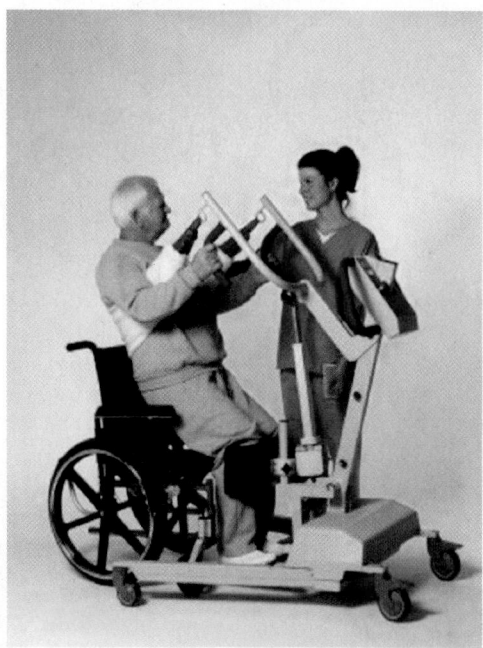

Figure 10–5 ■ A sit-to-stand power lift allows for client transfers from bed to chair. The client must be cognitive and provide some muscle tone in at least one leg and the trunk.
Courtesy of Stryker Instruments/Peterson.

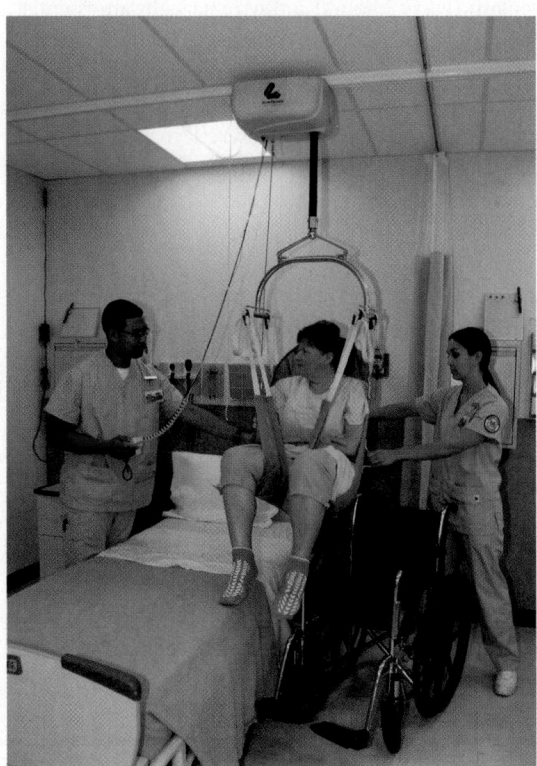

Figure 10–4 ■ A ceiling-mounted lift.

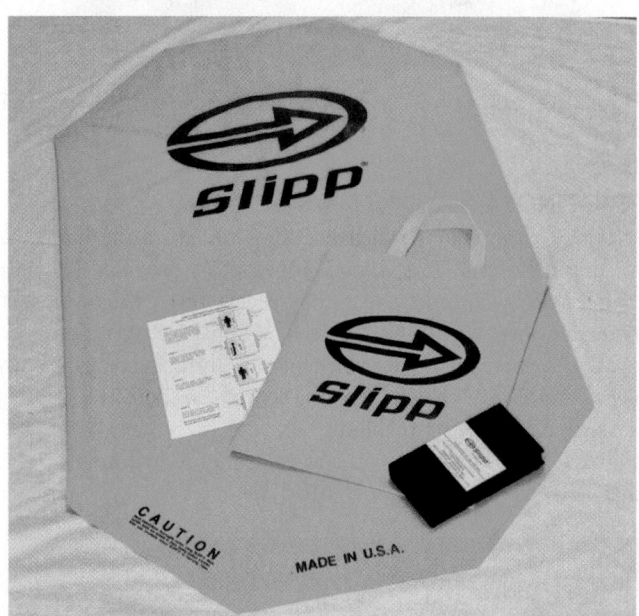

Figure 10–6 ■ The Slipp® Patient Mover is a client-moving device that decreases the nurse's exposure to back injuries and maximizes client comfort.
Courtesy Wright Products, Inc.

which the movement is to be produced or opposed. For example, when pushing an object, a person can increase the base of support by moving the front foot forward. When pulling an object, a person can increase the base of support by (a) moving the rear leg back if the person is facing the object or (b) moving the front foot forward if the person is facing away from the object. It is easier and safer to pull an object toward one's own center of gravity than to push it away, because a person can exert more control of the object's movement when pulling it.

CLINICAL ALERT!

Lateral-assist devices such as horizontal air transfer mattresses and transfer chairs are essential equipment for most client care areas. They help prevent acute and chronic back pain and disability. Observing principles of body mechanics is recommended even when using assistive equipment, because any lifting and forceful movements are potentially injurious, especially when repeated over time.

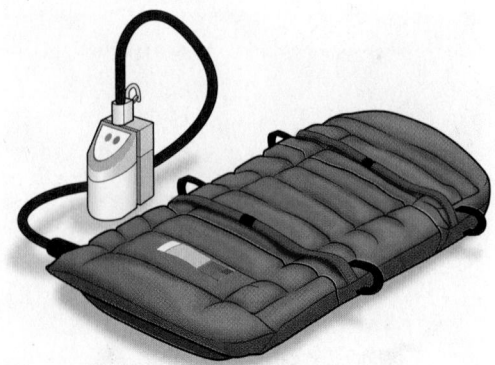

Figure 10–7 ■ An air transfer system. Once inflated, the client can be transferred laterally or repositioned on a frictionless air surface.

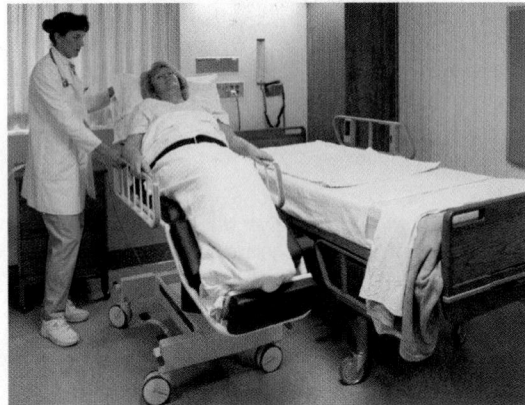

Figure 10–8 ■ Transfer chair that can transfer the client laterally from bed to stretcher without lifting and then can transport the client through the facility in a sitting or reclining position.

PIVOTING

Pivoting is a technique in which the body is turned in a way that avoids twisting of the spine. To **pivot**, place one foot ahead of the other, raise the heels very slightly, and put the body weight on the balls of the feet. When the weight is off the heels, the frictional surface is decreased and the knees are not twisted when the body turns. Keeping the body aligned, turn (pivot) about 90° in the desired direction. The foot that was forward will now be behind.

A summary of principles and guidelines related to body mechanics is in Table 10–1.

Preventing Back Injury

Nurses provide clients with the opportunity to change positions, expand their lungs, or change their environments as appropriate. It is important, however, that nurses not jeopardize their own health while caring for clients. Client positioning, lifting, and transferring are significant risk factors for back injuries. As mentioned earlier, 35 pounds of client weight should be the maximum a nurse should attempt.

Two movements to avoid because of their potential for causing back injury are twisting (rotation) of the thoracolumbar spine and acute flexion of the back with hips and knees straight (stooping). Undesirable twisting of the back can be prevented by squarely facing the direction of movement, whether pushing, pulling, or sliding, and moving the object directly toward or away from one's center of gravity. Guidelines for preventing back injuries are presented in Client Teaching Considerations.

POSITIONING CLIENTS IN BED

Positioning a client in good body alignment and changing the position regularly (every 2 hours) and systematically are essential aspects of nursing practice. Clients who can move easily automatically reposition themselves for comfort. Such clients generally require minimal positioning assistance from nurses, other than guidance about ways to maintain body alignment and to exercise their joints. However, clients who are weak, frail, in pain, paralyzed, or unconscious rely on nurses to provide or assist with position changes. For all clients, it is important to assess the skin and provide skin care before and after a position change.

Any position, correct or incorrect, can be detrimental if maintained for a prolonged period. Frequent position changes help to prevent muscle discomfort, undue pressure resulting in pressure ulcers, damage to superficial nerves and blood vessels, and contractures. A **contracture** is a permanent shortening of the muscle. Position changes also maintain muscle tone and stimulate postural reflexes.

When the client is not able to move independently or assist with moving, *the preferred method is for two or more nurses to move or turn the client using assistive equipment.* Appropriate assistance reduces the risk of muscle strain and body injury to both the client and nurse, and is likely to protect the dignity and comfort of the client.

CLIENT TEACHING CONSIDERATIONS

Preventing Back Injuries

- Understand that the use of body mechanics will not necessarily prevent injury if manually handling a load greater than 35 pounds without the use of assistive devices.
- Avoid lifting anything greater than 35 pounds. Use assistive equipment, get help from coworkers, and participate in the purchasing/ordering process of appropriate assistive equipment for your work setting.
- Become consciously aware of your posture and body mechanics.
- When standing for a period of time, periodically move legs and hips, and flex one hip and knee and rest your foot on an object if possible.
- When sitting, keep your knees slightly higher than your hips.

- Use a firm mattress and soft pillow that provide good body support at natural body curvatures.
- Exercise regularly to maintain overall physical condition and regulate weight; include exercises that strengthen the pelvic, abdominal, and spinal muscles.
- Avoid movements that cause pain or require spinal flexion with straight legs (e.g., toe-touching and sit-ups) or spinal rotation (twisting).
- When moving an object, spread your feet apart to provide a wide base of support.
- Wear comfortable low-heeled shoes that provide good foot support and reduce the risk of slipping, stumbling, or turning your ankle.

TABLE 10–1	Summary of Guidelines and Principles Related to Body Mechanics

Guidelines	Principles
Plan the move or transfer carefully. Free the surrounding area of obstacles.	Appropriate preparation prevents potential falls and injury.
Obtain the assistance of other people or use mechanical devices if the maximum weight for the manual lift exceeds 35 pounds. Encourage clients to assist as much as possible.	The maximum weight that should be lifted by a nurse under ideal conditions (load close to the body and vertical height at waist height) is 35 pounds. This weight limit decreases when the lift is less than ideal (e.g., arms extended).
Adjust the working area to waist level and keep the body close to the area. Put the bed at the correct height (waist level when providing care; hip level when moving a client). Lower the bedside rails to prevent stretching and reaching.	Objects that are close to the center of gravity are moved with the least effort.
Use proper alignment. Stand as close as possible to the object to be moved. Avoid stretching, reaching, and twisting, which may place the line of gravity outside the base of support.	Balance is maintained and muscle strain is avoided as long as the line of gravity passes through the base of support.
Before moving an object, widen your stance and flex your knees, hips, and ankles.	The wider the base of support and the lower the center of gravity, the greater the stability.
Before moving an object, contract your gluteal, abdominal, leg, and arm muscles to prepare them for action.	The greater the preparatory contraction of muscles before moving an object, the less the energy required to move it, and the lower the likelihood of musculoskeletal strain and injury.
Always face the direction of the movement.	Ineffective use of major muscle groups occurs when the spine is rotated or twisted.
Avoid working against gravity. Pull, push, roll, or turn objects instead of lifting them. Lower the head of the client's bed before moving the client up in bed.	Moving an object along a level surface requires less energy than moving an object up an inclined surface or lifting it against the force of gravity. Pulling creates less friction than pushing.
Use your gluteal and leg muscles rather than the sacrospinal muscles of your back to exert an upward thrust when lifting. Distribute the workload between both arms and legs to prevent back strain.	The synchronized use of as many large muscle groups as possible during an activity increases overall strength and prevents muscle fatigue and injury.
When *pushing* an object, enlarge the base of support by moving the front foot forward.	Balance is maintained with minimal effort when the base of support is enlarged in the direction in which the movement will occur.
When *pulling* an object, enlarge the base of support by either moving the rear leg back if facing the object or moving the front foot forward if facing away from the object.	
When moving or carrying objects, hold them as close as possible to your center of gravity.	The closer the line of gravity to the center of the base of support, the greater the stability.
Use the weight of the body as a force for pulling or pushing, by rocking on the feet or leaning forward or backward.	Body weight adds force to counteract the weight of the object and reduces the amount of strain on the arms and back.

When positioning clients in bed, the nurse can do a number of things to ensure proper alignment and promote client comfort and safety:

- Make sure the mattress is firm and level, yet has enough give to fill in and support natural body curvatures.
- Ensure that the bed is kept clean and dry. Wrinkled or damp sheets increase the risk of pressure ulcer formation. Make sure the client's extremities can move freely whenever possible. For example, the top bed linens need to be loose enough for clients to move their feet.
- Place support devices in specified areas according to the client's position. See Box 10–1 for commonly used support devices. Use only those support devices needed to maintain alignment and to prevent stress on the client's muscles and joints. If the client is capable of movement, too many devices limit mobility and increase the potential for muscle weakness and atrophy. Common

alignment problems that can be corrected with support devices include:

Flexion of the neck
Internal rotation of the shoulder
Adduction of the shoulder
Excessive abduction of the arm
Flexion of the wrist
Anterior convexity of the lumbar spine
External rotation of the hips
Hyperextension of the knees
Plantar flexion of the foot

Fowler's Position

Fowler's position, or a semisitting position, is a bed position in which the head and trunk are raised 45° to 60° relative to the bed (visualize a 90° right angle to orient your thinking) and the knees may

BOX 10–1 Support Devices

- *Pillows.* Different sizes are available. Used for support or elevation of an arm or leg. Specially designed dense pillows can be used to elevate the upper body. Pillows can also be used as a trochanter roll by placing the pillow from the client's iliac crest to midthigh. This prevents external rotation of the leg when the client is in a supine position.
- *Mattresses.* There are two types of mattresses: ones that fit on the bed frame (e.g., standard bed mattress) and mattresses that fit on the standard bed mattress (e.g., egg-crate mattress). Mattresses should be evenly supportive.
- *Suspension or heel guard boot.* These are made of a variety of substances. They usually have a firm exterior and padding

of foam to protect the skin. They prevent foot drop and relieve pressure on heels.
- *Footboard.* A flat panel often made of plastic or wood. It keeps the feet in dorsiflexion to prevent plantar flexion.
- *Hand roll.* Can be made by rolling a washcloth. Purpose is to keep hand in a functional position and prevent finger contractures.
- *Abduction pillow.* A triangular-shaped foam pillow that maintains hip abduction to prevent hip dislocation following total hip replacement.

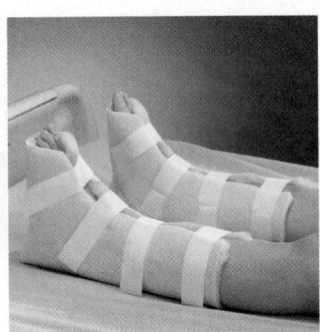
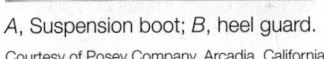
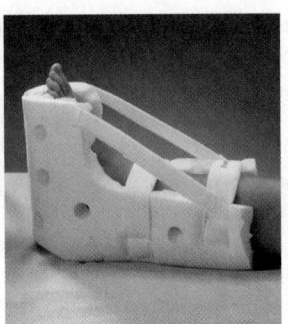

A, Suspension boot; *B*, heel guard.
Courtesy of Posey Company, Arcadia, California.

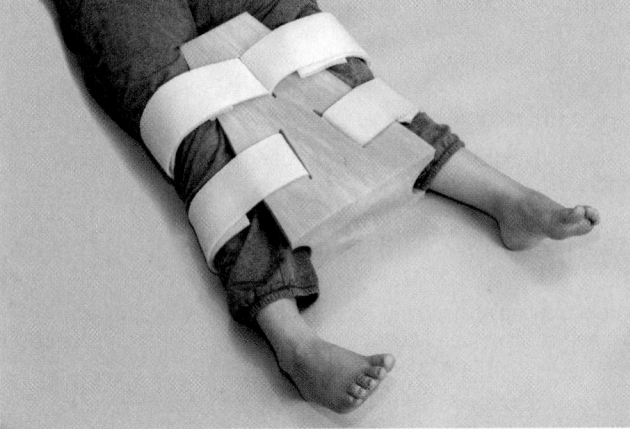

Maintaining postoperative abduction following total hip replacement.

or may not be flexed. Nurses may need to clarify the meaning of the term *Fowler's position* in their particular setting. Typically, Fowler's position refers to a 45° angle of elevation of the upper body.

Semi-Fowler's position is when the head and trunk are raised 15° to 45°. This position is sometimes called low Fowler's, and typically means 30° of elevation. In **high-Fowler's position**, the client's head and torso are raised 60° to 90°, and most often means the client is sitting upright at a right angle to the bed. See Box 10–2 and Skill 10–1 for information about positioning a client in semi-Fowler's position.

Fowler's position is the position of choice for people who have difficulty breathing and for some people with heart problems. Gravity pulls the diaphragm downward, allowing greater lung expansion. Clients who are confined to bed but are capable of eating, reading, watching television, or visiting find this position comfortable.

Orthopneic Position

An adaptation of high-Fowler's position is the **orthopneic position**. The client sits either in bed or on the side of the bed leaning over an overbed table across the lap (Figure 10–9 ■). This position facilitates respiration by allowing maximum chest expansion. It is particularly helpful to clients who have problems exhaling, such as those with chronic obstructive pulmonary disease (COPD), because they can press the lower part of the chest against the edge of the overbed table.

Dorsal Recumbent Position

In the **dorsal recumbent (back-lying) position**, the client's head and shoulders are slightly elevated on a small pillow. In some

agencies, the terms *dorsal recumbent* and *supine* are used interchangeably. Strictly speaking, however, in the supine or dorsal position, the head and shoulders are not elevated. The dorsal recumbent position is used to provide comfort and to facilitate healing following certain surgeries or anesthetics (e.g., spinal). See Box 10–3 and Skill 10–1 for information about positioning a client in dorsal recumbent position.

Prone Position

In the **prone position**, the client lies on his or her abdomen with the head turned to one side. The hips are not flexed. Both children and adults sleep in this position, sometimes with one or both arms flexed over their heads (see figure in Box 10–4).

This position has several advantages. It is the only bed position that allows full extension of the hip and knee joints. When used periodically, the prone position helps to prevent flexion contractures of the hips and knees, thereby counteracting a problem caused by all other bed positions. The prone position also promotes drainage from the mouth and is especially useful for clients recovering from surgery of the mouth or throat.

The prone position poses some distinct disadvantages, especially for the acutely ill client. The pull of gravity on the trunk produces a marked lordosis (forward curvature of the lumbar spine) in most people, and the neck is rotated laterally to a significant degree. For this reason, the prone position may not be recommended for clients with problems of the cervical or lumbar spine. This position also causes plantar flexion. Some clients with cardiac or respiratory

BOX 10–2 Supported Fowler's Positions (Semi and Full)

- *Semi-Fowler's or low Fowler's:* Bed-sitting position with upper part of body elevated 15 to 45° (most typically 30°) commencing at hips.
- *Fowler's:* Bed-sitting position with upper part of body elevated 45° to 60° (most typically 45°) commencing at the hips.

MEASURES TO PROMOTE ALIGNMENT AND COMFORT*
- Pillow at lower back to support lumbar region and prevent posterior flexion of lumbar curvature.
- Pillow to support head, neck, and upper back to prevent hyperextension of neck. Avoid too large a pillow or too many pillows because they may cause neck flexion contractures.

- Pillow under forearms to eliminate pull on shoulder and assist venous blood flow from hands and lower arms.
- Small pillow under thighs to flex knees to prevent hyperextension of knees.
- Trochanter roll or pillow lateral to femur to prevent external rotation of hips.
- Footboard or suspension boot to provide support for dorsiflexion and prevent plantar flexion of feet (foot drop).

* The amount of support depends on the needs of the individual client.

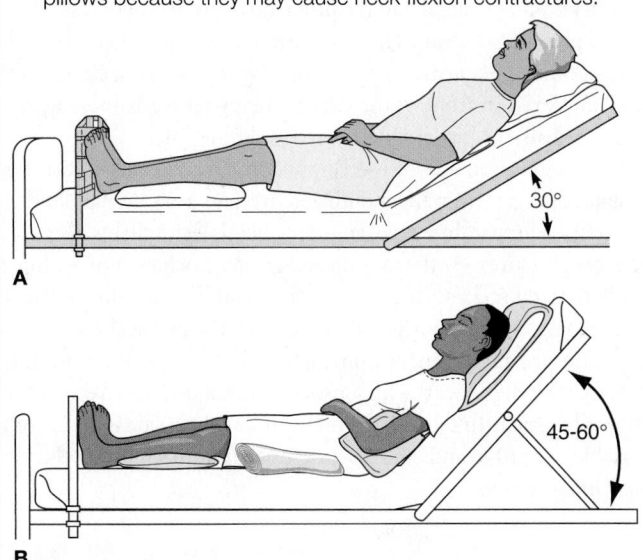

A

B

A, Low Fowler's (semi-Fowler's) position (supported); *B,* Fowler's position (supported). The amount of support depends on the needs of the individual client.

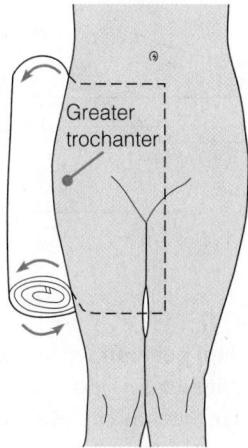

Making a trochanter roll: (1) Fold the towel in half lengthwise. (2) Roll the towel tightly, starting at one narrow edge and rolling within approximately 30 cm (1 ft) of the other edge. (3) Invert the roll. Then palpate the greater trochanter of the femur and place the roll with the center at the level of the greater trochanter; place the flat part of the towel under the client; then roll the towel snugly against the hip.

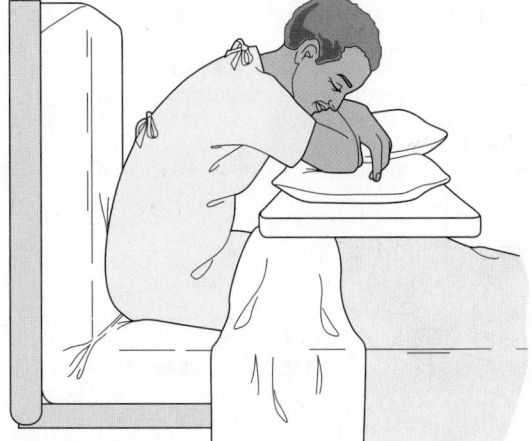

Figure 10–9 ■ Orthopneic position.

problems find the prone position confining and suffocating, because chest expansion is inhibited during respirations. *The prone position should be used only when the client's back is properly aligned, only for short periods, and only for individuals with no evidence of spinal abnormalities.* As a result, this position is not often used. Box 10–4 and Skill 10–1 describe how to support a client in the prone position.

BOX 10–3 Dorsal Recumbent Position (Supported)

MEASURES TO PROMOTE ALIGNMENT AND SUPPORT*
- Pillow of suitable thickness under head and shoulders if necessary for alignment and to prevent hyperextension of neck in thick-chested person.
- Roll or small pillow under lumbar curvature to prevent posterior flexion of lumbar curvature.
- Roll or sandbag placed laterally to trochanter of femur to prevent external rotation of legs.
- Small pillow under thigh to flex knee slightly and prevent hyperextension of knees.
- Footboard, suspension boots, or rolled pillow to support feet in dorsiflexion and to prevent plantar flexion (foot drop).
- Pillow under lower legs to prevent pressure on heels.

* The amount of support depends on the needs of the individual client.

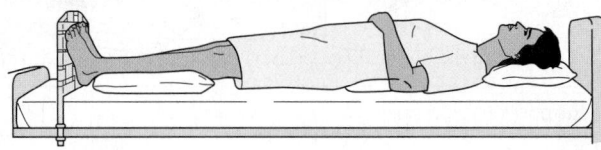

Dorsal recumbent position (supported).

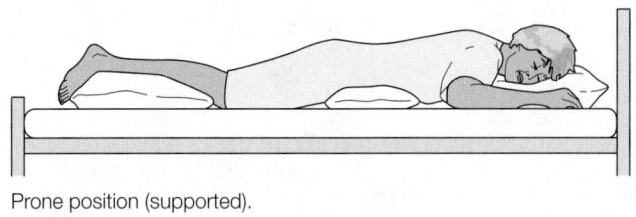

BOX 10–4 Prone Position (Supported)

MEASURES TO PROMOTE ALIGNMENT AND SUPPORT*
- Small pillow under head unless contraindicated because of promotion of mucous drainage from mouth—prevents flexion or hyperextension of neck.
- Small pillow or roll under abdomen just below diaphragm to prevent hyperextension of lumbar curvature; difficulty breathing; pressure on breasts (women); pressure on genitals (men).
- Allow feet to fall naturally over end of mattress or support lower legs on a pillow so that toes do not touch the bed to prevent plantar flexion (foot drop).

*The amount of support depends on the needs of the individual client.

Prone position (supported).

Lateral Position

In the **lateral (side-lying) position**, the client lies on one side of the body (see the figure in Box 10–5). Flexing the top hip and knee and placing this leg in front of the body creates a wider, triangular base of support and achieves greater stability. The greater the flexion of the top hip and knee, the greater the stability and balance in this position. This flexion reduces lordosis and promotes good back alignment. For this reason, the lateral position is good for resting and sleeping clients. The lateral position helps to relieve pressure on the sacrum and heels of clients who sit for much of the day or who are confined

BOX 10–5 Lateral Position (Supported)

MEASURES TO PROMOTE ALIGNMENT AND SUPPORT*
- Pillow under head and neck to provide good alignment and prevent lateral flexion and fatigue of sternocleidomastoid muscles.
- Pillow under upper arm to place it in good alignment; lower arm should be flexed comfortably. Avoids internal rotation and adduction of shoulder that could cause subsequent limited function, and prevents impaired chest expansion.
- Pillow under leg and thigh to place them in good alignment. Check that shoulders and hips are in straight alignment. These measures prevent internal rotation and adduction of femur and twisting of the spine.

*The amount of support depends on the needs of the individual client.

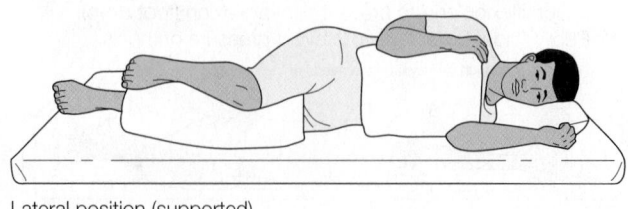

Lateral position (supported).

to bed and rest in the Fowler's or dorsal recumbent position much of the time. In the lateral position, most of the body's weight is borne by the lateral aspect of the lower scapula, the lateral aspect of the ilium, and the greater trochanter of the femur. Clients who have sensory or motor deficits on one side of the body, or have had surgery involving mostly one side of the body, usually find that lying on the uninvolved side is more comfortable. Box 10–5 and Skill 10–1 describe how to support a client in the lateral position.

Sims' Position

In **Sims' (semiprone) position**, the client assumes a posture halfway between the lateral and the prone positions (sometimes called a lateral oblique position). The lower arm is positioned behind the client, and the upper arm is flexed at the shoulder and the elbow. Both legs are flexed in front of the client. The upper leg is more acutely flexed at both the hip and the knee than the lower leg.

Sims' position may be used for unconscious clients because it facilitates drainage from the mouth and prevents aspiration of fluids. It is also used for paralyzed (paraplegic or hemiplegic) clients because it reduces pressure over the sacrum and greater trochanter of the hip. It is often used for clients receiving enemas and occasionally for clients undergoing examinations or treatments of the perineal area. Many people, especially pregnant women, find the Sims' position comfortable for sleeping. Clients with sensory or motor deficits on one side of the body usually find that lying on the uninvolved side is more comfortable. Box 10–6 and Skill 10–1 describe how to support a client in the Sims' position.

BOX 10–6 Sims' (Semiprone) Position (Supported)

MEASURES TO PROMOTE ALIGNMENT AND SUPPORT*
- Pillow to support head, maintaining it in good alignment unless drainage from the mouth is required.
- Pillow under upper arm to prevent internal rotation of shoulder and arm.
- Pillow under upper leg to support it in alignment and to prevent internal rotation and adduction of hip and leg.
- Sandbags (or rolled towels) to support feet in dorsiflexion to prevent foot drop.

*The amount of support depends on the needs of the individual client.

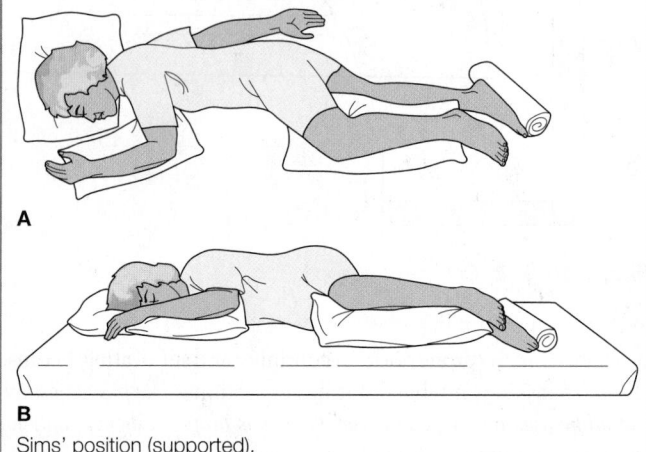

A

B

Sims' position (supported).

●○○● NURSING PROCESS: POSITIONING CLIENTS IN BED

Supporting the Client's Position in Bed

ASSESSMENT

Assess the client's strength, ability to move, and any special needs before the change of position. Factors to assess include:

- *Adipose tissue.* A client who has ample adipose (fatty) tissue generally requires less support and cushioning than the emaciated person while in a back-lying position, but greater support to maintain a lateral position.
- *Skeletal structure.* Both the amount and the type of support needed vary according to the individual's skeletal structure. A person with a marked lumbar lordosis requires more lumbar support than one with a slight lumbar curvature.
- *Health status.* A person who has flaccid (weak, soft) or spastic paralysis requires supportive devices. The support differs with the client's specific health status.
- *Discomfort.* A person who experiences pain during movement requires more support to prevent movement than one who can move without pain. A person who is unconscious is unable to indicate discomfort and will need appropriate support and change of position.
- *Skin condition.* People who have nutrition problems and/or impaired circulation require more cushioning of the pressure points to prevent skin breakdown than do healthy people.

- *Ability to move.* People who can move in bed can change position frequently. The client who is unable to move (e.g., the unconscious client) requires support so that muscles do not become strained.
- *Hydration.* Clients who are dehydrated are at greater risk of pressure ulcer formation than well-hydrated clients and therefore need more support under pressure areas.
- *Cultural issues.* Are there communication barriers, personal space issues, or caregiver gender issues that need to be taken into account? Depending on their background, some clients may feel very uncomfortable being touched by someone of the opposite gender, or by someone of the same gender. The only way to know is to ask, and to observe carefully for responses to the situation. Protect the client's modesty and personal space needs whenever possible, and offer reassurance throughout the movement. Some clients may respond well to a matter-of-fact approach; others may appreciate the use of good-natured humor. Most will appreciate kindness and a firm, gentle touch.

PLANNING

- Determine the client's need for supportive devices, such as pillows, rolled or folded towels, foam rubber supports, footboard, hand rolls, wrist splints, or sandbags.
- Determine the amount of assistance and the type of assistive device required to position the client. The risk of muscle strain and body injury, to both the client and nurse, is lowered when appropriate assistance and assistive devices are used.

DELEGATION

Positioning clients in bed can be delegated to unlicensed assistive personnel (UAP). The nurse must give specific directions to UAP about the appropriate positions for the client and the reporting of any changes in skin integrity. The UAP should be encouraged to have the client participate as much as possible in the position change. The nurse is responsible for evaluating the client's comfort and alignment after the repositioning and for assessing skin integrity, particularly at pressure points.

Equipment

The following equipment can be used when positioning clients:

- Pillows—one to six depending on client need
- Trochanter rolls
- Footboard or suspension boots
- Hand rolls or wrist splints, if needed
- Folded towel
- Sandbag or rolled towel

IMPLEMENTATION

Preparation

- Check the position-change schedule for the next time and type of position change.
- Administer an analgesic, if appropriate, before changing the client's position.
- Check if the client has toileting needs.
- Obtain required assistance, as needed.

Performance

1. Prior to performing the procedure, introduce self and verify the client's identity using agency protocol. Explain to the client what you are going to do, why it is necessary, and how he or she can participate.
2. Perform hand hygiene and observe other appropriate infection prevention procedures.
3. Provide for client privacy.
4. Raise the height of the bed to bring the client close to your center of gravity to avoid back strain.

Supporting a Client in Fowler's Position

1. Position the client.
   - Have the client flex the knees slightly before raising the head of the bed. **Rationale:** *Slight knee flexion prevents the person from sliding toward the foot of the bed as the bed is raised.* Be certain the client's hips are positioned directly over the point where the bed will bend when the head is raised. **Rationale:** *An appropriate hip position ensures that the client will be sitting upright when the head of the bed is raised.*
   - Raise the head of the bed to 45° or the angle required by or ordered for the client.
2. Provide supportive devices to align the client appropriately (see Box 10–1).
   - Place a small pillow or roll under the lumbar region of the back if you feel a space in the lumbar curvature. **Rationale:** *The pillow supports the natural lumbar curvature and prevents flexion of the lumbar spine.*

Continued on page 288

Supporting the Client's Position in Bed—*continued*

- Place a small pillow under the client's head. **Rationale:** *The pillow supports the cervical curvature of the vertebral column.* Alternatively, have the client rest the head against the mattress. **Rationale:** *Too many pillows beneath the head can cause neck flexion contracture and respiratory issues in obese clients.* Clients with a cervical collar should not use a pillow. **Rationale:** *This can lead to increased risk of pressure ulcers under the collar.*
- Place one or two pillows under the lower legs from below the knees to the ankles. **Rationale:** *The pillows provide a broad base of support that is soft and flexible, prevent uncomfortable hyperextension of the knees, and reduce pressure on the heels.* Make sure that no pressure is exerted on the popliteal space and that the knees are flexed. **Rationale:** *Pressure against the popliteal space can damage nerves and vein walls, predisposing the client to thrombus formation. Keeping the knees slightly flexed also prevents the person from sliding down in the bed.*
- Avoid using the knee gatch of a hospital bed to flex the client's knees. **Rationale:** *The position of the knee gatch rarely coincides with the position of the client's knees. Even when the knee gatch does bend at the client's knees, considerable pressure (due to the narrow base of support beneath the knees and the firm, unyielding mattress) can be exerted against the popliteal space and beneath the client's calves.*
- Put a trochanter roll or pillow lateral to each femur (optional) (see Box 10–2). **Rationale:** *This prevents external rotation of the hips.*
- Support the client's feet with heel boots, high-top tennis shoes, or a footboard. **Rationale:** *This prevents plantar flexion.* Routinely remove, provide range-of-motion (ROM) exercises, assess, and provide skin care. The footboard should protrude several inches above the toes. **Rationale:** *This protects the toes from pressure exerted by the top bedding.* The footboard should be placed 1 inch away from the heels. **Rationale:** *This prevents undue pull on the Achilles tendon and discomfort.*
- Place pillows to support both arms and hands if the client does not have normal use of them. **Rationale:** *These pillows prevent shoulder and muscle strain from the effects of downward gravitational pull, dislocation of the shoulder in paralyzed clients, edema of the hands and arms, and flexion contracture of the wrist.* Arrange the pillows to support only the forearms and hands, up to the elbow.

Supporting a Client in the Dorsal Recumbent Position
1. Assist the client to the supine position.
2. Provide supportive devices to align the client appropriately (see Box 10–3).
- Place a pillow of suitable thickness under the client's head and shoulders as needed. **Rationale:** *This prevents hyperextension of the neck. Too many pillows beneath the head may cause or worsen neck flexion contracture.*
- Place a pillow under the lower legs from below the knees to the ankles. **Rationale:** *This prevents hyperextension of the knees, keeps the heels off the bed, and reduces lumbar lordosis.*
- Place trochanter rolls or pillows laterally against the femurs (optional). **Rationale:** *These prevent external rotation of the hips.*
- Place a rolled towel or small pillow under the lumbar curvature if you feel a space between the lumbar area and

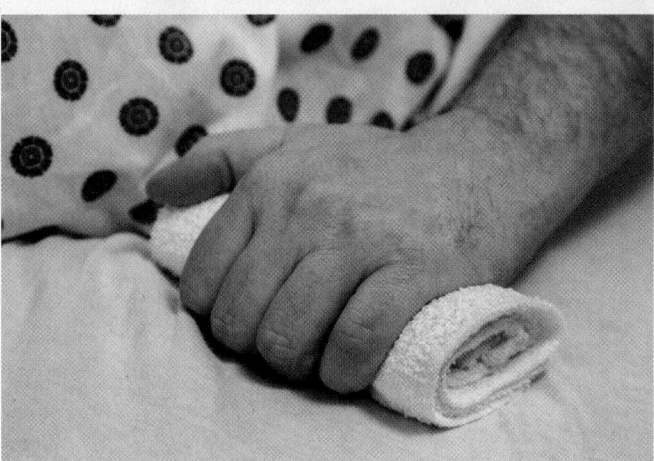

❶ A hand roll may be made from a folded and rolled washcloth. It is used to maintain functional position of the wrist and fingers and to prevent contractures.

the bed. **Rationale:** *This pillow supports the lumbar curvature and prevents flexion of the lumbar spine.*
- Put heel boots or high-top tennis shoes on the client or a footboard on the bed to support the feet. **Rationale:** *This prevents plantar flexion (foot drop).* Routinely remove, provide ROM, assess, and provide skin care.
- If the client is unconscious or has paralysis of the upper extremities, elevate the forearms and hands (*not* the upper arms) on pillows. **Rationale:** *This position promotes comfort and prevents edema. Pillows are not placed under the upper arms because they can cause shoulder flexion.*
- If the client has actual or potential finger and wrist flexion deformities, use hand rolls or wrist/hand splints. **Rationale:** *This prevents flexion contractures of the fingers.* Hand rolls, having a circumference of 13 to 15 cm (5 to 6 in.), exert even pressure over the entire flexor surface of the palm and fingers. ❶

Supporting a Client in the Prone Position
1. Assist the client to a prone position.
- See Skill 10–3 later in this chapter.
2. Provide supportive devices to position the client appropriately (see Box 10–4).
- Turn the client's head to one side, and either omit the pillow entirely if drainage from the mouth is being encouraged, or place a small pillow under the head to align the head with the trunk. **Rationale:** *This prevents flexion of the neck laterally.* Avoid placing the pillow under the shoulders. **Rationale:** *A pillow placed under the shoulders increases lumbar lordosis.*
- Place a small pillow or roll under the abdomen in the space between the diaphragm (or the breasts of a woman) and the iliac crests. **Rationale:** *The pillow prevents hyperextension of the lumbar curvature, difficulty breathing, and, for some women, pressure on the breasts. Supports placed too low can increase lumbar lordosis and pressure on bony prominences.*
- Place a pillow under the lower legs from below the knees to just above the ankles. **Rationale:** *This raises the toes off the bed surface and reduces plantar flexion. This pillow also*

Supporting the Client's Position in Bed—*continued*

flexes the knees slightly for comfort and prevents excessive pressure on the patellae. Or, position the client on the bed so that the feet are extended in a normal anatomic position over the lower edge of the mattress. **Rationale:** *There should be no pressure on the toes.*

Supporting a Client in the Lateral Position

1. Assist the client to a lateral position.
   - See Skill 10–3 later in this chapter.
2. Provide supportive devices to align the client appropriately (see Box 10–5).
   - Place a pillow under the client's head so that the head and neck are aligned with the trunk. **Rationale:** *The pillow prevents lateral flexion and discomfort of the major neck muscles (e.g., the sternocleidomastoid muscles).*
   - Have the client flex the lower shoulder and position it forward so that the body does not rest on it. Rotate it into any position of comfort. **Rationale:** *In this way, circulation is not disrupted.*
   - Place a pillow under the upper arm. **Rationale:** *This prevents internal rotation and adduction of the shoulder and downward pressure on the chest that could interfere with chest expansion during respiration.* If the client has respiratory difficulty, increase the shoulder flexion and position the upper arm in front of the body off the chest.
   - Place two or more pillows under the upper leg and thigh so that the extremity lies in a plane parallel to the surface of the bed. **Rationale:** *A position parallel to the bed most closely approximates correct standing alignment and prevents internal rotation of the thigh and adduction of the leg. The pillow also prevents pressure caused by the weight of the top leg resting on the lower leg. Such pressure can damage the vein walls in the lower leg and predispose the client to thrombus formation and can also lead to pressure ulcers.*
   - Ensure that the two shoulders are aligned in the same plane as the two hips. If they are not, pull one shoulder or hip forward or backward until all four joints are aligned in the same plane. **Rationale:** *Proper alignment prevents twisting of the spine.*
   - Place a folded towel under the natural hollow at the waistline (optional). **Rationale:** *This prevents postural scoliosis of the lumbar spine.* Take care to fill in only the space at the waistline. **Rationale:** *A towel support that extends too high or too low creates undue pressure against the rib cage or iliac crests.*
   - Place a rolled pillow (fold pillow lengthwise) alongside the client's back to stabilize the position. **Rationale:** *The pillow provides support for the client to stay on the side.* This pillow may not be needed when the client's upper hip and knee are appropriately flexed.

Supporting a Client in Sims' Position

1. Turn the client as for the prone position.
2. Provide supportive devices to align the client appropriately (see Box 10–6).
   - Place a small pillow under the client's head, unless drainage from the mouth is being encouraged. **Rationale:** *The pillow prevents lateral flexion of the neck and cushions the cranial and facial bones and the ear. It is contraindicated if drainage of mucus is required. Too large a pillow produces an uncomfortable lateral flexion of the neck.*
   - Place the lower arm behind and away from the client's body in a position that is comfortable and does not disrupt circulation. **Rationale:** *This position prevents damage to the nerves and blood vessels in the axillae.*
   - Position the upper shoulder so that it is abducted slightly from the body, and the shoulder and elbow are flexed. Place a pillow in the space between the chest and abdomen and the upper arm and bed. **Rationale:** *This position and support prevent internal shoulder rotation and adduction and maintain alignment of the upper trunk.*
   - Place a pillow in the space between the abdomen and pelvis and the upper thigh and bed. **Rationale:** *This position prevents internal rotation and adduction of the hip and also reduces lumbar lordosis.*
   - Ensure that the two shoulders are aligned in the same plane as the two hips. If they are not, pull one shoulder or hip forward or backward until all four joints are aligned in the same plane. **Rationale:** *This prevents twisting of the spine.*
   - Place a support device (e.g., foot boot on the client or a sandbag or rolled towel against the lower foot of the client). **Rationale:** *This device may prevent foot drop. Efforts to correct plantar flexion in this position, however, are usually unsuccessful.*

Document all position changes carefully, recording:
- Time and change of position moved from and position moved to (according to agency protocol).
- Number of personnel required for turning and positioning.
- Safety precautions and the use of any premedications.
- Ways the client is able to assist with positioning.
- Any signs of pressure areas or contractures.
- Any difficulty the client has with breathing (Fowler's, prone, and Sims' positions).
- Use of support/assistive devices and any special requirements.

SAMPLE DOCUMENTATION

10/15/2015 1030 Turned to (L) side by 2 staff. Pillows under head, upper arm & upper leg. Skin intact without redness over bony prominences. ——————————————— M. Foti, RN

EVALUATION

- Check the skin integrity of the pressure areas from the previous position. Relate findings to previous assessment data if available. Conduct follow-up assessment for previous and/or new skin breakdown areas and document.
- Check for proper alignment after the position change. Do a visual check and ask the client for a comfort assessment.
- Determine that all required safety precautions (e.g., side rails) are in place.
- Report significant changes to the primary care provider.

MOVING AND TURNING CLIENTS IN BED

Although healthy people usually take for granted that they can change body position and go from one place to another with little effort, people who are ill may have difficulty even moving in bed. How much assistance clients require depends on their ability to move and their health status. Nurses should be sensitive to both the need of clients to function independently and their need for assistance to move. Correct body alignment for the client must also be maintained so that undue stress is not placed on the musculoskeletal system.

When assisting a person to move, the nurse needs to use appropriate numbers of staff and **assistive devices** (such as those previously shown in Figures 10–3 through 10–8) to avoid injury to self and client. Having enough staff and assistive devices also helps to ensure client comfort and modesty. Hydraulic lifts are examples of assistive equipment that take the place of manual lifts and transfers. The lift can be used in transferring the client between the bed and a wheelchair, the bed and the bathtub, and the bed and a stretcher.

CLINICAL ALERT!

Studies confirm that repositioning clients in bed, specifically pulling a client toward the head of the bed, is one of the most significant causes of back injuries and back pain among caregivers in the health care industry (Fragala, 2011, p. 65).

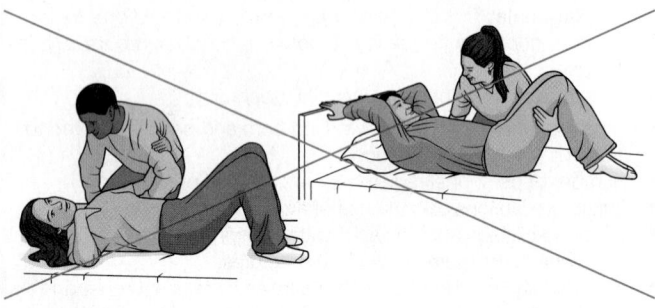

Actions and rationales common to the lifting and moving procedures that follow are outlined in Box 10–7. Correct body alignment for the client must also be maintained so that undue stress is not placed on the musculoskeletal system.

See Skills 10–2 through 10–5 on moving and turning clients in bed and helping them sit up on the edge of the bed.

BOX 10–7	**Actions and Rationales Applicable to Moving and Lifting Clients**

- Never lift or hold any client or client part greater than 35 pounds without assistive devices.
- Before moving a client, assess the degree of exertion required and the client's physical abilities (e.g., muscle strength, presence of paralysis) and ability to assist with the move, ability to understand instructions, degree of comfort or discomfort when moving, client's weight, presence of orthostatic hypotension (particularly important when client will be standing).
- If indicated, use pain-relief modalities or medication prior to moving the client.
- Prepare any needed assistive devices and supportive equipment (e.g., mechanical lifts, friction reducing slide sheet, pillows, trochanter roll).
- Plan around encumbrances to movement such as an IV or urinary catheter.
- Be alert to the effects of any medications the client takes that may impair alertness, balance, strength, or mobility.
- Obtain required assistance from other individuals.
- Explain the procedure to the client and listen to any suggestions the client or support people have.
- Provide privacy.
- Perform hand hygiene.
- Raise the height of the bed. **Rationale:** *This brings the client close to your center of gravity.*
- Lock the wheels on the bed, and raise the rail on the side of the bed opposite you *to ensure client safety.*
- Face in the direction of the movement. **Rationale:** *This prevents spinal twisting.*
- Assume a broad stance. **Rationale:** *This increases stability and provides balance.*
- Lean your trunk forward, and flex your hips, knees, and ankles. **Rationale:** *This lowers your center of gravity, increases stability, and ensures use of large muscle groups during movements.*
- Tighten your gluteal, abdominal, leg, and arm muscles. **Rationale:** *This prepares them for action and prevents injury.*
- Rock from the front leg to the back leg when pulling or from the back leg to the front leg when pushing. **Rationale:** *This overcomes inertia, counteracts the client's weight, and helps attain a balanced, smooth motion.*
- After moving the client, determine and document the client's comfort (presence of anxiety, dizziness, or pain), body alignment, tolerance of the activity (e.g., check pulse rate, blood pressure), ability to assist, use of support devices, and safety precautions required (e.g., side rails).

●○○● NURSING PROCESS: MOVING AND TURNING CLIENTS IN BED

Moving a Client Up in Bed

ASSESSMENT

Assess:
- Client's physical ability to assist with the move (e.g., muscle strength, presence of paralysis).
- Client's ability to understand instructions and willingness to participate.

- Client's degree of comfort or discomfort when moving. If needed, administer analgesics or perform other pain-relief measures prior to the move.
- Client's weight.
- The availability of assistive equipment and other personnel to assist you.

PLANNING

Review the client record to determine if previous nurses have recorded information about the client's ability to move. Use proper assistive equipment and additional personnel as needed. Ensure that the client understands instructions, and provide an interpreter as needed. Determine the number of personnel and type of equipment needed to safely perform the positional change to prevent injury to staff and client.

Moving a Client Up in Bed—*continued*

DELEGATION

The skills of moving and turning clients in bed can be delegated to UAP. The nurse should make sure that any needed equipment and additional personnel are available to reduce risk of injury to the health care personnel. Emphasize the need for the UAP to report changes in the client's condition that require assessment and intervention by the nurse.

Equipment

- Assistive devices such as an overhead trapeze, friction-reducing device, or a mechanical lift

IMPLEMENTATION

Preparation

Determine:

- Assistive devices that will be required.
- Encumbrances to movement such as an IV or an indwelling urinary catheter.
- Medications the client is receiving, because certain medications may hamper movement or alertness of the client.
- Assistance required from other health care personnel.

Performance

1. Prior to performing the procedure, introduce self and verify the client's identity using agency protocol. Explain to the client what you are going to do, why it is necessary, and how he or she can participate. Listen to any suggestions made by the client or support people.
2. Perform hand hygiene and observe other appropriate infection prevention procedures.
3. Provide for client privacy.
4. Adjust the bed and the client's position.
   - Adjust the head of the bed to a flat position or as low as the client can tolerate. **Rationale:** *Moving the client upward against gravity requires more force and can cause back strain.*
   - Raise the height of the bed appropriate to personnel safety (at the elbows).
   - Lock the wheels on the bed and raise the rail on the side of the bed opposite you.
   - Remove all pillows, then place one against the head of the bed. **Rationale:** *This pillow protects the client's head from inadvertent injury against the top of the bed during the upward move.*
5. For the client who is able to reposition without assistance:
   - Place the bed in flat or reverse Trendelenburg's position (as tolerated by the client). Stand by and instruct the client to move self. Assess if the client is able to move without causing friction to the skin.
   - Encourage the client to reach up and grasp the upper side rails with both hands, bend knees, and push off with the feet and pull up with the arms simultaneously.
   - Ask if a positioning device is needed (e.g., pillow).
6. For the client who is partially able to assist:
   - For a client who weighs less than 200 pounds: Use a friction-reducing device and two assistants. **Rationale:** *Moving a client up in bed is not a one-person task. During any client handling, if the caregiver is required to lift more than 35 lb of a client's weight, then the client should be considered fully dependent and assistive devices should be used. This reduces risk of injury to the caregiver.*
   - For a client who weighs between 201 and 300 pounds: Use a friction-reducing slide sheet and four assistants *OR* an air transfer system and two assistants. **Rationale:** *Moving a*

client up in bed is not a one-person task. During any client handling, if the caregiver is required to lift more than 35 lb of a client's weight, then the client should be considered fully dependent and assistive devices should be used. This reduces risk of injury to the caregiver.
   - For a client who weighs more than 300 pounds: Use an air transfer system and two assistants *OR* a total transfer lift.
   - Ask the client to flex the hips and knees and position the feet so that they can be used effectively for pushing. **Rationale:** *Flexing the hips and knees keeps the entire lower leg off the bed surface, preventing friction during movement, and ensures use of the large muscle groups in the client's legs when pushing, thus increasing the force of movement.*
   - Place the client's arms across the chest. Ask the client to flex the neck during the move and keep the head off the bed surface. **Rationale:** *This keeps the arms off the bed surface and minimizes friction during movement.*
   - Use a friction-reducing device and assistants to move the client up in bed. Ask the client to push on the count of three.
7. Position yourself appropriately, and move the client.
   - Face the direction of the movement, and then assume a broad stance with the foot nearest the bed behind the forward foot and weight on the forward foot. Lean your trunk forward from the hips. Flex hips, knees, and ankles.
   - Tighten your gluteal, abdominal, leg, and arm muscles and rock from the back leg to the front leg and back again. Then, shift your weight to the front leg as the client pushes with the heels and pulls with the arms so that the client moves toward the head of the bed.
8. For the client who is unable to assist:
   - Use a ceiling lift with supine sling or mobile floor-based lift and two or more caregivers. Follow the manufacturer's guidelines for using the lift. **Rationale:** *Moving a client up in bed is not a one-person task. During any client handling, if the caregiver is required to lift more than 35 lb of a client's weight, then the client should be considered fully dependent and assistive devices should be used. This reduces risk of injury to the caregiver.*
9. Ensure client comfort.
   - Elevate the head of the bed and provide appropriate support devices for the client's new position.
   - See the sections on positioning clients earlier in this chapter.
10. Document all relevant information. Record:
   - Time and change of position moved from and position moved to.
   - Any signs of pressure areas.
   - Use of support devices.
   - Ability of client to assist in moving and turning.
   - Response of client to moving and turning (e.g., anxiety, discomfort, dizziness).

Turning a Client to the Lateral or Prone Position in Bed

IMPLEMENTATION

Preparation

Determine:

- Assistive devices that will be required (e.g., friction-reducing device or mechanical lift).
- Encumbrances to movement such as an IV or an indwelling urinary catheter.
- Medications the client is receiving, because certain medications may hamper movement or alertness of the client.
- Assistance required from other health care personnel. **Rationale:** *Moving a client is not a one-person task. During any client handling, if the caregiver is required to lift more than 35 lb of a client's weight, then the client should be considered fully dependent and assistive devices should be used. This reduces risk of injury to the caregiver.*

Performance

1. Prior to performing the procedure, introduce self and verify the client's identity using agency protocol. Explain to the client what you are going to do, why it is necessary, and how he or she can participate.
2. Perform hand hygiene and observe other appropriate infection prevention procedures.
3. Provide for client privacy.
4. Position yourself and the client appropriately before performing the move. The other individual(s) stand on the opposite side of the bed.
   - Adjust the head of the bed to a flat position or as low as the client can tolerate. **Rationale:** *This provides a position of comfort for the client.*
   - Raise the height of the bed appropriate to personnel safety (i.e., at the elbows).
   - Lock the wheels on the bed.
   - Move the client closer to the side of the bed opposite the side the client will face when turned. **Rationale:** *This ensures that the client will be positioned safely in the center of the bed after turning.* Use a friction-reducing device or mechanical lift (depending on level of client assistance required) to pull the client to the side of the bed. Adjust the client's head and reposition the legs appropriately.
   - While standing on the side of the bed nearest the client, place the client's near arm across the chest. Abduct the client's far shoulder slightly from the side of the body and externally rotate the shoulder. ❶ **Rationale:** *Pulling the one arm forward facilitates the turning motion. Pulling the other arm away from the body and externally rotating the shoulder prevents that arm from being caught beneath the client's body during the roll.*
   - Place the client's near ankle and foot across the far ankle and foot. **Rationale:** *This facilitates the turning motion. Making these preparations on the side of the bed closest to the client helps prevent unnecessary reaching.*
   - The person on the side of the bed toward which the client will turn should be positioned directly in line with the client's waistline and as close to the bed as possible.
5. Roll the client to the lateral position. The second person(s) standing on the opposite side of the bed helps roll the client from the other side.
   - Place one hand on the client's hip and the other hand on the client's shoulder. **Rationale:** *This position of the hands supports the client at the two heaviest parts of the body, providing greater control in movement during the roll.*

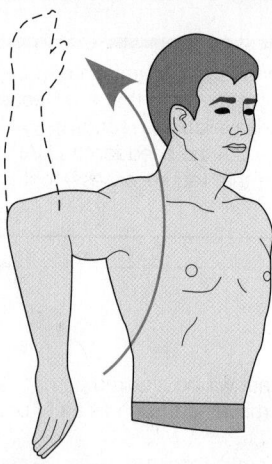

❶ External rotation of the shoulder prevents the arm from being caught beneath the client's body when the client is turned.

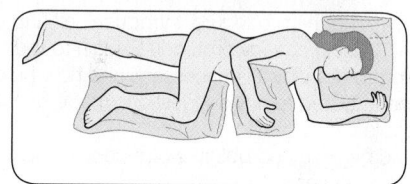

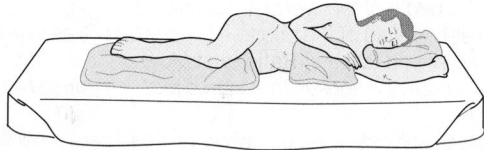

❷ Lateral position with pillows in place.

- Position the client on his or her side with arms and legs positioned and supported properly. ❷

Variation: Turning the Client to a Prone Position

To turn a client to the prone position, follow the preceding steps, with two exceptions:

- Instead of abducting the far arm, keep the client's arm alongside the body for the client to roll over. **Rationale:** *Keeping the arm alongside the body prevents it from being pinned under the client when the client is rolled.*
- Roll the client completely onto the abdomen. **Rationale:** *It is essential to move the client as close as possible to the edge of the bed before the turn so that the client will be lying on the center of the bed after rolling. Never pull a client across the bed while the client is in the prone position.* **Rationale:** *Doing so can injure a woman's breasts or a man's genitals.*

6. Document all relevant information. Record:
   - Time and change of position moved from and position moved to.
   - Any signs of pressure areas.
   - Use of support devices.
   - Ability of client to assist in moving and turning.
   - Response of client to moving and turning (e.g., anxiety, discomfort, dizziness).

Logrolling a Client

IMPLEMENTATION

Logrolling is a technique used to turn a client whose body must at all times be kept in straight alignment (like a log). An example is the client with back surgery or a spinal injury. Considerable care must be taken to prevent additional injury. This technique requires a minimum of two nurses or, if the client is large, three nurses. For the client who has a cervical injury, one nurse must maintain the client's head and neck alignment.

Preparation

Determine:

- Assistive devices that will be required.
- Encumbrances to movement such as an IV or an indwelling catheter.
- Medications the client is receiving, because certain medications may hamper movement or alertness of the client.
- Assistance required from other health care personnel. At least two to three additional people are needed to perform this skill safely.

Performance

1. Prior to performing the procedure, introduce self and verify the client's identity using agency protocol. Explain to the client what you are going to do, why it is necessary, and how he or she can participate.
2. Perform hand hygiene and observe other appropriate infection prevention procedures.
3. Provide for client privacy.
4. Position yourselves and the client appropriately before the move.
    - Place the client's arms across the chest. **Rationale:** *Doing so ensures that the arms will not be injured or become trapped under the body when the client is turned.*
5. Pull the client to the side of the bed.
    - Use a turn sheet or friction-reducing device to facilitate logrolling. First, stand with another nurse on the same side of the bed. Assume a broad stance with one foot forward, and grasp the rolled edge of the friction-reducing device. On a signal, pull the client toward both of you. ❶
    - One nurse counts: "One, two, three, go." Then, at the same time, all staff members pull the client to the side of the bed by shifting their weight to the back foot. **Rationale:** *Moving the client in unison maintains the client's body alignment.*

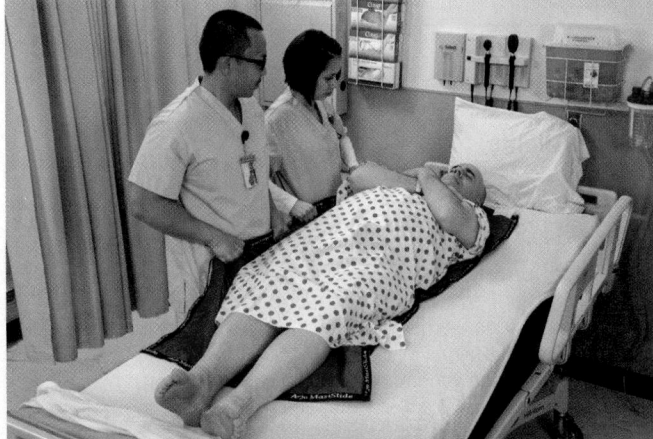

❶ Using a friction-reducing slide sheet, the nurses pull the sheet with the client on it to the edge of the bed.

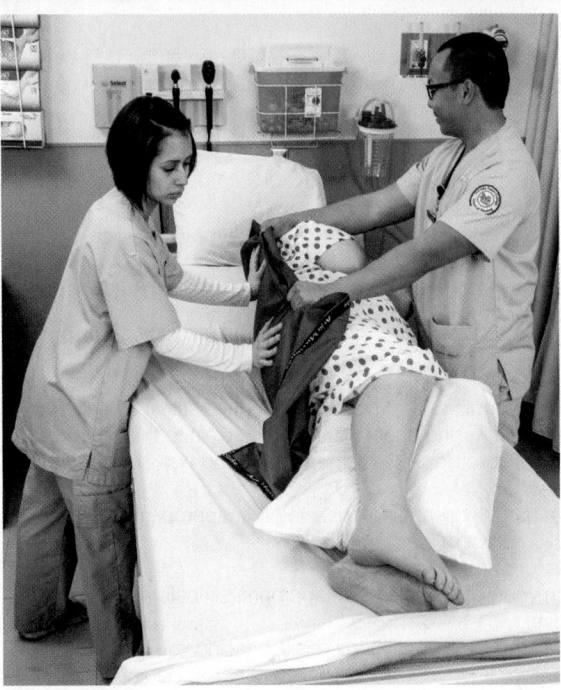

❷ The nurse on the right uses the far edge of the friction-reducing slide sheet to roll the client toward him; the nurse on the left remains behind the client and assists with turning.

6. One person moves to the other side of the bed and places supportive devices for the client when turned.
    - Place a pillow where it will support the client's head after the turn. **Rationale:** *The pillow prevents lateral flexion of the neck and ensures alignment of the cervical spine.*
    - Place one or two pillows between the client's legs to support the upper leg when the client is turned. **Rationale:** *This pillow prevents adduction of the upper leg and keeps the legs parallel and aligned.*
7. Roll and position the client in proper alignment.
    - The person farthest from the client assumes a stable stance.
    - This person reaches over the client and grasps the friction-reducing device. ❷
    - One nurse counts: "One, two, three, go." Then, at the same time, all nurses roll the client to a lateral position.
    - The nurse behind the client helps turn the client and provides pillow supports to ensure good alignment in the lateral position.
    - Support the client's head, back, and upper and lower extremities with pillows.
    - Raise the side rails and place the call bell within the client's reach.
8. Document all relevant information.
9. Record:
    - Time and change of position moved from and position moved to.
    - Any signs of pressure areas.
    - Use of support devices.
    - Ability of client to assist in moving and turning.
    - Response of client to moving and turning (e.g., anxiety, discomfort, dizziness).

Assisting a Client to Sit on the Side of the Bed (Dangling)

IMPLEMENTATION

The client assumes a sitting position on the edge of the bed before walking, moving to a chair or wheelchair, eating, or performing other activities.

Preparation

Determine:

- Assistive devices that will be required.
- Encumbrances to movement such as an IV or a heavy cast on one leg.
- Medications the client is receiving, because certain medications may hamper movement or alertness of the client.
- Assistance required from other health care personnel.

Performance

1. Prior to performing the procedure, introduce self and verify the client's identity using agency protocol. Explain to the client what you are going to do, why it is necessary, and how he or she can participate.
2. Perform hand hygiene and observe other appropriate infection prevention procedures.
3. Provide for client privacy.
4. Position yourself and the client appropriately before performing the move.
   - Assist the client to a lateral position facing you, using an assistive device dependent on client assistance needs.
   - Raise the head of the bed slowly to its highest position. **Rationale:** *This decreases the distance that the client needs to move to sit up on the side of the bed.*
   - Position the client's feet and lower legs at the edge of the bed. **Rationale:** *This enables the client's feet to move easily off the bed during the movement, and the client is aided by gravity into a sitting position.*
   - Stand beside the client's hips and face the far corner of the bottom of the bed (the angle in which movement will occur). Assume a broad stance, placing the foot nearest the client

forward. Lean your trunk forward from the hips. Flex your hips, knees, and ankles.

5. Move the client to a sitting position, using an assistive device depending on client assistance needs.
   - Place the arm nearest to the head of the bed under the client's shoulders and the other arm over both of the client's thighs near the knees. **Rationale:** *Supporting the client's shoulders prevents the client from falling backward during the movement. Supporting the client's thighs reduces friction of the thighs against the bed surface during the move and increases the force of the movement.*
   - Tighten your gluteal, abdominal, leg, and arm muscles.
   - Pivot on the balls of your feet in the desired direction facing the foot of the bed while pulling the client's feet and legs off the bed. **Rationale:** *Pivoting prevents twisting of the nurse's spine. The weight of the client's legs swinging downward increases downward movement of the lower body and helps make the client's upper body vertical.*
   - Keep supporting the client until the client is well balanced and comfortable. **Rationale:** *This movement may cause some clients to become light-headed or dizzy.*
   - Assess vital signs (e.g., pulse, respirations, and blood pressure) as indicated by the client's health status.
6. Document all relevant information. Record:
   - Ability of the client to assist in moving and turning.
   - Type of assistive device, if one was used.
   - Response of the client to moving and turning (e.g., anxiety, discomfort, dizziness).

Note: This skill describes the process to use for a client who is able to perform the task independently and only needs standby assistance for steadying, or a client who requires minimum assistance in which the client can perform the task with or without friction-reducing assistive devices and the health care worker provides 25% of the work. For clients who require moderate assistance (requiring no more than 50% assistance by caregiver) or maximum assistance (requiring more than 50% assistance by the caregiver), a lateral chair, or mobile or ceiling-mounted transfer system is required.

EVALUATION

- Check the skin integrity of the pressure areas from the previous position. Relate findings to previous assessment data if available. Conduct follow-up assessment for previous and/or new skin breakdown areas.
- Check for proper alignment after the position change. Do a visual check and ask the client for a comfort assessment.

- Determine that all required safety precautions (e.g., side rails) are in place.
- Determine the client's tolerance of the activity (e.g., vital signs before and after dangling), particularly the first time the client changes position.
- Report significant changes to the primary care provider.

LIFESPAN CONSIDERATIONS | Positioning, Moving, and Turning Clients

INFANTS

- Position infants on their backs for sleep, even after feeding. There is little risk of regurgitation and choking, and the rate of sudden infant death syndrome (SIDS) is significantly lower in infants who sleep on their backs.
- The skin of newborns can be fragile and may be abraded or torn (sheared) if the infant is pulled across a bed.

CHILDREN

- Carefully inspect the dependent skin surfaces of all infants and children confined to bed at least three times in each 24-hour period.

OLDER ADULTS

- In clients who have had cerebrovascular accidents (strokes), there is a risk of shoulder displacement on the paralyzed side from improper moving or repositioning techniques. Use care when moving, positioning in bed, and transferring. Pillows or foam devices are helpful to support the affected arm and shoulder and prevent injury.
- Decreased subcutaneous fat and thinning of the skin place older adults at risk for skin breakdown. Repositioning approximately every 2 hours (more or less, depending on the unique needs of the individual client) helps reduce pressure on bony prominences and avoid tissue trauma.

- Assess the height of the bed and the person's leg length to ensure that self-movements in and out of the bed are smooth.
- When making a home visit, it is particularly important to inspect the mattress for support. A sagging mattress, a mattress that is too soft, or an underfilled waterbed used over a prolonged period can contribute to the development of hip flexion contractures and low back strain and pain. Bed boards made of plywood and placed beneath a sagging mattress are increasingly recommended for clients who have back problems or are prone to them.
- Assess the caregivers' knowledge and application of body mechanics to prevent injury.
- Demonstrate how to turn and position the client in bed. Observe the caregiver performing a return demonstration. Reevaluate this technique periodically to reinforce correct application of body mechanics.

- Teach caregivers the basic principles of body alignment and how to check for proper alignment after the client has been changed to a new position.
- Warn caregivers of the dangers of lifting and repositioning and encourage the use of assistive devices and a "no manual lift" policy.
- Teach the caregiver to check the client's skin for redness and integrity after repositioning the client. Stress the importance of informing the nurse about the length of time skin redness remains over pressure areas after the person has been repositioned. Emphasize that reddened areas should not be massaged because doing so may lead to tissue trauma. Teach the caregiver that open areas must be inspected and treated by a health care professional.

TRANSFERRING CLIENTS

Many clients require some assistance in transferring between bed and chair or wheelchair, between wheelchair and toilet, and between bed and stretcher. Before transferring any client, however, the nurse must determine the client's physical and mental capabilities to participate in the transfer skill. In addition, the nurse must analyze and organize the activity.

A **gait belt**, sometimes called a walking or **transfer belt**, has traditionally been used to transfer a client from one position to another and for ambulation (Figure 10–10 ■). A gait belt can have handles that allow the nurse to control movement of the client during the transfer or during ambulation (Figure 10–11 ■). Rockefeller and Proctor (2011) point out that the long-held belief that the use of gait belts improves safety for both clients and caregivers is based on tradition and not on evidence-based research. The few studies that have been done indicate that using a gait belt for transfer falls into either a moderate or high-risk category for low back disorders. Gait belts are not appropriate for all clients. They are suitable for clients who can bear weight and require only minimal assistance. The gait belt with handles is easier to grasp. Gait belts should not be used to lift a client off the floor or for bariatric clients. In addition, they should not be relied on for clients who are at high risk for falls (Rockefeller and Proctor, 2011, p. 33).

A sliding board is another device that can be used for transferring a client between a bed and chair (Figure 10–12 ■). Boards are often made of low-friction materials or with movable sliding sections. Some clients may be able to transfer themselves using a sliding/transfer board. If a caregiver is needed, the client is either pushed or

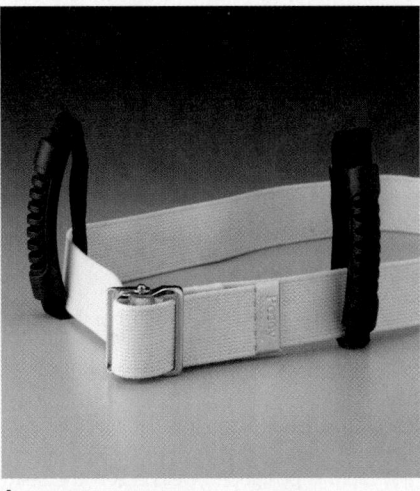

A

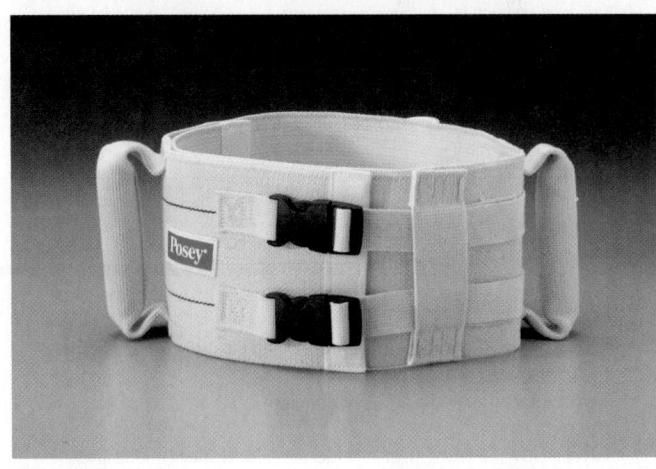

B

Figure 10–11 ■ *A*, Gait belt with add-on handles; *B*, gait belt with handles.
Courtesy of Posey Company, Arcadia, CA.

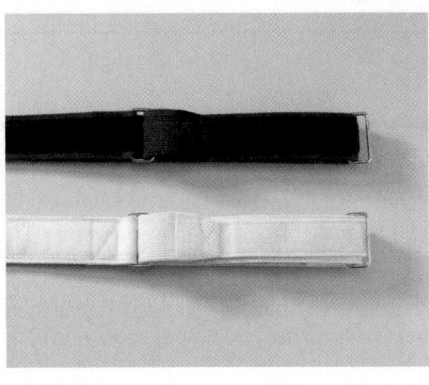

Figure 10–10 ■ Gait belt.
Courtesy of Posey Company, Arcadia, CA.

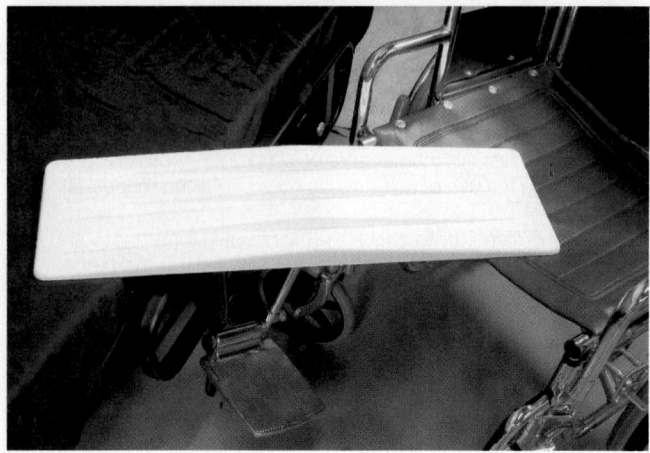

Figure 10–12 ■ Plastic transfer board.
Courtesy of Posey Company, Arcadia, CA.

pulled across the transfer board using a slide sheet. Clients must have sitting balance. See Skill 10–6 for transferring a client between a bed and a chair and Skill 10–7 for transferring a client between a bed and a stretcher.

General guidelines for transfer techniques include the following:

• Plan what to do and how to do it. Determine the space in which the transfer maneuver will take place (bathrooms, for instance, are usually cramped), the number of assistants (one or two) needed to accomplish the transfer safely, the skill and strength of the nurse(s), and the client's capabilities (e.g., size, weight, cognition, balance, cooperation).

• Obtain essential equipment before starting: gait/transfer belt, friction-reducing device (e.g., slide sheet, slide board, air transfer system), wheelchair, stretcher, lift, etc. Check that all equipment is functioning correctly. The gait/transfer belt is meant only to increase control of the client's movements; if the client requires lifting, a mechanical lifting device should be used.

• Remove obstacles from the area used for the transfer.

• Explain the transfer to the client, including what the client should do.

• Explain the transfer to the nursing personnel who are helping; specify who will give directions (one person needs to be in charge).

• Always support or hold the client rather than the equipment and ensure the client's safety and dignity.

• During the transfer, explain step by step what the client should do, for example, "Move your right foot forward."

• Make a written plan of the transfer, including the client's tolerance (e.g., pulse and respiratory rates).

Because wheelchairs and stretchers are unstable, they can predispose the client to falls and injury. Guidelines for the safe use of wheelchairs and stretchers are shown in Practice Guidelines.

Document all relevant information. Record:

• Time and change of position moved from and position moved to.

• Any signs of pressure areas.

• Use of support devices.

• Assistive devices, if used.

• Ability of client to assist in moving and turning.

• Response of client to moving and turning (e.g., anxiety, discomfort, dizziness).

PRACTICE GUIDELINES

Safe Use of Wheelchairs

• Always lock the brakes on both wheels of the wheelchair when the client transfers in or out of it.

• Raise the footplates before transferring the client into the wheelchair.

• Lower the footplates after the transfer, and place the client's feet on them.

• Ensure the client is positioned well back in the seat of the wheelchair.

• Use seat belts that fasten behind the wheelchair to protect confused clients from falls. *Note:* Seat belts are a form of restraint and must be used in accordance with policies and procedures that apply to the use of restraints.

• Back the wheelchair into or out of an elevator or a door, rear large wheels first.

• Place your body between the wheelchair and the bottom of an incline, even if this means pulling the wheelchair down a hill rather than pushing it.

CLINICAL ALERT!

Air, foam, and gel cushions that distribute weight evenly (not doughnut-type cushions) are essential for clients confined to a wheelchair and must be checked frequently to ensure they are intact. Strict continence management is also important for preventing skin breakdown. Maintaining wheelchair tire pressure will prevent added resistance and energy expenditure. Periodically monitor the client's upper extremities for pain and overuse syndromes.

PRACTICE GUIDELINES

Safe Use of Stretchers

• Lock the wheels of the bed and stretcher before the client transfers in or out of them.

• Fasten safety straps across the client on a stretcher, and raise the side rails.

• Never leave a client unattended on a stretcher unless the wheels are locked and the side rails are raised on both sides and/or the safety straps are securely fastened across the client.

• Always push a stretcher from the end where the client's head is positioned. This position protects the client's head in the event of a collision.

• If the stretcher has two swivel wheels and two stationary wheels:
  a. Always position the client's head at the end with the stationary wheels.
  b. Push the stretcher from the end with the stationary wheels. The stretcher is maneuvered more easily when pushed from this end.

• Maneuver the stretcher when entering the elevator so that the client's head goes in first.

●○● NURSING PROCESS: TRANSFERRING CLIENTS

Transferring Between Bed and Chair

ASSESSMENT

Assess:

- The client's body size.
- Ability to follow instructions.
- Ability to bear weight.
- Ability to position/reposition feet on floor.
- Ability to push down with arms and lean forward.
- Ability to achieve independent sitting balance.
- Activity tolerance.
- Muscle strength.
- Joint mobility.
- Presence of paralysis.
- Level of comfort.
- Presence of orthostatic hypotension.
- The technique with which the client is familiar.
- The space in which the transfer will need to be maneuvered (bathrooms, for example, are usually cramped).
- The number of assistants (one or two) needed to accomplish the transfer safely.

PLANNING

Review the client record to determine if previous nurses have recorded information about the client's ability to transfer. Implement pain-relief measures far enough ahead of time so that they are effective when the transfer begins. The decision must be made at this time regarding the client's ability to participate. If the client can safely participate in the transfer, a gait/transfer belt and/or sliding board can be used; if not, a powered standing assist lift or full body lift would be safer for the client and nurse (see Skill 10–8).

DELEGATION

The skill of transferring a client can be delegated to UAP who have demonstrated safe transfer technique for the involved client. It is important for the nurse to assess the client's capabilities and communicate specific information about what the UAP should report back to the nurse.

Equipment

- Robe or appropriate clothing
- Slippers or shoes with nonskid soles
- Gait/transfer belt
- Chair, commode, wheelchair as appropriate to client need
- Slide board, if appropriate
- Lift, if appropriate

IMPLEMENTATION

Preparation

- Plan what to do and how to do it.
- Obtain essential equipment before starting (e.g., gait/transfer belt, wheelchair) and check that all equipment is functioning correctly.
- Remove obstacles from the area so clients do not trip. Make sure there are no spills or liquids on the floor on which clients could slip.

Performance

1. Prior to performing the procedure, introduce self and verify the client's identity using agency protocol. Explain the transfer process to the client. During the transfer, explain step by step what the client should do, for example, "Move your right foot forward."
2. Perform hand hygiene and observe other appropriate infection prevention procedures.
3. Provide for client privacy.
4. Position the equipment appropriately.
   - Lower the bed to its lowest position so that the client's feet will rest flat on the floor. Lock the wheels of the bed.
   - Place the wheelchair parallel to the bed and as close to the bed as possible. ❶ Put the wheelchair on the side of the bed that allows the client to move toward his or her stronger side. Lock the wheels of the wheelchair and raise the footplate.
5. Prepare and assess the client.
   - Assist the client to a sitting position on the side of the bed (see Skill 10-5).
   - Assess the client for orthostatic hypotension before moving the client from the bed.
   - Assist the client in putting on a bathrobe and nonskid slippers or shoes.

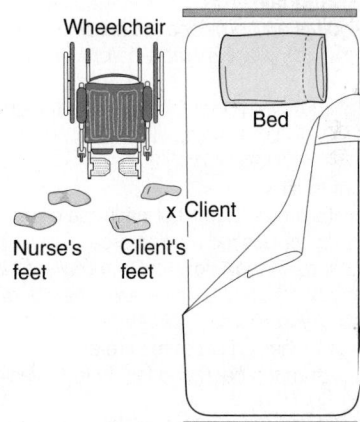

❶ The wheelchair is placed parallel to the bed and as close to the bed as possible. Note that placement of the nurse's feet mirrors that of the client's feet.

- Place a gait/transfer belt snugly around the client's waist. Check to be certain that the belt is securely fastened.
6. Give explicit instructions to the client. Ask the client to:
   - Move forward and sit on the edge of the bed (or surface on which the client is sitting) with feet placed flat on the floor. **Rationale:** *This brings the client's center of gravity closer to the nurse's.*
   - Lean forward slightly from the hips. **Rationale:** *This brings the client's center of gravity more directly over the base of support and positions the head and trunk in the direction of the movement.*

Continued on page 298

SKILL 10-6

Transferring Between Bed and Chair—*continued*

- Place the foot of the stronger leg beneath the edge of the bed (or sitting surface) and put the other foot forward. **Rationale:** *In this way, the client can use the stronger leg muscles to stand and power the movement. A broader base of support makes the client more stable during the transfer.*
- Place the client's hands on the bed surface (or available stable area) so that the client can push while standing. **Rationale:** *This provides additional force for the movement and reduces the potential for strain on the nurse's back.* The client should not grasp your neck for support. **Rationale:** *Doing so can injure the nurse.*

7. Position yourself correctly.
   - Stand directly in front of the client and to the side requiring the most support. Hold the gait/transfer belt with the nearest hand; the other hand supports the back of the client's shoulder. Lean the trunk forward from the hips. Flex the hips, knees, and ankles. Assume a broad stance, placing one foot forward and one back. Mirror the placement of the client's feet, if possible. **Rationale:** *This helps prevent loss of balance during the transfer.*

8. Assist the client to stand, and then move together toward the wheelchair or sitting area to which you wish to transfer the client.
   - Count to three or give the verbal instructions of "Ready—steady—stand." On the count of three or the word "stand," ask the client to push down against the mattress/side of the bed while you transfer your weight from one foot to the other (while keeping your back straight) and stand upright, moving the client forward (directly toward your center of gravity) into a standing position. (If the client requires more than a very small degree of pulling, even with the assistance of two nurses, a mechanical device should be obtained and used.)
   - Support the client in an upright standing position for a few moments. **Rationale:** *This allows the nurse and the client to extend the joints and provides the nurse with an opportunity to ensure that the client is stable before moving away from the bed.*
   - Together, pivot on your foot farthest from the chair, or take a few steps toward the wheelchair, bed, chair, commode, or car seat.

9. Assist the client to sit.
   - Move the wheelchair forward or have the client back up to the wheelchair (or desired seating area) and place the legs against the seat. **Rationale:** *Having the client place the legs against the wheelchair seat minimizes the risk of the client falling when sitting down.*
   - Make sure the wheelchair brakes are on.
   - Have the client reach back and feel/hold the arms of the wheelchair.
   - Stand directly in front of the client. Place one foot forward and one back.
   - Tighten your grasp on the transfer belt, and tighten your gluteal, abdominal, leg, and arm muscles.
   - Have the client sit down while you bend your knees/hips and lower the client onto the wheelchair seat.

10. Ensure client safety.
    - Ask the client to push back into the wheelchair seat. **Rationale:** *Sitting well back on the seat provides a broader base of support and greater stability and minimizes the risk of falling from the wheelchair. A wheelchair or bedside*

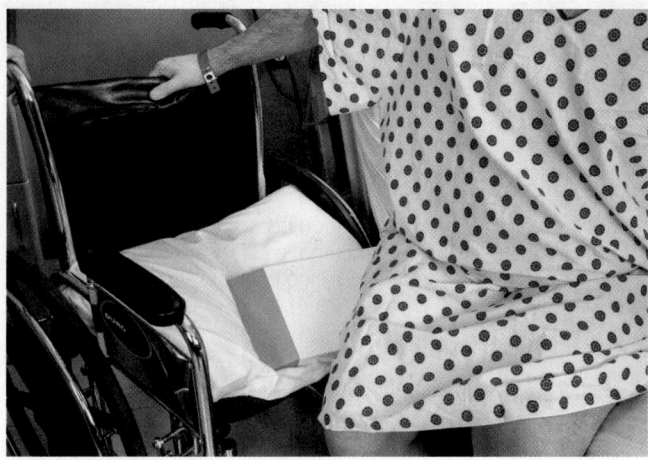

❷ Using a slide board.

commode can topple forward when the client sits on the edge of the seat and leans far forward.
- Remove the gait/transfer belt.
- Lower the footplates, and place the client's feet on them, if applicable.

Variation: Transferring with a Belt and Two Nurses
- Even if a client is able to partially bear weight and is cooperative, it still may be safer to transfer a client with the assistance of two nurses. If so, you should position yourselves on both sides of the client, facing the same direction as the client. Flex your hips, knees, and ankles. Grasp the client's transfer belt with the hand closest to the client, and with the other hand support the client's elbows.
- Coordinating your efforts, all three of you stand simultaneously, pivot, and move to the wheelchair. Reverse the process to lower the client onto the wheelchair seat.

Variation: Transferring a Client with an Injured Lower Extremity
When the client has an injured lower extremity, movement should always occur toward the client's unaffected (strong) side. For example, if the client's right leg is injured and the client is sitting on the edge of the bed preparing to transfer to a wheelchair, position the wheelchair on the client's left side. **Rationale:** *In this way, the client can use the unaffected leg most effectively and safely.*

Variation: Using a Slide Board
- For clients who cannot stand but are able to cooperate and possess sufficient upper body strength, use a slide board to help them move without nursing assistance. ❷ **Rationale:** *This method not only promotes the client's sense of independence but also preserves your energy.*

11. Document relevant information:
    - Client's ability to bear weight and pivot
    - Number of staff needed for transfer and safety measures/precautions used
    - Length of time up in chair
    - Client response to transfer and being up in chair or wheelchair.

Note: This skill describes the process to use for a client who is able to perform the task independently and only needs standby assistance for steadying. For clients who require moderate or maximum assistance, a lateral chair or a mobile or ceiling-mounted transfer system is required.

EVALUATION
- Check the skin integrity of the pressure areas from the previous position. Conduct follow-up assessment for previous and/or new skin breakdown areas.
- Check for proper alignment after the position change. Do a visual check and ask the client for a comfort assessment.
- Determine that all required safety precautions (e.g., locked wheels) are in place.
- Determine the client's tolerance of the activity (e.g., vital signs before and after transfer, particularly the first time the client is transferred).
- Report significant data to the primary care provider.

Transferring Between Bed and Stretcher

The stretcher, or gurney, is used to transfer supine clients from one location to another. Whenever the client is capable of accomplishing the transfer from bed to stretcher independently, either by lifting onto it or by rolling onto it, the client should be encouraged to do so. If the client cannot move onto the stretcher independently and weighs less than 200 pounds, a friction-reducing device (e.g., slide sheet) and/or a lateral transfer board (Figure 10–13 ■) or an air transfer system should be used and at least two caregivers are needed to assist with the transfer. Some friction-reducing devices have handles or long straps to avoid awkward stretching by the caregivers when pulling the client during the lateral transfer (Figure 10–14 ■). For clients between 201 and 300 pounds, a slide sheet or transfer board and four caregivers or an air transfer system and two caregivers should be used. For clients who weigh more than 300 pounds, two caregivers and either an air transfer system or a ceiling lift with supine sling should be used.

Depending on the client's condition (e.g., neck immobilizer, IVs, drains, chest tube), additional assistants may be needed.

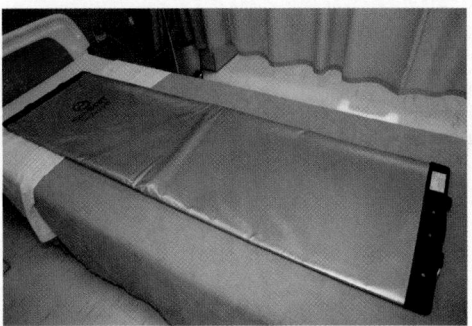

Figure 10–13 ■ A lateral transfer board. The friction-reducing material rolls when transferring clients in a supine position.

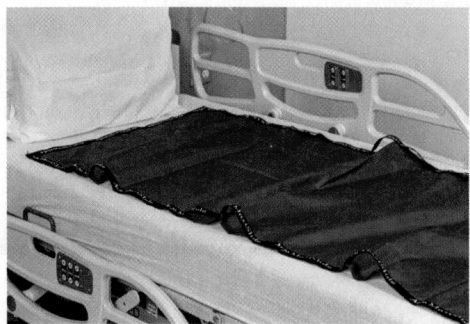

Figure 10–14 ■ Friction-reducing transfer device with handles.

WHAT IF   Transferring Between Bed and Chair

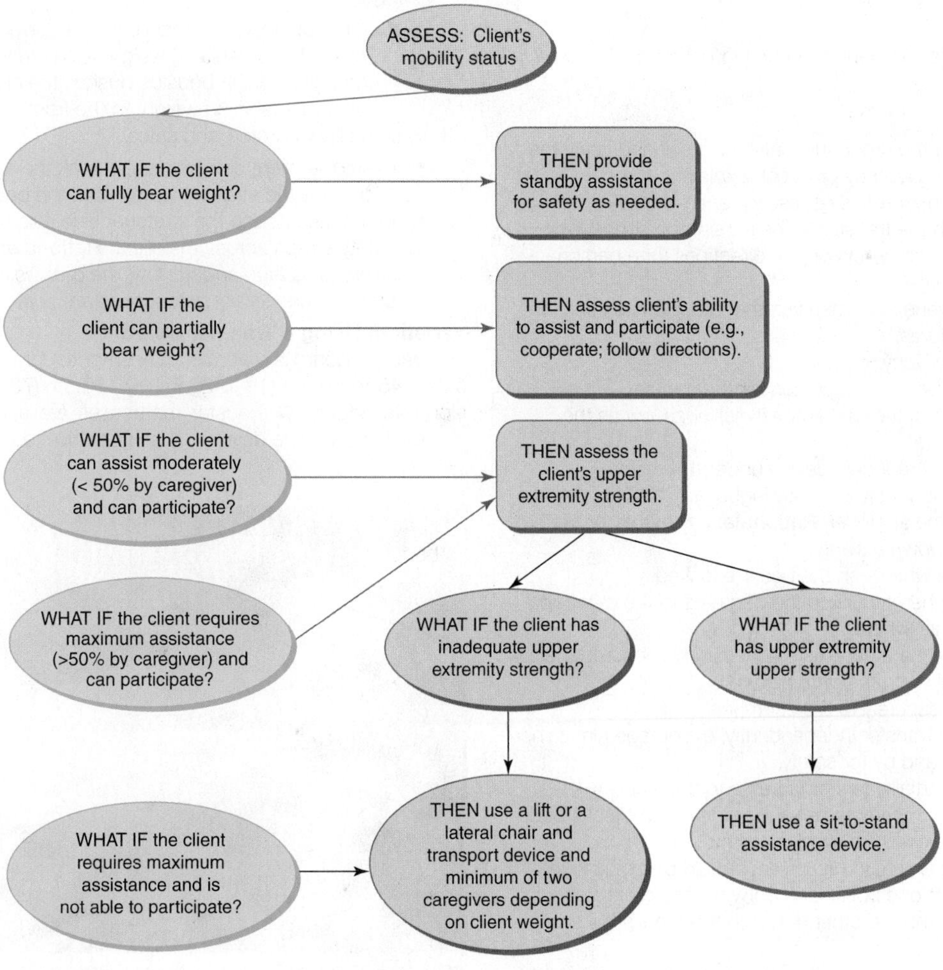

ASSESS: Client's mobility status

WHAT IF the client can fully bear weight? → THEN provide standby assistance for safety as needed.

WHAT IF the client can partially bear weight? → THEN assess client's ability to assist and participate (e.g., cooperate; follow directions).

WHAT IF the client can assist moderately (< 50% by caregiver) and can participate? → THEN assess the client's upper extremity strength.

WHAT IF the client requires maximum assistance (>50% by caregiver) and can participate?

WHAT IF the client has inadequate upper extremity strength?

WHAT IF the client has upper extremity upper strength?

WHAT IF the client requires maximum assistance and is not able to participate? → THEN use a lift or a lateral chair and transport device and minimum of two caregivers depending on client weight.

THEN use a sit-to-stand assistance device.

Adapted from *Navigating the New Safe Patient Handling and Mobility Interprofessional National Standards* (ANA webinar), by S. Harrington and C. Brigham, 2013. Retrieved from http://www.nursingworld.org/MainMenuCategories/WorkplaceSafety/Healthy-Work-Environment/SafePatient/SPHM-Standards-Media; *The Illustrated Guide to Safe Patient Handling and Movement*, by A. L. Nelson, K. Motacki, and N. Menzel, 2009. New York, NY: Springer; and *Algorithms for Safe Patient Handling and Movement*, U.S. Department of Veterans Affairs, 2012. Retrieved from http://www.visn8.va.gov/PatientSafetyCenter/safePtHandling

●○○● NURSING PROCESS: TRANSFERRING BETWEEN BED AND STRETCHER

Transferring Between Bed and Stretcher

ASSESSMENT
Assess:
- The client's body size and weight.
- Ability to follow instructions.
- Activity tolerance.
- Level of comfort.
- The space in which the transfer maneuver will take place.
- The number of assistants (one to four) needed to accomplish the transfer safely.

PLANNING
Review the client record to determine if previous nurses have recorded information about how the client tolerated similar transfers. If indicated, implement pain-relief measures so that they are effective when the transfer begins.

DELEGATION

The skill of transferring a client can be delegated to UAP who have demonstrated good body mechanics and safe transfer technique for the involved client. It is important for the nurse to assess the number of staff needed, assistive devices needed, and the client's ability to assist, and to communicate specific information about what the UAP should report to the nurse.

Equipment
- Stretcher
- Transfer assistive devices (e.g., slide sheet, transfer board, air transfer system, lift)

IMPLEMENTATION
Preparation
Obtain the necessary equipment and nursing personnel to assist in the transfer.

Performance
1. Prior to performing the procedure, introduce self and verify the client's identity using agency protocol. Explain to the client what you are going to do, why it is necessary, and how he or she can participate. Explain the transfer to the nursing personnel who are helping and specify who will give directions (one person needs to be in charge).
2. Perform hand hygiene and observe other appropriate infection prevention procedures.
3. Provide for client privacy.
4. Adjust the client's bed in preparation for the transfer.
   - Lower the head of the bed until it is flat or as low as the client can tolerate.
   - Place the friction-reducing device under the client.
   - Raise the bed so that it is slightly higher (i.e., 1/2 in.) than the surface of the stretcher. **Rationale:** *It is easier for the client to move down a slant.*
   - Ensure that the wheels on the bed are locked.
   - Place the stretcher parallel to the bed next to the client and lock the stretcher wheels.
   - *Optional:* Fill the gap that exists between the bed and the stretcher loosely with the bath blankets.
5. Transfer the client securely to the stretcher.
   - If the client can transfer independently, encourage him or her to do so and stand by for safety.
   - If the client is partially able or not able to transfer:
     - One caregiver needs to be at the side of the client's bed, between the client's shoulder and hip.
     - The second and third caregivers should be at the side of the stretcher: one positioned between the client's shoulder and hip and the other between the client's hip and lower legs.
     - All caregivers should position feet in a walking stance.
     - On a planned command, the caregivers at the stretcher's side pull (shifting weight to the rear foot) and the caregiver at the bedside pushes the client toward the stretcher (shifting weight to the front foot).
6. Ensure client comfort and safety.
   - Make the client comfortable, unlock the stretcher wheels, and move the stretcher away from the bed.
   - Immediately raise the stretcher side rails and/or fasten the safety straps across the client. **Rationale:** *Because the stretcher is high and narrow, the client is in danger of falling unless these safety precautions are taken.*

Variation: Using a Transfer Board
The transfer board is a lacquered or smooth polyethylene board measuring 45 to 55 cm (18 to 22 in.) by 182 cm (73 in.) with handholds along its edges. ❶ Transfer mattresses are also available, as are mechanical assistive devices. It is imperative to have enough people

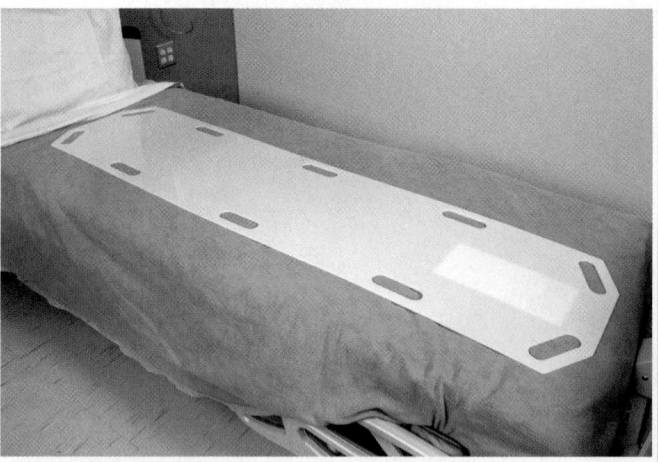

❶ A smooth polyethylene transfer board for transferring clients.

Transferring Between Bed and Stretcher—*continued*

assisting with the transfer to prevent injury to staff as well as clients. Turn the client to a lateral position away from you, position the board close to the client's back, and roll the client onto the board. Pull the client and board across the bed to the stretcher. Safety belts may be placed over the chest, abdomen, and legs.

EVALUATION
• Report any significant deviations from normal to the primary care provider.
• Note use of appropriate safety measures (e.g., locking wheels of bed and stretcher) by UAP during transfer process.

7. Document relevant information:
   • Equipment used
   • Number of people needed for transfer
   • Destination if reason for transfer is transport from one location to another.

SAMPLE DOCUMENTATION

7/22/2015 1030 Moved onto stretcher for transfer with the help of 2 staff and friction-reducing device. Became slightly dizzy. Vital signs remained stable, no c/o pain. Side rails on stretcher up and locked. ————————————————— E. Mitchell, RN

LIFESPAN CONSIDERATIONS   **Transferring Clients**

INFANTS
• The infant who is lying down, on the side or supine, can be placed in either a bassinet or crib for transport. If the bassinet has a bottom shelf, it can be used for carrying the IV pump or monitor.

CHILDREN
• The toddler should be transported in a high-top crib with the side rails up and the protective top in place. Stretchers should not be used because the mobile toddler may roll or fall off.

OLDER ADULTS
• Because the conditions of older clients can change from day to day, always assess the situation to ensure that you have the

right equipment and enough people to assist when transferring a client.
• Use special caution with older clients to prevent skin tears or bruising during a transfer or when using a hydraulic lift.
• Write the method used to transfer each client—equipment used, best position, and number of people needed to assist in the transfer. This can be part of the care plan and also be available in the client's room as a guide to all personnel caring for the client.
• Avoid sudden position changes. They can cause orthostatic hypotension and increase the risk of fainting and falls.

Ambulatory and Community Settings   **Transferring from Bed to a Chair** | **PATIENT-CENTERED CARE** |

• The caregiver and client should practice transfer skills in the hospital or long-term care setting before the client is discharged.
• Assess furniture in the home. Does the client's favorite chair have arms for ease of using and sitting? Examine the fabric—is

it rough? Will it cause skin abrasions? If the client will be using a wheelchair, is there enough space in the bedroom and bathroom for a safe transfer?
• Observe client and caregiver transfer skills in the home setting to reinforce prior teaching.

LIFTING DEVICES

Lifting devices, such as a mobile floor-based lift (see Figure 10–3), ceiling-mounted lift (see Figure 10–4), and sit-to-stand lift (see Figure 10–5) are used for clients who weigh more than 35 pounds and who cannot assist health care personnel in moving and transferring themselves. Floor-based and ceiling-mounted lifts can be used in transferring the client between the bed and a wheelchair, the bed and the bathtub, the bed and a stretcher, and the bed and toilet, or when lifting the client from the floor. The sit-to-stand lift can be used to assist a seated client to a standing position for dressing/undressing, and to transfer the client from the edge of the bed to a wheelchair. The mobile floor-based lift (Figure 10–3 ■) consists of a base on casters, a hydraulic mechanical pump, a mast

boom, and a sling, and its use is described in Skill 10–8. The sling may consist of a one-piece or two-piece canvas seat. The one-piece seat stretches from the client's head to the knees. The two-piece seat has one canvas strap to support the client's buttocks and thighs and a second strap extending up to the axillae to support the back. There are other types of slings depending on the client's needs (e.g., slings for clients with an amputation, clients with paraplegia, and large clients). Due to infection control standards, it is recommended that clients have their own sling. It is important to be familiar with the model used and the practices that accompany use. Before using the lift, the nurse ensures that it is in working order and that the hooks, chains, straps, and sling are in good repair. Most agencies recommend that two nurses operate a lift. Check agency policy.

●○○● NURSING PROCESS: HYDRAULIC LIFTS

Using a Mobile Floor-Based Hydraulic Lift

ASSESSMENT

Determine:

- Client's ability to comprehend instructions.
- Degree of physical disability.
- Weight of the client (to ensure that the lift can safely move the client).
- Presence of orthostatic hypotension.
- Pulse rate.

PLANNING
DELEGATION

The skill of using a hydraulic lift can be delegated to UAP who have demonstrated competent use of the equipment for the involved client.

Equipment

- Hydraulic lift (such as a mobile floor or ceiling-mounted lift) with any necessary accessories

IMPLEMENTATION

Preparation

Obtain the lift and put in the client's room. Arrange for assistance from others at a designated time.

Performance

1. Prior to performing the procedure, introduce self and verify the client's identity using agency protocol. Explain to the client what you are going to do, why it is necessary, and how he or she can participate. Explain the procedure and demonstrate the lift. **Rationale:** *Some clients may initially be anxious of being lifted and will be reassured by a demonstration.*
2. Perform hand hygiene and observe other appropriate infection prevention procedures.
3. Provide for client privacy.
4. Prepare the equipment.
   - Lock the wheels of the client's bed and raise the bed to the high position.
   - Put up the side rail on the opposite side of the bed, and lower the side rail near you.
   - Position the lift so that it is close to the client.
   - Place the chair that is to receive the client beside the bed. Allow adequate space to maneuver the lift.
   - Lock the wheels, if a chair with wheels is used.
5. Position the client on the sling. *The remaining steps of this procedure need to be performed by at least two health care personnel working together with the client.*
   - Roll the client away from you.
   - Place the canvas seat or sling under the client with the wide lower edge under the client's thighs to the knees and the more narrow upper edge up under the client's shoulders. **Rationale:** *This places the sling under the client's center of gravity and greatest part of body weight. Correct placement permits the client to be lifted evenly, with minimal shifting.*
   - With the help of your assistant, roll the client to the opposite side, and pull the canvas sling through.
   - Roll the client to the supine position, and center the client on top of the canvas sling.
6. Attach the sling to the swivel bar.
   - Wheel the lift into position, with the footbars under the bed on the side where the chair is positioned. Set the adjustable base at the widest position to ensure stability. Lock the wheels of the lifter.
   - Lower the side rail.
   - Move the lift arms directly over the client and lower the horizontal bar by releasing the hydraulic valve. Lock the valve.
   - Attach the lifter straps or hooks to the corresponding openings in the canvas seat. Check that the hooks are correctly placed and that matching straps or chains are of equal length. Face the hooks away from the client. **Rationale:** *This prevents the hooks from injuring the client.*
7. Lift the client gradually.
   - Elevate the head of the bed to place the client in a sitting position.
   - Ask the client to remove eyeglasses and put them in a safe place. **Rationale:** *The swivel bar may come close to the face and cause breakage of eyeglasses.*
   - *Nurse 1:* Close the pressure valve, and gradually pump the jack handle until the client is above the bed surface. **Rationale:** *Gradual elevation of the lift is less frightening to the client than a rapid rise.*
   - *Nurse 2:* Assume a broad stance, and guide the client with your hands as the client is lifted. **Rationale:** *This prepares the nurse to reassure the client and provide control during the movement.*
   - Check the placement of the sling before moving the client away from the bed.
8. Move the client over the chair.
   - *Nurse 1:* With the pressure valve securely closed, slowly roll the lift until the client is over the chair. Use the steering handle to maneuver the lift.
   - *Nurse 2:* Guide movement by hand until the client is directly over the chair. **Rationale:** *Slow movement decreases swaying and is less frightening. Guidance also decreases swaying and gives a sense of security.*
9. Lower the client into the chair.
   - *Nurse 1:* Release the pressure valve very gradually. **Rationale:** *Gradual release is less frightening than a quick descent.*
   - *Nurse 2:* Guide the client into the chair.

Using a Mobile Floor-Based Hydraulic Lift—*continued*

10. Ensure client comfort and safety.
- Remove the hooks from the canvas seat. Leave the seat in place. **Rationale:** *The seat is left in place in preparation for the lift back to bed.*
- Align the client appropriately in a sitting position and return the client's eyeglasses, if appropriate.

- Apply a seat belt as needed.
- Place the call bell within reach.

11. Document the type of equipment, number of assistants needed, safety precautions taken, and the client's physiological and psychological response.

EVALUATION
- Note safety precautions required for clients during and after the transfer.
- Check body alignment of the client in the sitting position.
- Relate vital signs, especially pulse rate and blood pressure, to determine response to the transfer.

- Compare the client's current response to previous responses to use of the hydraulic lift.
- Report any significant deviations from normal to the primary care provider.

SPECIALIZED BEDS

Therapeutic beds, also referred to as specialized or specialty beds, are bed units that provide a healing environment. Check agency policy to determine if an order by a primary care provider is needed. Specialty beds replace hospital beds. They provide pressure relief, eliminate shearing and friction, and decrease moisture. Examples are high-air-loss beds, low-air-loss beds, and beds that provide kinetic therapy. Kinetic beds provide continuous passive motion or oscillation therapy, which is intended to counteract the effects of a client's immobility. Five major types of therapeutic beds are commonly used today, as listed in Table 10–2.

Nurses should understand how to operate therapeutic beds before providing care. Operating instructions should be attached to the bed in a prominent place. Controls should be conveniently located for both the client and the nurse and have a lockout mechanism to prevent accidental activation. Mattress sections of therapeutic beds often require special sheets. Assess for skin irritation or pressure areas, discomfort, numbness or tingling in the extremities, and change in ability to move or motor strength of extremities.

Turning and positioning of clients in special beds requires training. UAP and other care providers who have been trained may perform these procedures for stable clients. The nurse should perform the first few turns when a client is initially placed on a specialty bed. The nurse also ensures that the UAP knows how to handle catheters and other tubing or equipment involved. In some particularly unstable situations, two individuals should perform the turn. If UAP turn the client without a nurse, any abnormal findings must be reported immediately to the nurse.

CLINICAL ALERT!

The long-held standard for turning clients who cannot turn themselves has been every 2 hours. Recent studies in select intensive care units in both the United States and the United Kingdom, however, have suggested that this standard is often not met. Some intensive care units use rotation therapy, specialized beds that can be programmed to turn a client up to eight times an hour.

LIFESPAN CONSIDERATIONS Specialized Beds

CHILD
- Spinal cord and other injuries requiring therapeutic beds are rare in children. Most orthopedic conditions can be treated with body casts and external braces.

OLDER ADULTS
- Older adults are at increased risk for skin and neurologic impairments. They may be less aware of or less able to report complications related to pressure areas.

Ambulatory and Community Settings Specialized Beds

PATIENT-CENTERED CARE

- Some clients with long-term disabilities may have specialized beds in the home. Ensure that all family and caregivers have been instructed in proper use of the bed and can demonstrate an appropriate level of care.

- If the bed is electric, assess adequacy and safety of the wiring in the home.
- Confirm that the caregivers are aware of emergency measures if the client arrests, a fire occurs in the home, or the electricity fails.

TABLE 10–2	Mechanical Devices for Reducing Pressure on Body Parts

Alternating pressure mattress	Composed of a number of cells in which the pressure alternately increases and decreases; uses a pump.
Water bed	Support surface filled with water. Water temperature can be controlled.
Static low-air-loss (LAL) bed	Consists of many air-filled cushions divided into four or five sections. Separate controls permit each section to be inflated to a different level of firmness; thus pressure can be reduced on bony prominences but increased under other body areas for support.
Active or second-generation LAL bed	Like the static LAL, but in addition gently pulsates or rotates from side to side, thus stimulating capillary blood flow and facilitating movement of pulmonary secretions.
Air-fluidized (AF) bed (static high-air-loss bed)	Forced temperature-controlled air is circulated around millions of tiny silicone-coated beads, producing a fluidlike movement. Provides uniform support to body contours. Decreases skin maceration by its drying effect. Moisture from the client penetrates the linens and soaks the beads. Airflow forces the beads away from the client and rapidly dries the sheet. A major disadvantage is that the head of the bed cannot be elevated. Some beds are a unique combination of air-fluidized therapy and low-air-loss therapy on an articulating frame. These are used with clients who require head elevation.

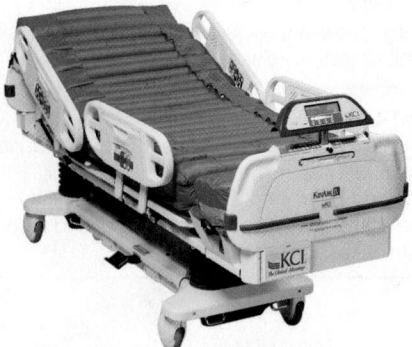

Low-air-loss bed KinAir IV.
Courtesy ArjoHuntleigh.

FOCUSING ON CLINICAL THINKING

Consider This

1. As a nurse, what can you do to prevent back injury to yourself and others?

2. You are providing nursing care for a client who has the following equipment: two IVs (one inserted into a central line and the other in a peripheral line), an indwelling catheter, a nasogastric tube connected to suction, and a Hemovac drain. The client is scheduled to go to the radiology department via stretcher. How will you facilitate the client being moved to the stretcher without injury to the client or yourself?

3. You and another nursing student have turned a client with right-sided paralysis to a left semiprone position. The client can understand what you say to him but he cannot express himself verbally. He can appropriately move his head for "yes" and "no." How will you determine that the client is comfortable and in correct alignment after positioning him?

4. What would you do if a client who needs to be transferred from the bed to a chair exhibits the following: expresses fear of falling, does not want to move because "it will hurt," and states "you are new and don't know what to do"?

See Focusing on Clinical Thinking answers on student resource website.

TEST YOUR KNOWLEDGE

1. A client is to be placed in a dorsal recumbent position. How should the nurse position this client?
   1. In a semisitting position in which the head and trunk are raised and flexed
   2. In a sitting position on the side of the bed with an overbed table across the lap
   3. In a back-lying position in which the client's head and shoulders are slightly elevated on a small pillow
   4. In a lying position on the abdomen with the head turned to one side

2. A nurse gathers three other people on the unit to assist in the transfer of a client. Which staff member needs to be corrected for use of proper body mechanics before the lift starts?
   1. The staff member who assumes a wide stance
   2. The staff member who is stretching to reach the client's transfer sheet
   3. The staff member who faces the direction of the movement
   4. The staff member who adjusts the work area to waist level

3. Which statement identifies correct safety information for nurses?
   1. Nurses who are physically fit sustain fewer injuries than their less active coworkers.
   2. A nurse should not lift over 35 pounds of client body weight.
   3. Back belts are likely to be effective in reducing back injury.
   4. Training nurses in body mechanics alone will prevent job-related injuries.

4. Which steps will the nurse need to perform to move a client up in bed? Select all that apply.
   1. Remove all pillows, then place one against the head of the bed.
   2. Elicit the client's help in lessening the workload when possible.
   3. Face opposite the direction of movement, and then assume a broad stance.
   4. Ensure client comfort.
   5. Use a friction-reducing device to help pull the client up in bed.

5. The nurse asks a nursing student to support the client's leg to prevent its external rotation while supine. Which assistive device should the student use?
   1. A trochanter roll
   2. A footboard
   3. A hand roll
   4. An abduction pillow

6. Which nursing action supports the nurse's intervention to align and support a client in the Sims' position?
   1. A sandbag to support feet in extension to prevent foot drop
   2. A pillow under the lower leg to prevent internal rotation and abduction of the hip and leg
   3. A pillow under the upper arm to prevent external rotation of shoulder and arm
   4. A pillow to support the head, maintaining it in good alignment

7. A nurse is attending an in-service on moving and lifting clients. Which statement by the nurse requires clarification by the in-service educator?
   1. "Appropriate numbers of staff should be used to perform the maneuver."
   2. "Appropriate assistive devices should be used to perform the maneuver."
   3. "The height of the bed should be raised to bring the client close to my center of gravity."
   4. "I should rock from my back leg to my front leg when pulling a client."

8. Which client who requires repositioning could be safely delegated to the UAP by the nurse?
   1. A client who is 6 hours post–lumbar laminectomy
   2. A client who was involved in a motor vehicle collision this morning and is being evaluated for a cervical injury
   3. A client in a chronic vegetative state
   4. A client who was intubated and placed on a ventilator this morning

9. The nurse is preparing to use a hydraulic lift to move the client into the bedside chair. What is the priority action for the nurse before beginning the skill?
  1. Position the client on the sling.
  2. Explain the procedure to the client.
  3. Lift the client gradually.
  4. Apply gloves.

10. The nurse is working in a long-term care facility and caring for a client in a chronic vegetative state. It is important for the nurse to document which of the following in the client's medical record? Select all that apply.
  1. When the client is repositioned and in which position the client is placed
  2. Any change in skin integrity
  3. Number of staff members participating in repositioning of clients
  4. The body mechanics used by the staff when repositioning the client
  5. Rationale for frequent repositioning

See Answers to Test Your Knowledge in Appendix A.

READINGS AND REFERENCES

References

American Nurses Association. (n.d.). *Safe patient handling and mobility (SPHM)*. Retrieved from http://nursingworld.org/MainMenuCategories/Policy-Advocacy/State/Legislative-Agenda-Reports/State-SafePatientHandling

American Nurses Association. (2011). *2011 ANA health and safety survey*. Retrieved from http://www.nursingworld.org/MainMenuCategories/WorkplaceSafety/Healthy-Work-Environment/Work-Environment/2011-HealthSafetySurvey.html

American Nurses Association. (2013). *Safe patient handling and mobility. Interprofessional national standards across the care continuum*. Silver Spring, MD: Author.

Bureau of Labor Statistics. (2013). *Nonfatal occupational injuries and illnesses requiring days away from work, 2012.* Retrieved from http://www.bls.gov/news.release/pdf/osh2.pdf

Fragala, G. (2011). Facilitating repositioning in bed. *AAOHN Journal, 59*(2), 63–68. doi:10.3928/08910162-20110117-01

Harrington, S., & Brigham, C. (2013). *Navigating the new safe patient handling and mobility interprofessional national standards* (ANA webinar). Retrieved from http://www.nursingworld.org/MainMenuCategories/WorkplaceSafety/Healthy-Work-Environment/SafePatient/SPHM-Standards-Media

Nelson, A. L., Motacki, K., & Menzel, N. (2009). *The illustrated guide to safe patient handling and movement*. New York, NY: Springer.

Rockefeller, K., & Proctor, R. B. (2011). Is there a role for gait belts in safe patient handling and movement programs? *American Journal of SPHM, 1*(1), 30–35.

Safe lifting becomes standard practice. (2013). *Hospital Case Management, 21*(2), 26–28.

U.S. Department of Veterans Affairs. (2012). *Algorithms for safe patient handling and movement*. Retrieved from http://www.visn8.va.gov/PatientSafetyCenter/safePtHandling/

Selected Bibliography

Asher, A. (2013). Equipment used for safe mobilization of the ICU patient. *Critical Care Nursing Quarterly, 36*, 101–108. doi:10.1097/CNQ.0b013e318275357e

Berman, A., Snyder, S., & Frandsen, G. (2016). *Kozier & Erb's fundamentals of nursing: Concepts, process, and practice* (10th ed.). Upper Saddle River, NJ: Pearson.

Darragh, A. R., Campo, M. A., Frost, L., Miller, M., Pentico, M., & Margulis, H. (2013). Safe-patient-handling equipment in therapy practice: Implications for rehabilitation. *American Journal of Occupational Therapy, 67*(1), 45–53. doi:10.5014/ajot.2013.005389

Edelstein, J. E. (2013). Assistive devices for ambulation. *Physical Medicine and Rehabilitation Clinics of North America, 24*, 291–303. doi:10.1016/j.pmr.2012.11.001

Hard to handle: Risk rises as obesity surges. (2013). *Hospital Employee Health, 32*(1), 5–6.

Pelczarski, K. (2012). Back in action: Design considerations for safe patient handling. *Health Facilities Management, 25*(8), 21–25.

Stevens, L., Rees, S., Lamb, K. V., & Dalsing, D. (2013). Creating a culture of safety for safe patient handling. *Orthopaedic Nursing, 32*, 155–164. doi:10.1097/NOR.0b013e318291dbc5

U.S. Food and Drug Administration. (2014). *Medical devices: Patient lifts*. Retrieved from http://www.fda.gov/MedicalDevices/ProductsandMedicalProcedures/GeneralHospitalDevicesandSupplies/ucm308622.htm

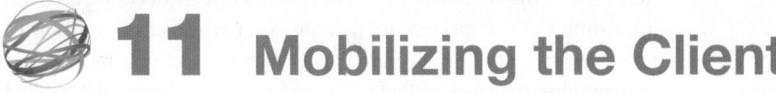

11 Mobilizing the Client

LEARNING OUTCOMES

At the completion of this chapter, the student will be able to:

1. Define the key terms used in the skills of client mobilization.
2. Describe appropriate safety measures to use when assisting clients to ambulate.
3. Recognize when it is appropriate to delegate client ambulation assistance to unlicensed assistive personnel.
4. Verbalize the steps used in assisting the client to:
   a. Use a wheelchair.
   b. Ambulate.
   c. Use a cane.
   d. Use crutches.
   e. Use a walker.
5. Demonstrate appropriate documentation and reporting of client mobilization activities.

SKILLS

Skill 11–1 Assisting the Client to Use a Wheelchair
Skill 11–2 Assisting the Client to Ambulate
Skill 11–3 Assisting the Client to Use a Cane

Skill 11–4 Assisting the Client to Use Crutches
Skill 11–5 Assisting the Client to Use a Walker

KEY TERMS

The importance of body movement to a person's health cannot be overemphasized. The overall benefits of exercise and the ability to carry out the activities of daily living (ADLs) by walking and moving are often taken for granted by a healthy person. Being ill and confined to bed weakens the body and can result in serious impairments not only to movement but also to the functioning of other body systems. Clients should be encouraged to keep moving, and they may require assistance through the use of walkers, canes, and crutches in order to do so. Some clients may require the use of a wheelchair for a short or an extended period of time. Clients and their families often need to learn how to use equipment that enhances mobility.

In the field of nursing, work-related musculoskeletal disorders (MSDs), such as back and shoulder injuries, persist as the leading and most costly U.S. occupational health problem. The American Nurses Association (ANA) has been involved in the effort to protect nurses from MSDs for many years and has taken the official position of supporting actions and policies that result in the elimination of manual handling of clients in order to establish a safe environment for nurses and clients (ANA, 2013). Safe patient handling and mobility (SPHM) programs can greatly reduce health care worker injuries. See Chapter 10 ∞ for additional information about preventing back injuries and using assistive devices for safe client handling.

ASSISTING CLIENTS TO USE WHEELCHAIRS

There are two general types of wheelchairs: manual and electric/power. This chapter focuses on manual wheelchairs because there

are significant variations in the design and operation of power wheelchairs. It is important to evaluate a client's ability to propel him- or herself manually by means of a wheelchair if independent use is desired. Otherwise, an electric wheelchair that can be manipulated by the client using whatever physical abilities are available must be chosen. Manual wheelchairs may be either folding or rigid framed and come in a variety of sizes (Figure 11–1 ■).

Manual wheelchairs come in different classifications. Normal wheelchairs are 16 kg (36 lb) or heavier, lightweight ones are 15 to 16 kg (34 to 36 lb), and high-strength lightweight types range from 13 to 15 kg (28 to 34 lb). Ultra-lightweight wheelchairs start at about 6 kg (14 lb) (Spinlife, 2013). The lighter the wheelchair, the easier the client can maneuver it around. The cost, however, increases as the weight of the wheelchair decreases. Folding wheelchairs have an X-shaped brace under the seat that allows the seat to fold arm to arm. Although the ability to fold the wheelchair for placement in a car or for compact storage may be desirable, folding wheelchairs have drawbacks. The brace makes the wheelchair heavy and possibly too heavy for one person to lift. In addition, the frame is not as strong as a rigid frame, and the moving joints are subject to wear. The rigid frame usually has a seat back that folds down and easily removable wheels. Armrests can be removed from most wheelchairs.

Footplates (footrests) and leg rests may be rigid or adjustable. Adjustable leg rests are more common in wheelchairs found in hospitals since they are used when the feet need to be raised to aid in circulation or for individuals who cannot bend their knees. Wheel locks are generally side mounted with short or long lever arms that

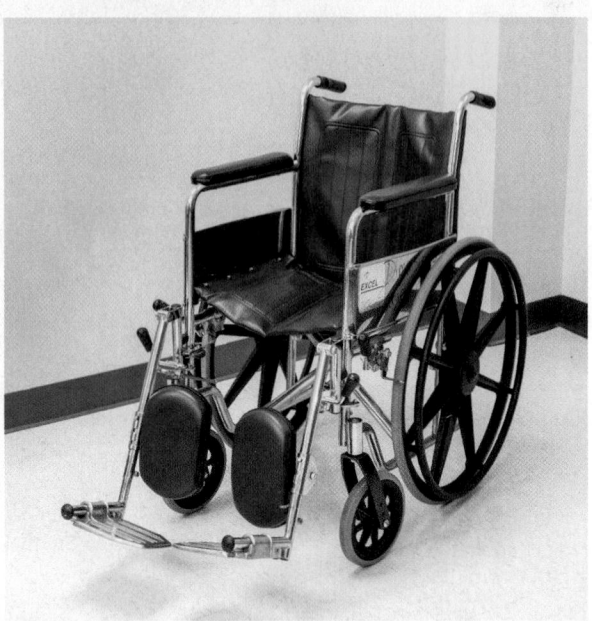

Figure 11–1 ■ Standard wheelchair.

are used to manually move the brake arm against the wheel. The size and type of the wheelchair's smaller front caster wheels are selected according to the expected use. Larger caster wheels roll over bumps more easily but are heavier, are harder to turn, and take more room to turn. Tires may be air filled (pneumatic) or solid (airless). Air-filled tires are light, smooth, and durable. Solid tires do not go flat, which makes them more reliable for power wheelchairs when the extra weight is less of a concern.

For individuals who spend a great deal of time in a wheelchair, proper seating is of utmost importance. If the seat does not adequately support the client, skin breakdown and adverse effects of poor posture can result. For temporary use, the sling seat that comes with most wheelchairs is acceptable. However, sling seats can cause internal rotation of the hips, flexion of the pelvis, and inadequate neck support. They may also cause skin breakdown if used for extended periods of time. For long-term use, a rigid back and a solid seat platform with a foam, air, gel, or honeycomb cushion are required. It may also be desirable to use a tilt, multi-positioning chair with the ability to assume a reclining position when the client is expected to remain in a wheelchair for lengthy amounts of time.

●○● NURSING PROCESS: WHEELCHAIRS

Assisting the Client to Use a Wheelchair

SKILL 11-1

ASSESSMENT
Determine the client's body size, ability to follow instructions, activity tolerance, muscle strength, joint mobility, presence of paralysis, level of comfort, and experience with the use of a wheelchair. It is important to use the right size wheelchair for the individual client, in consideration of the client's needs. Selections include pediatric, standard, or bariatric models.

PLANNING
Review the client's needs and the types of wheelchairs available. Wheelchairs vary in the ability to adjust the chair back, arms, legs, and foot supports, and to carry an intravenous (IV) pole, oxygen tank, or other supplies.

DELEGATION

Unlicensed assistive personnel (UAP) are qualified to transfer clients into and out of wheelchairs and to transport clients in wheelchairs if properly trained and supervised and if the client is in stable condition. If it is the first time the client has transferred into or out of a wheelchair, the nurse should assist and demonstrate as necessary, observe the performance of both the client and UAP, and reinforce proper technique with both.

Equipment
- Wheelchair
- Pillows (as needed)
- Chair alarm pads or other alerting devices if necessary for the safety of a confused client who may need help remembering to call for assistance when needed

IMPLEMENTATION
Performance
1. Prior to performing the procedure, introduce self and verify the client's identity using agency protocol. Explain to the client what you are going to do, why it is necessary, and how he or she can participate. Discuss how this activity relates to the overall plan of care.
2. Perform hand hygiene and observe other appropriate infection prevention procedures.
3. Provide for client privacy.
4. Lock the wheels of the wheelchair, raise the footplate, and transfer the client into the wheelchair (see Skill 10–6 in Chapter 10 ∞).
5. Examine the client's body alignment and provide support if the client cannot maintain proper alignment independently.

6. Place equipment (e.g., urinary catheter bags and oxygen tubing) safely on the wheelchair where they cannot get caught in the wheels. Keep the urinary catheter drainage bag below the level of the client's bladder. **Rationale:** *This prevents reflux of urine back into the bladder and potential infection.*
7. Instruct the client in the importance of periodic shifting of body weight. **Rationale:** *This reduces pressure on bony prominences and preserves intact skin.* If the client cannot perform these movements independently, establish a routine for assisting the client at least every hour.
8. Ensure client safety.
   - Ask the client to sit far back into the wheelchair seat.
     Rationale: *A wheelchair can topple forward if the client sits on the edge of the seat and leans far forward.*

Assisting the Client to Use a Wheelchair—*continued*

- Do not put overly heavy items on the back of the wheelchair.
- Position the calf supports. Lower the footplates, and place the client's feet on them. Adjust the leg height if needed.
- Apply a seat belt as required. Although a belt may be appropriate for transport in a wheelchair, the client cannot be left secured with a seat belt or a fixed table such as in a "gerichair" because this is considered a physical restraint (Centers for Medicare and Medicaid Services, 2008).

- Release the brakes and transport the client (see Practice Guidelines).
- Do not leave the client unattended if the client cannot mobilize the wheelchair independently.

9. Document the transfer and client teaching in the client record using forms or checklists supplemented by narrative notes when appropriate. If necessary, include a description of the positioning aids used.

EVALUATION
- Perform a detailed follow-up assessment based on the client's response to the transfer and ability to use the wheelchair.

- Report significant deviations from expected or normal for the client to the primary care provider.

LIFESPAN CONSIDERATIONS   Using a Wheelchair

Be sensitive to the significance that the wheelchair may have for the client. For some, it may mean an opportunity for some much-desired mobility. For an older client, it may signify a negative milestone of increasing dependence. For a young client who is undergoing a temporary lack of mobility (such as with a fractured femur), it might be necessary to emphasize safety precautions, because the temptation to try "tricks" with the wheelchair may arise.

CHILDREN
- Children learn quickly how to maneuver themselves in an appropriately sized wheelchair. They may view the wheelchair

almost as a special "toy" and disregard the dangers involved in, for instance, trying to balance the wheelchair on its back wheels only while moving rapidly. Ensure that proper education is performed and supervision is sufficient until it is clear that the child will be safe in the wheelchair.

OLDER ADULTS
- Some older adults may have incomplete sensation or control in their extremities. Clients who have had strokes may have lost their sense of what is truly "upright." Ensure that arms and legs are appropriately supported and protected from injury.

Ambulatory and Community Settings   Safety

Using a Wheelchair
- Many homes are not constructed to permit wheelchair access. Arrange for a home assessment prior to discharging a client who will need to use a wheelchair inside the home. A ramp may need to be constructed so that the person requiring the wheelchair can enter the home without negotiating stairs. Modifications inside the home as well may be necessary, especially for use of bathrooms. Sometimes bedrooms may need to be

relocated downstairs so that the client will be able to access a bed without difficulty.
- Teach the client and family how to use the wheelchair appropriately. This includes collapsing the wheelchair for transport in a car, proper wheeling down sidewalks and ramps (if a person in a wheelchair is being pushed down an incline, the person assisting should back down the incline), and using it with public transportation services (e.g., buses that accept wheelchairs, elevator access to transit loading areas).

PRACTICE GUIDELINES

Safely Transporting a Client in a Wheelchair

- Always lock the brakes on both wheels of the wheelchair when the client transfers in or out of it. Recognize that the wheel locks are not brakes. They will not stop a rolling wheelchair and may not prevent sliding.
- Raise the footplates and move the calf rests out of the way before transferring the client into the wheelchair.
- Lower the footplates after the transfer, put the calf rests back in place, and place the client's feet on the footrests.
- Ensure the client is positioned well back in the seat of the wheelchair.
- Use seat belts that fasten behind the wheelchair to protect confused clients from falls. Note:*Seat belts are a form of restraint and must be used in accordance with policies and procedures that apply to the use of restraints (see Chapter 12 ∞). The temporary use of a seat belt while actively transporting a client is generally not considered a restraint, but a safety precaution.*

- Back the wheelchair into and, if possible, out of an elevator, rear large wheels first. This allows the client to see the door and makes exiting the elevator easier.
- Place your body between the wheelchair and the bottom of an incline or curb. Proceed backward, using your body weight as a brake if needed.
- If it is appropriate to take a rest while going up or down a long slope, turn the wheelchair sideways, perpendicular to the slope, and lock the wheels while resting.
- When wheeling the client up or down steps, both the helper and the client should be facing up the steps. *Note: Clients should be wheeled up or down only long-tread, low-rise steps. Since adequate control cannot be ensured on steps where the entire back wheel cannot rest, the client must be carried up or down regular-sized steps. Ramps are always preferable to steps, even long-tread, low-rise steps.*

AMBULATION

Ambulation (the act of walking) is a function that most people take for granted. However, when people are ill, they are often confined to bed and are nonambulatory. The longer clients are in bed, the more difficulty they have walking. In fact, evidence continues to support that early, routine mobilization of critically ill clients is safe, improves muscle strength and functional independence, and reduces hospital length of stay (Dammeyer, Dickinson, Packard, Baldwin, & Ricklemann, 2013).

Even 1 or 2 days of bed rest can make a person feel weak, unsteady, and shaky when first getting out of bed. A client who has had surgery, is older, or has been immobilized for a longer time will feel more pronounced weakness. This is because a decrease in muscle size and strength, together with the risk for orthostatic hypotension, can develop quickly in the client who is confined to bed. The potential problems of immobility are far less likely to occur when clients become ambulatory as soon as possible. The nurse can assist clients to prepare for ambulation by helping them become as independent as possible while in bed. Nurses should encourage clients to perform ADLs, maintain good body alignment, and carry out active ROM exercises to the maximum degree possible yet within the limitations imposed by their illness and recovery program (see Chapter 13 ∞). Collaboration with physical therapy, when ordered, can also be very useful in strengthening the muscles needed for ambulation. Clients are taught exercises such as quadriceps muscle exercises, which can then be practiced with the nurse or on their own.

Clients who have been in bed for long periods often need a plan of muscle tone exercises to strengthen the muscles used for walking before attempting to walk. One of the most important muscle groups is the quadriceps femoris, which extends the knee and flexes the thigh. This group is also important for elevating the legs, for example, for walking upstairs. These exercises are frequently called quadriceps

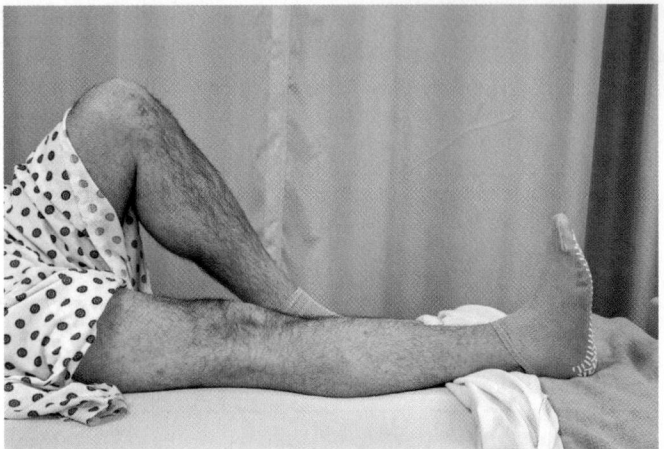

Figure 11–2 ■ Tensing the quadriceps femoris muscles before ambulating.

drills or sets (Figure 11–2 ■). To strengthen these muscles, the client consciously tenses them, drawing the kneecap upward and inward. The client pushes the popliteal space of the knee against the bed surface, relaxing the heels on the bed surface. On the count of 1, the muscles are tensed; they are held during the counts of 2, 3, 4; and they are relaxed at the count of 5. The exercise should be done within the client's tolerance, that is, without fatiguing the muscles. Carried out several times an hour during waking hours, this simple exercise significantly strengthens the muscles used for walking.

Common problems that affect walking include pathology of the muscles, disease or injury of the bones of the lower extremities, and impaired balance—such as from an inner ear infection or due to a cerebrovascular accident (CVA [stroke]) that produces **hemiplegia** (loss of movement on one side of the body). Nurses frequently need to assist clients in walking and in using a variety of devices.

●○○ NURSING PROCESS: AMBULATION

Assisting the Client to Ambulate

Clients who have been immobilized for even a few days may require assistance with ambulation. The amount of assistance will depend on the client's condition, including age, health status, and length of inactivity. Assistance may mean walking alongside the client while providing standby support for safety or providing instruction to the client about the use of assistive devices such as a cane, walker, or crutches or using a sit-to-stand lift with ambulation capability (see Figure 10–5 in Chapter 10 ∞) or a lift with an ambulation sling (Figure 11–3 ■).

Some clients experience postural (orthostatic) hypotension on assuming a vertical position from a lying position and may need information about ways to control this problem. The client may exhibit some or all of the following symptoms: pallor, diaphoresis, nausea, tachycardia, and dizziness. If any of these are present, the client should be assisted to a supine position in bed and closely assessed.

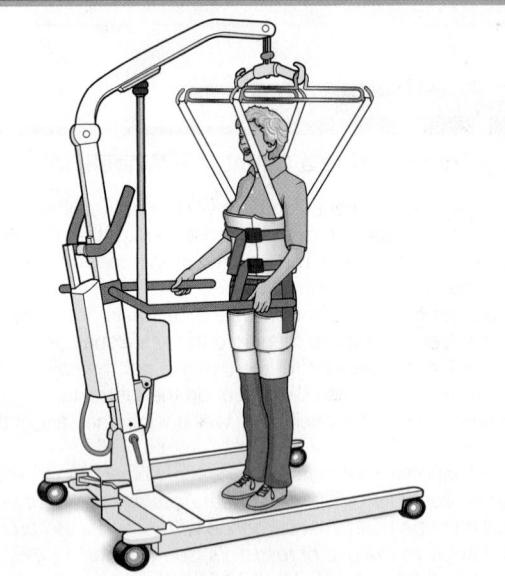

Figure 11–3 ■ Promoting ambulation by using a lift with an ambulation sling.

Assisting the Client to Ambulate—*continued*

ASSESSMENT
Assess:
- Length of time in bed and the amount and type of activity the client was last able to tolerate.
- Baseline vital signs.
- Range of motion of joints needed for ambulating (e.g., hips, knees, ankles).
- Muscle strength of lower extremities.
- Need for ambulation aids (e.g., cane, walker, crutches, sit-to-stand lift with ambulation capability, lift with ambulation sling).

- Client's intake of medications (e.g., narcotics, sedatives, antihypertensives, tranquilizers, and antihistamines) that may cause drowsiness, dizziness, weakness, and orthostatic hypotension and seriously hinder the client's ability to walk safely.
- Presence of joint inflammation, fractures, muscle weakness, or other conditions that impair physical mobility.
- Ability to understand directions.
- Level of comfort.

PLANNING
Implement pain-relief measures so that they are effective.

The amount of assistance needed while ambulating will depend on the client's age, health status, length of inactivity, and emotional readiness. Review any previous experiences with ambulation and the success of such efforts. Plan the length of the walk with the client in light of the nursing or primary care provider's orders and the medical condition of the client. Be prepared to shorten the walk according to the person's activity tolerance.

DELEGATION

Ambulation of clients is frequently delegated to UAP. However, the nurse should conduct an initial assessment of the client's abilities in order to direct other personnel and/or family members in providing appropriate assistance. Any unusual events that arise from assisting the client in ambulation must be validated and interpreted by the nurse.

INTERPROFESSIONAL PRACTICE

Assisting a client to ambulate may be within the scope of practice for specific health care providers. For example, in addition to nurses, physical therapists may help a client to ambulate. Although these providers may verbally communicate their findings and plan to the health care team members, the nurse must also know where to locate their documentation in the client's medical record.

Equipment
- Assistive devices required for safe ambulation of the client (e.g., gait/transfer belt, walker, cane, sit-to-stand assist device, lift with ambulation sling)
- Wheelchair for following the client, or chairs along the route if the client needs to rest
- Portable oxygen tank if the client needs it

IMPLEMENTATION
Preparation
- Be certain that others are available to assist you if needed. Also, plan the route of ambulation that has the fewest hazards and a clear path for ambulation.

Performance
1. Prior to performing the procedure, introduce self and verify the client's identity using agency protocol. Explain to the client what you are going to do, why ambulation is necessary, and how he or she can participate. Discuss how this activity relates to the overall plan of care. Stress that the client must keep the nurse informed as to how the activity is being tolerated as it progresses.
2. Perform hand hygiene and observe other appropriate infection prevention procedures.
3. Ensure that the client is appropriately dressed to walk and has shoes or slippers with nonskid soles.
4. Prepare the client for ambulation.
   - Have the client sit up in bed for at least 1 minute prior to preparing to dangle legs.
   - Assist the client to sit on the edge of the bed and allow dangling for at least 1 minute (see Skill 10–5).
   - Assess the client carefully for signs and symptoms of orthostatic hypotension (dizziness, light-headedness, or a sudden increase in heart rate) prior to leaving the bedside. **Rationale:** *Allowing for gradual adjustment can minimize drops in blood pressure (and fainting) that occur with shifts in position from lying to sitting, and sitting to standing.*
   - Assist the client to stand by the side of the bed for at least 1 minute until he or she feels secure.
   - Carefully attend to any IV tubing, catheters, or drainage bags. Keep urinary drainage bags below the level of the

client's bladder. **Rationale:** *This prevents backflow of urine into the bladder and risk of infection.*
   - If the client is a high safety risk (e.g., cannot follow commands, is medically unstable, lacks experience with assistive device, has neurologic deficits), use a lift with an ambulation sling and one or two caregivers.
   - If the client is a high safety risk, but has upper extremity strength and is able to grasp with at least one hand, use a lift with an ambulation sling or a sit-to-stand lift with ambulation capability and 1–2 caregivers.
   - If the client is a low safety risk (e.g., able to follow commands, medically stable, and experienced with assistive device), use a gait/transfer belt for standby assist as needed and assistive devices as needed (e.g., crutches, walker, cane) and 1–2 caregivers. Make sure the belt is pulled snugly around the client's waist and fastened securely. Grasp the belt at the client's back, and walk behind and slightly to one side of the client. ❶
5. Ensure client safety while assisting the client to ambulate.
   - Encourage the client to ambulate independently if he or she is able, but walk beside the client's weak side, if appropriate. If the client has a lightweight IV pole because of infusing fluids, he or she may find that holding onto the pole while ambulating helps with balance. If the pole or other equipment is cumbersome in any way, the nurse must push it to match the client's pace, securing any assistance necessary in order to move smoothly with the client.
   - Remain physically close to the client in case assistance is needed at any point.
   - If it is the client's first time out of bed following surgery, injury, or an extended period of immobility, or if the client is quite weak or unstable, have an assistant follow you and the client with a wheelchair in the event that it is needed quickly.

Continued on page 312

Assisting the Client to Ambulate—*continued*

- Encourage the client to assume a normal walking stance and gait as much as possible. Ask the client to straighten the back and raise the head so that the eyes are looking forward in a normal horizontal plane. **Rationale:** *Clients who are unsure of their ability to ambulate tend to look down at their feet, which makes them more likely to fall.*

6. Protect the client who begins to fall while ambulating.
   - If a client begins to experience the signs and symptoms of orthostatic hypotension or extreme weakness, quickly assist the client into a nearby wheelchair or other chair, and help the client to lower the head between the knees.
   - Stay with the client. **Rationale:** *A client who faints while in this position could fall head first out of the chair.*
   - When the weakness subsides, assist the client back to bed.
   - If a chair is not close by, assist the client to a horizontal position on the floor before fainting occurs.
     a. Assume a broad stance with one foot in front of the other. **Rationale:** *A broad stance widens your base of support. Placing one foot behind the other allows you to rock backward and use the femoral muscles when supporting the client's weight and lowering the center of gravity (see the next step), thus preventing back strain.*
     b. Bring the client backward so that your body supports the person. **Rationale:** *Clients who faint or start to fall usually pitch slightly forward because of the momentum of ambulating. Bringing the client's weight backward against your body allows gradual movement to the floor without injury to the client.*
     c. Allow the client to slide down your leg, and lower the person gently to the floor, making sure the client's head does not hit any objects.

Variation: Two Nurses
- Place a gait/transfer belt around the client's waist. Each nurse grasps the side handle with the near hand and the lower aspect of the client's upper arm with the other hand. **Rationale:** *This provides a secure grip for each nurse.*
- Walk in unison with the client, using a smooth, even gait, at the same speed and with steps the same size as the client's. **Rationale:** *This gives the client a greater feeling of security.*

7. Document distance and duration of ambulation and assistive devices, if used, in the client record using forms or checklists

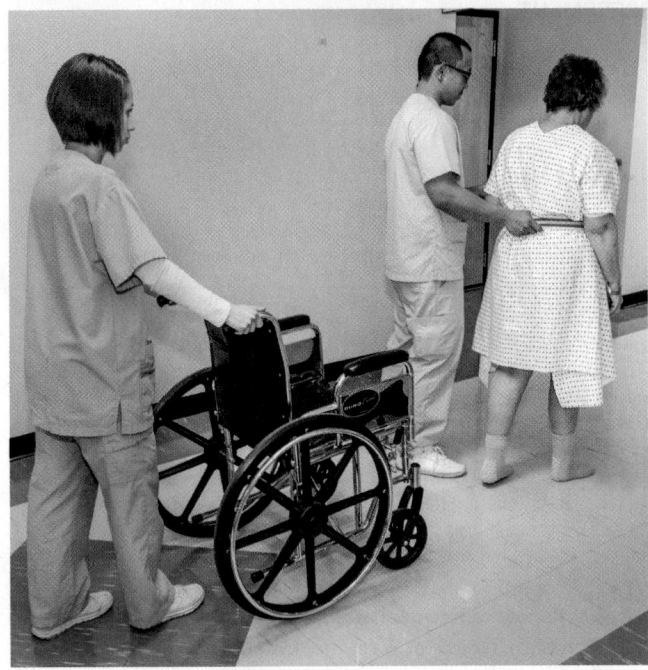

❶ Using a gait/transfer belt to support the client.

supplemented by narrative notes when appropriate. Include description of the client's gait (including body alignment) when walking, pace, activity tolerance when walking (e.g., pulse rate, facial color, any shortness of breath, feelings of dizziness, or weakness), degree of support required, and respiratory rate and blood pressure after initial ambulation to compare with baseline data.

SAMPLE DOCUMENTATION

8/22/2015 1030 Ambulated length of hall (120 ft) and returned with minimal assistance of 2 staff. Steady gait, no dyspnea, tolerated well. VS remain at baseline after walking. —————— B. Schneider, RN

EVALUATION
- Establish a plan for continued ambulation based on expected or normal ability for the client.

- Report significant deviations from normal to the primary care provider.

LIFESPAN CONSIDERATIONS   Assisting the Client to Ambulate

CHILDREN
- Children and adolescents who have sustained a sports injury (e.g., sprained ankle) may want to be more active than they should be. A cast, splint, or boot may be put in place to limit activity and assist in healing. Teach children the importance of appropriate activity and the use of assistive devices (e.g., crutches) if necessary. Help them focus on what they *can* do rather than what they cannot do (e.g., "You can stand at the free throw line and shoot baskets").

OLDER ADULTS
- Inquire how the client has ambulated previously and/or check any available chart notes regarding the client's abilities and modify assistance accordingly.

- Take into account a decrease in speed, strength, resistance to fatigue, reaction time, and coordination due to a decrease in nerve conduction, muscle strength, and the effects of aging on baroreceptors and proprioceptors.
- Be cautious when using a gait/transfer belt with a client with osteoporosis. Too much pressure from the belt can increase the risk of vertebral compression fractures. If a client has had abdominal surgery, it may be necessary to use a gait vest instead of a gait belt.
- If assistive devices such as a walker or cane are used, make sure clients are supervised as they begin to learn the proper method of using them. Crutches may be much more difficult for older adults due to decreased upper body strength. In general, older adults do much better with walkers than with crutches.

- Be alert to signs of activity intolerance, especially in older clients with cardiac and lung problems.
- Break up the eventual desired client mobility goal into shorter, more easily attained but progressively more ambitious client goals. Increase slowly to build endurance, strength, and flexibility.
- Be aware of any fall risks the older client may have, such as the following:
  - The normal effects of aging on the body's mobility abilities
  - Effects of medications

- Neurologic disorders
- Orthopedic problems
- Presence of equipment that must accompany the client when ambulating
- Environmental hazards
- Orthostatic hypotension
- In older adults, the body's responses return to normal more slowly. For instance, an increase in heart rate from exercise may stay elevated for hours before returning to normal.

Assisting the Client to Ambulate
- When making a home visit, assess carefully for safety issues concerning ambulation. Counsel the client and family about inadequate lighting, unfastened rugs, slippery floors, and loose objects on the floors.

- Check the surroundings for adequate supports such as railings and grab bars.
- Recommend that nonskid strips be placed on outside steps and inside stairs that are not carpeted.
- Ask to see the shoes the person intends to wear while ambulating. They should be in good repair and supportive of the foot.

ASSISTING CLIENTS TO USE MECHANICAL AIDS FOR WALKING

Mechanical aids for walking include canes, crutches, and walkers. Three types of **canes** are commonly used: the standard straight-legged cane; the tripod or crab cane, which has three feet; and the **quad cane**, which has four feet and provides the most support (Figure 11–4 ■).

Cane tips should have rubber caps to improve traction and prevent slipping. The standard cane is 91 cm (36 in.) long; some aluminum canes can be adjusted from 56 to 97 cm (22 to 38 in.). The length should permit the elbow to be slightly flexed, at a 25° to 30° angle. Clients may use either one or two canes, depending on how much support they require.

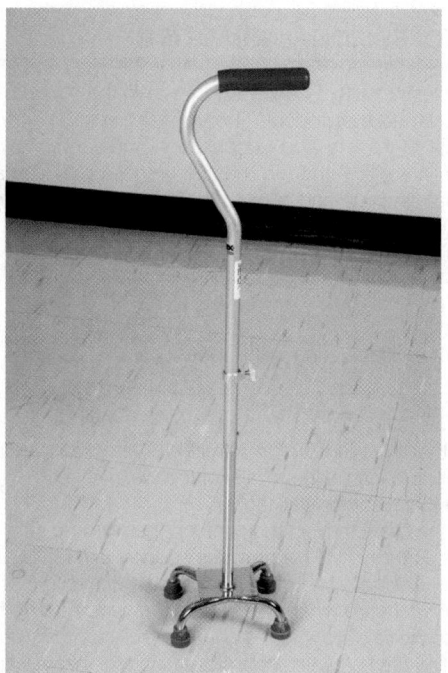

Figure 11–4 ■ A quad cane.

Crutches may be a temporary need for some people and a permanent one for others. Both crutches and canes should enable a person to ambulate independently; therefore, it is important to learn to use them properly. The most frequently used kinds of crutches are the underarm crutch, or **axillary crutch** with hand bars, and the **Lofstrand crutch**, which extends only to the forearm. On the Lofstrand crutch, the metal cuff around the forearm and the metal bar stabilize the wrists and thus make walking easier, especially on stairs. The platform or elbow extensor crutch also has a cuff for the upper arm to permit forearm weight-bearing. The platform crutch is helpful for clients who have damaged not only a lower extremity but also an upper one. All crutches require suction tips, usually made of rubber, which help to prevent slipping on a floor surface. In crutch walking, the client's weight is borne by the muscles of the shoulder girdle and the upper extremities. Before beginning crutch walking, exercises that strengthen the upper arms and hands are recommended.

Walkers are for clients who need more support than a cane provides and lack the strength and balance required for crutches. Walkers come in many different shapes and sizes, with devices suited to individual needs. The standard type is made of polished aluminum. It has four legs with rubber tips and plastic hand grips (Figure 11–5 *A* ■). Many walkers have adjustable legs.

The standard walker needs to be picked up to be used. The client therefore requires partial strength in both hands and wrists, strong elbow extensors, and strong shoulder depressors. The client also needs the ability to bear at least partial weight on both legs.

Four-wheeled and two-wheeled models of walkers (roller walkers) do not need to be picked up to be moved, but they are less stable than the standard walker. Clients who are too weak or unstable to pick up and move the walker with each step use a roller walker. Four-wheeled walkers allow the user some added stability as compared to using no assistive device, and the capability of rapid ambulation, but they are suitable only for a client who does not need a walker to bear weight. These walkers also have hand brakes. The client needs to demonstrate correct use of the hand brakes. Some roller walkers have a seat at the back so the client can sit down to rest when desired. An adaptation of the standard and four-wheeled walker is one that has

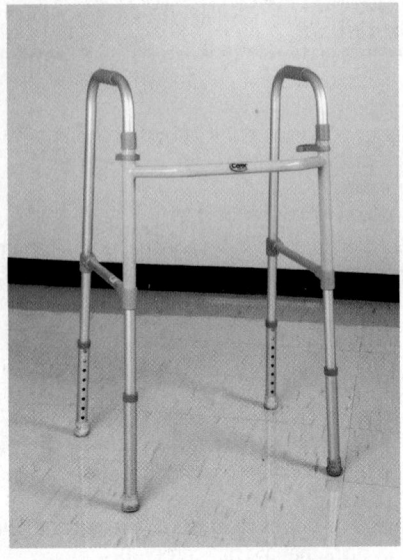

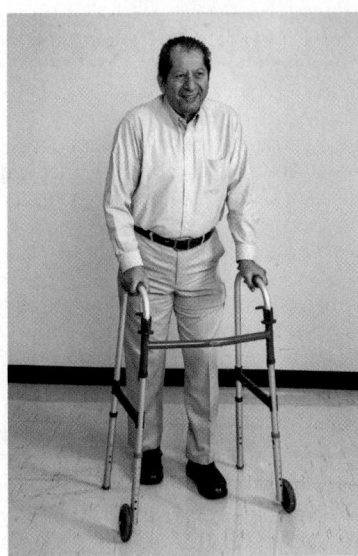

Figure 11–5 ■ *A,* Standard walker; *B,* two-wheeled walker.

two tips and two wheels (Figure 11–5 *B*). This type provides more stability than the four-wheeled model yet still permits the client to keep the walker in contact with the ground all the time. The legs with wheels allow the client to easily push the walker forward, and the legs without wheels prevent the walker from rolling away as the client steps forward. The nurse may need to adjust the height of a client's walker so that the hand bar is below the client's waist and the client's elbows are slightly flexed. This position helps the client assume a more normal stance. A walker that is too low causes the client to stoop; one that is too high makes the client stretch and reach.

●○● NURSING PROCESS: ASSISTING CLIENTS TO USE MECHANICAL AIDS FOR WALKING

SKILL 11-3

Assisting the Client to Use a Cane

ASSESSMENT
Inquire about the following: client's physical strength of the lower extremities, arms, and hands; ability to bear body weight; ability to keep balance in a standing position on one or both legs; and ability to hold the body erect.

PLANNING
Determine what type of ambulatory assistive device is most appropriate for the client. The primary care provider or physical therapist may specify this information.

DELEGATION

Due to the extent of knowledge required, teaching the client to use assistive devices is not delegated to UAP. The nurse or the physical therapist will teach the client initial use of the cane. However, once the client has demonstrated adequate skill, UAP may assist the client in ambulating with this equipment.

INTERPROFESSIONAL PRACTICE

Assisting a client to use a cane may be within the scope of practice for other health care providers. For example, in addition to nurses, both physical therapists and occupational therapists may assist a client to use a cane. Although these therapists may verbally communicate their findings and plan to the health care team members, the nurse must also know where to locate their documentation in the client's medical record.

Equipment
• Appropriately sized cane with rubber tips

IMPLEMENTATION
Preparation
• Ensure that the client's path is free from clutter and hazards.

Performance
1. Prior to performing the procedure, introduce self and verify the client's identity using agency protocol. Explain to the client what you are going to do, why it is necessary, and how he or she can participate. Discuss how this activity will be used in planning further care or treatments.
2. Perform hand hygiene and observe other appropriate infection prevention procedures.

3. Ensure that the client is appropriately dressed for walking, especially in regards to stability of footwear.
4. Prepare the client for walking.
   • Ask the client to hold the cane on the stronger side of the body. **Rationale:** *This provides support and body alignment when walking. The arm opposite the advancing foot normally swings forward when walking, so the hand holding the cane will come forward and the cane will support the weaker leg.*
   • Position the tip of a standard cane (and the nearest tip of other canes) about 15 cm (6 in.) to the side and 15 cm (6 in.) in front

Assisting the Client to Use a Cane—*continued*

of the near foot, so that the elbow is slightly flexed. **Rationale:** *This provides the best balance and prevents the person from leaning on the cane. In this position, the client stands erect, with the center of gravity within the base of support.*

5. When maximum support for a cane is required, instruct the client to move as follows:
   - Move the cane forward about 30 cm (1 ft), or a distance that is comfortable while the body weight is borne by both legs. ❶, *A*
   - Then, move the affected (weak) leg forward to the cane while the weight is borne by the cane and stronger leg. ❶, *B*
   - Next, move the unaffected (stronger) leg forward ahead of the cane and weak leg while the weight is borne by the cane and weak leg. ❶, *C*
   - Repeat the above three steps. **Rationale:** *This pattern of moving provides at least two points of support on the floor at all times.*

6. If the client requires minimal support from the cane, for instance, just a little assist with balance, instruct the client to follow these steps:
   - Move the cane and weak leg forward at the same time, while the weight is borne by the stronger leg. ❷, *A*
   - Move the stronger leg forward while the weight is borne by the cane and the weak leg. ❷, *B*

7. Ensure client safety.
   - Walk beside the client on the affected side. **Rationale:** *The client is most likely to fall toward the affected side.*

- Walk the client for the time or distance indicated in the plan of care, being prepared to revise this plan if the client's condition warrants it.
- If the client loses balance or strength and is unable to regain it, slide your hand up to the client's axilla, and take a broad stance to provide a base of support. If there was any indication that this situation might occur, the client should have had a gait belt placed before ambulation began. Have the client rest against your hip until assistance arrives, or gently lower yourself and the client to the floor.
- For stair climbing, the phrase "up with the good, down with the bad" can help clients remember which pattern of movement to use. This means that when climbing stairs the client should ascend first with the good leg, bringing the weaker leg up to that level afterward. The pattern is reversed when descending stairs. This is also the pattern used with crutches on stairs.

8. Document the client's progress in the client record using forms or checklists supplemented by narrative notes when appropriate. Describe the distance ambulated and any difficulties the client experienced.

CLINICAL ALERT!

Instruct clients to use the cane opposite the side of pain or weakness to facilitate balance and decrease weight on painful extremities.

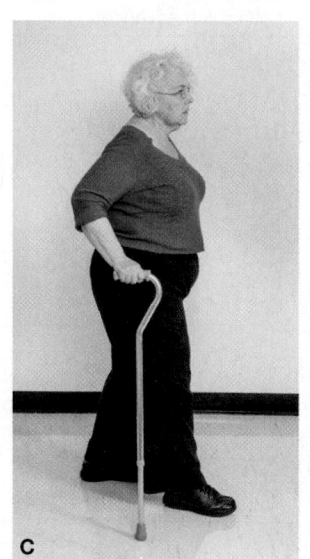

❶ Steps involved in using a cane to provide maximum support.

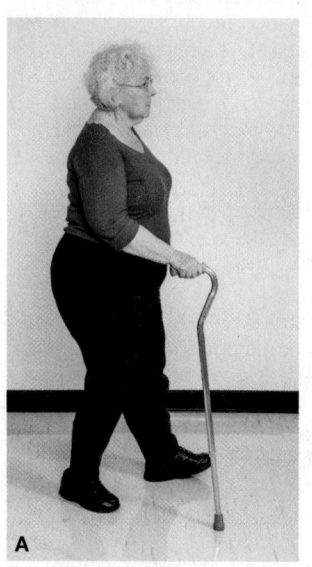
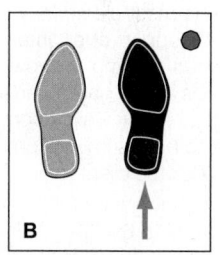

❷ Steps involved in using a cane when less than maximum support is required.

Assisting the Client to Use Crutches

IMPLEMENTATION

In a hospital facility, crutch walking and other forms of assisted ambulation are taught most often by physical therapy, but it is within the professional nurse's scope of practice to teach, and certainly to practice and reinforce, assisted ambulation with the client.

Preparation

Ensure that the crutches are the proper length (Box 11–1 on page 319).

Performance

1. Assist the client to assume the tripod (triangle) position, the basic crutch stance used before crutch walking.
   - Ask the client to stand and place the tips of the crutches 15 cm (6 in.) in front of the feet and out laterally about 15 cm (6 in.). This is the starting position for all the different variations of ambulation with crutches. ❶ **Rationale:** *The tripod position provides a wide base of support and enhances both stability and balance.*

Continued on page 316

SKILL 11-3

SKILL 11-4

Assisting the Client to Use Crutches—*continued*

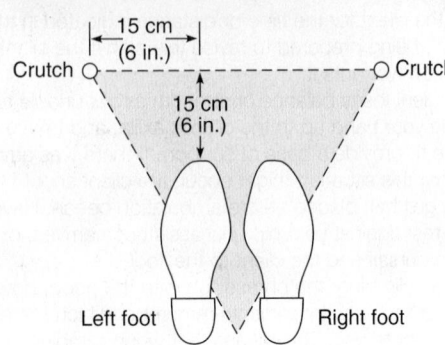

❶ The tripod position.

- Make sure the feet are slightly apart. A tall person requires a wider base than a short person.
- Ensure that posture is erect; that is, the hips and knees should be extended, the back straight, and the head held straight and high. There should be no hunch to the shoulders and thus no weight borne by the axillae. The elbows should be extended sufficiently to allow weight bearing on the hands.
- Stand slightly behind and on the client's affected side. **Rationale:** *By standing behind the client and toward the affected side, the nurse can provide support if the client loses balance.*
- If the client is unsteady, place a gait belt around the client's waist, and grasp the belt from above, not from below. **Rationale:** *A fall can be prevented more effectively if the belt is held from above. In addition, this manner of holding the belt is less likely to result in a twisting injury to the nurse's hands.*

2. Teach the client the appropriate crutch gait. Specific gaits are chosen based on client capabilities and ability to bear weight. This varies from client to client.

Four-Point Alternate Gait
This is the most elementary and safest gait, providing at least three points of support at all times, but it requires coordination. It can be used when walking in crowds because it does not require much space. It is a slow gait because it requires the client to move crutches and legs and shift weight constantly. To use this gait, the client has to be able to bear some weight on both legs (**❷**, reading from bottom to top). Ask the client to:

- Move the right crutch ahead a suitable distance (e.g., 10 to 15 cm [4 to 6 in.]).
- Move the left foot forward, preferably to the level of the crutch.
- Move the left crutch forward.
- Move the right foot forward.

Three-Point Gait
To use this gait, the person must be able to bear entire body weight on the unaffected leg. It is a fast gait that requires strength in the three unaffected extremities. The two crutches and the unaffected leg bear weight alternately (**❸**, reading from bottom to top).

Ask the client to:
- Move both crutches and the weaker leg forward.
- Move the stronger leg forward.

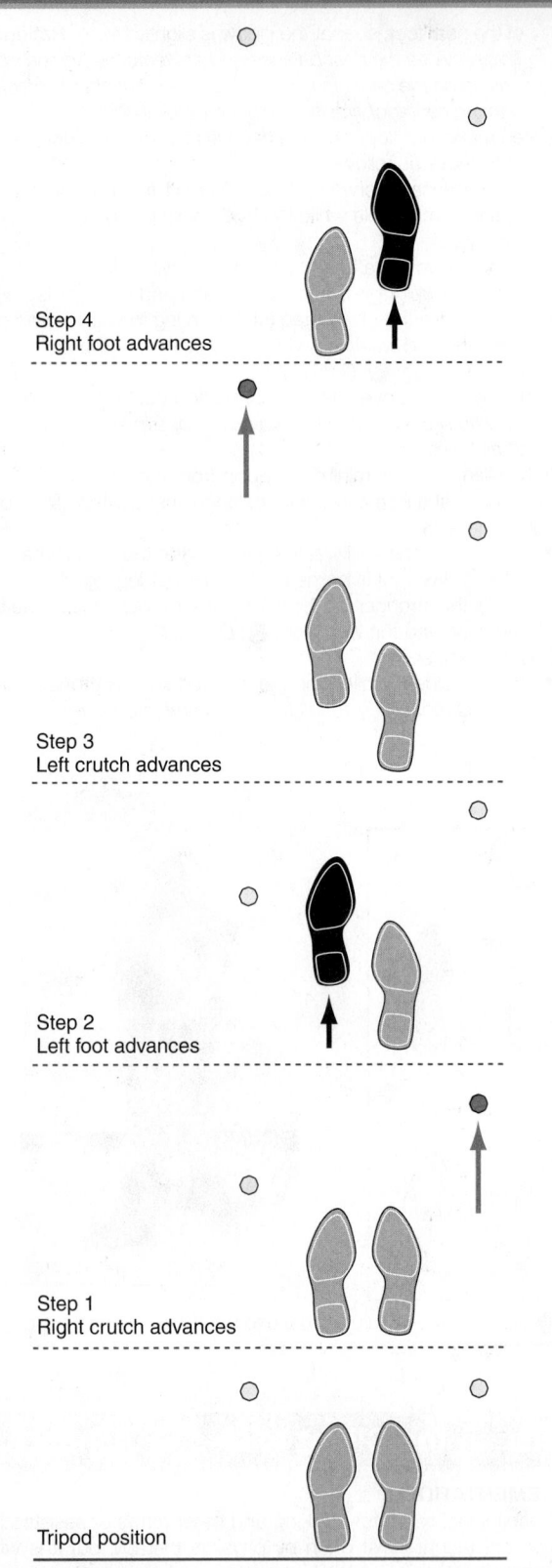

Step 4
Right foot advances

Step 3
Left crutch advances

Step 2
Left foot advances

Step 1
Right crutch advances

Tripod position

❷ The four-point alternate crutch gait.

Assisting the Client to Use Crutches—*continued*

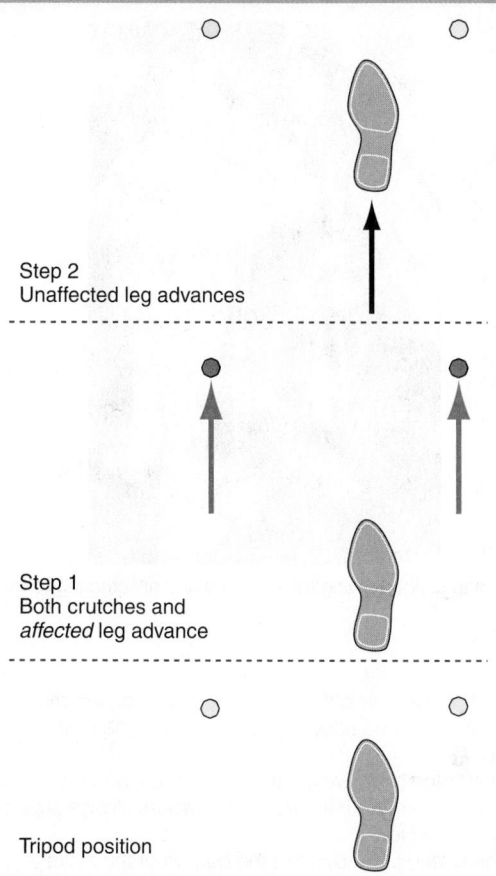

Step 2
Unaffected leg advances

Step 1
Both crutches and *affected* leg advance

Tripod position

❸ The three-point crutch gait.

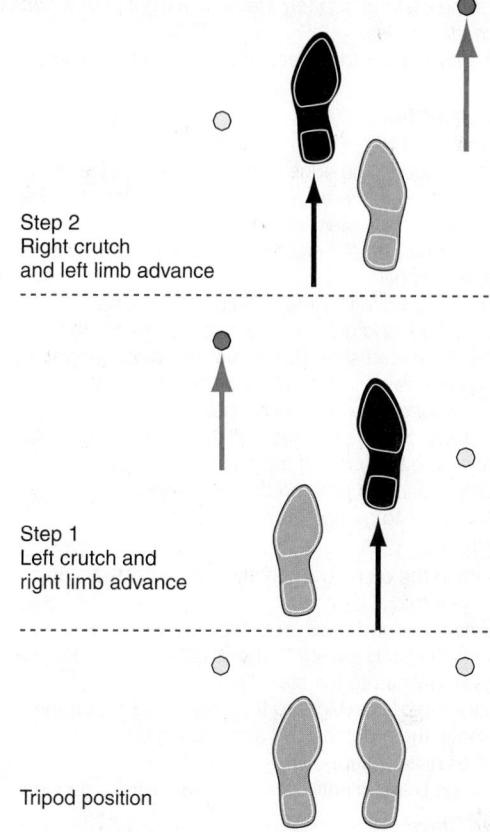

Step 2
Right crutch
and left limb advance

Step 1
Left crutch and
right limb advance

Tripod position

❹ The two-point alternate crutch gait.

Two-Point Alternate Gait

This gait is intermediate in pace and in required strength between the four-point gait and the three-point gait. It requires more balance than the four-point gait, because only two points support the body at one time; it also requires at least partial weight bearing on each foot. In this gait, arm movements with the crutches are similar to the arm movements during normal walking (❹, reading from bottom to top).

Ask the client to:

• Move the left crutch and the right foot forward together.
• Move the right crutch and the left foot ahead together.

Swing-To Gait

People with paralysis of the legs and hips use the swing gaits. Prolonged use of these gaits results in atrophy of the unused muscles. The swing-to gait is the easier of these two gaits.

Ask the client to:

• Move both crutches ahead together.
• Lift body weight by the arms and swing *to* the crutches.

Swing-Through Gait

This gait requires considerable client skill, strength, and coordination.

Ask the client to:

• Move both crutches forward together.
• Lift body weight by the arms and swing through and beyond the crutches.

3. Teach the client to get into and out of a chair.

Getting Into a Chair

• Teach the client to always leave the crutches within arms' reach when sitting or reclining, as they are needed for safe ambulation.
• Ensure that the chair has armrests and is secure or braced against a wall.

• Instruct the client to:
  a. Stand with the back of the unaffected leg centered against the chair.
  b. Transfer the crutches to the hand on the affected side, hold the crutches by the hand bars, and then grasp the arm of the chair with the hand on the unaffected side. ❺ **Rationale:** *This*

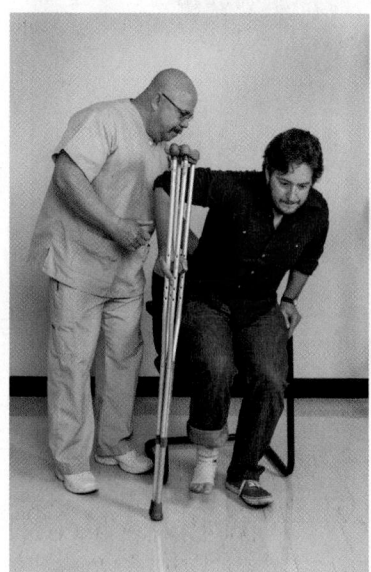

❺ A client using crutches getting into a chair.

Continued on page 318

Assisting the Client to Use Crutches—*continued*

allows the client to support the body weight on the arms and the unaffected leg.

  c. Lean forward, flex the knees and hips, and lower into the chair.

Getting Out of a Chair

- Instruct the client to:

  a. Move forward to the edge of the chair and place the unaffected leg at the edge of the chair. **Rationale:** *This position helps the client stand up from the chair and achieve balance, because the unaffected leg is supported against the edge of the chair.*

  b. Grasp the crutches by the hand bars in the hand on the affected side, and grasp the arm of the chair with the hand on the unaffected side. **Rationale:** *The body weight is placed on the crutches and the hand on the armrest to support the unaffected leg when the client rises to stand.*

  c. Push down on the crutches and the chair armrest while elevating the body out of the chair.

  d. Assume the tripod position before moving.

4. Teach the client to go up and down stairs.

Going Up Stairs

- Stand behind the client and slightly to the affected side.
- Ask the client to:

  a. Assume the tripod position at the bottom of the stairs.

  b. Transfer the body weight to the crutches and move the unaffected leg onto the step. ❻

  c. Transfer the body weight to the unaffected leg on the step and move the crutches and affected leg up to the step. The crutches always support the affected leg.

- Repeat steps b and c until the top of the stairs is reached.

Going Down Stairs

- Stand one step below the person on the affected side.
- Ask the client to:

  a. Assume the tripod position at the top of the stairs.

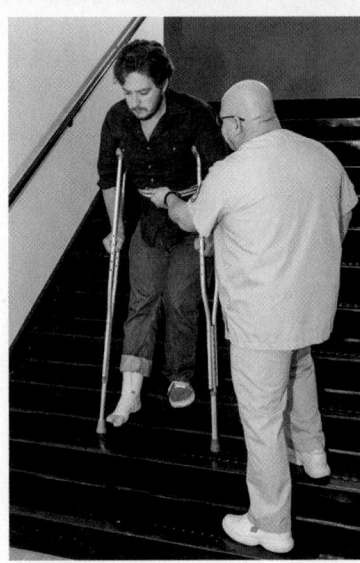

❼ Descending stairs: Moving the crutches and affected leg to the next step.

  b. Shift the body weight to the unaffected leg, and move the crutches and affected leg down onto the next step. ❼

  c. Transfer the body weight to the crutches, and move the unaffected leg to that step. The crutches always support the affected leg.

  d. Repeat steps b and c until the bottom of the stairs is reached.

    or

- Ask the client to:

  a. Hold both crutches in the outside hand and grasp the handrail with the other hand for support.

  b. Move as in steps b and c, above.

5. Reinforce client teaching (see Client Teaching Considerations).

6. Document the client's progress in the client record using forms or checklists supplemented by narrative notes when appropriate. Describe the distance ambulated and any difficulties the client experienced, including changes in vital signs as compared to baseline.

SAMPLE DOCUMENTATION

8/22/2015 1500 Attempted crutch walking up steps. Unable to lift affected leg to next step, balance remained stable. Became dyspneic and upset. Vital signs (when seated) at baseline after activity. Reassured that this skill takes time. Encouraged to continue seated leg exercises and frequent ambulation. Will re-try tomorrow. —————————————————————— B. Schneider, RN

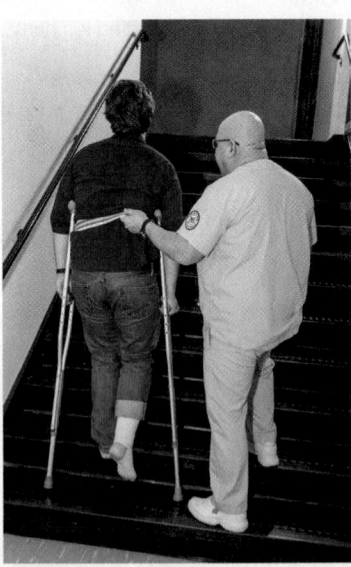

❻ Climbing stairs: Placing weight on the crutches while first moving the unaffected leg onto a step.

BOX 11–1   Measuring Clients for Crutches

When nurses measure clients for axillary crutches, it is most important to obtain the correct length for the crutches and the correct placement of the hand piece. There are two methods for measuring crutch length:

1. The client lies in the supine position, and the nurse measures from the anterior fold of the axilla to a point 2.5 cm (1 in.) lateral from the heel of the foot.
2. The client stands erect and positions the crutch tips 5 cm (2 in.) in front of and 15 cm (6 in.) to the side of the feet. The nurse makes sure the shoulder rest of the crutch is at least three fingerwidths, that is, 2.5 to 5 cm (1 to 2 in.), below the axilla.

To determine the correct placement of the hand bar:

1. The client stands upright and supports the body weight by the hand grips of the crutches.
2. The nurse measures the angle of elbow flexion. It should be about 30°. A goniometer (a handheld instrument used to measure joint angles) may be used to verify the correct angle.

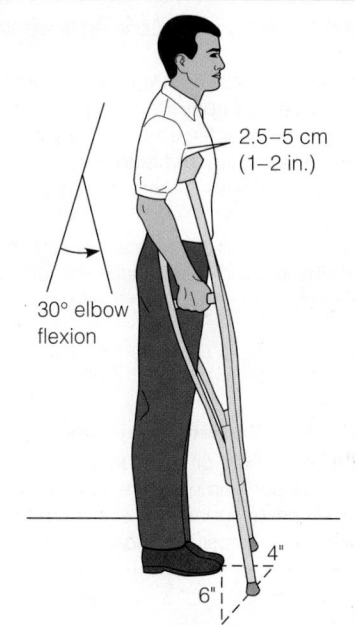

2.5–5 cm
(1–2 in.)

30° elbow
flexion

4"

6"

The standing position for measuring the correct length for crutches.

CLIENT TEACHING CONSIDERATIONS

Teaching the Client to Use Crutches

- If you have been given a plan of exercises developed for you to strengthen your arm muscles, follow this plan.
- It is necessary for a health care professional to establish the correct length for your crutches and the correct placement of the hand pieces. Crutches that are too long force your shoulders upward and make it difficult for you to push your body off the ground. Crutches that are too short will make you hunch over and develop an improper body stance.
- The weight of your body should be borne by the arms rather than the axillae (armpits). Continual pressure on the axillae can injure the radial nerve and eventually cause crutch palsy, a weakness of the muscles of the forearm, wrist, and hand. Injuries to the radial nerve may cause pain, numbness and tingling, and muscle atrophy, but these problems are reversible by using crutches correctly so weight is not borne by the axillae.

- Maintain an erect posture as much as possible to prevent strain on muscles and joints and to maintain balance.
- Each step taken with crutches should be a comfortable distance for you. It is wise to start with a small rather than large step.
- Inspect the crutch tips regularly, and replace them if worn.
- Keep the crutch tips dry and clean to maintain their surface friction. If the tips become wet, dry them well before use.
- Wear a shoe with a low heel that grips the floor. Rubber soles decrease the chances of slipping. Adjust shoelaces so they cannot come untied or reach the floor where they might catch on the crutches. Consider shoes with alternative forms of closure (e.g., Velcro), especially if you cannot easily bend to tie laces. Slip-on shoes are acceptable only if they are snug and the heel does not come loose when the foot is bent.

Assisting the Client to Use a Walker

IMPLEMENTATION
Preparation
- Ensure the client has adequate arm strength to use a walker.
- Ensure the walker is at the correct height. The walker should reach to the level of the client's hip joint, and the elbows should be bent at about a 30° angle while using it.
- Ensure the client has a clear path free from obstacles.
- Ensure that the client wears shoes that support the feet and are resistant to skidding and slipping.

Performance
1. Give the client these instructions when maximum overall support is required:
   - Move the walker ahead about 15 cm (6 in.) while your body weight is put on both legs.
   - Then move the right foot up to the walker while your body weight remains on the left leg and both arms.
   - Next, move the left foot up to the right foot while your body weight shifts to the right leg and both arms.

SKILL 11-5

Continued on page 320

Assisting the Client to Use a Walker—*continued*

2. Give the client these instructions if one leg is weaker than the other:
- Move the walker and the weak leg ahead together about 15 cm (6 in.) while your body weight is put on the stronger leg.
- Then move the stronger leg ahead while your weight is shifted to the affected leg and both arms.

3. Document the client's progress in the client record using forms or checklists supplemented by narrative notes when appropriate. Describe the distance ambulated, any difficulties the client experienced, and changes in vital signs in relation to baseline.

EVALUATION

- Perform a detailed follow-up assessment based on the client's response and ability in using mechanical aids for walking.

- Report significant deviations from expected or normal for the client to the primary care provider.

SAFETY ALERT!

SAFETY

When rising from a bed, chair, or bedside commode and intending to use a walker, clients sometimes overestimate the stability of the walker, which typically has a lightweight aluminum frame and sometimes wheels. Teach clients to use the more stable surface or arms of the furniture from which they are arising to push up from and to use the walker only for stabilizing balance during the transfer once they are upright until they are actually ready to begin ambulating with it.

LIFESPAN CONSIDERATIONS Assisting Clients to Use Mechanical Aids for Walking

CHILDREN
- Children learn and adapt quickly to the use of assistive devices. Care should be taken to check regularly that they are using proper technique. They may reach the point where they prematurely believe they no longer need them.

OLDER ADULTS
- Older adults' conditions can change rapidly. Check regularly to see that the current assistive device is the most appropriate one and that it fits the client properly.

- Reinforce teaching regarding proper use of mechanical aids. Clients can easily fall into bad habits such as leaning the axillae on the crutches.
- Be aware that there may be a social stigma attached to the use of walkers in the minds of older adults. They may avoid using needed devices because of a need to perceive themselves as other than "old."

Ambulatory and Community Settings Safety

Assisting Clients to Use Mechanical Aids for Walking
- When making a home visit, assess carefully for safety issues for ambulation with mechanical devices. Counsel the client and family about poor lighting, unfastened rugs, slippery floors, and loose objects on the floors.
- Recommend nonskid strips be placed on outside steps and inside stairs that are not carpeted.
- Check that appropriate chairs are available. Such chairs should be high enough to sit on and rise from comfortably, with sturdy arms from which to push oneself up.

- Reinforce client teaching about proper gaits with canes, crutches, and walkers. Ask the client to demonstrate how the appliance is normally used, because inappropriate gaits and transferring techniques can develop.
- Ensure that the equipment is properly maintained and stored out of the way when not in use.
- Tennis balls with a cross cut in them may be applied over walker tips to make sliding easier.

FOCUSING ON CLINICAL THINKING

Consider This

1. Your client has been in bed on a ventilator for a week following a motor vehicle crash with broken ribs and a broken arm. He has become very weak. He is now off the ventilator and his broken ribs and arm are healing well. What actions will you take to prepare him for ambulating?

2. Your client has a weak right leg and arm secondary to a stroke. What modifications in usual techniques would be appropriate when assisting this client when using a wheelchair?

3. An 84-year-old client is recovering from a severe episode of the flu and is very weak. The primary care provider has ordered that the client be ambulated in the hall three times a day. The client complains of dizziness when standing and is fearful of falling. What may be causing the dizziness? What precautions should you take?

4. A client who uses a walker lives in a two-story house. What advice would you provide regarding how to use the walker at home?

See Focusing on Clinical Thinking answers on student resource website.

TEST YOUR KNOWLEDGE

1. The nurse is caring for a client who uses a mechanical aid for walking. The device extends only to the forearm. The device stabilizes the wrists and this makes walking safer and easier. Which device is this client using?
   1. An axillary crutch
   2. A walker
   3. A Lofstrand crutch
   4. A quad cane

2. A home care nurse is assessing a new client regarding safety issues for ambulation in the home. Which statement, if made by the client's wife, indicates the need for further teaching?
   1. "My husband should wear nonskid shoes to ambulate."
   2. "I should help my husband to stand up in the shower."
   3. "I should remove any loose objects on the floor."
   4. "My husband should not ambulate on unfastened rugs."

3. The nurse is assessing the client's technique after teaching the client how to use crutches. Which situation would require intervention by the nurse?
   1. The weight of the client's body is put on the axillae.
   2. The client maintains an erect posture.
   3. The client is wearing rubber-soled shoes.
   4. The shoulder rest is three fingerwidths below the axillae.

4. A nurse is assisting a client into a wheelchair. Which practice guidelines are important to follow for this client? Select all that apply.
   1. The nurse locks the brakes on both wheels of the wheelchair when the client transfers in and out of it.
   2. The nurse lowers the footplates before transferring the client into the wheelchair.
   3. The nurse raises the footplates after transferring the client into the wheelchair.
   4. The nurse ensures that the client is positioned toward the front of the wheelchair seat.
   5. The nurse backs the wheelchair into or out of the elevator, rear large wheels first.

5. A nurse is deciding which client to assign to the unlicensed assistive personnel (UAP) for ambulation. Which client would be most suited for ambulation by the UAP?
   1. A client who has just been admitted for syncope
   2. A client with orthostatic hypotension
   3. A client just returned from the recovery room after surgery
   4. A client who had surgery 2 days ago

6. The nurse is preparing to document the client's ambulation. Which components are important to include in the documentation? Select all that apply.
   1. The distance of ambulation
   2. The duration of ambulation
   3. The client's gait
   4. The baseline blood pressure only
   5. The degree of support needed

7. The nurse working in a long-term care facility is assigned a client who requires three people to transfer. The unit has been extremely busy, and everyone is busy at this time. The nurse needs to assist the client back into bed now because the client is complaining of discomfort and wants to return to bed. Which action should the nurse take?
   1. Assist the client back to bed without assistance.
   2. Encourage the client to wait until help is available.
   3. Transfer the client with one other person assisting.
   4. Use a hydraulic lift to transfer the client with the assistance of another person.

8. The nurse is caring for a client who is required to remain in bed for an extended period of time while in traction for a fractured femur. How can the nurse prepare the client for ambulation?
   1. Place the bed in reverse Trendelenburg position so the client can put some weight on the feet in bed.
   2. Encourage the client to be as independent as possible while in bed.
   3. Encourage the client to exercise both legs while in bed.
   4. Perform range of motion of all extremities every 4 hours.

9. The nurse observes an unlicensed assistive personnel (UAP) pushing a client in a wheelchair. Which action would require the nurse to correct the UAP's performance?
   1. The UAP raises the footrests for the client to get into the wheelchair.
   2. The UAP pushes the wheelchair into the elevator with the client facing forward so they can see where they are going.
   3. The UAP locks the brakes and holds the wheelchair while the client sits in the seat.
   4. The UAP holds the handle of the wheelchair while unlocking the brakes before moving the chair forward.

10. The nurse assesses a client newly fitted for a cane and recognizes that the cane is well fitted when observing which action?
    1. The client's arm is straight and the client is standing upright.
    2. The client's elbow is flexed and the client is flexing the knees.
    3. The client's elbow is flexed slightly and the client is standing upright.
    4. The client's elbow is flexed 45° and the client is standing upright.

See Answers to Test Your Knowledge in Appendix A.

READINGS AND REFERENCES

References

American Nurses Association. (2013). *Safe patient handling and mobility. Interprofessional national standards across the care continuum.* Silver Spring, MD: Author.

Centers for Medicare and Medicaid Services. (2008). *Hospitals—Restraint/seclusion interpretive guidelines & updated state operations manual (SOM) Appendix A.* Baltimore, MD: Author.

Dammeyer, J., Dickinson, S., Packard, D., Baldwin, N., & Ricklemann, C. (2013). Building a protocol to guide mobility in the ICU. *Critical Care Nursing Quarterly, 36,* 37–49. doi:10.1097/CNQ.0b013e3182750acd

Spinlife. (2013). *Ultralight wheelchairs.* Retrieved from http://www.spinlife.com/category.cfm?categoryID=38&adv=googleads&tar=slink-UltralightWheelchairs-lightweight%20wheelchairs-e&utm_medium=cpc&utm_content=12263372124&utm_campaign=Wheelchairs

Selected Bibliography

American Nurses Association. (n.d.). *Safe patient handling and mobility.* Retrieved from http://www.nursingworld.org/MainMenuCategories/WorkplaceSafety/Healthy-Work-Environment/SafePatient

Berman, A., Snyder, S., & Frandsen, G. (2016). *Kozier & Erb's fundamentals of nursing: Concepts, process, and practice* (10th ed.). Upper Saddle River, NJ: Pearson.

Clark, D. E., Lowman, J. D., Griffin, R. L., Matthews, H. M., & Reiff, D. A. (2013). Effectiveness of an early mobilization protocol in a trauma and burns intensive care unit: A retrospective cohort study. *Physical Therapy, 93,* 186–196. doi:10.2522/ptj.20110417

Dang, M. T. (2010). Walking away the blues: Exercise for depression in older adults. *Nursing, 40*(11), 33–36. doi:10.1097/01.NURSE.0000389023.26136.b3

Divo, M., & Pinto-Plata, V. (2012). Role of exercise in testing and in therapy of COPD. *Medical Clinics of North America, 96,* 753–766. doi:10.1016/j.mcna.2012.05.004

Edelstein, J. E. (2013). Assistive devices for ambulation. *Physical Medicine and Rehabilitation Clinics of North America, 24,* 291–303. doi:10.1016/j.pmr.2012.11.001

Farinatti, P., Borges, J., Gomes, R., Lima, D., & Fleck, S. (2010). Effects of a supervised exercise program on the physical fitness and immunological function of HIV-infected patients. *Journal of Sports Medicine and Physical Fitness, 50,* 511–518.

Rockefeller, K., & Proctor, R. B. (2011). Is there a role for gait belts in safe patient handling and movement programs? *American Journal of SPHM, 1,* 30–35.

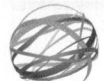 # 12 Fall Prevention and Restraints

LEARNING OUTCOMES

At the completion of this chapter, the student will be able to:

1. Define key terms used in the skills of preventing falls and restraining clients.
2. Explain measures to prevent falls in hospital, long-term care, and ambulatory settings.
3. Identify indications and contraindications for restraining clients.
4. Describe various kinds of restraints and how each may be used.
5. Recognize when it is appropriate to delegate safety measures to unlicensed assistive personnel.
6. Verbalize steps used in:
   a. Using a bed or chair exit safety monitoring device.
   b. Applying restraints.
   c. Implementing seizure precautions.
7. Demonstrate appropriate documentation and reporting of fall prevention, restraints, and seizure precautions.

SKILLS

Skill 12–1 Using a Bed or Chair Exit Safety Monitoring Device
Skill 12–2 Applying Restraints

Skill 12–3 Implementing Seizure Precautions

KEY TERMS

chemical restraints, 328
limb restraints, 330
magnetic box mobility monitor, 325

mitt (hand) restraints, 330
physical restraints, 328
restraint-free environment, 328

restraints, 328
safety monitoring devices, 325
seclusion, 328

seizure, 334
seizure precautions, 334
vest restraints, 330

A safe physical environment is one in which people can function without injury and feel a sense of security. Box 12–1 delineates areas of particular importance for the nurse to assess in order to ensure a safe environment. The skills in this chapter focus on those measures the nurse can take to reduce the risk of client injury as a result of unsafe movement within and out of a bed or chair. These include measures that are taken in anticipation of and in the event of a seizure during which the client cannot control physical movement and is at risk of sustaining an injury. Attention to the dignity and well-being of clients must be maintained at all times. Many clients will have strong emotional responses around issues of falling, being restrained, and having a seizure. Embarrassment, fear, and a decreased sense of autonomy and control can all compromise a client's healing potential. The holistic nurse will demonstrate therapeutic presence while providing the skills presented in this chapter.

PREVENTING FALLS

Falls are common among older adults and clients who are ill, injured, or weak. Falls are the leading cause of injuries among older adults. More than one third of adults ages 65 and older experience falls and in this group, falls are the leading cause of injury-related deaths and the most common cause of injuries and hospital admissions (Jorgensen, 2011, p. 2).

Health care facilities have strong incentives to reduce the number of client falls. As of 2008, the Centers for Medicare and Medicaid Services (CMS) stopped paying for injuries caused by in-hospital falls (Titler, Shever, Kanak, Picone, & Qin, 2011). In 2010, The Joint Commission added two required standards relating to client safety and hospital falls (Jorgensen, 2011): (1) The hospital must assess and manage the client's risks for falls and (2) the hospital must implement interventions to reduce falls based on the client's assessed risk. Therefore, identifying clients at risk for falling can improve a hospital's fall rate.

It is important to assess clients for fall risk on admission, whenever a change in physical or mental status occurs, on transfer, and before discharge (Kulik, 2011, p. 6). Many assessment tools to determine a client's risk of falling are available. Most assess for age, number of diseases, medications, environment, mobility problems, mental status, continence, and history of falls. Assessing the client for fall risks gives the nurse information needed to develop an individualized care plan.

The nurse can complete a 2- to 5-minute assessment tool called the "Timed Up and Go" (TUG) test in a hospital, long-term care, or home setting. This assessment requires the client to complete a series of tasks that are important for independent mobility: standing, walking, turning, and sitting (Picone, 2013, p. 57). The test consists of asking the client to stand up from a standard chair, walk at a comfortable

---

BOX 12–1 Safety Assessment

Assess the client (in institutional as well as home care settings) upon admission and on an ongoing basis by determining the following:

- Level of awareness or consciousness, specifically, orientation to time, place, and person; ability to concentrate and make judgments; ability to assimilate many kinds of information at one time; and ability to perceive reality accurately and act on those perceptions. Consider clients whose judgment and motor function are altered by medications, such as narcotics, tranquilizers, hypnotics, and sedatives.
- Cardiac status, and the presence of low blood pressure and postural hypotension.
- Lifestyle factors, such as polypharmacy (taking many medications), risk-taking behavior, and substance use.
- Environmental factors such as lighting, types of flooring surfaces, clutter, proximity of personal items, and safety/maintenance/fit of wheelchair or ambulatory devices.
- Use of safety equipment such as railings, adaptive bathroom features such as hand rails, stools, and skid-prevention strips.
- Sensory alterations, such as impaired vision, hearing, smell, tactile perception, and taste.

- Mobility status. Note in particular individuals who have muscle weakness, poor balance or coordination, or paralysis; those weakened by illness or surgery; and those who use ambulatory aids such as canes and walkers. Assess safety of footwear (e.g., fit, heel height, slip potential of sole).
- Emotional state, which can alter the ability to perceive environmental hazards. Individuals who are acutely anxious, angry, in pain, or depressed, or who have insomnia may have reduced perceptual awareness or may think and react to environmental stimuli more slowly.
- Ability to communicate. Individuals with diminished ability to receive and convey information (e.g., clients with aphasia) and those with language barriers may not be able to read such safety signs as "Wet Floor" or "Out of Order."
- Previous accidents and frequency or predisposition to accidents.
- Safety knowledge about use of potentially dangerous equipment and precautions to take to prevent injury (e.g., fire safety, water safety, oxygen precautions, radiation protection, accident prevention).

---

pace for a distance of 3 m (10 ft) to a spot marked with a piece of tape, turn, walk back, and sit down. The client is allowed to use their routine walking aid. The client is instructed not to use their arms to stand up from the chair and no physical assistance is given. The time to complete the test is measured with a stopwatch. Usually the test is performed twice and the better time is used. A time of 14 seconds or more indicates a high risk of falling (Herman, Giladi, & Hausdorff, 2011; Picone, 2013). This quick assessment, along with an assessment of the client's environment, can help the nurse recommend safety measures to the client and family.

Health agencies have protocols to help prevent client falls. The Agency for Healthcare Research and Quality (AHRQ) (2013) strongly encourages health agencies to have "universal fall precautions" as part of the hospital's fall prevention program. Universal fall precautions keep *all* client environments safe (see Box 12–2).

BOX 12–2 Sample Universal Fall Precautions

- Familiarize the client with the environment.
- Have the client "teach back" how to use the call light.
- Keep the call light within reach at all times.
- Keep the client's personal possessions within safe reach.
- Provide sturdy hand rails in client bathrooms, rooms, and hallways.
- Keep the hospital bed in the low position with brakes locked when client is resting in bed.
- Provide nonslip, well-fitting footwear.
- Use night lights or supplemental light.
- Keep floor surfaces clean and dry. Clean up all spills promptly.
- Keep client area uncluttered.

From *Preventing Falls in Hospitals: A Toolkit for Improving Quality of Care*, by Agency for Healthcare Research and Quality, 2013. Retrieved from http://www.ahrq.gov/professionals/systems/long-term-care/resources/injuries/fallpxtoolkit/index.html; and *Institute for Clinical Systems Improvement: Prevention of Falls (Acute Care)*, by J. Degelau et al., 2012. Retrieved from https://www.icsi.org/_asset/dcn15z/Falls-Interactive0412.pdf#page=19.

As older adults age, they experience a decrease in muscle strength that affects their balance and increases their risk of falling. The majority of falls in the acute hospital setting occur in the client's room, generally around the bed and in the bathroom, with the majority of falls not being observed. The major reason for these falls relates to toileting and a client's fear of having "an accident." Evidence reveals an association between being in a hurry to get to the bathroom and falls. AHRQ (2013) recommends a proactive approach called *scheduled rounding*. In this approach the nurse conducts hourly visits between 6 AM and 10 PM and visits every 2 hours between 10 PM and 6 AM. The hourly rounding can be alternated between the nurse and unlicensed assistive personnel. The rounding usually includes pain assessment, offering help with toileting, offering hydration or nutrition, positioning the client if needed, making sure the client's call light and personal items are within safe reach, and asking the client and family to use the call light if the client needs to get out of bed. For information on preventing falls and subsequent injury of clients, see the Practice Guidelines.

Although it may seem that raising the side rails on a bed is an effective method of preventing falls, do not routinely raise rails for this purpose. Research has shown that clients with memory impairment, altered mobility, nocturia, and other sleep disorders are prone to becoming entrapped in side rails and may, in fact, be more likely to fall trying to get out around raised rails (Nowicki, Fulbrook & Burns, 2010). Clients may even become entrapped between the mattress and side rails, leading to asphyxiation deaths. In some settings, side rails are not used at all. Instead, beds are lowered fully, and long pads are placed on each side of the bed.

Health care environments should be safety oriented with systems in place to allow objective evaluation of outcomes. Environments should be designed with many safety features to reduce the risk of falls, such as regular toileting and orientation of clients who are confused or impaired; the use of fall risk alerts such as client ID wrist bands of a specific color; railings along corridors; call bells at

PRACTICE GUIDELINES

Preventing Falls in Health Care Settings

- On admission, orient clients to their surroundings and explain the call system.
- Carefully assess clients' ability to ambulate and transfer. Provide walking aids and assistance as required.
- Encourage clients to wear nonskid footwear.
- Encourage clients to use grab bars mounted in toilet and bathing areas and railings along corridors.
- Closely supervise clients at risk for falls, especially at night.
- Encourage clients to use the call bell to request assistance. Ensure that the bell is within easy reach.
- Place bedside tables and overbed tables near the bed or chair so that clients do not overreach and consequently lose their balance.

- Always keep hospital beds in the low position and wheels locked when not providing care so that clients can move in or out of bed easily.
- Make sure nonskid bath mats are available in tubs and showers.
- Keep the environment tidy; in particular, keep light cords from underfoot and furniture out of the way.
- Use individualized interventions (e.g., alarm sensitive to client position) rather than side rails for clients who are confused.
- Attach side rails to the beds of sedated, restless, and unconscious clients, and keep the rails in place when the client is unattended.

each bedside; safety bars in toilet areas; locks on beds, wheelchairs, and stretchers; well-maintained and appropriately sized wheelchairs; one-quarter to one-half length side rails on beds or pads beside beds; night-lights; freedom from clutter; and so on.

Older adults are at particularly high risk for falls (see Lifespan Considerations). Risk factors for falls and associated preventive measures are shown in Table 12–1.

CLINICAL ALERT!

Bed and chair alarms can be triggered by normal positional changes. However, the nurse should never assume an alarm is false if the client is out of sight.

Electronic **safety monitoring devices** are available to detect when clients are attempting to move or get out of bed. For example, a bed or chair safety monitor has a position-sensitive switch that triggers an audio alarm when the client attempts to get out of the bed or chair. A **magnetic box mobility monitor** mounted on a bed or chair connects with a clip to clothing. It will pull apart should the client try to move away from the chair or bed, triggering an alarm. There are also dual-sensor systems that include a pressure-sensitive sensor combined with an infrared beam detector. These monitors, however, can alarm with normal position changes, so nurses must be careful to assess whether the client is actually trying to exit the bed or chair. See Skill 12–1 for using a safety monitoring device.

LIFESPAN CONSIDERATIONS **Preventing Falls**

INFANTS/CHILDREN
- Assess risk for falls (age, mental status, medications, physical and mental impairments).
- Encourage parents to change the infant's diaper on a soft towel placed on the floor.
- Use changing tables and cribs with properly padded sides and rails.
- Use home safety devices, such as guards on windows that are above ground level, stair gates, and guard rails to help keep an active child from taking a dangerous fall.

OLDER ADULTS
- Assess for potential personal causes of falls: hypotension, unsteady gait, altered mental responsiveness (such as from medications), poor vision, foot pathology, unsafe footwear (loose, poorly fitting, slippery bottoms, high heels, rough edges), cognitive changes, and fear.

- In the home or community setting, assess for potential environmental causes of falls:
  - *Lighting:* inadequate amount, inaccessible or inconvenient switches
  - *Floors:* presence of electrical cords, loose rugs, clutter, slippery surfaces
  - *Stairs:* absent or unsteady railings, uneven step height or surfaces
  - *Furniture:* unsteady base, lack of armrests, cabinets too high or too low
  - *Bathroom:* inappropriate toilet height, slippery floors or tub, absence of grab bars.
- In the home, consider alternatives to a hospital or regular bed if the client is extremely prone to falling out of bed:
  - Place the mattress directly onto the floor.
  - Use a water mattress.
  - Place padding on the floor next to the bed or between the client and side rails.

| TABLE 12–1 | Risk Factors and Preventive Measures for Falls |

Risk Factor	Preventive Measures
Poor vision	Ensure eyeglasses are functional. Ensure appropriate lighting. Mark doorways and edges of steps as needed. Keep the environment tidy.
Cognitive dysfunction (confusion, disorientation, impaired memory or judgment)	Set safe limits to activities. Remove unsafe objects.
Impaired gait or balance and difficulty walking because of lower extremity dysfunction (e.g., arthritis)	Wear shoes or well-fitted slippers with nonskid soles. Use ambulatory devices as necessary (cane, crutches, walker, braces, wheelchair). Provide assistance with ambulation as needed. Monitor gait and balance. Adapt living arrangements to one floor if necessary. Encourage exercise and activity as tolerated to maintain muscle strength, joint flexibility, and balance. Ensure uncluttered environment with securely fastened rugs.
Difficulty getting in and out of chair or in and out of bed	Encourage the client to request assistance. Keep the bed in the low position. Install grab bars in the bathroom. Provide a raised toilet seat.
Orthostatic hypotension	Instruct client to rise slowly from a lying to sitting to standing position, and to stand in place for several seconds before walking.
Urinary frequency or receiving diuretics	Provide a bedside commode. Assist with voiding on a frequent and scheduled basis.
Weakness from disease process or therapy	Encourage the client to summon help. Monitor activity tolerance.
Current medication regimen that includes anticonvulsants, sedatives, anxiolytics (especially benzodiazepines), hypnotics, tranquilizers, narcotic analgesics, diuretics	Attach side rails to the bed if appropriate. Keep the rails in place when the bed is in the lowest position, or place pads beside the bed. Monitor orientation and alertness status. Discuss how alcohol contributes to fall-related injuries. Encourage the client not to mix alcohol and medications and to avoid alcohol when necessary. Encourage annual or more frequent review of all medications prescribed.

●○● NURSING PROCESS: PREVENTING FALLS

Using a Bed or Chair Exit Safety Monitoring Device

SKILL 12–1

ASSESSMENT
Assess:
- Mobility status.
- Judgment about ability to get out of bed safely.
- Client's pattern of exiting the bed (e.g., using the upper extremities to pull self up before lowering the feet and legs to the floor or leaning toward the edge of the bed prior to dropping the legs over the side).
- Proximity of the client's room to the nurses' station.
- Position of side rails.
- Functioning status of the call light.

PLANNING
Determine the best type of device and appropriate location for the device. If the device is applied to the body, choose a location where skin is intact.

DELEGATION

Risk factors for falls may be observed and recorded by individuals other than the nurse. The nurse is responsible for assessing the client and confirming that there is a risk of the client falling when getting out of a chair or bed unassisted. The nurse develops a plan of care that includes a variety of interventions that will protect the client. If indicated, use of a safety monitoring device may be delegated to unlicensed assistive personnel (UAP) who have been trained in its application and monitoring.

INTERPROFESSIONAL PRACTICE

Assessing a client's risk for falls is within the scope of practice for several health care providers. For example, in addition to nurses, both physical therapists and occupational therapists assess for fall risk. Although these therapists may verbally communicate their findings and plan to the health care team members, the nurse must also know where to locate their documentation in the client's medical record.

Equipment
- Alarm and control device
- Sensor
- Connection to nurse call system

Using a Bed or Chair Exit Safety Monitoring Device—*continued*

IMPLEMENTATION
Performance

1. Prior to performing the procedure, introduce self and verify the client's identity using agency protocol. Explain to the client and family the purpose and procedure of using a safety monitoring device. Explain that the device does not limit mobility in any manner; rather, it alerts the staff when the client is about to get out of bed or a chair. Explain that the nurse must be called when the client needs to get out of bed or a chair.
2. Perform hand hygiene and observe other appropriate infection prevention procedures.
3. Provide for client privacy.
4. Test the battery device and alarm sound. **Rationale:** *Testing ensures that the device is functioning properly prior to use.*
5. Apply the leg band or sensor pad.
   - Place the leg band according to the manufacturer's recommendation. Place the client's leg in a straight horizontal position. **Rationale:** *The alarm device is position sensitive; that is, when it approaches a near-vertical position (such as in walking, crawling, or kneeling as the client attempts to get out of bed), the audio alarm will be triggered.*
   - For the bed or chair device, the sensor is usually placed under the buttocks area. ❶
   - For a bed or chair device, set the time delay to 1 to 12 seconds for determining the client's movement patterns.
   - Connect the sensor pad to the control unit and the nurse call system.
6. Instruct the client to call the nurse when the client wants or needs to get up, and assist as required.
   - When assisting the client up, deactivate the alarm.
   - Assist the client back to bed or chair, and reattach the alarm device.
7. Ensure client safety with additional safety precautions.
   - Place the call light within client reach, lift side rails per agency policy, and lower the bed to its lowest position. **Rationale:** *The alarm device is not a substitute for other precautionary measures.*
   - Place fall risk or fall precaution signs on the client's door, chart, and other relevant locations.
8. Document the type of alarm used, where it was placed, and its effectiveness in the client record using forms or checklists supplemented by narrative notes when appropriate. Record all additional safety precautions and interventions discussed and employed.

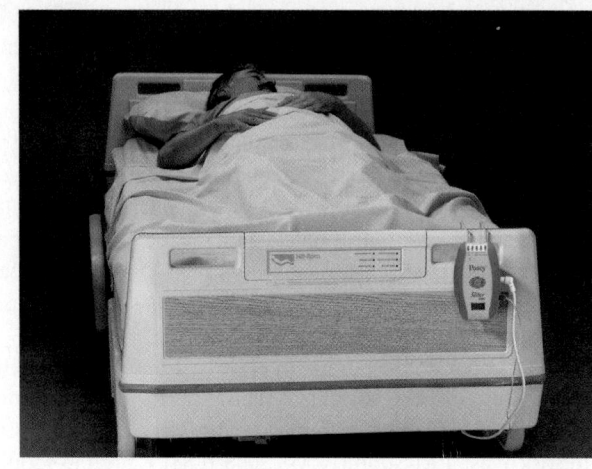

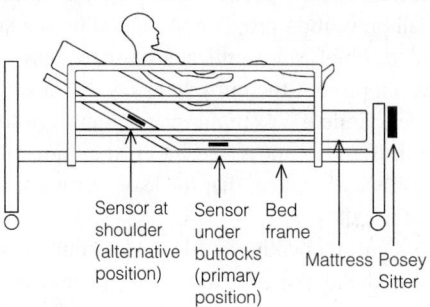

❶ Placement of a bed exit monitoring device.

Images courtesy J. T. Posey Company, Arcadia, California.

Sensor at shoulder (alternative position) Sensor under buttocks (primary position) Bed frame Mattress Posey Sitter

SAMPLE DOCUMENTATION

7/2/2015 1130 Found out of bed despite frequent verbal reminders to use call light for assistance. Explained about using a magnetic box mobility alarm to ensure own safety from possible fall. Verbalized agreement. Alarm device applied. Reminded again of importance to call the nurse for assistance. Call light placed within client's reach.
—————————————————————— J. Wallace, RN

EVALUATION

- If the alarm is too sensitive to client movement that is not an attempt to move from bed or chair, reassess and modify alarm controls accordingly.
- Conduct appropriate follow-up relating to effectiveness of safety precautions.
- Report any difficulties using the device or any falls to the primary care provider.

Ambulatory and Community Settings Safety

Using a Bed or Chair Exit Safety Monitoring Device

If a monitoring device is used in the home, instruct caregivers to do the following:
- Test the monitoring device every 12 to 24 hours to ensure that it is working.
- Check the volume of the alarm to ascertain they can hear it.

- Although these devices are sensitive and alarms can be triggered by normal movement, instruct family to investigate all alarms, and not to assume a false alarm. They may, however, adjust the alarm controls.

Use of the device does not take the place of proper supervision of clients at risk for falling. Assessment of the reasons for falling, especially among older adults, can lead to effective prevention.

RESTRAINING CLIENTS

Restraints are devices used to limit the physical activity of the client or a part of the body. The CMS states "all patients have the right to be free from physical or mental abuse, and corporal punishment. All patients have the right to be free from restraint or seclusion, of any form, imposed as a means of coercion, discipline, convenience, or retaliation by staff. Restraint or seclusion may only be imposed to ensure the immediate physical safety of the patient, a staff member, or others and must be discontinued at the earliest possible time" (2008, p. 83). In general, the shift in attitudes about the use of restraints has been toward using other means for controlling behaviors that may pose a threat to self or others. This desired outcome is referred to as a **restraint-free environment**.

The decision to use a restraint must be based on a comprehensive, individualized client assessment. This assessment needs to determine whether the use of less restrictive measures is a greater risk than the risk of using a restraint (CMS, 2008, p. 83). Restraints should not be considered a part of routine client care and should not be included in a fall prevention program. A request from a family member to apply a restraint is not sufficient cause to apply a restraint. It should, however, prompt the nurse to assess the client and current situation to determine if a restraint intervention is needed. The assessments and, if a restraint is needed must be documented. This documentation should reflect that the least restrictive intervention was used (CMS, 2008, p. 86).

Restraints are frequently used for older adults with dementia who are confused and may pose a threat to themselves. It is important to screen such clients on admission using available standardized instruments (e.g., the Mini Cog for cognitive function, the Confusion Assessment Method [CAM] for level of confusion, and the Katz ADL to assess mobility and transfer ability). Any deviation from the admission baseline signals a need to rescreen the client.

Restraints can be classified as physical, chemical, or seclusion. **Physical restraints** include "any manual method, physical or mechanical device, material, or equipment that immobilizes or reduces the ability of a patient to move his or her arms, legs, body, or head freely" (CMS, 2008, p. A184;). Examples can include leather or cloth wrist and ankle restraints, soft belts or vests, hand mitts, pelvic ties, gerichairs, and overchair tables). They cannot be removed easily and they restrict the client's movement. Generally, if a client

can easily remove a device, the device would not be considered a restraint. **Chemical restraints** involve using medication to control behavior or to restrict the client's freedom of movement and is *not* a standard treatment for the client's medical or psychological condition (CMS, 2008). **Seclusion** is the involuntary confinement of a client alone in a room or area from which the client is physically prevented from leaving (CMS, 2008).

Improper use of restraints and lack of monitoring can lead to injury and death and to psychological harm. Restraints can cause injury to clients through the hazards of immobility (e.g., muscle atrophy, bone loss, contractures, pressure ulcers, constipation, decreased appetite, and so on), confusion, boredom and loneliness, depression, and loss of dignity. Death can result due to strangulation, suffocation, broken necks, burns, pneumonia, and sepsis. Cases have been documented in which restrained individuals did not receive proper care related to hygiene, skin assessments, hydration, nutritional requirements, elimination, pain assessment, and appropriate assessments and monitoring of vital signs. The recent focus in health care safety is to explore ways to prevent, reduce, and hopefully eliminate the use of restraints while still protecting a client's safety, rights, and dignity. Attention to the legal and ethical rights of clients has fueled movement toward restraint-free environments.

Increasingly, determining the need for safety measures is viewed as an independent nursing function. However, because restraints restrict the individual's freedom, their use has legal implications. Nurses need to know their agency's policies and the state laws about restraining clients. The CMS (2008) revised standards for use of restraints effective January 2007, and these standards apply to all health care organizations. See Box 12–3 for standards of use of restraint and seclusion.

The standards address two types of behaviors in which restraints might be necessary: nonviolent, non–self-destructive behavior and violent or self-destructive behavior. For the nonviolent, non–self-destructive behavior, restraints may be necessary to directly support medical healing. For example, a client attempting to seriously interfere with a physical treatment or device (e.g., an IV line, respirator, or a dressing) may require a restraint when less restrictive approaches do not work to prevent this interference. For violent or self-destructive behavior, restraint or seclusion may be used to protect the client from injury to self or others. Seclusion may *only* be used for the

---

| **BOX 12–3** | **Standards for Use of Restraints and Seclusion** |

- Restraint may be used to ensure the client's immediate physical safety, even if the client is not violent or self-destructive.
- Seclusion may *only* be used for the management of violent or self-destructive behavior that is an immediate threat to the client's physical safety.
- Restraint or seclusion may only be used when less restrictive interventions have been determined to be ineffective to protect the client, a staff member, or others from harm.
- The type or technique of restraint or seclusion used must be the least restrictive intervention that will be effective to protect the client, a staff member, or others from harm.

- The use of restraint or seclusion must be implemented in accordance with safe and appropriate restraint and seclusion techniques per hospital policy.
- Restraint or seclusion must be discontinued at the earliest possible time.

From: *Hospitals—Restraint/Seclusion Interpretive Guidelines & Updated State Operations Manual (SOM)* Appendix A, by Centers for Medicare and Medicaid Services, 2008, Baltimore, MD: Author.

BOX 12–4 Alternatives to Restraints

- Assess for pain and treat appropriately.
- Ask family members or significant others to stay with the client.
- Reduce stimulation (e.g., noise, lights); play soothing music.
- Assign nurses in pairs to act as "buddies" so that one nurse can observe the client when the other leaves the unit.
- Place unstable clients in an area that is constantly or closely supervised.
- Prepare clients before a move to limit relocation shock and resultant confusion.
- Stay with a client using a bedside commode or bathroom if the client is confused or sedated or has a gait disturbance or a high-risk score for falling.
- Provide frequent toileting, if needed; provide a bedside commode.
- Monitor all the client's medications and, if possible, attempt to lower or eliminate dosages of sedatives or psychotropics.
- Position beds at their lowest level to facilitate getting in and out of bed.
- Replace full-length side rails with half- or three-quarter-length rails to prevent confused clients from climbing over rails or falling from the end of the bed.

- Use rocking chairs to help confused clients expend some of their energy so that they will be less inclined to wander.
- Wedge pillows or pads against the sides of wheelchairs to keep clients well positioned safely.
- Place a removable lap tray on a wheelchair to provide support and help keep the client in place.
- To quiet agitated clients, try a warm beverage, soft lights, a back rub, or a walk.
- Use "environmental restraints," such as pieces of furniture or large plants as barriers, to keep clients from wandering beyond appropriate areas.
- Place a picture or other personal item on the door to clients' rooms to help them identify their room.
- Try to determine the causes of the client's sundowner syndrome (nocturnal wandering and disorientation as darkness falls, associated with dementia). Possible causes include poor hearing, poor eyesight, or pain.
- Allow restless clients to walk after determining the safety of the environment.
- Establish ongoing assessment to monitor changes in physical and cognitive functional abilities and risk factors.

management of violent or self-destructive behavior that jeopardizes the immediate physical safety of the client, a staff member, or others. In both cases, a nurse may apply restraints but a physician or other licensed independent practitioner (LIP) who is responsible for the care of the client must order the use of restraint or seclusion. In addition, a face-to-face evaluation of the client must occur within 1 hour and be conducted by the physician or LIP, or an RN or physician assistant (PA) who has been trained according to the new requirements (CMS, 2008). If an RN or PA performs the evaluation, the attending physician or LIP responsible for the client's care must be consulted as soon as possible after the evaluation is performed. A written restraint order for an adult with violent or self-destructive behavior, following evaluation, is valid for only 4 hours for up to a total of 24 hours. If the client must be restrained and secluded, there must be continual visual and audio monitoring of the client's status. All orders must be renewed daily. Each order for restraint used to ensure the physical safety of the nonviolent or non–self-destructive client is renewed per hospital policy.

Restrained clients must be monitored regularly, and the new standards allow hospital policies to guide staff in determining appropriate intervals for assessment and monitoring. However, in the case of clients in seclusion, continual, ongoing monitoring is required.

Standards require that a primary care provider's order for restraints include delineation of the reason for, specific time frame (only for violent or self-destructive behavior), and type of restraint necessary. Restraint or seclusion must be discontinued at the earliest possible time, regardless of the length of time identified in the order. "As-needed" (prn) orders for restraints are prohibited. *In all cases, restraints should be used only after every other possible means of ensuring safety have been unsuccessful and documented.* See alternatives to the use of restraints in Box 12–4. Restrained clients often become more restless and anxious as a result of the loss of self-control. Nurses must

document that the need for the restraint was made clear both to the client and to support people such as family members.

Clients have the right to be free from restraints that are not medically necessary. As a result, there must be justification that the use of restraints will protect the client and that less restrictive measures were attempted and found not effective. Restraints *cannot* be used for staff convenience or client punishment. Given that the above conditions are met and restraints are needed, it is important for the nurse to be able to correctly apply restraints without endangering client safety.

Before selecting a restraint, nurses need to understand its purpose clearly and measure it against the following five criteria:

1. It restricts the client's movement as little as possible. If a client needs to have one arm restrained, do not restrain the entire body.
2. It is safe for the particular client. Choose a restraint with which the client cannot self-inflict injury. For example, a client who is physically restrained could incur injury trying to climb out of bed if one wrist is tied to the bed frame. A vest restraint would restrain the client more safely.
3. It does not interfere with the client's treatment or health problem. If a client has poor blood circulation to the hands, apply a restraint that will not aggravate that circulatory problem.
4. It is readily changeable. Restraints need to be changed frequently, especially if they become soiled. Keeping other guidelines in mind, choose a restraint that can be changed with minimal disturbance to the client.
5. It is as discreet as possible. Both clients and visitors are often embarrassed by a restraint, even though they understand why it is being used. The less obvious the restraint, the more comfortable people feel.

Selecting a Restraint

There are several kinds of restraints. Among the most common are vest restraints, belt restraints, mitt or hand restraints, and limb restraints.

There are several types of **vest restraints**. All are essentially sleeveless jackets or vests with straps (tails) that can be tied to fixed parts of the bed frame under the mattress or wheelchair frame. These body restraints are used to ensure the safety of confused or sedated clients in beds or wheelchairs. The U.S. Food and Drug Administration (FDA) advises that manufacturers place "front" and "back" labels on vest restraints.

Belt or safety strap body restraints are used to ensure the safety of all clients who are being moved on stretchers or in wheelchairs. Some wheelchairs have a soft, padded safety bar that attaches to side brackets that are installed under the armrests. To prevent the person from slumping forward, the nurse then attaches a shoulder "Y" strap to the bar and over the client's shoulders to the rear handles. Other safety belt models have a three-loop design. One loop surrounds the person's waist and attaches to the rear handles. If such restraints are unavailable, the nurse can place a folded towel or small sheet around the client's waist and fasten it at the back of the wheelchair. Belt restraints may also be used for certain clients confined to bed or to chairs.

A **mitt** or **hand restraint** (Figure 12–1 ■) is used to prevent clients of any age from using their hands or fingers to scratch and injure themselves. For example, a client who is confused may need to be prevented from pulling at IV tubing or a head bandage following brain surgery. Hand or mitt restraints allow the client to be ambulatory and/or to move the arm freely rather than be confined to a bed or a chair. Mitts need to be removed on a regular basis to permit the client to wash and exercise the hands. The nurse also needs to remove the mitt to check the circulation to the hand.

Limb restraints (Figure 12–2 ■), which are generally made from cloth, may be used to immobilize a limb, primarily for therapeutic reasons (e.g., to maintain IV infusion). Commonly used with

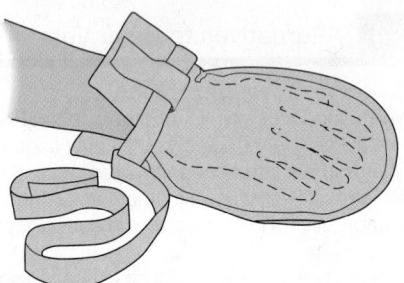

Figure 12–1 ■ A mitt restraint.

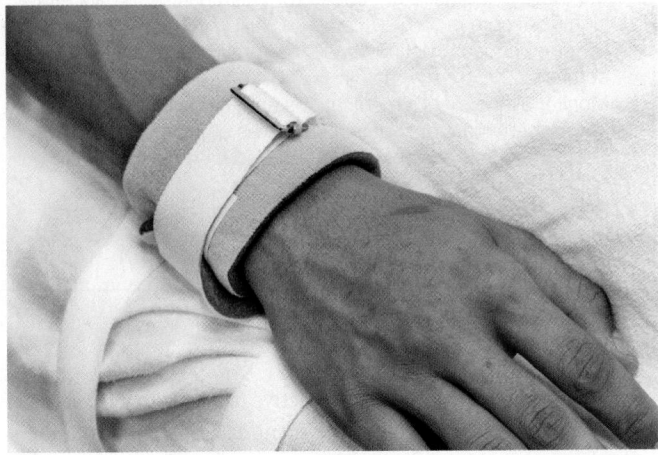

Figure 12–2 ■ A limb restraint.

children, elbow restraints (e.g., no-nos) prevent flexion of the joint so that tubing, connections, catheters, and bandages cannot be reached. Restraints for infants and children include mummy restraints, elbow restraints, and crib nets (see Lifespan Considerations on page 333).

PRACTICE GUIDELINES

Applying Restraints

- Use restraints only when other measures have not worked. The goal is to provide a restraint-free or least restrictive environment.
- Obtain consent from the client or guardian before applying restraints if possible.
- Ensure that a primary care provider, properly trained RN, or a PA performs a face-to-face evaluation within 1 hour of initiating the restraints.
- Ensure that a primary care provider's order has been provided.
- Assure the client and the client's support people that the restraint is temporary and protective. Need for ongoing restraint must be reevaluated according to agency policy. A restraint must never be applied as punishment for any behavior or merely for the nurse's convenience.
- Pad bony prominences (e.g., wrists and ankles) before applying a restraint over them. The movement of a restraint without padding over such prominences can quickly abrade the skin.
- Apply the restraint in such a way that the client can move as freely as possible without defeating the purpose of the restraint.
- Ensure that limb restraints are applied securely but not so tightly that they impede blood circulation to any body area or extremity.
- Always tie a limb restraint with a knot (e.g., a half-bow) that will not tighten when pulled.
- Tie the ends of a body restraint to the part of the bed that moves to elevate the head. Never tie the ends to a side rail or to the fixed frame of the bed if the bed position is to be changed.
- Assess the restraint per agency protocol time frame. Some facilities have specific forms to be used to record ongoing

- assessment. This may be a visual check to ensure client safety and no signs of injury.
- Assess skin integrity per agency protocol (e.g., every 2 hours), and provide range-of-motion (ROM) exercises (see Chapter 13 ⚭) and skin care (see Chapter 31 ⚭) when restraints are removed.
- Assess and assist with basic needs: nutrition, hydration, hygiene, elimination.
- Reassess the continued need for the restraint. Include an assessment of the underlying cause of the behavior necessitating use of the restraints. Whenever possible, try to avoid the use of restraints, and discontinue them as soon as possible.
- When a restraint is temporarily removed, do not leave the client unattended.
- Immediately report to the nurse in charge and record on the client's chart any persistent reddened or broken skin areas under the restraint.
- At the first indication of cyanosis or pallor, coldness of a skin area, or a client's complaint of a tingling sensation, pain, or numbness, loosen the restraint and exercise the limb.
- Apply a restraint so that it can be released quickly in case of an emergency and with the body part in a normal anatomic position.
- Provide multisensory soothing measures and emotional support verbally, with relaxation music or a small fountain, with a calming scent such as lavender (if tolerated by the client), with something beautiful to look at such as artwork, and through touch.

When evaluating if a device is a restraint or not, determine the intended use (e.g., physical restriction), its involuntary application, and/or the client need for the restraint. For example, if all of the bed's side rails are up and restrict the client's freedom to leave the bed, and the client did not voluntarily request all rails to be up, they are a restraint. If, however, one side rail is up to assist the client to get in and out of the bed, it is not a restraint because it is helping the client to exit the bed. Also, if the client can release or remove a device, it would not be considered a restraint.

See Skill 12–2 for applying restraints.

●○○● NURSING PROCESS: RESTRAINING CLIENTS

Applying Restraints

ASSESSMENT
Assess:
- The behavior indicating the possible need for a restraint.
- Underlying cause for assessed behavior.
- What other protective measures may be implemented before applying a restraint.
- Status of skin to which restraint is to be applied.
- Circulatory status distal to restraints and of extremities.
- Effectiveness of other available safety precautions.

PLANNING
Review institutional policy for restraints and seek consultation as appropriate before obtaining an order to apply a restraint. All other possible interventions that are less restrictive *must* have been tried and their failure documented. The primary care provider must be notified prior to using a restraint, unless there is a danger to self or others. In that case, the primary care provider must be notified within the prescribed time frame per agency protocol.

Equipment
- Appropriate type and size of restraint

DELEGATION

The nurse must make the determination that restraints are appropriate in specific situations, select the proper type of restraints, evaluate the effectiveness of the restraints, and assess for potential complications from their use. Application of ordered restraints and their temporary removal for skin monitoring and care may be delegated to UAP who have been trained in their use.

IMPLEMENTATION
Performance
1. Prior to performing the procedure, introduce self and verify the client's identity using agency protocol. Explain to the client and family what you are going to do, why it is necessary, and how they can participate. Allow time for the client to express feelings about being restrained. Provide needed emotional reassurance that the restraints will be used only when absolutely necessary and that there will be close contact with the client in case assistance is required.
2. Perform hand hygiene and observe other appropriate infection prevention procedures.
3. Provide for client privacy if indicated.
4. Apply the selected restraint.

Belt Restraint (Safety Belt)
- Determine that the safety belt is in good order. If a Velcro safety belt is to be used, make sure that both pieces of Velcro are intact.
- If the belt has a long portion and a shorter portion, place the long portion of the belt behind (under) the client who is confined to bed and secure it to the movable part of the bed frame. **Rationale:** *The long attached portion will then move up when the head of the bed is elevated and will not tighten around the client.* Place the shorter portion of the belt around the client's waist, over the gown. There should be one fingerwidth between the belt and the client.

  or
- Attach the belt around the client's waist, and fasten it at the back of the chair.

  or
- If the belt is attached to a fixed part of the stretcher, secure the belt firmly over the client's hips or abdomen. **Rationale:** *Belt restraints must be applied to all clients on stretchers even when the side rails are up.*

Vest Restraint
- Place the vest on the client, with the opening at the front or the back, depending on the type.
- Pull the tie on the end of the vest flap across the chest, and place it through the slit in the opposite side of the chest.
- Repeat for the other tie.

Use a half-bow (a type of quick-release) knot to secure each tie around the movable bed frame or behind the chair to a chair leg.

Continued on page 332

SKILL 12–2

Applying Restraints—*continued*

❶ **Rationale:** *A half-bow knot does not tighten or slip when the attached end is pulled, but unties easily when the loose end is pulled.*

or

• Fasten the ties together behind the chair using a slip or quick-release knot.
• Ensure that the client is positioned appropriately to enable maximum chest expansion for breathing.

Mitt Restraint

• Apply the commercial thumbless mitt (see Figure 12–1) to the hand to be restrained. Make sure the fingers can be slightly flexed and are not caught under the hand. Ensure that the restraint is not too tight by checking that one to two fingers can fit under the strap before securing around the client's wrist. **Rationale:** *This avoids impaired circulation.*
• Follow the manufacturer's directions for securing the mitt.
• Assess the client's circulation to the hands shortly after the mitt is applied and at regular intervals. **Rationale:** *Client complaints of numbness, discomfort, or inability to move the fingers could indicate impaired circulation to the hand.*
• If a mitt is to be worn for several days, remove it at regular intervals per agency protocol. Wash and exercise the client's hand, then reapply the mitt. Check agency practices about recommended intervals for removal.

Wrist or Ankle Restraint

• Pad bony prominences on the wrist or ankle if needed to prevent skin breakdown.
• Apply the padded portion of the restraint around the ankle or wrist.
• Pull the tie of the restraint through the slit in the wrist portion or through the buckle and ensure the restraint is not too tight. ❷
• Using a half-bow knot, attach the other end of the restraint to the movable portion of the bed frame. **Rationale:** *If the ties are attached to the movable portion, the wrist or ankle will not be pulled when the bed position is changed.*

5. Adjust the plan of care as required, for example, to include releasing the restraint, providing skin care and ROM exercises, and attending to the client's physical needs by providing fluids, nutrition, and toileting.

6. Document on the client's chart the behavior(s) indicating the need for the restraint, all other interventions implemented in an attempt to avoid the use of restraints and their outcomes, and the time the primary care provider was notified of the need for restraint. Also record:

• The type of restraint applied, the time it was applied, and the goal for its application.
• The client's response to the restraint, including a rationale for its continued use.
• The times that the restraints were removed and skin care given.
• Any other assessments and interventions.
• Explanations given to the client and significant others.

SAMPLE DOCUMENTATION

7/10/2015 1200 Confused. Disoriented to time and place. Reoriented frequently. Pulling at central IV line, NG tube and chest tube. Medicated for pain relief. Lights dimmed ———————— M. Murray, RN
1245 Continues to pull at IV and tubes. Dr. Jones notified. Received an order to apply mitt restraints. Family notified and situation explained. Family member to come and sit with client. Mitt restraints applied, relaxation music initiated ———————— M. Murray, RN
1330 Son arrived and sitting with client. Calm though still disoriented. Mitts removed, skin intact, hands warm with good color and mobility. Vital signs stable ———————— M. Murray, RN

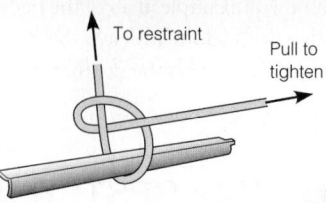
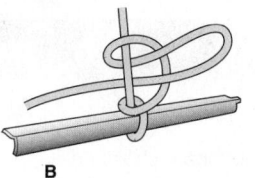
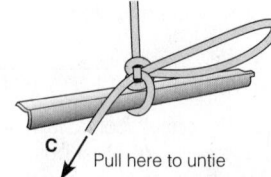

❶ To make a half-bow (quick-release) knot, first place the restraint tie under the side frame of the bed (or around a chair leg). *A,* Bring the free end up, around, under, and over the attached end of the tie and pull it tight. *B,* Again take the free end over and under the attached end of the tie, but this time make a half-bow loop. *C,* Tighten the free end of the tie and the bow until the knot is secure. To untie the knot, pull the end of the tie and then loosen the first cross over the tie.

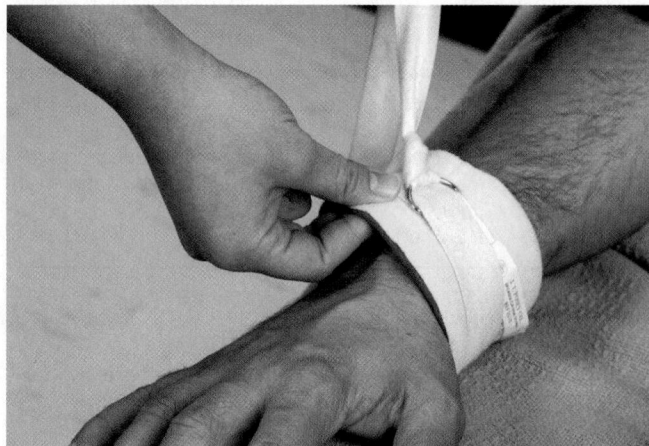

A

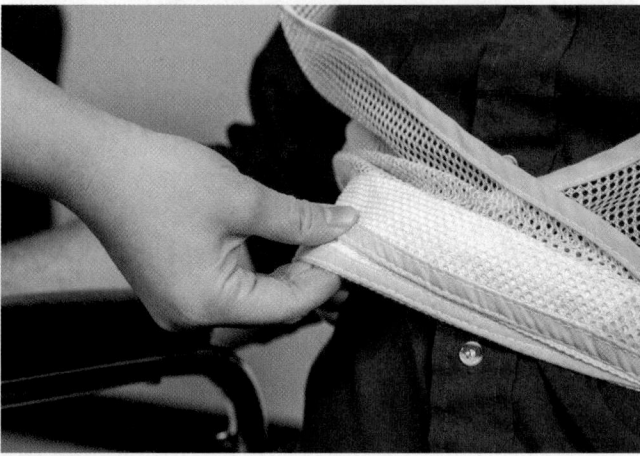

B

❷ Ensure that a finger can be inserted between the restraint and *A,* the wrist, and *B,* the chest.

Applying Restraints—*continued*

EVALUATION
- Perform a detailed follow-up of the need for the restraints and the client's response. Relate these findings to previous data if available.
- Evaluate circulatory status of restrained limbs.
- Evaluate skin status beneath restraints.

- Remove the restraints as soon as they are no longer needed and document.
- Report significant deviations from normal to the primary care provider.

LIFESPAN CONSIDERATIONS Applying Restraints

INFANTS
Elbow restraints are used to prevent infants or small children from flexing their elbows to touch or reach their face or head, especially after surgery. Ready-made elbow restraints are available commercially (e.g., no-nos).

A mummy restraint is made by folding a blanket or sheet around the infant in a certain way to prevent movement during a procedure such as gastric washing, eye irrigation, or collection of a blood specimen.

- Obtain a blanket or sheet large enough so that the distance between opposite corners is about twice the length of the infant's body. Lay the blanket or sheet on a flat, dry surface.
- Fold down one corner, and place the baby on it in the supine position.
- Fold the right side of the blanket over the infant's body, leaving the left arm free (see figure, part *A*1). The right arm is in a natural position at the side.
- Fold the excess blanket at the bottom up under the infant (see figure, part *B*2).
- With the left arm in a natural position at the baby's side, fold the left side of the blanket over the infant, including the arm, and tuck the blanket under the body (see figure, part *B*3).

- Remain with the infant who is in a mummy restraint until the specific procedure is completed.

CHILDREN
- A human restraint (parent or assistant) can be used during intramuscular injections.
- A papoose board immobilizer can be used for toddlers and larger children.
- A crib net is simply a device placed over the top of a crib to prevent active young children from climbing out of the crib. At the same time, it allows them freedom to move about in the crib. The crib net or dome is not attached to the movable parts of the crib so that the caregiver can have access to the child without removing the dome or net.
  - Place the net over the sides and ends of the crib.
  - Secure the ties to the springs or frame of the crib. The crib sides can then be freely lowered without removing the net.
  - Test with your hand that the net will stretch if the child stands against it in the crib.

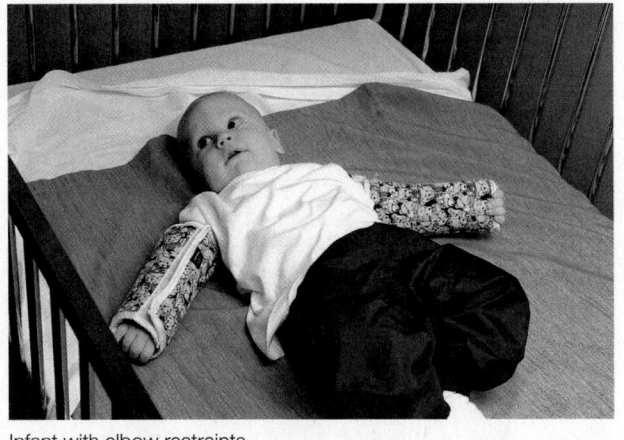

Infant with elbow restraints.

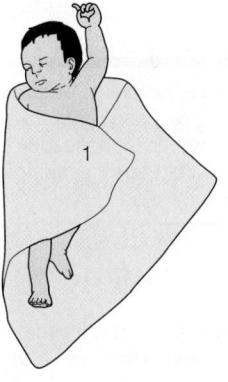
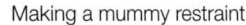
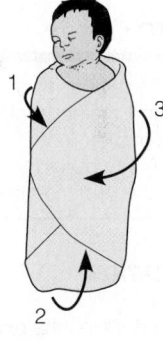

A   **B**

Making a mummy restraint.

Ambulatory and Community Settings Safety

Applying Restraints

Although other measures should always be tried first, restraints may be necessary for clients in wheelchairs or in the home. Safety guidelines apply in all cases. Assess the knowledge and skill of all caregivers in the use of restraints and educate as indicated.

- Use means other than restraints as much as possible, and stay with the client. Remember that the goal is a restraint-free environment.

- Pad bony prominences, such as wrists and ankles, if needed before applying a restraint over them.
- Tie restraints with half-bow (quick-release) knots that will not tighten when pulled and that release quickly in case of emergency. Tie to parts of the wheelchair that do not move.
- Assess restrained limbs for signs of impaired blood circulation.
- Always stay with a client whose restraint is temporarily removed.

Many institutions use a restraint monitoring and intervention flow sheet to ensure careful documentation.

CLINICAL ALERT!

Multidisciplinary staff teams should evaluate the clinical environment on an ongoing basis to prevent injuries to clients and staff. An environment of safety means that staff are accountable for analyzing reasons for falls without shame or blame. Assess and plan for each client upon admission and on an ongoing basis to provide the least restrictive approach to safety.

SEIZURE PRECAUTIONS

A **seizure** is a single temporary event that consists of uncontrolled electrical neuronal discharge of the brain that interrupts normal brain function (Osborn, Wraa, Watson, & Holleran, 2014, p. 543). The etiology or cause of the seizure can be different based on the age of the client. Trauma during birth is the leading cause of seizures in newborns. Infants and children develop seizures as a result of fever, trauma, and infections of the central nervous system. The

development of seizures in the adult population is most commonly related to structural abnormalities of the brain such as tumors, strokes, and trauma.

Seizures are classified into two categories: partial and generalized. Partial seizures (also called focal) involve electrical discharges from one area of the brain. In contrast, generalized seizures affect the whole brain. Each of these seizure categories includes different types of seizures, depending on the characteristics of the seizure activity (e.g., loss of consciousness versus no impairment to consciousness). Thus, it is important for nurses to thoroughly describe their observations before, during, and after a client's seizure episode. Clients are at risk for injury if they experience seizures that involve the entire body such as *grand mal* (tonic-clonic) seizures or any seizure that includes loss of consciousness. **Seizure precautions** are safety measures taken by the nurse to protect clients from injury should they have a seizure. Skill 12–3 describes how to implement seizure precautions.

●○●● NURSING PROCESS: SEIZURE PRECAUTIONS

Implementing Seizure Precautions

ASSESSMENT

Assess the history of seizures during the admission assessment. If the client has experienced a seizure previously, ask for detailed information, including characteristics of an aura or warning symptoms that indicate the seizure is beginning, duration and frequency of the seizures, consequences of the seizures (e.g., incontinence or difficulty breathing), and actions that should be taken to prevent or reduce seizure activity.

PLANNING

Review emergency procedures because respiratory arrest or other injury can result from a seizure.

DELEGATION

UAP should be familiar with establishing and implementing seizure precautions and methods of obtaining assistance during a client's seizure. Care of the client during a seizure, however, is the responsibility of the nurse due to the importance of careful assessment of respiratory status and the potential need for intervention.

Equipment

- Blankets or other linens to pad side rails
- Oral suction equipment and clean gloves
- Oxygen equipment

IMPLEMENTATION

Performance

1. Prior to performing the procedure, introduce self and verify the client's identity using agency protocol. Explain to the client what you are going to do, why it is necessary, and how he or she can participate.
2. Perform hand hygiene and observe other appropriate infection prevention procedures. If the client is actively seizing, apply clean gloves in preparation for performing respiratory care measures.
3. Provide for client privacy.
4. Pad the bed of any client who might have a seizure. Secure blankets or other linens around the head, foot, and side rails of the bed. ❶
5. Put oral suction equipment in place and test to ensure that it is functional. **Rationale:** *Suctioning may be needed to prevent aspiration of oral secretions.*
6. If a seizure occurs:
   - Remain with the client and call for assistance. Do not restrain the client.
   - If the client is not in bed, assist the client to the floor and protect the client's head by holding it in your lap or on a pillow. Loosen any clothing around the neck and chest.

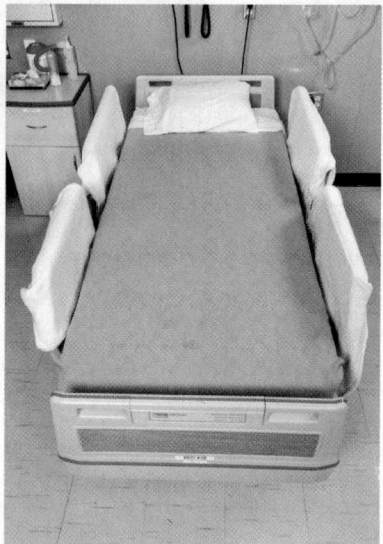
❶ Padding a bed for seizure precautions.

Implementing Seizure Precautions—*continued*

- Turn the client to a lateral position if possible. **Rationale:** *Turning to the side allows secretions to drain out of the mouth, decreasing the risk of aspiration, and helps keep the tongue from occluding the airway.*
- Move items in the environment to ensure the client does not experience an injury.
- Do not insert anything into the client's mouth.
- Time the seizure duration.
- Observe the progression of the seizure, noting the sequence and type of limb involvement. Observe skin color. When the seizure allows, check pulse and respirations.
- Apply gloves and use equipment to suction the mouth if the client vomits or has excessive oral secretions.
- Apply oxygen via mask or nasal cannula.
- Administer anticonvulsant medications, as ordered.
- When the seizure has subsided, assist the client to a comfortable position. Reorient. Explain what happened. Reassure the client. Provide hygiene as necessary. Allow the client to verbalize feelings about the seizure.
- If applied, remove and discard gloves.
- Perform hand hygiene.

7. Document the event in the client record using forms or checklists supplemented by narrative notes when appropriate.

SAMPLE DOCUMENTATION

7/8/2015 1815 Upon entering room, observed generalized muscle spasms/contractions of arms and legs lasting 25 seconds. Seizure padding previously placed on bed. Incontinent of urine. Cyanotic. Placed on left side. Suctioned. Airway clear. Respirations 14/min with irregular pattern. Oxygen applied at 4 L/min via mask. Oxygen saturation 90% on O$_2$. Not currently responding to verbal stimuli. Dr. Smith notified. Diazepam 10 mg given IV per order. VS taken every 15 min. See neuro flow sheet.————————— M. Faustino, RN

1835 Respirations 15/min, regular. Responding to verbal stimuli, oriented to person, place and time. Oxygen saturation 97% on O$_2$. O$_2$ discontinued per doctor's order. VS continue every 15 min. See neuro flow sheet.————————— M. Faustino, RN

EVALUATION

- Perform a detailed follow-up examination of the client. Administer medications if indicated and ordered.

- Report significant deviations from normal to the primary care provider.

LIFESPAN CONSIDERATIONS   **Implementing Seizure Precautions**

INFANTS
- The most common cause of seizures in young infants is birth injury (e.g., intracranial trauma, hemorrhage, anoxia) or congenital brain defects.

CHILDREN
- In children over 3 years of age, the most common cause of seizures is idiopathic epilepsy.
- Febrile seizures associated with acute infections occur more commonly in children than in adults and are usually preventable through the use of antipyretics and tepid baths.

- Determine oxygenation. Apply oxygen if the pulse oximetry reading is less than 95% (see Chapter 25 ∞). Oxygen can be applied via head hood, tent, nasal cannula, or mask, depending on the age and response of the child. Oxygen is drying and must be humidified. Tents are cooling, and the child's thermal balance must be monitored. The concentration of oxygen in tents is more difficult to regulate.
- Children who have frequent seizures may need to wear helmets for protection.
- Children on anticonvulsant medications should wear a medical identification tag (bracelet or necklace).

Ambulatory and Community Settings   **Safety**

Implementing Seizure Precautions
- Discuss with the client and family the factors that may precipitate a seizure.
- If clients have frequent or recurrent seizures or take anticonvulsant medications, they should wear a medical identification tag (bracelet or necklace) and carry a card delineating any medications they take.
- When making home visits, inspect anticonvulsant medications and confirm that clients are taking them correctly. Blood level measurements may be required periodically.

- Discuss safety precautions for inside and out of the home. If seizures are not well controlled, activities that may require restriction or direct supervision by others include tub bathing, swimming, cooking, using electric equipment or machinery, and driving.
- Assist clients in determining which individuals in the community should or must be informed of their seizure disorder (e.g., employers, health care providers such as dentists, motor vehicle department if driving, and companions).

FOCUSING ON CLINICAL THINKING

Consider This

1. In spite of repeated reminders to ask a family member for assistance before trying to go to the bathroom at night at home, your unsteady client insists on attempting the trip alone. The primary care provider suggests trying an activity-monitoring device. How would you explain this device to the client and family?

2. Your older client picks at her IV line and dressings, and has already pulled one IV out, necessitating a restart. When you remind her not to touch them, she sweetly replies: "I just forgot." You have obtained an order to apply a mitt restraint to the one hand she uses for these activities. What safety measures would be needed when using such a restraint?

3. When you walk into a client's room, you find the client alternately flexing and extending the arms but the rest of the body is not moving. The head is arched back and the client does not appear to be conscious. There is an oral airway, a suction machine, and oxygen equipment in the room. What are the most important things you should do at this time?

See Focusing on Clinical Thinking answers on student resource website.

TEST YOUR KNOWLEDGE

1. The nurse is caring for a client who is on "fall precautions." The nurse has placed a bed alarm under the client. Which term will the nurse correctly use in the documentation of client care?
   1. A physical restraint
   2. A chemical restraint
   3. A safety monitoring device
   4. A seizure monitoring device

2. A nurse is offering client teaching related to fall prevention at a local senior center. Which learning points would be important to review as part of this teaching plan? Select all that apply.
   1. Wear shoes or well-fitting slippers with nonskid soles.
   2. Have an uncluttered environment with securely fastened rugs.
   3. Ensure that proper lighting is available.
   4. Do not mix alcohol and medications, and avoid alcohol when necessary.
   5. Void on a frequent and scheduled basis.

3. A nurse is caring for a client who is acutely confused and agitated. The client has repeatedly attempted to get out of bed, and has also been trying to pull out all of his postoperative tubes and intravenous lines. The nurse intervenes by restraining the client with wrist restraints. Why are restraints indicated for this client?
   1. To prevent the client from injuring self
   2. To prevent the nurse from having extra work
   3. To prevent the client from being embarrassed later
   4. To prevent the primary care provider from having to order more medications

4. The nurse is applying a belt restraint on a client. Which statement, if made by the nurse, indicates the need for further teaching?
   1. "Before applying the belt restraint, I need to make sure that the Velcro is intact."
   2. "If the client is going to a test on a stretcher, then I am able to remove the restraint."
   3. "If I am restraining the client in the chair, I will fasten the belt restraint at the back of the chair."
   4. "After I restrain the client, there should be a finger's width between the belt and the client."

5. A home care nurse is meeting a client who has been discharged from the hospital with a new diagnosis of seizure disorder. Which action will the nurse implement?
   1. Assure the client that stress at home will not be a precipitating factor for the seizures.
   2. Discuss the need to inform the Department of Motor Vehicles of the seizure disorder.
   3. Inform the client that she may drive to work, bathe, and cook at home as usual.
   4. Tell the client that the monitoring of her medications will be done by her primary care provider.

6. A client is beginning to exhibit seizure activity. Unlicensed assistive personnel (UAP) are in the room to provide assistance. Which safety measure may the nurse assign to the UAP?
   1. Assess respiratory status and rate.
   2. Determine if the primary care provider needs to be called.
   3. Evaluate the type and length of seizure.
   4. Obtain blankets or other linens with which to pad the side rails.

7. The nurse has just applied hand mitts to a child with the goal of preventing self-harm because the child was pulling at intravenous lines and tubes. The nurse must assess and document which of the following related to the use of restraints? Select all that apply.
   1. Skin status beneath the restraints
   2. Circulation in the restrained arm
   3. Intravenous site condition
   4. Frequency of restraint assessment performed
   5. Urine output

8. The nurse accidentally spills a water pitcher in the unit hallway. What is the priority action the nurse should take to prevent falls?
   1. Go get towels or something to clean up the spill.
   2. Stay at the site of the spill and send someone else to call housekeeping to clean the spill.
   3. Call housekeeping from the nursing station to clean up the spill.
   4. Refill the water pitcher and take it to the client, and then return to clean up the spill.

9. The nurse admitted an older client with a new diagnosis of syncope (dizziness) to the hospital. The client was previously healthy and vigorous. When performing a safety assessment of this client, the nurse determines which is the most significant factor in the client's risk for falls?
   1. Hospital environment
   2. Safe equipment
   3. History of previous accidents and frequency of past accidents
   4. Medical diagnosis

10. The nurse is caring for a client who is confused and disoriented, has pulled out the urinary catheter twice, and now has hematuria. The primary care provider orders restraints. What type of restraint would the nurse choose initially?
    1. Mitt restraints
    2. Limb restraints
    3. Waist restraints
    4. Vest restraint

See Answers to Test Your Knowledge in Appendix A.

READINGS AND REFERENCES

References

Agency for Healthcare Research and Quality. (2013). *Preventing falls in hospitals: A toolkit for improving quality of care.* Retrieved from http://www.ahrq.gov/professionals/systems/long-term-care/resources/injuries/fallpxtoolkit/index.html

Centers for Medicare and Medicaid Services. (2008). *Hospitals—Restraint/seclusion interpretive guidelines & updated state operations manual (SOM) Appendix A.* Baltimore, MD: Author.

Degelau, J., Belz, M., Bungum, L., Flavin, P. L., Harper, C., Leys, K., . . . Webb, B. (2012). *Institute for Clinical Systems Improvement: Prevention of falls (acute care).* Retrieved from https://www.icsi.org/_asset/dcn15z/Falls-Interactive0412.pdf#page=19

Herman, T., Giladi, N., & Hausdorff. (2011). Properties of the "timed up and go" test: More than meets the eye. *Gerontology, 57*(3), 203–210. doi:10.1159/000314963

Jorgensen, J. (2011). Reducing patient falls: A call to action. *American Nurse Today Supplement: Best Practices for Falls Reduction, 6*(2), 2–3.

Kulik, C. (2011). Components of a comprehensive fall-risk assessment. *American Nurse Today Supplement: Best Practices for Falls Reduction, 6*(2), 6–7.

Nowicki, T., Fulbrook, P., & Burns, C. (2010). Bed safety off the rails. *Australian Nursing Journal, 18*(1), 31–34.

Osborn, K. S., Wraa, C. E., Watson, A. B., & Holleran, R. (2014). *Medical–surgical nursing: Preparation for practice* (2nd ed.). Upper Saddle River, NJ: Prentice Hall.

Picone, E. N. (2013). The timed up and go test. Assessing gait speed and balance in older adults. *American Journal of Nursing, 113*(3), 56–59.

Titler, M. G., Shever, L. L., Kanak, M. F., Picone, D. M., & Qin, R. (2011). Factors associated with falls during hospitalization in an older adult population. *Research and Theory for Nursing Practice, 25*(2), 127–152. doi:10.1891/1541-6577.25.2.127.

Selected Bibliography

Aranda-Gallardo, M., Asencio, J. M., Canca-Sanchez, J. C., Mora-Banderas, A. M., & Moya-Suarez, A. B. (2013). Instruments for assessing the risk of falls in acute hospitalized patients: A systematic review protocol. *Journal of Advanced Nursing, 69*, 185–193. doi:10.1111/j.1365-2648.2012.06104.x

Berman, A., Snyder, S., & Frandsen, G. (2016). *Kozier & Erb's fundamentals of nursing: Concepts, process, and practice* (10th ed.). Upper Saddle River, NJ: Pearson.

Gray-Miceli, D. (2014). *Five easy steps to prevent falls. The comprehensive guide to keeping patients of all ages safe.* Silver Spring, MD: American Nurses Association.

Haut, A., Kolbe, N., Strupeit, S., Mayer, H., & Meyer, G. (2010). Attitudes of relatives of nursing home residents toward physical restraints. *Journal of Nursing Scholarship, 42*, 448–456. doi:10.1111/j.1547-5069.2010.01341.x

Heaton, C. (2012). Creating a protocol to reduce inpatient falls. *Nursing Times, 108*(12), 16–18.

The Joint Commission (2013). *Hospital: 2014 National Patient Safety Goals.* Retrieved from http://www.jointcommission.org/hap_2014_npsgs

The Joint Commission (2013). *Long term care (Medicare/Medicaid): 2014 National Patient Safety Goals.* Retrieved from http://www.jointcommission.org/lt2_2014_npsgs

Ludwick, R., O'Toole, R., & Meehan, A. (2012). Restraints or alternatives: Safety work in care of older persons. *International Journal of Older People Nursing, 7*, 11–19. doi:10.1111/j.1748-3743.2010.00244.x.

McCabe, D. E., Alvarez, C. D., McNulty, R., & Fitzpatrick, J. J. (2011). Perceptions of physical restraints use in the elderly among registered nurses and nurse assistants in a single acute care hospital. *Geriatric Nursing, 32*, 39–45. doi:10.1016/j.gerinurse.2010.10.010

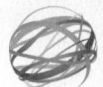

13 Maintaining Joint Mobility

LEARNING OUTCOMES

At the completion of this chapter, the student will be able to:

1. Define the key terms used in the skills of maintaining joint mobility.
2. Identify indications for various types of range-of-motion exercises:
   a. Active
   b. Passive
   c. Active-assistive.
3. Identify normal range of motion for joints throughout the body.
4. Describe the purpose of a continuous passive motion mechanical device.
5. Recognize when it is appropriate to delegate maintenance of joint mobility to unlicensed assistive personnel.
6. Verbalize the steps used in:
   a. Performing passive range-of-motion exercises.
   b. Using a continuous passive motion device.
7. Demonstrate appropriate documentation and reporting of joint mobility.

SKILLS

Skill 13–1 Performing Passive Range-of-Motion Exercises

Skill 13–2 Using a Continuous Passive Motion Device

KEY TERMS

Physical activity is essential to a human's biopsychosocial well-being. Many clients, however, have disease processes that impair mobility. Some of these disease processes, such as musculoskeletal trauma, paralysis, burns, and severe pain, impose immobility; others, such as myocardial infarction, require immobility to conserve oxygen and other important body nutrients. Historically, bed rest was considered part of the treatment plan for severe illness and recovery after surgery. In the early 20th century, physicians and researchers began to recognize the adverse effects of complete bed rest, such as neuromuscular weakness and contractures (permanent shortening of a muscle). Indeed, recent studies have documented the safety of progressive mobility even in clients who are critically ill (Dammeyer, Dickinson, Packard, Baldwin, & Ricklemann, 2013; Lipshutz & Gropper, 2013).

Nurses assist clients to restore optimal mobility and rest in order to ensure metabolic, physical, and social function. Maintaining joint mobility is clearly related to optimal rehabilitation. Nurses are often independent providers with respect to this goal. However, in select clients, this is an interdependent function. Nurses should ensure that the primary care provider has ordered appropriate medication (e.g., analgesics, antispasmodics) and that consultations with physical, occupational, and recreational therapists and physiatrists are conducted based on client needs. This is particularly important in those clients with pain or upper motor neuron diseases that result in **spasticity** (sudden, prolonged involuntary muscle contraction) and **rigidity** (resistance of a relaxed limb to passive movement) who may benefit from antispasmodics and splinting. Additionally, therapists have expertise in nonpharmacologic pain-relief measures and the application of heat or cold. In this chapter, we will examine the means in which nurses assist clients to retain and regain joint mobility and strengthen attached muscles in order to ensure or restore normal movement.

Clients who experience restrictions in activity are at risk for impaired joint mobility. Joints are the functional units of the musculoskeletal system. The bones of the skeleton articulate at the joints, and most of the skeletal muscles attach at two bones of a joint. These muscles are categorized according to the type of joint movement they produce on contraction (e.g., flexors and extensors). The flexor muscles are stronger than the extensor muscles. Thus, when a person is inactive, the joints are pulled into a flexed (bent) position. If this tendency is not counteracted with exercise and position changes, the muscles, tendons, ligaments, and soft tissues can permanently shorten and the joint becomes fixed in a flexed position, producing a joint contracture. Contractures begin within hours of immobility. Joint contractures limit the passive range of motion of a joint and compromise the functional status and comfort of clients. The types of joint movement are shown in Table 13–1.

TABLE 13–1	Types of Joint Movements

Movement	Action
Flexion	Decreasing the angle of the joint (e.g., bending the elbow)
Extension	Increasing the angle of the joint (e.g., straightening the arm at the elbow)
Hyperextension	Further extension or straightening of a joint (e.g., bending the head backward)
Abduction	Movement of the bone *away from* the midline of the body
Adduction	Movement of the bone *toward* the midline of the body
Rotation	Movement of the bone around its central axis
Circumduction	Movement of the distal part of the bone in a circle while the proximal end remains fixed
Eversion	Turning the sole of the foot outward by moving the ankle joint
Inversion	Turning the sole of the foot inward by moving the ankle joint
Pronation	Moving the bones of the forearm so that the palm of the hand faces downward when held in front of the body
Supination	Moving the bones of the forearm so that the palm of the hand faces upward when held in front of the body

RANGE-OF-MOTION EXERCISES

The **range of motion (ROM)** of a joint is the maximum movement that is possible for each joint. Joint ROM varies from individual to individual and is determined by genetic makeup, developmental patterns, the presence or absence of disease, and the amount of physical activity in which the person normally engages.

When people are ill, ROM exercises are taught to the client or performed passively on the client until normal activity levels are restored. ROM exercises may be active, passive, or active-assistive.

Active Range of Motion

Active range-of-motion exercises are isotonic exercises in which the client independently moves each joint in the body through its complete range of movement, maximally stretching all muscle groups, attached tendons, ligaments, and soft tissues within each plane over the joint. These exercises maintain or increase muscle strength and endurance and help to maintain cardiorespiratory function in a client who is immobilized. They also prevent deterioration of joint capsules, **ankylosis** (fusion), and contractures. Instructions for the client performing active ROM exercises are shown in Client Teaching Considerations.

Full ROM does not occur spontaneously in the immobilized client, even if the person can independently perform activities of daily living (ADLs). It also does not occur in those who independently move about in bed, independently transfer between bed and wheelchair or chair, or independently ambulate a short distance. This

---

CLIENT TEACHING CONSIDERATIONS

Active ROM Exercises

- Perform each ROM exercise as taught to the point of slight resistance, but not beyond, and never to the point of pain.
  - If necessary, premedicate the client for pain prior to performing exercises.
  - Perform the movements systematically, using the same sequence during each session.
  - Try to control the movement, making it as smooth and gentle as possible.
  - Perform each exercise at least five times.
  - Perform each series of exercises twice daily.
- Performing ADLs is beneficial to maintaining mobility, but ADLs are not sufficient to maintain adequate ROM for all joints. Performing the ROM exercises is essential.

OLDER ADULTS

- For older adults, full range of motion in all joints may not be possible. Prior functional status, not age, should guide the nurse in goal setting. Emphasis should be placed on the achievement of a sufficient range of motion to carry out ADLs, such as bathing, dressing, and grooming, as well as instrumental ADLs such as meal preparation, shopping, managing finances, and travel. These functions are lost quickly, particularly in the hospitalized client, and may result in discharge to an extended care facility instead of home.

- Maintaining or improving functional ability is critical for older adults. Ask them to assist as much as possible with all bathing and transfer activities in order to maintain muscle strength, tone, and functional ability.
- Refer clients to occupational and physical therapists in developing a plan for maintaining or increasing mobility.

CHILDREN

- "Tummy time" is important for babies while they are awake and supervised. Parents are aware of the need for their babies to sleep on their backs to avoid sudden infant death syndrome (SIDS). However, the American Physical Therapy Association (APTA) (2013) informs parents that too much time on their backs can cause babies to have flattening of the skull and tightening of the neck muscles, causing torticollis or a "wry neck. Increasing the amount of time the baby spends on its tummy helps promote muscle development in the neck and shoulders, which the baby needs to roll, sit, and crawl, and prevents the development of flat areas on the back of the baby's head.
- Children can engage in ROM exercises through active play that involves kicking, running, climbing, throwing, dancing, jumping, twisting, and wiggling. A consult with a recreational therapist will facilitate these activities.

is because only a few muscle groups are maximally stretched during these activities. Although clients may successfully achieve some active ROM movements of the upper extremities while combing their hair, bathing, and dressing, they continue to be at risk for muscle weakness, atrophy, and joint contracture. Furthermore, it is highly unlikely that a client who is confined to bed or a client who uses a wheelchair will achieve full ROM of the lower extremities without teaching or assistance. This lack of full ROM will ultimately limit the ability to stand and walk, which will further limit mobility and independence. For this reason, clients who are confined to bed, as well as most clients who use wheelchairs and many ambulatory clients, need active ROM exercises until they regain their normal activity levels. The teaching of these exercises is often a collaborative approach, with the physical therapist teaching the client to perform the exercises and nurses reinforcing the continued mobility. Eventually, the client may be able to accomplish these exercises independently.

Passive Range of Motion

During **passive range-of-motion exercises**, *another* person moves each of the client's joints through their complete range of movement in order to fully stretch all muscle groups, attached tendons, ligaments, and soft tissues within each plane over each joint.

Because the client does not contract the muscles independently, passive ROM exercises are of no value in maintaining muscle strength but are useful in maintaining joint flexibility. For this reason, passive ROM exercises should be performed only when the client is unable to accomplish the movements actively.

Passive ROM exercises should be accomplished for each movement of the arms, legs, and neck that the client is unable to achieve actively. As with active ROM exercises, passive ROM exercises should be accomplished to the point of slight resistance, but not beyond, and never to the point of discomfort. The movements should be systematic, and the same sequence should be followed during each exercise session. Each stretch should be gradually applied for 15 to 20 seconds. Although there is no research that demonstrates the effectiveness of a certain number of repetitions, the practice in nursing has been that each exercise is repeated at least five times and each session lasts approximately 20 minutes, at the client's tolerance. Each exercise is usually done at least twice daily. Performing one series of exercises along with the bath is helpful. Passive ROM exercises are accomplished most effectively when the client lies supine in bed.

General guidelines for providing passive ROM exercises are shown in the Practice Guidelines. Skill 13–1 explains how to perform these exercises.

PRACTICE GUIDELINES

Providing Passive ROM Exercises

- At the request of the client, provide music selected by the client to promote relaxation. ROM exercises are an invaluable opportunity to spend quality time with the client, to convey caring touch, and to listen to the client's thoughts and feelings.
- Ensure that the client understands the reason for doing ROM exercises.
- Clothe the client in loose (stretchy) clothing, and cover the body with a blanket.
- Position the bed at an appropriate height and use correct body mechanics when providing ROM exercise to avoid muscle strain or injury to self and client (see Chapter 10 ∞).
- Expose only the limb being exercised to maintain the client's thermal comfort and protect modesty.
- Support the client's limbs above and below the joint as needed to sense resistance and prevent muscle strain or injury. This may also be accomplished by cupping joints in the palm of your hand or cradling limbs along your forearm. If a joint is painful (e.g., arthritic), support the limb in the muscular areas above and below the joint.
- Use a firm, comfortable grip when handling the limb.
- Move the body parts smoothly, slowly, and rhythmically. Jerky movements cause discomfort and, possibly, injury.
- Avoid moving or forcing a body part beyond the existing range of motion. Muscle strain, pain, and injury can result. This is particularly important for clients with flaccid (limp) paralysis, whose muscles can be stretched and joints dislocated without their awareness, and clients with rigidity.

- If muscle spasticity occurs during movement, stop the movement temporarily and attempt to apply slow, gentle pressure on the part until the muscle relaxes; then proceed with the motion. Never force a movement.
- If a contracture is present, apply slow firm pressure, without causing pain, to stretch the muscle fibers.
- If rigidity is present, apply pressure against the rigidity, and continue the exercise slowly.
- Teach the client's caregiver the purposes and techniques of performing passive ROM at home if appropriate.
- Avoid hyperextension of joints.
- Use the exercises as an opportunity to assess the client's skin condition.
- Use the exercises as an opportunity to engage in therapeutic communication and touch with the client.

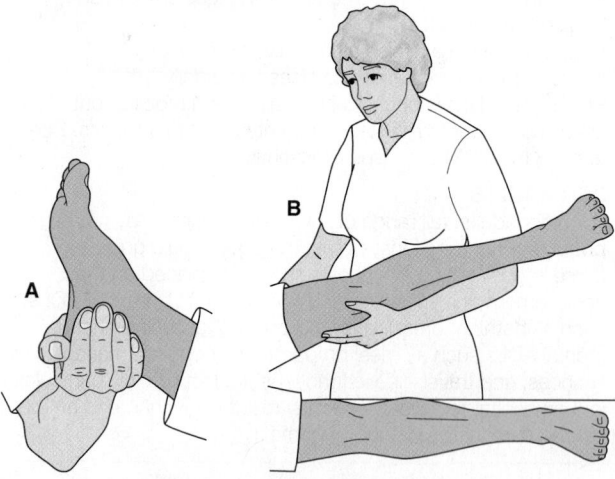

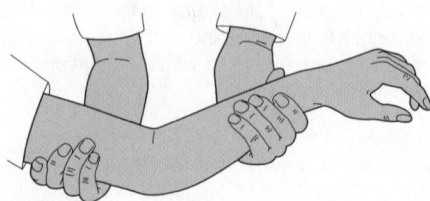

Supporting a limb above and below the joint for passive exercise.

Holding limbs for support during passive exercise: *A,* cupping; *B,* cradling.

Active-Assistive Range of Motion

During **active-assistive range-of-motion exercises**, the client uses the stronger, opposite arm or leg to move each of the joints of a limb incapable of active motion. The client learns to support and move the weak arm or leg with the strong arm or leg as far as possible. Then the nurse continues the movement passively to its maximal degree. This activity increases active movement on the strong side of the client's body and maintains joint flexibility on the weak side. Such exercise is especially useful for clients who have had a stroke and are hemiplegic (paralyzed on one half of the body). Some clients who begin with passive ROM exercises after a disability progress to active-assistive ROM exercises and, finally, to active ROM exercises.

CLINICAL ALERT!

If a joint is traumatized (inflamed, swollen, painful), it is best to avoid ROM exercises without first consulting with the primary care provider. If ROM exercises are indicated, proceed with caution and do not "range" the joint to a point of resistance or pain. In such cases, consultation with a physical therapist (who may recommend modalities such as heat and cold) is indicated.

●○● NURSING PROCESS: RANGE-OF-MOTION EXERCISES

Performing Passive Range-of-Motion Exercises

SKILL 13-1

ASSESSMENT

- Review the client's chart for nursing admission assessment, primary care provider's orders for activity status, medical diagnosis, physical examination, primary care provider's progress notes, and physical and occupational therapy evaluations to determine limitations to joint mobility.
- Determine the client's ability to perform active, passive, or active-assistive ROM exercises (e.g., level of consciousness, cognitive function, and ability to move independently).
- Assess current ROM as baseline data.
- Note the presence of any joint contractures, swelling, redness, or pain that may limit the client's ROM. It is important to address pain in a timely manner (e.g., with premedication) to facilitate full ROM exercise (see Chapter 9 ∞).
- Note any cultural considerations that may apply such as comfort with touch and personal space issues; client comfort with the gender of the nurse, caregiver, or unlicensed assistive personnel; or linguistic barriers. When possible, try to accommodate the client's preference for gender. When this is not possible, a sensitive, matter-of-fact approach that acknowledges the client's feelings may facilitate client comfort. Provide linguistically appropriate verbal and written instructions as needed.

PLANNING
DELEGATION

Performing passive ROM exercises can be delegated to unlicensed assistive personnel (UAP). Some agencies may have specially trained nursing assistants who perform restorative activities, such as ROM, for clients. For UAP who do not have this special training, however, it is important for the nurse to review the general guidelines for performing passive ROM exercises to avoid injury to the UAP or client (see earlier Practice Guidelines). Encourage the UAP to perform ROM during the bath. Emphasize the importance of reporting anything unusual to the nurse. If a client has a recent spinal cord injury or some form of orthopedic trauma, the nurse or a physical therapist should do the ROM exercises.

INTERPROFESSIONAL PRACTICE

Performing ROM exercises may be within the scope of practice for other health care providers. For example, in addition to nurses, physical therapists and occupational therapists may perform ROM exercises. Although these therapists may verbally communicate their findings and plan to the health care team members, the nurse must also know where to locate their documentation in the client's medical record.

Equipment
- No special equipment is needed other than a bed.

IMPLEMENTATION
Preparation
- Prior to initiating the exercises, review any possible restrictions with the primary care provider or physical therapist. Also refer to the agency's protocol.

Performance
1. Prior to performing the skill, introduce self and verify the client's identity using agency protocol. Explain to the client what you are going to do, why it is necessary, and how he or she can participate. Listen to any suggestions made by the client or support people. Discuss the importance of ROM exercises in the plan of care. **Rationale:** *The more a client can assist, the better. Whenever possible, progress should be made toward active ROM exercise.*
2. Perform hand hygiene and observe other appropriate infection prevention procedures.
3. Provide for client privacy, and use client-selected music if requested. **Rationale:** *The ROM session is an opportunity to use touch with the client in a relaxing and therapeutic manner. Any measures that will enhance relaxation are warranted, such as privacy, scent, and sound.*
4. Assist the client to a supine position near you and expose only the body parts requiring exercise. **Rationale:** *This ensures thermal comfort and protects modesty.*
5. Place the client's feet together, place the arms at the sides, and leave space around the head and the feet. **Rationale:** *Positioning the client close to you prevents excessive reaching.*
6. Perform exercises in a head-to-toe format. Follow a repetitive pattern and return to the starting position after each motion. Repeat each motion at least five times on the appropriate limb. **Rationale:** *This ensures thoroughness in the movement and reduces chances of forgetting any part of the body.*
7. Support the limb being ranged above and below the joint. **Rationale:** *This facilitates support and comfort. It also allows the nurse to detect ease/resistance to movement.*

Continued on page 342

SKILL 13–1

Performing Passive Range-of-Motion Exercises—*continued*

8. Assess for pain by eliciting client self-report before, throughout, and after the session. Observe the client for nonverbal/behavioral cues of discomfort or pain, as well as verbal. Accept the client's self-report or behavioral cues and address pain fully in a timely manner (see Chapter 9 ∞). **Rationale:** *Monitoring for pain is an essential nursing responsibility. Using verbal self-report and observing behavior will enable the nurse to respond therapeutically to any clients who experience pain, whether or not they are able to verbalize for themselves.*

9. Assess the client for changes in cardiopulmonary status (e.g., dyspnea, fatigue, change in vital signs). **Rationale:** *Weak or debilitated clients may have decreased tolerance for activity when beginning the ROM exercises.*

If a change occurs, stop and note the length of the recovery time for the client. **Rationale:** *A decrease in recovery time can indicate improved activity tolerance.*

10. Perform ROM slowly, gently, and smoothly. **Rationale:** *This will encourage relaxation and lengthening of muscles so they can be ranged further.*

11. Neck (pivot joint)
  * Remove the client's pillow.
  * Flex and extend the neck (ROM: 45° from midline):
    * Place the palm of one hand under the client's head and the palm of the other hand on the client's chin.
    * Move the head from the upright midline position forward until the chin rests on the chest. ❶
    * Move the head from the flexed position back to the resting supine position without the head pillow. ❶

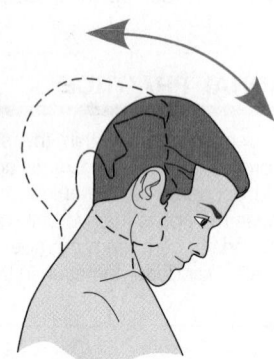

❶ Flexion/extension of the neck.

  * Lateral flexion of the neck (ROM: 40° from midline):
    * Place the heels of the hands on each side of the client's cheeks.
    * Move the head laterally toward the right and left shoulders. ❷

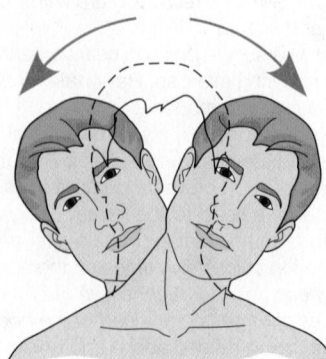

❷ Lateral flexion of the neck.

  * Rotation (ROM: 70° from midline):
    * Place the heels of the hands on each side of the client's cheeks.
    * Turn the face as far as possible to the right and left. ❸

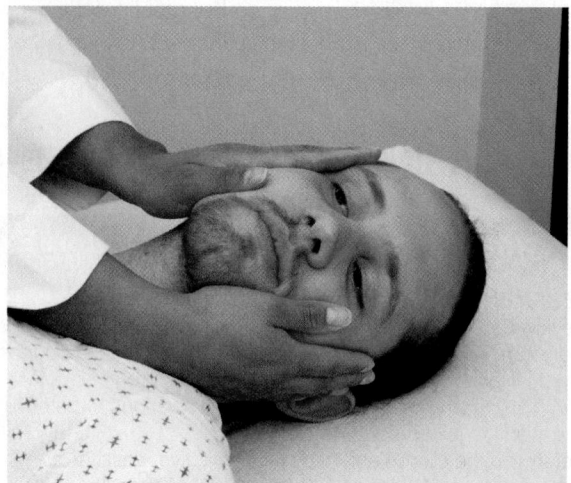

❸ Rotation of the neck.

12. Shoulder (ball-and-socket joint)
  * Flexion (ROM: 180° from the side):
    * Begin with the client's arm at the side. Grasp the arm beneath the elbow with one hand and beneath the wrist with the other hand unless otherwise indicated.
    * Raise the arm from a position by the side forward and upward to a position beside the head. ❹ The elbow may need to be flexed if the headboard is in the way.
  * Extension (ROM: 180° from vertical position beside the head):
    * Move the arm from a vertical position beside the head forward and down to a resting position at the side of the body. ❹

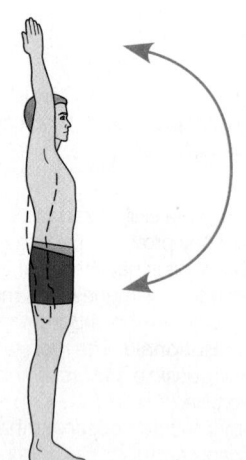

❹ Flexion/extension of the shoulder.

Performing Passive Range-of-Motion Exercises—*continued*

- Abduction (ROM: 180°):
  - Move the arm laterally from the resting position at the side to a side position above the head, palm of the hand either toward or away from the head. ⑤

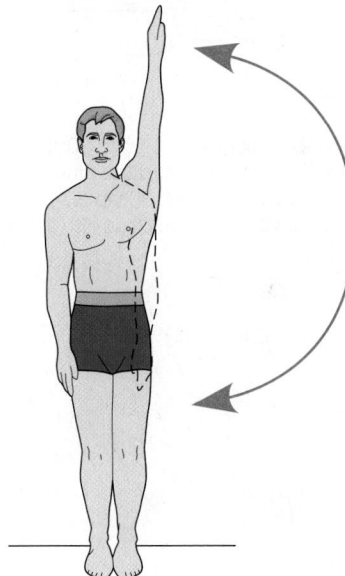

⑤ Abducting the shoulder.

- Adduction (ROM: 230°):
  - Move the arm laterally from the position beside the head downward laterally and *across* the front of the body as far as possible. The elbow may be straight or bent. ⑥

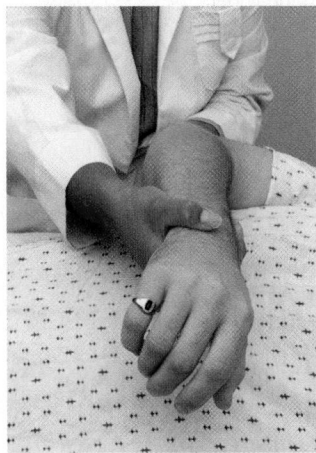

⑥ Adducting the shoulder.

- External rotation (ROM: 90°):
  - With the arm held out to the side at shoulder level and the elbow bent to a right angle, fingers pointing down, move the arm upward so that the fingers point up and the back of the hand touches the mattress. ⑦
- Internal rotation (ROM: 90°):
  - With the arm held out to the side at shoulder level and the elbow bent to a right angle, fingers pointing up, bring the arm forward and down so that the palm touches the mattress. ⑦

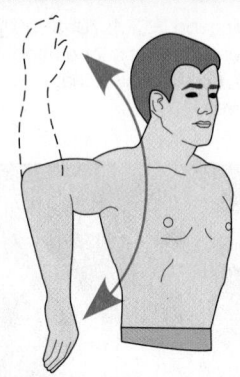

⑦ External/internal rotation of the shoulder.

- Circumduction (ROM: 360°):
  - Move the arm forward, up, back, and down in a full circle. ⑧

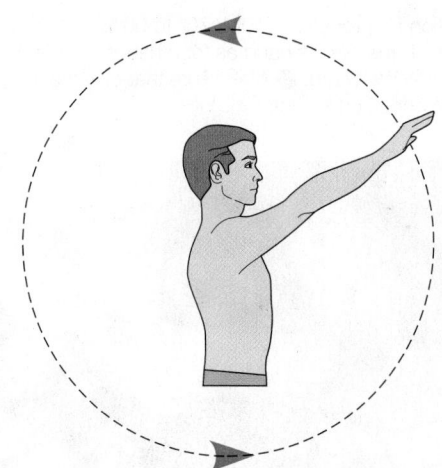

⑧ Circumduction of the shoulder.

13. Elbow (hinge joint)
- Flexion (ROM: 150°):
  - Bring the lower arm forward and upward so that the hand is level with the shoulder. ⑨
- Extension (ROM: 150°):
  - Bring the lower arm forward and downward, straightening the arm. ⑨

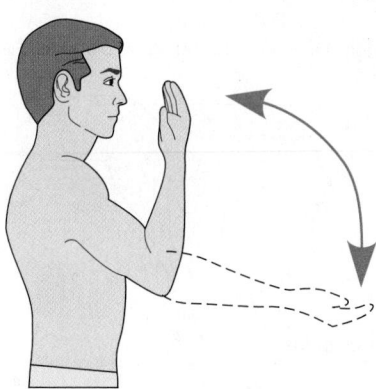

⑨ Flexion/extension of the elbow.

Continued on page 344

Performing Passive Range-of-Motion Exercises—*continued*

- Rotation for supination (ROM: 70° to 90°):
  - Grasp the client's hand as for a handshake and turn the palm upward. ❿ Make sure that only the forearm (not the shoulder) moves.

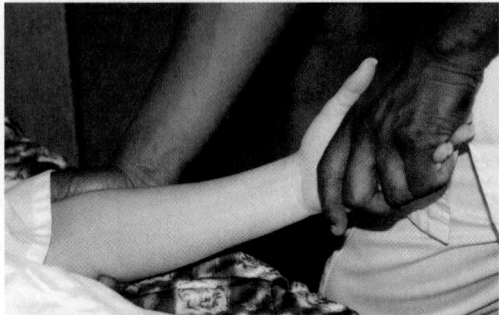

❿ Supinating the forearm.

- Rotation for pronation (ROM: 70° to 90°):
  - Grasp the client's hand as for a handshake and turn the palm downward. ⓫ Make sure that only the forearm (not the shoulder) moves.

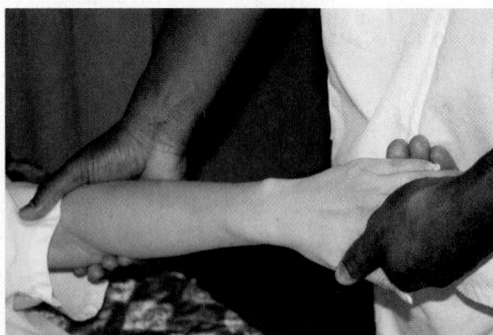

⓫ Pronating the forearm.

14. Wrist (condyloid joint)
- Flexion (ROM: 80° to 90°):
  - Flex the client's arm at the elbow until the forearm is at a right angle to the mattress. Support the wrist joint with one hand while your other hand manipulates the joint.
  - Bring the fingers of the hand toward the inner aspect of the forearm. ⓬
- Extension (ROM: 80° to 90°):
  - Straighten the hand to the same plane as the arm. ⓬

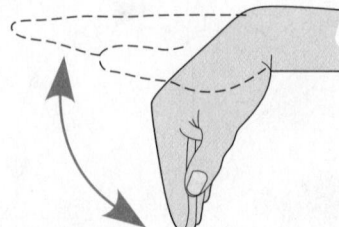

⓬ Flexion/extension of the wrist.

- Hyperextension (ROM 70° to 90°):
  - Bend the fingers of the hand back as far as possible. ⓭

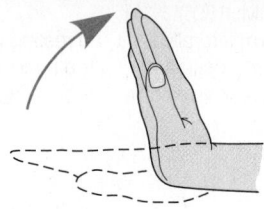

⓭ Hyperextension of the wrist.

- Radial flexion (abduction) (ROM: 0° to 20°):
  - Bend the wrist laterally toward the thumb side. ⓮
- Ulnar flexion (adduction) (ROM: 30° to 50°):
  - Bend the wrist laterally toward the fifth finger. ⓮

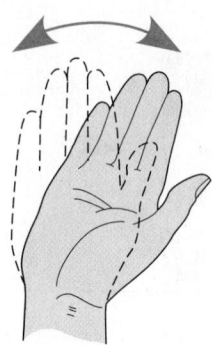

⓮ Radial and ulnar flexion.

15. Hand and fingers (metacarpophalangeal joints—condyloid; interphalangeal joints—hinge)
- Flexion (ROM: 90°):
  - Make a fist. ⓯
- Extension (ROM: 90°):
  - Straighten the fingers. ⓯
- Hyperextension (ROM: 30°):
  - Gently bend fingers back.

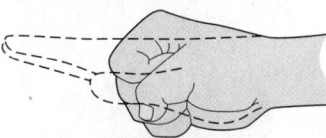

⓯ Flexion/extension of the fingers.

- Abduction (ROM: 20°):
  - Spread the fingers of the hand apart. ⓰
- Adduction (ROM: 20°):
  - Bring fingers together. ⓰

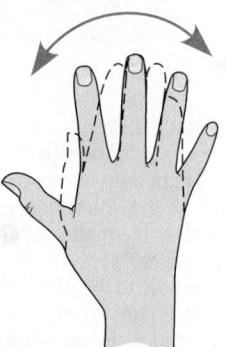

⓰ Abduction/adduction of the fingers.

Performing Passive Range-of-Motion Exercises—*continued*

16. Thumb (saddle joint)
- Flexion (ROM: 90°):
  - Move the thumb across the palmar surface of the hand toward the fifth finger. ⑰
- Extension (ROM: 90°):
  - Move the thumb away from the hand. ⑰

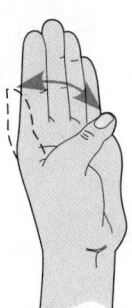

⑰ Flexion/extension of the thumb.

- Abduction (ROM: 30°):
  - Extend the thumb laterally (can be done when placing fingers in abduction and adduction). ⑱
- Adduction (ROM: 30°):
  - Move the thumb back to the hand. ⑱

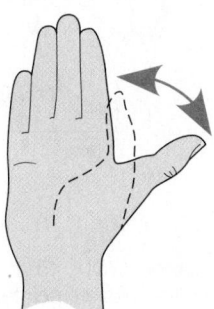

⑱ Abduction/adduction of the thumb.

- Opposition:
  - Touch thumb to the top of each finger of the same hand. The thumb joint movements involved are abduction, rotation, and flexion. ⑲

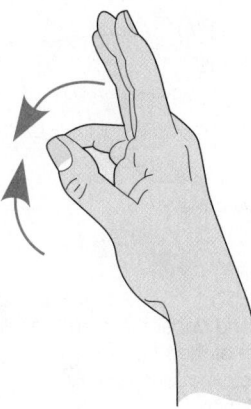

⑲ Opposition.

17. Hip (ball-and-socket joint)
- To carry out hip and leg exercises, place one hand under the client's knee and the other under the ankle. ⑳

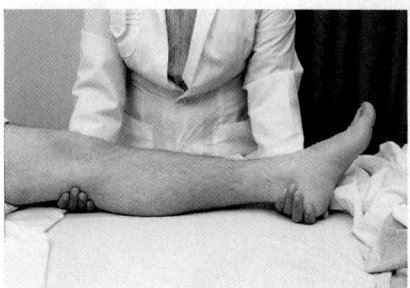

⑳ Position for knee and hip movements.

- Flexion (ROM: knee extended, 90°; knee flexed, 120°):
  - Lift the leg and bend the knee, moving the knee up toward the chest as far as possible. ㉑

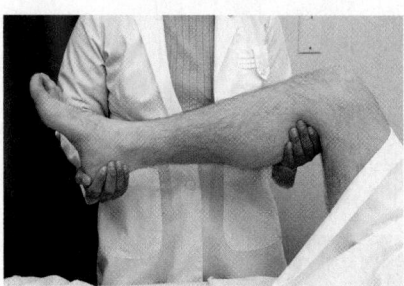

㉑ Flexing the knee and the hip.

- Extension (ROM: 90° to 120°):
  - Bring the leg down, straighten the knee, and lower the leg to the bed.
- Abduction (ROM: 45° to 50°):
  - Move the leg to the side away from the client. ㉒

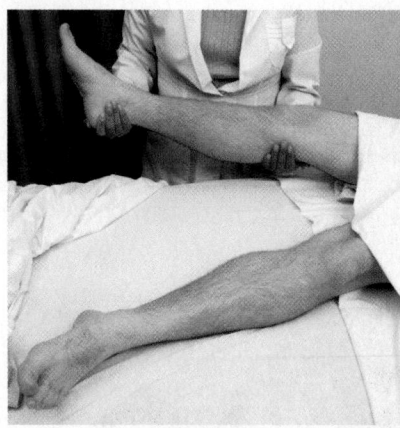

㉒ Abducting the leg.

- Adduction (ROM: 20° to 30° beyond other leg):
  - Move the leg back across and in front of the other leg. ㉓

Continued on page 346

Performing Passive Range-of-Motion Exercises—*continued*

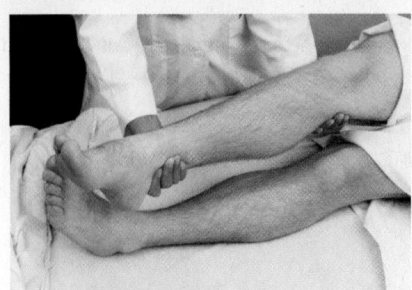

㉓ Adducting the leg.

- Circumduction (ROM: 360°):
  - Move the leg in a circle. ㉔

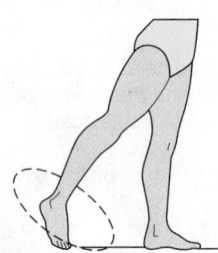

㉔ Circumduction of the hip.

- Internal rotation (ROM: 90°):
  - Roll the foot and leg inward. ㉕

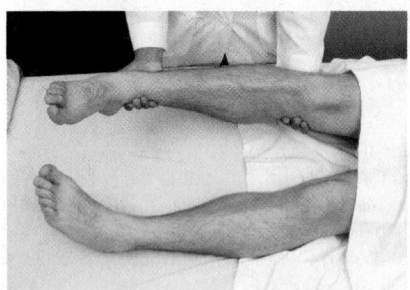

㉕ Internal rotation of the hip.

- External rotation (ROM: 90°):
  - Roll the foot and leg outward. ㉖ *Note:* An alternative method is to flex the knee and hip to 90°. Place the foot away from the midline. Move the thigh and knee toward the midline for internal rotation (ROM: 40°). Place the foot toward the midline and move the thigh and knee away from the midline for external rotation (ROM: 45°). ㉗

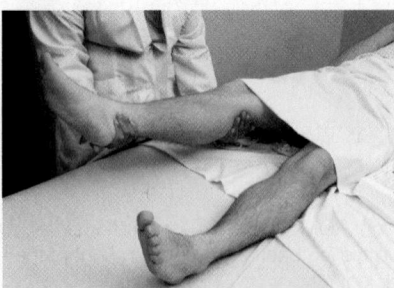

㉖ External rotation of the hip.

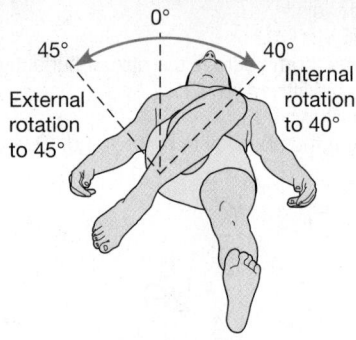

㉗ Internal and external hip rotation.

18. Knee (hinge joint)
    - Flexion (ROM: 120° to 130°):
      - Bend the leg, bringing the heel toward the back of the thigh (done with hip flexion). ㉘
    - Extension (ROM: 120° to 130°):
      - Straighten the leg, returning the foot to the bed. ㉘

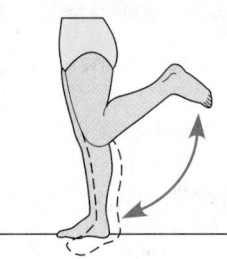

㉘ Flexion/extension of the knee.

19. Ankle (hinge joint)
    - Extension (plantar flexion) (ROM: 45° to 50°):
      - Move the foot so the toes are pointed downward. ㉙
    - Flexion (dorsiflexion) (ROM: 20°):
      - Move the foot so the toes are pointed upward. ㉙

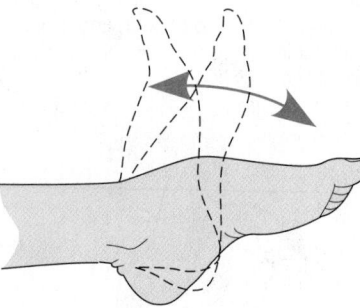

㉙ Extension/flexion of the ankle.

20. Foot (gliding)
    - Eversion (ROM: 5°):
      - Place one hand under the client's ankle and the other over the arch of the foot.
      - Turn the whole foot outward. ㉚
    - Inversion (ROM: 5°):
      - Use the same hand placement as above, and turn the whole foot inward. ㉛

Performing Passive Range-of-Motion Exercises—*continued*

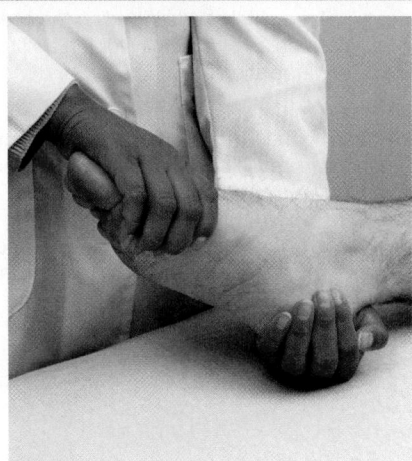

㉚ Everting the foot.

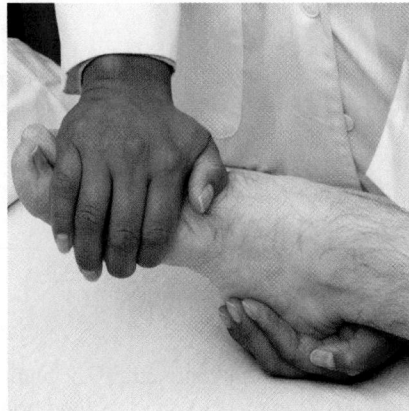

㉛ Inverting the foot.

21. Toes (interphalangeal joints—hinge; metatarsophalangeal joints—hinge; intertarsal joints—gliding)
    • Flexion (ROM: 35° to 60°):
      • Place one hand over the arch of the foot.
      • Place the fingers of the other hand over the toes to curl the toes downward. ㉜

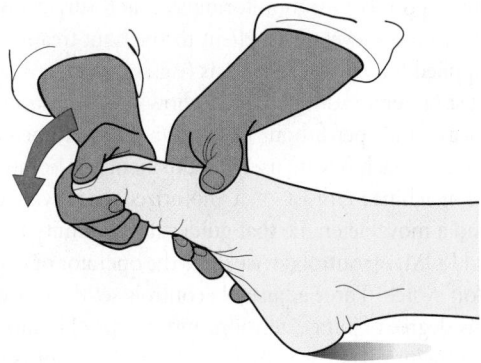

㉜ Flexing the toes.

• Extension (ROM: 35° to 60°):
  • Place one hand over the arch of the foot.
  • Place the fingers of the other hand under the toes to bend the toes upward. ㉝
• Abduction (ROM: 0° to 15°):
  • Spread the toes apart.
• Adduction (ROM: 0° to 15°):
  • Bring the toes together.

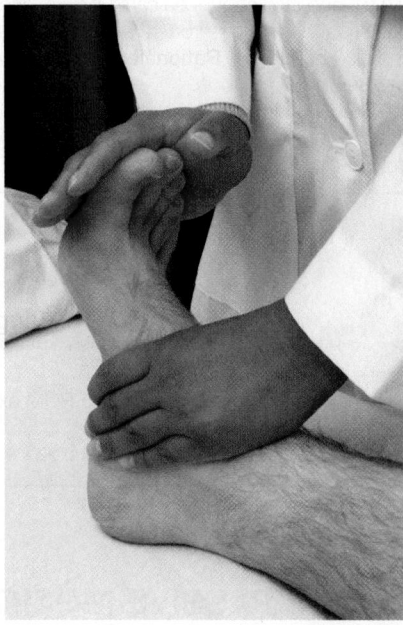

㉝ Extending the toes.

22. Move to the other side of the bed and repeat exercises for the other arm and leg.
23. Document
    • Type of ROM exercise (e.g., active, passive, active-assistive).
    • Joints exercised and their degree of joint motion.
    • Length of exercise.
    • Client's tolerance level to the activity.
    • Any abnormalities.

SAMPLE DOCUMENTATION

8/16/2015 1000 Passive ROM performed with bath. All joints ranged fully with 5 reps each. Resistance in shoulders resolved when pace slowed. Tolerated well, no c/o pain ———————— M. Foti, RN

EVALUATION
• Relate current ROM of joints to baseline ROM: Is there a pattern of improvement? Determine the client's pulse and endurance for the exercise. Is the client progressing from passive ROM to active ROM? If so, ask the client to demonstrate active ROM exercises.
• Observe UAP performing passive ROM exercises. Provide appropriate feedback.

• Report unexpected or notable changes, for example, joint laxity, resistance to ROM, pain, redness, swelling of joint, rigidity, spasticity, or contractures, to the primary care provider. Consult with an occupational or a physical therapist for guidance with ROM as needed.

CHILDREN
- Perform exercises gently and with full ROM, avoiding hyperextension of joints. **Rationale:** *Some children may have lax ligaments, and overstretching can cause injury and pain.*
- A small roll can be made of soft cloth to place in the palms. **Rationale:** *The roll is used to prevent contractures of the fingers. Ensure that the thumb is adducted with finger opposition.* Consult an occupational therapist for a well-fitting splint if needed.
- Special boots (ankle-foot orthotics, often ordered by a physical therapist) or high-top sneakers can be used. These should be properly fitted, and skin should be carefully examined for pressure areas. Usually, there is an on/off schedule to follow. Footboards can also be placed. **Rationale:** *This helps prevent foot drop(plantar flexion of the foot).*
- In some children with impaired mobility, splinting of the wrist, knees, or ankles may be necessary. **Rationale:** *Splinting helps prevent severe contractures(Hockenberry & Wilson, 2012).*

- Children have developmental needs including the need to play. Performing ROM can be an opportunity for fun and for enhancing the child–caregiver relationship.

OLDER ADULTS
- Avoid hyperextending the joints of older adults. **Rationale:** *Such movements can cause pain or nerve damage because joints become less flexible with age.*
- Work slowly and assess for pain when working with older adults, especially those who have arthritis. **Rationale:** *Arthritis changes can cause contractures and enlarged, painful joints.*
- Assess for skin breakdown or reddened areas during the ROM procedure. **Rationale:** *Older adults are at risk for skin breakdown due to decreased subcutaneous fat and increased thinning of the skin.*

Teach the client's caregiver:
- The purpose and importance of performing ROM exercises at home.
- To move gently and slowly through each exercise.

- To perform the exercises at least twice daily and to do five repetitions of each exercise.
- How to use correct body mechanics to prevent muscle strain while performing the exercises.

CONTINUOUS PASSIVE MOTION DEVICES

Continuous passive motion (CPM) is a postoperative treatment method that has been in use for more than 25 years and has been thought to promote recovery after joint surgery. CPM devices are available for the shoulder, elbow, wrist, hand, knee, ankle, jaw, and toe. The CPM machine has been used most frequently on clients who have undergone total knee replacement. In recent years, early mobilization and ambulation have become more widely accepted in this client population. Therefore, not all surgeons may choose to use CPM. In fact, the usefulness of CPM following total knee replacement has recently been questioned because of the results of randomized controlled clinical trials. The CPM machine has not been shown to improve outcomes when compared to today's early mobilization and ambulation protocols (Alkire & Swank, 2010; Viswanathan & Kidd, 2010). CPM continues to be used for joint surgeries and is also being evaluated in other populations such as clients who have had a cerebrovascular accident (stroke) and clients who are immobilized and critically ill. Therefore, it remains an important skill for nurses.

After extensive joint surgery, muscle contraction and joint motion usually cause pain in most clients and, as a result, they fail to move the joint. With CPM, however, the pain of movement can be reduced because a machine is providing the joint motion passively, and

the client's muscle is not actively contracting. The pumping action of continuous movement can serve to prevent blood from accumulating in the joint after surgery. As a result, the client can experience decreased edema and pain.

Because the motion is provided mechanically and passively, there is no fatigue factor. The machine flexes and extends the limb repetitively, and can be applied continuously (usually 12 to 14 hours a day). Sometimes it is applied in intervals, for example, for 2 hours three times a day, depending on the primary care provider's orders. Nurses are responsible for monitoring skin and surgical wound integrity and comfort level of the client throughout treatment. When CPM is applied for extended sessions (e.g., more than 3 hours), the device must be removed regularly to allow skin and wound assessment (at least twice per 8-hour shift). In addition to being used in hospitals, CPM machines are used in outpatient and home settings.

CPM machines consist of a motorized base with a nonslip surface and a movable cradle that guides the extremity through the prescribed ROM. A control device gives the operator or client access to an on/off switch. Three adjustable controls set the degree of joint flexion, the degree of joint extension, and the speed of movement as ordered by the primary care provider. Physical therapists should be consulted to ensure proper initial setup.

Skill 13–2 explains the steps involved in applying a CPM device for the knee.

●○○● NURSING PROCESS: CONTINUOUS PASSIVE MOTION DEVICES

Using a Continuous Passive Motion Device

ASSESSMENT
- Review the client's chart for orders and notes from the primary care provider and notes from physical therapists.
- Assess the client's complaints of discomfort or pain, and address these in a timely manner, premedicating when needed.
- Assess the appearance of the client's joint (e.g., size and color, character, and amount of drainage).
- Determine the client's baseline ROM.
- Assess the client's ability and willingness to learn about and use the CPM device.
- Check the safety test date (this is the date that the machine was tested for electrical safety) and ensure that it is within the guidelines established at the agency.

PLANNING
DELEGATION

The initial application and setting up of the CPM device should not be delegated to UAP because application of scientific and nursing knowledge and potential problem solving are needed. The UAP, however, can assist the client with ADLs (e.g., bathing) while the CPM device is being used. The UAP can also assist the nurse in placing the client's limb in the CPM device. The nurse needs to discuss with the UAP what observations to report to the nurse (e.g., client complaint of increased pain, swelling, and/or skin breakdown).

INTERPROFESSIONAL PRACTICE

Applying a CPM device may be within the scope of practice for other health care providers. For example, in addition to nurses, physical therapists may perform the initial application and setting up of the CPM device as well as assess how the client is tolerating the device. Although these providers may verbally communicate their findings and plan to the health care team members, the nurse must also know where to locate their documentation in the client's medical record.

Equipment
- CPM device
- Padding for the cradle
- Restraining straps
- **Goniometer** (a handheld device used to measure the angle of a joint in degrees)

IMPLEMENTATION
Preparation
- Verify the primary care provider's orders and agency protocol.
- Determine the degrees of flexion, extension, and speed initially prescribed.
- Check agency protocol and the primary care provider's orders about increases in degrees and speed for subsequent treatments.
- Have another person ready to assist in placing the client's limb in the CPM device.

Performance
1. Prior to performing the skill, introduce self and verify the client's identity using agency protocol. Explain to the client what you are going to do, why it is necessary, and how he or she can participate. Listen to any suggestions made by the client or support people. Discuss the importance of CPM in the plan of care.
2. Perform hand hygiene and observe other appropriate infection prevention procedures.
3. Provide for client privacy.
4. Make sure the client has been assisted in toileting prior to beginning.
5. Address client reports of pain prior to beginning, and premedicate if necessary.
6. Set up the machine.
   - Place the machine on the bed. Remove an egg-crate mattress, if indicated. **Rationale:** *Doing so provides a stable surface.*
   - Connect the control box to the CPM machine.
7. Set the prescribed levels of flexion, extension, and speed.
   - Most postoperative clients are started on 10° to 45° of flexion and 0° to 10° of extension.
     - Adjust the speed control to the slow to moderate range for the first postoperative day, and then increase the speed as ordered and tolerated.

- Place padding on the CPM cradle. **Rationale:** *This prevents rubbing and pressure.*
- Run the machine through a complete cycle. **Rationale:** *This ensures that the machine is functioning properly.*
- Stop the machine in full extension.
8. Position the client and place the leg in the machine.
   - Place the client in a supine position with the head of the bed elevated 15° to 25°.
   - Support the leg and, with the client's help (or another staff member if the client is unable to assist), lift the leg and place it in the padded cradle.
   - Adjust the device to the client's extremity. Lengthen or shorten appropriate sections of the frame to fit the machine to the client.
   - Center the client's leg on the frame. **Rationale:** *This avoids the development of pressure areas.*
   - Align the client's knee joint with the hinged joint of the machine.
   - Adjust the foot support so that the foot is supported in either a neutral position or slight dorsiflexion (e.g., 20°). **Rationale:** *This prevents foot drop.* Check agency protocol.
   - Ensure that the leg is neither internally nor externally rotated. **Rationale:** *Neutral alignment prevents injury.*
   - Secure straps around the thigh and top of the foot and cradle to allow enough space to fit several fingers under the strap.
9. Start the machine.
   - When the machine reaches the fully flexed position, stop the machine, and verify the degree of flexion with a goniometer. **Rationale:** *This is a double check of the setting and helps prevent possible complications.*
   - Restart the machine, and observe a few cycles of flexion and extension to ensure proper functioning.

Continued on page 350

Using a Continuous Passive Motion Device—*continued*

10. Ensure continued client safety and comfort.
  - Make sure that the client is comfortable. Observe for non-verbal signs of discomfort.
    - Place within the client's reach the call light, the bedside table, and any items frequently used by the client.
    - Turn off the electric bed controls. **Rationale:** *This prevents the client from inadvertently changing the alignment of the extremity.*
    - Instruct a mentally alert client how to operate the on/off switch.
  - Loosen the straps and check the client's skin at least twice every 4 hours.

11. Document the degree of flexion, the degree of extension, the speed, the duration of the therapy, the client's activity tolerance, circulation, sensation (feeling), and skin condition.

SAMPLE DOCUMENTATION

8/17/2015 1230 CPM removed. Skin intact, incision without redness or drainage. Reports pain at 3/10. Given Percocet 2.5 mg per order.————————————K. Armor, RN

1300 Rates pain at 0/10. Resting comfortably. ———— K. Armor, RN
1400 CPM resumed @ 30° flexion, 10° extension. Denies pain.————————————K. Armor, RN

EVALUATION

- Conduct appropriate follow-up: increase in tolerance and current ROM; degree of discomfort; and skin integrity of feet, elbows, sacrum, and groin.
- Relate baseline ROM data to the client's response to therapy.
- Report any resistance to joint motion, increased pain with CPM, or joint abnormality to the primary care provider.

LIFESPAN CONSIDERATIONS **CPM Device**

CHILDREN
- Explain the use of the CPM device in terms that the child will understand and will not increase the child's anxiety. Use of dolls or stuffed animals may help.
- Arrange for social or creative activities that are developmentally appropriate for the child during the CPM treatment.

OLDER ADULTS
- Older clients may have limited joint flexibility.
- Older clients may need to balance periods of activity with periods of rest.
- If the older client is apprehensive, teach techniques for muscle relaxation and pain control such as guided imagery and progressive relaxation (see Chapter 9 ∞).
- Provide distractions (such as music or TV) and opportunities for socialization.

Ambulatory and Community Settings **CPM Device**   **PATIENT-CENTERED CARE**

The CPM machine can be used at home if the client or caregiver demonstrates competence. Teach the client or caregiver:
- How to set the controls and progressively increase the adjustment as the client's tolerance builds.
- To get assistance from another person and use proper body dynamics to prevent injury to self and client.

- To report excessive pain, swelling, or redness of the affected joints.
- To provide skin care and check for skin breakdown every 4 hours.
- How to clean and care for the equipment.

Chapter **13** Review

FOCUSING ON CLINICAL THINKING

Consider This

1. The nursing assistant reports to you that an older adult client is complaining of pain during the passive ROM exercises. What will you do?

2. After the nursing report, the UAP tells you that she has never taken care of a client who is on a CPM device. She is clearly nervous about the machine and says she is "afraid of hurting the client." What actions will you take?

See Focusing on Clinical Thinking answers on student resource website.

TEST YOUR KNOWLEDGE

1. Which statement pertaining to joint movements indicates the need for further teaching?
   1. "Abduction is movement of the bone toward the midline of the body."
   2. "Rotation is movement of the bone around its central axis."
   3. "Inversion is turning the sole of the foot inward by moving the ankle joint."
   4. "Supination is moving the bones of the forearm so that the palm of the hand faces upward when held in front of the body."

2. A nurse is teaching a client about active range-of-motion (ROM) exercises. The nurse then watches the client demonstrate these principles. The nurse would evaluate that teaching was successful with which client action?
   1. Exercises past the point of resistance.
   2. Performs each exercise one time.
   3. Performs each series of exercises once a day.
   4. Performs the movements systematically, using the same sequence during each session.

3. The nurse indicates an understanding of passive range of motion when which statement is made?
   1. "Passive ROM exercises are isotonic exercises in which the client moves independently."
   2. "Passive ROM exercises are helpful in maintaining muscle strength."
   3. "Passive ROM exercises are useful in maintaining joint flexibility."
   4. "Passive ROM exercises are best accomplished when performed quickly."

4. The student nurse is performing passive range of motion while the instructor observes. Which movement made by the student nurse indicates an understanding of normal ROM for the body joints?
   1. Flex the elbow 180°.
   2. Flex the wrist 80° to 90°.
   3. Abduct the hip 90°.
   4. Extend the knee 45° to 90°.

5. The nurse would do which of the following when caring for a client receiving continuous passive range of motion (CPM) following surgery? Select all that apply.
   1. Remove the CPM apparatus once per 8-hour shift to assess skin integrity.
   2. Apply the CPM for 2 hours at a time, or up to 14 hours, depending on the primary care provider's order.
   3. Carefully document the degree of flexion and extension as well as the speed of the CPM.
   4. Never change the settings on the CPM once they are initially set by the primary care provider.
   5. Give the client a remote control device so the machine can be stopped as needed.

6. The nurse on a rehabilitation unit could safely delegate passive ROM exercises to the unlicensed assistive personnel (UAP) to perform on which client?
   1. The client who has sustained a spinal cord injury due to a motor vehicle crash yesterday
   2. The client who had a cerebrovascular accident 10 days ago
   3. The client whose intracranial pressure increases during procedures
   4. The client who has recently sustained an orthopedic trauma

7. The nurse anticipates the use of a continuous passive motion (CPM) mechanical device on which client?
   1. The client who recently fractured cervical vertebrae 6 (C_6) and has quadriplegia
   2. The client diagnosed to be in a chronic vegetative state
   3. The client who has had total joint replacement surgery
   4. The athlete attempting to improve muscle strength

8. The nurse should notify the primary care provider immediately for which observation while the client performs active range of motion?
   1. The client tolerates the procedure well in the morning but then complains of fatigue in the evening.
   2. The client's wrist is noted to be suddenly edematous and painful.
   3. The client's right elbow remains resistant to movement.
   4. The client declines range of motion while family members are visiting.

9. The nurse is preparing to perform passive range-of-motion exercises. Which sequence is best?
   1. Elbow, neck, ankle, foot
   2. Hip, knee, ankle, neck
   3. Neck, elbow, hip, knee, ankle
   4. Ankle, hip, elbow, knee

10. The nurse moves the client's right arm laterally from the position beside the head downward laterally and across the front of the body as far as possible. What movement has the nurse done to the arm?
    1. Adduction
    2. External rotation
    3. Internal rotation
    4. Circumduction

See Answers to Test Your Knowledge in Appendix A.

READINGS AND REFERENCES

References

Alkire, M. R., & Swank, M. L. (2010). Use of inpatient continuous passive motion versus no CPM in computer-assisted total knee arthroplasty. *Orthopaedic Nursing, 29*, 36–40. doi:10.1097/NOR.0b013e3181c8ce23

American Physical Therapy Association. (2013). *New moms: Tummy time tools.* Retrieved from http://www.moveforwardpt.com/resources/detail.aspx?cid=d62e1e58-3b3c-484a-abfc-c9f5f7060968

Dammeyer, J., Dickinson, S., Packard, D., Baldwin, N., & Ricklemann, C. (2013). Building a protocol to guide mobility in the ICU. *Critical Care Nursing Quarterly, 36*, 37–49. doi:10.1097/CNQ.0b013e3182750acd

Hockenberry, M., & Wilson, D. (2012). *Wong's nursing care of infants and children* (9th ed.). St. Louis, MO: Mosby/Elsevier.

Lipshutz, A. K. M., & Gropper, M. A. (2013). Acquired neuromuscular weakness and early mobilization in the intensive care unit. *Anesthesiology, 118*(1), 202–215. doi:10.1097/ALN.0b013e31826be693

Viswanathan, P., & Kidd, M. (2010). Effect of continuous passive motion following total knee arthroplasty on knee range of motion and function: A systematic review. *New Zealand Journal of Physiotherapy, 38*, 14–22.

Selected Bibliography

Berman, A., Snyder, S., & Frandsen, G. (2016). *Kozier & Erb's fundamentals of nursing: Concepts, process, and practice* (10th ed.). Upper Saddle River, NJ: Pearson.

Clark, D. E., Lowman, J. D., Griffin, R. L., Matthews, H. M., & Reiff, D. A. (2013). Effectiveness of an early mobilization

protocol in a trauma and burns intensive care unit: A retrospective cohort study. *Physical Therapy, 93*, 186–196. doi:10.2522/ptj.20110417

Lee, D., & Higgins, P. A. (2010). Adjunctive therapies for the chronically critically ill. *AACN Advanced Critical Care, 21*, 92–106. doi:10.1097/NCI.0b013e3181c9dec5

Letzkus, L., Hengartner, M., Yeago, D., & Crist, P. (2013). The immobile pediatric population: Can progressive mobility hasten recovery. *Journal of Pediatric Nursing, 28*, 296–299. doi:10.1016/j.pedn.2013.02.029

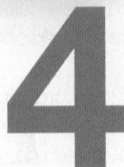

UNIT

4

Applying the Nursing Process

This unit explores skills related to client mobility and safety including positioning, mobilizing, fall prevention and use of restraints, and maintaining joint mobility. The client's mobility level is closely associated with autonomy. By helping the client to maintain, regain, or improve mobility, the nurse helps the client maximize his or her independence. While optimum mobility is the goal, it is important that safety be maintained to prevent injury to the client and the nurse.

CLIENT: Bertha   AGE: 91 Years   CURRENT MEDICAL DIAGNOSIS: Cerebral Vascular Accident (stroke)

Medical History: Bertha was eating dinner at home when she suddenly lost all motor and sensory function on the left side of her body. An ambulance was called and she was transported to the acute care facility. An MRI revealed a cerebral vascular accident (commonly referred to as a stroke). Following acute care, she is being transferred to the rehabilitation facility to help her maximize mobility. Bertha has a history of hypertension and type 2 diabetes mellitus.

Personal and Social History: Bertha is a widow and lives with her 70-year-old son who never married. She lives in a farmhouse that

has been in her family for three generations. She has sold most of the land around her home because neither she nor her son is able to farm the land. The house has running water and an indoor bathroom, but they rely on a coal stove and wood-burning fireplaces for heat. One of her daughters and another son live in their own homes on the property, and she has another daughter who lives in the nearest big city about 60 miles away but visits several times a year. Her children have tried to convince her to sell her home and move, but she wants to live in her house until she dies, and refuses to move.

Questions

Assessment

1. What additional data would the nurse need in creating the care plan?

Analysis

2. List two possible nursing diagnoses that can be identified from the medical/personal history and assessment data above.

Planning

3. Develop two expected outcomes for Bertha related to regaining mobility.

Implementation

4. When assisting this client to transfer from bed to the chair, where will the nurse position the chair to provide the most support to the client's weak side?

5. The nurse assesses that Bertha is highly motivated to regain full mobility when she tells the nurse, "I want to exercise more

than just when I go to physical therapy. I'm in a hurry to get back home." What recommendations might the nurse make that will help Bertha achieve her goals of restoring mobility through exercise?

6. When performing passive range of motion on Bertha's left side, how will the nurse know that maximum joint movement has been reached?

7. Bertha becomes confused and disoriented at night. What interventions might the nurse include in her plan of care to avoid the use of restraints?

Evaluation

8. How will the nurse know if the expected outcomes have been achieved?

See Applying the Nursing Process suggested answers on student resource website.

Medication Administration

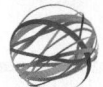

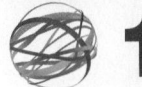 **14** Drug Calculations

LEARNING OUTCOMES

At the completion of this chapter, the student will be able to:

1. Define key terms used in the calculation of drug dosages.
2. State the basic units of measurement in the following systems:
   a. Metric
   b. Apothecaries'
   c. Household
3. Convert weights within the metric system.
4. Convert weights and measures between systems.
5. Convert units of volume.
6. Convert units of weight.
7. Calculate drug dosages using the following formulas:
   a. Basic
   b. Ratio and proportion
   c. Fractional equation
   d. Dimensional analysis
8. Calculate individualized drug dosages using the following methods:
   a. Body weight
   b. Body surface area
9. Calculate IV flow rates by:
   a. Calculating milliliters per hour.
   b. Calculating drops per minute.
   c. Calculating flow rates based on time or on body weight and time.

KEY TERMS

apothecaries' system, *354*
basic formula, *356*
dimensional analysis method, *358*
drop factor, *360*
fractional equation method, *358*
household measures, *355*
macrodrip infusion set, *360*
metric system, *354*
microdrip infusion set, *360*
ratio and proportion method, *357*

Calculating drug dosages safely and accurately is an important nursing responsibility in medication administration. Careful and accurate calculations are essential in the prevention of medication errors. This chapter includes a basic overview of the systems of measurement, conversion of units of weight and measures, four possible methods of drug calculation, and how to calculate intravenous flow rates.

SYSTEMS OF MEASUREMENT

Three systems of measurement are used in North America: the metric system, the apothecaries' system, and the household system, which is similar to the apothecaries' system.

Metric System

The metric system, devised by the French in the latter part of the 18th century, is the system prescribed by law in most European countries and in Canada. The **metric system** is logically organized into units of 10; it is a decimal system. Basic units can be multiplied or divided by 10 to form secondary units. Multiples are calculated by moving the decimal point to the right, and division is accomplished by moving the decimal point to the left.

Basic units of measurement are the *meter*, the *liter*, and the *gram*. Prefixes derived from Latin designate subdivisions of the basic unit: *deci* (1/10 or 0.1), *centi* (1/100 or 0.01), and *milli* (1/1,000 or 0.001). Multiples of the basic unit are designated by prefixes derived from Greek: *deka* (10), *hecto* (100), and *kilo* (1,000). Only the measurements of volume (the liter) and of weight (the gram) are discussed in this chapter. These are the measures used in medication administration (Figure 14–1 ■). The *kilogram* (kg) is the only multiple of the gram used, and the *milligram* (mg) and *microgram* (mcg) are subdivisions. Fractional parts of the liter are usually expressed in *milliliters* (mL), for example, 600 mL; multiples of the liter are usually expressed as *liters* or milliliters, for example, 2.5 liters or 2,500 mL. In nursing practice it is important to understand the difference between weight and volume. A drug dosage may be ordered by weight (i.e., grams, mg, mcg) and administered by volume (mL). For example, a primary care provider prescribes 20 mg (weight) of codeine in an elixir (liquid) form. The codeine elixir bottle is labeled 10 mg per 5 mL. The nurse administers 10 mL (volume) of codeine elixir.

Apothecaries' System

The **apothecaries' system** is older than the metric system and was brought to the United States from England during the colonial period. Many now consider the apothecaries' system out of date and have replaced it with the metric system.

The basic unit of weight in the apothecaries' system is the *grain* (gr), likened to a grain of wheat, and the basic unit of volume is the *minim*, a volume of water equal in weight to a grain of wheat. The word *minim* means "the least." In ascending order, the other units of *weight* are the *scruple*, the *dram*, the *ounce*, and the *pound*. Today, the scruple is seldom used. The units of *volume* are, in ascending order, the fluid dram, the fluid ounce, the pint, the quart, and the gallon.

Volume   **Weight**

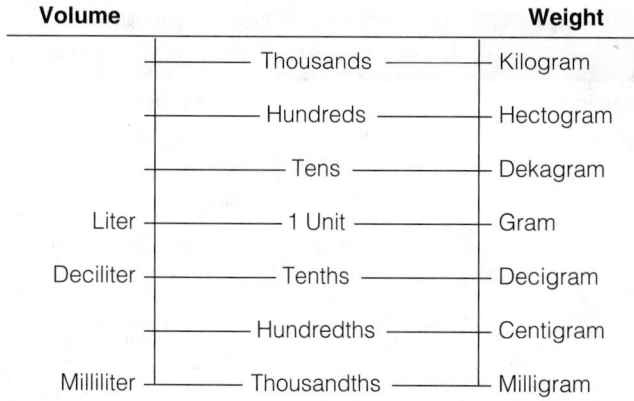

Figure 14–1 ■ Basic metric measurements of volume and weight.

Quantities in the apothecaries' system are often expressed by lowercase Roman numerals, particularly when the unit of measure is abbreviated. Unlike other measurement systems, the Roman numeral follows the unit of measure. For example, two grains are written as gr ii. Quantities less than 1 are expressed as a fraction, for example, gr 1/6. As stated earlier, apothecaries' units are unfamiliar to many practitioners and they may be confused with metric units. Therefore, nurses are advised *not* to use apothecaries' units. Use metric units instead to avoid medication errors.

Household System

Household measures may be used when more accurate systems of measure are not required. Included in **household measures** are drops, teaspoons, tablespoons, cups, and glasses. Although pints and quarts are often found in the home, they are defined as apothecaries' measures.

CONVERTING UNITS OF WEIGHT AND MEASURE

Sometimes drugs are dispensed from the pharmacy in grams when the order specifies milligrams, or they are dispensed in milligrams though ordered in grains. For example, a primary care provider orders morphine gr 1/4. The medication is available labeled only in milligrams. The nurse knows that 1 mg = 1/60 gr or 60 mg = 1 grain. To convert the ordered dose to milligrams, the nurse calculates as follows:

$$\text{If } 60 \text{ mg} = 1 \text{ gr}$$
$$\text{Then } x \text{ mg} = 1/4 \text{ gr } (0.25 \text{ gr})$$
$$x = \frac{(60 \times 0.25)}{1}$$
$$x = 15 \text{ mg}$$

Converting Weights Within the Metric System

It is relatively simple to arrive at equivalent units of weight within the metric system because the system is based on units of 10. Only three metric units of weight are used for drug dosages, the gram (g), milligram (mg), and microgram (mcg): 1,000 mg or 1,000,000 mcg equal 1 gram (g). Equivalents are computed by dividing or multiplying; for example, to change milligrams to grams, the nurse divides the

number of milligrams by 1,000. The simplest way to divide by 1,000 is to move the decimal point three places to the left:

$$500 \text{ mg} = ? \text{ g}$$

Move the decimal point three places to the *left*:

$$\text{Answer} = 0.5 \text{ g}$$

Conversely, to convert grams to milligrams, multiply the number of grams by 1,000, or move the decimal point three places to the right:

$$0.006 \text{ g} = ? \text{ mg}$$

Move the decimal point three places to the *right*:

$$\text{Answer} = 6 \text{ mg}$$

PRACTICE A
Perform the calculations below and check your answers in Appendix A.

1. 0.125 mg = _____ mcg
2. 0.008 g = _____ mg
3. 200 mcg = _____ mg
4. 50 mg = _____ g
5. 0.3 mg = _____ mcg

Converting Weights and Measures Between Systems

When preparing client medications, a nurse may need to convert weights or volumes from one system to another. As an example, the pharmacy may dispense milligrams or grams of chloral hydrate, yet the nurse must administer an order that reads "chloral hydrate gr v." To prepare the correct dose, the nurse must convert from the apothecaries' to the metric system. To give clients a useful, realistic measure for home use, the nurse may have to convert from the apothecaries' or metric system to the household system. All conversions are approximate, that is, not totally precise.

Converting Units of Volume

Commonly used approximate equivalents are shown in Table 14–1. By learning these equivalents, the nurse can make many conversions readily. For example, 15 minims = approximately 15 drops (gtt); therefore, 1 minim is approximately 1 drop. Similarly, 1 quart approximates 1,000 mL, and 1 gallon approximates 4,000 mL.

TABLE 14–1	Approximate Volume Equivalents: Metric, Apothecaries', and Household Systems		

Metric	Apothecaries'		Household	
1 mL	=	15 minims (min or m)	=	15 drops (gtt)
4–5 mL	=	1 fluid dram	=	1 teaspoon (tsp)
15 mL	=	4 fluid drams	=	1 tablespoon (Tbsp)
30 mL	=	1 fluid ounce	=	Same
500 mL	=	1 pint (pt)	=	Same
1,000 mL	=	1 quart (qt)	=	Same
4,000 mL	=	1 gallon (gal)	=	Same

The following are some situations in which nurses need to apply knowledge of volume conversion:

- Fluid ounces are sometimes used in prescribing liquid medications, such as cough syrups, laxatives, antacids, and antibiotics for children. The fluid ounce is frequently converted to milliliters when measuring a client's fluid intake or output.
- Liters and milliliters are the volumes commonly used in preparing solutions for enemas, irrigating solutions for bladder irrigations, and solutions for cleaning open wounds. In some situations, the nurse needs to convert the volumes of such solutions.

PRACTICE B

Perform the calculations below and check your answers in Appendix A.

1. 6.75 L = _____ mL
2. 2,850 mL = _____ L
3. 1 ounce (oz) = _____ mL
4. 120 mL = _____ oz
5. 8 oz = _____ mL

Converting Units of Weight

The units of weight most commonly used in nursing practice are the gram, milligram, and kilogram, and the grain and the pound. Household units of weight are generally not applicable.

Table 14–2 shows metric and apothecaries' approximate equivalents. Learning these equivalents helps the nurse make weight conversions readily, as for example in the following situations:

- Converting milligrams to grains and vice versa, for example, when preparing medications.
- Converting pounds to kilograms and vice versa, as in a person's weight.

When converting units of weight from the metric system to the apothecaries' system, the nurse should keep in mind that a milligram is smaller than a grain (1 mg = 1/60 grain and 1 grain = 60 mg). The result of converting a smaller unit (milligram) to a larger unit (grain) is a smaller number. Thus, the nurse must divide (by 60 if converting from milligrams to grains). Conversely, when converting from a larger unit to a smaller unit, the nurse multiplies (by 60 if converting from grains to milligrams), and the product is a larger number. In other words:

Small units (mg) to large units (grains) = a smaller number
Large units (grains) to small units (mg) = a larger number

$$\frac{3,000 \text{ mg}}{60} = 50 \text{ grains}$$

$$50 \text{ grains} \times 60 = 3,000 \text{ mg}$$

When converting pounds to kilograms, the nurse applies the same rule. The pound is a smaller unit than the kilogram, and the nurse converts by dividing or multiplying by 2.2:

$$2.2 \text{ lb} = 1 \text{ kg}$$

$$110 \text{ lb} = x \text{ kg}$$

$$x = \frac{110 \times 1}{2.2}$$

$$= 50 \text{ kg}$$

TABLE 14–2	Approximate Weight Equivalents: Metric and Apothecaries' Systems	
Metric		**Apothecaries'**
1 mg	=	1/60 grain
60 mg	=	1 grain (gr)
1 g	=	15 grains
4 g	=	1 dram
30 g	=	1 ounce
500 g	=	1.1 pound (lb)
1,000 g (1 kg)	=	2.2 lb

or

$$50 \text{ kg} = x \text{ lb}$$

$$1 \text{ kg} = 2.2 \text{ lb}$$

$$x = \frac{2.2 \times 50}{1}$$

$$= 110 \text{ lb}$$

The conversion of milligrams to grams was previously discussed. The decimal point is moved three spaces to the left:

$$3,000 = 3 \text{ g}$$

PRACTICE C

Perform the following calculations and check your answers in Appendix A.

1. gr 1 1/2 = _____ mg
2. 145 lb = _____ kg
3. 30 mg = _____ gr
4. 45 kg = _____ lb
5. gr 3 3/4 = _____ mg

METHODS OF CALCULATING DOSAGES

Four common formulas are used to calculate drug dosages. Any of the formulas can be used. Nursing students are encouraged to review all four and to choose the method that works best for them. It is important to use one method consistently to avoid confusion in calculations and, thus, promote client safety. When calculating drug dosages, there are times when the nurse may need to round numbers. Box 14–1 reviews general guidelines for rounding.

Basic Formula

The **basic formula** for calculating drug dosages is commonly used and easy to remember:

D = desired dose (i.e., dose ordered by primary care provider)
H = dose on hand (i.e., dose on label of bottle, vial, ampule)
V = vehicle (i.e., form in which the drug comes, such as tablet or liquid)

$$\text{Formula} = \frac{D \times V}{H} = \text{amount to administer}$$

BOX 14–1	Guidelines for Rounding Numbers in Drug Calculations

Generally . . .

- Quantities *greater than 1* are rounded to the nearest *tenth.*
- Quantities *less than 1* are rounded to the nearest *hundredth* (Giangrasso & Shrimpton, 2013, p. 11).

To round to the nearest tenth:

- Look at the number in the hundredths place. If this number is 5 or greater, add 1 to the tenths place number. For example, 1.67 = 1.7. If the number in the hundredths place is less than 5, leave the number in the tenths place as is. For example, 1.63 = 1.6.

To round to the nearest hundredth:

- Look at the number in the thousandths place. If this number is 5 or greater, add 1 to the hundredths place number. For example, 0.825 = 0.83. If the number in the thousandths place is less than 5, leave the number in the hundredths place as is. For example, 0.823 = 0.82.

ORAL MEDICATIONS

- A capsule cannot be divided.
- Tablets that are scored (a line marked on the tablet) may be divided. A tablet must be scored by the manufacturer to be divided properly.
- For tablets that are *not* scored and capsules, it may not be realistic to administer the exact amount as calculated. For example, if the calculation for *x* results in 1.9 tablets or capsules, the nurse gives 2 tablets or capsules because it is unrealistic to accurately administer 1.9 tablets or capsules.
- If the oral medication is a liquid, the nurse checks to see if it is possible to administer an accurate dosage. This often depends on the syringes used to draw up the medication. For example, a tuberculin (TB) syringe is a 1-mL syringe that includes markings for hundredths of a milliliter. These syringes are often used in pediatrics because they can measure medications given in very small amounts. The nurse needs to pay attention to the markings on the syringe. Some syringes (e.g., 3-mL) have

calibrations where each line indicates one tenth of a milliliter. In contrast, the calibration lines for larger syringes (e.g., 10-mL) indicate a 0.2-mL increment. The nurse must select the proper size syringe for the calculated volume of medication.

PARENTERAL MEDICATIONS

- Rounding depends on the amount (i.e., less than or more than 1) and the syringe used. As indicated above, a TB syringe can be used for very small amounts (e.g., to the hundredth of a mL) and larger syringes would be used for rounding to a tenth of a milliliter.

IV INFUSION

- By gravity:
  - Round to the nearest whole number. For example, if the flow rate calculation equals 37.5 drops/minute, the nurse adjusts the flow rate to 38 drops/minute.
- By IV pump:
  - If the IV pump uses only whole numbers, round to the nearest whole number.
  - Some IV pumps used in critical care units can be set to a tenth of a rate (e.g., 11.1 mL/h). Round to the nearest tenth decimal point.

ROUNDING DOWN

- Rounding down may be used in pediatrics or when administering high-alert medications to adults. This type of rounding is done to avoid the danger of an overdose (Giangrasso & Shrimpton, 2013, p. 11).
- To round down to hundredths, drop all of the numbers after the hundredth place. For tenths, drop all of the numbers after the tenth place, and for whole numbers, all of the numbers after the decimal. For example, 6.6477 rounded down to the nearest
  - Hundredth = 6.64.
  - Tenth = 6.6.
  - Whole number = 6.

EXAMPLE

Order: erythromycin 500 mg

On hand: 250 mg in 5 mL

$$D = 500 \text{ mg} \quad H = 250 \text{ mg} \quad V = 5 \text{ mL}$$

$$\frac{500 \text{ mg}}{250 \text{ mg}} \times 5 \text{ mL} = \frac{2{,}500}{250} = 10 \text{ mL}$$

ANOTHER EXAMPLE

Order: phenobarbital gr ii

On hand: phenobarbital 30 mg tablets

Note: Before doing the drug calculation, the nurse needs to convert to one system and unit of measurement. In this case, the nurse converts the grains (order) to the measurement on hand (mg):

$$1 \text{ gr} = 60 \text{ mg}$$

$$2 \text{ gr} = 120 \text{ mg}$$

$$D = 120 \text{ mg} \quad H = 30 \text{ mg} \quad V = \text{tablet}$$

$$\frac{120 \text{ mg}}{30 \text{ mg}} \times 1 \text{ tablet} = 4 \text{ tablets}$$

Ratio and Proportion Method

The **ratio and proportion method** is considered the oldest method used for calculating dosage problems. The equation is set up with the known quantities on the left side (i.e., H [dose on hand] and V [form in which the drug comes]). The right side of the equation consists of the desired dose (i.e., D) and the unknown amount to administer (i.e., *x*). The equation looks like this:

$$H : V :: D : x$$

Once the equation is set up, multiply the extremes (i.e., H and *x*) and the means (i.e., V and D). Then solve for *x*.

EXAMPLE

Order: Keflex 750 mg

On hand: Keflex, 250 mg capsules

$$H = 250 \text{ mg} : V = 1 \text{ capsule} :: D = 750 \text{ mg} : x$$

$$250 : 1 :: 750 : x$$

Multiply the extremes (i.e., H and *x*) and the means (V and D):

$$250x = 750$$

$$x = 3 \text{ tablets}$$

ANOTHER EXAMPLE

Order: aspirin gr 10

On hand: aspirin, 325-mg tablets

Note: Before doing the drug calculation, the nurse needs to convert to one system and unit of measurement. In this case, the nurse converts the grains to milligrams:

$$1 \text{ gr} = 60 \text{ mg}$$
$$10 \text{ gr} = 600 \text{ mg}$$
$$H = 325 \text{ mg} : V = \text{tablet} :: D = 600 \text{ mg} : x$$
$$325 : 1 :: 600 : x$$

Multiply the extremes (i.e., H and x) and the means (V and D):

$$\frac{325x}{325} = \frac{600}{325}$$

$x = 1.8 = 2$ tablets since a tablet cannot be accurately cut into 0.8.

Fractional Equation Method

The **fractional equation method** is similar to the ratio and proportion method, except it is written as a fraction:

$$\frac{H}{V} = \frac{D}{x}$$

The formula consists of cross multiplying and solving for x:

$$\frac{H}{V} = \frac{D}{x}$$
$$Hx = DV$$
$$x = \frac{DV}{H}$$

EXAMPLE

Order: Lanoxin 0.25 mg

On hand: Lanoxin, 0.125 mg tablets

$$\frac{0.125 \text{ mg}}{1 \text{ tablet}} = \frac{0.25 \text{ mg}}{x \text{ tablets}}$$

Cross multiply:

$$0.125 \, x = 0.25$$

Solve for x:

$$\frac{0.125x}{0.125} = \frac{0.25}{0.125}$$
$$x = 2 \text{ tablets}$$

EXAMPLE REQUIRING CONVERSION

Order: atropine gr 1/100

On hand: atropine 0.4 mg/mL

Note: Before doing the drug calculation, the nurse must convert from two systems to one system and unit of measurement. In this case, because the dosage on hand is in milligrams, the nurse converts the grains to milligrams:

$$1 \text{ gr} = 60 \text{ mg}$$
$$1/100 \text{ gr} = 0.6 \text{ mg}$$
$$\frac{0.4 \text{ mg}}{1 \text{ mL}} = \frac{0.6 \text{ mg}}{x \text{ mL}}$$

Cross multiply:

$$0.4 \, x = 0.6$$

Solve for x:

$$\frac{0.4x}{0.4} = \frac{0.6}{0.4}$$
$$x = 1.5 \text{ mL}$$

Dimensional Analysis Method

The **dimensional analysis method** is often used in the physical sciences where a quantity in one unit of measurement is converted to an equivalent quantity in a different unit of measurement by canceling matching units of measurement. In some of the previous examples, the nurse needed to convert from one or two systems to one system and unit of measurement. This involved extra steps or equations. One advantage of dimensional analysis is that only one equation is needed. The three components (D, H, and V) are still needed to solve the problem. However, when the units of measurement differ for D and H, the dimensional analysis method includes the conversion factor in the equation. Springhouse (2010, p. 77) outlines six steps when using dimensional analysis:

1. Identify the dose on hand.
2. Identify the desired dose.
3. Write down the conversion factor, if needed.
4. Set up the equation.
5. Cancel units that appear in the numerator and denominator.
6. Multiply the numerator. Multiply the denominator. Divide the products.

EXAMPLE

Order: valsartan 120 mg

On hand: valsartan, 40 mg tablets

1. Identify the dose on hand: 40 mg.
2. Identify the desired dose: 120 mg.
3. No conversion is needed.
4. Set up the equation. Remember to put V (the form in which the drug comes) in the *numerator*:

$$\frac{1 \text{ tablet}}{40 \text{ mg}} \times \frac{120 \text{ mg}}{1}$$

5. Cancel units:

$$\frac{1 \text{ tablet}}{40 \text{ mg}} \times \frac{120 \text{ mg}}{1}$$

6. Multiply the numerator and denominator and then divide:

$$\frac{1 \text{ tablet}}{40} \times \frac{120}{1} = \frac{120}{40} \times = 3 \text{ tablets}$$

EXAMPLE USING A CONVERSION FACTOR

Order: dofetilide 0.5 mg

On hand: dofetilide, 125 mcg capsules

1. Identify the dose on hand: 125 mcg capsule.
2. Identify the desired dose: 0.5 mg.
3. Write down the conversion:

$$\frac{1,000 \text{ mcg}}{1 \text{ mg}}$$

4. Set up the equation. Remember (a) to put the form of the drug in the numerator and (b) to set up the conversion factor so that units that need to cancel appear in both numerator and denominator:

$$\frac{1 \text{ capsule}}{125 \text{ mcg}} \times \frac{1,000 \text{ mcg}}{1 \text{ mg}} \times \frac{0.5 \text{ mg}}{1}$$

5. Cancel units:

$$\frac{1 \text{ capsule}}{125 \text{ mcg}} \times \frac{1,000 \text{ mcg}}{1 \text{ mg}} \times \frac{0.5 \text{ mg}}{1}$$

6. Multiply numerator and denominator and divide:

$$\frac{1 \text{ capsule}}{125} \times \frac{1,000}{1} \times \frac{0.5}{1} = \frac{500}{125} = 4 \text{ capsules}$$

ANOTHER EXAMPLE REQUIRING CONVERSION

Order: Tylenol gr xv

On hand: Tylenol, 325 mg tablets

1. Identify the dose on hand: 325 mg tablet
2. Identify the desired dose: gr xv
3. Write down the conversion:

$$\frac{60 \text{ mg}}{1 \text{ gr}}$$

4. Set up the equation. Remember (a) to put the form of the drug in the numerator and (b) to set up the conversion factor so that units that need to cancel appear in both numerator and denominator:

$$\frac{1 \text{ tablet}}{325 \text{ mg}} \times \frac{60 \text{ mg}}{1 \text{ gr}} \times \frac{15 \text{ gr}}{1}$$

5. Cancel units:

$$\frac{1 \text{ tablet}}{325 \text{ mg}} \times \frac{60 \text{ mg}}{1 \text{ gr}} \times \frac{15 \text{ gr}}{1}$$

6. Multiply numerator and denominator and divide:

$$\frac{1 \text{ tablet}}{325} \times \frac{60}{1} \times \frac{15}{1} = \frac{900}{325} = 2.76 \text{ tablets} = 3 \text{ tablets}$$

because a tablet cannot be accurately cut into 0.76

Calculation for Individualized Drug Dosages

Nurses often need to individualize the dosage of a medication for pediatric clients. Other clients who may require an individualized dosage include those receiving chemotherapy and clients who are critically ill. The two methods for individualizing drug dosages are body weight and body surface area.

BODY WEIGHT

Unlike adult dosages, children's dosages are not always standard. Body weight significantly affects dosage; therefore, dosages are calculated. In some settings (e.g., critical care), adult dosages may also be based on a client's weight. Dosages based on weight use kilograms of body weight and per kilogram medication recommendations to arrive at appropriate and safe doses.

The steps involved in calculating an individualized dose are as follows:

1. Convert pounds to kilograms.

2. Determine the drug dose per body weight by multiplying drug dose × body weight × frequency.
3. Choose a method of drug calculation to determine the amount of medication to administer.

EXAMPLE

Order: Keflex 20 mg/kg/day in three divided doses. The client weighs 20 pounds.

On hand: Keflex oral suspension 125 mg per 5 mL

1. Convert pounds to kilograms:

$$20 \div 2.2 = 9 \text{ kg}$$

2. Multiply drug dose × body weight × frequency:

$$20 \text{ mg} \times 9 \text{ kg} = 1 \text{ day} = 180 \text{ mg/day}$$
$$180 \div 3 \text{ divided doses} = 60 \text{ mg per dose}$$

3. The nurse chooses his or her preferred method of calculation (e.g., basic formula, ratio and proportion, fractional, dimensional analysis) to determine how many milliliters per dose of medication. (The answer is 2.4 mL per dose.)

BODY SURFACE AREA

Sometimes the body surface calculation may be used instead of body weight to individualize the medication dosage. It is considered to be the most accurate method of calculating a child's dose. Body surface area is determined by using a nomogram and the child's height and weight. Figure 14–2 ■ shows a standard nomogram that will give a child's body surface area based on the weight and height of the child. The formula is the ratio of the child's body surface area to the surface area of an average adult (1.7 square meters, or 1.7 m²), multiplied by the normal adult dose of the drug:

$$\frac{\text{Child's dose} = \text{surface area of child (m}^2)}{1.7 \text{ m}^2} \times \text{normal adult dose}$$

For example, a child who weighs 10 kg and is 50 cm tall has a body surface area of 0.4 m². Therefore, the child's dose of tetracycline corresponding to an adult dose of 250 mg would be as follows:

$$\text{Child's dose} = \frac{0.4 \text{ m}^2}{1.7 \text{ m}^2} \times 250 \text{ mg}$$
$$= 0.2 \times 250 = 50 \text{ mg}$$

CALCULATING INTRAVENOUS FLOW RATES

An important nursing function is to regulate the flow of an intravenous (IV) infusion. Because equipment varies according to the manufacturer, the nurse must become familiar with the equipment used in each particular agency. Equipment for IV infusions includes the IV solution and an infusion set, which usually includes the IV tubing, a drip chamber, at least one injection port, a roller clamp, and an IV pump or other infusion controlling device (Figure 14–3 ■).

The nurse initiating the IV calculates the correct flow rate, regulates the infusion, and monitors the client's responses. If an electronic infusion control device is not used, the nurse manually regulates the drops per minute of flow using the IV roller clamp (Figure 14–4 ■) to ensure that the prescribed amount of solution will be infused by gravity in the correct time span. If the flow is incorrect, problems such as hypervolemia, hypovolemia, excessive medication administration,

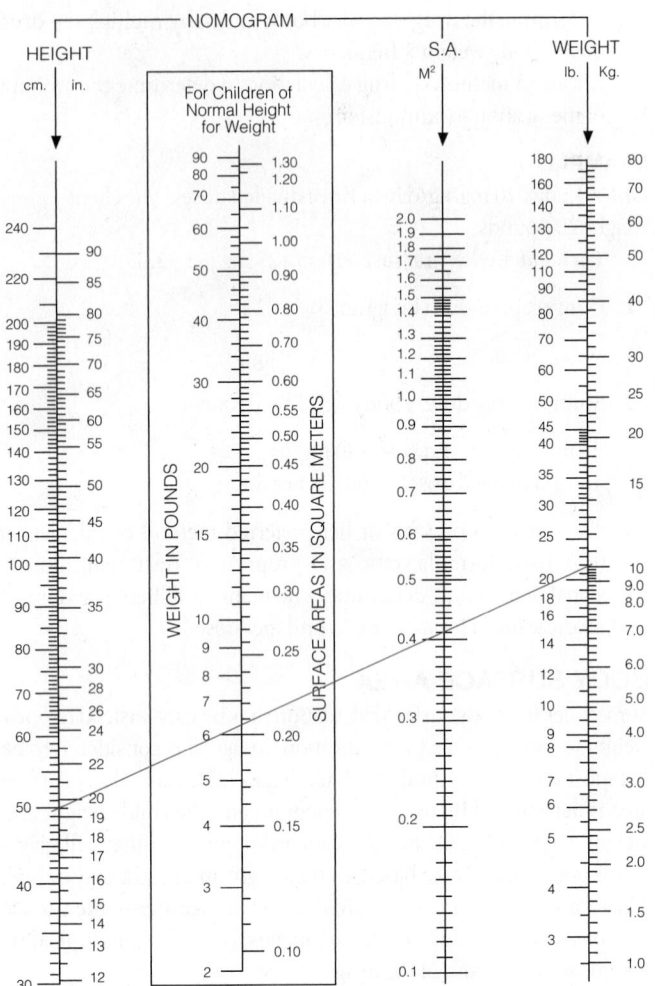

Figure 14–2 ■ Nomogram with estimated body surface area. A straight line is drawn between the child's height (on the left) and the child's weight (on the right). The point at which the line intersects the surface area column is the estimated body surface area.

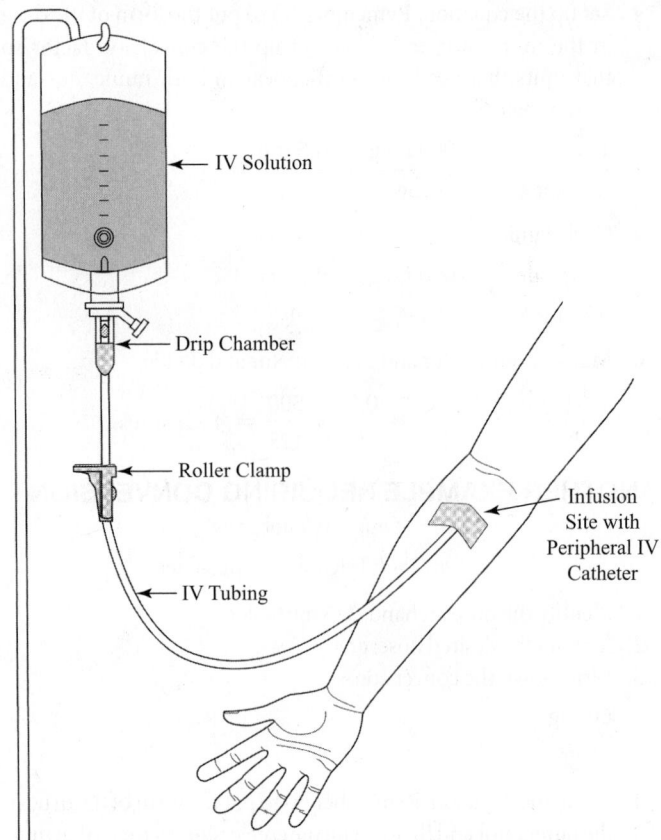

Figure 14–3 ■ Equipment for IV infusion (gravity flow).
From *Dosage Calculations: A Multi-Method Approach*, by A. P. Giangrasso and D. M. Shrimpton, 2013, Upper Saddle River, NJ: Pearson.

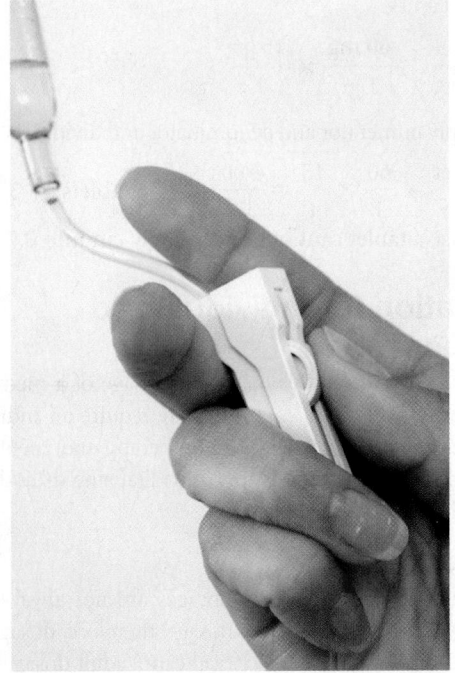

Figure 14–4 ■ IV roller clamp.

or inadequate medication administration can result. Most facilities use some form of infusion controller to avoid these problems.

Intravenous tubing sets have their own type of drip chamber, so it is important to know the number of drops per milliliter of solution for the IV tubing before calculating a drip rate. The size of the drop that the IV tubing delivers varies with different brands and types of IV tubing. Manufacturers specify the number of drops that equal 1 mL on the package of the IV tubing (Figure 14–5 ■). The number of drops that equal 1 mL is called the **drop factor**. A **macrodrip infusion set** can have drop factors of 10, 15, or 20 drops/mL. The drop factor for a **microdrip infusion set** is always 60 drops/mL.

Orders for IV infusions may take several forms: "3,000 mL over 24 hours"; "1 liter every 8 hours × 3 bags"; "125 mL/h until oral intake is a minimum of 500 mL every 8 hours." To calculate flow rates, the nurse must know the volume of fluid to be infused and the specific time for the infusion. The commonly used method of indicating flow rate designates the number of milliliters to be administered in 1 hour (mL/h) and the number of drops delivered in 1 minute (gtt/min).

Calculating Milliliters per Hour

Hourly rates of infusion can be calculated by dividing the total infusion volume by the total infusion time in hours. For example,

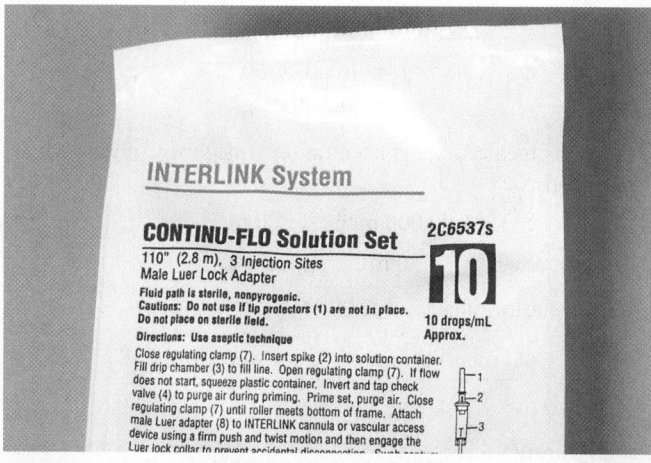

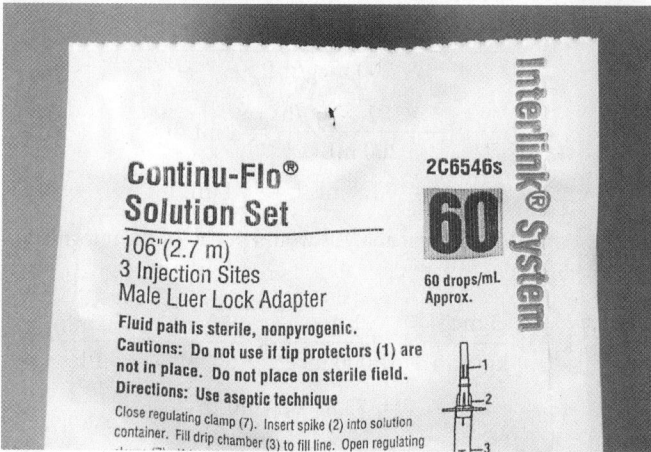

Figure 14–5 ■ Samples of IV tubing containers with drop factors of 10 and 60.

if 3,000 mL is infused in 24 hours, the number of milliliters per hour is

$$\frac{3{,}000 \text{ mL (total infusion volume)}}{24 \text{ h (total infusion time)}} = 125 \text{ mL/h}$$

Electronic infusion devices are commonly used for IV management. The nurse calculates the volume of IV solution to be delivered per hour and programs this information into the machine (Figure 14–6 ■). For the above example, the nurse would set the infusion pump to deliver 125 mL/h. IV pumps can only be set to deliver a specific amount of mL/h. They cannot be set to deliver drops/min or mL/min.

Electronic infusion pumps are designed to infuse fluid/medication in milliliters per hour. This is true even if the amount of fluid needs to be infused in less than 1 hour. A common example is when an IV medication needs to be infused in 30 minutes.

EXAMPLE

Order: oxacillin 250 mg in 100 mL D_5W IV every 4 hours. Infuse over 30 minutes.

Using the ratio and proportion method:

$$100 \text{ mL} : 30 \text{ min} :: x \text{ mL} : 1 \text{ hour (60 minutes)}$$

$$30x = 6{,}000$$

$$x = 200 \text{ mL}$$

The nurse will set the infusion pump at 200 mL/h and the medication will be infused in 30 minutes.

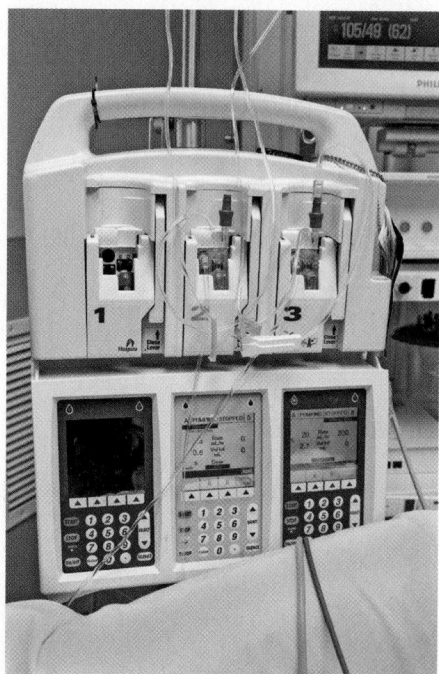

Figure 14–6 ■ Programmable multichannel infusion pumps.

Calculating Drops per Minute

The nurse initiating and monitoring an infusion that is by gravity flow must regulate the drops per minute to ensure that the prescribed amount of solution will infuse. Following is a common formula used for calculating drops per minute:

$$\text{Drops per minute} = \frac{\text{total infusion volume} \times \text{drop factor}}{\text{number of hours} \times 60 \text{ minutes}}$$

If the requirements are 1,000 mL in 8 hours and the drop factor is 20 drops/mL, the drops per minute should be:

$$\frac{1{,}000 \text{ mL} \times 20 \text{ drops/mL}}{8 \text{ h} \times 60 \text{ min (480 min)}} = 41.6 \text{ drops/min}$$

$$= 42 \text{ drops/min}$$

For this rate of 42 drops/min, the nurse regulates the drops per minute by tightening or releasing the IV roller clamp and counting the drops for 15 seconds, then multiplying that number by 4.

Calculating IV Flow Rates Based on Time

IV medications can be administered per a unit of time; for example, milligrams, micrograms, or units of a medication per a unit of time such as per minute or per hour. These IV solutions usually come premixed from the pharmacy and an IV infusion pump is used for administration of the solution. The nurse needs to accurately set the infusion rate on the IV pump.

For example, an order of 10,000 units of heparin is to be added to 500 mL of D_5W. The client is to receive 1,200 units of heparin per hour via an infusion pump. The nurse needs to calculate how many mL/h to set the IV pump. Following are examples of converting to mL/h using different formulas:

RATIO AND PROPORTION METHOD

$$10,000 \text{ units} : 500 \text{ mL} :: 1,200 \text{ units} : x \text{ mL}$$

Cross multiply:

$$10,000\, x = 600,000 (1,200 \times 500)$$
$$x = \frac{600,000}{10,000}$$
$$x = 60 \text{ mL/h}$$

BASIC FORMULA METHOD

$$\frac{1,200 \text{ units}}{10,000 \text{ units}} \times 500 \text{ mL}$$

Cancel:

$$\frac{1,200 \text{ units}}{10,000 \text{ units} \times 500 \text{ mL}}$$
$$\frac{1,200}{20} = 60 \text{ mL}$$

DIMENSIONAL ANALYSIS METHOD

$$x \text{ mL} = \frac{500 \text{ mL}}{10,000 \text{ units}} \times \frac{1,200 \text{ units}}{1 \text{ h}} = \frac{600,000}{10,000} = \frac{60 \text{ mL}}{\text{h}}$$

Calculating IV Flow Rates Based on Body Weight and Time

Some IV medications are prescribed not only based on a client's body weight as discussed earlier, but also based on the amount of drug the client receives over time. For example, an order for 50 mg of a medication is to be added to 250 mL of normal saline. This IV solution is to be administered at 3 mcg/kg/min. The client weighs 82 kg. The amount of medication that the client is to receive is based on both body weight and time. The nurse needs to calculate how many mL/h to set the IV pump for. One formula for determining the mL/h rate is as follows:

$$\frac{\text{Ordered mcg/kg/min} \times \text{client's weight in kg} \times 60 \text{ min/h}}{\text{Medication concentration (mcg/mL)}}$$

The answer will be in mL/h because the mcg, min, and kg cancel. First, the nurse must convert the milligrams in the IV bag (50) to micrograms:

$$1 \text{ mg} : 1,000 \text{ mcg} :: 50 \text{ mg} : x \text{ mcg}$$

Cross multiply:

$$x = 1,000 \times 50$$
$$x = 50,000 \text{ mcg}$$

Next, the medication concentration (mcg/mL) needs to be determined:

$$\frac{50,000 \text{ mcg}}{250 \text{ mL}} = \frac{200 \text{ mcg}}{1 \text{ mL}}$$

Complete the formula:

$$\frac{3 \text{ mcg/kg/min} \times 82 \text{ kg} \times 60 \text{ min/h}}{200 \text{ mcg/mL}}$$

Cancel pairs of values:

$$\frac{3 \text{ mcg/kg/min} \times 82 \text{ kg} \times 60 \text{ min/h}}{200 \text{ mcg/mL}}$$
$$\frac{3 \times 82 \times 60/\text{h}}{200 \text{ mL}} = x \text{ mL/h}$$
$$x = 73.8 \text{ mL/h} = 74 \text{ mL/h}$$

Nurses using dimensional analysis would put all of the information into one formula:

$$82 \text{ kg} \times \frac{3 \text{ mcg}}{\text{kg/min}} \times \frac{1 \text{ mg}}{1,000 \text{ mcg}} \times \frac{250 \text{ mL}}{50 \text{ mg}} \times \frac{60 \text{ min}}{1 \text{ h}}$$
$$= 73.8 = 74 \text{ mL/h}$$

As shown in this chapter, drug calculations can range from a simple conversion to a complex calculation for a drug administered by mcg/kg/minute. Likewise, the understanding of and comfort level with math varies among nurses. Safe practices for nurses who may be unsure of their calculations include the following:

- Avoid distractions when performing drug calculations. Staying focused is essential, particularly when several steps are involved in the calculation.
- Ask themselves "Does this make sense?" For example, if the result of the calculation is to administer 0.001 tablet or 20 tablets, the nurse needs to critically think and ask why a client would receive so little or so many tablets for one dose.
- Ask another nurse to double-check the calculations, particularly if the result of the calculation does not make sense. Some institutions have policies requiring a second nurse to confirm the calculation result when high-risk medications are being given.

FOCUSING ON CLINICAL THINKING

Consider This

A client with a history of chronic obstructive pulmonary disease (COPD) is admitted with a deep venous thrombosis (DVT) of the lower left leg. The orders include the following:

  Vital signs q4 hours
  Albuterol 4 mg, po, three (3) times daily
  Tagamet 200 mg, po, with meals
  Potassium chloride (KCl) 15 mEq, po, two (2) times daily
  Heparin 12,500 units in 250 mL D_5W at 1,200 units/hour

1. The albuterol is available in 2 mg/5 mL. How many mL will the nurse give per dose?

2. The label on the single-dose unit of Tagamet states 300 mg/5 mL. How many mL will the nurse give per dose?
3. The KCl is available as 10 mEq/15 mL. How many mL of KCl will the nurse give per dose?
4. How many mEq of KCl will the client receive per day?
5. How many mL of KCl will the client receive per day?
6. The nurse will set the heparin drip to infuse at how many mL per hour?
7. The client will be receiving what concentration of heparin (units) each minute?

See Focusing on Clinical Thinking answers on student resource website.

TEST YOUR KNOWLEDGE

1. Which system of measurement includes teaspoons and tablespoons?
   1. Apothecaries'
   2. Ratio and proportion
   3. Household
   4. Fractional equation
2. Which of the following units of measurement belongs to the apothecaries' system?
   1. Minim
   2. Meter
   3. Gram
   4. Liter
3. A nurse needs to medicate a client with 1 gram of metformin. If the medication is available only in milligrams, how many milligrams will this client receive?
   1. 10 mg
   2. 100 mg
   3. 500 mg
   4. 1,000 mg
4. A nursing student is preparing to give medications with a clinical instructor. The order is written for 60 mg of phenobarbital, and the medication dose available is in the apothecaries' system. How much medication will the nursing student administer?
   1. 1/60 grain
   2. 1 grain
   3. 15 grains
   4. 1 dram
5. Which of the following statements, if made by the nursing student, demonstrates correct understanding of the different units of volume in the metric, apothecaries', and household systems?
   1. "1 milliliter is the same as 15 minims or 15 drops."
   2. "15 milliliters is the same as 15 minims or 1 tablespoon."
   3. "500 milliliters is the same as 1 pint or 6 quarts."
   4. "4,000 milliliters is the same as 1 gallon or 20 pints."

6. The nurse is weighing the client. The client weighs 165 lb. How much is this weight in kilograms (kg)?
   Fill in the blank _____
7. The nurse needs to administer Keflex 500 mg twice a day. The medication available is Keflex 250 mg capsules. How many capsules will the client receive at each dose?
   1. 2 capsules
   2. 3 capsules
   3. 4 capsules
   4. 5 capsules
8. The medication order for a client is Medrol 75 mg. The label on the vial indicates Medrol 125 mg per 2 mL. How many mL will the nurse administer?
   Fill in the blank _____
9. The primary care provider has written the following order: nitroglycerin IV drip of 100 mg in 250 mL D_5W. Begin the infusion at 20 mcg/min. At what rate will the nurse set the infusion pump?
   1. 1 mL/h
   2. 2 mL/h
   3. 3 mL/h
   4. 4 mL/h
10. The primary care provider has written the following order: dopamine 400 mg in 250 mL D_5W at 3 mcg/kg/min IV. The client weighs 91 kg. At what flow rate will the nurse set the IV pump?
    1. 10 mL/h
    2. 20 mL/h
    3. 30 mL/h
    4. 40 mL/h

See Answers to Test Your Knowledge in Appendix A.

READINGS AND REFERENCES

References

Giangrasso, A. P., & Shrimpton, D. M. (2013). *Dosage calculations: A multi-method approach.* Upper Saddle River, NJ: Pearson.
Springhouse. (2010). *Dosage calculations made incredibly easy!* (4th ed.). Ambler, PA: Lippincott Williams & Wilkins.

Selected Bibliography

Berman, A., Snyder, S., & Frandsen, G. (2016). *Kozier & Erb's fundamentals of nursing: Concepts, process, and practice* (10th ed.). Upper Saddle River, NJ: Pearson.
Giangrasso, A. P., & Shrimpton, D. (2010). *Ratio & proportion dosage calculations.* Upper Saddle River, NJ: Pearson.

Gray, M. (2010). *Calculate with confidence* (5th ed.). St. Louis, MO: Elsevier.
Olsen, J. L., Giangrasso, A. P., & Shrimpton, D. M. (2012). *Medical dosage calculations: A dimensional analysis approach* (10th ed.). Upper Saddle River, NJ: Pearson
Wright, K. (2012). How to ensure patient safety in drug dose calculation. *Nursing Times, 108*(42), 12–13.

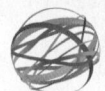

15 Administering Oral and Enteral Medications

LEARNING OUTCOMES

At the completion of this chapter, the student will be able to:

1. Define the key terms used in the skills of administering oral and enteral medications.
2. Describe the legal aspects of administering medications.
3. Identify indications for the various types of drug preparations.
4. Provide examples of various types of medication orders.
5. Identify the essential parts of a medication order.
6. Discuss strategies to increase medication administration safety.
7. Describe the various medication dispensing systems.
8. State the "rights" to accurate medication administration.
9. Recognize when it is appropriate to delegate aspects of administering oral and enteral medications to unlicensed assistive personnel.
10. Verbalize the steps used in administering:
    a. Oral medications.
    b. Medications by enteral tube.
11. Demonstrate appropriate documentation and reporting of oral and enteral medication administration.

SKILLS

Skill 15–1 Administering Oral Medications
Skill 15–2 Administering Medications by Enteral Tube

KEY TERMS

adverse effects, *366*
brand name, *364*
buccal, *366*
chemical name, *364*
desired effect, *366*
drug, *364*
gastrostomy tube, *381*

generic name, *364*
medication, *364*
medication history, *370*
medication reconciliation, *371*
meniscus, *378*
nasogastric (NG) tube, *381*
NPO, *375*

official name, *364*
oral, *366*
orogastric (OG) tube, *381*
prescription, *364*
prn order, *367*
side effect, *366*
single order, *367*

standing order, *367*
stat order, *367*
sublingual, *366*
therapeutic effect, *366*
trade name, *364*

A **medication** is a substance administered for the diagnosis, cure, treatment, or relief of a symptom or for prevention of disease. In the health care context, the words *medication* and **drug** are generally used interchangeably. The term *drug* also has the connotation of an illicitly obtained substance such as heroin, cocaine, or amphetamine. Medications have been known and used since antiquity. Crude drugs, such as opium, castor oil, and vinegar, were used in ancient times. Over time the number of drugs available has increased greatly, and knowledge about these drugs has become correspondingly more accurate and detailed.

In the United States, medications are usually dispensed on the order of physicians and dentists. In some U.S. states, qualified nurse practitioners or other advanced practice nurses and physician assistants may prescribe drugs. The written direction for the preparation and administration of a drug is called a **prescription**. One drug can have as many as four kinds of names: its generic name, official name, chemical name, and trade name or brand name. The **generic name** is given before a drug officially becomes an approved medication. The generic name is generally used throughout the drug's lifetime. The **official name** is the name under which the drug is listed in

one of the official publications (e.g., the *United States Pharmacopeia*). The **chemical name** is the name by which a chemist knows it; this name describes the constituents of the drug precisely. A drug's **trade name** is the name given to it by the drug manufacturer. The name is usually selected to be short and easy to remember. The trade name is sometimes called the **brand name**. Because one drug may be manufactured by several companies, it can have several trade names; for example, the drug hydrochlorothiazide (official name) is known by the trade names Esidrix and HydroDIURIL.

Medications are often available in a variety of forms. See Table 15–1 for examples of types of drug preparations or forms. It is important for the nurse to administer the correct form of medication.

LEGAL ASPECTS OF DRUG ADMINISTRATION

The administration of drugs in the United States is controlled by law. See Table 15–2 for a summary of U.S. drug legislation.

Nurses need to (a) know how nurse practice acts in their areas define and limit their functions and (b) recognize the limits of their

TABLE 15–1	Types of Drug Preparations

Type	Description
Aerosol spray or foam	A liquid, powder, or foam deposited in a thin layer on the skin by air pressure
Aqueous solution	One or more drugs dissolved in water
Aqueous suspension	One or more drugs finely divided in a liquid such as water
Caplet	A solid form, shaped like a capsule, coated and easily swallowed
Capsule	A gelatinous container that holds a drug in powder, liquid, or oil form
Cream	A nongreasy, semisolid preparation used on the skin
Elixir	A sweetened and aromatic solution of alcohol used as a vehicle for medicinal agents
Extract	A concentrated form of a drug made from vegetables or animals
Gel or jelly	A clear or translucent semisolid that liquefies when applied to the skin
Liniment	A medication mixed with alcohol, oil, or soapy emollient and applied to the skin
Lotion	A medication in a liquid suspension applied to the skin
Lozenge (troche)	A flat, round, or oval preparation that dissolves and releases a drug when held in the mouth
Ointment (salve, unction)	A semisolid preparation of one or more drugs used for application to the skin and mucous membrane
Paste	A preparation like an ointment, but thicker and stiff, that penetrates the skin less than an ointment
Pill	One or more drugs mixed with a cohesive material, in oval, round, or flattened shapes
Powder	A finely ground drug or drugs; some are used internally, others externally
Suppository	One or several drugs mixed with a firm base such as gelatin and shaped for insertion into the body (e.g., the rectum); the base dissolves gradually at body temperature, releasing the drug
Syrup	An aqueous solution of sugar often used to disguise unpleasant-tasting drugs
Tablet	A powdered drug compressed into a hard small disk; some are readily broken along a scored line; others are enteric coated to prevent them from dissolving in the stomach
Tincture	An alcohol or water-and-alcohol solution prepared from drugs derived from plants
Transdermal patch	A semipermeable membrane shaped like a disk or patch that contains a drug to be absorbed through the skin over a long period of time

own knowledge and skill. Every nurse is responsible for adhering to their state's nurse practice act and following legal provisions when administering medications. Under the law, nurses are responsible for their own actions even when there is a written order. If a primary care provider writes an incorrect order (e.g., morphine 100 mg instead of morphine 10 mg), *a nurse who administers the written incorrect dosage is responsible for the error as well as the primary care provider.* Therefore, nurses should question any order that appears unreasonable and refuse to give the medication until the order is clarified.

Another aspect of nursing practice governed by law is the use of controlled substances. In hospitals, controlled substances are kept in a locked drawer, cupboard, medication cart, or computer-controlled dispensing system. Agencies may have special inventory forms for recording the use of controlled substances. The information required usually includes the name of the client, the date and time of administration, the name of the drug, the dosage, and the signature of the person who administered the drug. The name of the primary care provider who ordered the drug may also be a part of the record. Some agencies may require a verifying signature of another registered nurse for administration of a controlled substance. Most health care agencies maintain a list of high-alert medications, including controlled substances, that require verification by two registered nurses. Before

TABLE 15–2	U.S. Drug Legislation

Legislation	Content
Food, Drug, and Cosmetic Act (1938)	Implemented by the U.S. Food and Drug Administration (FDA); requires that labels be accurate and that all drugs be tested for harmful effects.
Durham–Humphrey Amendment (1952)	Clearly differentiates drugs that can be sold only with a prescription, those that can be sold without a prescription, and those that should not be refilled without a new prescription.
Kefauver–Harris Amendment (1962)	Requires proof of safety and efficacy of a drug for approval.
Comprehensive Drug Abuse Prevention and Control Act (1970) (Controlled Substances Act)	Categorizes controlled substances and limits how often a prescription can be filled; established government-funded programs to prevent and treat drug dependence.

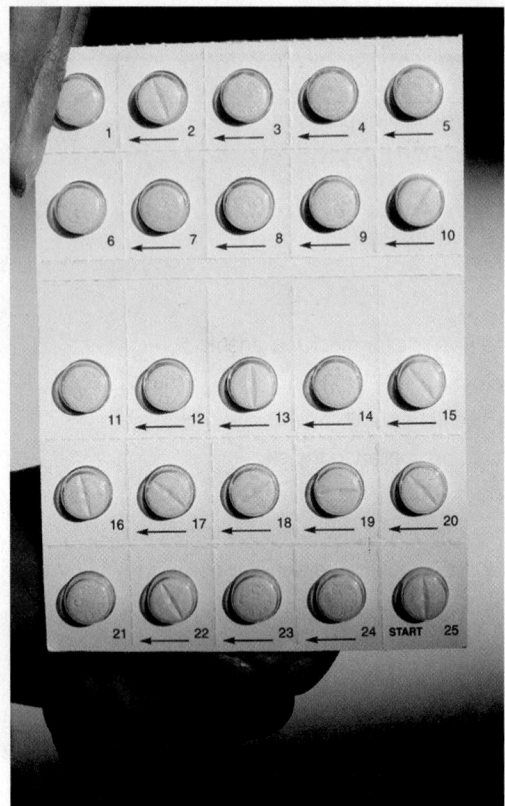

Figure 15–1 ■ Some narcotics are kept in specially designed packages or plastic containers that are sectioned and numbered.

removing a controlled substance, the nurse verifies the number actually available with the number indicated on the narcotic or controlled substance inventory record (Figure 15–1 ■). If the number is not the same, the nurse must investigate and correct the discrepancy.

Included on the record are the controlled substances wasted during preparation. When a portion or all of a controlled substance dose is discarded, the nurse must ask a second nurse to witness the discarding of the unused medication. Both nurses must sign the control inventory form.

In most agencies, counts of controlled substances are taken at the end of each shift. The count total should balance with the total at the end of the last shift minus the number used. If the totals do not balance and the discrepancy cannot be resolved, it must be reported immediately to the nurse manager, nursing supervisor, and pharmacy according to agency policy. In facilities that use a computerized dispensing system, manual counts are not required, because the dispensing system runs a continuous count; however, discrepancies must be reported and accounted for.

EFFECTS OF DRUGS

The **therapeutic effect** of a drug, also referred to as the **desired effect**, is the primary effect intended, that is, the reason the drug is prescribed. For example, the therapeutic effect of morphine sulfate is analgesia, and the therapeutic effect of diazepam is relief of anxiety.

A **side effect**, or secondary effect, of a drug is one that is unintended. Side effects are usually predictable and may be either harmless or potentially harmful. For example, digitalis increases the strength of myocardial contractions (desired effect), but it can have the side effect of inducing nausea and vomiting. Some side effects are tolerated for the drug's therapeutic effect; more severe side effects, also called **adverse effects** or reactions, may justify the discontinuation of a drug. The nurse should monitor for dose-related side or adverse effects and report these to the health care provider who may discontinue the medication or change the dosage.

ROUTES OF ADMINISTRATION

Pharmaceutical preparations are generally designed for one or two specific routes of administration. The route of administration should be indicated when the drug is ordered. When administering a drug, the nurse should ensure that the pharmaceutical preparation is appropriate for the route specified. Numerous routes exist for medication administration. This chapter describes the oral route, and subsequent chapters discuss other routes.

Oral

Oral administration is the most common, least expensive, and most convenient route for most clients. In oral administration, the drug is swallowed. Because the skin is not broken as it is for an injection, oral administration is also a safe method.

The major disadvantages are possible unpleasant taste of the drugs, irritation of the gastric mucosa, irregular absorption from the gastrointestinal tract, slow absorption, and in some cases, harm to the client's teeth. For example, the liquid preparation of ferrous sulfate (iron) can stain the teeth.

Sublingual

In **sublingual** administration, a drug is placed under the tongue, where it dissolves (Figure 15–2 ■). In a relatively short time, the drug is largely absorbed into the blood vessels on the underside of the tongue. The medications should not be swallowed. Nitroglycerin is one example of a drug commonly given in this manner.

Buccal

Buccal means "pertaining to the cheek." In buccal administration, a medication (e.g., a tablet) is held in the mouth against the mucous

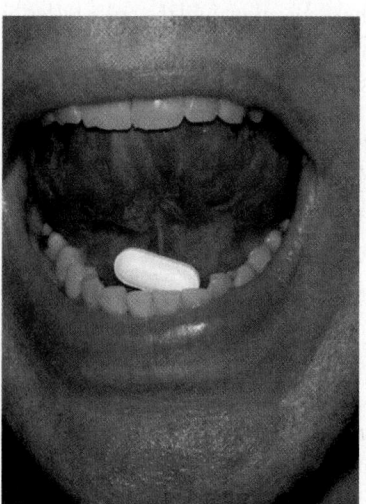

Figure 15–2 ■ Sublingual administration of a tablet.

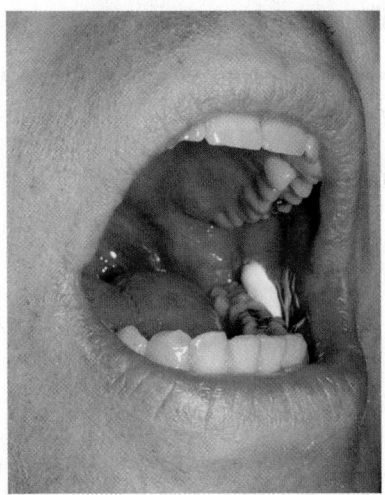

Figure 15–3 ■ Buccal administration of a tablet.

membranes of the cheek until the drug dissolves (Figure 15–3 ■). The drug may act locally on the mucous membranes of the mouth or systemically when it is swallowed in the saliva.

Enteral

Oral medications can also be administered into feeding or enteral tubes. See Skill 15–2.

MEDICATION ORDERS

A physician usually determines the client's medication needs and orders medications, although in some settings nurse practitioners and physician assistants (PAs) now order some drugs. State law determines whether nurse practitioners and PAs have prescriptive ability and the class of drug for which they may prescribe. Also, each health agency will have its own policies. Usually the order is written, although telephone and verbal orders are acceptable in a number of agencies. Nursing students need to know the agency policies about medication orders. In some hospitals, for example, only licensed nurses are permitted to accept telephone and verbal orders. Patient Safety Solutions (2012), a health care consulting service that focuses on client safety, strongly recommends that health organizations have solid guidelines in place to reduce or eliminate errors stemming from verbal orders. For example, for all verbal or telephone orders the nurse must first write down the order and then read it back, verbatim, to the prescribing care provider.

SAFETY ALERT!   SAFETY

Encourage the prescribing care provider to provide correct spelling of a drug, using aids such as "B as in boy." It is also important for the provider to pronounce numbers separately. For example, the number 16 should be stated as "one six" to avoid confusion with the number 60.

Policies about primary care providers' orders vary considerably from agency to agency. For example, a client's orders may be automatically canceled after surgery or an examination involving an anesthetic agent. The primary care provider must then write new orders. Most agencies also have lists of abbreviations officially accepted for use

in the agency. To prevent medication errors, The Joint Commission has mandated that agencies must standardize abbreviations, acronyms, and symbols used throughout the organization and *must* list abbreviations that are never to be used (The Joint Commission, 2012). The Institute for Safe Medication Practices (ISMP) has a comprehensive list of error-prone abbreviations, symbols, and dose designations that should not be used when communicating medical information (2013a). See Table 15–3 for the list of unacceptable abbreviations.

Types of Medication Orders

Four common medication orders are the stat order, the single order, the standing order, and the prn order:

1. A **stat order** indicates that the medication is to be given immediately and only once (e.g., morphine 10 mg IV stat).
2. The **single order**, or *one-time order*, is for medication to be given once at a specified time (e.g., Seconal 100 mg at bedtime before surgery).
3. The **standing order** may or may not have a termination date. A standing order may be carried out indefinitely (e.g., multiple vitamins daily) until an order is written to cancel it, or it may be carried out for a specified number of days (e.g., KCl twice daily × 2 days). In some agencies, standing orders are automatically canceled after a specified number of days and must be reordered.
4. A **prn order**, or *as-needed order*, permits the nurse to give a medication when, in the nurse's judgment, the client requires it (e.g., Amphojel 15 mL prn). The nurse must use good judgment about when the medication is needed and when it can be safely administered.

Essential Parts of a Drug Order

A drug order has seven essential parts, as listed in Box 15–1. In addition, unless it is a standing order it should state the number of doses or the number of days the drug is to be administered.

The *client's full name*, that is, the first and last names and middle initials or names, should always be used to avoid confusion between two clients who have the same last name. In some agencies, the client's identification number and primary care provider's name are put on the order as further identification. Some hospitals imprint the client's name, identification number, and room number on all forms; some agencies use stickers with similar information.

In addition to the *day*, the *month*, and the *year* the order was written, some agencies also require that the time of day be written. Writing the *time of day* on the order can eliminate errors when the nursing shifts change and makes clear when certain orders automatically terminate. For example, in some settings narcotics can be ordered only for 48 hours after surgery. Therefore, a drug that is ordered at 1600 hours November 1, 2015, is automatically canceled at 1600 hours November 3, 2015. Many health agencies use the 24-hour clock, which eliminates confusion between morning and afternoon times. Time with the 24-hour clock starts at midnight, which is 0000 hours (Figure 15–4 ■).

The *name of the drug to be administered* must be clearly written. In some settings only generic names are permitted; however, trade names are widely used in hospitals and health agencies.

TABLE 15–3	Unacceptable Abbreviations—"Do Not Use" List from The Joint Commission and Institute for Safe Medication Practices (ISMP)		
Abbreviation	**Potential Problem**		**Use Instead**
**U, u (unit)	Mistaken for "0" (zero), the number "4" (four), or "cc"		Write "unit"
**IU (international unit)	Mistaken for IV (intravenous) or the number 10 (ten)		Write "International Unit"
**Q.D., QD, q.d., qd (daily)	Mistaken for each other		Write "daily"
**Q.O.D., QOD, q.o.d., qod (every other day)	Period after the Q mistaken for "I" and the "O" mistaken for "I"		Write "every other day"
**Trailing zero (X.0 mg)	Decimal point is missed		Write X mg
**Lack of leading zero (.X mg)	Decimal point is missed		Write 0.X mg
**MS	Can mean morphine sulfate or magnesium sulfate Confused for one another		Write "morphine sulfate"
**MSO_4 and $MgSO_4$	Can mean morphine sulfate or magnesium sulfate Confused for one another		Write "magnesium sulfate"
> (greater than) < (less than)	Opposite of intended; mistakenly use incorrect symbol		Write "greater than" Write "less than"
@	Mistaken for the number "2" (two)		Write "at"
cc	Mistaken for U (units) when poorly written		Write "mL" or "milliliters"
μg	Mistaken for mg (milligrams) resulting in one thousand-fold overdose		Write "mcg" or "micrograms"
TIW (three times a week)	Has been misinterpreted as "two times a week" or "three times a day" resulting in misdosing		Write "three times weekly"
AS (left ear) AD (right ear) AU (both ears) OD (right eye) OS (left eye) OU (each eye)	Mistaken for OS (left eye), OD (either "overdose" or "optic density"), and OU ("each eye" or "both eyes") Mistaken as AD, AS, AU (right ear, left ear, each ear)		Write "left ear," "right ear," or "both ears," as appropriate Use "right eye," "left eye," or "each eye"
HS	Has been used to indicate "half strength" and "bedtime" or "hour of sleep"		Write out "half strength" or "at bedtime," as appropriate
SC and SQ (subcutaneous) Apothecary units	Have been read as "SL" (sublingual) and as "5 every hour" Unfamiliar to many practitioners Confused with metric units		Write "subq" or "subcutaneous" Use metric units
Abbreviations for drug names	Misinterpreted due to similar abbreviations for multiple drugs		Write drug names in full

**These abbreviations are from The Joint Commission's official *Do Not Use* List; the others are from *ISMP's List of Error-Prone Abbreviations, Symbols, and Dose Designations*.
From *Facts about the Official "Do Not Use" List*, by The Joint Commission, 2012. Retrieved from http://www.jointcommission.org/facts_about_the_official_/; and *ISMP's List of Error-Prone Abbreviations, Symbols, and Dose Designations*, by the Institute for Safe Medication Practices, 2013a. Retrieved from http://www.ismp.org/tools/errorproneabbreviations.pdf.

Culturally Responsive Care

PATIENT-CENTERED CARE

Ethnopharmacology

Drug response can be affected by ancestry. Until recently, clinical drug research was conducted on Caucasian males even when the health disorder being studied was prevalent in other ethnic groups. Research has shown that one size does *not* fit all.

IMPLICATIONS FOR NURSING INTERVENTIONS

- Remember that there may be differences in medication responses among different ethnic groups and differences *within* ethnic groups.
- Avoid profiling and stereotyping.
- Ask about health beliefs, values, and customs/practices.
- Be accepting of differences in cultural beliefs and practices.

- Conduct a cultural assessment with each client.
- Learn about drug effects (including adverse effects) that are related to ancestry.
- Ask the client direct, specific questions to reveal the presence or absence of potential adverse effects of medications.
- Monitor the client and document findings carefully, because it may be possible to maintain therapeutic benefit at a lower dosage of a given drug.
- Implement a treatment plan with the client and family that is consistent with their cultural and traditional beliefs while incorporating the necessary modern treatments.
- Keep cultural context in mind when planning education for clients and families.

BOX 15–1	Essential Parts of a Drug Order

- Full name of the client
- Date and time the order is written
- Name of the drug to be administered
- Dosage of the drug
- Frequency of administration
- Route of administration
- Signature of the person writing the order

BOX 15–2	Parts of a Prescription

- Descriptive information about the client: name, address, and sometimes age
- Date on which the prescription was written
- The Rx symbol, meaning "take thou"
- Medication name, dosage, and strength
- Route of administration
- Dispensing instructions for the pharmacist, for example, "dispense 30 capsules"
- Directions for administration to be given to the client, for example, "one tablet with meals"
- Refill and/or special labeling, for example, "refill × 1"
- Prescriber's signature
- Permission to use generics or stipulation of "brand only"
- Prescriber's license number and DEA number if required

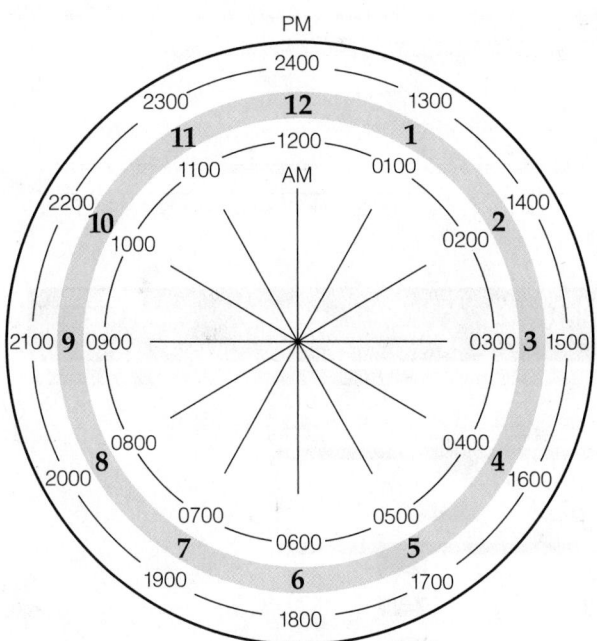

Figure 15–4 ■ The 24-hour clock.

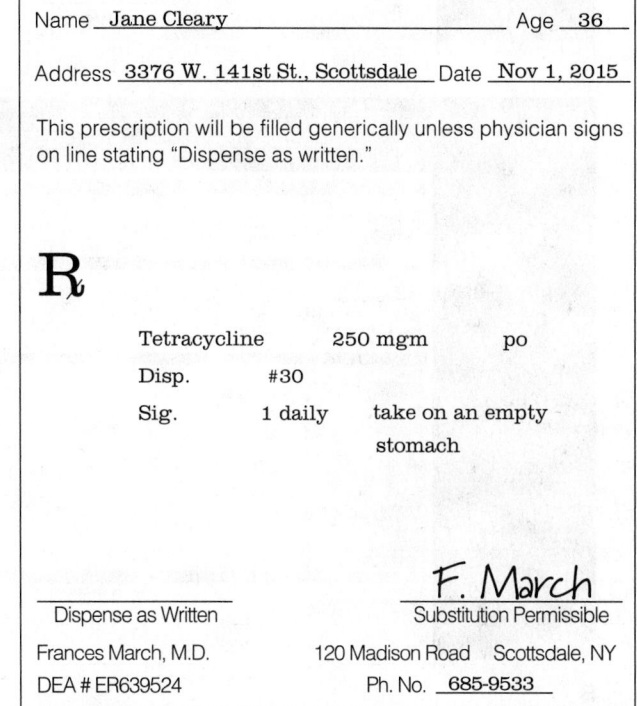

Figure 15–5 ■ A prescription filled out by a primary care provider.

The *dosage of the drug* includes the amount or the strength of the medication, and the times or *frequency of administration*—for example, tetracycline 250 mg (amount) four times a day (frequency) and potassium chloride 10% (strength) 5 mL (amount) three times a day with meals (time and frequency). Dosages can be written in the apothecaries' system or the metric system. The metric system, however, is strongly suggested for safety reasons because many practitioners are unfamiliar with apothecaries' units.

Also included in the order is the *route of administration* of the drug. This part of the order, like other parts, is frequently abbreviated. It is not unusual for a drug to have several possible routes of administration; therefore, it is important that the route be included in the order.

The *signature* of the ordering primary care provider or nurse (if receiving a verbal or telephone order) makes the drug order a legal request. *An unsigned drug order is not valid,* and the ordering health care practitioner needs to be notified if the order is unsigned.

When a primary care provider writes a prescription for a client, the prescription also includes information for the pharmacist. Therefore, a prescription's content differs from that of a medication order in a hospital. Compare the parts of a prescription listed in Box 15–2 with those shown in Figure 15–5 ■.

Communicating a Medication Order

A drug order is written on the client's chart by a primary care provider or by a nurse receiving a telephone or verbal order from a primary care

provider. Most acute care agencies have a specified time frame (e.g., 24 or 48 hours) in which the primary care provider issuing the telephone or verbal order must cosign the order written by the nurse. The medication order is then copied by a nurse or clerk to a Kardex or medication administration record. Increasingly, nurses receive computer printouts of a client's medications instead of a copy of the primary care provider's order. This method avoids errors and saves nursing time.

CLINICAL ALERT!

If your assigned client receives new medication orders, double-check the transcribed information with the primary care provider's order. This ensures client safety.

Medication administration records (MARs) vary in form, but all include the client's name, room, and bed number; drug name and dose; and times and method of administration (Figure 15–6 ■). In

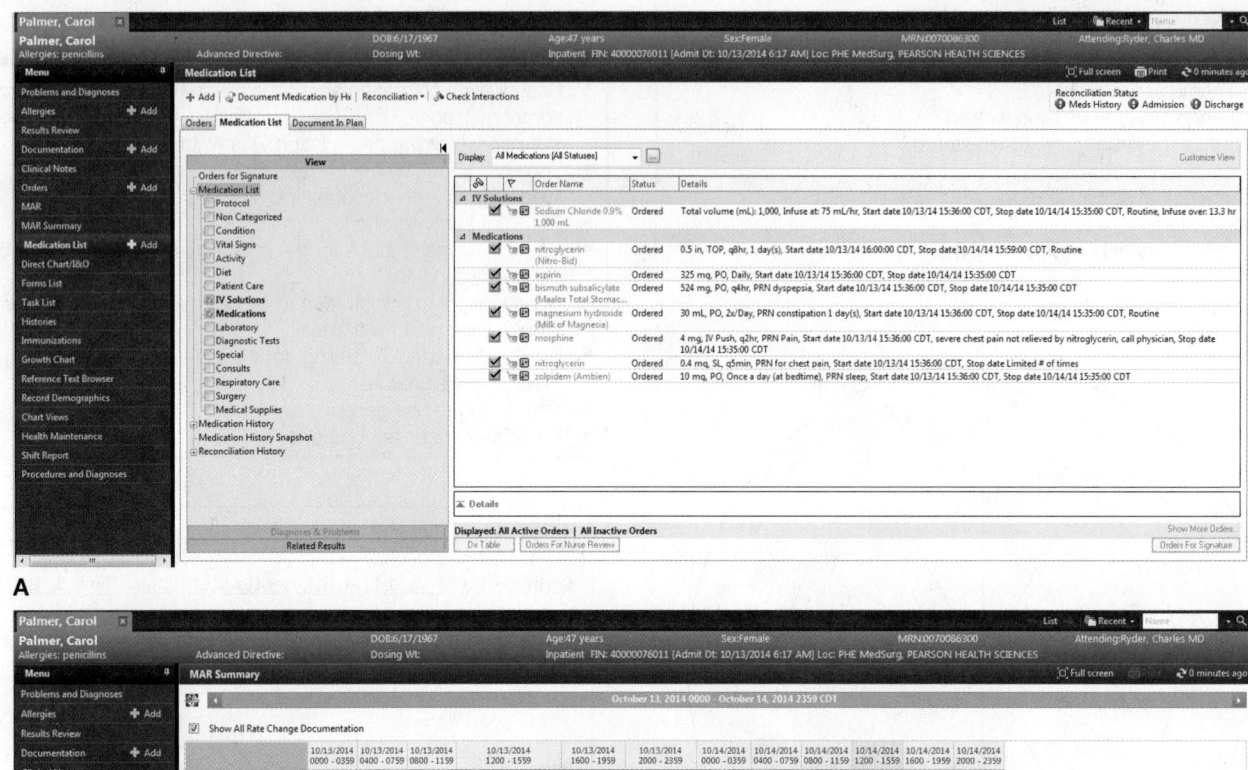

Figure 15–6 ■ Sample EHR forms: *A,* Medication list; *B,* medication administration record (MAR) summary.
"Sample EHR Components" from Cerner Electronic Health Record. Copyright © by Cerner Corporation. Used by permission of Cerner Corporation.

some agencies, the date the order was prescribed and the date the order expires are also included.

The nurse should always question the primary care provider about any order that is illegible, ambiguous, unusual (e.g., an abnormally high dosage of a medication), or contraindicated by the client's condition. When the nurse judges a primary care provider–ordered medication inappropriate, the following actions are required:

- Contact the primary care provider and discuss the rationale for believing the medication order to be inappropriate.
- Document the following in notes: when the primary care provider was notified, what was conveyed to the primary care provider, and how the primary care provider responded.
- If the primary care provider cannot be reached, document all attempts to contact the primary care provider and the reason for withholding the medication.
- If someone else gives the medication, document data about the client's condition before and after the medication.

- If an incident report is indicated, clearly document factual information.

ADMINISTERING MEDICATIONS SAFELY

The nurse should always assess a client's health status and obtain a medication history prior to giving any medication. The extent of the assessment depends on the client's illness or current condition, the intended drug, and the route of administration. For example, if a client has dyspnea, the nurse assesses respirations carefully before administering any medication that might affect breathing. It is also important to determine whether the route of administration is suitable. For example, a client who is nauseated may not be able to retain a drug taken orally. In general, the nurse assesses the client *prior* to administering any medication to obtain baseline data by which to evaluate the effectiveness of the medication.

The **medication history** includes information about the drugs the client is taking currently or has taken recently. This includes

PRACTICE GUIDELINES

Administering Medications

- Nurses who administer medications are responsible for their own actions. Question any order that is illegible or that you consider incorrect. Call the person who prescribed the medication for clarification.
- Be knowledgeable about the medications you administer. You need to know why the client is receiving the medication. Look up the necessary information if you are not familiar with the medication.
- Federal laws govern the use of narcotics and barbiturates. Keep these medications in a locked place.
- Use only medications that are in a clearly labeled container.
- Do not use liquid medications that are cloudy or have changed color.
- Calculate drug doses accurately. If you are uncertain, ask another nurse to double-check your calculations.
- Administer only medications you have personally prepared.
- Before administering a medication, verify the client's identity using appropriate means of identification, such as checking the identification bracelet.

- Do not leave medications at the bedside, with certain exceptions (e.g., nitroglycerin, cough syrup). Check agency policy.
- If a client vomits after taking an oral medication, report this to the nurse in charge, or the primary care provider, or both.
- Take special precautions when administering certain medications; for example, have another nurse check the dosages of anticoagulants, insulin, and certain IV preparations.
- Most hospital policies require new orders from the primary care provider for a client's postsurgery care.
- When a medication is omitted for any reason, record the fact together with the reason.
- When a medication error is made, report it immediately to the nurse in charge, the primary care provider, or both. In addition, an incident report will need to be completed per agency policy.
- Always check the medication's expiration date.
- Wash hands between clients. Hand antiseptic gels are appropriate if hands are not visibly soiled. Hand washing with soap and water is required for visibly soiled hands.

---

prescription drugs; over-the-counter (OTC) drugs such as herbals, antacids, alcohol, and tobacco; and nonsanctioned drugs such as marijuana. Sometimes an incompatibility with one or more of these drugs affects the choice of a new medication.

Older adults often take vitamins, herbs, and food supplements, and/or use folk remedies that they do not list in their medication history. Because many of these have unknown or unpredictable actions and side effects, they need to be noted, with attention paid to possible incompatibilities with prescribed medications.

An important part of the history is the client's knowledge of his or her drug allergies. Some clients can tell a nurse, "I am allergic to penicillin, adhesive tape, and curry." The nurse should clarify with the client any side effects, adverse reactions, or allergic responses due to medications. Other clients may not be sure about allergic reactions. An illness occurring after a drug was taken may not be identified as an allergy, but the client may associate the drug with an illness or unusual reaction. The client's primary care provider can often give information about allergies. During the history, the nurse tries to elicit information about drug dependencies. How often drugs are taken and the client's perceived need for them are measures of dependence.

Also included in the history are the client's normal eating habits. Sometimes the medication schedule needs to be coordinated with mealtimes or the ingestion of foods. Where a medication must be taken with food on a specified schedule, clients can often adjust their mealtime or have a snack (e.g., with a bedtime medication). In addition, certain foods are incompatible with certain medications; for example, milk is incompatible with tetracycline.

It is also important for the nurse to identify any problems the client may have in self-administering a medication. A client with poor eyesight, for example, may require special labels for the medication container; older clients with unsteady hands may not be able to hold a syringe or to inject themselves or another person. Obtaining information as to how and where clients store their medications is also important. If clients have difficulty opening certain containers, they may change containers but fail to remove old labels, which increases the risk of medication errors.

The nurse needs to consider socioeconomic factors for all clients, but especially for older clients. Two common problems are lack

of transportation to obtain medications and inadequate finances to purchase medications. When aware of these problems, the nurse can refer the client to appropriate social service agencies to ensure that medications are purchased.

Clinical guidelines for administering medications are given in Practice Guidelines.

Medication Administration Errors

The National Coordinating Council for Medication Error Reporting and Prevention (NCC MERP) (2013) estimates that 98,000 people die annually from medical errors that occur in hospitals and that a significant number of those deaths are due to medication errors. The NCC MERP defines a medication error as "any preventable event that may cause or lead to inappropriate medication use or patient harm while the medication is in the control of the health care professional, patient, or consumer. Such events may be related to professional practice, health care products, procedures, and systems, including prescribing; order communication; product labeling, packaging, and nomenclature; compounding; dispensing; distribution; administration; education; monitoring; and use" (para. 2).

Medication errors can occur at all stages of the medication administration process. Tzeng, Yin, and Schneider (2013, p. 14) describe the four main types of medication errors in hospitalized clients: (1) prescription errors (e.g., wrong drug or dose), (2) transcription/interpretation error (e.g., misinterpretation of abbreviations), (3) preparation errors (e.g., calculation error), and (4) administration errors (e.g., wrong dose, wrong time, omission or additional dose). Most medication errors occur during the administration stage.

Medication administration errors result from system and individual factors. Individual factors include fatigue and stress. Many studies report medication errors related to the system factor of interruptions and distractions that occur during medication administration. Research has demonstrated that interruptions create a greater risk for and severity of errors in medication administration (Flanders & Clark, 2010, p. 282). Interruptions and distractions hinder the ability of the nurse to stay focused on the task. In addition, after an interruption, the nurse needs additional time to refocus their concentration and determine what has been done and remains to be done—all of which increase the risk for error (Clark &

Flanders, 2012; Lewis, Smith, & Williams-Jones, 2012). Many nurses pride themselves on being able to multitask. Scientists who study short-term memory, however, agree that the less a person tries to hold in mind at one time, the better. Clark and Flanders (2012) report that "research into the effects of interruptions and multitasking is accumulating and has a consistent theme—the brain is not capable of multitasking" (p. 242). This is especially true during medication administration.

Of interest are the studies that investigated the sources of interruption during medication administration. Sources include overhead pages, monitor alarms, telephone calls, and family inquiries, with the most common source being questions from nursing colleagues and other health care team members (Flanders & Clark, 2010; Hall et al., 2010; Lewis et al., 2012). As a result, some studies have evaluated the effectiveness of interventions to reduce interruptions and distractions during medication administration. Strategies to reduce interruptions include using a medication safety checklist, placing signs outside and within medication rooms to promote a quiet environment, having others take nonurgent telephone calls for the nurse who is administering medications, creating a "No Interruption" or "Quiet Zone" by placing red duct tape around the medication cart and/or medication dispensing machines. The red-taped area indicates "do not disturb with nonurgent matters" to others. Another approach is where the nurse wears a bright, colorful *Do Not Disturb* sash or vest during medication administration (Flanders & Clark, 2010; Klejka, 2012). All the studies have shown that one or more of these strategies has resulted in reduced medication errors.

Nurses play an important role in medication safety because they perform the last safety checks before a medication is administered to a client. Therefore, it is important for health care leaders to recognize the complexity of the nurse's environment and the importance of medication administration, and examine ways to reduce system factors that impact client safety, such as interruptions during medication administration.

Medication Reconciliation

Another safety issue that affects the nurse is the need to ensure that clients receive the appropriate medications and dosages as they move or transition through a facility. The Institute for Healthcare Improvement (IHI) (2011b) defines **medication reconciliation** as "the process of creating the most accurate list possible of all medications a patient is taking—including drug name, dosage, frequency, and route—and comparing that list against the physician's admission, transfer, and/or discharge orders, with the goal of providing correct medications to the patient at all transition points within the hospital." Preventing adverse drug events (ADEs) is the incentive behind the idea of medication reconciliation. More than half of hospital medication errors occur when clients transition in care both within and outside of the organization (IHI, 2011a; The Joint Commission, 2013b).

All facilities accredited by The Joint Commission must have protocols and processes in place for medication reconciliation, particularly in the following transition areas: on admission, during transfer between units, and at discharge. See Box 15–3 for an overview of the elements of medication reconciliation. The nurse needs to make a complete list of the client's medications (including prescriptions, vitamins, supplements, and OTC medications) on admission. This current list needs to be compared to any new medications ordered by the primary care provider on admission and during the client's hospital stay. Medications that are to be administered around the time of shift report need to be discussed at the report. For example, insulin is a common medication scheduled between night and day shifts. It is important for the oncoming nurse to know if the medication was given or not. If a client is

---

BOX 15–3 Elements of Medication Reconciliation

The Joint Commission (2013a) requires that medication reconciliation occur:

- *At admission:* Collect a list of the medications the client is currently taking when he or she is admitted to the hospital or seen in an outpatient setting (p. 5).
- *At discharge:* Consult the client's home medication list and current medication orders, and compare them with the discharge medication orders to ensure that medications are appropriately continued, resumed, or discontinued. Provide the client (or family) with written information about the medications the client should be taking when discharged from the hospital or outpatient setting. Explain the importance of managing medication information to the client upon discharge (p. 6).

The Institute for Health Care Improvement (2011a) recommends medication reconciliation also occur when transferring the client from one level of care to another. That is, compare the medication information the client brought to the hospital with the current medications ordered for the client by the hospital, and the transfer orders to identify and resolve any discrepancies (p. 9).

---

transferred to another setting, within or outside the facility, a complete list of the client's medications must be communicated to the next provider of care. This list is also provided to clients on discharge from the facility. In addition, the client should receive, at discharge, written and oral information on each medication to be taken at home. It is important for the nurse to emphasize to clients the importance of keeping the list of their medications and taking it with them to their follow-up visits and to future hospitalizations, if any. Maintaining their list of current medications helps improve communication and avoid potential errors in medication administration. The U.S. Food and Drug Administration (2011) developed a form called "My Medicine Record" to help consumers keep track of their prescription medications, OTC drugs, and dietary supplements. This form is available online and can be downloaded. Individuals can then complete it by either writing in the information or entering the information on their computers and printing it.

Medication Dispensing Systems

Medical facilities vary in their medication dispensing systems. The systems can include the following:

- *Medication cart.* The medication cart is on wheels, allowing the nurse to move the cart to outside the client's room. The cart contains small numbered drawers that correlate with the room numbers on the nursing unit (Figure 15–7 ■). The drawer holds the client's medications for the shift or 24 hours. The medication is usually in unit-dose packaging; that is, the individual drug package states the drug name, dose, and expiration date (Figure 15–8 ■).

SAFETY ALERT! | SAFETY

2014 The Joint Commission National Patient Safety Goals (2013a)

GOAL 3: MAINTAIN AND COMMUNICATE ACCURATE CLIENT MEDICATION INFORMATION.
Rationale: *There is evidence that medication discrepancies can affect client outcomes.* Medication reconciliation is intended to identify and resolve discrepancies—it is a process of comparing the medications a client is taking (and should be taking) with newly ordered medications. The comparison addresses duplication, omissions, and interactions, and the need to continue current medications.

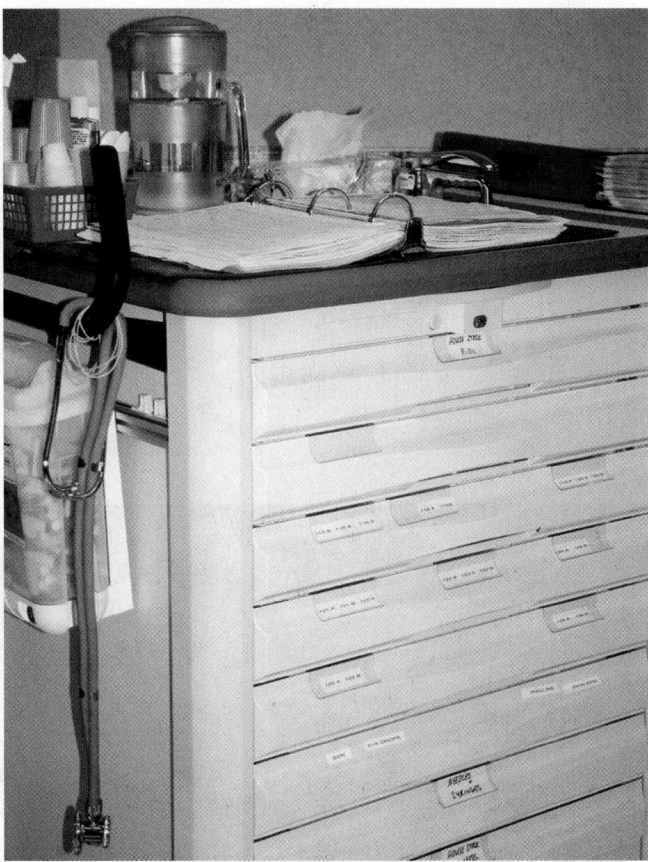

Figure 15–7 ■ Medication cart.

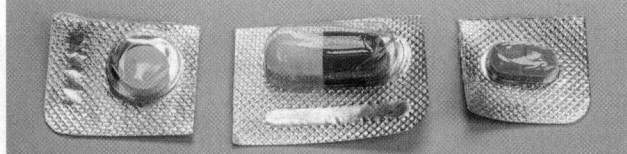

Figure 15–8 ■ Unit-dose medication packages.

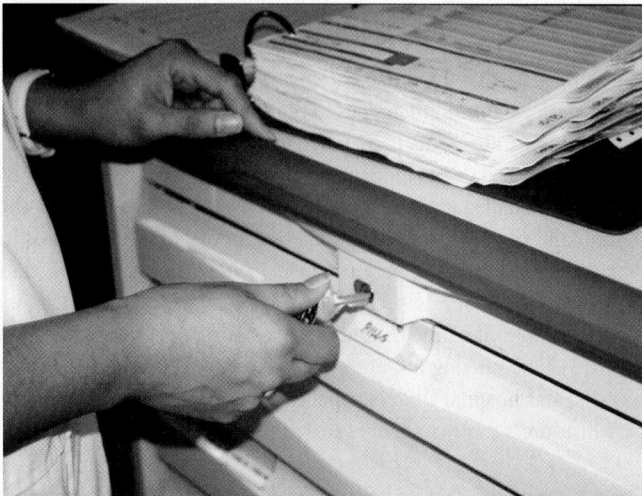

Figure 15–9 ■ The medication cart is kept locked when not in use. The nurse is using a key to access client medications.

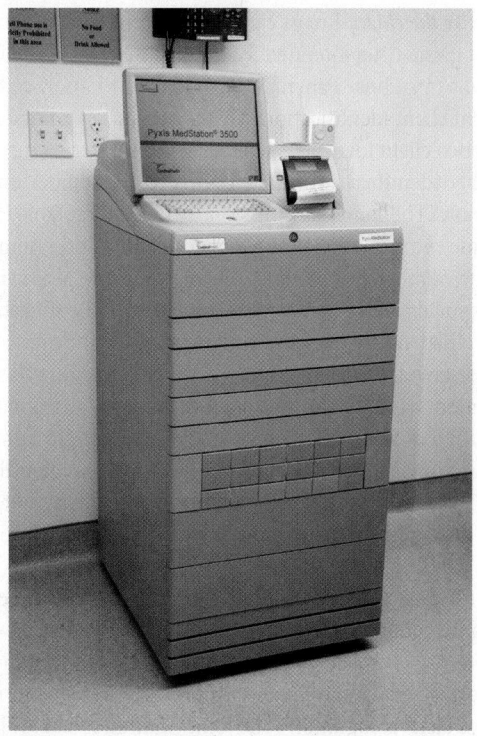

Figure 15–10 ■ Automated dispensing cabinet (ADC).

A larger locked drawer in the cart contains the controlled substances rather than keeping them in the client's individual drawer. The cart may also include a supply drawer that contains client-labeled bulk containers, such as Metamucil, and/or supplies such as syringes. The MAR is usually located in a binder or a computer located on top of the medication cart. The medication cart must be kept locked when not in use, so the nurse either carries a key for the medication cart or enters a special code to open it (Figure 15–9 ■).

- *Medication cabinet.* Some facilities have a locked cabinet in the client's room. This cabinet holds the client's unit-dose medications and MAR. Controlled substances are not kept in this cabinet but at another location on the nursing unit. The nurse uses either a key or a special code for opening the client's medication cabinet, because it must be locked when not in use.
- *Medication room.* Depending on the facility, a medication room may be used for a variety of purposes. For example, the medication carts, when not in use, may be placed in this room. The medication room may also be the central location for stock medications, controlled medications, and/or drugs used for emergencies. The medication room may have a refrigerator for intravenous and other medications needing a cold environment. The room may also contain other

medication administration supplies (syringes, needles, etc.). Nurses access the medication room with either a key or a special code because the room is often kept locked. Check agency policy.

- *Automated dispensing cabinet (ADC).* This computerized access system (Figure 15–10 ■) automates the distribution, management, and control of medications. Similar to automated teller machines, the nurse uses a password to access the system, selects the client's name from an on-screen list, and selects the medication(s). More than 80% of hospitals use ADCs (Stachowiak, 2013). The benefit of using ADCs is the reduction in the risk for medication errors. These benefits include improved drug security, inventory control, computerized alerts, and the potential to limit access to certain high-alert drugs (Mandrack et al., 2012, p. 135). To further promote safety, many facilities have instituted a pharmacy profiling system as part of the ADC. This means that a nurse cannot remove a medication from an ADC unless a pharmacist has reviewed the order and released the medication. The expectation of the ISMP is that the nurse obtains the medications for one client from the ADC and then goes to the client's bedside to administer the medications. This is a challenge for nurses because of the increased time it would take to administer medications to six clients. Another challenge is that there are often not enough ADCs on the unit and the nurses wait in line to access the ADC. This leads to rushed medication selection, errors in medication removal, and unsafe workarounds such as removing more than one client's medications at a time (Mandrack et al., 2012, p. 138; Stachowiak, 2013). The nursing literature recommends that nurses, pharmacists, and hospital leaders collaborate and discuss a process that will address these challenges and improve ADC safety.

Process of Administering Medications

When administering any drug, regardless of the route of administration, the nurse must do the following:

1. *Identify the client.* Errors can and do occur, usually because one client gets a drug intended for another. One of The Joint Commission's National Patient Safety Goals is to improve the accuracy of client identification. This goal requires a nurse to use at least two client identifiers whenever administering medications. Neither identifier can be the client's room number or physical location (The Joint Commission, 2013a). Acceptable identifiers include the person's name, assigned identification number, telephone number, photograph, or other person-specific identifier. In hospitals, most clients wear some sort of identification, such as a wristband with name and hospital identification number. Before giving the client any drug, always check the client's identification band. Some hospitals use bar-code technology for medication administration. A nurse preparing to administer a medication using bar-code technology scans or enters the nurse's own ID, the client's wristband, and each package of medication to be administered. Bar coding often includes two or more person-specific identifiers, which meets the identifier requirement (Figure 15–11 ■). In the long-term care and home care settings, the requirement for two identifiers is appropriate at the first encounter. Thereafter, and in any situation of continuing one-to-one care in which the clinician knows the resident, one identifier can be facial recognition (The Joint Commission, 2013b).

2. *Inform the client.* If the client is unfamiliar with the medication, the nurse should explain the intended action as well as any side effects or adverse effects that might occur. Listen to the client. It

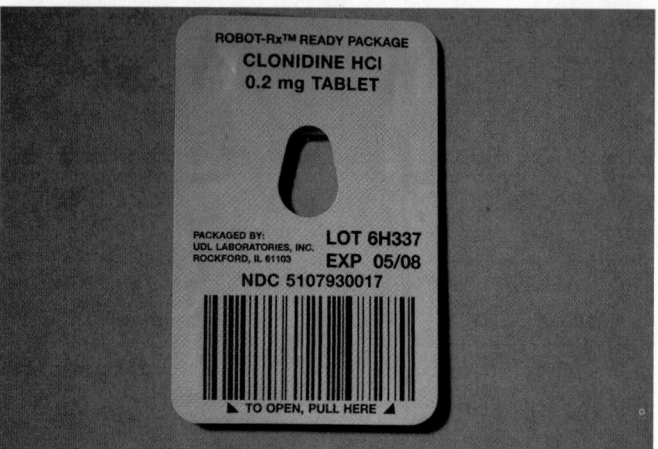

A

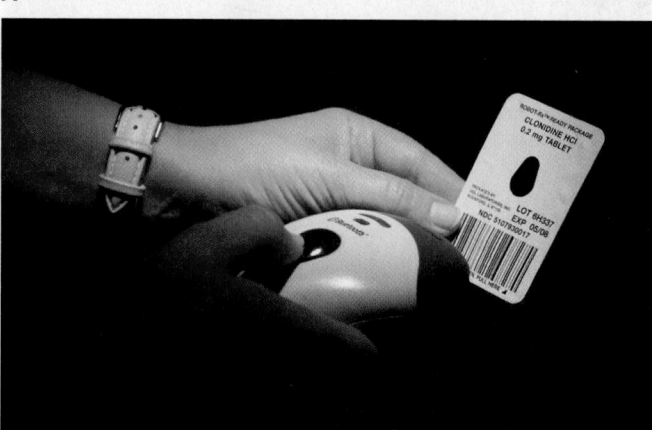

B

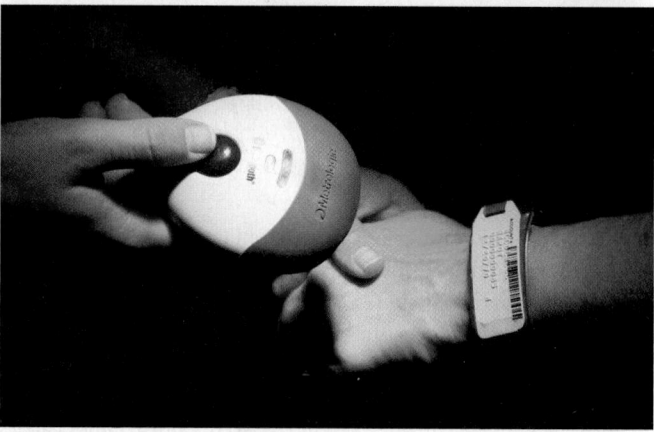

C

Figure 15–11 ■ *A,* A sample bar code. *B,* The nurse scans the bar code on the medication package and *C,* the bar code on the client's wristband before administering the medication.

CLINICAL ALERT!

Do not ask "Are you John Jones?" because the client may answer "yes" to the wrong name. Ask "What is your name?"

is easy to get so focused on the task of timely medication administration that the nurse may miss relevant information provided by the client. For example, if the client says that he doesn't take a pill for high blood pressure, this should be an "alert" for the nurse to stop and check if this is the correct medication for that client.

SAFETY ALERT!   SAFETY

2014 The Joint Commission National Patient Safety Goals (2013a)

GOAL 1: IMPROVE THE ACCURACY OF PATIENT IDENTIFICATION.

- Use at least two patient identifiers when providing care, treatment, and services. **Rationale:** *Wrong-patient errors occur in virtually all stages of diagnosis and treatment. The intent for this goal is twofold: first, to reliably identify the individual as the person for whom the service or treatment is intended; second, to match the service or treatment to that individual.* Acceptable identifiers may be the individual's name, an assigned identification number, telephone number, or other person-specific identifier.

Check Three Times for Safe Medication Administration

FIRST CHECK

- Read the MAR and remove the medication(s) from the client's drawer. Verify that the client's name and room number match the MAR.
- Compare the label of the medication against the MAR.
- If the dosage does not match the MAR, determine if you need to do a math calculation.
- Check the expiration date of the medication.

SECOND CHECK

- While preparing the medication (e.g., pouring, drawing up, or placing unopened package in a medication cup), look at the medication label and check against the MAR.

THIRD CHECK

- Recheck the label on the container (e.g., vial, bottle, or unused unit-dose medications) against the MAR before returning to its storage place *OR* before giving the medication to the client.

3. *Administer the drug.* Read the MAR carefully and perform three checks with the labeled medications (Box 15–4). Then administer the medication in the prescribed dosage, by the route ordered, and at the correct time. There has recently been a change in what is considered the correct time. Historically, there has been the "30-minute rule" (i.e., administer medications within 30 minutes before or after the scheduled time). In medication error research, one third of reported medication errors were wrong-time errors (Stokowski, 2012). Moreover, the ISMP conducted an extensive survey in 2010 and the 18,000 nurses who responded clearly stated that the "30-minute rule" was unsafe, impossible to follow given the current complex nature of medication administration, and created pressure to take shortcuts, which led to errors (ISMP, 2011). The ISMP maintains that "timely medication administration is a multifaceted issue that cannot be managed appropriately with a single standard" (Stokowski, 2012). Subsequently, the ISMP developed new guidelines for timely administration of scheduled medications. These guidelines are to be used as a resource for hospitals as they develop their own specific guidelines for their facility through an interdisciplinary team that includes nurses. The underlying principle of the guidelines is that medication administration still has to be timely; however, hospitals can determine which medications should be on a tight time

schedule and which can be administered with greater flexibility at the discretion of the nurse (ISMP, 2011; Stokowski, 2012). See Table 15–4 for the ISMP guidelines for timely medication administration.

Certain aspects of medication administration are important for the nurse to check each time a medication is administered. These are referred to as the "rights." Traditionally, there were five rights to medication administration. More rights have been added during the past few years with the most comprehensive being the ten rights (Bryant, 2011; Elliott & Liu, 2010). See Box 15–5.

4. *Provide adjunctive interventions as indicated.* Clients may need help when receiving medications. They may require physical assistance, for instance, in assuming positions for intramuscular injections, or they may need guidance about measures to enhance drug effectiveness and prevent complications, such as drinking fluids. Some clients convey fear about their medications. The nurse can relieve fears by listening carefully to clients' concerns and giving correct information.

5. *Record the drug administered.* The facts recorded in the chart, in ink or by computer printout, are the name of the drug, dosage, method of administration, specific relevant data such as pulse rate (taken in most settings prior to the administration of digitalis), and any other pertinent information. The record should also include the exact time of administration and the signature of the nurse providing the medication. Many medication records are designed so that the nurse signs once on the page and initials each medication administered. Often, medications that are given regularly are recorded on a special flow record. The prn (as-needed) or stat (at once) medications are recorded separately.

6. *Evaluate the client's response to the drug.* The kinds of behavior that reflect the action or lack of action of a drug and its untoward effects (both minor and major) are as variable as the purpose of the drug. The anxious client may show the desired effects of a tranquilizer by behavior that reflects a lowered stress level (e.g., slower speech or fewer random movements). How well a client slept can often measure the effectiveness of a sedative, and the effectiveness of an analgesic can be measured by how much pain the client feels. In all nursing activities, nurses need to be aware of the medications that a client is taking and record their effectiveness as assessed by the client and the nurse on the client's chart. The nurse may also report the client's response directly to the nurse manager and primary care provider.

TABLE 15–4 **Acute Care Guidelines for Timely Administration of Scheduled Medications**

Type of Scheduled Medication	Goals for Timely Administration
Time-Critical Scheduled Medications	
Hospital-defined time-critical medications* * Limited number of drugs where delayed or early administration of more than 30 minutes may cause harm or sub-therapeutic effect Includes but not limited to: Medications with a dosing schedule more frequent than every 4 hours	Administer at the **exact time indicated when necessary** (e.g., rapid-acting insulin), **otherwise, within 30 minutes** before or after the scheduled time
Non-Time-Critical Scheduled Medications	
Daily, weekly, monthly medications	**Within 2 hours** before or after the scheduled time
Medications prescribed more frequently than daily, but no more frequently than every 4 hours	**Within 1 hour** before or after the scheduled time

BOX 15–5   Ten "Rights" of Medication Administration

RIGHT MEDICATION
- The medication given was the medication ordered.

RIGHT DOSE
- The dose ordered is appropriate for the client.
- Give special attention if the calculation indicates multiple pills/tablets or a large quantity of a liquid medication. This can be an indication that the math calculation may be incorrect.
- Double-check calculations that appear questionable.
- Know the usual dosage range of the medication.
- Question a dose outside of the usual dosage range.

RIGHT TIME
- Give the medication at the right frequency and at the time ordered according to agency policy.
- Medications should be given within the agency guidelines.

RIGHT ROUTE
- Give the medication by the ordered route.
- Make certain that the route is safe and appropriate for the client.

RIGHT CLIENT
- Make sure medication is given to the intended client.
- Check the client's identification band with each administration of a medication.
- Know the agency's name alert procedure when clients with the same or similar last names are on the nursing unit.

RIGHT CLIENT EDUCATION
- Explain information about the medication to the client (e.g., why receiving, what to expect, any precautions).

RIGHT DOCUMENTATION
- Document medication administration after giving it, not before.
- If time of administration differs from prescribed time, note the time on the MAR and explain reason and follow-through activities (e.g., pharmacy states medication will be available in 2 hours) in nursing notes.
- If a medication is not given, follow the agency's policy for documenting the reason why.

RIGHT TO REFUSE
- Adult clients have the right to refuse any medication.
- The nurse's role is to ensure that the client is fully informed of the potential consequences of refusal and to communicate the client's refusal to the health care provider.

RIGHT ASSESSMENT
- Some medications require specific assessments prior to administration (e.g., apical pulse, blood pressure, lab results).
- Medication orders may include specific parameters for administration (e.g., do not give if pulse less than 60 or systolic blood pressure less than 100).

RIGHT EVALUATION
- Conduct appropriate follow-up (e.g., Was the desired effect achieved or not? Did the client experience any side effects or adverse reactions?).

Oral Medications

The oral route is the most common route by which medications are given. As long as a client can swallow and retain the drug in the stomach, this is the route of choice (see Skill 15–1). Oral medications are contraindicated when a client is vomiting, has gastric or intestinal suction, or is unconscious and unable to swallow. Such clients in a hospital are usually on orders for "nothing by mouth" (Latin *nil per os*: **NPO**).

●○● NURSING PROCESS: ORAL MEDICATIONS

Administering Oral Medications

SKILL 15–1

ASSESSMENT
Assess:
- Allergies to medication(s).
- Client's ability to swallow the medication.
- Presence of vomiting or diarrhea that would interfere with the ability to absorb the medication.
- Specific drug action, side effects, interactions, and adverse reactions.
- Client's knowledge of and learning needs about the medication.

- Perform appropriate assessments (e.g., vital signs, laboratory results) specific to the medication.
- Determine if the assessment data influence administration of the medication (i.e., is it appropriate to administer the medication or does the medication need to be held and the prescriber notified?).

PLANNING
DELEGATION

In acute care settings, administration of oral/enteral medications is performed by the nurse and is not delegated to unlicensed assistive personnel (UAP). The nurse can inform the UAP of the intended therapeutic effects and/or specific side effects of the medication and request the UAP to report specific client observations to the nurse for follow-up. In some states, trained UAP may administer certain medications to stable clients in long-term care settings. It is important, however, for the nurse to remember that the medication knowledge of the UAP is limited and *assessment and evaluation of the effectiveness of the medication remain the responsibility of the nurse*.

Equipment
- Dispensing system
- Disposable medication cups: small paper or plastic cups for tablets and capsules, waxed or plastic calibrated medication cups for liquids
- MAR or computer printout
- Pill crusher/cutter
- Straws to administer medications that may discolor the teeth or to facilitate the ingestion of liquid medication for certain clients
- Drinking glass and water or juice
- Soft foods such as applesauce or pudding to use for crushed medications for clients who may choke on liquids

Administering Oral Medications—*continued*

IMPLEMENTATION
Preparation

- Know the reason why the client is receiving the medication, the drug classification, contraindications, usual dosage range, side effects, and nursing considerations for administering and evaluating the intended outcomes for the medication.
- Check the MAR.
- Check for the drug name, dosage, frequency, route of administration, and expiration date for administering the medication, if appropriate. **Rationale:** *Orders for certain medications (e.g., narcotics, antibiotics) expire after a specified time frame, and they need to be reordered by the primary care provider.*
  - If the MAR is unclear or pertinent information is missing, compare the MAR with the prescriber's most recent written order.
  - Report any discrepancies to the charge nurse or the prescriber, as agency policy dictates.
- Verify the client's ability to take medication orally.
  - Determine whether the client can swallow, is NPO, is nauseated or vomiting, has gastric suction, or has diminished or absent bowel sounds.
- Organize the supplies.
  - Gather the MAR(s) for each client so that medications can be prepared for one client at a time. **Rationale:** *Organization of supplies saves time and reduces the chance of error.*

Performance

1. Perform hand hygiene and observe other appropriate infection prevention procedures.
2. Unlock the dispensing system.
3. Obtain appropriate medication.
   - Read the MAR and take the appropriate medication from the shelf, drawer, or refrigerator. The medication may be dispensed in a bottle, box, or unit-dose package.
   - Compare the label of the medication container or unit-dose package against the order on the MAR or computer printout. **Rationale:** *This is a safety check to ensure that the right medication is given.* If these are not identical, recheck the prescriber's written order in the client's chart. If there is still a discrepancy, check with the nurse in charge or the pharmacist. ❶
   - Check the expiration date of the medication. Return expired medications to the pharmacy. **Rationale:** *Outdated medications are not safe to administer.*
   - Use only medications that have clear, legible labels. **Rationale:** *This ensures accuracy.*
4. Prepare the medication.
   - Calculate the medication dosage accurately.

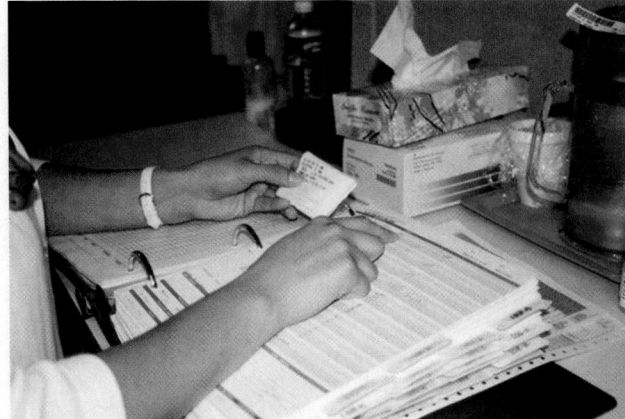

❶ Compare the medication label to the MAR.

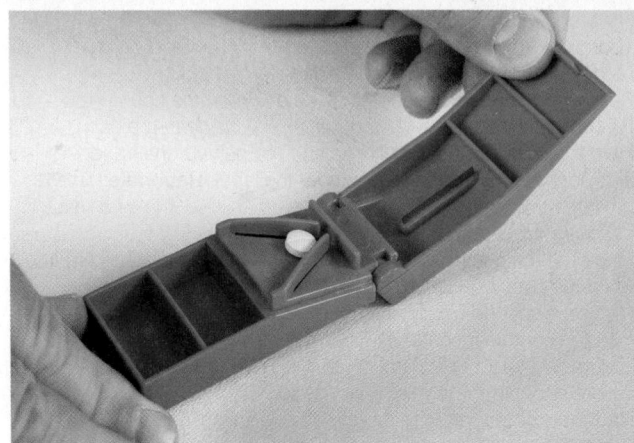

❷ A cutting device can be used to divide tablets.

- Prepare the correct amount of medication for the required dose, without contaminating the medication. **Rationale:** *Aseptic technique maintains drug cleanliness.*
- While preparing the medication, recheck each prepared drug and container with the MAR again. **Rationale:** *This second safety check reduces the chance of error.*

Tablets or Capsules

- Place packaged unit-dose capsules or tablets directly into the medicine cup. Do not remove the medication from the package until at the bedside. **Rationale:** *The wrapper keeps the medication clean. Not removing the medication facilitates identification of the medication in the event the client refuses the drug or assessment data indicate to hold the medication. Unopened unit-dose packages can usually be returned to the medication cart.*
- If using a stock container, pour the required number into the bottle cap, and then transfer the medication to the disposable cup without touching the tablets.
- Keep narcotics and medications that require specific assessments, such as pulse measurements, respiratory rate or depth, or blood pressure, separate from the others. **Rationale:** *This reminds the nurse to complete the needed assessment(s) in order to decide whether to give the medication or to withhold the medication if indicated.*
- Break only scored tablets if necessary to obtain the correct dosage. Use a cutting or splitting device if needed. ❷ Check agency policy to determine how unused portions of a medication are to be discarded.
- If the client has difficulty swallowing, check if the medication can be crushed. Some drug handbooks have an appendix that lists the "do not crush" medications. The ISMP (2013b) provides on its website an updated list of medications that should not be crushed. Some medications that should not be crushed include time-released and enteric-coated medications. An example of a tablet that should not be crushed is oxycodone (OxyContin), a long-acting narcotic that normally lasts 12 hours after administration. Tablet disruption may cause a potentially fatal overdose of oxycodone.
- If it is acceptable, crush the tablets to a fine powder with a pill crusher or between two medication cups. Then, mix the powder with a small amount of soft food (e.g., custard, applesauce).

CLINICAL ALERT!

Check with the pharmacy before crushing tablets. Sustained-action, enteric-coated, buccal, or sublingual tablets should not be crushed.

Continued on page 378

Administering Oral Medications—*continued*

Liquid Medication

- Thoroughly mix the medication before pouring. Discard any medication that has changed color or turned cloudy.
- Remove the cap and place it upside down on the countertop. **Rationale:** *This avoids contaminating the inside of the cap.*
- Hold the bottle so the label is next to the palm of the hand and pour the medication away from the label. **Rationale:** *This prevents the label from becoming soiled and illegible as a result of spilled liquids.* ❸
- Place the medication cup on a flat surface at eye level and fill it to the desired level, using the bottom of the **meniscus** (crescent-shaped upper surface of a column of liquid) to align with the container scale. ❹ **Rationale:** *This method ensures accuracy of measurement.*
- Before capping the bottle, wipe the lip with a paper towel. **Rationale:** *This prevents the cap from sticking.*
- When giving small amounts of liquids (e.g., less than 5 mL), prepare the medication in a sterile syringe without the needle or in a specially designed oral syringe. ❺ Label the syringe with the name of the medication and the route (PO). **Rationale:** *Any oral solution removed from the original container and placed into a syringe should be labeled to avoid medications being given by the wrong route (e.g., IV). This practice facilitates client safety and avoids tragic errors.*
- Keep unit-dose liquids in their package and open them at the bedside.

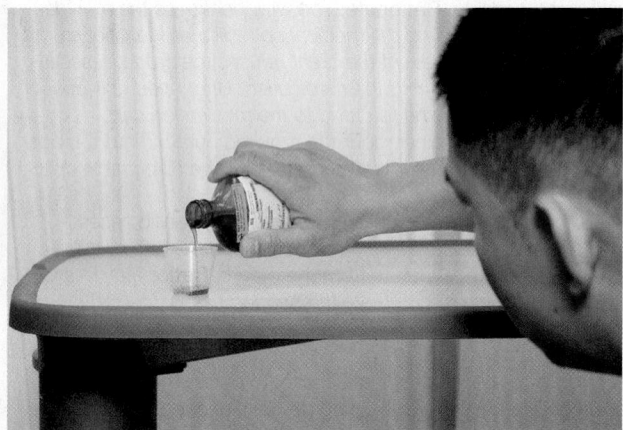

❸ Pouring a liquid medication from a bottle.

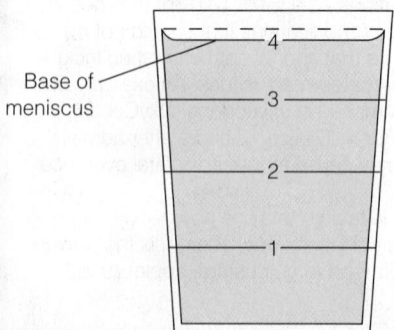

Base of meniscus

❹ The *bottom* of the curved meniscus is the measuring guide.

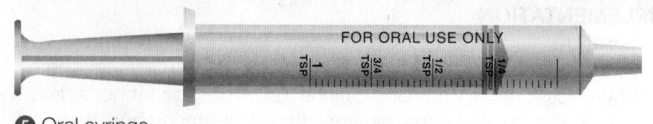

FOR ORAL USE ONLY

❺ Oral syringe.

SAFETY ALERT! [SAFETY]

2014 The Joint Commission National Patient Safety Goals (2013a)

GOAL 3: IMPROVE THE SAFETY OF USING MEDICATIONS.

- Label all medications, medication containers, and other solutions on and off the sterile field in perioperative and other procedural settings.
- Medication containers include syringes, medicine cups, and basins. **Rationale:** *Medications or other solutions in unlabeled containers are unidentifiable. Errors, sometimes tragic, have resulted from medications and other solutions being removed from their original containers and placed into unlabeled containers. This unsafe practice neglects basic principles of safe medication management, yet it is routine in many organizations. The labeling of all medications, medication containers, and other solutions is a risk-reduction activity consistent with safe medication management. This practice addresses a recognized risk point in the administration of medications in perioperative and other procedural settings.*

Oral Narcotics

- If an agency uses a manual recording system for controlled substances, check the narcotic record for the previous drug count and compare it with the supply available. Some medications, including narcotics, are kept in plastic containers that are sectioned and numbered.
- Remove the next available tablet and drop it in the medicine cup.
- After removing a tablet, record the necessary information on the appropriate narcotic control record and sign it.
- *Note:* Computer-controlled dispensing systems allow access only to the selected drug and automatically record its use.

All Medications

- Place the prepared medication and MAR together on the medication cart.
- Recheck the label on the container before returning the bottle, box, or envelope to its storage place. **Rationale:** *This third check further reduces the risk of error.*
- Avoid leaving prepared medications unattended. **Rationale:** *This precaution prevents potential mishandling errors.*
- Lock the medication cart before entering the client's room. **Rationale:** *This is a safety measure because medication carts are not to be left open when unattended.*
- Check the room number against the MAR if agency policy does not allow the MAR to be removed from the medication cart. **Rationale:** *This is another safety measure to ensure that the nurse is entering the correct client room.*

5. Provide for client privacy.
6. Prepare the client.
   - Introduce self and verify the client's identity using agency protocol. **Rationale:** *This ensures that the right client receives the medication.*
   - Assist the client to a sitting position or, if not possible, to a side-lying position. **Rationale:** *These positions facilitate swallowing and prevent aspiration.*

Administering Oral Medications—*continued*

- If not previously assessed, take the required assessment measures, such as pulse and respiratory rates or blood pressure. Take the apical pulse rate before administering digitalis preparations. Take the blood pressure before giving antihypertensive drugs. Take the respiratory rate prior to administering opioids. **Rationale:** *Opioids depress the respiratory center. If any of the findings are above or below the predetermined parameters, consult the primary care provider before administering the medication.*

7. Explain the purpose of the medication and how it will help, using language that the client can understand. Include relevant information about effects; for example, tell the client receiving a diuretic to expect an increase in urine output. **Rationale:** *Information can facilitate acceptance of and compliance with the therapy.*

8. Administer the medication at the correct time.
   - Take the medication to the client within the guidelines of the agency.
   - Give the client sufficient water or preferred juice to swallow the medication. Before using juice, check for any food and medication incompatibilities. **Rationale:** *Fluids ease swallowing and facilitate absorption from the gastrointestinal tract. Grapefruit juice may not be safe for clients who take certain medications.* Liquid medications other than antacids or cough preparations may be diluted with 15 mL (1/2 oz) of water to facilitate absorption.
   - If the client is unable to hold the pill cup, use the pill cup to introduce the medication into the client's mouth, and give only one tablet or capsule at a time. **Rationale:** *Putting the cup to the client's mouth maintains the cleanliness of the nurse's hands. Giving one medication at a time eases swallowing.*
   - If an older child or adult has difficulty swallowing, ask the client to place the medication on the back of the tongue before taking the water. **Rationale:** *Stimulation of the back of the tongue produces the swallowing reflex.*
   - If the medication has an objectionable taste, ask the client to suck a few ice chips beforehand, or give the medication with juice, applesauce, or pudding if there are no contraindications. **Rationale:** *The cold temperature of the ice chips will desensitize the taste buds, and juice, applesauce, or pudding may mask the taste of the medication.*
   - If the client says that the medication you are about to give is different from what the client has been receiving, do not give the medication without first checking the original order. **Rationale:** *Most clients are familiar with the appearance of medications taken previously. Unfamiliar medications may signal a possible error.*
   - Stay with the client until all medications have been swallowed. **Rationale:** *The nurse must see the client swallow the medication before the drug administration can be recorded.* The nurse may need to check the client's mouth to ensure that the medication was swallowed and not hidden inside the cheek. A primary care provider's order or agency policy is required for medications left at the bedside.

9. Document each medication given.
   - Record the medication given, dosage, time, any complaints or assessments of the client, and your signature.
   - If medication was refused or omitted, record this fact on the appropriate record; document the reason, when possible, and the nurse's actions according to agency policy.

10. Dispose of all supplies appropriately.
   - Replenish stock (e.g., medication cups) and return the cart to the appropriate place.
   - Discard used disposable supplies.

EVALUATION

- Return to the client when the medication is expected to take effect (usually 30 minutes) to evaluate the effects of the medication on the client.
- Observe for desired effect (e.g., relief of pain or decrease in body temperature).
- Note any adverse effects or side effects (e.g., nausea, vomiting, skin rash, change in vital signs).
- Relate to previous findings, if available.
- Report significant deviations from normal to the primary care provider.

LIFESPAN CONSIDERATIONS Administering Oral Medications

- Knowledge of growth and development is essential for the nurse administering medications to infants and children.
- Nurses must know the range of safe medication dosages for infants and children.

INFANTS

- Oral medications can be effectively administered in several ways:
  - A syringe or dropper
  - A medication nipple, which allows the infant to suck the medication
  - Mixed in small amounts of food
  - A spoon or medication cup, for older children.
- Never mix medications into foods that are essential, since the infant may associate the food with an unpleasant taste and refuse that food in the future. Never mix medications with formula.
- Place a small amount of liquid medication along the inside of the baby's cheek and wait for the infant to swallow before giving more to prevent aspiration or spitting out.
- When using a spoon, retrieve and refeed medication that is thrust outward by the infant's tongue.

CHILDREN

- Whenever possible, give children a choice between the use of a spoon, dropper, or syringe.
- Dilute the oral medication, if indicated, with a small amount of water. Many oral medications are readily swallowed if they are diluted with a small amount of water. If large quantities of water are used, the child may refuse to drink the entire amount and receive only a portion of the medication.
- Oral medications for children are usually prepared in sweetened liquid form to make them more palatable. Crush medications that are not supplied in liquid form and mix them with substances available on most pediatric units, such as honey, flavored syrup, jam, or a fruit puree.
- Necessary foods such as milk or orange juice should not be used to mask the taste of medications because the child may develop unpleasant associations and refuse that food in the future.

Continued on page 381

WHAT IF **Administering Oral Medications**

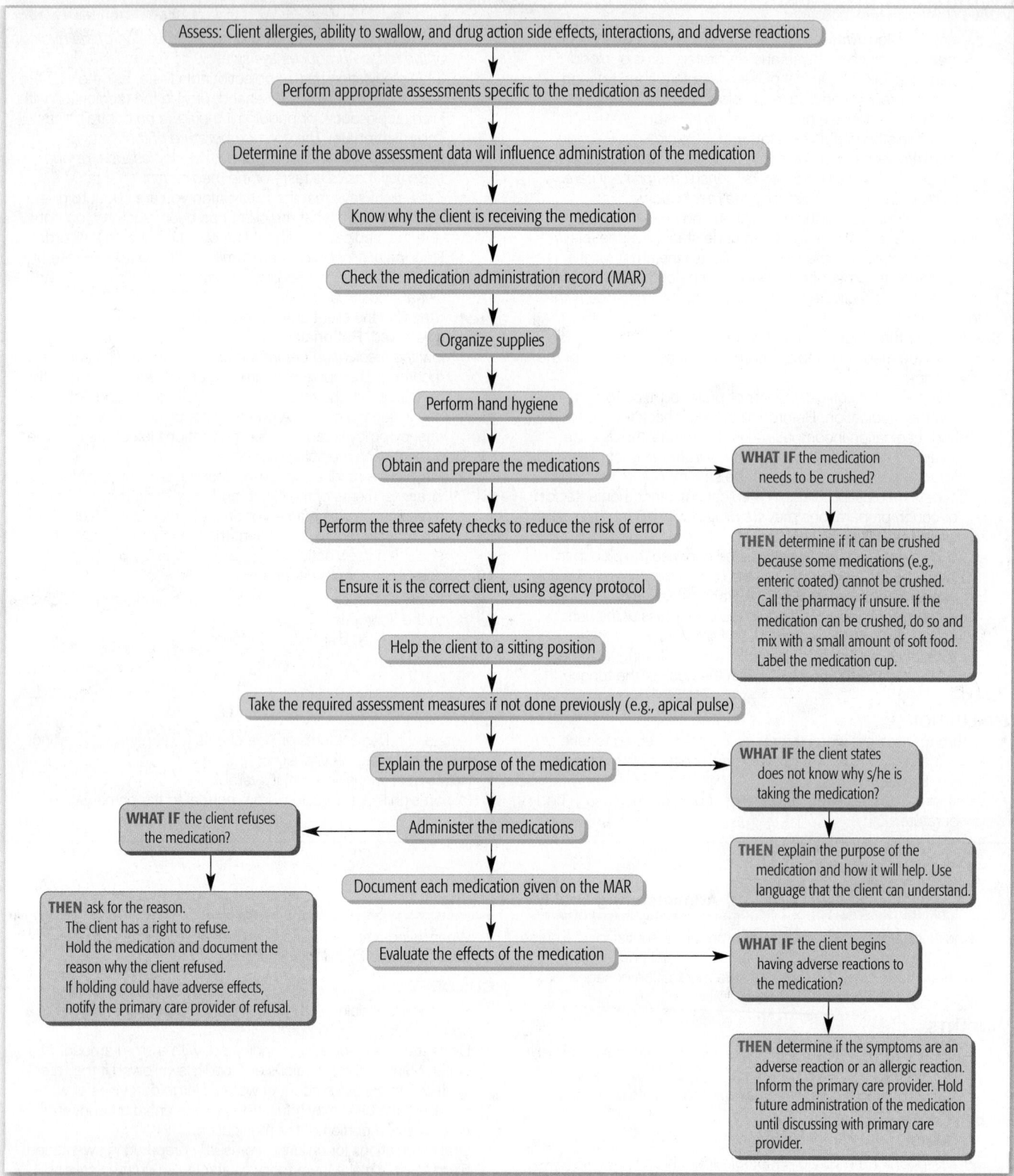

Assess: Client allergies, ability to swallow, and drug action side effects, interactions, and adverse reactions

Perform appropriate assessments specific to the medication as needed

Determine if the above assessment data will influence administration of the medication

Know why the client is receiving the medication

Check the medication administration record (MAR)

Organize supplies

Perform hand hygiene

Obtain and prepare the medications

Perform the three safety checks to reduce the risk of error

Ensure it is the correct client, using agency protocol

Help the client to a sitting position

Take the required assessment measures if not done previously (e.g., apical pulse)

Explain the purpose of the medication

Administer the medications

Document each medication given on the MAR

Evaluate the effects of the medication

WHAT IF the medication needs to be crushed?

THEN determine if it can be crushed because some medications (e.g., enteric coated) cannot be crushed. Call the pharmacy if unsure. If the medication can be crushed, do so and mix with a small amount of soft food. Label the medication cup.

WHAT IF the client states does not know why s/he is taking the medication?

THEN explain the purpose of the medication and how it will help. Use language that the client can understand.

WHAT IF the client begins having adverse reactions to the medication?

THEN determine if the symptoms are an adverse reaction or an allergic reaction. Inform the primary care provider. Hold future administration of the medication until discussing with primary care provider.

WHAT IF the client refuses the medication?

THEN ask for the reason.
The client has a right to refuse.
Hold the medication and document the reason why the client refused.
If holding could have adverse effects, notify the primary care provider of refusal.

- Disguise disagreeable-tasting medications with sweet-tasting substances mentioned previously. However, present any altered medication to the child honestly and not as a food or treat.
- Place the young child or toddler on your lap or a parent's lap in a sitting position.
- Administer the medication slowly with a measuring spoon, plastic syringe, or medicine cup.
- To prevent nausea, pour a carbonated beverage over finely crushed ice and give it before or immediately after the medication is administered.
- Follow medication with a drink of water, juice, a soft drink, or a Popsicle or frozen juice bar. This removes any unpleasant aftertaste.
- For children who take sweetened medications on a long-term basis, follow the medication administration with oral hygiene. These children are at high risk for dental caries.

OLDER ADULTS

- The physiological changes associated with aging influence medication administration and effectiveness. Examples include altered memory, less acute vision, decrease in renal function, less complete and slower absorption from the gastrointestinal tract, and decreased liver function. Many of these changes enhance the possibility of cumulative effects and toxicity.
- Older adults usually require smaller dosages of drugs, especially sedatives and other central nervous system depressants.
- Older adults are mature adults capable of reasoning. The nurse, therefore, needs to explain the reasons for and the effects of the client's medications.
- Socioeconomic factors such as lack of transportation and decreased finances may influence obtaining medications when needed.
- An increase in marketing and availability of vitamins, herbs, and supplements alerts the nurse to include this information in a medication history.

The nurse should instruct the client to:

- Learn the names of the medications as well as their actions and possible adverse effects. Carry a complete list of all prescriptions, OTC medications, and home remedies at all times.
- Keep all medications out of reach of children and pets.
- If using a syringe to administer the medication to an infant or child, remove and dispose of the plastic cap that fits on the end of the syringe. Infants and small children have been known to choke on these caps.
- Take the medications only as prescribed. Know which medications need to be taken on an empty stomach and which can be taken with food/meals. Immediately consult the nurse, pharmacist, or primary care provider about any problems with the medication.
- Always check the medication label to make sure the correct medication is being taken.
- Request labels printed with larger type on medication containers if there is difficulty reading the label.
- Check the expiration date and discard outdated medications. Previously, most people discarded old medicines by flushing them down the toilet. The Environmental Protection Agency (EPA) no longer recommends this. Inform clients to check with their local government. Many cities and towns have household hazardous waste facilities where they can take their old medicines. The expired medications may be placed in the trash if the following precautions are used: Keep the medication in the original container and mark out the person's name. Add a nontoxic but bad tasting product (e.g., cayenne pepper, mustard) to the container to keep individuals or animals from eating it. Place in a sturdy container, tape the container shut, and have this container be the last thing put in the garbage can.
- Ask the pharmacist to substitute childproof caps with ones that are more easily opened, as necessary.
- If a dose or more is missed, do not take two or more doses; ask the pharmacist or primary care provider for directions.
- Do not crush or cut a tablet or capsule without first checking with the primary care provider or pharmacist. Doing so may affect the medication's absorption.
- Never stop taking the medication without first discussing it with the primary care provider.
- Always check with the pharmacist before taking any nonprescription medications. Some OTC medications can interact with the prescribed medication.

Additionally, the nurse can set up a medication plan to assist clients and family members to remember a schedule. Weekly pill containers (available at pharmacies) or a written plan may be helpful.

Nasogastric and Gastrostomy Medications

For clients who cannot take anything by mouth (NPO) and have a nasogastric or gastrostomy tube in place, an alternative route for administering medications is through these tubes. A **nasogastric (NG) tube** is inserted by way of the nasopharynx or oropharynx and is placed into the client's stomach for the temporary purpose of feeding the client or to remove gastric secretions. An **orogastric (OG) tube** is an NG tube inserted through the mouth. Orogastric tubes are commonly used in newborns and young infants because they are nose breathers. A **gastrostomy tube** is surgically placed directly into the client's stomach and provides another route for administering nutrition and medications. See Chapter 19 ∞ for further discussion of nasogastric and gastrostomy tubes.

When administering medications by nasogastric/orogastric or gastrostomy tube, use the following guidelines:

- Always check with the pharmacist to see if the client's medications come in a liquid form because these are less likely to cause tube obstruction.
- If medications do not come in liquid form, check to see if they may be crushed. (Note that enteric-coated, sustained-action, buccal, and sublingual medications should never be crushed.)
  - Do not add medication directly to an enteral feeding formula because of potential incompatibility.

- Do not crush two or more medications at the same time because the chemical reaction that can occur is much greater than when combining drugs orally.
- Liquid medication must be further diluted with sterile water, especially if the liquid form is viscous.
- Each medication should be administered separately.
- Use only oral/enteral syringes labeled "for oral use only" to measure and administer medication through an enteral feeding tube.
- Crush a tablet into a fine powder and dissolve in at least 30 mL of warm sterile water. Cold liquids may cause client discomfort. Use only water for mixing and flushing. Some medications are mixed with other fluids, such as normal saline, in order to maximize dissolution. Nurses are encouraged to consult with a pharmacist.
- Sterile water is recommended for use in adult and neonatal/pediatric clients before and after medication administration (American Society for Parenteral and Enteral Nutrition [ASPEN], 2009, p. 156). ISMP (2010) advises not to use tap water because it often contains chemical contaminants that might interact with the drug.
  - Flushing the enteral feeding tube between medications decreases the incidence of enteral tube occlusions (ASPEN, 2009, p. 160; ISMP, 2010). Flush only with sterile water (no carbonated beverages, juices, coffee, or other liquids).
  - Read medication labels carefully before opening a capsule. Open hard gelatin capsules and mix the powder with sterile water.
- Do not administer whole or undissolved medications because they will clog the tube.
- Assess tube placement prior to administration of medications. (See Chapter 19 ∞ for methods to verify tube placement.)
- Before giving the medication, aspirate all stomach contents and measure the residual volume. Check agency policy if residual volume is greater than 100 mL.
- When administering the medication(s):
  - Remove the plunger from the syringe and connect the syringe to a pinched or folded-over tube. **Rationale:** *Pinching or folding over the tube prevents excess air from entering the stomach and causing distention.*
  - Put 15 to 30 mL (5 to 10 mL for children) of sterile water into the syringe barrel to flush the tube before administering the first

medication. Raise or lower the barrel of the syringe to adjust the flow as needed. Pinch or clamp the tubing before all the water is instilled. **Rationale:** *This avoids excess air entering the stomach.*
  - Pour liquid or dissolved medication into the syringe barrel and allow to flow by gravity into the enteral tube.
  - If you are giving several medications, administer each one separately and flush with at least 15 mL (5 mL for children) of sterile water between each medication.
  - When you have finished administering all medications, flush with another 15 to 30 mL (5 to 10 mL for children) of sterile warm water. **Rationale:** *Flushing clears the tube and prevents medication from adhering to the lining of the tube.*
- If the tube is connected to suction, disconnect the suction and keep the tube clamped for 20 to 30 minutes after giving the medication to allow for absorption of the medication(s).

Tube occlusion or clogging is a common complication of enteral feeding tubes. Clogging of an enteral tube results in delayed administration of medication and nutrition. If it cannot be corrected, the tube will need to be replaced. The two most common causes of clogged tubes are the use of protein formulas and administration of crushed medication into the tube (Kenny & Goodman, 2010). Prevention is the preferred solution. Several irrigants including carbonated soda, cranberry juice, and water have been studied to resolve an existing clog. Water was found to be better than cranberry juice, and there are no data to show that carbonated beverages are more effective than water (ASPEN, 2009; Dandeles, 2010). Water is the preferred flush solution, and if an occlusion does occur, sterile water should be used first. Commercial products are available. A "clog zapper" is a product that includes a syringe filled with powder consisting of papain and digestive enzymes that is reconstituted with water and instilled into the clogged tube through a catheter (Dandeles, 2010). Mechanical products also exist. One is a "PEG cleaning brush," which is a flexible catheter with a feather cut brush at the distal end to break up the clog. Another is an "enteral feeding tube declogger," which is a flexible plastic probe with a special screw-and-thread design that is inserted into the feeding tube and rotated to dislodge the obstruction.

Skill 15–2 provides guidelines for administering medications by enteral tube.

●○● NURSING PROCESS: NASOGASTRIC AND GASTROSTOMY MEDICATIONS

Administering Medications by Enteral Tube

SKILL 15-2

ASSESSMENT
Assess:
- Allergies to medication(s).
- Specific drug action, side effects, interactions, and adverse reactions.
- Client's knowledge of and learning needs about the medication.
- Whether fluid restriction or fluid overload is a concern for the client.

- Perform appropriate assessments (e.g., vital signs, laboratory results) specific to the medication.
- Determine if the assessment data influence administration of the medication (i.e., is it appropriate to administer the medication or does the medication need to be held and/or the primary care provider notified?).

Administering Medications by Enteral Tube—*continued*

SKILL 15-2

PLANNING
DELEGATION

The administration of medications through an enteral tube is performed by the nurse and is not delegated to UAP. The nurse can inform the UAP of the intended therapeutic effects and/or specific side effects of the medication and request the UAP to report specific client observations to the nurse for follow-up.

Equipment
- Medication to be administered
- Disposable medication cups: small paper or plastic calibrated medication cups for liquids
- 60-mL syringe with catheter tip for large-bore tube or Luer-Lok tip for small-bore tube
- Pill crusher for medications that need to be crushed
- Tongue blade or straw to stir dissolved medication
- pH test strip
- Sterile water to dissolve crushed medications
- Sterile water for flushing tube (check agency policy)
- Emesis basin
- Clean gloves
- MAR or computer printout

IMPLEMENTATION
Preparation
- Know the reason why the client is receiving the medication, the drug classification, contraindications, usual dosage range, side effects, and nursing considerations for administering and evaluating the intended outcomes for the medication.
- Check the MAR.
- Check for the drug name, dosage, frequency, route of administration, and expiration date for administration of the medication, if appropriate. **Rationale:** *Orders for certain medications (e.g., narcotics, antibiotics) expire after a specified time frame, and they need to be reordered by the primary care provider.*
  - If the MAR is unclear or pertinent information is missing, compare the MAR with the prescriber's most recent written order.
  - Report any discrepancies to the charge nurse or the prescriber, as agency policy dictates.
- Organize the supplies.
  - Gather the MAR(s) for each client so that medications can be prepared for one client at a time. **Rationale:** *Organization of supplies saves time and reduces the chance of error.*
- Prepare the client.
  - Assist the client to a Fowler's position in bed or a sitting position in a chair. If a sitting position is contraindicated, a slightly elevated right side-lying position is acceptable. **Rationale:** *These positions enhance gravitational flow and prevent aspiration of fluid into the lungs.*

Performance
1. Perform hand hygiene and observe other appropriate infection prevention procedures.
2. Prepare medications for appropriate administration by enteral tube (e.g., use liquids or crush and dissolve tablets). Calculate medication dosage accurately.
3. Provide for client privacy.
   - Introduce self and verify the client's identity using agency protocol. **Rationale:** *This ensures that the right client receives the medication.*
   - If not previously assessed, take the required assessment measures, such as pulse and respiratory rates or blood pressure. Take the apical pulse rate before administering digitalis preparations. Take the blood pressure before giving antihypertensive drugs. Take the respiratory rate prior to administering narcotics. If any of the findings are above or below the predetermined parameters, consult the primary care provider before administering the medication.
4. Explain the purpose of the medication and how it will help, using language that the client can understand. Include relevant information about effects; for example, tell the client receiving an analgesic to expect a decrease in pain. **Rationale:** *Information can facilitate acceptance of and compliance with the therapy.*

5. Apply clean gloves.
6. If the client is receiving a continuous tube feeding, press the "HOLD" button on the enteric feeding pump. **Rationale:** *Pausing or holding the pump temporarily stops the administration of the tube feeding. This prevents potential drug and formula incompatibility or interaction problems (ASPEN, 2009).*

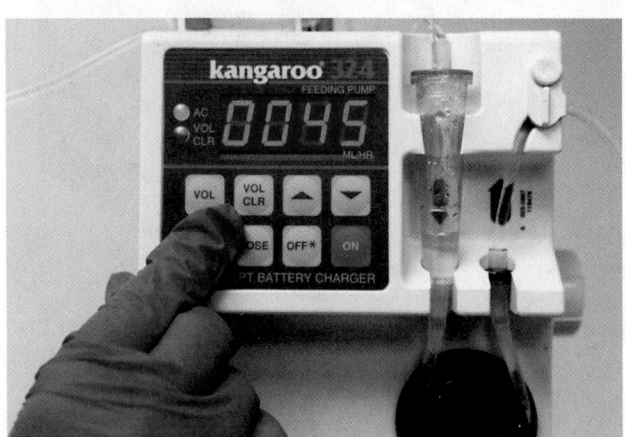

A

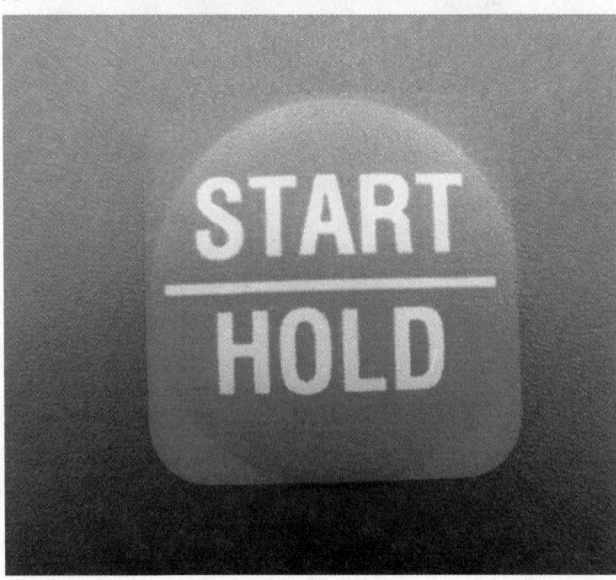

B

 A, Pausing the enteral feeding pump prior to administering medications by *B*, pressing the "HOLD" button.

Continued on page 384

SKILL 15–2

Administering Medications by Enteral Tube—*continued*

7. Disconnect tubing that is being used for suction or feeding from the gastric tube. Place a cap on the end of the tubing. **Rationale:** *Putting a cap on the end of the tubing prevents contamination.*

8. Assess tube placement (see Chapter 19 ∞ for methods to verify tube placement).

9. Pinch or fold over the gastric tube. ❷ **Rationale:** *Pinching or folding over the tubing prevents gastric contents from flowing out of the tube.*

10. Gently aspirate all the stomach contents and measure the residual volume. ❸

11. Return residual back to the stomach. **Rationale:** *Returning the residual prevents loss of fluids and electrolytes.* Pinch or fold over the gastric tube and remove the syringe.
    - Check agency policy if the residual volume is greater than 100 mL.

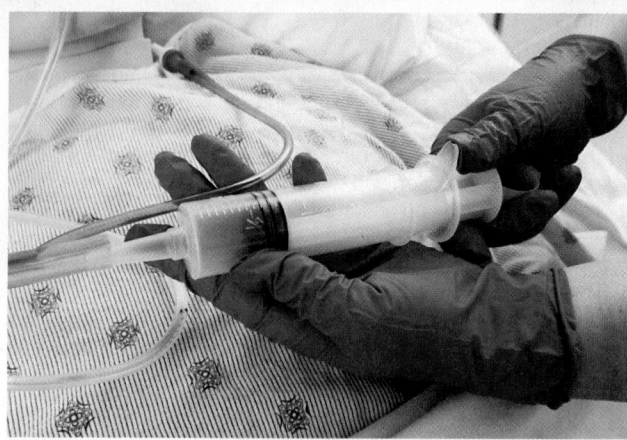

❸ Gently aspirate for residual volume prior to medication administration.

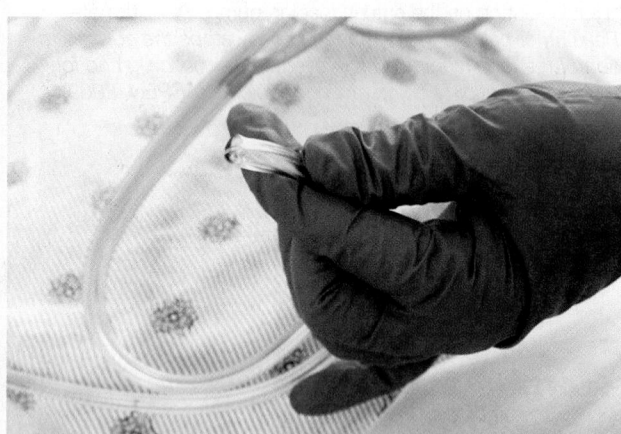

A

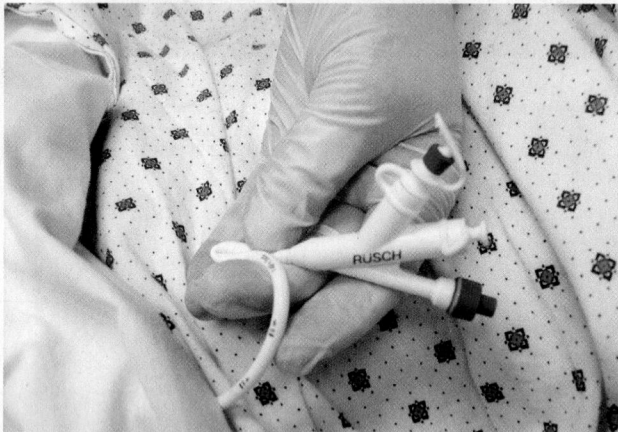

B

❷ Pinching or folding over *A,* a nasogastric tube, and *B,* a gastrostomy tube.

12. Administer the medication(s).
    - Remove the plunger from the syringe and connect the syringe to a pinched or folded-over tube. **Rationale:** *Pinching or folding over the tube prevents excess air from entering the stomach and causing distention.*
    - Put 15 to 30 mL of sterile water into the syringe barrel to flush the tube before administering the first medication. Raise or lower the barrel of the syringe to adjust the flow as needed. Pinch or clamp the tubing before all of the water is instilled. **Rationale:** *This avoids excess air entering the stomach.*
    - Pour liquid or dissolved medication into the syringe barrel and allow to flow by gravity into the enteral tube.
    - If administering more than one medication, flush with a minimum of 15 mL of sterile water between each medication.
    - After administering the last medication, flush the tube with 30 mL of sterile water. **Rationale:** *Flushing clears the tube and decreases clogging of the tube (ASPEN, 2009; ISMP, 2010).*
    - Pinch or fold over the gastric tube and reconnect to tubing for continuous tube feeding. If the client was previously connected to suction, keep the gastric tube clamped for 20 to 30 minutes after giving the medication. **Rationale:** *Keeping the tube clamped for that time will help ensure that the medication is absorbed before restarting the suction.*
    - Remove and discard gloves.
    - Perform hand hygiene.

13. Document each medication given.
    - Record the medication given, dosage, time, any complaints or assessments of the client, and your signature.
    - If medication was refused or omitted, record this fact on the appropriate record; document the reason, when possible, and the nurse's actions according to agency policy.
    - Record fluid intake accurately if the client is on intake and output.

14. Dispose of all supplies appropriately.
    - Replenish stock (e.g., medication cups) and return the cart to the appropriate place.
    - Discard used disposable supplies.

EVALUATION
- Return to the client when the medication is expected to take effect (usually 30 minutes) to evaluate the effects of the medication on the client.
- Observe for desired effect (e.g., relief of pain or decrease in body temperature).
- Note any adverse effects or side effects (e.g., nausea, vomiting, skin rash, change in vital signs).

- Compare tube patency before and after medication administration.
- Relate to previous findings, if available.
- Report deviations from normal to the primary care provider.

WHAT IF   Administering Enteral Medications

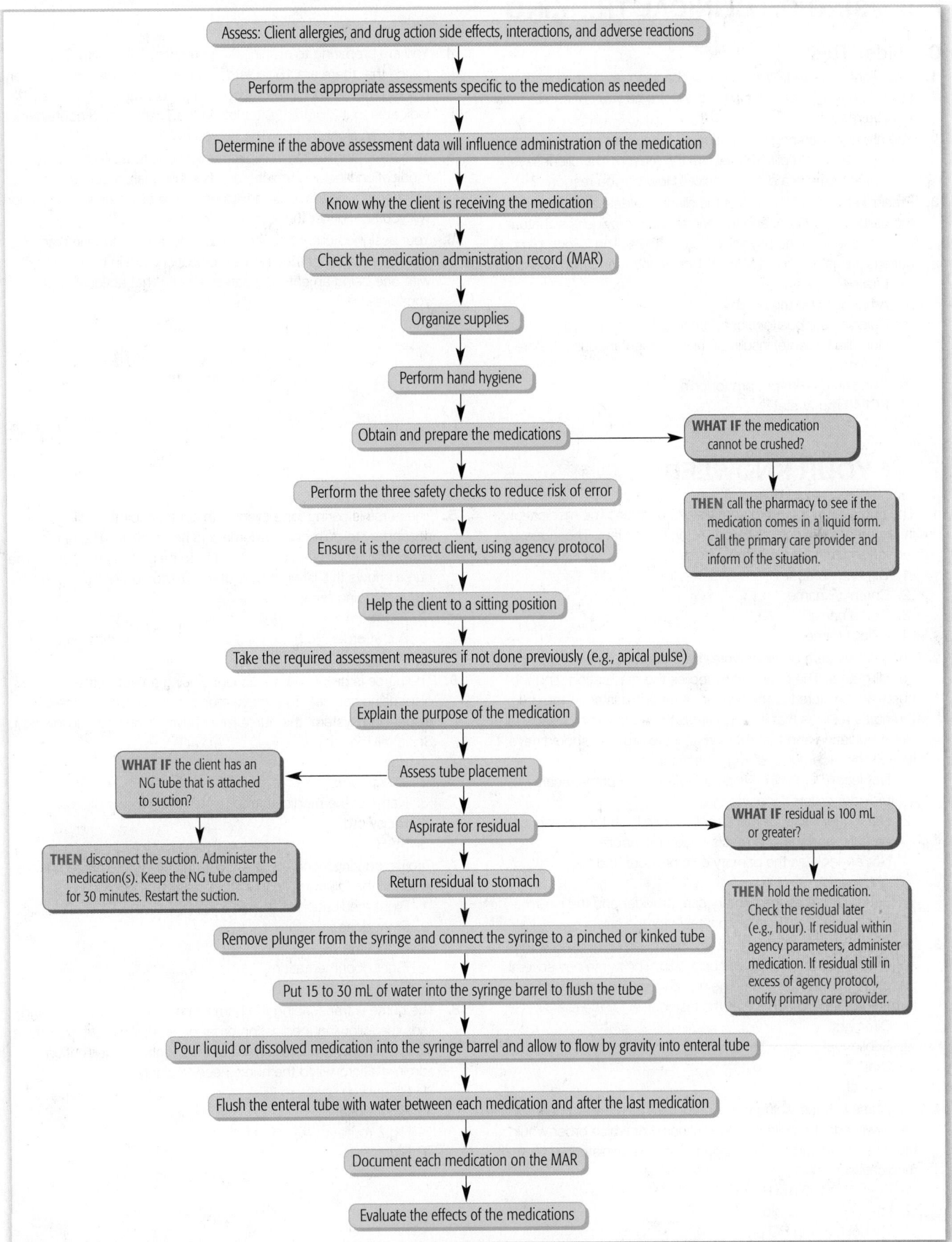

Assess: Client allergies, and drug action side effects, interactions, and adverse reactions

Perform the appropriate assessments specific to the medication as needed

Determine if the above assessment data will influence administration of the medication

Know why the client is receiving the medication

Check the medication administration record (MAR)

Organize supplies

Perform hand hygiene

Obtain and prepare the medications

WHAT IF the medication cannot be crushed?

THEN call the pharmacy to see if the medication comes in a liquid form. Call the primary care provider and inform of the situation.

Perform the three safety checks to reduce risk of error

Ensure it is the correct client, using agency protocol

Help the client to a sitting position

Take the required assessment measures if not done previously (e.g., apical pulse)

Explain the purpose of the medication

WHAT IF the client has an NG tube that is attached to suction?

Assess tube placement

THEN disconnect the suction. Administer the medication(s). Keep the NG tube clamped for 30 minutes. Restart the suction.

Aspirate for residual

WHAT IF residual is 100 mL or greater?

Return residual to stomach

THEN hold the medication. Check the residual later (e.g., hour). If residual within agency parameters, administer medication. If residual still in excess of agency protocol, notify primary care provider.

Remove plunger from the syringe and connect the syringe to a pinched or kinked tube

Put 15 to 30 mL of water into the syringe barrel to flush the tube

Pour liquid or dissolved medication into the syringe barrel and allow to flow by gravity into enteral tube

Flush the enteral tube with water between each medication and after the last medication

Document each medication on the MAR

Evaluate the effects of the medications

FOCUSING ON CLINICAL THINKING

Consider This

1. The client asks you, "Why are you checking my name band again? I haven't changed since the last time you checked!" How will you respond?

2. You are administering medication and the client asks you why he is getting a certain pill. You tell him the reason. The client says, "My pill at home is a different color." How do you respond?

3. Presume that the full name of the client, the date and time that the order was written, and the primary care provider's signature are all present on the physician's order sheet. The following medications are listed on the MAR. Which, if any, would you question?
   a. Lasix 40 mg stat
   b. Ampicillin 500 mg IVPB
   c. Dulcolax suppository, one, prn if no bm for 3 days
   d. Humulin L (Lente) insulin 36 units, subcutaneously, before breakfast
   e. Codeine q4–6h, po, prn for pain
   f. KCl 40 mg IV stat

4. You are preparing to administer a narcotic, Tylenol No. 3. You notice that there are 16 tablets remaining in the plastic container holding the narcotic. The narcotic inventory record, however, indicates that 3 of the 20 tablets in the Tylenol No. 3 container have been signed out. What do you do?

5. You are to administer multiple medications to a client. These medications include tablets (one is sublingual), a capsule, and a powder that needs to be mixed with juice or water. In what order will you administer these medications?

6. Your assigned client has a gastrostomy feeding tube in place. You note that all of the client's medications are in tablet form, with one being an enteric-coated tablet. What action(s) will you take?

TEST YOUR KNOWLEDGE

1. The nurse is preparing to administer ibuprofen. The medication in the client's drawer is labeled Motrin (ibuprofen). The nurse recognizes that Motrin is the drug's:
   1. Generic name.
   2. Chemical name.
   3. Brand name.
   4. Official name.

2. The primary care provider writes an order for Lanoxin (digoxin) 25 milligrams. The pharmacy supplies the medication, and the nurse administers the medication. After administering the drug the nurse realizes that it is 100 times the acceptable dosage for this medication and that the primary care provider should have written the order for 0.25 mg. The nurse is:
   1. Not legally liable for this error because the primary care provider ordered the wrong dose.
   2. Not legally liable for this error because both the primary care provider and the pharmacist made the error.
   3. Not as liable as the primary care provider and the pharmacist.
   4. Equally liable as the primary care provider and the pharmacist because all were accountable for the error.

3. The nurse is caring for a client who has been diagnosed with angina and is complaining of chest pain. The nurse has several prn orders for nitroglycerin. The nurse would administer what form of the medication to get the faster relief for the client?
   1. Ointment
   2. Sublingual
   3. Oral
   4. Buccal

4. The nurse is transcribing the primary care provider's orders for the newly admitted client's medications. For which order would the nurse need further clarification prior to administering the medication?
   1. Digoxin 0.125 mg PO qd
   2. Lasix 40 mg PO bid
   3. Tylenol 650 mg PO prn
   4. Lipitor 20 mg PO at bedtime

5. The nurse is caring for a client with acute respiratory distress secondary to pulmonary edema and heart failure. The primary care provider orders Lasix 40 mg IV to be given immediately. The nurse knows this is what type of medication order?
   1. A standing order
   2. A prn order
   3. A stat order
   4. A single order

6. The nurse is preparing medications using an automated dispensing cabinet. To retrieve medications from this type of dispensing system, the nurse must have which of the following? Select all that apply.
   1. Key
   2. Client name
   3. Name of the medication to be administered
   4. Password
   5. MAR

7. Prior to administering medication to the client, the nurse checks which of the following "rights"? Select all that apply.
   1. Right medication
   2. Right dose
   3. Right time
   4. Right documentation
   5. Right evaluation

8. The nurse is transcribing the primary care provider's orders and finds the following medication order on a client's chart: morphine 8 mg prn every 2 hours. Which of the "rights" of medication administration would the nurse need to clarify?
   1. Right drug
   2. Right dose
   3. Right route
   4. Right time

9. The nurse is preparing to administer a medication via the oral route. Place the following steps the nurse would take in the correct order of implementation.
1. Pour medication.
2. Check the medication administration record.
3. Check the client's ID band.
4. Perform hand hygiene.
5. Determine allergies.

10. The nurse is preparing to administer a medication via an enteral tube. Which medication would the nurse be unable to administer via this route?
1. Enteric-coated aspirin
2. Benadryl liquid
3. Tylenol tablet
4. Simethicone drops

See Answers to Test Your Knowledge in Appendix A.

READINGS AND REFERENCES

References

American Society for Parenteral and Enteral Nutrition. (2009). Enteral nutrition practice recommendations. *Journal of Parenteral and Enteral Nutrition, 33*, 122–167. doi:10.1177/0148607108330314

Bryant, S. L. (2011). Nursing's national treasure: The five (5) plus five (5) rights of medication administration. Can you dig it? *Clinical Simulation in Nursing, 7*(6), e247. doi:10.1016/j.ecns.2011.09.013

Clark, A. P., & Flanders, S. (2012). Interruptions and medication errors. Part II. *Clinical Nurse Specialist, 26*(5), 239–243. doi:10.1097/NUR.0b013e31825e5be4

Dandeles, L. (2010). *What products can be used to unclog feeding tubes?* Retrieved from http://dig.pharm.uic.edu/faq/Jul10/feedingtube.aspx

Elliott, M., & Liu, Y. (2010). The nine rights of medication administration: An overview. *British Journal of Nursing, 19*, 300–305.

Flanders, S., & Clark, A. P. (2010). Interruptions and medication errors. Part I. *Clinical Nurse Specialist, 24*(6), 281–285. doi:10.1097/NUR.0b013e3181faf78b

Food and Drug Administration. (2011). *My medicine record.* Retrieved from http://www.fda.gov/downloads/AboutFDA/Reports ManualsForms/Forms/UCM095018.pdf

Hall, L. M., Ferguson-Pare, M., Peter, E., White, D., Besner, J., Chisholm, A., . . . Hemingway, A. (2010). Going blank: Factors contributing to interruptions to nurses' work and related outcomes. *Journal of Nursing Management, 18*, 1040–1047. doi:10.1111/j.1365-2834.2010.01166.x

Institute for Healthcare Improvement. (2011a). *How-to-guide: Prevent adverse drug events (medication reconciliation).* Retrieved from http://www.ihi.org/knowledge/Pages/Tools/HowtoGuidePreventAdverseDrugEvents.aspx

Institute for Healthcare Improvement. (2011b). *Reconcile medications at all transition points.* Retrieved from http://www.ihi.org/knowledge/Pages/Changes/ReconcileMedicationsatAllTransitionPoints.aspx

Institute for Safe Medication Practices. (2010). *Preventing errors when administering drugs via an enteral feeding tube.* Retrieved from http://www.ismp.org/newsletters/acutecare/articles/20100506.asp

Institute for Safe Medication Practices. (2011). *ISMP acute care guidelines for timely administration of scheduled medications.* Retrieved from http://www.ismp.org/tools/guidelines/acutecare/tasm.pdf

Institute for Safe Medication Practices. (2013a). *ISMP's list of error-prone abbreviations, symbols, and dose designations.* Retrieved from http://www.ismp.org/tools/errorproneabbreviations.pdf

Institute for Safe Medication Practices. (2013b). *Oral dosage forms that should not be crushed.* Retrieved from http://www.ismp.org/tools/

The Joint Commission. (2012). *Facts about the official "do not use" list of abbreviations.* Retrieved from http://www.jointcommission.org/facts_about_the_official_/

The Joint Commission. (2013a). *National Patient Safety Goals effective January 1, 2014: Hospital accreditation program.* Retrieved from http://www.jointcommission.org/hap_2013_npsg

The Joint Commission. (2013b). *National Patient Safety Goals effective January 1, 2014: Long term accreditation program.* Retrieved from http://www.jointcommission.org/ltc_2013_nspg/

Kenny, D. J., & Goodman, P. (2010). Care of the patient with enteral tube feeding: An evidence-based practice protocol. *Nursing Research, 59*(1), S22–S31. doi:10.1097/NNR.0b013e3181c3bfe9

Klejka, D. E. (2012). Shhh! Conducting a quiet zone pilot study for medication safety. *Nursing, 42*(9), 18–21. doi:10.1097/01.NURSE.0000418623.06842.59

Lewis, T., Smith, C. B., & Williams-Jones, P. (2012). Tips to reduce dangerous interruptions by healthcare staff. *Nursing, 42*(11), 65–67. doi:10.1097/01.NURSE.0000421387.36112.e0

Mandrack, M., Cohen, M. R., Featherling, J., Gellner, L., Judd, K., Kienle, P. C., & Vanderveen, T. (2012). Nursing best practices using automated dispensing cabinets: Nurses' key role in improving medication safety. *MEDSURG Nursing, 21*(3), 134–139, 144.

National Coordinating Council for Medication Error Reporting and Prevention. (2013). *Consumer information for safe medication use.* Retrieved from http://www.nccmerp.org/consumerInfo.html

Patient Safety Solutions. (2012). *Patient safety tip of the week: Verbal orders.* Retrieved from http://patientsafetysolutions.com/docs/January_10_2012_Verbal_Orders.htm

Stachowiak, M. E. (2013). Automated dispensing cabinets: Curse or cure? *American Journal of Nursing, 113*(5), 11. doi:10.1097/01.NAJ.0000430215.97411.8f

Stokowski, L. A. (2012). *Timely medication administration guidelines for nurses: Fewer wrong-time errors?* Retrieved from http://www.medscape.com/viewarticle/772501_print

Tzeng, H., Yin, C., & Schneider, T. E. (2013). Medication error-related issues in nursing practice. *MEDSURG Nursing, 22*(1), 13–16, 50.

Selected Bibliography

Anderson, P., & Townsend, T. (2010). Medication errors: Don't let them happen to you. *American Nurse Today, 5*(3), 23–27.

Berman, A., Snyder, S., & Frandsen, G. (2016). *Kozier & Erb's fundamentals of nursing: Concepts, process, and practice* (10th ed.). Upper Saddle River, NJ: Pearson.

Blank, L. J., Benyo, E. M., & Glover, J. U. (2012). Bridging the gap in transitional care: A closer look at medication reconciliation. *Geriatric Nursing, 33*(5), 401–409. doi:10.1016/j.gerinurse.2012.07.007

Flora, D. S., Parsons, P. L., & Slattum, P. W. (2012). Managing medications for improved care transitions. *Journal of the American Society on Aging, 35*(4), 37–42.

Flynn, L., Liang, Y., Dickson, G. L., Xie, M., & Suh, D. (2012). Nurses' practice environments, error interception practices, and inpatient medication errors. *Journal of Nursing Scholarship, 44*(2), 180–186. doi:10.1111/j.1547-5069.2012.01443.x

Hall, D. (2010). Med reconciliation: Do the right thing. *Nursing Management, 41*(2), 32–36. doi:10.1097/01.NUMA.0000368566.67102.9e

Hicks, R. W., Wanzer, L. J., & Denholm, B. (2012). Implementing AORN recommended practices for medication safety. *AORN Journal, 96*(6), 605–622. doi:10.1016/j.aorn.2012.09.012

Simons, S., & Remington, R. (2013). The percutaneous endoscopic gastrostomy tube: A nurse's guide to PEG tubes. *MEDSURG Nursing, 22*(2), 77–83.

Yoder, M., & Schadewald, D. (2012). The effect of a safe zone on nurse distractions, interruptions, and medication administration errors. *Western Journal of Nursing Research, 34*, 1068–1069. doi:10.1177/0193945912453687

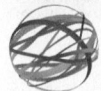 **16** Administering Topical Medications

LEARNING OUTCOMES

At the completion of this chapter, the student will be able to:

1. Define the key terms used in the skills of administering topical medications.
2. Recognize when it is acceptable to delegate aspects of administering topical medications to unlicensed assistive personnel.
3. Verbalize the steps used in administering the following topical medications:
   a. Dermatologic
   b. Ophthalmic
   c. Otic
   d. Nasal
   e. Metered-dose inhalers
   f. Vaginal
   g. Rectal.
4. Demonstrate appropriate documentation and reporting of topical medication administration.

SKILLS

KEY TERMS

aerosolization, *397*
atomization, *397*
dermatologic, *388*
instillations, *391*
irrigation, *391*
metered-dose inhaler (MDI), *397*
nebulizers, *397*
ophthalmic, *391*
otic, *394*
pruritus, *388*
suppositories, *401*
transdermal patch, *388*

A topical medication is applied locally to the skin or to the mucous membranes of the eye, ear, nose, lungs, vagina, and rectum. Many drugs are applied topically to produce a local effect (e.g., an antibiotic cream for a skin infection, corticosteroid nasal spray to reduce inflammation of nasal mucosa from allergies). Some medications are applied topically for a systemic effect such as slow absorption of the medication into the general circulation. Examples include a nitroglycerin patch to treat coronary artery disease or a medication in a suppository form to treat nausea. Topical skin or **dermatologic** preparations include ointments, pastes, creams, lotions, powders, sprays, and patches. See Practice Guidelines for applying dermatologic medications.

Before applying a dermatologic preparation, thoroughly clean the area with soap and water and dry it with a patting motion. Skin encrustations (i.e., crusts or scabs) harbor microorganisms, and these as well as previously applied applications can prevent the medication from coming in contact with the area to be treated. Nurses should wear gloves when administering skin applications and always use surgical asepsis when an open wound is present.

CLINICAL ALERT!

The nurse should wear gloves when applying a transdermal patch to avoid getting any of the medication on his or her skin, which can result in the nurse receiving the effect of the medication.

DERMATOLOGIC MEDICATIONS

Medications applied to the skin may be used for a variety of reasons. Examples include:

- Decrease itching (**pruritus**).
- Lubricate and soften the skin.
- Cause local vasoconstriction or vasodilation.
- Increase or decrease secretions from the skin.
- Provide a protective coating to the skin.
- Apply an antibiotic or antiseptic to treat or prevent infection.
- Reduce local inflammation.
- Provide an entry for medications that will be absorbed into the systemic circulation.

Transdermal Medications

A particular type of dermatologic medication delivery system is the **transdermal patch**. This system administers sustained-action medications (e.g., pain relievers, nitroglycerin, estrogen, and nicotine) via multilayered films containing the drug and an adhesive layer. Technology is expanding the use of drug patches. For example, researchers are working on transdermal patches that will include ultrasound and electrical charges to force larger drug molecules through the skin. One potential example of these "active patches" may permit the delivery of insulin to people with diabetes (MRIsafety.com, 2012, para. 2).

PRACTICE GUIDELINES

Dermatologic Medication Administration

POWDER

Make sure the skin surface is dry. Spread apart any skinfolds, and sprinkle the site until the area is covered with a fine *thin* layer. Cover the site with a dressing if ordered.

SUSPENSION-BASED LOTION

Shake the container before use to distribute suspended particles. Put a little lotion on a small gauze dressing or pad, and apply the lotion to the skin by stroking it evenly in the direction of the hair growth.

CREAMS, OINTMENTS, PASTES, AND OIL-BASED LOTIONS

Warm and soften the preparation in gloved hands to make it easier to apply and to prevent chilling (if a large area is to be treated). Smear it evenly over the skin using long strokes that follow the direction of the hair growth. Explain that the skin may feel somewhat greasy after application. Apply a sterile dressing if ordered by the primary care provider.

AEROSOL SPRAY

Shake the container well to mix the contents. Hold the spray container at the recommended distance from the area (usually about 15 to 30 cm [6 to 12 in.] but check the label). Cover the client's face with a towel if the upper chest or neck is to be sprayed. Spray the medication over the specified area.

TRANSDERMAL PATCHES

Select a clean, dry area that is free of hair and matches the manufacturer's recommendations. Remove the patch from its protective covering, holding it without touching the adhesive edges, and apply it by pressing firmly with the palm of the hand for about 10 seconds. Advise the client to avoid using a heating pad over the area to prevent an increase in circulation and the rate of absorption. Remove the patch at the appropriate time, folding it so that the sticky, medicated sides are together. Some patches contain nonvisible metal in their backing. This may cause burning in the area of the patch. Inform clients to tell MRI personnel that they are wearing a transdermal patch (MRIsafety.com, 2012).

The rate of delivery of the drug is controlled and varies with each product (e.g., from 12 hours to 1 week). Generally, the patch is applied to a hairless, clean area of skin that is not subject to excessive movement, friction (e.g., bra strap or waistline areas), or wrinkling (i.e., the lower abdomen). It may be applied on the upper arm, side, chest, lower back, or buttocks (Figure 16–1 ■). Remove lotion, sunscreen, powder, or any other product that may impair absorption of the medication in the patch. Use mild, nonirritating soap and water to cleanse, if necessary. Patches should not be applied to areas with cuts, burns, or abrasions, or on distal parts of extremities (e.g., the forearms). Women who use a patch containing estrogen or nicotine should not apply the patch to the breasts, per the manufacturer's instructions (Association of Reproductive Health Professionals, 2011). If hair is likely to interfere with patch adhesion or removal, clipping (not shaving) may be necessary before application.

Reddening of the skin with or without mild local itching or burning, as well as allergic contact dermatitis, may occasionally occur. Upon removal of the patch, any slight reddening of the skin usually disappears within a few hours. All applications should be changed regularly to prevent local irritation, and each successive application should be placed on a different site. The transdermal patch should be dated, timed, and initialed by the nurse before it is applied to the client.

All clients need to be assessed for allergies to the drug and to materials in the patch before the patch is applied. If a client has a transdermal patch on and develops a fever, it may be because the medication is being absorbed and metabolizing at a faster rate than normal. The client will need to be monitored for changes in effects of the medication.

When transdermal patches are removed, care needs to be taken as to how and where they are discarded. In the home environment, if they are simply discarded into a trash can, pets or children can be exposed to them, causing effects from any drug remaining on the patch. When removed, they should be folded with the medication side to

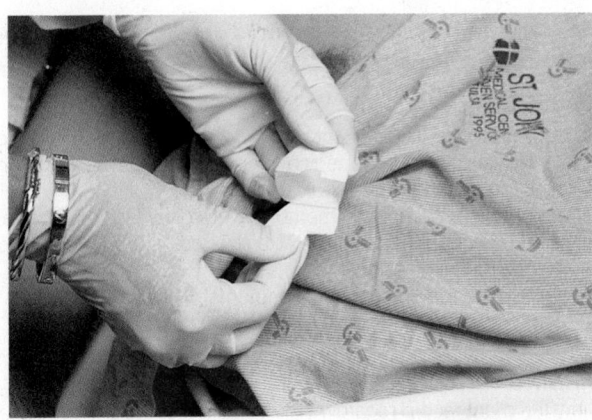

A

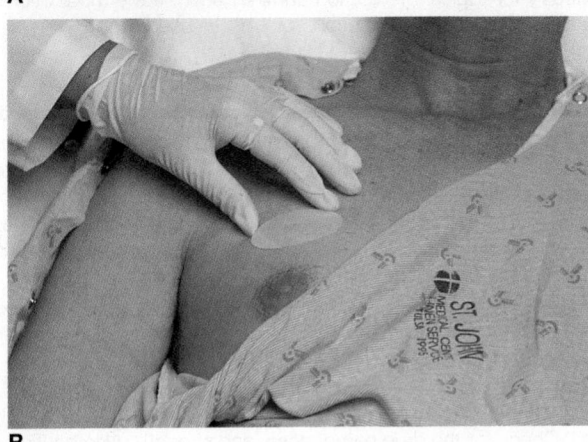

B

Figure 16–1 ■ Transdermal patch administration: *A,* protective coating removed from patch; *B,* patch immediately applied to clean, dry, hairless skin.

the inside, put into a closed container, and kept out of reach of children and pets.

Transdermal ointment is another form of transdermal medication. A common example is nitroglycerin ointment, which is used to prevent chest pain. The nurse squeezes out the ordered dose onto a paper dose-measuring applicator (Figure 16–2 ■). This paper applicator is placed with the ointment side down onto a dry, hairless area of skin, similar to the transdermal patch. Using the paper applicator, lightly spread the ointment (do not rub) and tape the paper applicator into place. Clients at home may want to cover the paper applicator with plastic wrap to avoid staining their clothing.

CLINICAL ALERT!

It is important to keep track of transdermal patches. Some patches are clear and may be difficult to see and, as a result, be overlooked. If the client is obese, patches may be difficult to find in the skinfolds. Check under the breasts and groin areas. Duplication of patches may cause adverse reactions. Remove the old patch and clean the skin thoroughly before applying a new one.

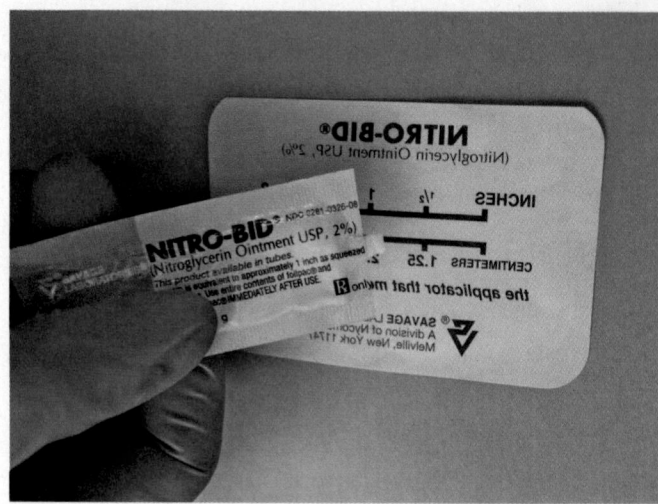

Figure 16–2 ■ Using premeasured paper to measure medication dosage.

●○● NURSING PROCESS: DERMATOLOGIC MEDICATIONS

Administering Dermatologic Medications

ASSESSMENT

- In addition to the assessment performed by the nurse related to the administration of any medication (see Chapter 15 ∞), prior to applying dermatologic medications:
  - Inspect skin or mucous membrane areas for lesions, rashes, erythema, and breakdown. Note size, color, distribution, and configuration of lesions.
  - Determine the presence of symptoms of skin irritation (e.g., pruritus, burning sensation, pain).

- Note the presence of excessive body hair that may require clipping before the application of a topical medication.
- If a transdermal patch is to be applied, ask clients if they are already wearing a patch, and if so, where it is located.
- Determine if assessment data influence administration of the medication (i.e., is it appropriate to administer the medication or does the medication need to be held and the primary care provider notified?).

PLANNING

Review the client record regarding the condition of the skin area used previously for topical medication administration. If the medication is intended for systemic absorption, rotate sites used.

Equipment
- Clean gloves (sterile for nonintact skin)
- Solution to wash area if indicated
- 2×2 gauze pads for cleaning
- Medication (e.g., lotion, cream, ointment, patch)
- Application tube (if required)

DELEGATION

Due to the need for assessment and interpretation of client status, topical medication administration is generally not delegated to unlicensed assistive personnel (UAP). In some agencies, UAP may apply lotions and creams used primarily for relieving itching or dry skin. However, responsibility for periodically assessing the area remains with the nurse and agency policy.

IMPLEMENTATION
Preparation
- Check the medication administration record (MAR).
  - Check for the drug name, dose, and strength. Also confirm the prescribed frequency.
  - Check client allergy status.
  - If the MAR is unclear or pertinent information is missing, compare it with the most recent primary care provider's written order.
  - Report any discrepancies to the charge nurse or primary care provider, as agency policy dictates.

- Know the reason why the client is receiving the medication, the drug classification, contraindications, usual dose range, side effects, and nursing considerations for administering and evaluating the intended outcomes of the medication.
- Determine whether the area is to be washed or the hair clipped before applying medication.

Administering Dermatologic Medications—*continued*

Performance
1. Compare the label on the medication tube or jar with the medication record and check the expiration date.
2. If necessary, calculate the medication dosage.
3. Introduce self and explain to the client what you are going to do, why it is necessary, and how he or she can participate. Discuss how the results will be used in planning further care or treatments.
4. Perform hand hygiene and observe other appropriate infection prevention procedures. Apply clean gloves. **Rationale:** *This protects the nurse's hands from contact with the medication.*
5. Prepare the client.
   - Prior to performing the procedure, verify the client's identity using agency protocol. **Rationale:** *This ensures that the right client receives the right medication.*
   - Assist the client to a comfortable position, either sitting or lying. Expose the area to be treated but provide for client privacy.
6. Apply the medication and dressing as ordered.
   - Place a small amount of cream or ointment on the gloved hand, and spread it evenly on the skin.

   or

   - Apply sterile gloves if indicated (i.e., nonintact skin). Pour some lotion on the gauze, and pat the skin area with it.
   - Repeat the application until the area is completely covered.
   - Apply a sterile dressing as necessary.

   or

   - Apply a prepackaged transdermal patch.

- Write the date and time on the label *before* application. **Rationale:** *Knowing the date and time ensures safety and communication when there are multiple caregivers. Writing on the patch after application could puncture it.*

   or

- Squeeze out transdermal ointment onto premeasured medication administration paper.
- Place the applicator paper with ointment side down onto the skin.
- Lightly spread the ointment.
- Tape the paper applicator into place.
7. Remove and discard clean (or sterile if used) gloves.
   - Perform hand hygiene.
8. Provide for client comfort.
   - Provide a clean gown or pajamas after the application if the medication will come in contact with the clothing.
9. Document all relevant assessments and interventions.
   - Record the type of preparation used, the site to which it was applied, the time, and the response of the client, including data about the appearance of the site, discomfort, itching, and so on.
   - For transdermal patches, document both removal of the previous patch and application of the new patch. Include location of the patch in documentation and at change-of-shift report.
   - Return at a time by which the preparation should have absorbed to assess the reaction (e.g., relief of itching, burning, swelling, or discomfort).

EVALUATION
- Perform follow-up based on findings of the effectiveness of the medication or outcomes that deviated from expected or normal for the client. Relate findings to previous data if available.

- Report significant deviations from normal to the primary care provider.

OPHTHALMIC MEDICATIONS

Medications may be administered to the eye using **instillations** (slowly pouring or dropping a liquid onto a surface). **Ophthalmic** medications (for the eyes) are applied in the form of liquids or ointments. Eyedrops are packaged in monodrip plastic containers that are used to administer the preparation. Ointments are usually supplied in small tubes. All containers must state that the medication is for ophthalmic use. Sterile preparations and sterile technique are indicated. Prescribed liquids are usually diluted, for example, to less than 1% strength. An eye **irrigation** is administered to wash out the conjunctival sac to remove secretions or foreign bodies or to remove chemicals that may injure the eye.

●○● NURSING PROCESS: OPHTHALMIC MEDICATIONS

Administering Ophthalmic Medications

ASSESSMENT
- In addition to the assessment performed by the nurse related to the administration of any medication (see Chapter 15 ∞), prior to applying ophthalmic medications, assess:
  - Appearance of the eye and surrounding structures for lesions, exudate, erythema, or swelling.
  - The location and nature of any discharge, lacrimation, and swelling of the eyelids or of the lacrimal gland.

- Client complaints (e.g., itching, burning pain, blurred vision, and photophobia).
- Client behavior (e.g., squinting, blinking excessively, frowning, or rubbing the eyes).
- Determine if assessment data influence administration of the medication (i.e., is it appropriate to administer the medication or does the medication need to be held and the primary care provider notified?).

Continued on page 392

Administering Ophthalmic Medications—*continued*

PLANNING
DELEGATION

Due to the need for assessment, interpretation of client status, and use of sterile technique, ophthalmic medication administration is not delegated to UAP.

Equipment
- Clean gloves
- Sterile absorbent sponges soaked in sterile normal saline

- Medication
- Sterile eye dressing (pad) as needed and paper tape to secure it

For irrigation, add:
- Irrigating solution (e.g., normal saline) and irrigating syringe or tubing
- Dry sterile absorbent sponges
- Moisture-resistant towel
- Basin (e.g., emesis basin)

IMPLEMENTATION
Preparation
- Check the MAR.
  - Check for the drug name, dose, and strength. Also confirm the prescribed frequency of the instillation and which eye is to be treated.
  - Check client allergy status.
  - If the MAR is unclear or pertinent information is missing, compare it with the most recent primary care provider's written order.
  - Report any discrepancies to the charge nurse or primary care provider, as agency policy dictates.
- Know the reason why the client is receiving the medication, the drug classification, contraindications, usual dose range, side effects, and nursing considerations for administering and evaluating the intended outcomes of the medication.

Performance
1. Compare the label on the medication tube or bottle with the medication record and check the expiration date.
2. If necessary, calculate the medication dosage.
3. Introduce self and explain to the client what you are going to do, why it is necessary, and how he or she can participate. The administration of an ophthalmic medication is not usually painful. Ointments are often soothing to the eye, but some liquid preparations may sting initially. Discuss how the results will be used in planning further care or treatments.
4. Perform hand hygiene and observe other appropriate infection prevention procedures.
5. Provide for client privacy.
6. Prepare the client.
   - Prior to performing the procedure, verify the client's identity using agency protocol. **Rationale:** *This ensures that the right client receives the right medication.*
   - Assist the client to a comfortable position, usually lying.
7. Clean the eyelid and the eyelashes.
   - Apply clean gloves.
   - Use sterile cotton balls moistened with sterile irrigating solution or sterile normal saline, and wipe from the inner canthus to the outer canthus. **Rationale:** *If not removed, material on the eyelid and lashes can be washed into the eye. Cleaning toward the outer canthus prevents contamination of the other eye and the lacrimal duct.*
8. Administer the eye medication.
   - Check the ophthalmic preparation for the name, strength, and number of drops if a liquid is used. **Rationale:** *Checking medication data is essential to prevent a medication error.* Draw the correct number of drops into the shaft of the dropper if a dropper is used. If ointment is used, discard the first bead. **Rationale:** *The first bead of ointment from a tube is considered to be contaminated.*
   - Instruct the client to look up to the ceiling. Give the client a dry sterile absorbent sponge. **Rationale:** *The person is*

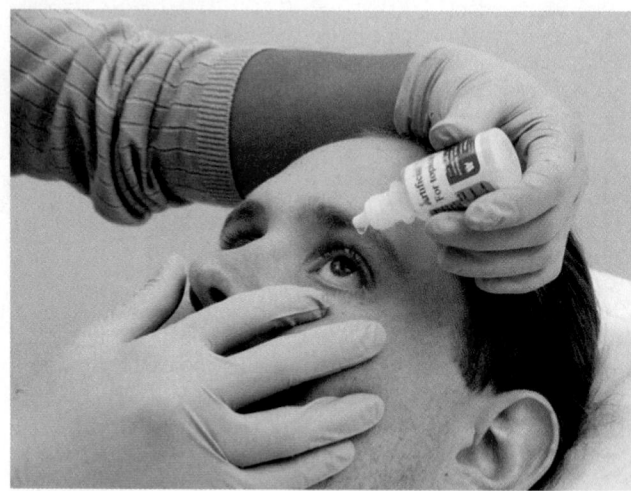

❶ Instilling an eyedrop into the lower conjunctival sac.

less likely to blink if looking up. While the client looks up, the cornea is partially protected by the upper eyelid. A sponge is needed to press on the nasolacrimal duct after a liquid instillation to prevent systemic absorption or to wipe excess ointment from the eyelashes after an ointment is instilled.
- Expose the lower conjunctival sac by placing the thumb or fingers of your nondominant hand on the client's cheekbone just below the eye and gently drawing down the skin on the cheek. If the tissues are edematous, handle the tissues carefully to avoid damaging them. **Rationale:** *Placing the fingers on the cheekbone minimizes the possibility of touching the cornea, avoids putting any pressure on the eyeball, and prevents the person from blinking or squinting.*
- Holding the medication in the dominant hand, place the hand on the client's forehead to stabilize the hand. Approach the eye from the side and instill the correct number of drops onto the outer third of the lower conjunctival sac. Hold the dropper 1 to 2 cm (0.4 to 0.8 in.) above the sac. ❶ **Rationale:** *The client is less likely to blink if a side approach is used. When instilled into the conjunctival sac, drops will not harm the cornea as they might if dropped directly on it. The dropper must not touch the sac or the cornea.*

or

- Holding the tube above the lower conjunctival sac, squeeze 2 cm (0.8 in.) of ointment from the tube into the lower conjunctival sac from the inner canthus outward. ❷
- Instruct the client to close the eyelids but not to squeeze them shut. **Rationale:** *Closing the eye spreads the medication over the eyeball. Squeezing can injure the eye and push out the medication.*

Administering Ophthalmic Medications—*continued*

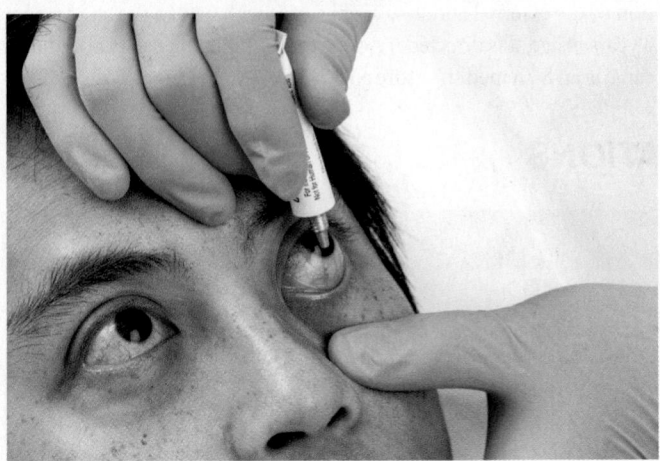

❷ Instilling an eye ointment into the lower conjunctival sac.

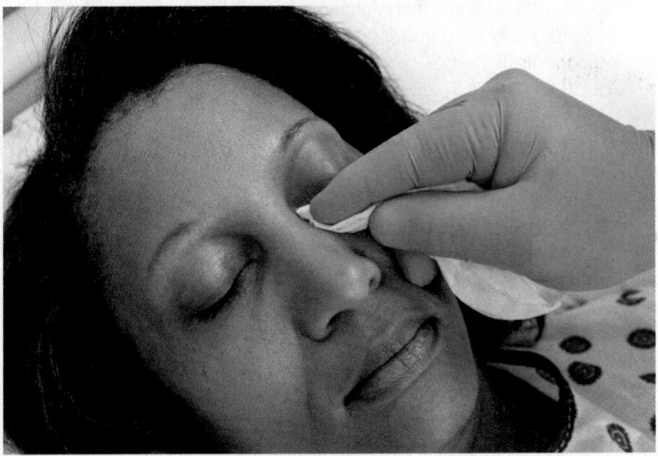

❸ Pressing on the nasolacrimal duct.

- For liquid medications, press firmly or have the client press firmly on the nasolacrimal duct for at least 30 seconds. ❸ **Rationale:** *Pressing on the nasolacrimal duct prevents the medication from running out of the eye and down the duct, preventing systemic absorption.*
- Remove and discard gloves.
- Perform hand hygiene.

Variation: Eye Irrigation
- Place absorbent pads under the head, neck, and shoulders. Place an emesis basin next to the eye to catch drainage. Some eye medications cause systemic reactions such as confusion or a decrease in heart rate and blood pressure if the eyedrops go down the nasolacrimal duct and get into the systemic circulation.
- Expose the lower conjunctival sac. Or, to irrigate in stages, first hold the lower lid down, then hold the upper lid up. Exert pressure on the bony prominences of the cheekbone and beneath the eyebrow when holding the eyelids. **Rationale:** *Separating the lids prevents reflex blinking. Exerting pressure on the bony prominences minimizes the possibility of pressing the eyeball and causing discomfort.*
- Fill and hold the eye irrigator about 2.5 cm (1 in.) above the eye. **Rationale:** *At this height the pressure of the solution will not damage the eye tissue, and the irrigator will not touch the eye.*
- Irrigate the eye, directing the solution onto the lower conjunctival sac and from the inner canthus to the outer canthus. **Rationale:** *Directing the solution in this way prevents possible injury to the cornea and prevents fluid and contaminants from flowing down the nasolacrimal duct.*
- Irrigate until the solution leaving the eye is clear (no discharge is present) or until all the solution has been used.
- Instruct the client to close and move the eye periodically. **Rationale:** *Eye closure and movement help to move secretions from the upper to the lower conjunctival sac.*

9. Clean and dry the eyelids as needed. Wipe the eyelids gently from the inner to the outer canthus to collect excess medication.
10. Remove and discard gloves.
    - Perform hand hygiene.
11. Apply an eye pad if needed, and secure it with paper eye tape.
12. Assess the client's response immediately after the instillation or irrigation and again after the medication should have acted.
13. Document all relevant assessments and interventions. Include the name of the drug or irrigating solution, the strength, the number of drops if a liquid medication, the time, and the response of the client.

EVALUATION
- Perform follow-up based on findings of the effectiveness of the administration or outcomes that deviated from expected or normal for the client. Relate findings to previous data if available.

- Report significant deviations from normal to the primary care provider.

LIFESPAN CONSIDERATIONS Administering Ophthalmic Medications

INFANTS/CHILDREN
- Explain the technique to the parents of an infant or child.
- For a young child or infant, obtain assistance to immobilize the arms and head. The parent may hold the infant or young child. **Rationale:** *This prevents accidental injury during medication administration.*

- For a young child, use a doll to demonstrate the procedure. **Rationale:** *This facilitates cooperation and decreases anxiety.*
- Children may tolerate drops better than ointment because drops are less likely to cause blurred vision.
- An intravenous (IV) bag and tubing may be used to deliver irrigating fluid to the eye.

OTIC MEDICATIONS

Instillations or irrigations of the external auditory canal are referred to as **otic** instillations and are generally carried out for cleaning purposes. Sometimes instillations involving applications of heat and antiseptic solutions are prescribed. Irrigations performed in a hospital require aseptic technique so that microorganisms will not be introduced into the ear. Sterile technique is used if the eardrum is perforated. The position of the external auditory canal varies with age. In the child under 3 years of age, it is directed upward. In the adult, the external auditory canal is an S-shaped structure about 2.5 cm (1 in.) long.

●○● NURSING PROCESS: OTIC MEDICATIONS

Administering Otic Medications

SKILL 16–3

ASSESSMENT

- In addition to the assessment performed by the nurse related to the administration of any medications (see Chapter 15 ∞), prior to applying otic medications, assess:
  - Appearance of the pinna of the ear and meatus for signs of redness and abrasions.
  - Type and amount of any discharge.
- Determine if assessment data influence administration of the medication (i.e., is it appropriate to administer the medication or does the medication need to be held and the primary care provider notified?).

PLANNING
DELEGATION

Due to the need for assessment, interpretation of client status, and use of sterile technique, otic medication administration is not delegated to UAP.

Equipment
- Clean gloves
- Cotton-tipped applicator
- Correct medication bottle with a dropper
- Flexible rubber tip (optional) for the end of the dropper, which prevents injury from sudden motion, for example, by a client who is disoriented
- Cotton fluff

For irrigation, add:
- Moisture-resistant towel
- Basin (e.g., emesis basin)
- Irrigating solution at 37°C (98.6°F) temperature, about 500 mL (16 oz) or as ordered. **Rationale:** *A solution that is not at body temperature may induce dizziness.*
- Container for the irrigating solution
- Syringe (rubber bulb or Asepto syringe is frequently used)

IMPLEMENTATION
Preparation
- Check the MAR.
  - Check for the drug name, strength, number of drops, and prescribed frequency.
  - Check client allergy status.
  - If the MAR is unclear or pertinent information is missing, compare it with the most recent primary care provider's written order.
  - Report any discrepancies to the charge nurse or primary care provider, as agency policy dictates.
- Know the reason why the client is receiving the medication, the drug classification, contraindications, usual dose range, side effects, and nursing considerations for administering and evaluating the intended outcomes of the medication.

Performance
1. Compare the label on the medication container with the medication record and check the expiration date.
2. If necessary, calculate the medication dosage.
3. Introduce self and explain to the client what you are going to do, why it is necessary, and how he or she can participate. The administration of an otic medication is not usually painful. Discuss how the results will be used in planning further care or treatments.
4. Perform hand hygiene and observe other appropriate infection prevention procedures.
5. Provide for client privacy.
6. Prepare the client.
   - Prior to performing the procedure, verify the client's identity using agency protocol. **Rationale:** *This ensures that the right client receives the right medication.*
   - Assist the client to a comfortable position for eardrop administration, usually lying with the ear being treated uppermost.

7. Clean the pinna of the ear and the meatus of the ear canal.
   - Apply gloves if infection is suspected.
   - Use cotton-tipped applicators and solution to wipe the pinna and auditory meatus. **Rationale:** *This removes any discharge present before the instillation so that it won't be washed into the ear canal.* Ensure that the applicator does *not* go into the ear canal. **Rationale:** *This avoids damage to the tympanic membrane or wax becoming impacted within the canal.*
8. Administer the ear medication.
   - Warm the medication container in your hand, or place it in warm water for a short time. **Rationale:** *This promotes client comfort and prevents nerve stimulation and pain.*
   - Partially fill the ear dropper with medication.
   - Straighten the auditory canal. Pull the pinna upward and backward for clients over 3 years of age. ❶ **Rationale:** *The auditory canal is straightened so that the solution can flow the entire length of the canal.*

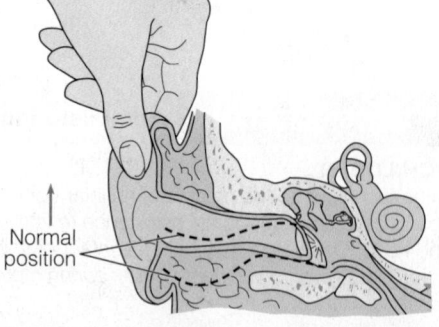

Normal position

❶ Straightening the adult ear canal by pulling the pinna upward and backward.

Administering Otic Medications—*continued*

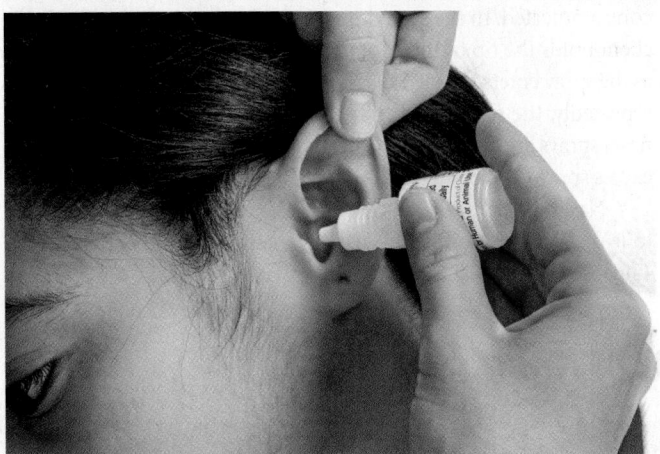

❷ Instilling eardrops.

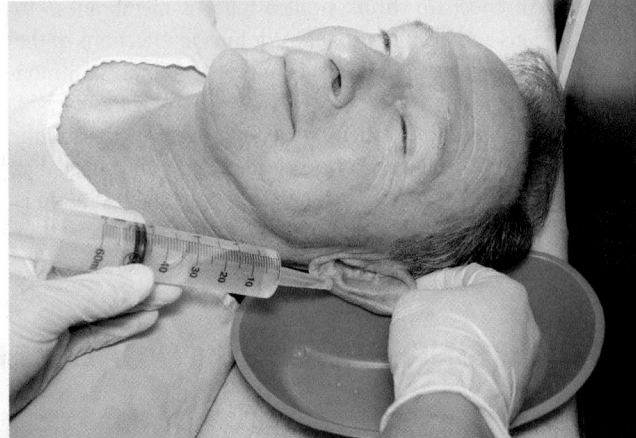

❸ Ear irrigation.

- Instill the correct number of drops along the side of the ear canal. ❷
- Press gently but firmly a few times on the tragus of the ear (the cartilaginous projection in front of the exterior meatus of the ear). **Rationale:** *Pressing on the tragus assists the flow of medication into the ear canal.*
- Ask the client to remain in the side-lying position for about 5 minutes. **Rationale:** *This prevents the drops from escaping and allows the medication to reach all sides of the canal cavity.*
- Insert a small piece of cotton fluff loosely at the meatus of the auditory canal for 15 to 20 minutes. Do not press it into the canal. **Rationale:** *The cotton helps retain the medication when the client is up. If pressed tightly into the canal, the cotton would interfere with the action of the drug and the outward movement of normal secretions.*

Variation: Ear Irrigation

- Explain that the client may experience a feeling of fullness, warmth, and, occasionally, discomfort when the fluid comes in contact with the tympanic membrane.
- Assist the client to a sitting or lying position with head tilted toward the affected ear. ❸ **Rationale:** *The solution can then flow from the ear canal to a basin.*
- Place the moisture-resistant towel around the client's shoulder under the ear to be irrigated, and place the basin under the ear to be irrigated.
- Fill the syringe with solution.

  or

- Hang up the irrigating container, and run solution through the tubing and the nozzle. **Rationale:** *Solution is run through to remove air from the tubing and nozzle.*
- Straighten the ear canal.
- Insert the tip of the syringe into the auditory meatus, and direct the solution gently upward against the top of the canal. **Rationale:** *The solution will flow around the entire canal and out at the bottom. The solution is instilled gently because strong pressure from the fluid can cause discomfort and damage the tympanic membrane.*
- Continue instilling the fluid until all the solution is used or until the canal is cleaned, depending on the purpose of the irrigation. Take care not to block the outward flow of the solution with the syringe.
- Assist the client to a side-lying position on the affected side. **Rationale:** *Lying with the affected side down helps drain the excess fluid by gravity.*
- Place a cotton fluff in the auditory meatus to absorb the excess fluid.
- Remove and discard gloves.
  - Perform hand hygiene.

9. Assess the client's response and the character and amount of discharge, appearance of the canal, discomfort, and so on, immediately after the instillation and again when the medication is expected to act. Inspect the cotton ball for any drainage.
10. Document all nursing assessments and interventions relative to the procedure. Include the name of the drug or irrigating solution, the strength, the number of drops if a liquid medication, the time, and the response of the client.

EVALUATION

- Perform follow-up based on findings of the effectiveness of the administration or outcomes that deviated from expected or normal for the client. Relate findings to previous data if available.

- Report significant deviations from normal to the primary care provider.

LIFESPAN CONSIDERATIONS   Administering Otic Medications

INFANTS/CHILDREN

- Obtain assistance to immobilize an infant or young child. **Rationale:** *This prevents accidental injury due to sudden movement during the procedure.*

- In infants and children under 3 years of age, the ear canal is directed upward. For this reason, to administer medication, gently pull the pinna down and back. For a child *older* than 3 years of age, pull the pinna upward and backward.

NASAL MEDICATIONS

Nasal instillations (nose drops and sprays) usually are instilled for their astringent effect (to shrink swollen mucous membranes), to loosen secretions and facilitate drainage, or to treat infections of the nasal cavity or sinuses. Nasal decongestants are the most common nasal instillations. Many of these products are available without a prescription. Clients need to be taught to use these agents with caution. Chronic use of nasal decongestants may lead to a rebound effect, that is, an increase in nasal congestion. If excess decongestant solution is swallowed, serious systemic effects may also develop, especially in children. Saline drops are safer as a decongestant for children.

Usually clients self-administer nasal sprays. It is suggested that clients blow their noses prior to administration of nasal sprays unless contraindicated. In the seated position with the head tilted back, the client holds the tip of the container just inside the naris and inhales as the spray enters the nasal passages. For clients who use nasal sprays repeatedly, the nares need to be assessed for irritation. In children, nasal sprays are given with the head in an upright position to prevent excess spray from being swallowed.

Nasal drops may be used to treat sinus infections. Clients need to learn ways to position themselves to effectively treat the affected sinus (see Skill 16–4).

●○○● NURSING PROCESS: NASAL MEDICATIONS

Administering Nasal Medications

ASSESSMENT

- If nasal secretions are excessive, ask the client to blow the nose to clear the nasal passages.
- Inspect the discharge on the tissues for color, odor, and thickness.
- In addition to the assessment performed by the nurse related to the administration of any medications (see Chapter 15 ∞), prior to applying nasal medications, assess:
  - Appearance of nasal cavities.
  - Congestion of the mucous membranes and any obstruction to breathing. Ask the client to hold one nostril closed and blow out gently through the other nostril. Listen for the sound of any obstruction to airflow. Repeat for the other nostril.

- Assess signs of distress when nares are occluded. Block each naris and observe for signs of greater distress when the naris is obstructed.
- Facial discomfort with or without palpation. An infected or congested sinus can cause an aching, full feeling over the area of the sinus and facial tenderness on palpation.
- Assess any crusting, redness, bleeding, or discharge of the mucous membranes of the nostrils. Use a nasal speculum. The membrane normally appears moist, pink, and shiny.
- Determine if assessment data influence administration of the medication (i.e., is it appropriate to administer the medication or does the medication need to be held or the primary care provider notified?).

PLANNING
DELEGATION

Due to the need for assessment and interpretation of client status, nasal medication administration is not delegated to UAP.

Equipment
- Tissues
- Clean gloves
- Correct medication bottle with a dropper

IMPLEMENTATION
Preparation
- Check the MAR.
  - Check for the drug name, strength, and number of drops. Also confirm the prescribed frequency of the instillation and which side of the nose is to be treated.
  - Check client allergy status.
  - If the MAR is unclear or pertinent information is missing, compare it with the most recent primary care provider's written order.
  - Report any discrepancies to the charge nurse or primary care provider, as agency policy dictates.
- Know the reason why the client is receiving the medication, the drug classification, contraindications, usual dose range, side effects, and nursing considerations for administering and evaluating the intended outcomes of the medication.

Performance
1. Compare the label on the medication container with the MAR and check the expiration date.
2. If necessary, calculate the medication dosage.
3. Introduce self and explain to the client what you are going to do, why it is necessary, and how he or she can participate. The administration of nasal medication is not usually painful. Discuss how the results will be used in planning further care or treatments.

4. Perform hand hygiene and observe other appropriate infection prevention procedures.
5. Provide for client privacy.
6. Prepare the client.
   - Prior to performing the procedure, verify the client's identity using agency protocol. **Rationale:** *This ensures that the right client receives the right medication.*
7. Assist the client to a comfortable position.
   - To treat the opening of the eustachian tube, have the client assume a back-lying position. **Rationale:** *The drops will flow into the nasopharynx, where the eustachian tube opens.*
   - To treat the ethmoid and sphenoid sinuses, have the client take a back-lying position with the head over the edge of the bed or a pillow under the shoulders so that the head is tipped backward. ❶
   - To treat the maxillary and frontal sinuses, have the client assume the same back-lying position, with the head turned toward the side to be treated. ❷ If only one side is to be treated, be sure the person is positioned so that the correct side is accessible. If the client's head is over the edge of the bed, support it with your hand so that the neck muscles are not strained.
8. Administer the medication.
   - Apply clean gloves.

Administering Nasal Medications—*continued*

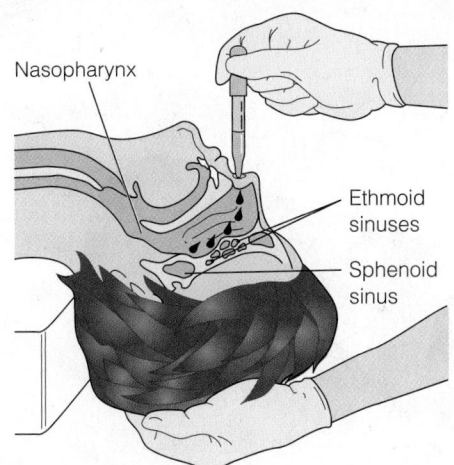

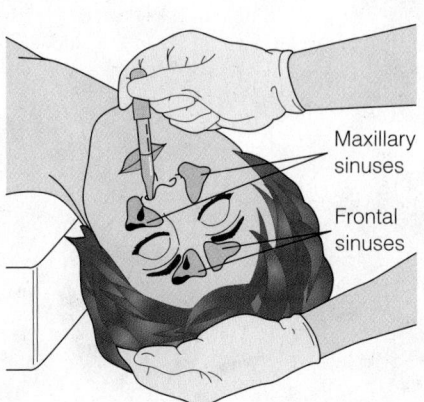

① Position of the head to instill drops into the ethmoid and sphenoid sinuses.

② Position of the head to instill drops into the maxillary and frontal sinuses.

- Draw up the required amount of solution into the dropper.
- Hold the tip of the dropper just above the nostril, and direct the solution laterally toward the midline of the superior concha of the ethmoid bone as the client breathes through the mouth. Do not touch the mucous membrane of the nostril. **Rationale:** *If the solution is directed toward the base of the nasal cavity, it will run down the eustachian tube. Touching the mucous membrane with the dropper could damage the membrane and cause the client to sneeze.*
- Repeat for the other nostril if indicated.

- Ask the client to remain in the position for 5 minutes. **Rationale:** *The client remains in the same position to help the solution come in contact with all of the nasal surface or flow into the desired area.*
- Discard any remaining solution in the dropper, and dispose of soiled supplies appropriately.
- Remove and discard gloves.
- Perform hand hygiene.
9. Document all nursing assessments and interventions relative to the procedure. Include the name of the drug or irrigating solution, the strength, the number of drops if a liquid medication, the time, and the response of the client.

EVALUATION
- Perform follow-up based on findings of the effectiveness of the administration or outcomes that deviated from expected or normal for the client. Relate findings to previous data if available.

- Report significant deviations from normal to the primary care provider.

INHALED MEDICATIONS

Nebulizers deliver most medications administered through the inhaled route. A nebulizer is used to deliver a fine spray (fog or mist) of medication or moisture to a client.

There are two kinds of nebulization: atomization and aerosolization. In **atomization**, a device called an *atomizer* produces rather large droplets for inhalation. In **aerosolization**, the droplets are suspended in a gas, such as oxygen. The smaller the droplets, the farther they can be inhaled into the respiratory tract. When a medication is intended for the nasal mucosa, it is inhaled through the nose; when it is intended for the trachea, bronchi, and/or lungs, it is inhaled through the mouth.

A *large-volume nebulizer* can provide a heated or cool mist. It is used for long-term therapy, such as that following a tracheostomy. The *ultrasonic nebulizer* provides 100% humidity and can provide particles small enough to be inhaled deeply into the respiratory tract.

The **metered-dose inhaler (MDI)**, a handheld nebulizer (Figure 16–3 ■), is a pressurized container of medication that can be used by the client to release medication through a mouthpiece. The force with which the air moves through the nebulizer causes the large particles of medicated solution to break up into finer particles, forming a mist or fine spray. MDIs can deliver accurate doses, provide for target action at the needed sites, and sustain fewer systemic effects than medication delivered by other routes.

To ensure correct delivery of the prescribed medication by MDIs, nurses need to instruct clients to use aerosol inhalers correctly. The client compresses the medication canister by hand to release medication through a mouthpiece. An extender or spacer (Figure 16–3*B*) may be attached to the mouthpiece to facilitate medication absorption for better results (Figure 16–4 ■). Spacers are holding chambers into which the medication is fired and from which the client inhales, so that the dose is not lost by exhalation.

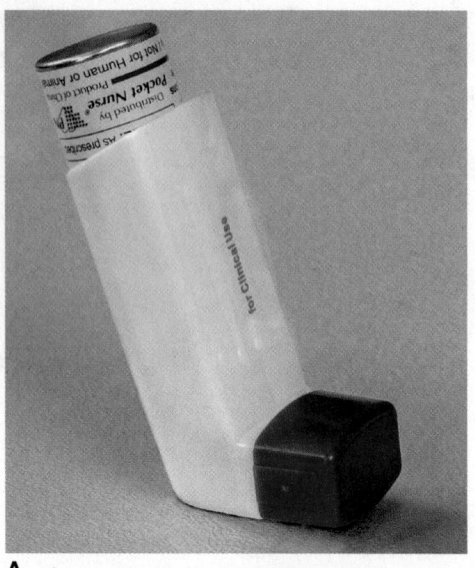

A

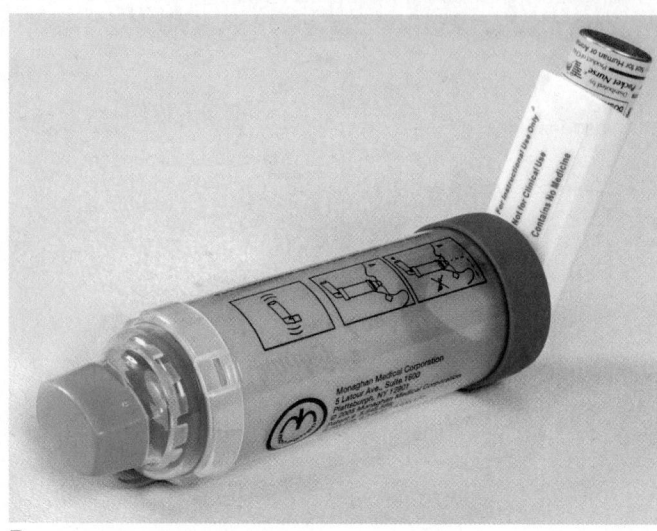

B

Figure 16–3 ■ *A*, Metered-dose inhaler; *B*, metered-dose inhaler with spacer.

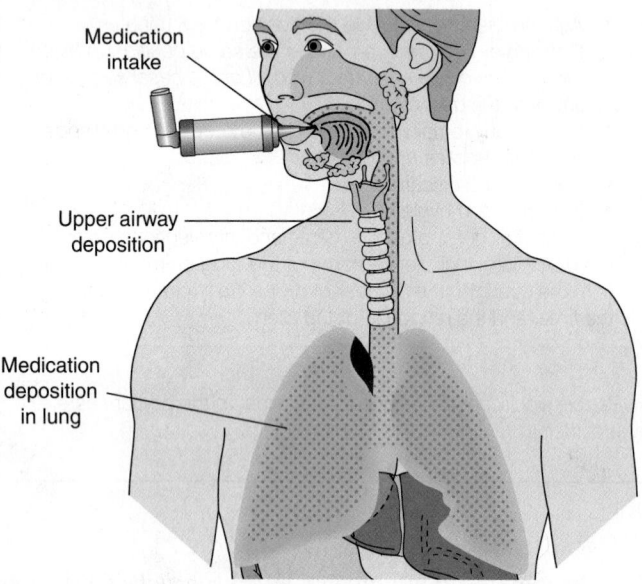

Medication intake

Upper airway deposition

Medication deposition in lung

Figure 16–4 ■ Delivery of medication to the lungs using a metered-dose inhaler extender.

Breath-activated MDIs are being produced in which inhalation triggers the release of a premeasured dose of medication. Their main advantage is that they decrease the problem that some clients have of coordinating the actuating (releasing) of the medication and inhaling of the medication. There are also dry powder inhalers (DPIs). A capsule is inserted into the center of the chamber of the inhalation device. A piercing device punctures the capsule, which allows the medication to be released upon inhalation by the client.

CLINICAL ALERT!

It is important for the nurse to assess if the client is using the MDI correctly. A client's ability to use an MDI correctly can decrease over time.

●○● NURSING PROCESS: INHALED MEDICATIONS

Administering Metered-Dose Inhaler Medications

SKILL 16–5

ASSESSMENT
- In addition to the assessment performed by the nurse related to the administration of any medications (see Chapter 15 ∞), prior to administering medications with an MDI, assess:
  - Lung sounds.
  - Respiratory rate and depth.
  - Cough (productive or nonproductive); amount, color, and character of expectorations.

- Presence of dyspnea.
- Vital signs for baseline data.
See Chapter 3 ∞ for assessment of the chest lung sounds.
- Determine if assessment data influence administration of the medication (i.e., is it appropriate to administer the medication or does the medication need to be held or the primary care provider notified?).

Administering Metered-Dose Inhaler Medications—*continued*

PLANNING
DELEGATION

Due to the need for assessment, teaching, and interpretation of client status, inhaled medication administration is not delegated to UAP.

Equipment
- Metered-dose nebulizer with medication canister and extender if indicated

SKILL 16-5

IMPLEMENTATION
Preparation
- Check the MAR.
  - Check for the drug name, strength, and prescribed frequency.
  - Check client allergy status.
  - If the MAR is unclear or pertinent information is missing, compare it with the most recent primary care provider's written order.
  - Report any discrepancies to the charge nurse or primary care provider, as agency policy dictates.
- Know the reason why the client is receiving the medication, the drug classification, contraindications, usual dose range, side effects, and nursing considerations for administering and evaluating the intended outcomes of the medication.

Performance
1. Compare the label on the medication container with the MAR and check the expiration date.
2. Introduce self and explain to the client what you are going to do, why it is necessary, and how he or she can participate. Discuss how the results will be used in planning further care or treatments.
3. Perform hand hygiene and observe other appropriate infection prevention procedures.
4. Provide for client privacy.
5. Prepare the client.
   - Prior to performing the procedure, verify the client's identity using agency protocol. **Rationale:** *This ensures that the right client receives the right medication.*
   - Explain that this nebulizer delivers a measured dose of drug with each push of the medication canister, which fits into the top of the nebulizer.
6. Instruct the client to use the metered-dose nebulizer as follows:

Metered-Dose Inhaler
- Ensure that the canister is firmly and fully inserted into the inhaler.
- Remove the mouthpiece cap. Holding the inhaler upright, shake the inhaler vigorously for 3 to 5 seconds to mix the medication evenly.
- Exhale comfortably (as in a normal full breath).
- Hold the inhaler with the canister on top and the mouthpiece at the bottom.
   a. Hold the MDI 2 to 4 cm (1 to 2 in.) from the open mouth. ❶
   or
   b. Put the mouthpiece far enough into the mouth with its opening toward the throat such that the lips can tightly close around the mouthpiece. ❷

Metered-Dose Inhaler with Spacer
- Insert the MDI mouthpiece into the spacer.
- Holding the inhaler and spacer, shake vigorously for 3 to 5 seconds to mix the medication evenly.
- An MDI with a spacer or extender is always placed in the mouth. ❸

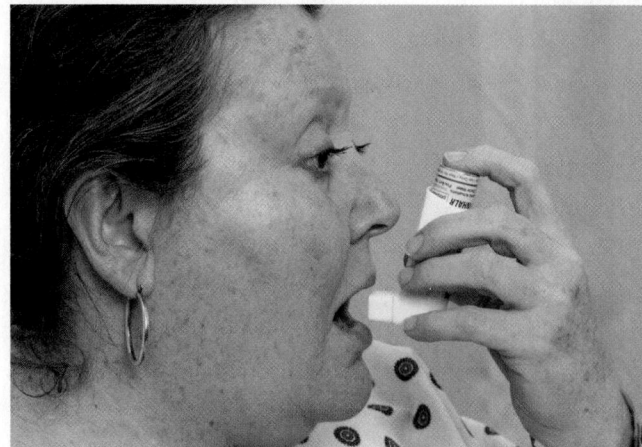

❶ Inhaler positioned 2 to 4 cm (1 to 2 in.) away from the open mouth.

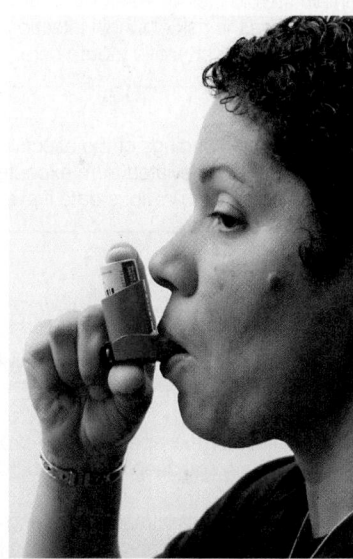

❷ Placing the MDI in the mouth with lips sealed around the mouthpiece.

Administering the Medication
- Press down *once* on the MDI canister (which releases the dose) and inhale slowly (for 3 to 5 seconds) and deeply through the mouth.
- Hold your breath for 10 seconds or as long as possible. **Rationale:** *This allows the aerosol to reach deeper airways.*
- Remove the inhaler from or away from the mouth.

Continued on page 400

Administering Metered-Dose Inhaler Medications—*continued*

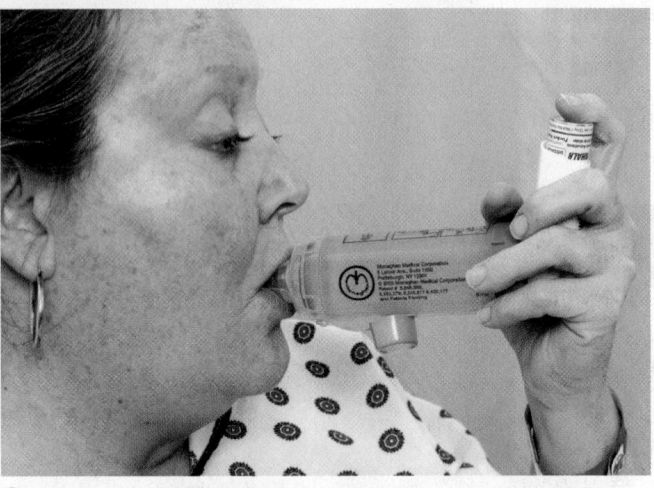

❸ An extender spacer attached to a mouthpiece placed in the mouth.

- Exhale slowly through *pursed* lips. **Rationale:** *Controlled exhalation keeps the small airways open during exhalation.*
- Repeat the inhalation if ordered. Wait 1 to 2 minutes between inhalations of bronchodilator medications. **Rationale:** *Waiting gives the first inhalation a chance to work so the subsequent dose can reach deeper into the lungs.*
- Many MDIs contain steroids for an anti-inflammatory effect. Prolonged use increases the risk of fungal infections in the mouth, indicating a need for attentive mouth care.

EVALUATION
- Perform follow-up based on findings of the effectiveness of the medication or outcomes that deviated from expected or normal for the client. Relate findings to previous data if available.

CLINICAL ALERT!

If two inhalers are to be used, the bronchodilator medication (which opens the airways) should be given prior to other medications. A mnemonic to help remember this is *B before C* (i.e., *B*ronchodilator before *C*orticosteroid).

- Following use of the inhaler, rinse the mouth with water and spit it out. **Rationale:** *Rinsing the mouth removes any remaining medication and reduces irritation and risk of infection.*
- Clean the MDI mouthpiece, and spacer if appropriate, daily. Use mild soap and water, rinse it, and let it air-dry before reusing.

CLINICAL ALERT!

Inhaled steroids may not be correctly used by clients because they do not associate these medications with immediate symptom relief. The bronchodilators act to open the airways in the short term. However, it is the inhaled steroids that keep airway inflammation under control.

- Store the canister at room temperature. Avoid extremes of temperature.
- Report adverse reactions such as restlessness, palpitations, nervousness, or rash to the primary care provider.
7. Document all nursing assessments and interventions relative to the procedure. Include the name of the drug, the strength, the time, and the response of the client.

- Report significant deviations from normal to the primary care provider.

LIFESPAN CONSIDERATIONS   Administering Metered-Dose Inhalers and Nebulizers

CHILDREN
- Spacers hold a medication in suspension and provide the child an opportunity to take several deep breaths in order to inhale all the medication.
- A mask is used for nebulizer treatments, allowing the child to breathe naturally. Some infants and children may be frightened or uncomfortable with the mask and become resistant. Use a doll or stuffed animal to demonstrate its use, and allow them to play with the equipment before putting it in place. Having the child sit in a parent's lap during the procedure can help the child relax and be more cooperative.

Ambulatory and Community Settings   Metered-Dose Inhalers   PATIENT-CENTERED CARE

- Disinfect the MDI mouthpieces weekly by soaking for 20 minutes in 1 pint of water with 2 ounces of vinegar added.
- Teach clients how to determine the amount of medication remaining in an MDI canister:
  - Calculate the number of days' doses in a canister. Divide the number of doses (puffs) in the canister (on the label) by the number of puffs taken per day. The previous method of floating the canister in water is not considered accurate because some of the propellant may remain (even after the medication is gone), which leads the client to incorrectly believe he or she is receiving medication.
- Review instructions and periodically assess the client's techniques for using an inhaler spacer or chamber correctly. Research shows that these devices assist in delivering the medication deeply into the lungs rather than only to the oropharynx.

VAGINAL MEDICATIONS

Vaginal medications are inserted as creams, jellies, foams, or suppositories to treat infection or to relieve vaginal discomfort (e.g., itching or pain). Medical aseptic technique is usually used. Vaginal creams, jellies, and foams are applied by using a tubular applicator with a plunger. **Suppositories** are inserted with the index finger of a gloved hand. Suppositories are designed to melt at body temperature, so they are generally stored in the refrigerator to keep them firm for insertion. See Skill 16–6 for administering vaginal instillations.

A vaginal irrigation (douche) is the washing of the vagina by a liquid at a low pressure. Vaginal irrigations are not necessary for ordinary female hygiene but are used to prevent infection by applying an antimicrobial solution that discourages the growth of microorganisms, to remove an offensive or irritating discharge, and to reduce inflammation or prevent hemorrhage by the application of heat or cold. In hospitals, sterile supplies and equipment are used; in a home, sterility is not usually necessary because people are accustomed to the microorganisms in their environments. Sterile technique, however, is indicated if there is an open wound.

●○● NURSING PROCESS: VAGINAL MEDICATIONS

Administering Vaginal Medications

SKILL 16–6

ASSESSMENT

- In addition to the assessment performed by the nurse related to the administration of any medications (see Chapter 15 ∞), prior to applying vaginal medications, assess:
  - The vaginal orifice for inflammation; amount, character, and odor of vaginal discharge.
  - For complaints of vaginal discomfort (e.g., burning or itching).

- Determine if assessment data influence administration of the medication (i.e., is it appropriate to administer the medication or does the medication need to be held and the primary care provider notified?).

PLANNING
DELEGATION

Due to the need for assessment and interpretation of client status, vaginal medication administration is not delegated to UAP.

Equipment
- Drape
- Correct vaginal suppository or cream
- Applicator for vaginal cream
- Clean gloves

- Lubricant for a suppository
- Disposable towel
- Clean perineal pad

For an irrigation, add:
- Moisture-proof pad
- Vaginal irrigation set (these are often disposable) containing a nozzle, tubing and a clamp, and a container for the solution
- Irrigating solution (It is recommended that the solution be warmed to a temperature of 37.8°C to 43.3°C [100°F to 110°F] if not specified, to minimize discomfort caused by cooler solutions.)

IMPLEMENTATION
Preparation
- Check the MAR.
- Check for the drug name, strength, and prescribed frequency.
  - Check client allergy status.
  - If the MAR is unclear or pertinent information is missing, compare it with the most recent primary care provider's written order.
  - Report any discrepancies to the charge nurse or primary care provider, as agency policy dictates.
- Know the reason why the client is receiving the medication, the drug classification, contraindications, usual dose range, side effects, and nursing considerations for administering and evaluating the intended outcomes of the medication.

Performance
1. Compare the label on the medication container with the medication record and check the expiration date.
2. If necessary, calculate the medication dosage.
3. Introduce self and explain to the client what you are going to do, why it is necessary, and how she can participate. Explain to the client that a vaginal instillation is normally a painless procedure, and in fact may bring relief from itching and burning if an infection is present. Many people feel embarrassed about this procedure, and some may prefer to perform the procedure themselves if instruction is provided. Discuss how the results will be used in planning further care or treatments.

4. Perform hand hygiene and observe other appropriate infection prevention procedures.
5. Provide for client privacy.
6. Prepare the client.
   - Prior to performing the procedure, verify the client's identity using agency protocol. **Rationale:** *This ensures that the right client receives the right medication.*
   - Ask the client to void. **Rationale:** *If the bladder is empty, the client will have less discomfort during the treatment, and the possibility of injuring the vaginal lining is decreased.*
   - Assist the client to a back-lying position with the knees flexed and the hips rotated laterally.
   - Drape the client appropriately so that only the perineal area is exposed.
7. Prepare the equipment.
   - Unwrap the suppository, and put it on the opened wrapper.
   or
   - Fill the applicator with the prescribed cream, jelly, or foam. Directions are provided with the manufacturer's applicator.
8. Assess and clean the perineal area.
   - Apply gloves. **Rationale:** *Gloves prevent contamination of the nurse's hands from vaginal and perineal microorganisms.*
   - Inspect the vaginal orifice, note any odor or discharge from the vagina, and ask about any vaginal discomfort.

Continued on page 402

Administering Vaginal Medications—*continued*

SKILL 16–6

- Provide perineal care to remove microorganisms. **Rationale:** *This decreases the chance of moving microorganisms into the vagina.*

9. Administer the vaginal suppository, cream, foam, jelly, or irrigation.

Suppository

- Lubricate the rounded (smooth) end of the suppository, which is inserted first. **Rationale:** *Lubrication facilitates insertion.*
- Lubricate your gloved index finger.
- Expose the vaginal orifice by separating the labia with your non-dominant hand.
- Insert the suppository about 8 to 10 cm (3 to 4 in.) along the posterior wall of the vagina, or as far as it will go. ❶ **Rationale:** *The posterior wall of the vagina is about 2.5 cm (1 in.) longer than the anterior wall because the cervix protrudes into the uppermost portion of the anterior wall.*
- Ask the client to remain lying in the supine position for 5 to 10 minutes following insertion. The hips may also be elevated on a pillow. **Rationale:** *This position allows the medication to flow into the posterior fornix after it has melted.*

Vaginal Cream, Jelly, or Foam

- Gently insert the applicator about 5 cm (2 in.).
- Slowly push the plunger until the applicator is empty. ❷
- Remove the applicator and place it on the towel. **Rationale:** *The applicator is placed on the towel to prevent the spread of microorganisms.*
- Discard the applicator if disposable or clean it according to the manufacturer's directions.
- Ask the client to remain lying in the supine position for 5 to 10 minutes following the insertion.

Irrigation

- Place the client on a bedpan.
- Clamp the tubing. Hold the irrigating container about 30 cm (12 in.) above the vagina. **Rationale:** *At this height, the pressure of the solution should not be great enough to injure the vaginal lining.*
- Run fluid through the tubing and nozzle into the bedpan. **Rationale:** *Fluid is run through the tubing to remove air and to moisten the nozzle.*
- Insert the nozzle carefully into the vagina. Direct the nozzle toward the sacrum, following the direction of the vagina.
- Insert the nozzle about 7 to 10 cm (3 to 4 in.), start the flow, and rotate the nozzle several times. **Rationale:** *Rotating the nozzle irrigates all parts of the vagina.*
- Use all of the irrigating solution, permitting it to flow out freely into the bedpan.
- Remove the nozzle from the vagina.

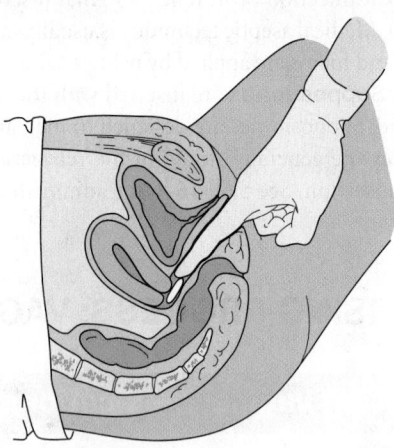

❶ Instilling a vaginal suppository.

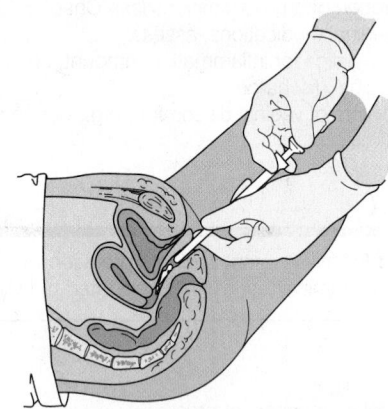

❷ Using an applicator to instill a vaginal cream.

- Assist the client to a sitting position on the bedpan. **Rationale:** *Sitting on the bedpan will help drain the remaining fluid by gravity.*

10. Ensure client comfort.
    - Dry the perineum with tissues as required.
    - Apply a clean perineal pad if there is excessive drainage.
    - Remove and discard gloves.
    - Perform hand hygiene.

11. Document all nursing assessments and interventions relative to the skill. Include the name of the drug or irrigating solution, the strength, the time, and the response of the client.

EVALUATION

- Perform follow-up based on findings of the effectiveness of the administration or outcomes that deviated from expected or normal for the client. Relate findings to previous data if available.

- Report significant deviations from normal to the primary care provider.

RECTAL MEDICATIONS

Insertion of medications into the rectum in the form of suppositories is a frequent practice. Rectal administration is a convenient and safe method of giving certain medications. Advantages include the following:

- It avoids irritation of the upper gastrointestinal tract in clients who encounter this problem (e.g., in clients who are nauseated or vomiting).

- It is advantageous when the medication has an objectionable taste or odor.
- The drug is released at a slow but steady rate.
- Rectal suppositories are thought to provide higher bloodstream levels (titers) of medication, because the venous blood from the lower rectum is not transported through the liver.

●○● NURSING PROCESS: RECTAL MEDICATIONS

Administering Rectal Medications

ASSESSMENT

- In addition to the assessment performed by the nurse related to the administration of any medications (see Chapter 15 ∞), prior to administering rectal medications, assess:
  - Client's need for the medication if prn (e.g., abdominal distention and/or discomfort if the suppository is intended to stimulate defecation).
  - Whether the client desires to defecate or time of last defecation (suppositories that are given for a systemic effect should be given when the rectum is free of feces to enhance absorption of the drug).

- Any side effects; any contraindications to the rectal route (e.g., recent rectal surgery or rectal pathology, such as bleeding).
- Determine if assessment data influence administration of the medication (i.e., is it appropriate to administer the medication or does the medication need to be held and the primary care provider notified?).

PLANNING
DELEGATION

Due to the need for assessment and interpretation of client status, rectal medication administration is not delegated to UAP.

Equipment
- Correct suppository
- Clean glove
- Lubricant

IMPLEMENTATION
Preparation
- Check the MAR.
  - Check for the drug name, strength, and prescribed frequency.
  - Check client allergy status.
  - If the MAR is unclear or pertinent information is missing, compare it with the most recent primary care provider's written order.
  - Report any discrepancies to the charge nurse or primary care provider, as agency policy dictates.
- Know the reason why the client is receiving the medication, the drug classification, contraindications, usual dose range, side effects, and nursing considerations for administering and evaluating the intended outcomes of the medication.

Performance
1. Compare the label on the medication container with the medication record and check the expiration date.
2. Introduce self and explain to the client what you are going to do, why it is necessary, and how he or she can participate. Discuss how the results will be used in planning further care or treatments.
3. Perform hand hygiene and observe other appropriate infection prevention procedures.
4. Provide for client privacy.
5. Prepare the client.
   - Prior to performing the procedure, verify the client's identity using agency protocol. **Rationale:** *This ensures that the right client receives the right medication.*

   - Assist the client to a left lateral or left Sims' position, with the upper leg acutely flexed. **Rationale:** *The left lateral or Sims' position is preferred because it positions the sigmoid colon downward, which allows gravity to help retain the suppository.*
   - Fold back the top bedclothes to expose only the buttocks.
6. Prepare the equipment.
   - Unwrap the suppository, and leave it on the opened wrapper.
   - Apply glove on the hand used to insert the suppository. **Rationale:** *The glove prevents contamination of the nurse's hand by rectal microorganisms and feces.*
   - Lubricate the smooth, rounded end of the suppository, or see the manufacturer's instructions. **Rationale:** *The smooth, rounded end is inserted first. Lubrication prevents anal friction and tissue damage on insertion.*
   - Lubricate the gloved index finger.
7. Insert the suppository.
   - Ask the client to breathe through the mouth. **Rationale:** *This usually relaxes the external anal sphincter.*
   - Insert the suppository gently into the anus, rounded end first (or according to the manufacturer's instructions) and along the wall of the rectum with the gloved index finger. ❶ For an adult, insert the suppository 10 cm (4 in.) or after passing the sphincter. **Rationale:** *The rounded end facilitates insertion. The suppository needs to be placed along the wall of the rectum, rather than within feces, in order to be absorbed effectively.*

Continued on page 404

SKILL 16–7

Administering Rectal Medications—*continued*

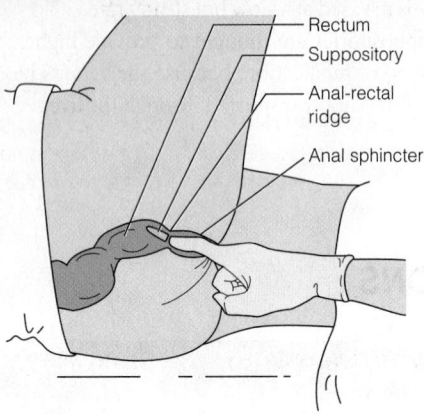

- Rectum
- Suppository
- Anal-rectal ridge
- Anal sphincter

❶ Inserting a rectal suppository beyond the internal sphincter and along the rectal wall.

- Withdraw the finger. Press the client's buttocks together for a few minutes. **Rationale:** *This helps minimize any urge to expel the suppository.*
- Remove the glove by turning it inside out and discard. **Rationale:** *Turning the glove inside out contains the rectal microorganisms and prevents their spread.*
- Perform hand hygiene.
- Ask the client to remain flat or in the left lateral position for at least 5 minutes. **Rationale:** *This helps prevent expulsion of the suppository.* The suppository should be retained at least 30 to 40 minutes or according to the manufacturer's instructions.
- If the client has been given a laxative suppository, place the call light within easy reach to summon assistance for the bedpan or toilet.

8. Document all nursing assessments and interventions relative to the procedure. Include the type of suppository given/name of the drug, the time it was given, the amount of time it was retained if it was expelled, the results or effects, and the response of the client.

EVALUATION
- Perform follow-up based on findings of the effectiveness of the administration or outcomes that deviated from expected or normal for the client. Relate findings to previous data if available.
- Report significant deviations from normal to the primary care provider.

LIFESPAN CONSIDERATIONS **Administering Rectal Medications**

INFANTS/CHILDREN
- Obtain assistance to immobilize an infant or young child. **Rationale:** *This prevents accidental injury due to sudden movement during the procedure.*
- For a child under 3 years, the nurse should use the gloved fifth finger for insertion. After this age, the index finger can usually be used.
- For a child or infant, insert a suppository 5 cm (2 in.) or less.

Chapter **16** Review

FOCUSING ON CLINICAL THINKING

Consider This

1. The client observes you putting on gloves before applying ordered topical cream. You are asked why you wear them since the client doesn't wear gloves at home when applying the cream. What would be your response?
2. Your client is scheduled for cataract surgery on the right eye. You have an order for antibiotic eyedrops OS q1h × 4 before surgery at 10 am. Would you question any of these orders? If so, why?
3. Eardrops are administered with the affected ear facing upward, whereas ear irrigations are performed with the affected ear facing downward. Explain the rationale for this.
4. Would sterile or clean technique be indicated for administration of nose drops? Explain your answer.
5. The client has been using vaginal cream at home for a yeast infection but the infection remains. What questions would you ask to determine if the client has been performing the cream application properly?
6. The client has just started using a bronchodilator metered-dose inhaler for asthma. After a few days, the client reports the inhaler is not providing any relief—just making the client jittery. What might explain this? What would you suggest?
7. Your client requires a rectal suppository but is unable to lie on the left side. How will you administer the suppository?

See Focusing on Clinical Thinking answers on student resource website.

TEST YOUR KNOWLEDGE

1. A nurse is reading the primary care provider's progress note for a client. The progress note recommends to continue use of dermatologic preparations. The nurse knows that which products fall into this category? Select all that apply.
   1. Ointments
   2. Pastes
   3. Sprays
   4. Patches
   5. Lotions

2. The nurse is teaching the client how to administer a nicotine transdermal patch prior to discharge from the hospital. Which statement, made by the client, indicates the need for further teaching by the nurse?
   1. "I should apply the patch to an area on my body that is hairless and clean."
   2. "I should avoid placing the patch on areas with cuts, burns, or abrasions."
   3. "I should apply the patch to my forearm."
   4. "I should be careful when discarding the patch because some medication may still be present on it."

3. A nurse is administering an ophthalmic medication for a child with conjunctivitis. Which nursing action demonstrates an understanding of the principles of administering an ophthalmic preparation?
   1. When using an ointment, the nurse administers the first bead for optimal effectiveness.
   2. The nurse uses sterile cotton balls to remove material on the eyelid.
   3. When using a sterile cotton ball, the nurse wipes from the outer canthus to the inner canthus.
   4. The nurse instructs the client to look straight ahead.

4. A nurse is teaching the parents of a 2-year-old how to administer an otic medication. The parents are performing a return demonstration. Which action would require immediate intervention by the nurse?
   1. The mother is gently pulling the child's pinna upward and backward.
   2. The father is assisting with the immobilization of the child's head.
   3. The mother uses a cotton-tipped applicator and solution to wipe the pinna and auditory meatus.
   4. The father warms the medication container in his hand.

5. A nurse is teaching a teenager how to administer nasal drops for allergies. Which technique, if done by the teenager, demonstrates effective teaching by the nurse?
   1. Directs the solution medially toward the midline of the superior concha.
   2. Touches the mucous membranes of the nares with the solution.

3. Knows that immediate movement is permitted after administration.
4. Breathes through the mouth while administering the medication.

6. A nurse is teaching the mother of a client with asthma about proper use of a metered-dose inhaler. Which statement, if made by the mother, indicates that teaching has been effective?
   1. "Since my child does not like the spacer, I don't have to use it at all."
   2. "I only need to shake the inhaler if it is a new one."
   3. "I should have my child hold his breath for 5 seconds after taking the inhaler."
   4. "I need to give my child the bronchodilator before the steroid medication."

7. A nurse is assisting a client with the administration of a vaginal suppository. Which action is necessary with the administration of this medication?
   1. Have the client gently insert the applicator about 5 cm (2 in.).
   2. Ask the client to remain lying in the supine position for 5 to 10 minutes following the administration.
   3. Slowly push the plunger until the applicator is empty.
   4. Remove the applicator and place it on a towel.

8. The nurse is teaching the mother of a 1-year-old how to administer a rectal suppository for when the child is febrile. Which technique demonstrates an understanding of the principles of rectal medication administration?
   1. The mother prepares to use the index finger for insertion.
   2. The mother administers the medication without assistance to avoid frightening the child.
   3. The mother inserts the suppository 5 cm (2 in.) or less.
   4. The mother prepares to use the ring finger for insertion.

9. The nurse is administering a medication that has small droplets suspended in a gas. The nurse recognizes that this indicates the medication is:
   1. Heated nebulized.
   2. Cool mist nebulized.
   3. Atomized.
   4. Aerosolized.

10. The nurse learns that the client began experiencing pruritus after beginning a new medication. Which question would the nurse want to ask the client?
    1. "Are you still scratching this morning?"
    2. "Are you still having difficulty swallowing this morning?"
    3. "Do you still have purple spots on your arm?"
    4. "Are you still having pain with breathing?"

See Answers to Test Your Knowledge in Appendix A.

READINGS AND REFERENCES

References

Association of Reproductive Health Professionals. (2011). *Transdermal contraceptive patch*. Retrieved from http://www.arhp.org/Publications-and-Resources/Quick-Reference-Guide-for-Clinicians/choosing/Transdermal-Patch

MRIsafety.com. (2012). Transdermal medication patches and other drug delivery patches. Retrieved from http://www.mrisafety.com/safety_article.asp?subject=56

Selected Bibliography

Berman, A., Snyder, S., & Frandsen, G. (2016). *Kozier & Erb's fundamentals of nursing: Concepts, process, and practice* (10th ed.). Upper Saddle River, NJ: Pearson.

Cohen, M. (2013). Medication errors: Fentanyl overdose: Off with the old. *Nursing, 43*(1), 12. doi:10.1097/01.NURSE.0000423966.16024.e7

Corjulo, M. T. (2011). Mastering the metered-dose inhaler: An essential step toward improving asthma control in school. *NASN School Nurse, 26*, 285–290. doi:10.1177/1942602X11416989.

Rawles, Z. (2010). Ear irrigation: Anatomy, process and patient care. *British Journal of Healthcare Assistants, 4*, 580–582.

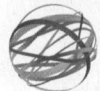# 17 Administering Parenteral Medications

LEARNING OUTCOMES

At the completion of this chapter, the student will be able to:

1. Define the key terms used in the skills of administering parenteral medications.
2. Describe the types of equipment required for parenteral medications:
   a. Syringes
   b. Needles
   c. Ampules
   d. Vials.
3. Identify sites used for intradermal, subcutaneous, and intramuscular injections.
4. Describe the various methods used to administer medications intravenously.

5. Verbalize the steps used in:
   a. Preparing medications from ampules.
   b. Preparing medications from vials.
   c. Mixing medications using one syringe.
   d. Administering an intradermal injection.
   e. Administering a subcutaneous injection.
   f. Administering an intramuscular injection.
   g. Adding medications to intravenous fluid containers.
   h. Administering intermittent intravenous medications using a secondary set.
   i. Administering intravenous medications using IV push.
6. Demonstrate appropriate documentation and reporting of parenteral medication administration.

SKILLS

KEY TERMS

ampule, *411*
bevel, *409*
deltoid site, *425*
diluent, *412*
filter needle, *411*
filter straw, *411*
gauge, *409*
hub, *409*

insulin syringe, *408*
intradermal (ID) injection, *417*
intramuscular (IM) injections, *422*
intravenous push (IVP), *438*
parenteral, *406*
piggyback, *433*
prefilled unit-dose systems, *407*
primary port, *436*

reconstitution, *412*
rectus femoris site, *425*
secondary port, *436*
shaft, *409*
syringe pump, *434*
tandem, *433*
tuberculin syringe, *409*
vastus lateralis site, *424*

ventrogluteal site, *423*
vial, *411*
volume-control infusion set, *434*
wheal, *418*
Z-track technique, *426*

Parenteral administration of medications involves using a medication route other than topically or via the alimentary or digestive tract. Nurses give parenteral medications intradermally (just beneath the dermis or skin), subcutaneously (in subcutaneous tissue between skin and muscle), intramuscularly (into a muscle), or intravenously (into a vein). Because these medications are absorbed more quickly than oral medications and are irretrievable once injected, the nurse must prepare and administer them carefully and accurately. Administering parenteral drugs requires the same nursing knowledge as for oral and topical drugs; however, because injections are invasive procedures, aseptic technique must be used to minimize the risk of infection.

EQUIPMENT

To administer parenteral medications, nurses use syringes and needles to withdraw medication from ampules and vials.

Syringes

Syringes have three parts: the tip, which connects with the needle; the barrel, or outside part, on which the scales are printed; and the plunger, which fits inside the barrel (Figure 17–1 ■). When handling a syringe, the nurse may touch the outside of the barrel and the handle of the plunger; however, the nurse must *avoid letting any unsterile object contact the tip or inside of the barrel, the shaft of the plunger, or the shaft or tip of the syringe.*

There are several kinds of syringes differing in size, shape, and material. Syringes range in sizes from 1 to 60 mL. A nurse typically uses a syringe ranging from 1 to 3 mL in size for injections (e.g., subcutaneous or intramuscular). The choice of syringe depends on many factors, such as medication, location of injection, and type of tissue. Syringes ranging from 1 to 3 mL may have two scales marked on them: the minim and the milliliter. The milliliter scale is

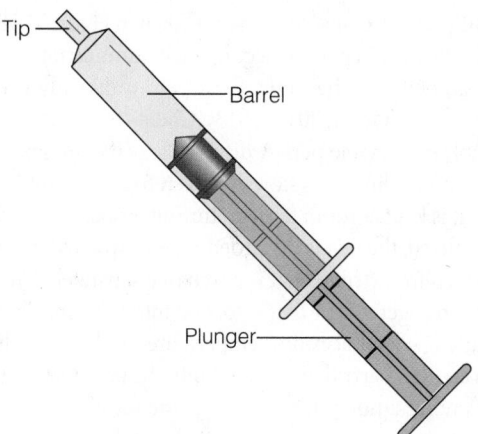

Figure 17–1 ■ The three parts of a syringe.

the one normally used; the minim scale is used for very small dosages (Figure 17–2 ■). The larger sized syringes (e.g., 10, 20, and 60 mL) are not used to administer drugs directly but can be useful for adding medications to intravenous (IV) solutions, pushing medication through an IV line, or irrigating wounds.

The tip of a syringe varies and is classified as either a Luer-Lok (sometimes spelled Luer-Lock) or non–Luer-Lok, also known as a Slip Tip syringe. A Luer-Lok syringe has a tip that requires the needle to be twisted onto it to avoid accidental removal of the needle (Figure 17–3A ■). A non–Luer-Lok or Slip Tip syringe has a smooth graduated tip, and needles are slipped onto it (Figure 17–3B). The larger 60-mL, non–Luer-Lok syringe (Figure 17–4 ■) is often used for irrigation purposes (e.g., wounds, tubes).

Most syringes used today are made of plastic, are individually packaged for sterility in a paper wrapper or a rigid plastic container (Figure 17–5 ■), and are disposable. The syringe and needle may be packaged together or separately. Needleless systems are also available in which the needle is replaced by a plastic cannula or a more rigid blunt tip instead of a sharp tip.

Injectable medications are frequently supplied in disposable **prefilled unit-dose systems**. These are available as (a) prefilled syringes ready for use or (b) prefilled sterile cartridges and needles that require the attachment of a reusable holder (injection system) before use (Figure 17–6 ■). Examples of the latter system are the Tubex and Carpuject injection systems. The manufacturers provide specific

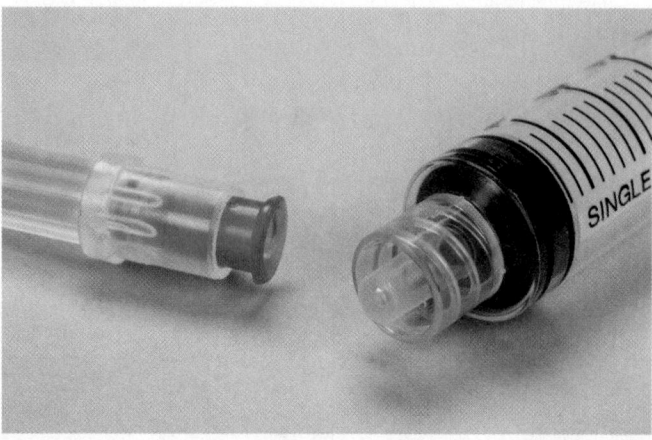

A

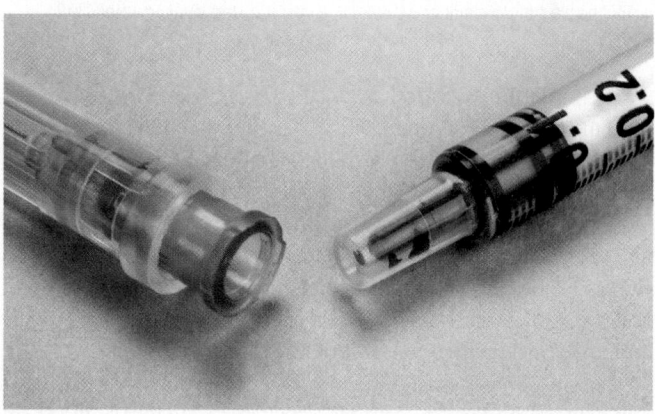

B

Figure 17–3 ■ Tips of syringes: *A*, Luer-Lok syringe (note threaded tip); *B*, non–Luer-Lok or Slip Tip syringe (note the smooth graduated tip).

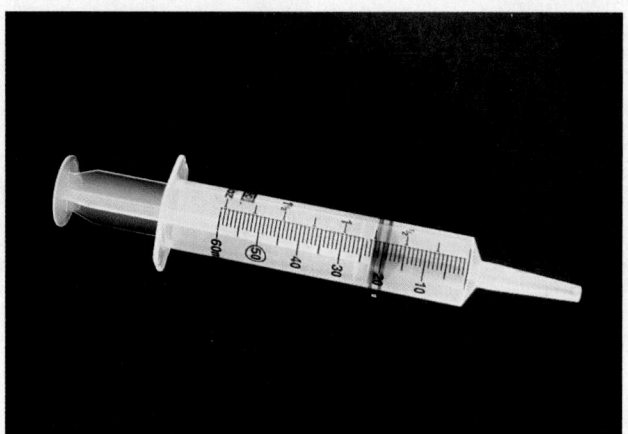

Figure 17–4 ■ A 60-mL non–Luer-Lok (Slip Tip) syringe, which can be used for irrigation of tubes or wounds.

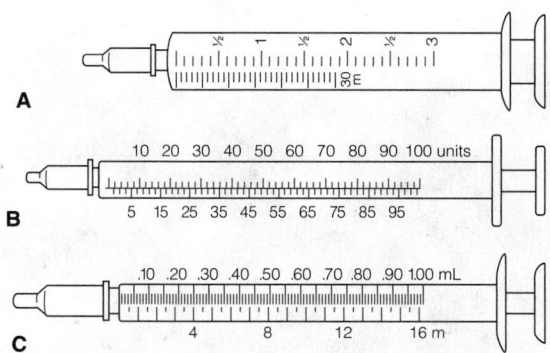

Figure 17–2 ■ Three kinds of syringes: *A*, 3-mL syringe marked in tenths (0.1) of a milliliter and in minims; *B*, insulin syringe marked in 100 units; *C*, tuberculin syringe marked in tenths and hundredths (0.01) of 1 mL and in minims.

directions for use. Because most prefilled cartridges are overfilled, excess medication must be ejected before the injection to ensure the right dosage. Because the needle is fused to the syringe, the nurse cannot change the gauge or length of the needle. The nurse, however, can transfer the medication into a regular syringe if the assessment of the client necessitates a different needle gauge or length. The Carpuject has a removable protective cap that allows the prefilled cartridge to become a vial so that the nurse can withdraw the medication.

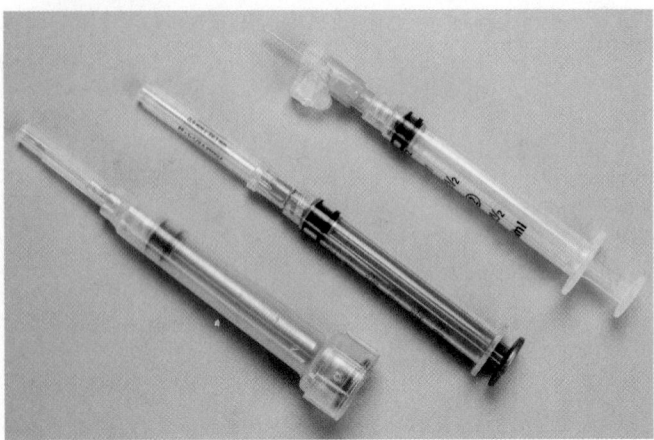

Figure 17–5 ■ Disposable plastic syringes and needles: *Top*, syringe with needle safety device; *Middle*, with plastic cap over the needle; *Bottom*, with plastic case over the needle and syringe.

An **insulin syringe** has a scale specially designed for insulin administration: a 100-unit calibrated scale is intended for use with U-100 insulin. This corresponds to the universal 100 units per 1 mL concentration of insulin. This is the only syringe that should be used to administer insulin. Several low-dose insulin syringes are also available (e.g., 30-unit and 50-unit). These syringes frequently have a nonremovable needle. All insulin syringes are calibrated on the 100-unit scale in North America. The correct choice of syringe is based on the amount of insulin required (Figure 17–7 ■).

An insulin pen is an insulin injector device that looks like a pen and contains an insulin cartridge. The pen is easy to use: the client attaches a new needle for each injection, dials in a dose, inserts the needle, and presses the injection button to deliver the insulin (Gebel,

2012). The parts of an insulin pen are shown in Figure 17–8 ■. Many clients use the insulin pen for accurate self-administration of insulin.

Not all pens are the same. Each pen works only with specific types of insulins (Gebel, 2012, 2013). Clients have a choice between a disposable or reusable pen. A disposable pen comes prefilled with a cartridge of insulin and is stored in the refrigerator until the time of use when it is kept at room temperature after opening. When the insulin is depleted, the pen is discarded. Clients who use a reusable pen insert an insulin cartridge that is purchased separately. The cartridge is kept in a refrigerator until it is loaded into the pen. The pen, after being loaded, is kept at room temperature until the insulin is gone and then another cartridge is loaded into the pen (Gebel, 2012). Another difference among insulin pens is the insulin dose. Some pens allow clients to inject half units of insulin and others can only dose in whole units.

Increasingly, many hospitals have considered the advantages of insulin pens and subsequently changed from nurses using a vial and syringe to an insulin pen for subcutaneous administration of insulin (Edgeworth, 2011). Some common problems have been encountered with the use of insulin pens in hospitals. These problems, however, can be corrected with training for all practitioners before they use insulin pen devices. Grissinger (2011) and Edgeworth (2011) describe the following common problems:

- ***Needlestick injuries.*** Nurses who held the insulin pen at an angle other than the correct 90° angle were found to be at a higher risk of an accidental needlestick. Also, the area of the client's skin that needs to be pinched between the nurse's fingers should be approximately 2.5 cm (1 in.) wide to avoid a needlestick.
- ***Errors in technique.*** Sometimes the nurse may see a "wet spot" on the skin after injection and then wonders if the client received the

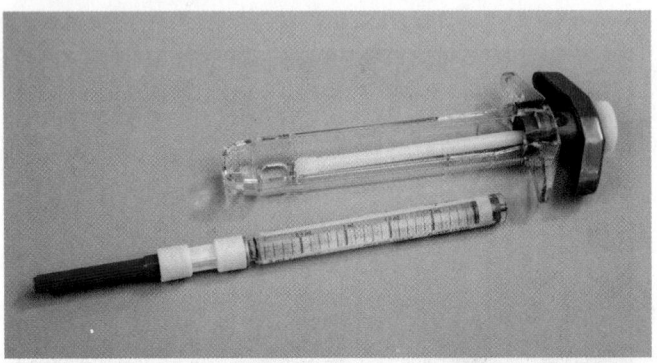

A

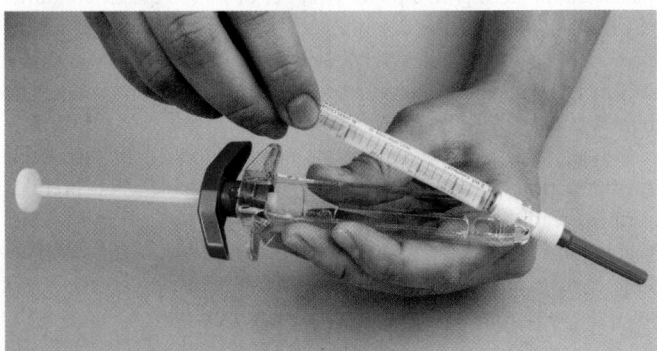

B

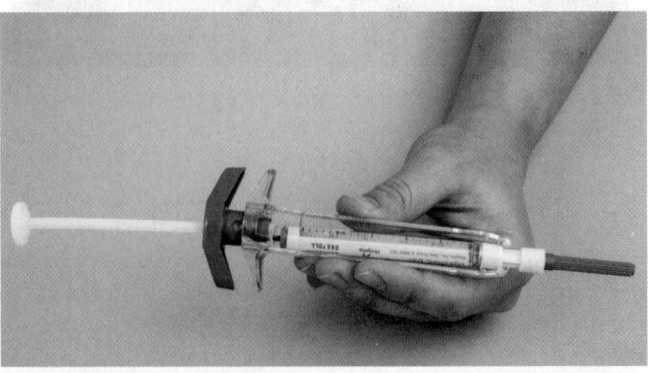

C

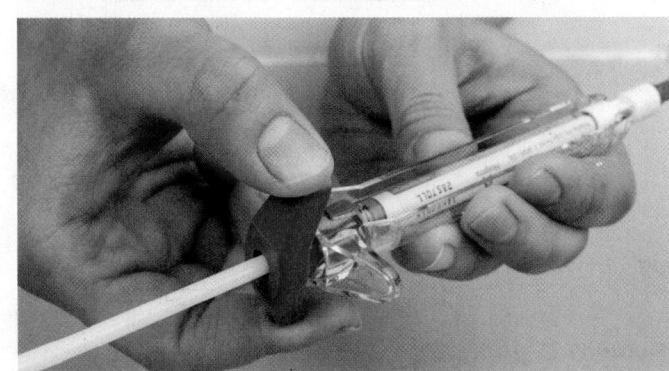

D

Figure 17–6 ■ *A,* Carpuject syringe and prefilled sterile cartridge with needle; *B,* assembling the device; *C,* the cartridge slides into the syringe barrel; *D,* the top twists, securing the cartridge into the unit.

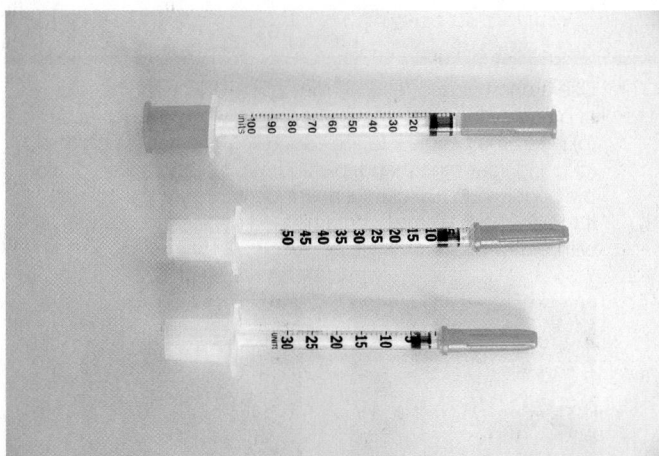

Figure 17–7 ■ Different insulin syringes based on the amount of insulin required. Note the difference in the number of units of insulin per line.

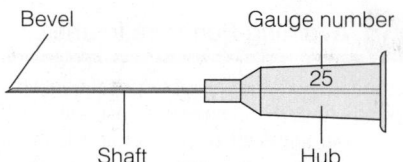

Figure 17–9 ■ The parts of a needle.

Needles

Needles are made of stainless steel, and most are disposable. A needle has three discernible parts: the **hub**, which fits onto the syringe; the **shaft**, which is attached to the hub; and the **bevel**, which is the slanted part at the tip of the needle (Figure 17–9 ■). A disposable needle has a plastic hub. Needles used for injections have three variable characteristics:

1. *Slant or length of the bevel.* The bevel of the needle may be short or long. Longer bevels provide the sharpest needles and cause less discomfort. They are commonly used for subcutaneous and intramuscular injections. Short bevels are used for intradermal and intravenous injections because a long bevel can become occluded if it rests against the side of a blood vessel.
2. *Length of the shaft.* The shaft length of *commonly* used needles varies from 3/8 to 1 1/2 inches. The appropriate needle length is chosen according to the client's muscle development, the client's weight, and the type of injection.
3. **Gauge** *(or diameter) of the shaft.* The gauge varies from #18 to #30. The larger the gauge number, the smaller the diameter of the shaft. Smaller gauges produce less tissue trauma, but larger gauges are necessary for viscous medications, such as penicillin.

   For an adult requiring a subcutaneous injection, it is appropriate to use a needle of #24 to #26 gauge and 3/8 to 5/8 inch long. Clients with obesity may require a 1-inch needle. For intramuscular injections, a longer needle (e.g., 1 to 1 1/2 inches) with a larger gauge (e.g., #20 to #22 gauge) is used. Slender adults and children usually require a shorter needle. The nurse must assess the client to determine the appropriate needle length.

full dose. The buttons of some pens are difficult to push down, causing the nurse to inadvertently lift the needle out of the skin and leave a wet spot. The Institute for Safe Medication Practices (ISMP) (2013) directs users to remove the needle immediately after injection to decrease the risk of air entering the cartridge (p. 2). It is also important for the nurse and/or client to remember to roll the insulin suspension (i.e., NPH and regular mixture), if appropriate. Not doing so can result in inaccurate doses.

- *Using the pen like a vial.* Insulin should not be withdrawn from the pen cartridge as if it were a vial. This can produce an air bubble into the cartridge and cause an inaccurate dose for the next injection.
- *Using the same pen for more than one client.* The Centers for Disease Control and Prevention (CDC) (2012a) has received an increasing number of reports about improper use of insulin pens in hospitals. Specifically, that there has been inappropriate reuse and sharing of insulin pens. Insulin pens are designed for *single-person* use only. They are **never** to be used for more than one person because this creates a risk of bloodborne pathogen transmission. ISMP (2013) states that "placing a new sterile needle on a pen previously used for one client is not enough to ensure pen sterility for delivery of a dose of insulin to another client" (p. 1).

   The **tuberculin syringe** was originally designed to administer tuberculin solution. It is a narrow syringe, calibrated in tenths and hundredths of a milliliter (up to 1 mL) on one scale and in sixteenths of a minim (up to 1 minim) on the other scale. This type of syringe can also be used for administering other drugs, particularly when small or precise measurement is indicated (e.g., pediatric dosages, allergy testing).

PREVENTING NEEDLESTICK INJURIES

One of the most potentially hazardous procedures that health care personnel face is using and disposing of needles and sharps. Needlestick injuries present a major risk for infection with hepatitis B and C virus, human immunodeficiency virus (HIV), and many other

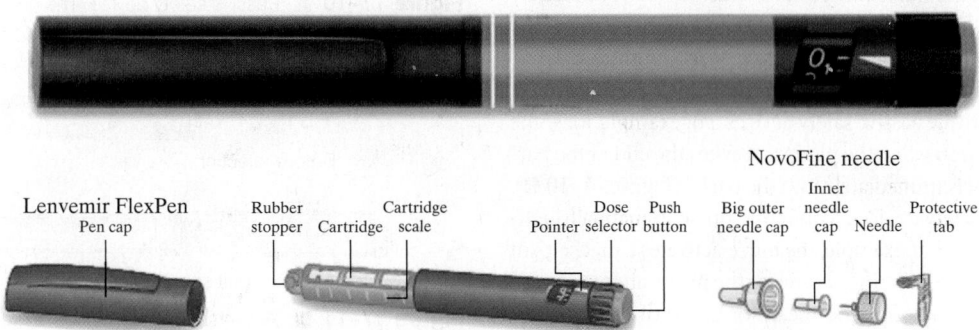

Figure 17–8 ■ Insulin pen. The dose selector knob dials the desired dose of insulin. Pressing the injection button administers the insulin.

BOX 17-1 Avoiding Puncture Injuries

- Use appropriate puncture-proof disposal containers to dispose of uncapped needles and sharps. These are provided in all client areas. Never throw sharps in wastebaskets. Sharps include any items that can cut or puncture skin such as:
  - Needles
  - Surgical blades
  - Lancets
  - Razors
  - Broken glass
  - Broken capillary pipettes
  - Exposed dental wires
  - Reusable items (e.g., large-bore needles, hooks, rasps, drill points)
  - ANY SHARP INSTRUMENT!
- Never bend or break needles before disposal.
- Never recap *used* needles (i.e., ones that have been inserted into clients) except under specified circumstances (e.g., when transporting a syringe to the laboratory for an arterial blood gas or blood culture).
- When recapping a needle (i.e., drawing up a medication into a syringe *prior* to administration):
  - Use a safety mechanical device that firmly grips the needle cap and holds it in place until it is ready to recap.

- Use a one-handed "scoop" method: (a) Place the needle cap and syringe with needle horizontally on a flat surface; (b) insert the needle into the cap, using one hand; and then (c) using your other hand, pick up the cap and tighten it to the needle hub. Be careful not to contaminate the needle. If the needle becomes contaminated, replace the needle with a new one.

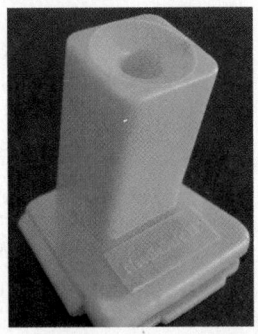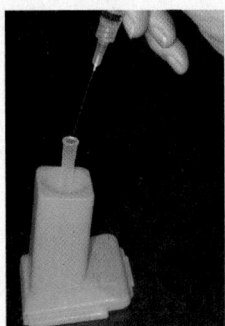

A mechanical safety device that holds the needle cap in place until the nurse is ready to recap.

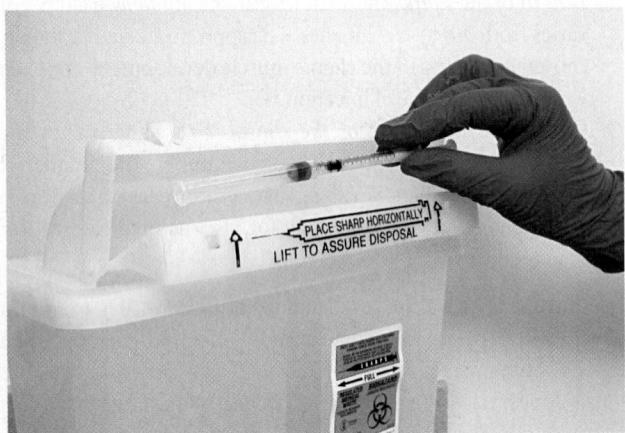

Dispose of a used syringe and needle in a sharps container.

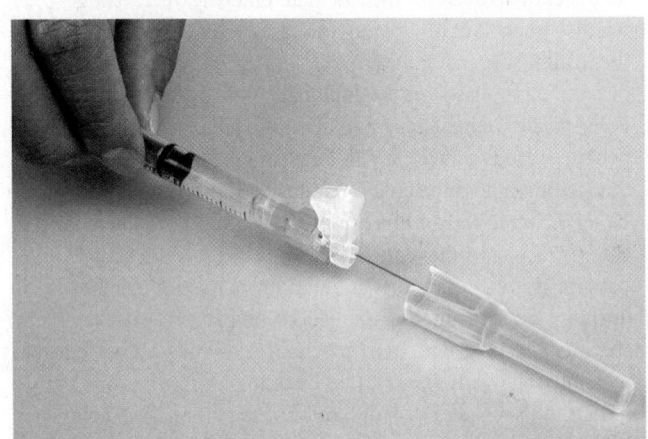

Recapping a needle using the one-handed scoop method.

pathogens. Standards have been set by the Occupational Safety and Health Administration (OSHA) to prevent such injuries. Some of these are summarized in Box 17–1. In addition, the Needlestick Safety and Prevention Act is a federal law that requires safer needle devices to prevent exposure to bloodborne pathogens and requires documentation of all needlestick injuries. If an accidental needlestick injury occurs, the nurse must follow specific steps outlined by the agency.

Safety syringes have been designed to protect health care workers. Safety devices are categorized as either *passive* or *active*. The nurse does not need to activate passive safety devices. For example, for some syringes, after injection when the plunger reaches the end of the barrel, the needle retracts immediately into the barrel (Figure 17–10 ■). In contrast, active safety devices require the nurse to manually activate the safety feature. For example, the nurse activates a mechanism to retract a needle into the syringe barrel, or the nurse, after injection, manually pulls or pushes a plastic sheath or guard over the needle (Figure 17–11 ■).

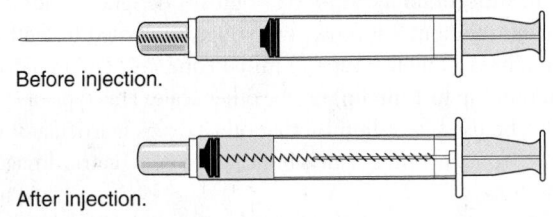

Before injection.

After injection.

Figure 17–10 ■ Passive safety device. The needle retracts immediately into the barrel after injection.

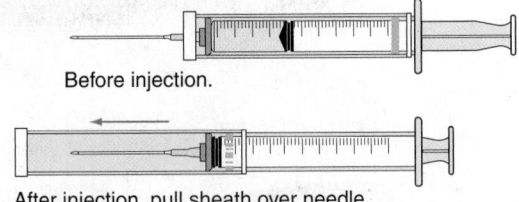

Before injection.

After injection, pull sheath over needle.

Figure 17–11 ■ Active safety device. The nurse manually pulls the sheath or guard over the needle after injection.

PREPARING INJECTABLE MEDICATIONS

Injectable medications can be prepared by withdrawing the medication from an ampule or vial into a sterile syringe, by using prefilled syringes, or by using needleless injection systems. Figure 17–12 ■ shows an example of a needleless system used to access medication from a vial.

Ampules and Vials

Ampules and vials (Figure 17–13 ■) are frequently used to package sterile parenteral medications. An **ampule** is a glass container usually designed to hold a single dose of a drug. It is made of clear glass and has a distinctive shape with a constricted neck. Ampules vary in size from 1 to 10 mL or more. Most ampule necks have colored marks around them, indicating where they are prescored for easy opening.

To access the medication in an ampule, the ampule must be broken at its constricted neck. Traditionally, files have been used to score the ampule. Today plastic ampule openers are available that prevent injury from broken glass. The device consists of a plastic cap that fits over the top of an ampule. The head of the ampule, when broken, remains inside the cap and is placed into a sharps container (Figure 17–14 ■). If an ampule opener is not available, the nurse can clean the ampule neck with an alcohol swab and, using dry sterile gauze, snap off the top of the ampule. Once the ampule is broken, the fluid is aspirated into a syringe using a **filter needle** or **filter straw** (Figure 17–15 ■). Both prevent aspiration of any glass particles.

CLINICAL ALERT!

It is important to replace the filter needle with a regular needle. Filter needles should not be used for injection.

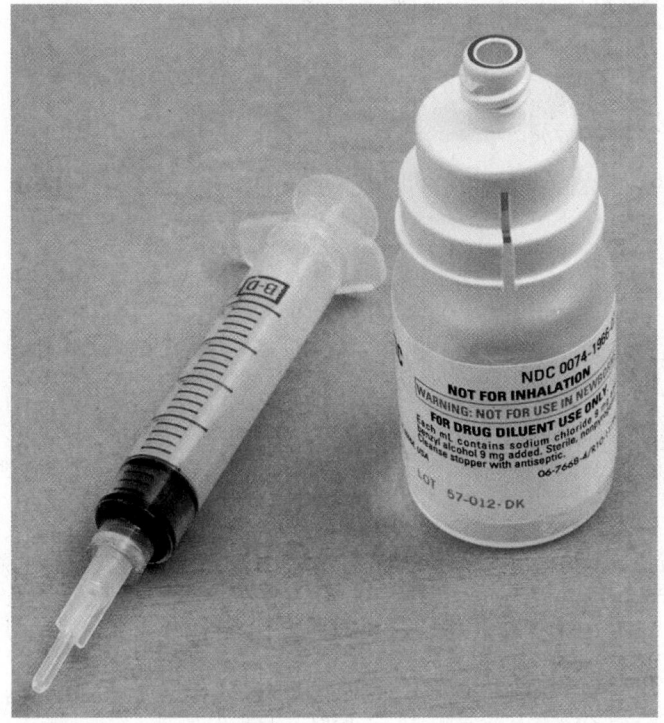

Figure 17–12 ■ A needleless system can extract medicine from a vial.

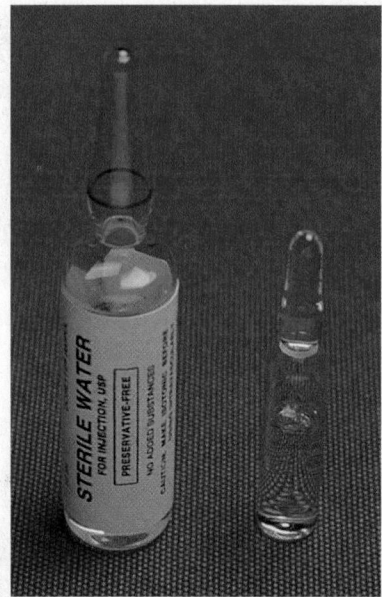

A

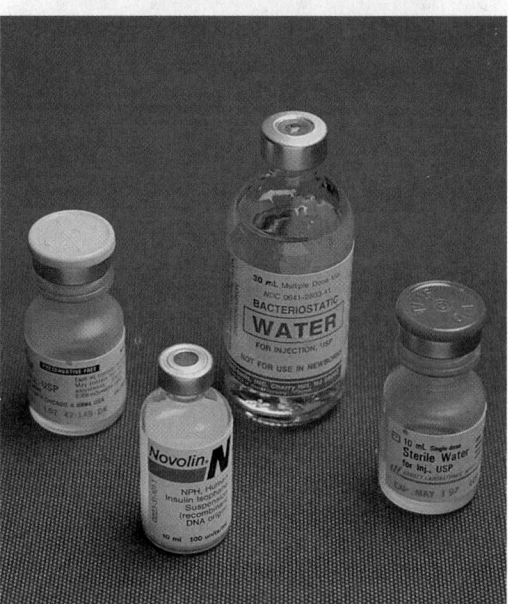

B

Figure 17–13 ■ A, Ampules; B, vials.

A **vial** is a small glass bottle with a sealed rubber cap. Vials come in different sizes, from single to multiple-dose vials. They usually have a metal or plastic cap that protects the rubber seal and must be removed to access the medication. To access the medication in a vial, the vial must be pierced with a needle. In addition, air must be injected into a vial before the medication can be withdrawn. Failure to inject air before withdrawing the medication leaves a vacuum within the vial that makes withdrawal difficult.

A single-use vial contains only one dose of medication and should be used only once. In contrast, a multidose vial is a bottle of liquid medication that contains more than one dose. Examples of these are insulin or vaccination vials. Recent investigations by the CDC (2012b) have identified improper uses of syringes, needles, and medication vials that have resulted in transmission of diseases such as hepatitis B. Whenever possible, use of single-dose vials is preferred over multidose vials, especially when medications will be administered to multiple clients. If multidose vials must be used, both the

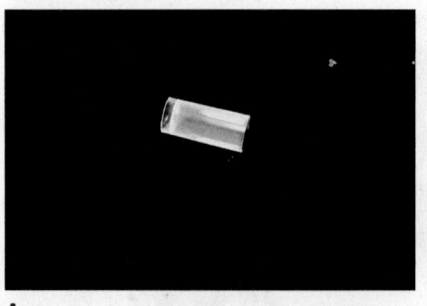
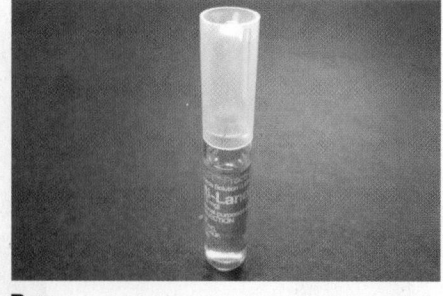
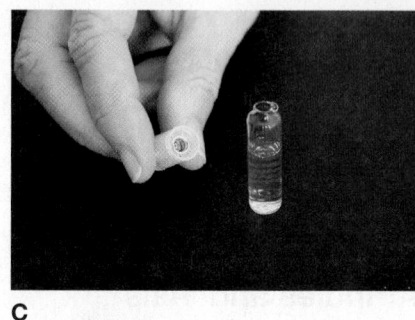

A   B   C

Figure 17–14 ■ *A,* Ampule opener; *B,* plastic opener is placed over top of ampule; *C,* top of ampule remains in opener after ampule is broken open.

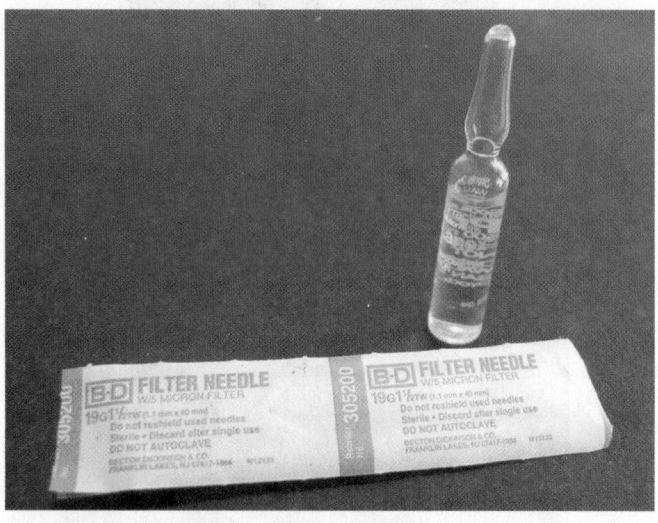
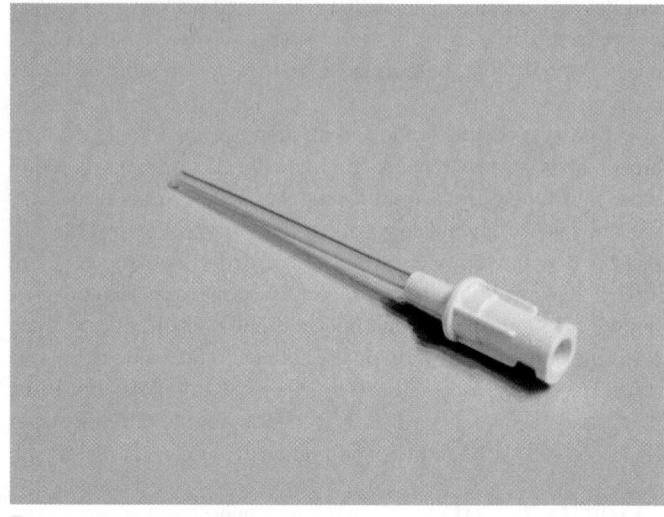

A   B

Figure 17–15 ■ A filter needle, *A,* or a filter straw, *B,* prevents glass from being withdrawn with the medication.

needle or cannula and syringe used to access the vial must be sterile. The *One and Only* health campaign is aimed at raising awareness about safe injection practice. The slogan is "One needle, One syringe, Only One time."

Several drugs (e.g., penicillin) are dispensed as powders in vials. A liquid called a **diluent** must be added to a powdered medication before it can be injected. The technique of adding a diluent to a powdered drug to prepare it for administration is called **reconstitution**. Powdered drugs usually have printed instructions (enclosed with each packaged vial) that describe the amount and kind of diluent to be added. Commonly used diluents are sterile water or sterile normal saline. Some preparations are supplied in individual-dose vials; others come in multidose vials. The following are two examples of the preparation of powdered drugs:

1. *Single-dose vial.* Instructions for preparing a single-dose vial state that 1.5 mL of sterile water be added to the sterile dry powder, thus providing a single dose of 2 mL. The volume of the drug powder is 0.5 mL. Therefore, the 1.5 mL of water plus the 0.5 mL of powder results in 2 mL of solution. In other instances, the addition of a solution does not increase the volume. Therefore, it is important to follow the manufacturer's directions.
2. *Multidose vial.* A dose of 750 mg of a certain drug is ordered for a client. On hand is a 10-gram multidose vial. The directions for preparation read: "Add 8.5 mL of sterile water, and each milliliter

will contain 1 g or 1,000 mg." To determine the amount to inject, the nurse calculates as follows:

$1 \text{ mL} = 1,000 \text{ mg}$
$x \text{ mL} = 750 \text{ mg}$
Cross multiply:
$x = 0.75$

The nurse will give 0.75 mL of the medication.

Glass and rubber particulates have been found in medications withdrawn from ampules and vials using a regular needle. To prevent withdrawing glass and rubber particles, it is strongly recommended that the nurse use a filter needle or straw when withdrawing medications from ampules and a filter needle when withdrawing from vials. After drawing the medication into the syringe, the filter needle or straw, whichever is appropriate, is replaced with the regular needle for injection. This prevents tracking of the medication through the client's tissues during the insertion of the needle, which minimizes discomfort. Using a new needle following the withdrawal of the medication from the vial also minimizes discomfort that can result from minor "dulling" of the needle tip from passing through the vial stopper. Also, if the client has a latex allergy, changing the needle would be important when using a vial with a rubber stopper/cap.

Skills 17–1 and 17–2 describe how to prepare medications from ampules and vials, respectively. Additionally, it is important to remember that when powdered drugs have been reconstituted, or a multidose vial is used, the date, time, and nurse's initials should be written on the label of the vial. Many of these drugs have to be used within a certain time period following reconstitution, so nurses need to know the expiration time after the drugs have been reconstituted or the vial punctured.

●○● NURSING PROCESS: PREPARING INJECTABLE MEDICATIONS

Preparing Medications from Ampules

ASSESSMENT
Assess:
- Client allergies to medication.
- Specific drug action, side effects, interactions, and adverse reactions.
- Client's knowledge of and learning needs about the medication.
- Intended route of parenteral medication to determine appropriate size of syringe and needle for the client.
- Ordered medication for clarity and expiration date.

- Perform appropriate assessments (e.g., vital signs, laboratory results) specific to the medication.
- Determine if the assessment data influence administration of the medication (i.e., is it appropriate to administer the medication or does the medication need to be held and/or the primary care provider notified?).

PLANNING
DELEGATION

Preparing medications from ampules involves knowledge and use of sterile technique. Therefore, these skills are not delegated to unlicensed assistive personnel (UAP).

Equipment
- Client's medication administration record (MAR) or computer printout
- Ampule of sterile medication

- File (if ampule is not scored) and small gauze square or plastic ampule opener
- Antiseptic swabs
- Syringe
- Needle for administering the medication
- Filter needle or straw for withdrawing medication from the ampule

IMPLEMENTATION
Preparation
- Check the MAR.
  - Check the label on the ampule carefully against the MAR to make sure that the correct medication is being prepared.
  - Follow the three checks for administering medications. Read the label on the medication (1) when it is taken from the medication cart, (2) before withdrawing the medication, and (3) after withdrawing the medication.
- Organize the equipment.

Performance
1. Perform hand hygiene and observe other appropriate infection prevention procedures.

2. Prepare the medication ampule for drug withdrawal.
   - Flick the upper stem of the ampule several times with a fingernail. **Rationale:** *This will bring all medication down to the main portion of the ampule.*
   - Use an ampule opener, or place a piece of gauze or an unopened alcohol wipe between your thumb and the ampule neck or around the ampule neck, and break off the top by bending it *toward* you to ensure the ampule is broken away from yourself and others. **❶ Rationale:** *The gauze protects the fingers from the broken glass, and any glass fragments will spray away from the nurse.*
   - Dispose of the top of the ampule in the sharps container.

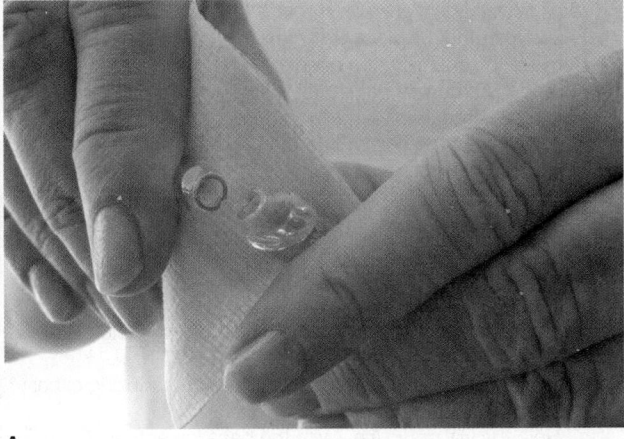

A

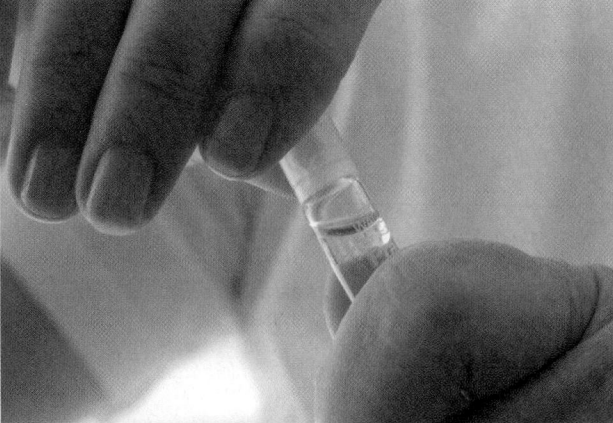

B

❶ *A*, Breaking the neck of an ampule using a gauze pad; *B*, breaking the neck of an ampule using an ampule opener.

Continued on page 414

SKILL 17–1

Preparing Medications from Ampules—*continued*

3. Withdraw the medication.
- Place the ampule on a flat surface.
- Attach the filter needle or straw to the syringe. **Rationale:** *The filter needle or straw prevents glass particles from being withdrawn with the medication.*
- Remove the cap from the filter needle or straw and insert the needle into the center of the ampule. If not using a filter needle or straw, do not touch the rim of the ampule with the needle tip or shaft. **Rationale:** *This will keep the needle sterile.* Withdraw all of the drug.

- Hold the ampule slightly on its side, if necessary, to obtain all of the medication. ❷
- Dispose of the filter needle or straw by placing it in a sharps container.
- Replace the filter needle or straw with a regular needle, tighten the cap at the hub of the needle, and push solution into the needle, to the prescribed amount.
- Discard excess medication into an acceptable receptacle, depending on ordered amount.

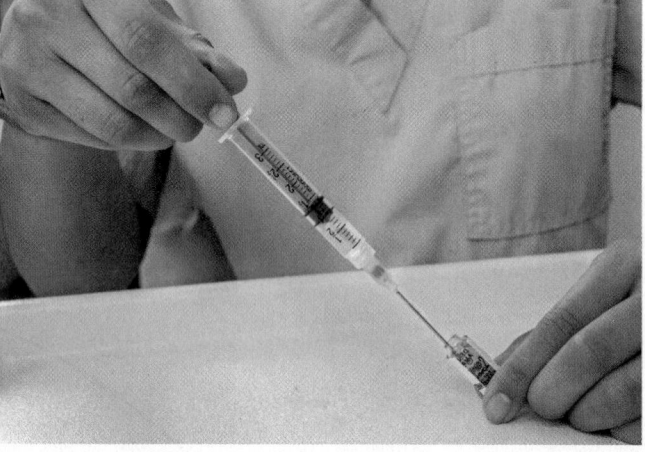

A

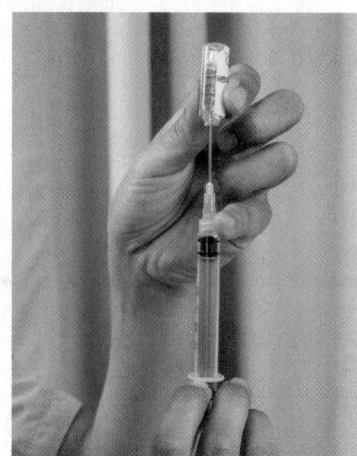

B

❷ Withdrawing a medication *A,* from an ampule on a flat surface, or *B,* from an inverted ampule.

SKILL 17–2

Preparing Medications from Vials

PLANNING
DELEGATION

Preparing medications from vials involves knowledge and use of sterile technique. Therefore, these techniques are not delegated to UAP.

Equipment
- Client's MAR or computer printout
- Vial of sterile medication
- Antiseptic swabs
- Safety needle and syringe
- Filter needle (check agency policy)
- Sterile water or normal saline, if drug is in powdered form

IMPLEMENTATION
Preparation
- Follow the same preparation as described in Skill 17–1.

Performance
1. Perform hand hygiene and observe other appropriate infection prevention procedures.
2. Prepare the medication vial for drug withdrawal.
- Mix the solution, if necessary, by rotating the vial between the palms of the hands, not by shaking. **Rationale:** *Some vials contain aqueous suspensions, which settle when they stand. In some instances, shaking is contraindicated because it may cause the mixture to foam.*
- Remove the protective cap, or clean the rubber cap of a previously opened vial with an antiseptic wipe by rubbing in a circular motion. **Rationale:** *The antiseptic cleans the rubber cap and reduces the number of microorganisms.*
3. Withdraw the medication.
- Attach a filter needle, as agency practice dictates, to draw up premixed liquid medications from multidose vials.

Rationale: *Using the filter needle prevents any solid particles from being drawn up through the needle.*
- Ensure that the needle is firmly attached to the syringe.
- Remove the cap from the needle, then draw up into the syringe the amount of air equal to the volume of the medication to be withdrawn.
- Carefully insert the needle into the upright vial through the center of the rubber cap, maintaining the sterility of the needle.
- Inject the air into the vial, keeping the bevel of the needle above the surface of the medication. ❶ **Rationale:** *The air will allow the medication to be drawn out easily because negative pressure will not be created inside the vial. The bevel is kept above the medication to avoid creating bubbles in the medication.*
- Withdraw the prescribed amount of medication using either of the following methods:
  a. Hold the vial down (i.e., with the base lower than the top), move the needle tip so that it is below the fluid level, and

Preparing Medications from Vials—*continued*

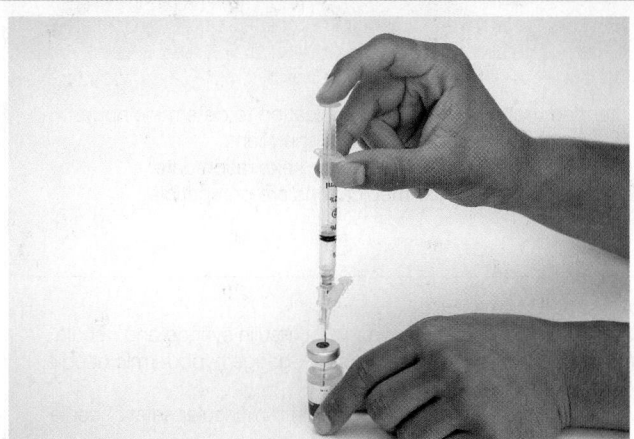

❶ Injecting air into a vial.

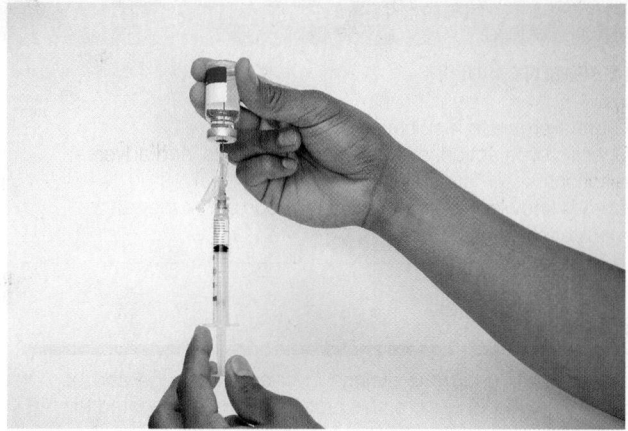

❸ Withdrawing a medication from an inverted vial.

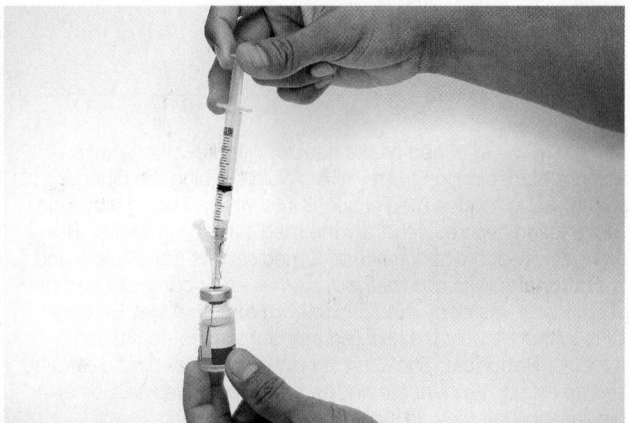

❷ Withdrawing a medication from a vial that is held with the base down.

withdraw the medication. ❷ Avoid drawing up the last drops of the vial. **Rationale:** *Proponents of this method say that keeping the vial in the upright position while withdrawing the medication allows particulate matter to precipitate out of the solution. Leaving the last few drops reduces the chance of withdrawing foreign particles.*

or

b. Invert the vial, ensure the needle tip is *below* the fluid level, and gradually withdraw the medication. ❸
Rationale: *Keeping the tip of the needle below the fluid level prevents air from being drawn into the syringe.*

● Hold the syringe and vial at eye level to determine that the correct dosage of drug is drawn into the syringe. Eject air remaining at the top of the syringe into the vial.

● When the correct volume of medication plus a little more (e.g., 0.25 mL [in case of air bubbles]) is obtained, withdraw the needle from the vial, and replace the cap over the needle using the one-hand scoop method, thus maintaining its sterility and preventing possible needlestick.

● If necessary, gently tap the syringe barrel with a finger or pen while holding the syringe with the needle end pointing up to dislodge any air bubbles present in the syringe. Carefully and slowly expel the air and any excess medication from the syringe, maintaining the "needle up" position. **Rationale:** *The tapping motion will cause the air bubbles to rise to the top of the syringe where they can be ejected out of the syringe. Sometimes when ejecting the air bubbles, the resulting amount of medication is less than ordered. Drawing up a little extra medication, as in the previous step, helps avoid this.*

● If giving an injection, replace the filter needle, if used, with a regular or safety needle of the correct gauge and length. Eject air from the new needle and verify correct medication volume before injecting the client.

Variation: Preparing and Using Multidose Vials

● Read the manufacturer's directions.
● Withdraw an equivalent amount of air from the vial before adding the diluent, unless otherwise indicated by the directions.
● Add the amount of sterile water or saline indicated in the directions.
● If a multidose vial is reconstituted, label the vial with the date and time it was prepared, the amount of drug contained in each milliliter of solution, and your initials. **Rationale:** *Time is an important factor to consider in the expiration of these medications.*
● Once the medication is reconstituted, store it in a refrigerator or as recommended by the manufacturer.

Mixing Medications in One Syringe

Frequently, clients need more than one drug injected at the same time. To spare the client the experience of being injected twice, two drugs (if compatible) are often mixed together in one syringe and given as one injection. Keep in mind that the absolute maximum volume of one injection is 3 mL if given by the intramuscular route and less when given subcutaneously. It is common, for example, to combine two types of insulin in this manner or to combine injectable preoperative medications such as morphine with atropine or scopolamine. When uncertain about drug compatibilities, the nurse should consult a pharmacist or check a compatibility chart before mixing the drugs.

The nurse must also exercise caution when mixing short- and long-acting insulins, because they vary in content. Chemically, insulin is a protein that, when hydrolyzed in the body, yields a number of amino acids. Some insulin preparations contain an additional modifying protein, such as globulin or protamine, which slows absorption. This fact is particularly relevant to mixing two insulin preparations for injection because many insulin syringes have needles that cannot be changed. A vial of insulin that does not have the added protein (i.e., regular insulin) should *never* be contaminated with insulin that does have the added protein (i.e., Lente or neutral protamine Hagedorn [NPH] insulin). Skill 17–3 describes how to mix medications in one syringe.

SKILL 17-3

●○● NURSING PROCESS: MIXING MEDICATIONS IN ONE SYRINGE

Mixing Medications Using One Syringe

ASSESSMENT
Assess:
- Client allergies to medications.
- Specific drug action, side effects, interactions, and adverse reactions.
- Client's knowledge of and learning needs about the medications.

- Intended route of parenteral medication to determine appropriate size of syringe and needle for the client.
- Ordered medications for clarity and expiration date.
- Determine that the two medications are compatible.

PLANNING
DELEGATION

Mixing medications in one syringe involves knowledge and use of aseptic technique. Therefore, this procedure is not delegated to UAP.

Equipment
- Client's MAR or computer printout
- Two vials of medication; one vial and one ampule; two ampules; or one vial or ampule and one cartridge

- Antiseptic swabs
- Sterile syringe and safety needle or insulin syringe and needle (If insulin is being given, use a small-gauge hypodermic needle, e.g., #26 gauge.)
- Additional sterile subcutaneous or intramuscular safety needle (optional)

IMPLEMENTATION
Preparation
- Check the MAR.
  - Check the label on the medications carefully against the MAR to make sure that the correct medication is being prepared.
  - Follow the three checks for administering medications. Read the label on the medication (1) when it is taken from the medication cart, (2) before withdrawing the medication, and (3) after withdrawing the medication.
  - Before preparing and combining the medications, ensure that the total volume of the injection is appropriate for the injection site.
- Organize the equipment.

Performance
1. Perform hand hygiene and observe other appropriate infection prevention procedures.
2. Prepare the medication ampule or vial for drug withdrawal.
   - See Skill 17–1, step 2, for an ampule.
   - Inspect the appearance of the medication for clarity. Note, however, that some medications are always cloudy. **Rationale:** *Preparations that have changed in appearance should be discarded.*
   - If using insulin, thoroughly mix the solution in each vial prior to administration. Rotate the vials between the palms of the hands. **Rationale:** *Mixing ensures an adequate concentration and thus an accurate dose. Shaking insulin vials can make the medication frothy, making precise measurement difficult.*
   - Clean the tops of the vials with antiseptic swabs.
3. Withdraw the medications.

Mixing Medications from Two Vials
- Take the syringe and draw up a volume of air equal to the volume of medications to be withdrawn from both vials A *and* B.
- Inject a volume of air equal to the volume of medication to be withdrawn into vial A. Make sure the needle does not touch the solution. **Rationale:** *This prevents cross contamination of the medications.*
- Withdraw the needle from vial A and inject the remaining air into vial B.
- Withdraw the required amount of medication from vial B. **Rationale:** *The same needle is used to inject air into and withdraw medication from the second vial. It must not be contaminated with the medication in vial A.*

- Using a newly attached sterile needle, withdraw the required amount of medication from vial A. Avoid pushing the plunger as that will introduce medication B into vial A. If using a syringe with a fused needle, withdraw the medication from vial A. The syringe now contains a mixture of medications from vials A and B. **Rationale:** *With this method, neither vial is contaminated by microorganisms or by medication from the other vial.* Be careful to withdraw only the ordered amount and not to create air bubbles. **Rationale:** *The syringe now contains two medications, and an excess amount cannot be returned to the vial.* See also the variation later in this skill.

Mixing Medications from One Vial and One Ampule
- First prepare and withdraw the medication from the vial. **Rationale:** *The ampule does not require the addition of air prior to withdrawal of the drug because it is an open container.*
- Then withdraw the required amount of medication from the ampule.

Mixing Medications from One Cartridge and One Vial or Ampule
- First ensure that the correct dose of the medication is in the cartridge. Discard any excess medication and air.
- Draw up the required medication from the vial or ampule into the cartridge. Note that when withdrawing medication from a vial, an equal amount of air must first be injected into the vial.
- If the total volume to be injected exceeds the capacity of the cartridge, use a syringe with sufficient capacity to withdraw the desired amount of medication from the vial or ampule, and transfer the required amount from the cartridge to the syringe.

Variation: Mixing Insulins
The following is an example of mixing 10 units of regular insulin and 30 units of NPH insulin, which contains protamine.
- Inject 30 units of air into the NPH vial and withdraw the needle. (There should be no insulin in the needle.) The needle should not touch the insulin. ❶
- Inject 10 units of air into the regular insulin vial and immediately withdraw 10 units of regular insulin. ❷ and ❸ Always withdraw the regular insulin first. **Rationale:** *This minimizes the possibility of the regular insulin becoming contaminated with the additional protein in the NPH.*
- Reinsert the needle into the NPH insulin vial and withdraw 30 units of NPH insulin. ❹ (The air was previously injected into the vial.) Be careful to withdraw only the ordered amount and not to create air bubbles. If excess medication has been drawn up,

Mixing Medications Using One Syringe—*continued*

discard the syringe and begin the procedure over again. **Rationale:** *The syringe now contains two medications, and an excess amount cannot be returned to the vial because the syringe contains regular insulin, which, if returned to the NPH vial, would dilute the NPH with regular insulin. The NPH vial would not provide accurate future dosages of NPH insulin.*

By using this method, you avoid adding NPH insulin to the regular insulin.

CLINICAL ALERT!

One way to determine which insulin to *withdraw* first is to remember the saying "Clear before cloudy." (Regular insulin is clear and NPH is cloudy due to the proteins in the insulin.)

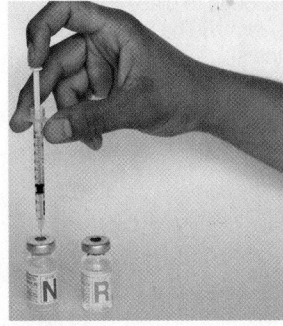

❶ Mixing two types of insulin.

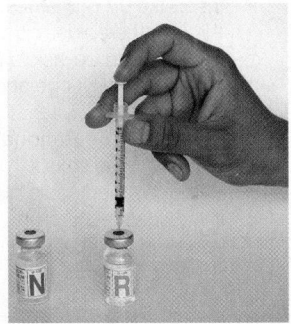

❷

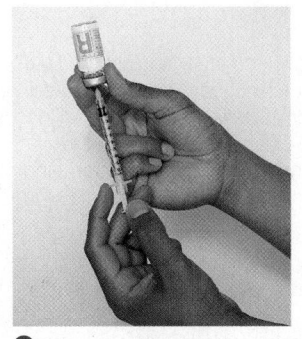

❸

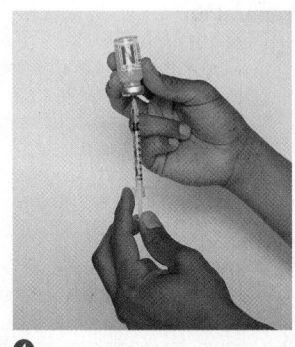

❹

Intradermal Injections

An **intradermal (ID) injection** is the administration of a drug into the dermal layer of the skin just beneath the epidermis. Usually, only a small amount of liquid is used, for example, 0.1 mL. This method of administration is frequently used for allergy testing and tuberculosis (TB) screening. Common sites for intradermal injections are the inner lower arm, the upper chest, and the back beneath the scapulae (Figure 17–16 ■). The left arm is commonly used for TB screening, and the right arm is used for all other tests. The steps for administering an intradermal injection are described in Skill 17–4.

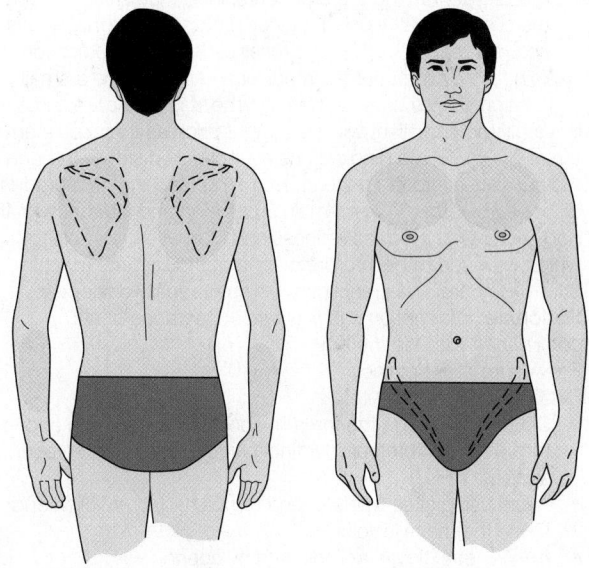

Figure 17–16 ■ Body sites commonly used for intradermal injections.

●○● NURSING PROCESS: INTRADERMAL INJECTIONS

Administering an Intradermal Injection for Skin Tests

ASSESSMENT
Assess:
- Appearance of injection site.
- Specific drug action and expected response.
- Client's knowledge of drug action and response.
- Check agency protocol about sites to use for skin tests.

PLANNING
DELEGATION

The administration of ID injections is an invasive technique that involves the application of nursing knowledge, problem solving, and sterile technique. Therefore, this skill is not delegated to UAP. The nurse, however, can inform the UAP about symptoms of allergic reactions and other desired and undesired responses and the necessity to report those observations immediately to the nurse.

Continued on page 418

Administering an Intradermal Injection for Skin Tests—*continued*

Equipment
- Vial or ampule of the correct medication
- Sterile 1-mL syringe calibrated into hundredths of a milliliter (i.e., tuberculin syringe) and a #25- to #27-gauge safety needle that is 1/4 to 5/8 inch long
- Alcohol swabs
- 2×2 sterile gauze square (optional)
- Clean gloves (according to agency protocol)
- Bandage (optional)
- Epinephrine on hand in case of allergic anaphylactic reaction

IMPLEMENTATION
Preparation
- Check the MAR.
  - Check the label on the medication carefully against the MAR to make sure that the correct medication is being prepared.
  - Follow the three checks for administering medications. Read the label on the medication (1) when it is taken from the medication cart, (2) before withdrawing the medication, and (3) after withdrawing the medication.
- Organize the equipment.

Performance
1. Perform hand hygiene and observe other appropriate infection prevention procedures.
2. Prepare the medication from the ampule or vial for drug withdrawal.
   - See Skill 17–1 (ampule) or 17–2 (vial).
3. Prepare the client.
   - Prior to performing the procedure, introduce self and verify the client's identity using agency protocol. **Rationale:** *This ensures that the right client receives the right medication.*
4. Explain to the client that the medication will produce a small wheal, sometimes called a *bleb*. A **wheal** is a small raised area, like a blister. The client will feel a slight prick as the needle enters the skin. Some medications are absorbed slowly through the capillaries into the general circulation, and the bleb gradually disappears. Other drugs remain in the area and interact with the body tissues to produce redness and induration (hardening), which will need to be interpreted at a particular time (e.g., in 24 or 48 hours). This reaction will also gradually disappear. **Rationale:** *Information can facilitate acceptance of and compliance with the therapy.*
5. Provide for client privacy.
6. Select and clean the site.
   - Select a site (e.g., the forearm about a hand's width above the wrist and three or four fingerwidths below the antecubital space).
   - Avoid using sites that are tender, inflamed, or swollen and those that have lesions.
   - Apply clean gloves as indicated by agency policy.
   - Cleanse the skin at the site using a firm circular motion starting at the center and widening the circle outward. Allow the area to dry thoroughly.
7. Prepare the syringe for the injection.
   - Remove the needle cap while waiting for the antiseptic to dry.
   - Expel any air bubbles from the syringe. Small bubbles that adhere to the plunger are of no consequence. **Rationale:** *A small amount of air will not harm the tissues.*
   - Grasp the syringe in your dominant hand, close to the hub, holding it between your thumb and forefinger. Hold the needle almost parallel to the skin surface, with the bevel of the needle up. **Rationale:** *The possibility of the medication entering the subcutaneous tissue increases when using an angle greater than 15°.*
8. Inject the fluid.
   - With the nondominant hand, pull the skin at the site until it is taut. For example, if using the ventral forearm, grasp the client's dorsal forearm and gently pull it to tighten the ventral skin. **Rationale:** *Taut skin allows for easier entry of the needle and less discomfort for the client.*

- Insert the tip of the needle far enough to place the bevel through the epidermis into the dermis. The outline of the bevel should be visible under the skin surface.
- Stabilize the syringe and needle. Inject the medication carefully and slowly so that it produces a small wheal or bleb on the skin. ❶ **Rationale:** *This verifies that the medication entered the dermis.*
- Withdraw the needle quickly at the same angle at which it was inserted. Activate the needle safety device. Apply a bandage if indicated.

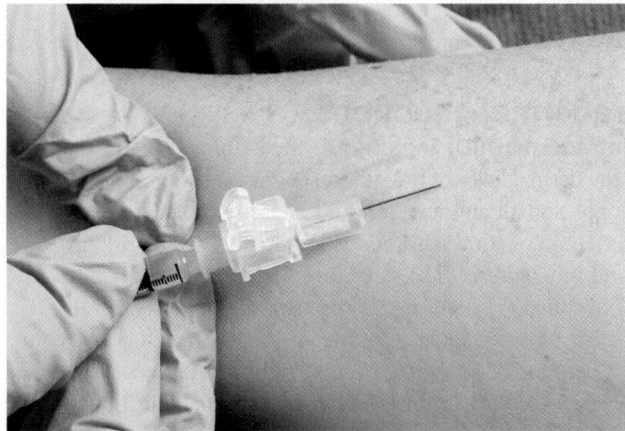

A

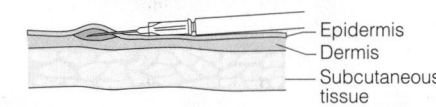
Epidermis
Dermis
Subcutaneous tissue

B

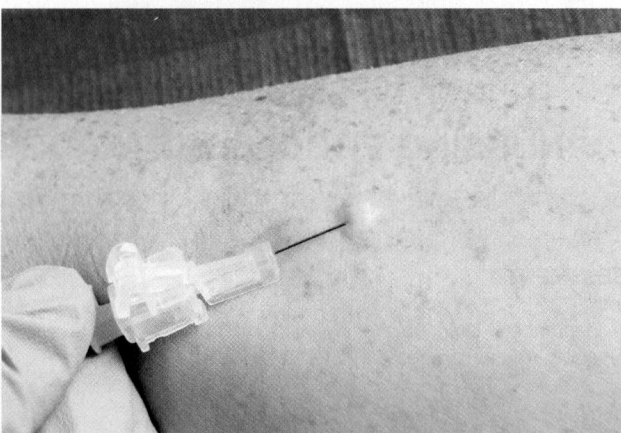

C

❶ For an intradermal injection: *A*, the needle enters the skin at a 15° or less angle; *B, C*, the medication forms a wheal or bleb under the epidermis.

Administering an Intradermal Injection for Skin Tests—*continued*

- Do not massage the area. **Rationale:** *Massage can disperse the medication into the tissue or out through the needle insertion site.*
- Dispose of the syringe and needle into the sharps container. **Rationale:** *Do not recap the needle in order to prevent needlestick injuries.*
- Remove and dispose of gloves.

- Perform hand hygiene.
- Circle the injection site with ink to observe for redness or induration (hardening), per agency policy.

9. Document all relevant information.
- Record the testing material given, the time, dosage, route, site, and nursing assessments.

EVALUATION
- Evaluate the client's response to the testing substance. **Rationale:** *Some medications used in testing may cause allergic reactions.* Epinephrine may need to be used.

- Evaluate the condition of the site in 24 or 48 hours, depending on the test. Measure the area of redness and induration in millimeters at the largest diameter and document findings.

LIFESPAN CONSIDERATIONS | **Administering an Intradermal Injection**

CHILDREN
- Children should be gently restrained during the procedure to prevent injury from a sudden movement.
- Make sure the child understands that the injection is not a punishment. Consider having parents or guardians step out of the room during the procedure to have them return immediately

after the procedure and "rescue" their child, thus promoting trust in the parents as perceived by the child.
- Ask the child not to rub or scratch the injection site. **Rationale:** *Rubbing the site can interfere with test results by irritating the underlying tissue.*

Ambulatory and Community Settings | **Administering an Intradermal Injection** | PATIENT-CENTERED CARE

- Assess the client's knowledge about the intradermal injection and the reason for follow-up with the health care professional. Set up an appointment for the visit.

- Instruct and explain why the injection site should not be washed, rubbed, or scratched.

Subcutaneous Injections

Among the many kinds of drugs administered subcutaneously are vaccines, insulin, and heparin. Common sites for subcutaneous injections are the outer aspect of the upper arms and the anterior aspect of the thighs. These areas are convenient and normally have good blood circulation. Other areas that can be used are the abdomen, the scapular areas of the upper back, and the upper ventrogluteal and dorsogluteal areas (Figure 17–17 ■). Only small doses (0.5 to 1 mL) of medication are usually injected via the subcutaneous route. Check agency policy.

The type of syringe used for subcutaneous injections depends on the medication to be given. Generally a 1- or 2-mL syringe is used for most subcutaneous injections. However, if insulin is being administered, an insulin syringe is used; if heparin is being administered, a tuberculin syringe or prefilled cartridge may be used.

Needle sizes and lengths are selected based on the client's body mass, the intended angle of insertion, and the planned site. Generally a #25-gauge, 5/8-inch needle is used for adults of normal weight, and the needle is inserted at a 45° angle; a 3/8-inch needle is used at a 90° angle. A child may need a 1/2-inch needle inserted at a 45° angle.

One method nurses use to determine length of needle is to pinch the tissue at the site and select a needle length that is half the width of the skinfold. To determine the angle of insertion, a general rule to follow relates to the amount of tissue that can be pinched or grasped at the site. A 45° angle is used when 2.5 cm (1 in.) of tissue can be grasped at the site; a 90° angle is used when 5 cm (2 in.) of tissue can be grasped.

When administering insulin to adults, the current standard needle gauge is #30 gauge with a short needle (4 to 6 mm [0.16 to 0.24 in.]). Most clients prefer the shorter and thinner needles because they are

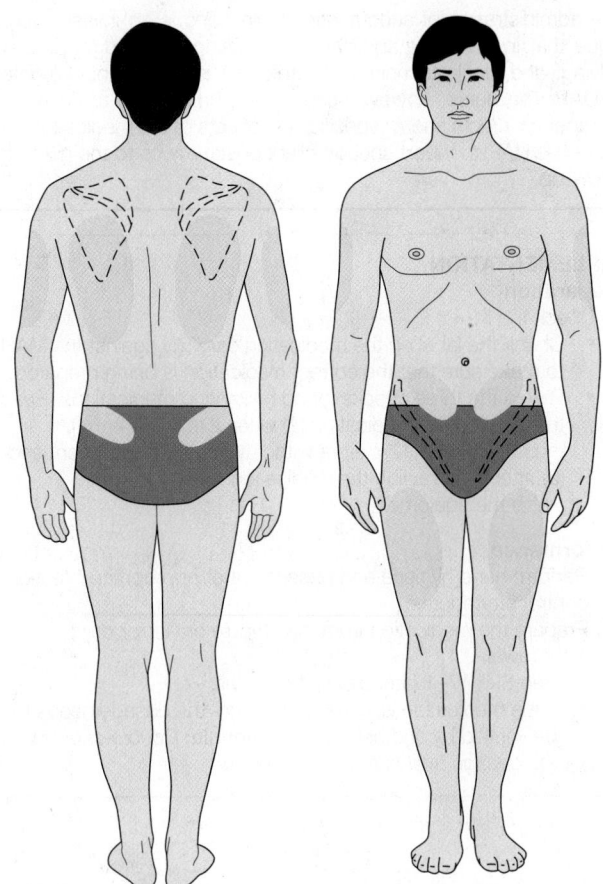

Figure 17–17 ■ Body sites commonly used for subcutaneous injections.

less painful. The risk of injecting into the muscle is lessened with the shorter needle.

Subcutaneous injection sites need to be rotated in an orderly fashion to minimize tissue damage, aid absorption, and avoid discomfort. This is especially important for clients who must receive repeated injections, such as clients with diabetes. Because insulin is absorbed at different rates in different parts of the body, blood glucose levels can vary in the client with diabetes when various sites are used. Insulin is absorbed most quickly when injected into the abdomen and then into the arms, and most slowly when injected into the thighs and buttocks. Rotate the injection sites weekly to prevent lipoatrophy and lipohypertrophy (Adams & Urban, 2013).

Nurses have traditionally been taught to aspirate by pulling back on the plunger after inserting the needle and before injecting the medication. The nurse could then determine whether the needle had entered a blood vessel. Absence of blood was believed to indicate that the needle was in subcutaneous tissue and not in the more vascular muscular tissue. According to the American Diabetes Association (ADA) (2004), routine aspiration is no longer recommended with insulin administration. Crawford and Johnson (2012) completed a recent review of evidence to answer the question of the need to aspirate for blood when administering an IM or subcutaneous injection. Their answer is "clearly 'no' for the injection of vaccines, immunizations, heparin, and insulin" (p. 25). Students, however, are likely to observe that the practice of aspirating subcutaneous injections will vary among nurses.

The steps for administering a subcutaneous injection are described in Skill 17–5.

●○○● NURSING PROCESS: SUBCUTANEOUS INJECTIONS

Administering a Subcutaneous Injection

SKILL 17–5

ASSESSMENT

Assess:
- Allergies to medication.
- Specific drug action, side effects, and adverse reactions.
- Client's knowledge and learning needs about the medication.
- Status and appearance of subcutaneous site for lesions, erythema, swelling, ecchymosis, inflammation, and tissue damage from previous injections.
- Ability of client to cooperate during the injection.
- Previous injection sites used.

PLANNING
DELEGATION

The administration of subcutaneous injections is an invasive technique that involves the application of nursing knowledge, problem solving, and sterile technique. Therefore, this skill is not delegated to UAP. The nurse, however, can inform the UAP of the intended therapeutic effects and/or specific side effects of the medication and direct the UAP to report specific client observations to the nurse for follow-up.

Equipment
- Client's MAR or computer printout
- Vial or ampule of the correct sterile medication
- Syringe and needle (e.g., 3-mL syringe, #25-gauge needle or smaller, 3/8 or 5/8 inch long)
- Antiseptic swabs
- Dry sterile gauze for opening an ampule, or ampule-opening device, or a small file if neck is not scored
- Clean gloves

IMPLEMENTATION
Preparation
- Check the MAR.
  - Check the label on the medication carefully against the MAR to make sure that the correct medication is being prepared.
  - Follow the three checks for administering medications. Read the label on the medication (1) when it is taken from the medication cart, (2) before withdrawing the medication, and (3) after withdrawing the medication.
- Organize the equipment.

Performance
1. Perform hand hygiene and observe other appropriate infection control procedures.
2. Prepare the medication from the ampule or vial for drug withdrawal.
   - See Skill 17–1 (ampule) or 17–2 (vial).
   - If the medication is insulin or heparin, the dosage needs to be verified by another nurse. **Rationale:** *Double-checking the dosage avoids medication errors.*

CLINICAL ALERT!

When asking another nurse to verify the dosage of insulin or heparin, leave the needle and syringe in the vial and ask, "What dosage do I have in the syringe?" The nurse needs to then check the vial medication name and concentration as well as calculate the dosage. This is a safer and more accurate method of double-checking than saying to another nurse, "I have 10 units of insulin," which "presets" the other nurse's checking of the medication dosage and can lead to an error. If the client is on a sliding scale, the capillary blood glucose (CBG) result and sliding scale also need to be part of the verification process.

3. Provide for client privacy.
4. Prepare the client.
   - Prior to performing the procedure, introduce self and verify the client's identity using agency protocol. **Rationale:** *This ensures that the right client receives the right medication.*

Administering a Subcutaneous Injection—*continued*

- Assist the client to a position in which the arm, leg, or abdomen can be relaxed, depending on the site to be used. **Rationale:** *A relaxed position of the site minimizes discomfort.*
- Obtain assistance in holding an uncooperative client. **Rationale:** *This prevents injury due to sudden movement after needle insertion.*

5. Explain the purpose of the medication and how it will help, using language that the client can understand. Include relevant information about effects of the medication. **Rationale:** *Information can facilitate acceptance of and compliance with the therapy.*

6. Select and clean the site.
   - Select a site free of tenderness, hardness, swelling, scarring, itching, burning, or localized inflammation. Select a site that has not been used frequently. **Rationale:** *These conditions could hinder the absorption of the medication and may also increase the likelihood of injury and discomfort at the injection site.*
   - Apply clean gloves.
   - As agency protocol indicates, clean the site with an antiseptic swab. Start at the center of the site and clean in a widening circle to about 5 cm (2 in.). Allow the area to dry thoroughly. **Rationale:** *The mechanical action of swabbing removes skin secretions, which contain microorganisms.*
   - Place and hold the swab between the third and fourth fingers of the nondominant hand, or position the swab on the client's skin above the intended site. **Rationale:** *Using this technique keeps the swab readily accessible when the needle is withdrawn.*

7. Prepare the syringe for injection.
   - Remove the needle cap while waiting for the antiseptic to dry. Pull the cap straight off to avoid contaminating the needle by the outside edge of the cap. **Rationale:** *The needle will become contaminated if it touches anything but the inside of the cap, which is sterile.*
   - Dispose of the needle cap.

8. Inject the medication.
   - Grasp the syringe in your dominant hand by holding it between your thumb and fingers. With palm facing to the side or upward for a 45° angle of insertion, or with the palm downward for a 90° angle of insertion, prepare to inject. ❶
   - Using the nondominant hand, pinch or spread the skin at the site, and insert the needle using the dominant hand and a firm steady push. Recommendations vary about whether to pinch or spread the skin and at what angle to administer subcutaneous injections. The most important consideration is the depth of the subcutaneous tissue in the area to be injected. If the client has more than 1.3 cm (1/2 in.) of adipose tissue in the injection site, it would be safe to

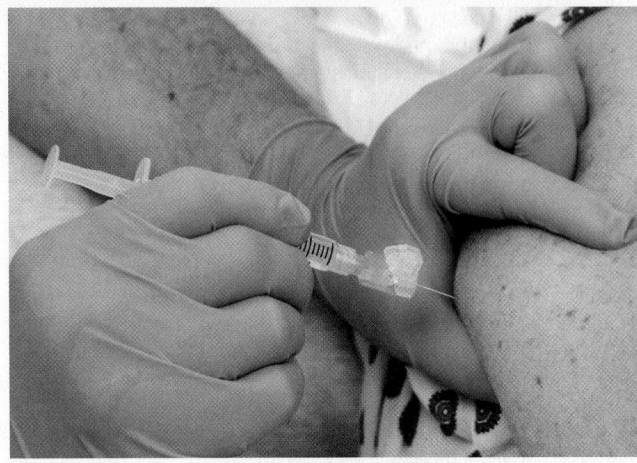

❷ Administering a subcutaneous injection into pinched tissue.

administer the injection at a 90° angle with the skin spread. If the client is thin or lean and lacks adipose tissue, the subcutaneous injection should be given with the skin pinched and at a 45° to 60° angle. One way to check that the pinch of skin is subcutaneous tissue is to ask the client to flex and extend the elbow. If any muscle is being held in the pinch, you will feel it contract and relax. If so, release the pinch and try again. ❷
   - When the needle is inserted, move your nondominant hand to the barrel of the syringe and the dominant hand to the end of the plunger.
   - Inject the medication by holding the syringe steady and depressing the plunger with a slow, even pressure. **Rationale:** *Holding the syringe steady and injecting the medication at an even pressure minimizes discomfort for the client.*
   - It is recommended that with many subcutaneous injections, especially insulin, the needle should be embedded within the skin for 5 seconds after complete depression of the plunger. **Rationale:** *This ensures complete delivery of the dose.*

9. Remove the needle.
   - Remove the needle smoothly, pulling along the line of insertion while depressing the skin with your nondominant hand. **Rationale:** *Depressing the skin places countertraction on it and minimizes the client's discomfort when the needle is withdrawn.* If you have a passive safety syringe, the needle will be in the barrel of the syringe after administering the medication.
   - If bleeding occurs, apply pressure to the site with dry sterile gauze until it stops. **Rationale:** *Bleeding rarely occurs after subcutaneous injection.*

10. Dispose of supplies appropriately.
    - Activate the needle safety device or discard the *uncapped* needle and attached syringe into designated receptacles. **Rationale:** *Proper disposal protects the nurse and others from injury and contamination. The CDC recommends not recapping the needle before disposal to reduce the risk of needlestick injuries.*
    - Remove and dispose of gloves.
    - Perform hand hygiene.

11. Document all relevant information.
    - Document the medication given, dosage, time, route, and any assessments.

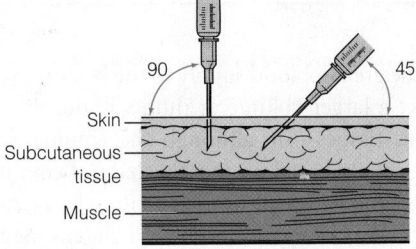

❶ Inserting a needle into the subcutaneous tissue using 90° and 45° angles.

Continued on page 422

Administering a Subcutaneous Injection—*continued*

- Many agencies prefer that medication administration be recorded on the medication record. The nurse's notes are used when prn medications are given or when there is a special problem.
12. Assess the effectiveness of the medication at the time it is expected to act and document it.

Variation: Administering a Heparin Injection

The subcutaneous administration of heparin requires special precautions because of the drug's anticoagulant properties.

- Select a site on the abdomen at least 5 cm (2 in.) inches *away* from the umbilicus and above the level of the iliac crests. Some agencies support the practice of subcutaneous injection of heparin in the thighs or arms as alternate sites to the abdomen. Avoid injecting into bruises, scars, masses, or areas of tenderness.
- Use a 3/8-inch, #25- or #26-gauge needle or smaller, and insert it at a 90° angle. If a client is very lean or debilitated, use a needle longer than 3/8 inch and insert it at a 45° angle. The arms or thighs may be used as alternate sites.
- Do *not* aspirate when giving heparin by subcutaneous injection. **Rationale:** *Aspiration can possibly damage the surrounding tissue and cause bleeding, as well as ecchymoses (bruises).*

- Do not massage the site after the injection. **Rationale:** *Massaging could cause bleeding and ecchymoses and hasten drug absorption.*
- Alternate the sites of subsequent injections.

Variation: Administering Enoxaparin (Lovenox)

Lovenox is a low molecular weight heparin that is used to prevent deep venous thrombosis (DVT). Administration of Lovenox has special considerations also.

- Choose an area on the abdomen at least 5 cm (2 in.) from the umbilicus and above the level of the iliac crests.
- Lovenox syringes come prefilled. Check that the syringe is for the correct dosage. Every syringe comes with a small air bubble. Do *not* expel the air bubble unless you have to adjust the dose.
- Pinch an inch of the cleansed area on the abdomen to make a fold in the skin. Insert the full length of the needle at a 90° angle into the fold of the skin.
- Press the plunger with your thumb until the syringe is empty.
- Pull the needle straight out at the same angle that it was inserted and release the skinfold.
- Point the needle down and away from yourself and others and push down on the plunger to activate the safety shield (Sanofi-Aventis, 2012).

EVALUATION

- Conduct appropriate follow-up such as desired effect of medication (e.g., relief of pain, sedation, lowered blood sugar, a prothrombin time within preestablished limits), any adverse reactions or side effects (e.g., nausea, vomiting, skin rash).

- Relate to previous findings if available.
- Report deviations from normal to the primary care provider.

Ambulatory and Community Settings   **Subcutaneous Injections**

- Store current bottle of insulin at room temperature to avoid painful injections, but keep extra supply in the refrigerator (ADA, 2013).
- If the client has impaired vision, consider prefilling syringes and storing them in an appropriate environment (e.g., the refrigerator) or obtaining prefilled medication syringes from pharmaceutical companies.
- For frequent injections, develop a plan for site rotation with the client and explain the reason for injection site rotation.
- For cost-saving measures, teach able clients to safely reuse disposable syringes. Clients with diabetes can be taught to use the same syringe two to three times. They should be instructed to change syringes when the needle appears dull. Clients should be encouraged to maintain needle asepsis, practice safe recapping, and assess for needle dullness with each injection (ADA, 2013). However, clients with poor personal hygiene, acute concurrent illness, open wounds on the hands, or decreased resistance to infection should be discouraged from reusing syringes.

- Explore with the client and primary care provider the appropriateness of the new inhaled version of insulin in place of the injectable version.
- For insulin-dependent clients, ensure that at least one knowledgeable support person can correctly inject insulin in an emergency situation and recognize and treat hypoglycemia.
- Teach the client and family how to safely dispose of needles. Do not throw needles in the garbage or flush used needles down the toilet. Put needles in recycling containers. The U.S. Environmental Protection Agency (2012) recommends finding out what services are offered in the client's community. For example, some communities offer collection sites or have a disposal site set up that will accept used needles. Some even offer a pickup service that collects the container of used needles.
- The CDC website includes a list of needle disposal rules and needle disposal programs for each state.

Intramuscular Injections

Many articles have been written about intramuscular injection techniques in nursing journals during the past four decades. Much of the literature has been in the form of opinions without sound research or evidence base. Unfortunately, the administration of intramuscular injections has been historically influenced by tradition and ritual, and new techniques (i.e., using the ventrogluteal site) are slow to be incorporated into clinical practice (Cocoman & Murray, 2010).

Injections into muscle tissue, or **intramuscular (IM) injections**, are absorbed more quickly than subcutaneous injections

because of the greater blood supply to the body muscles. Muscles can also take a larger volume of fluid without discomfort than subcutaneous tissues can, although the amount varies among individuals, chiefly based on muscle size and condition and the site used. An adult with well-developed muscles can usually safely tolerate up to 3 mL of medication in the gluteus medius and gluteus maximus muscles (Figure 17–18 ■). A maximum volume of 1 to 2 mL is usually recommended for adults with less developed muscles. In the deltoid muscle, volumes of 0.5 to 1 mL are recommended.

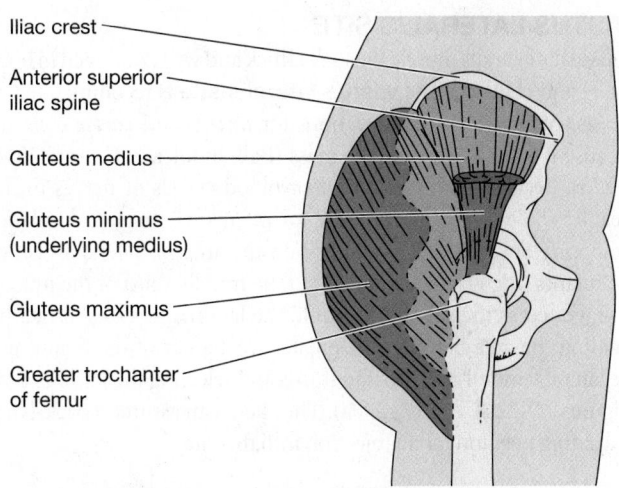

Figure 17–18 ■ Lateral view of the right buttock showing the three gluteal muscles used for intramuscular injections.

Labels: Iliac crest; Anterior superior iliac spine; Gluteus medius; Gluteus minimus (underlying medius); Gluteus maximus; Greater trochanter of femur

Usually a 3- to 5-mL syringe is needed. The size of syringe used depends on the amount of medication being administered. The standard prepackaged IM needle is 1 1/2 inches and #21, #22, or #23 gauge. Several factors indicate the size and length of the needle to be used:

- The muscle
- The type of solution
- The amount of adipose tissue covering the muscle
- The age of the client.

For example, a smaller needle such as a #23- to #25-gauge needle 1 inch long is commonly used for the deltoid muscle. More viscous solutions require a larger gauge (e.g., #20 gauge). Clients who are very obese may require a needle longer than 1 1/2 inches (e.g., 2 inches), and clients who are emaciated may require a shorter needle (e.g., 1 inch). Needle length must be long enough to penetrate the subcutaneous fat layer and be injected into the muscle. See Table 17–1 for a comparison of injection information.

A major consideration in the administration of IM injections is the selection of a safe site located away from large blood vessels, nerves, and bone. Choosing which injection site to use has often been based on the nurse's personal preference, tradition, or convenience rather than the result of an evidence-based approach (Cocoman & Murray, 2010, p. 1171). Several body sites can be used for IM injections, and these sites are discussed in detail next. Contraindications for using a specific site include tissue injury and the presence of nodules, lumps, abscesses, tenderness, or other pathology.

VENTROGLUTEAL SITE

The **ventrogluteal site** is in the gluteus medius muscle, which lies over the gluteus minimus (see Figure 17–18). The ventrogluteal site is the *preferred* site for IM injections because the area:

- Contains no large nerves or blood vessels.
- Provides the greatest thickness of gluteal muscle consisting of both the gluteus medius and gluteus minimus.
- Is sealed off by bone.
- Contains consistently less fat than the buttock area, thus eliminating the need to determine the depth of subcutaneous fat.

TABLE 17–1 **Comparison of Injection Information**

	Syringe Size	Needle Size	Needle Length	Volume of Fluid	Aspiration?	Common Sites	Common Uses
Intradermal (ID)	TB syringe	#25–#27 gauge	1/4–5/8 in.	0.1 mL	No	Inner lower arm Upper chest Back beneath scapulae	Allergy testing TB screening
Subcutaneous	1- to 2-mL syringe Insulin syringe	#25 gauge #30 gauge for insulin	Adult of normal weight: 5/8-in. needle inserted at 45° angle *or* 3/8-in. needle inserted at 90° angle Insulin needle: 4–6 mm	0.5–1 mL	No	Outer aspect of upper arms Anterior aspect of thigh Abdomen	Vaccines Insulin Heparin
Intramuscular (IM)	Deltoid: 1-mL syringe Ventrogluteal: 3- to 5-mL syringes *Note:* Size depends on amount of medication being administered.	Deltoid: #23–#25 gauge Ventrogluteal: #21 or #22 gauge	Deltoid: 1 in. Ventrogluteal: 1.5 in.	Deltoid: 0.5–1 mL Ventrogluteal: 3 mL max for adult with well-developed gluteal muscle 1–2 mL for adults with less-developed gluteal muscle	Deltoid: no Ventrogluteal: no scientific evidence confirming or rejecting aspiration	Deltoid Ventrogluteal	Deltoid: immunizations Ventrogluteal: medication that requires large muscle for absorption and/or volume greater than 1 mL

The ventrogluteal site is the safest site of choice for an IM injection of more than 1 mL in clients older than 7 months (Zimmerman, 2010). This is because it provides the greatest thickness of gluteal muscle and is free of penetrating nerves. Research on the ventrogluteal site being the best site spans several decades, but the use of this site for IM injections in clinical practice is infrequent.

The client position for the injection can be a back, prone, or side-lying position. The side-lying position, however, helps locate the ventrogluteal site more easily. Position the client on his or her side with the knee bent and raised slightly toward the chest. The trochanter will protrude, which facilitates locating the ventrogluteal site. To establish the exact site, the nurse places the heel of the hand on the client's greater trochanter, with the fingers pointing toward the client's head. The right hand is used for the left hip, and the left hand for the right hip. With the index finger on the client's anterior superior iliac spine, the nurse stretches the middle finger dorsally (toward the buttocks), palpating the crest of the ilium and then pressing below it. The triangle formed by the index finger, the third finger, and the crest of the ilium is the injection site (Figure 17–19 ■) and Figure 17–20 ■ shows administering an IM injection into the ventrogluteal site while using the preferred Z-track method shown in Skill 17–6.

VASTUS LATERALIS SITE

The vastus lateralis muscle is usually thick and well developed in both adults and children. The **vastus lateralis site** is recommended as the site of choice for IM injections for infants and young children because it is the largest muscle mass (Ball, Bindler, & Cowen, 2012, p. 273). Because there are no major blood vessels or nerves in the area, it is a desirable injection site for infants whose gluteal muscles are poorly developed. It is situated on the anterior lateral aspect of the infant's thigh (Figure 17–21 ■). The middle third of the muscle is suggested as the site. In the adult, the landmark is established by dividing the area between the greater trochanter of the femur and the lateral femoral condyle into thirds and selecting the middle third (Figures 17–22 ■ and 17–23 ■). The client can assume a back-lying or a sitting position for an injection into this site.

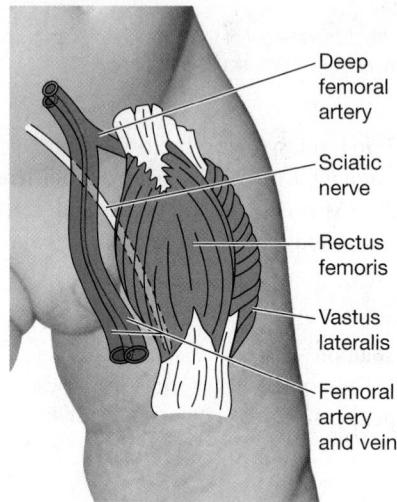

Deep femoral artery

Sciatic nerve

Rectus femoris

Vastus lateralis

Femoral artery and vein

Figure 17–21 ■ The vastus lateralis muscle of an infant's upper thigh, used for intramuscular injections.

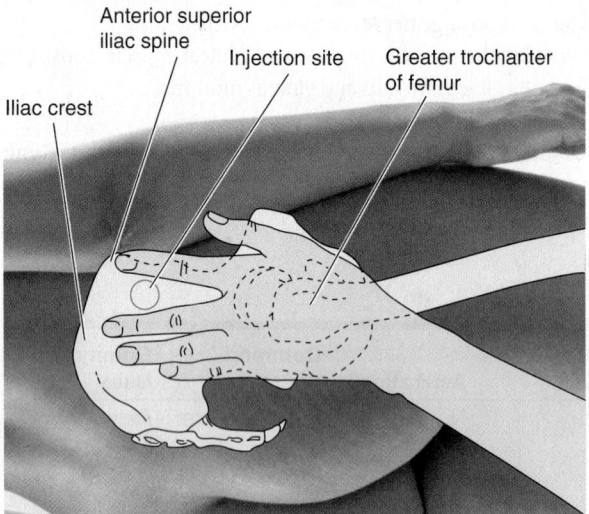

Anterior superior iliac spine

Injection site

Greater trochanter of femur

Iliac crest

Figure 17–19 ■ Landmarks for the ventrogluteal site for an intramuscular injection.

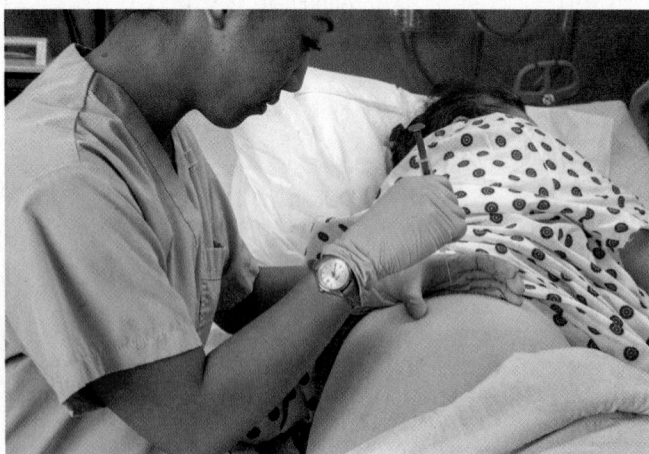

Figure 17–20 ■ Administering an intramuscular injection into the ventrogluteal site using the Z-track method.

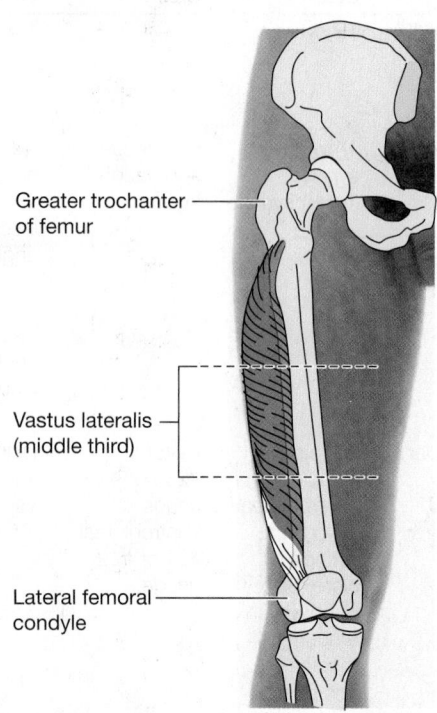

Greater trochanter of femur

Vastus lateralis (middle third)

Lateral femoral condyle

Figure 17–22 ■ Landmarks for the vastus lateralis site of an adult's right thigh, used for an intramuscular injection.

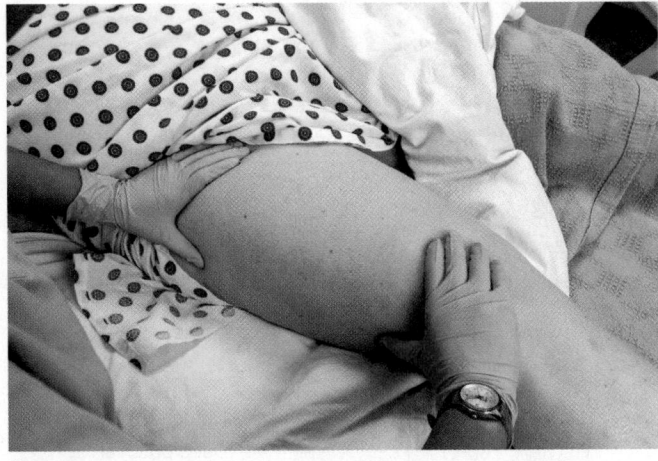

A

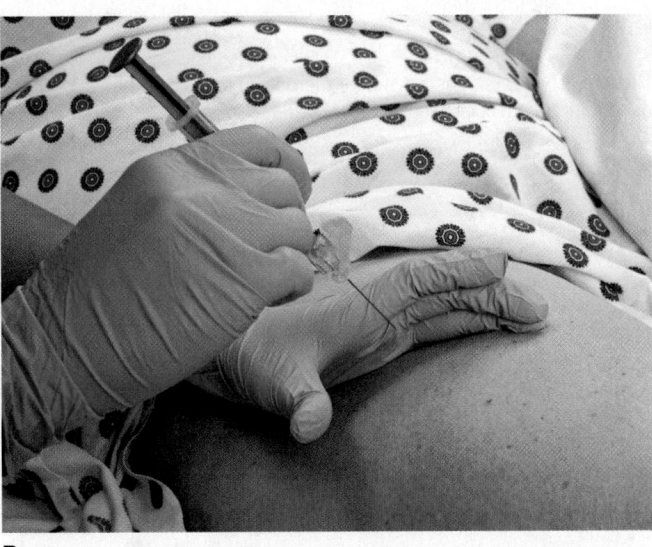

B

Figure 17–23 ■ *A*, Determining landmarks; *B*, administering an intra-muscular injection using the Z-track method into the vastus lateralis site.

DORSOGLUTEAL SITE

Historically, the dorsogluteal site was primarily used for IM injections. However, this site is close to the sciatic nerve and the superior gluteal nerve and artery. As a result, complications (e.g., numbness, pain, paralysis) occurred if the nurse injected a medication near or into the sciatic nerve. In addition, there tends to be more subcutaneous tissue at the dorsogluteal site. As a result, the medication may be injected into the subcutaneous tissue instead of the muscle, which can then affect the intended therapeutic effect.

Cocoman and Murray (2010), based on a review of nursing literature and research, stated that use of the dorsogluteal site should be avoided from injection practice because it presents an unacceptable risk for clients. Potera (2011) noted, however, that many nurses still use the dorsogluteal site. Several reasons for this preference include ease of site identification, more experience with using the dorsogluteal site, less confidence using the ventrogluteal site, and lack of emphasis to use the ventrogluteal site over the dorsogluteal site when learning about IM injections. In contrast, younger nurses follow the recommended clinical practice of using the ventrogluteal site.

It is important for nurses to know all potential sites for IM injections in order to make the best decision for the safety of the client. If

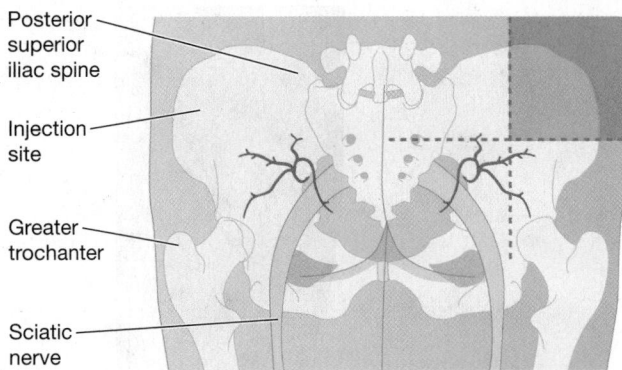

Figure 17–24 ■ Intramuscular dorsogluteal injection site. Artwork showing the correct site (red square) for a dorsogluteal injection. The dorsogluteal muscle is in the upper outside quadrant of the buttock. The dorsogluteal site is not often used due to the danger of damaging the sciatic nerve (yellow), or hitting the superior gluteal artery (red lines).
Peter Gardiner/Science Source.

a nurse decides to use the dorsogluteal site because other, safer sites are unavailable, it is imperative for the nurse to palpate the correct landmarks and choose the injection site carefully to avoid striking the sciatic nerve, major blood vessels, or bone. The nurse palpates the posterior superior iliac spine, then draws an imaginary line to the greater trochanter of the femur. This line is lateral to and parallel to the sciatic nerve. The injection site is lateral and superior to this line (Figure 17–24 ■). Palpating the ilium and the trochanter is important; visual calculations alone can result in an injection that is placed too low and injures other structures. The client needs to assume a prone position with the toes pointed inward or a side-lying position with the upper knee flexed and in front of the lower leg. These positions promote muscle relaxation and therefore minimize discomfort from the injection.

Sciatic nerve injury is associated with use of the dorsogluteal site and if that injury occurs, it provides the basis for nursing professional negligence suits. This is particularly true when there is wide agreement in the literature that the ventrogluteal site is the preferred site.

RECTUS FEMORIS SITE

The rectus femoris muscle, which belongs to the quadriceps muscle group, is used *only occasionally* for IM injections. The **rectus femoris site** is situated on the anterior aspect of the thigh (Figure 17–25 ■). Its chief advantage is that clients who administer their own injections can reach this site easily. Its main disadvantage is that an injection here may cause considerable discomfort for some people.

DELTOID SITE

The deltoid muscle is found on the lateral aspect of the upper arm. It is not used often for IM injections because it is a relatively small muscle and is very close to the radial nerve and radial artery. The **deltoid site** is sometimes considered for use in adults because of rapid absorption from the deltoid area, but no more than 1 mL of solution can be administered. This site is recommended for the administration of hepatitis B vaccine in adults.

The upper landmark for the deltoid site is located by the nurse placing four fingers across the deltoid muscle with the first finger on the acromion process. The top of the axilla is the line that marks the lower border landmark (Figure 17–26 ■). A triangle within these boundaries indicates the deltoid muscle about 5 cm (2 in.) below the acromion process (Figures 17–27 ■ and 17–28 ■).

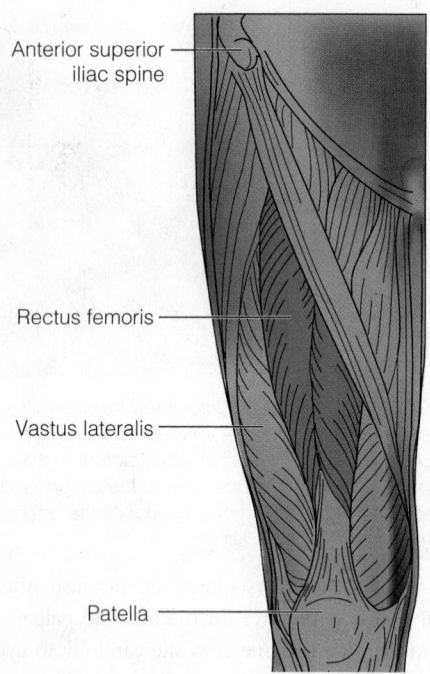

Figure 17–25 ■ Landmarks for the rectus femoris muscle of the upper right thigh, used for intramuscular injections.

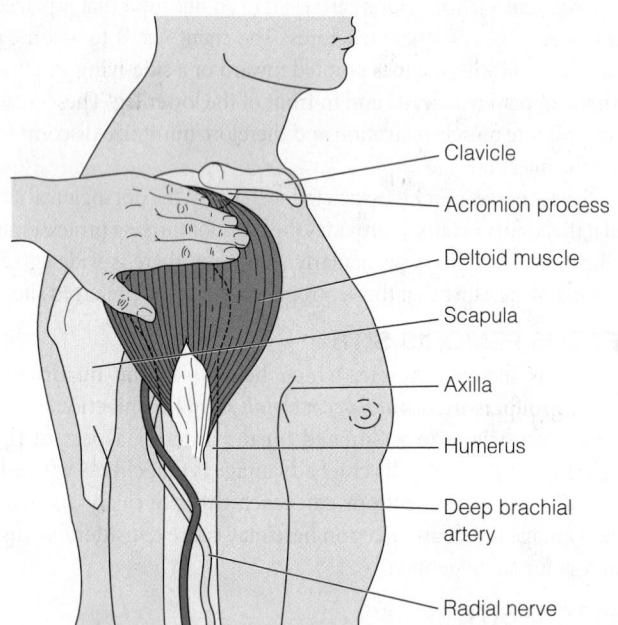

Figure 17–26 ■ A method of establishing the deltoid muscle site for an intramuscular injection.

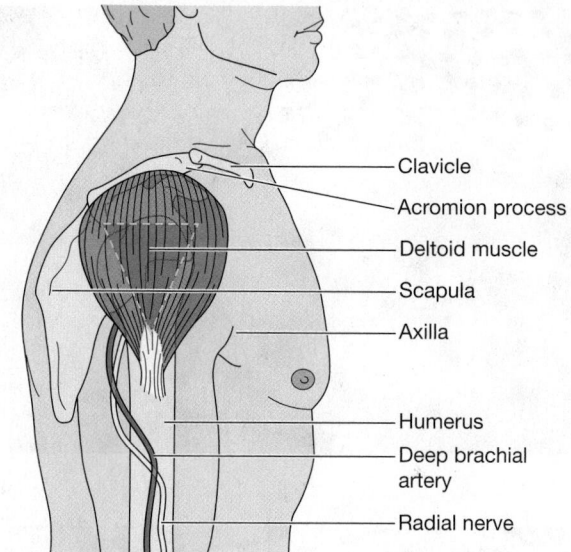

Figure 17–27 ■ Landmarks for the deltoid muscle of the upper arm, used for intramuscular injections.

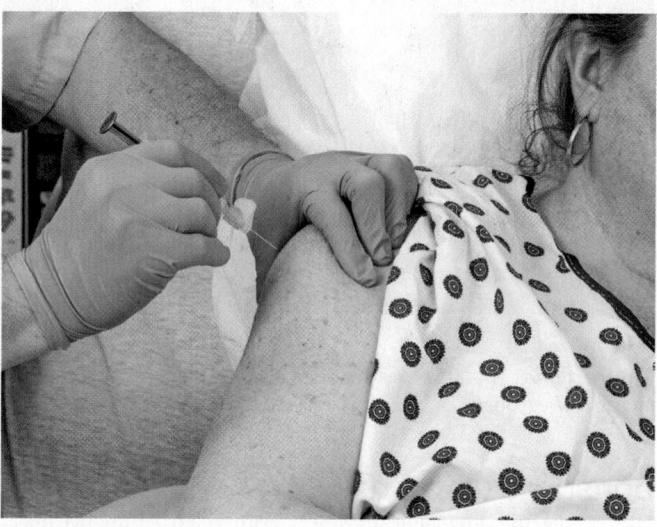

Figure 17–28 ■ Administering an intramuscular injection into the deltoid site.

Intramuscular Injection Technique

Skill 17–6 describes how to administer an IM injection using the **Z-track technique**, which is recommended for all IM injections (Carter-Templeton & McCoy, 2008; Cocoman & Murray, 2008; Hunter, 2008; Malkin, 2008; Nicoll & Hesby, 2002). The Z-track method has been found to be less painful than the traditional injection technique and decreases leakage of irritating and discoloring medications into the subcutaneous tissue (Barron & Cocoman, 2008;

Nicoll & Hesby, 2002; Zimmerman, 2010). Although the Z-track technique is not always used in practice, research evidence supports its effectiveness and recommends its routine use.

Another aspect of IM injection technique is the practice of aspirating for blood prior to administering the injection. Is this practice based on tradition or evidence? Historically, nurses have been taught to aspirate for blood before all IM injections to prevent accidently injecting the medication into a blood vessel. Aspiration technique consists of pulling the syringe plunger back for 5 to 10 seconds to create negative pressure in the tissue and looking for blood return. One study, however, found that only 3% of the nurses in that study aspirated long enough to have the action be of benefit (Hensel & Springmyer, 2011). Literature and integrative reviews of evidence indicate that the practice of aspiration before vaccination injections into the deltoid has no basis in scientific evidence (Crawford & Johnson, 2012;

Hensel & Springmyer, 2011). Moreover, the American Academy of Pediatrics, the American Council on Immunization Practices, and the World Health Organization have stated that the practice of aspiration is unnecessary for vaccinations because there are no large vessels located at the recommended vaccination sites (Crawford & Johnson, 2012; Hensel & Springmyer, 2011).

The evidence, however, is not clear regarding aspiration at IM sites *other* than the deltoid (i.e., ventrogluteal). What is currently known is that there has been no major complication connected to the ventrogluteal site because this site avoids all major nerves and blood vessels (Zimmerman, 2010, p. 60). Hensel and Springmyer (2011) state that "the practice of aspirating for blood return with any IM injection may cease as the use of the ventrogluteal site increases" (p. 592). Further research is needed to examine the practice of aspirating with medications other than vaccinations.

●○● NURSING PROCESS: INTRAMUSCULAR INJECTIONS

Administering an Intramuscular Injection

SKILL 17–6

ASSESSMENT
Assess:
- Client allergies to medication(s).
- Specific drug action, side effects, and adverse reactions.
- Client's knowledge of and learning needs about the medication.
- Tissue integrity of the selected site.
- Client's age and weight to determine site and needle size.
- Client's ability or willingness to participate.

- Determine whether the size of the muscle is appropriate to the amount of medication to be injected. An average adult's deltoid muscle can usually absorb 0.5 mL of medication, although some authorities believe 1 mL can be absorbed by a well-developed deltoid muscle. The gluteus medius muscle can often absorb 1 to 4 mL, although 4 mL may be very painful and may be contraindicated by agency protocol.

PLANNING
DELEGATION

The administration of IM injections is an invasive technique that involves the application of nursing knowledge, problem solving, and sterile technique. Therefore, delegation to UAP would be inappropriate. The nurse, however, can inform the UAP of the intended therapeutic effects and/or specific side effects of the medication and direct the UAP to report specific client observations to the nurse for follow-up.

Equipment
- Client's MAR or computer printout
- Sterile medication (usually provided in an ampule or vial or prefilled syringe)
- Syringe and needle of a size appropriate for the amount and type of solution to be administered
- Antiseptic swabs
- Clean gloves

IMPLEMENTATION
Preparation
- Check the MAR.
  - Check the label on the medication carefully against the MAR to make sure that the correct medication is being prepared.
  - Follow the three checks for administering the medication and dose. Read the label on the medication (1) when it is taken from the medication cart, (2) before withdrawing the medication, and (3) after withdrawing the medication.
  - Confirm that the dose is correct.
- Organize the equipment.

Performance
1. Perform hand hygiene and observe other appropriate infection prevention procedures.
2. Prepare the medication from the ampule or vial for drug withdrawal.
   - See Skill 17–1 (ampule) or 17–2 (vial).
   - Whenever feasible, change the needle on the syringe before the injection. **Rationale:** *Because the outside of a new needle is free of medication, it does not irritate subcutaneous tissues as it passes into the muscle.*
   - Invert the syringe needle uppermost and expel all excess air.
3. Provide for client privacy.
4. Prepare the client.
   - Prior to performing the procedure, introduce self and verify the client's identity using agency protocol. **Rationale:** *This ensures that the right client receives the right medication.*

- Assist the client to a supine, lateral, prone, or sitting position, depending on the chosen site. If the target muscle is the gluteus medius (ventrogluteal site), have the client in the supine position and flex the knee(s); in the lateral position, flex the upper leg; and in the prone position, toe in. **Rationale:** *Appropriate positioning promotes relaxation of the target muscle.*
- Obtain assistance in holding an uncooperative client. **Rationale:** *This prevents injury due to sudden movement after needle insertion.*
5. Explain the purpose of the medication and how it will help, using language that the client can understand. Include relevant information about effects of the medication. **Rationale:** *Information can facilitate acceptance of and compliance with the therapy.*
6. Select, locate, and clean the site.
   - Select a site free of skin lesions, tenderness, swelling, hardness, or localized inflammation and one that has not been used frequently.
   - If injections are to be frequent, alternate sites. Avoid using the same site twice in a row. **Rationale:** *This is to reduce the discomfort of IM injections.* If necessary, discuss with the prescribing primary care provider an alternative method of providing the medication.
   - Locate the exact site for the injection. See the discussion of sites earlier in this chapter.

Continued on page 428

Administering an Intramuscular Injection—*continued*

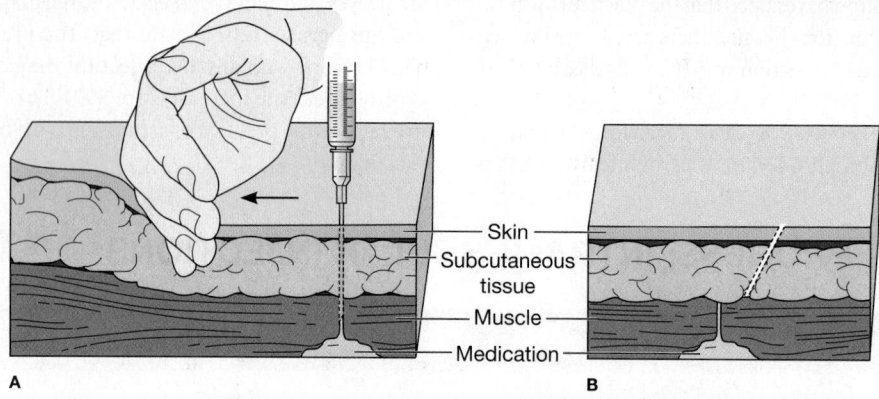

A   **B**

❶ Inserting an intramuscular needle at a 90° angle using the Z-track method: *A*, skin pulled to the side; *B*, skin released.
Note: When the skin returns to its normal position after the needle is withdrawn, a seal is formed over the intramuscular site. This prevents seepage of the medication into the subcutaneous tissues and subsequent discomfort.

- Apply clean gloves.
- Clean the site with an antiseptic swab. Using a circular motion, start at the center and move outward about 5 cm (2 in.). **Rationale:** *This will prevent entry of bacteria into the injection site (Hunter, 2008).*
- Transfer and hold the swab between the third and fourth fingers of your nondominant hand in readiness for needle withdrawal, or position the swab on the client's skin above the intended site. Allow skin to dry prior to injecting medication. **Rationale:** *This will reduce the stinging sensation from the antiseptic upon injection.*

7. Prepare the syringe for injection.
- Remove the needle cover and discard without contaminating the needle.
- If using a prefilled unit-dose medication, take caution to avoid dripping medication on the needle prior to injection. If this does occur, wipe the medication off the needle with a sterile gauze. Some sources recommend changing the needle if possible. **Rationale:** *Medication left on the needle can cause pain when it is tracked through the subcutaneous tissue (Nicoll & Hesby, 2002).*

8. Inject the medication using a Z-track technique.
- Use the ulnar side of the nondominant hand to pull the skin approximately 2.5 cm (1 in.) to the side. ❶ Under some circumstances, such as for an emaciated client or an infant, the muscle may be pinched. **Rationale:** *Pulling the skin and subcutaneous tissue or pinching the muscle makes it firmer and facilitates needle insertion.*
- Holding the syringe between the thumb and forefinger (as if holding a pencil), pierce the skin quickly and smoothly at a 90° angle ❷ and insert the needle into the muscle. **Rationale:** *Using a quick motion lessens the client's discomfort. Holding the syringe like a pen or pencil reduces accidental depression of the plunger and inadvertent administration of the medication while the needle is being inserted.*
- Hold the barrel of the syringe steady with your nondominant hand and aspirate by pulling back on the plunger with your dominant hand. ❸ Aspirate for 5 to 10 seconds. **Rationale:** *If the needle is in a small blood vessel, it takes time for the blood to appear.* If blood appears in the syringe, withdraw the needle, discard the syringe, and prepare a new injection. **Rationale:** *This step determines whether the needle has been inserted into a blood vessel.* As stated previously, the practice of aspiration immediately before the administration of an IM vaccine injection is not necessary. Aspiration should be used with the dorsogluteal site (last resort) because nee-

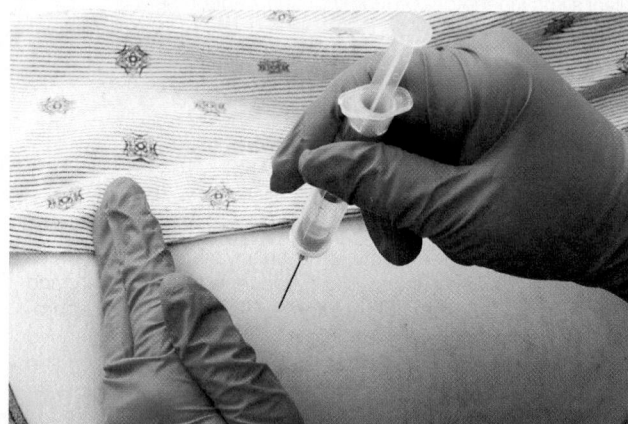

❷ Holding the syringe between the thumb and forefinger. Note that the nurse is using the Z-track technique.

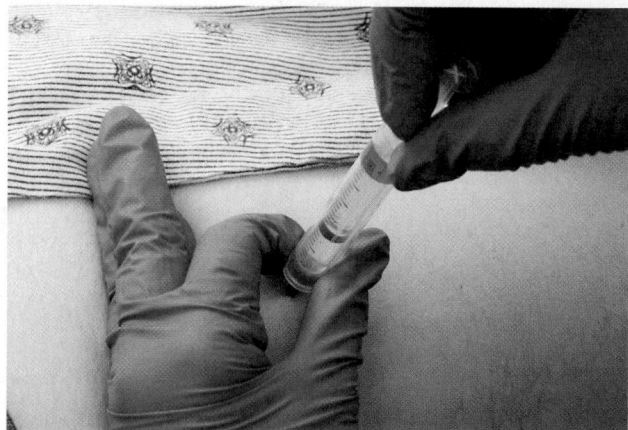

❸ In addition to pulling the skin to the side, the nondominant hand is holding the barrel of the syringe to prevent it from moving while the dominant hand aspirates by pulling back on the plunger.

dle insertion is close to the gluteal artery. Currently there is no clear evidence with other sites. Thus, it is recommended that nursing students consult the policy manual at the institution where they are practicing to determine the recommended guidelines for IM injection technique.

Administering an Intramuscular Injection—*continued*

- If blood does not appear, inject the medication steadily and slowly (approximately 10 seconds per milliliter) while holding the syringe steady if using the ventrogluteal site. **Rationale:** *Injecting medication slowly promotes comfort and allows time for tissue to expand and begin absorption of the medication* (Malkin, 2008; Zimmerman, 2010). *Holding the syringe steady minimizes discomfort.* One study found that rapidly injecting vaccinations without aspiration caused less pain (Hensel & Springmyer, 2011).
- After injection, if using the ventrogluteal site, wait 10 seconds. **Rationale:** *Waiting permits the medication to disperse into the muscle tissue, thus decreasing the client's discomfort.*

9. Withdraw the needle.
   - Withdraw the needle smoothly at the same angle of insertion. **Rationale:** *This minimizes tissue injury.* Release the skin.
   - Apply gentle pressure at the site with a dry sponge. **Rationale:** *Use of an alcohol swab may cause pain or a burning sensation.*

- If bleeding occurs, apply pressure with a dry sterile gauze until it stops.
- It is not necessary to massage the area at the site of injection. **Rationale:** *Massaging the site may cause leakage of medication from the site and result in irritation.*

10. If not using a passive safety syringe, activate the needle safety device or discard the uncapped needle and attached syringe into the proper sharps receptacle.
    - Remove and dispose of gloves.
    - Perform hand hygiene.
11. Document all relevant information.
    - Include the time of administration, drug name, dose, route, and the client's reactions.
12. Assess effectiveness of the medication at the time it is expected to act.

EVALUATION

- Conduct appropriate follow-up such as desired effect of medication (e.g., relief of pain or nausea/vomiting), any adverse reactions or side effects, local skin or tissue reactions at injection site (e.g., redness, swelling, pain, or other evidence of tissue damage).

- Relate to previous findings, if available.
- Report significant deviation from normal to the primary care provider.

LIFESPAN CONSIDERATIONS | **Intramuscular Injections**

INFANTS
- The vastus lateralis site is recommended as the site of choice for IM injections for infants. There are no major blood vessels or nerves in this area, and it is the infant's largest muscle mass. It is situated on the anterior lateral aspect of the thigh.
- Obtain assistance to immobilize an infant or young child. The parent may hold the child. **Rationale:** *This prevents accidental injury* during *the procedure.*

CHILDREN
- Use needles that will place medication in the main muscle mass; infants and children usually require smaller, shorter needles (#22 to #25 gauge, 5/8 to 1 in. long) for IM injections.

- The vastus lateralis is recommended as the site of choice for toddlers and children.
- For the older child and adolescent, the recommended sites are the same as for the adult: ventrogluteal or deltoid. Ask which arm they would like the injection in.

OLDER ADULTS
- Older clients may have decreased muscle mass or muscle atrophy. A shorter needle may be needed. Assessment of appropriate injection site is critical. Absorption of medication may occur more quickly than expected.

INTRAVENOUS MEDICATIONS

Because IV medications enter the client's bloodstream directly by way of a vein, their use is appropriate when a rapid effect is required. The IV route is also appropriate when medications are too irritating to tissues to be given by other routes. When an IV line is already established, this route is desirable because it avoids the discomfort of other parenteral routes. Methods used to administer medications intravenously include the following:

- Large-volume infusion of IV fluid
- Intermittent IV infusion (piggyback or tandem setups)
- Volume-controlled infusion (often used for children)
- Intravenous push (IVP)
- Intermittent injection ports (device).

In all of these methods, the client has an existing IV line or an IV access site such as a saline or heparin lock. Most agencies have procedures and policies about who may administer an IV medication. Chapter 18 ∞ describes the technique for performing a venipuncture and establishing an IV line.

With all IV medication administration, it is very important to observe clients closely for signs of adverse reactions. Because the drug enters the bloodstream directly and acts immediately, there is no way it can be withdrawn or its action terminated. Therefore, the nurse must take special care to avoid any errors in the preparation of the drug and the calculation of the dosage. When the administered drug is particularly potent, an antidote to the drug should be available. In addition, assess the vital signs before, during, and after infusion of the drug.

Before adding any medications to an existing intravenous infusion, the nurse must check for all of the "rights" and verify compatibility of the drug and the existing intravenous fluid. Be aware of any incompatibilities of the drug and the fluid that is infusing. For example, the drug phenytoin (Dilantin) is incompatible with glucose and will form a precipitate if injected through a port in an intravenous line with glucose/dextrose infusing.

Large-Volume Infusions

Mixing a medication into a large-volume IV container is the safest and easiest way to administer a drug intravenously. The drugs are diluted in volumes of 250, 500, or 1,000 mL of compatible fluids. It may be necessary to consult a pharmacist to confirm compatibility. Fluids such as IV normal saline or Ringer's lactate are frequently used. These are commonly called crystalloid fluids and are used for fluid replacement as well as medication administration. Commonly added drugs are potassium chloride and vitamins. It may also be necessary to ensure the

WHAT IF **Administering an Intramuscular Injection Using Z-Track Technique**

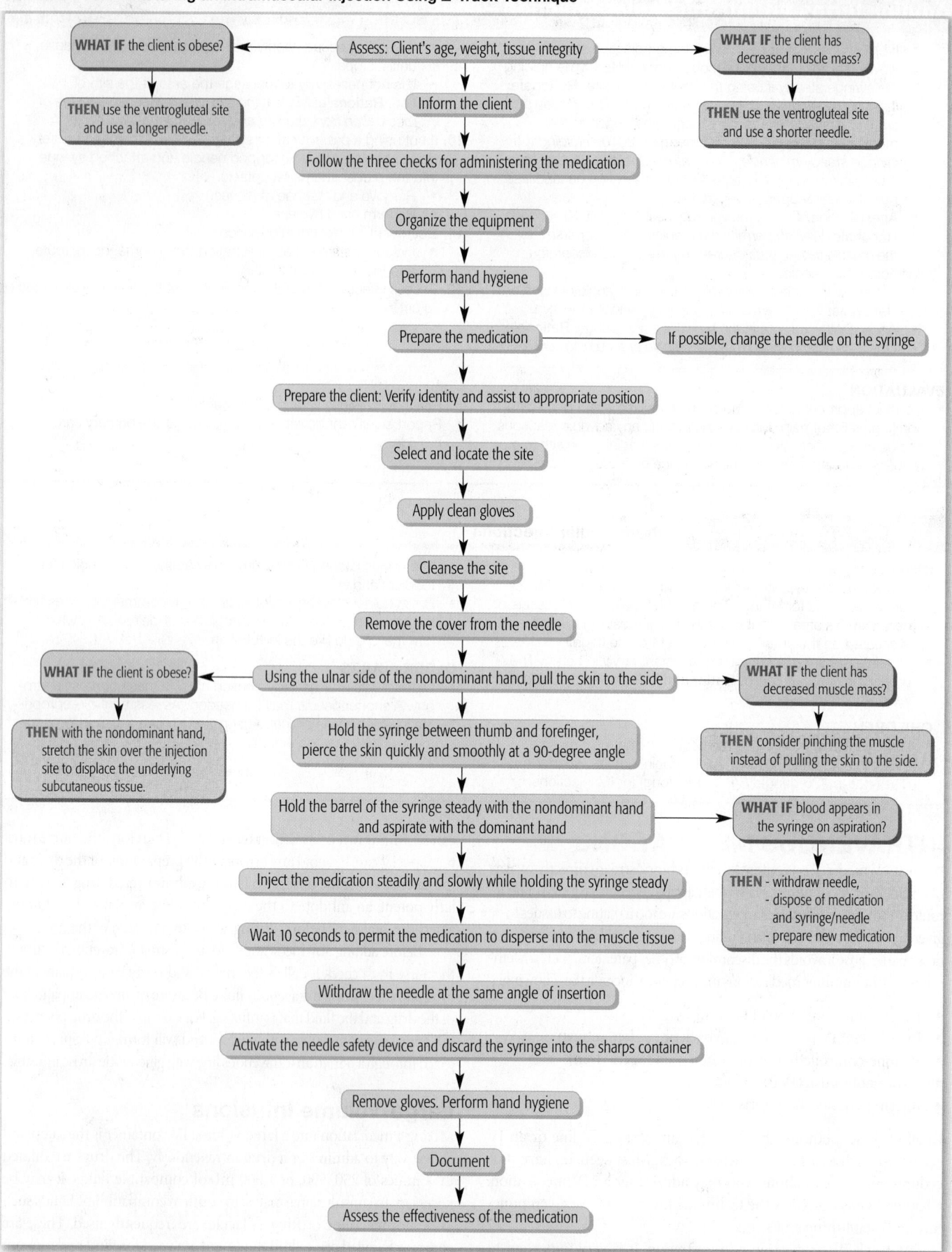

WHAT IF the client is obese?

THEN use the ventrogluteal site and use a longer needle.

Assess: Client's age, weight, tissue integrity

WHAT IF the client has decreased muscle mass?

THEN use the ventrogluteal site and use a shorter needle.

Inform the client

Follow the three checks for administering the medication

Organize the equipment

Perform hand hygiene

Prepare the medication → If possible, change the needle on the syringe

Prepare the client: Verify identity and assist to appropriate position

Select and locate the site

Apply clean gloves

Cleanse the site

Remove the cover from the needle

WHAT IF the client is obese?

THEN with the nondominant hand, stretch the skin over the injection site to displace the underlying subcutaneous tissue.

Using the ulnar side of the nondominant hand, pull the skin to the side

WHAT IF the client has decreased muscle mass?

THEN consider pinching the muscle instead of pulling the skin to the side.

Hold the syringe between thumb and forefinger, pierce the skin quickly and smoothly at a 90-degree angle

Hold the barrel of the syringe steady with the nondominant hand and aspirate with the dominant hand

WHAT IF blood appears in the syringe on aspiration?

THEN - withdraw needle,
- dispose of medication and syringe/needle
- prepare new medication

Inject the medication steadily and slowly while holding the syringe steady

Wait 10 seconds to permit the medication to disperse into the muscle tissue

Withdraw the needle at the same angle of insertion

Activate the needle safety device and discard the syringe into the sharps container

Remove gloves. Perform hand hygiene

Document

Assess the effectiveness of the medication

compatibility of some drugs with the plastic IV bag and tubing. A glass IV bottle and special tubing may be used in special situations.

The nurse adds the medication to the currently infusing fluid container or to a new container of fluid before it is hung for infusion. However, in many hospitals, the pharmacist adds the medication to the IV container. It is still the nurse's responsibility to check the IV label against the orders of the primary care provider.

●○● NURSING PROCESS: LARGE-VOLUME INFUSIONS

Adding Medications to Intravenous Fluid Containers

SKILL 17-7

ASSESSMENT
- Inspect and palpate the IV insertion site for signs of infection, infiltration, or a dislocated catheter.
- Inspect the surrounding skin for redness, pallor, or swelling.
- Palpate the surrounding tissues for coldness, tenderness, and the presence of edema, which could indicate leakage of the IV fluid into the tissues.
- Take vital signs for baseline data for medication that is particularly potent.
- Determine if the client has allergies to the medication(s).
- Check the compatibility of the medication(s) and IV fluid.

PLANNING
DELEGATION

Adding medications to IV fluid containers involves the application of nursing knowledge and critical thinking. Therefore, the nurse does not delegate this procedure to UAP. The nurse, however, can inform the UAP of the intended therapeutic effects and/or specific side effects of the medication(s) in the IV and direct the UAP to report specific client observations to the nurse for follow-up.

Equipment
- Client's MAR or computer printout
- Correct sterile medication
- Diluent for medication in powdered form (see manufacturer's instructions)
- Correct solution container, if a new one is to be attached
- Antiseptic swabs
- Sterile syringe of appropriate size (e.g., 5 or 10 mL) and a 1- to 1 1/2-inch, #20- or #21-gauge sterile safety needle if not using a needleless system
- IV additive label

IMPLEMENTATION
Preparation
- Check the medication administration record.
  - Check the label on the medication carefully against the MAR to make sure that the correct medication is being prepared.
  - Follow the three checks for administering medications. Read the label on the medication (1) when it is taken from the medication cart, (2) before withdrawing the medication, and (3) after withdrawing the medication.
  - Confirm that the dosage and route are correct.
  - Verify which infusion solution is to be used with the medication.
  - Consult a pharmacist, if required, to confirm compatibility of the drugs and solutions being mixed.
- Organize the equipment.

Performance
1. Perform hand hygiene and observe other appropriate infection prevention procedures.
2. Prepare the medication ampule or vial for drug withdrawal.
   - See Skill 17–1 (ampule) or 17–2 (vial).
   - Check the agency's practice for using a filter needle to withdraw premixed liquid medications from multidose vials or ampules.
3. Add the medication.

To New IV Container
- Locate the injection port. Clean the port with the antiseptic or alcohol swab. ❶ **Rationale:** *This reduces the risk of introducing microorganisms into the container when the needle is inserted.*
- Remove the needle cap from the syringe, insert the needle through the center of the injection port, and inject the medication into the bag. ❷ Activate the needle safety device.

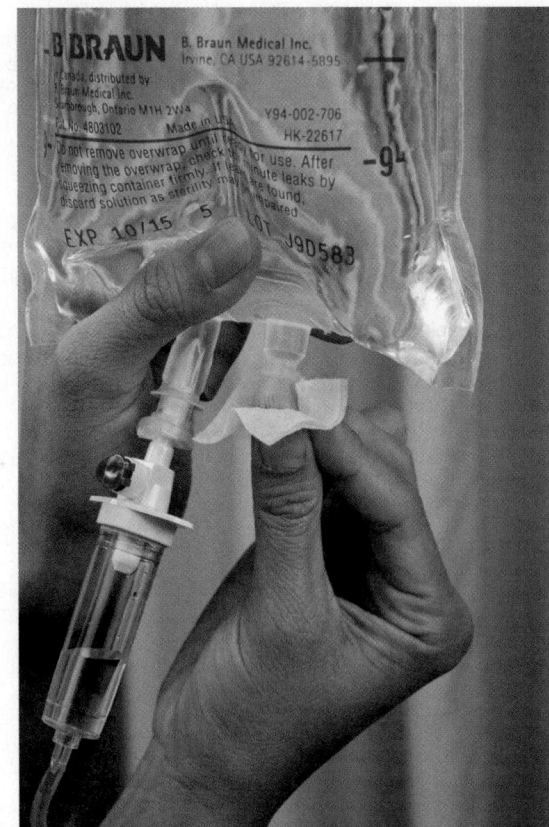

❶ Cleanse the injection port with an alcohol swab.

Continued on page 432

Adding Medications to Intravenous Fluid Containers—*continued*

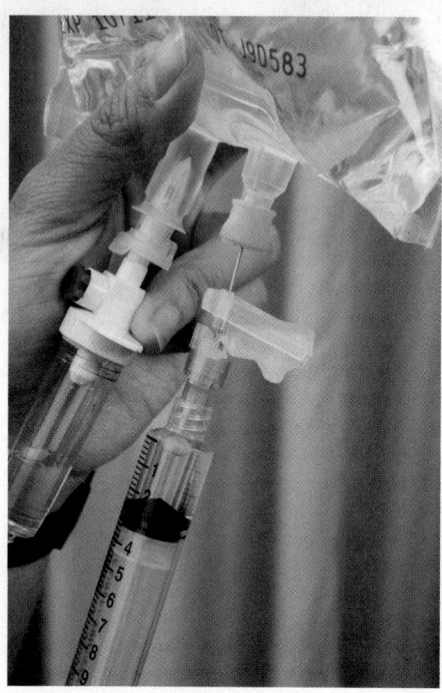

❷ Inserting a medication through the injection port of an infusing container.

- Mix the medication and solution by gently rotating or slowly inverting the bag or bottle several times. ❸ **Rationale:** *This should disperse the medication throughout the solution.*
- Complete the IV additive label with the client's name and room number (if appropriate), name and dose of medication, date, time, and nurse's initials. Attach it on the bag or bottle. ❹ **Rationale:** *This documents that medication has been added to the solution. The label should be easy to read when the bag is hanging.*
- Clamp the IV tubing. Remove the spike from the current IV container, taking care not to touch anything with the exposed spike. Place the used IV container in a sink or basin temporarily while attaching the new IV container. Spike the bag or bottle with IV tubing and hang the IV. If no IV infusion was running, be sure to fully flush the IV solution through the new tubing and verify that no air bubbles are present in the tubing prior to connecting to the IV access. **Rationale:** *Clamping prevents rapid infusion of the solution.*
- Regulate infusion rate as ordered. Often a controller device such as an IV pump is used to ensure accurate rate of infusion.

To an Existing Infusion

- Determine that the IV solution in the container is sufficient for adding the medication. **Rationale:** *Sufficient volume is necessary to dilute the medication adequately.*
- Confirm the desired dilution of the medication, that is, the amount of medication per milliliter of solution.
- Close the infusion clamp. **Rationale:** *This prevents the medication from infusing directly into the client as it is injected into the bag or bottle.*
- Wipe the medication port of the IV bag or bottle with the alcohol or disinfectant swab. **Rationale:** *This reduces the risk of introducing microorganisms into the container when the needle is inserted.* Remove the needle cover from the medication syringe.
- While supporting and stabilizing the bag with your thumb and forefinger, carefully insert the syringe needle through the port and inject the medication. **Rationale:** *The bag is supported dur-*

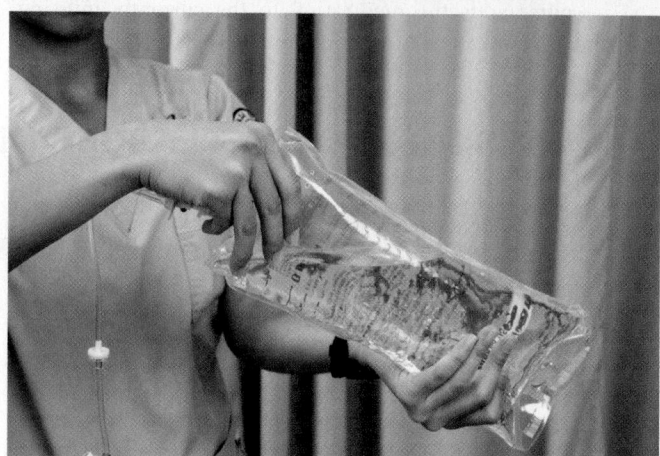

❸ Rotating an IV bag to distribute a medication.

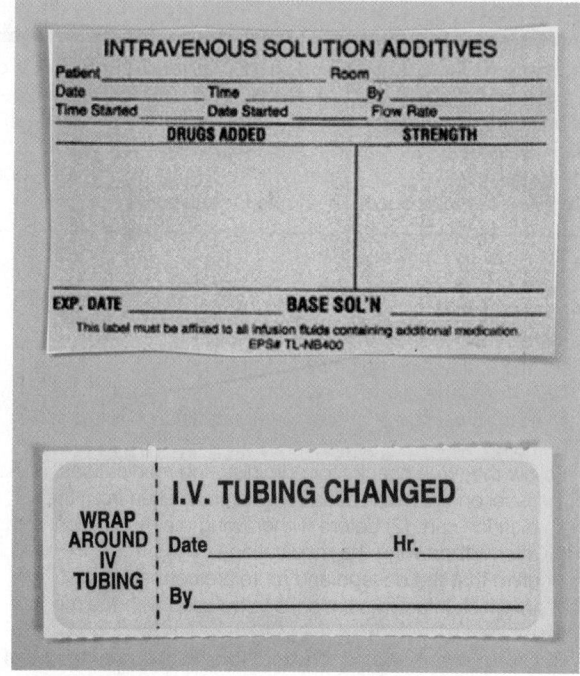

❹ *Top,* Label indicating a medication added to an IV infusion; *Bottom,* label indicating time when the IV tubing was changed.

ing the injection of the medication to avoid punctures. If the bag is too high to reach easily, lower it from the IV pole. Activate the needle safety device.
- Remove the bag from the pole and gently rotate or invert the bag. **Rationale:** *This will mix the medication and solution.*
- Rehang the container and regulate the flow rate, making sure that no air has entered the tubing during the procedure. **Rationale:** *This establishes the correct flow rate.*
- Complete the medication label and apply to the IV container.
4. Dispose of the equipment and supplies according to agency practice. **Rationale:** *This prevents inadvertent injury to others and the spread of microorganisms.*
5. Document the medication(s) on the appropriate form in the client's record.

EVALUATION

- Conduct appropriate follow-up such as desired effect of medication, any adverse reactions or side effects, or change in vital signs.
- Reassess status of IV site and patency of IV infusion.
- Relate to previous findings, if available.
- Report significant deviations from normal to the primary care provider.

Intermittent Intravenous Infusions

An intermittent infusion is a method of administering a medication mixed in a small amount of IV solution, such as 50 or 100 mL. It is important for the label on an IV intermittent medication to be designed to prevent medication errors. The ISMP (2010) developed recommended principles for these medication labels. See Figure 17–29 ■ for a sample label. The drug is administered at regular intervals, such as every 4 hours, with the drug being infused for a short period of time such as 30 to 60 minutes. Two commonly used additive or secondary IV setups are the tandem and the piggyback.

In a **tandem** setup, a second container is attached to the line of the first container at the lower, secondary port (Figure 17–30A ■). This setup permits medications to be administered intermittently or simultaneously with the primary solution.

In the **piggyback** alignment, a second set connects the second container to the tubing of the primary container at the upper port (Figure 17–30B). This setup is used solely for intermittent drug administration. Various manufacturers describe these sets differently, so the nurse must check the manufacturer's labeling and directions carefully. Most IV tubing has a one-way valve a short distance from

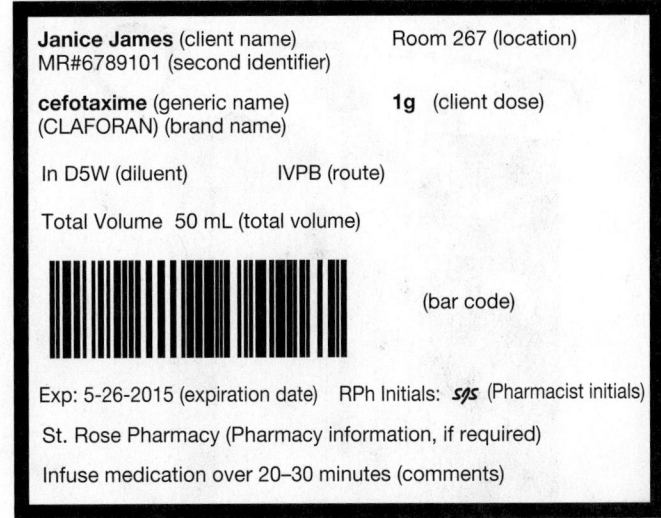

Janice James (client name)	Room 267 (location)
MR#6789101 (second identifier)	
cefotaxime (generic name)	**1g** (client dose)
(CLAFORAN) (brand name)	
In D5W (diluent) IVPB (route)	
Total Volume 50 mL (total volume)	

(bar code)

Exp: 5-26-2015 (expiration date)   RPh Initials: *sjs* (Pharmacist initials)

St. Rose Pharmacy (Pharmacy information, if required)

Infuse medication over 20–30 minutes (comments)

Figure 17–29 ■ Sample label for an IV piggyback medication using ISMP recommendations.

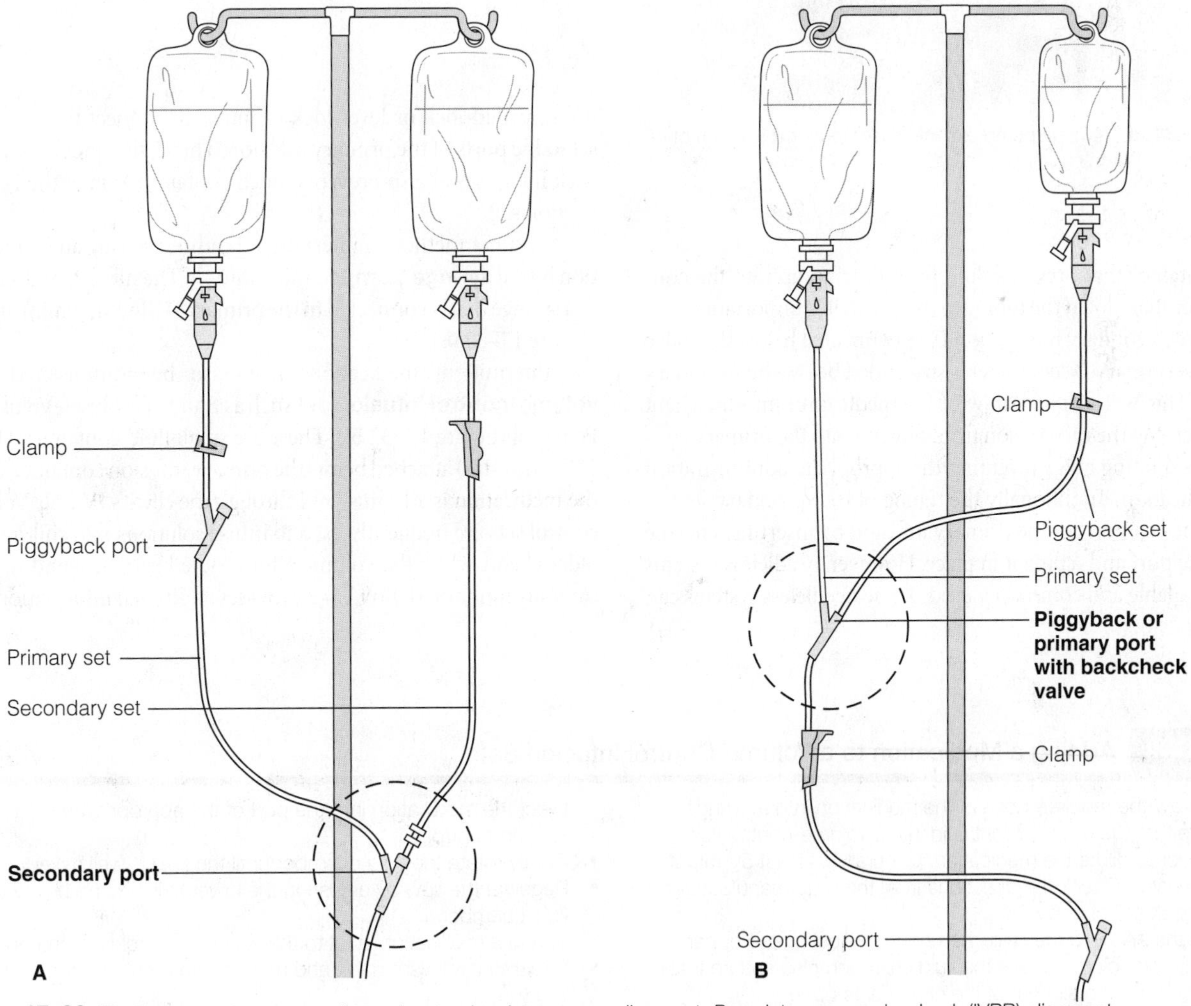

Clamp

Piggyback port

Primary set

Secondary set

Secondary port

A

Clamp

Piggyback set

Primary set

Piggyback or primary port with backcheck valve

Clamp

Secondary port

B

Figure 17–30 ■ Secondary intravenous lines: *A*, a tandem intravenous alignment; *B*, an intravenous piggyback (IVPB) alignment.

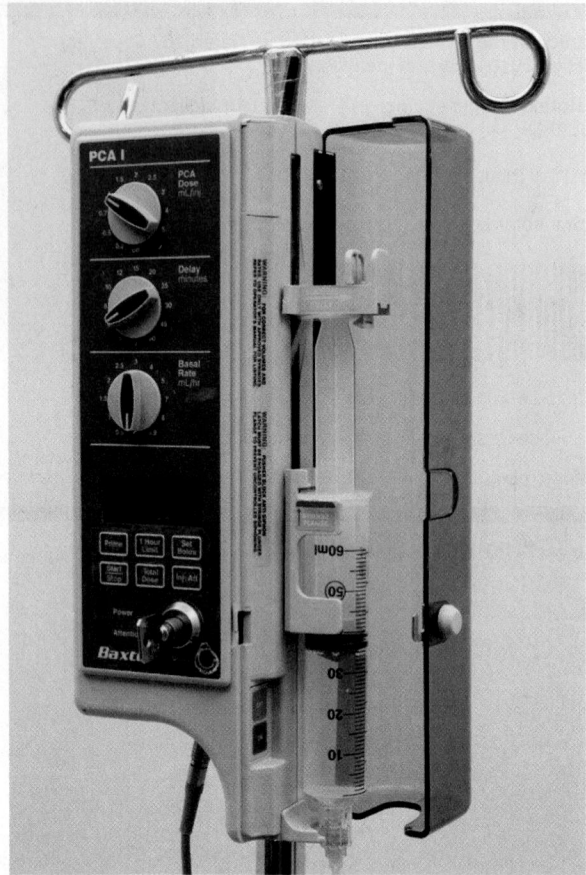

Figure 17–31 ■ Syringe pump or mini-infuser for administration of IV medications.

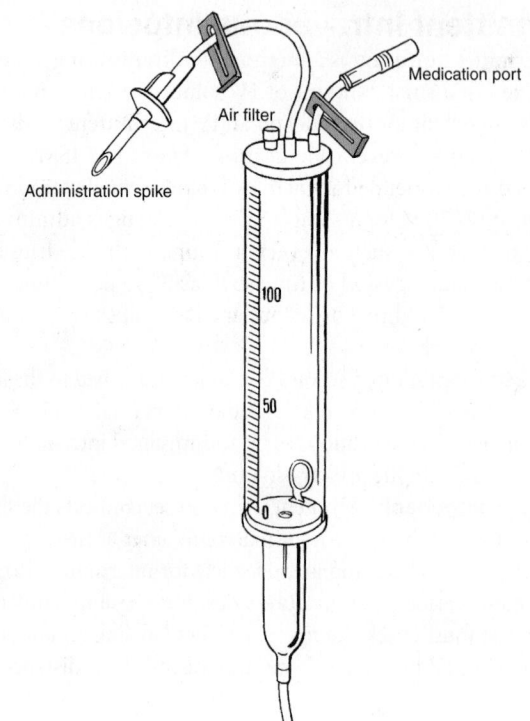

Figure 17–32 ■ A volume-control infusion set.

the IV container that prevents fluid from flowing up into the container rather than down the tubing to the client. It is important to ensure that any secondary medication IV is connected below this valve and that the primary IV container is suspended below the secondary container. This will facilitate flow of the medication into the client while preventing the medication from flowing into the primary container, thus diluting and preventing the appropriate administration of the medication. Traditionally the tubing of the secondary set has been attached to ports of the primary infusion by inserting a needle through the port and taping it in place. However, needleless systems are now available and commonly used. These needleless systems can

use threaded-lock or lever-lock cannulas to connect the secondary set to the ports of the primary infusion. This design prevents needle-stick injuries and also prevents touch contamination at the IV connection site.

Another method of intermittently administering an IV medication is by a **syringe pump** or mini-infuser. The medication is mixed in a syringe that is connected to the primary IV line via a mini-infuser (Figure 17–31 ■).

Intermittent medications may also be administered by a **volume-control infusion set** such as Buretrol, Soluset, Volutrol, or Pediatrol (Figure 17–32 ■). These are small fluid containers (100 to 150 mL in size) attached below the primary infusion container so that the medication is administered through the client's IV line. Volume-control sets are frequently used to infuse solutions into children and older clients when the volume administered is critical and must be carefully monitored. Box 17–2 provides additional information.

BOX 17–2   Adding a Medication to a Volume-Control Infusion Set

- Withdraw the required dose of the medication into a syringe.
- Ensure that there is sufficient fluid in the volume-control fluid chamber to dilute the medication. Generally, at least 50 mL of fluid is used. Check the directions from the drug manufacturer or consult the pharmacist.
- Close the inflow to the fluid chamber by adjusting the upper roller or slide clamp above the fluid chamber; also ensure that the clamp on the air vent of the chamber is open.
- Clean the medication port on the volume-control fluid chamber with an antiseptic swab.

- Inject the medication into the port of the appropriately filled volume-control set.
- Gently rotate the fluid chamber until the fluid is well mixed.
- Regulate the flow by adjusting the lower roller clamp below the fluid chamber.
- Attach a medication label to the volume-control fluid chamber.
- Document relevant data, and monitor the client and the infusion.

●○● NURSING PROCESS: INTERMITTENT INTRAVENOUS INFUSIONS

Administering Intermittent Intravenous Medications Using a Secondary Set

ASSESSMENT

- Inspect and palpate the IV insertion site for signs of infection, infiltration, or a dislocated catheter.
- Inspect the surrounding skin for redness, pallor, or swelling.
- Palpate the surrounding tissues for tenderness, coldness, and the presence of edema, which could indicate leakage of the IV fluid into the tissues.
- Take vital signs for baseline data if the medication being administered is particularly potent.

- Determine if the client has allergies to the medication(s).
- Check the compatibility of the medication, primary IV fluid, and any medication(s) in the primary IV bag.
- Determine specific drug action, side effects, normal dosage, recommended administration time, and peak action time.
- Check patency of the IV line by assessing flow rate.

PLANNING
DELEGATION

The administration of intermittent IV medications involves the application of nursing knowledge and critical thinking. Check the state's nurse practice act to verify the scope of practice for the LPN/LVN as it relates to IV medication administration. Agency policy also must be checked and followed. This skill is not delegated to UAP. The nurse, however, can inform the UAP of the intended therapeutic effects and/or specific side effects of the medication and direct the UAP to report specific client observations to the nurse for follow-up.

Equipment

- Client's MAR or computer printout
- 50- to 250-mL infusion bag with medication (most medication infusion bags are prepared by the pharmacist)
- Secondary administration set
- Antiseptic swabs
- Sterile needle if system is not needleless
- Tape
- Sterile needle or needleless adapter, syringe, and saline if medication is incompatible with the primary infusion

IMPLEMENTATION
Preparation

- Check the MAR.
  - Check the label on the medication carefully against the MAR to make sure that the correct medication is being prepared.
  - Confirm that the dosage is correct.
  - Ensure medication compatibility with the primary infusion solution.
  - Consult a pharmacist, if required, to confirm compatibility of the drugs and solutions being mixed.
- Organize the equipment.
- Remove the medication bag from the refrigerator 30 minutes before administration, if appropriate.

Performance

1. Perform hand hygiene and observe other appropriate infection prevention procedures.
2. Provide for client privacy.
3. Prepare the client.
   - Prior to performing the procedure, introduce self and verify the client's identity using agency protocol. **Rationale:** *This ensures that the right client receives the right medication.*
   - If not previously assessed, take the appropriate assessment measures necessary for the medication.
4. Explain the purpose of the medication and how it will help, using language that the client can understand. Include relevant information about the effects of the medication. **Rationale:** *Information can facilitate acceptance of and compliance with the therapy.*
5. Assemble the secondary infusion:
   - Close the clamp on the secondary infusion tubing.
   - Spike the secondary medication infusion bag and fully flush the tubing, making sure no air is trapped in the tubing. Do not allow more than one or two drops of the solution to exit the tubing to ensure that the client receives the full dose of medication.

- Hang the secondary container at or above the level of the primary infusion. Use the extension hook to lower the primary infusion if a piggyback setup is required. Some infusion pumps do not require this.
- Attach the needleless cannula to the tubing.
- Attach the appropriate label to the secondary tubing. *Secondary tubing is usually changed every 24 to 48 hours. Check agency policy.*
- If the secondary tubing remains from a prior medication administration, attach a new needleless cannula. **Rationale:** *Changing the needleless cannula will reduce the risk of transmission of microorganisms.*

CLINICAL ALERT

Each IV medication bag requires its own secondary tubing. Medication from the IV infusion bag remains in the secondary tubing. It is important, therefore, when hanging subsequent IV infusion bags to hang the same medication on the same secondary tubing. This avoids the mixing of incompatible medications.

6. Attach the secondary infusion to the primary infusion.
   - Clean the Y-port on the primary IV line with an antiseptic swab. Clean the **primary port** (the port farthest from the client) for a piggyback alignment and the **secondary port** (the port closest to the client) for a tandem setup.
   - If the medication is *not* compatible with the primary infusion, temporarily discontinue the primary infusion. Flush the primary line with a sterile saline solution before attaching the secondary set. To flush the line, wipe the port with an

Continued on page 436

SKILL 17-8

Administering Intermittent Intravenous Medications Using a Secondary Set—*continued*

antiseptic swab, clamp the primary line, and, using a sterile syringe and needleless adapter, instill sufficient sterile saline solution through the port to flush any primary fluid out of the infusion tubing.
- Insert the needleless cannula of the secondary line into the primary tubing port. ❶

7. Back prime the secondary tubing if primary and secondary fluids are compatible.
- Lower the medication infusion bag below the primary IV bag.
- Open the clamp of the medication bag.
- Allow the solution from the primary IV bag to backfill the secondary IV tubing and one third to one half of the secondary tubing chamber. ❷ **Rationale:** *This method of priming the secondary tubing allows for no loss of medication.*
- Clamp the secondary IV tubing.
- Hang the secondary IV bag on the IV pole. ❸

8. Program the IV pump for the infusion rate of the IV medication bag.

9. Unclamp the secondary IV tubing and check that the secondary solution is infusing. ❹

10. After infusion of the secondary IV medication bag, regulate the rate of the primary solution by adjusting the clamp or IV pump infusion rate. Some infusion pumps will do this automatically.

11. Leave the secondary bag and tubing in place for future administration or discard as appropriate.

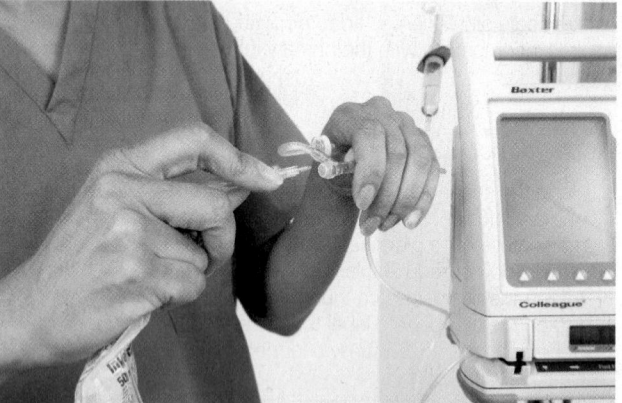

❶ Insert the needleless cannula of the secondary line into the primary tubing port.

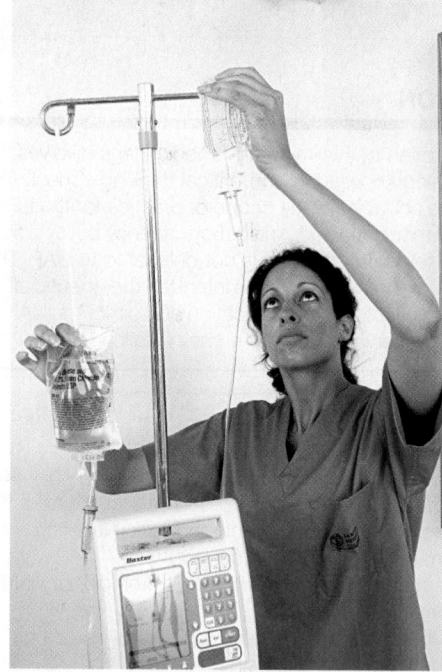

❸ Hang the IV medication bag on the IV pole.

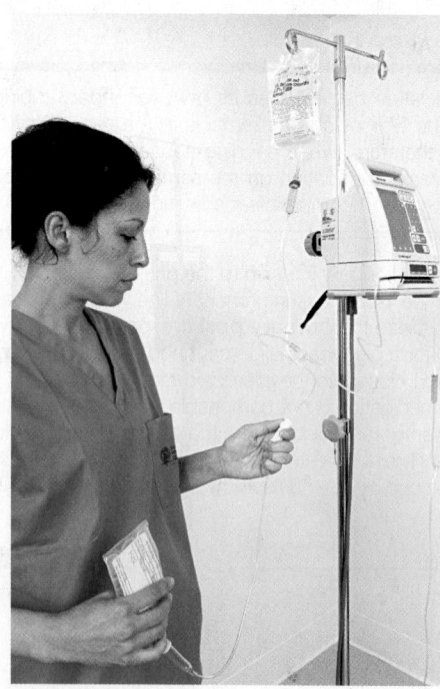

❷ Lower the IV medication bag to back prime the secondary tubing.

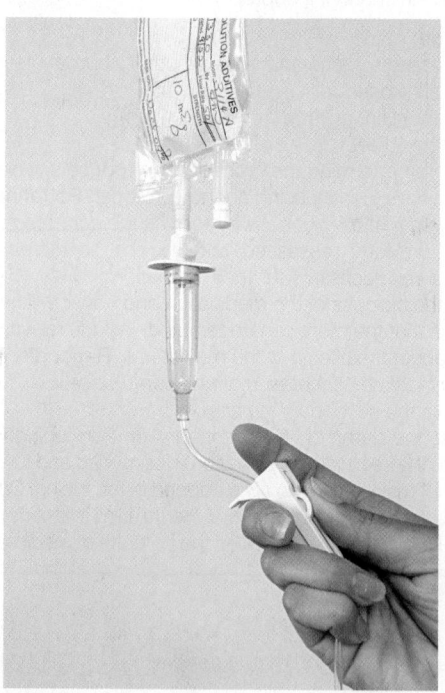

❹ Open the clamp on the secondary tubing.

Continued on page 437

Administering Intermittent Intravenous Medications Using a Secondary Set—*continued*

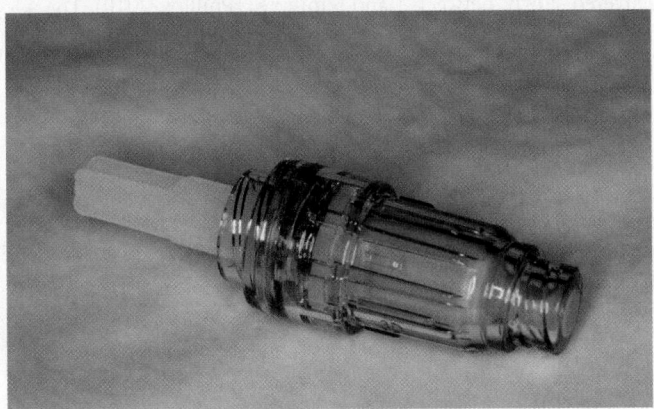

⑤ Intermittent infusion device with an injection port.

R.A. Penne-Casanova/Science Source.

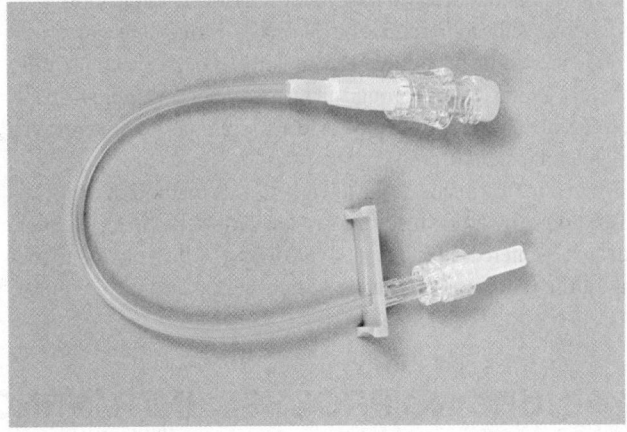

⑥ Intermittent infusion device with an injection port and extension tubing.

12. Document relevant data.
- Record the date, time, medication, dose, route, and solution; assessment of the IV site, if appropriate; and the client's response.
- Record the volume of fluid of the medication infusion bag on the client's intake and output record.

Variation: Using a Saline Lock
Intermittent infusion devices ⑤ may be attached to an intravenous catheter to allow medications to be administered intravenously without requiring a continuous IV infusion. The device may also have a port at one end of the lock and a needleless injection cap at the other end with the extension tubing between the two ends. ⑥

- Prepare two normal saline prefilled syringes (1 mL each).
- Spike the medication bag with minidrip (60 gtt/mL) IV tubing.
- Attach the needleless adapter to the tubing, prime the tubing, and close the clamp.
- Clean the needleless injection port of the saline lock with an antiseptic swab. Open the saline lock clamp, if appropriate.
- Insert the first saline syringe into the port and gently aspirate to check for patency. Flush slowly noting any resistance, swelling, pain, or burning. **Rationale:** *This ensures placement of the IV in the vein.*
- After connecting the IV tubing to the injection port of the lock, administer the medication, regulating the drip rate to allow medication to infuse for the appropriate time period. Macrodrip (10 to 20 gtt/mL) tubing may also be used if using an IV pump to regulate the flow.

- When the medication has been infused, disconnect the IV tubing, maintaining sterility of the end of the IV tubing.
- Insert the second saline syringe into the port and gently flush the saline lock. **Rationale:** *This clears the tubing and maintains patency.* Clamp the saline lock after flushing, if appropriate.
- Dispose of syringes in the appropriate container.

Variation: Adding a Medication to a Volume-Control Infusion
- Withdraw the required dose of the medication into a syringe.
- Ensure that there is sufficient fluid in the volume-control fluid chamber to dilute the medication. Generally, at least 50 mL of fluid is used. Check the directions from the drug manufacturer or consult the pharmacist.
- Close the inflow to the fluid chamber by adjusting the upper roller or slide clamp above the fluid chamber; also ensure that the clamp on the air vent of the chamber is open.
- Clean the medication port on the volume-control fluid chamber with an antiseptic swab.
- Inject the medication into the port of the appropriately filled volume-control set (i.e., the ordered amount of solution).
- Gently rotate the fluid chamber until the fluid is well mixed.
- Regulate the flow by adjusting the lower roller clamp below the fluid chamber.
- Attach a medication label to the volume-control fluid chamber.
- Document relevant data and monitor the client and the infusion.

EVALUATION
- Conduct appropriate follow-up such as desired effect of medication, any adverse reactions or side effects, or change in vital signs.

- Reassess status of the IV lock site and patency of the IV infusion.
- Relate to previous findings, if available.
- Report significant deviations from normal to the primary care provider.

Intravenous Push

Intravenous push (IVP), or IV push, is the intravenous administration of an undiluted drug directly into the systemic circulation. It is used when a medication cannot be diluted or in an emergency situation. An IVP can be introduced directly into a vein by venipuncture or into an existing IV line through an injection port or through an IV lock (see Skill 17–9). The purpose is to achieve rapid serum concentrations (Phillips, 2010, p. 641).

There are two major disadvantages to this method of drug administration: Any error in administration cannot be corrected after the drug has entered the client, and the drug may be irritating to the lining of the blood vessels. Before administering an IVP, the nurse should look up the maximum concentration recommended for the particular drug and the rate of administration. Most medications are delivered slowly, between 1 and 5 minutes (Phillips, 2010). The administered medication takes effect immediately.

CLINICAL ALERT!

Never administer a medication IVP into an IV line that is infusing blood, blood products, or parenteral nutrition. Check the compatibility of the IV solution and what to do if it is incompatible with the IVP medication. Check if the IVP medication needs to be diluted before administration.

●○● NURSING PROCESS: INTRAVENOUS PUSH

Administering Intravenous Medications Using IV Push

ASSESSMENT

- Inspect and palpate the IV insertion site for signs of infection, infiltration, or a dislocated catheter.
- Inspect the surrounding skin for redness, pallor, or swelling.
- Palpate the surrounding tissues for tenderness, coldness, and the presence of edema, which could indicate leakage of the IV fluid into the tissues.
- Take vital signs for baseline data if the medication being administered is particularly potent.

- Determine if the client has allergies to the medication(s).
- Check the compatibility of the medication(s) and IV fluid.
- Determine specific drug action, side effects, normal dosage, recommended administration time, and peak action time.
- Check patency of the IV.

PLANNING
DELEGATION

The administration of intravenous medication via IV push involves the application of nursing knowledge and critical thinking. Therefore, this procedure is not delegated to UAP. The nurse, however, can inform the UAP of the intended therapeutic effects and/or specific side effects of the medication and direct the UAP to report specific client observations to the nurse for follow-up. **Note:** *Administration of IV push medications varies by state nurse practice acts. For example, some states may allow the RN to delegate certain medications to be given by an LPN/LVN, whereas other states may allow only the RN to administer IV push medications. Nurses need to know their scope of practice according to their state's nurse practice act and agency policies.*

Equipment
IV Push for an Existing Line
- Client's MAR
- Medication in a prefilled syringe, vial, or ampule
- Sterile syringe (3 to 5 mL) (to prepare the medication)

- Sterile needles #21 to #25 gauge, 2.5 cm (1 in.) (needle is not needed if using a needleless system)
- Antiseptic swabs
- Watch with a digital readout or second hand
- Clean gloves

IV Push for an IV Lock
- Client's MAR
- Medication in a prefilled syringe, vial, or ampule
- Sterile syringe (3 to 5 mL) (to prepare the medication)
- Sterile syringe (3 mL) (for the saline or heparin flush)
- Vial of preservative-free normal saline to flush the IV catheter or vial of heparin flush solution or both depending on agency practice **Rationale:** *These maintain the patency of the IV lock. Saline is frequently used for peripheral locks.*
- Sterile needles (#21 gauge) (needle is not needed if using a needleless system)
- Antiseptic swabs
- Watch with a digital readout or second hand
- Clean gloves

IMPLEMENTATION
Preparation
- Check the MAR.
  - Check the label on the medication carefully against the MAR to make sure that the correct medication is being prepared.
  - Follow the three checks for correct medication and dose. Read the label on the medication (1) when it is taken from the medication cart, (2) before withdrawing the medication, and (3) after withdrawing the medication.
  - Calculate medication dosage accurately and the recommended delivery rate (e.g., 20 mg over 1 minute).
  - Confirm that the route is correct.
- Organize the equipment.

Performance
1. Perform hand hygiene and observe other appropriate infection prevention procedures.
2. Prepare the medication.

Existing Line
- Prepare the medication according to the manufacturer's directions. **Rationale:** *It is important to have the correct dose and the correct dilution.*

IV Lock
- Flushing with saline:
  a. Prepare two syringes, each with 1 mL of sterile normal saline.

SKILL 17-9

Administering Intravenous Medications Using IV Push—*continued*

- Flushing with heparin (if indicated by agency policy) and saline:
    a. Prepare one syringe with 1 mL of heparin flush solution (if indicated by agency policy).
    b. Prepare two syringes with 1 mL each of sterile normal saline.
    c. Draw up the medication into a syringe.
3. Put a small-gauge needle on the syringe if using a needle system.
4. Perform hand hygiene and apply clean gloves. **Rationale:** *This reduces the transmission of microorganisms and reduces the likelihood of the nurse's hands contacting the client's blood.*
5. Provide for client privacy.
6. Prepare the client.
    - Prior to performing the procedure, introduce self and verify the client's identity using agency protocol. **Rationale:** *This ensures that the right client receives the right medication.*
    - If not previously assessed, take the appropriate assessment measures necessary for the medication. If any of the findings are above or below the predetermined parameters, consult the primary care provider before administering the medication.
7. Explain the purpose of the medication and how it will help, using language that the client can understand. Include relevant information about the effects of the medication. **Rationale:** *Information can facilitate acceptance of and compliance with the therapy.*
8. Administer the medication by IV push.

IV Lock with Needle
- Clean the injection port with the antiseptic swab. **Rationale:** *This prevents microorganisms from entering the circulatory system during the needle insertion.*
- Insert the needle of the syringe containing normal saline through the center of the injection port and aspirate for blood. ❶ **Rationale:** *The presence of blood confirms that the catheter or needle is in the vein. In some situations, blood will not return even though the lock is patent.*
- Flush the lock by injecting 1 mL of saline slowly. **Rationale:** This removes blood and heparin (if present) from the needle and the lock.
- Observe the area above the IV catheter for puffiness or swelling, which indicates infiltration into tissue, which would require removal of the IV catheter.
- Remove the needle and syringe. Activate the needle safety device.
- Clean the lock's injection port with an antiseptic swab. **Rationale:** *This prevents the transfer of microorganisms.*
- Insert the needle of the syringe containing the prepared medication through the center of the injection port.
- Inject the medication slowly at the recommended rate of infusion. Use a watch or digital readout to time the injection. ❷. **Rationale:** *Injecting the drug too rapidly can have a serious untoward reaction.*
- Observe the client closely for adverse reactions. Remove the needle and syringe when all medication has been administered
- Activate the needle safety device.
- Clean the injection port of the lock.
- Attach the second saline syringe, and inject 1 mL of saline. **Rationale:** *The saline injection flushes the medication through the catheter and prepares the lock for heparin if this medication is used. Heparin is incompatible with many medications.*
- If heparin is to be used, insert the heparin syringe and inject the heparin slowly into the lock.

IV Lock with Needleless System
- Clean the injection port of the lock.
- Insert the syringe containing normal saline into the injection port.

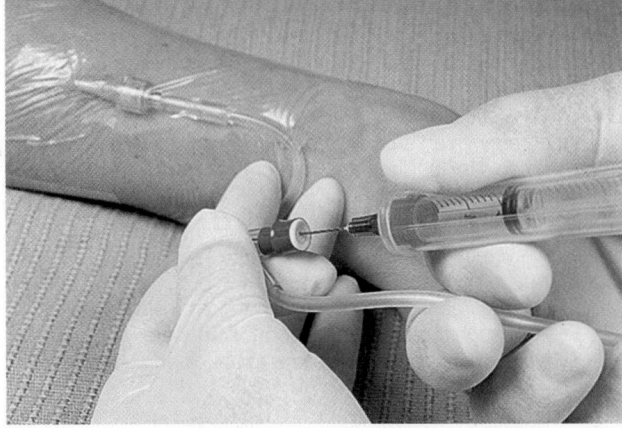

❶ Inserting a needle through the injection port of an IV lock.

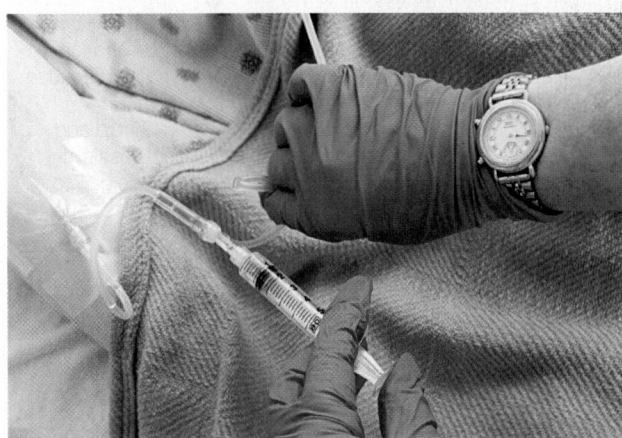

❷ Using a watch to time the rate of a medication injection.

- Flush the lock with 1 mL of sterile saline. **Rationale:** *This clears the lock of blood.*
- Remove the syringe.
- Insert the syringe containing the medication into the port. ❸
- Inject the medication following the precautions described previously.
- Withdraw the syringe.
- Repeat injection of 1 mL of saline.

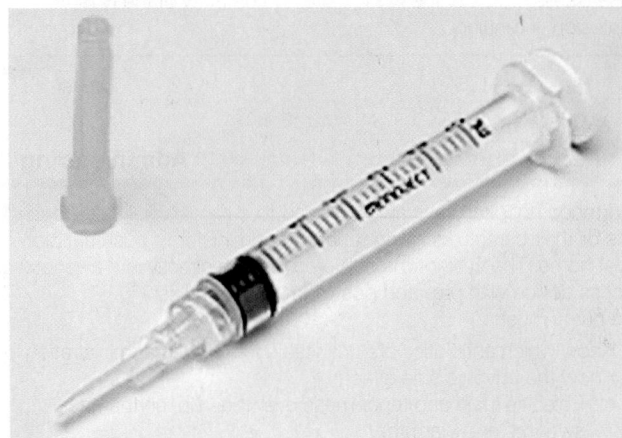

❸ A blunt plastic cannula replaces the sharp steel needle.
Courtesy Covidien.

Continued on page 440

SKILL 17-9

Administering Intravenous Medications Using IV Push—*continued*

Existing Line
- Identify the injection port closest to the client. Some ports have a circle indicating the site for the needle insertion. **Rationale:** *An injection port must be used because it is self-sealing. Any puncture to the plastic tubing will leak.*
- Clean the port with an antiseptic swab.
- Stop the IV flow by closing the clamp or pinching the tubing above the injection port. ❹
- Connect the syringe to the IV system.
  a. Needle system:
     - Hold the port steady.
     - Insert the needle of the syringe that contains the medication through the center of the port. **Rationale:** *This prevents damage to the IV line and to the diaphragm of the port.*
  b. Needleless system:
     - Remove the cap from the needleless syringe. Connect the tip of the syringe directly to the port. ❺
     - Inject the medication at the ordered rate. Use the watch or digital readout to time the medication administration. **Rationale:** *This ensures safe drug administration because a too rapid injection could be dangerous.*
     - After injecting the medication, withdraw the needle and activate the needle safety device. For a needleless system, detach the syringe and attach a new sterile cap to the port.
     - Release the clamp or tubing. Resume IV flow as ordered.
9. Dispose of equipment according to agency practice. **Rationale:** *This reduces needlestick injuries and the spread of microorganisms.*
10. Remove and dispose of gloves.
    - Perform hand hygiene.
11. Observe the client closely for adverse reactions.
12. Determine agency policy about recommended times for changing the IV lock. Some agencies advocate a change every 48 to 72 hours for peripheral IV devices.
13. Document all relevant information.
    - Record the date, time, drug, dose, and route; client response; and assessments of the infusion or heparin lock site if appropriate.

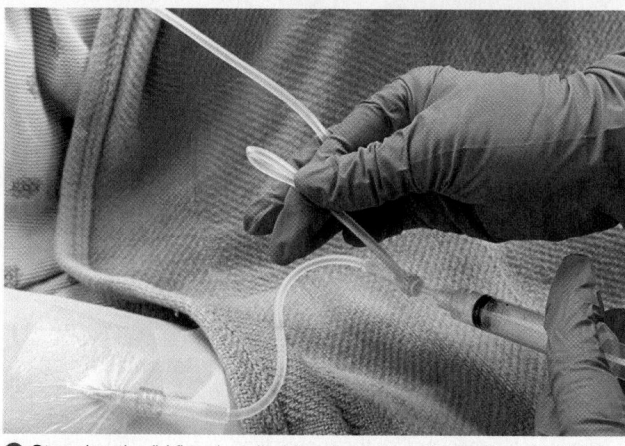

❹ Stopping the IV flow by pinching the tubing above the injection port.

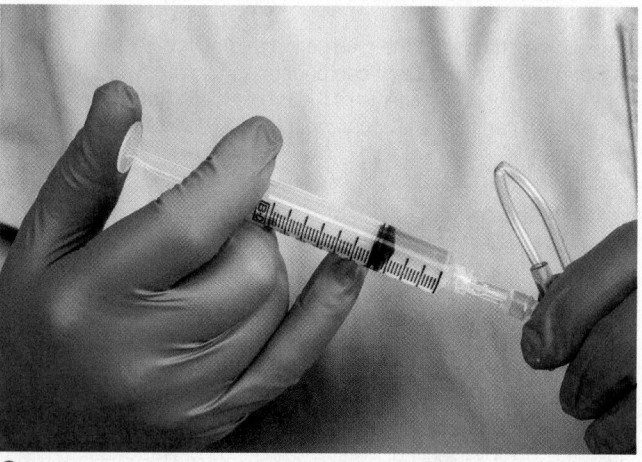

❺ Injecting a medication by IV push to an existing IV using a needleless system.

EVALUATION
- Conduct appropriate follow-up such as desired effect of medication, any adverse reactions or side effects, or change in vital signs.
- Reassess status of the IV lock site and patency of the IV infusion, if running.
- Relate to previous findings, if available.
- Report significant deviations from normal to the primary care provider.
- Inspect appearance of the medication and check the expiration date.

Ambulatory and Community Settings   **Administering IV Push Antibiotics** | PATIENT-CENTERED CARE |

Shortened hospital stays and the need to cut costs have led to clients or their caregivers being taught to administer IV push antibiotics at home. The antibiotic is delivered IV push directly into a venous access device with pre- and post-administration flushing. The nurse must:
- Know which antibiotics are unsuitable for IV push administration.
- Know the adverse side effects:
  - Phlebitis (pain and tenderness over the vein, erythema, swelling, and warmth)
  - Speed shock (systemic reaction when a drug is given too rapidly)
  - Venous spasm (cramping and pain above the infusion site)
  - Infiltration

- Assess the caregiver or client's eyesight and manual dexterity. Both are needed for safe administration of the antibiotic.
- Provide thorough teaching about:
  - Venous access device.
  - Administration rate (minutes/dose).
  - Schedule for medication administration.
  - Flushing technique.
  - Adverse reactions.
  - Signs that indicate an emergency and the need to call 911.
  - Proper storage of medication.
- Inspect the appearance of the medication and check the expiration date.

Chapter 17 Review

FOCUSING ON CLINICAL THINKING

Consider This

1. What size syringe, needle gauge, and needle length would you consider for the following situations?
   a. Administer a tuberculin test to a 22-year-old male who is 6 feet tall and weighs 180 pounds.
   b. The order is for 5 mL of a medication to be given deep IM. The client is a 40-year-old female who weighs 135 pounds and is 5 feet 7 inches tall.
   c. Administer 0.75 mL subcutaneously in the upper arm to a 50-year-old, 300-pound client. The nurse can grasp approximately 2 inches of the client's tissue at the upper arm.
   d. Administer 0.5 mL of a medication by IM injection to an older adult client who is emaciated.

2. The nurse needs to draw up two compatible medications into one syringe. In the following situations, describe the process for drawing up the medication and indicate which medication you would draw up first and why.
   a. One medication is a single-dose prefilled sterile cartridge that uses a Tubex syringe, and the other is in a multiple-dose vial.
   b. One medication is in a multiple-dose vial, and the other is in an ampule.
   c. Each medication is in an ampule.

3. The nurse needs to mix two insulins to equal a total of 24 units. The nurse checks the amount with another nurse, who states that the total indicates 25 units. What would you do if you were the nurse who needed to administer the insulin?

4. No bleb forms when you administer a tuberculin test. What would you do?

5. The primary care provider has ordered a medication to be added to an existing IV solution. You look up the medication in a drug handbook and read that a minimum of 500 mL is required. There is 475 mL remaining in the current IV that is infusing at 100 mL/h. What do you do?

6. You administered an intermittent IV medication via a saline lock approximately 10 minutes ago. The UAP reports to you that the client is complaining of a burning sensation at the site of the peripheral IV lock. What do you do?

7. The nurse calculates the amount of medication needed for the prescribed order to be 2 mL. The medication is to be given subcutaneously. The nurse checks with the drug handbook and the pharmacist, and the amount is within normal parameters. What would you do?

See Focusing on Clinical Thinking answers on student resource website.

TEST YOUR KNOWLEDGE

1. The nurse is preparing medication from an ampule. To prevent client injury, which item would the nurse use?
   1. Filter needle
   2. Alcohol swab
   3. Large-gauge needle
   4. Insulin syringe

2. The nurse is preparing to administer a thick and viscous medication via the intramuscular route. The nurse decides to use which needle?
   1. #18 gauge
   2. #20 gauge
   3. #22 gauge
   4. #24 gauge

3. The nurse is preparing a medication that is supplied in a vial. Place the following steps in the correct order for the nurse to prepare the medication.
   1. Inject air into the vial.
   2. Withdraw the medication.
   3. Clean the top with alcohol.
   4. Remove the plastic cap.
   5. Perform hand hygiene.

4. The nurse is preparing to administer a subcutaneous injection of heparin to a client who has had bilateral mastectomies. What site would the nurse use?
   1. The upper arm
   2. The area of the vastus lateralis
   3. The deltoid area
   4. The abdomen

5. The nurse is assisting with the resuscitation of a client and is preparing to administer a drug that needs to take effect quickly. Which administrative method is the best?
   1. Intramuscular
   2. Subcutaneous
   3. Intravenous push
   4. Volume-controlled intravenous infusion

6. The nurse is preparing to administer an intradermal injection. Which is the best angle for the nurse to hold the needle when inserting it into the client's skin?
   1. 90°
   2. 45°
   3. 30°
   4. 15°

7. The nurse is preparing to administer an intramuscular injection to a 10-month-old client. Which is the best site for the nurse to choose?
   1. The deltoid muscle
   2. The vastus lateralis muscle
   3. The ventrogluteal muscle
   4. The dorsogluteal site

8. The nurse is preparing to administer IV phenytoin (Dilantin) into an IV site that has a continuous dextrose and water infusion. Which action is the nurse's priority before administering the medication?
   1. Flush the line with normal saline.
   2. Clamp the running solution and crimp the tubing.
   3. Start a new IV site.
   4. Administer the medication through the closest port.

9. The nurse is preparing a medication to be administered subcutaneously. Which needle will the nurse choose for an average-sized young adult?
    1. #20 to #22 gauge
    2. #22 to #24 gauge
    3. #24 to #26 gauge
    4. #21 to #23 gauge

10. A nursing student is preparing to administer insulin to a client with diabetes. Indicate the correct order of the following steps for the administration of this medication:
    1. Cleanse the site with alcohol.
    2. Insert the needle quickly into the subcutaneous tissue.

3. Mix the insulins.
4. Assess the skin for the injection.
5. Pinch the skin lightly.
6. Inject the medication.
7. Count to five.
8. Remove the syringe.
Correct sequence: _____

See Answers to Test Your Knowledge in Appendix A.

READINGS AND REFERENCES

References

Adams, M. P., & Urban, C. (2013). *Pharmacology: Connections to nursing practice* (2nd ed.). Upper Saddle River, NJ: Pearson.

American Diabetes Association. (2004). Insulin administration. *Diabetes Care, 27*(1), S106–S109. doi:10.2337/diacare.27.2007.S106

American Diabetes Association. (2013). *Insulin storage and syringe safety.* Retrieved from http://www.diabetes.org/living-with-diabetes/treatment-and-care/medication/insulin/insulin-storage-and-syringe.html

Ball, J. W., Bindler, R. C., & Cowen, K. J. (2012). *Principles of pediatric nursing, caring for children* (5th ed.). Upper Saddle River, NJ: Pearson.

Barron, C., & Cocoman, A. (2008). Administering intramuscular injections to children: What does the evidence say? *Journal of Children's and Young People's Nursing, 2*, 138–143.

Carter-Templeton, H., & McCoy, T. (2008). Are we on the same page? A comparison of intramuscular injection explanations in nursing fundamental texts. *MEDSURG Nursing, 17*, 237–240.

Centers for Disease Control and Prevention. (2012a). *CDC clinical reminder: Insulin pens should never be used for more than one person.* Retrieved from http://www.cdc.gov/injectionsafety/clinical-reminders/insulin-pens.html

Centers for Disease Control and Prevention. (2012b). *Injection safety: Information for providers.* Retrieved from http://www.cdc.gov/injectionsafety/providers.html

Cocoman, A., & Murray, J. (2008). Intramuscular injections: A review of best practice for mental health nurses. *Journal of Psychiatric and Mental Health Nursing, 15*, 424–434. doi:10.1111/j.1365-2850.2007.01236.x

Cocoman, A., & Murray, J. (2010). Recognizing the evidence and changing practice on injection sites. *British Journal of Nursing,19*, 1170–1174.

Crawford, C. L., & Johnson, J. A. (2012). To aspirate or not: An integrative review of the evidence. *Nursing, 42*(3), 20–25. doi:10.1097/01.NURSE.0000411417.91161.87

Edgeworth, N. (2011). *Hospitals moving toward greater use of insulin pens.* Retrieved from http://diabeteshealth.com/read/2011/11/10/7342/hospitals-moving-toward-greater-use-of-insulin-pens

Gebel, E. (2012). Insulin pens. *Diabetes Forecast, 65*(1), 56–57.

Gebel, E. (2013). Insulin pens. *Diabetes Forecast, 66*(1), 60–61.

Grissinger, M. (2011). Avoiding problems with insulin pens in the hospital. *Pharmacy and Therapeutics (P&T), 36*, 615–616.

Hensel, D., & Springmyer, J. (2011). Do perinatal nurses still check for blood return when administering the Hepatitis B vaccine? *Journal of Obstetric, Gynecologic, and Neonatal Nursing, 40*, 589–594. doi:10.1111/j.1552-6909.2011.01277.x

Hunter, J. (2008). Intramuscular injection techniques. *Nursing Standard, 22*(24), 35–40. doi.org/10.7748/ns2008.02.22.24.35.c6413

Institute for Safe Medication Practices. (2010). *Principles of designing a medication label for intravenous piggyback medication for patient specific, inpatient use.* Retrieved from http://www.ismp.org/tools/guidelines/labelFormats/Piggyback.asp

Institute for Safe Medication Practices. (2013). Ongoing concern about insulin pen reuse shows hospitals need to consider transitioning away from them. *Nurse Advise-ERR, 11*(2), 1–2.

The Joint Commission. (2013). *National Patient Safety Goals effective January 1, 2014. Hospital accreditation program.* Retrieved from http://www.jointcommission.org/assets/1/6/HAP_NPSG_Chapter_2014.pdf

Malkin, B. (2008). Are techniques used for intramuscular injection based on research evidence? *Nursing Times, 104*(50/51), 48–51.

Nicoll, L. H., & Hesby, A. (2002). Intramuscular injection: An integrative research review and guideline for evidence-based practice. *Applied Nursing Research, 15*, 149–162. doi:10.1053/apnr.2002.34142

Phillips, L. D. (2010). *Manual of I.V. therapeutics: Evidence-based practice for infusion therapy* (5th ed.). Philadelphia, PA: F.A. Davis.

Potera, C. (2011). Most nurses don't follow guidelines on IM injections. *American Journal of Nursing, 111*(8), 16. doi:10.1097/01.NAJ.0000403344.05116.1c

Sanofi-Aventis. (2012). *How to self-inject LOVENOX®.* Retrieved from http://www.lovenox.com/consumer/prescribed-lovenox/self-inject/inject-lovenox.aspx

U.S. Environmental Protection Agency. (2012). *Disposal of medical sharps.* Retrieved from http://www.epa.gov/wastes/nonhaz/industrial/medical/disposal.htm

Zimmerman, P. G. (2010). Revisiting IM injections. *American Journal of Nursing, 110*(2), 60–61. doi:10.1097/01.NAJ.0000368058.72729.c6

Selected Bibliography

Berman, A., Snyder, S., & Frandsen, G. (2016). *Kozier & Erb's fundamentals of nursing: Concepts, process, and practice* (10th ed.). Upper Saddle River, NJ: Pearson.

Centers for Disease Control and Prevention. (2011). *The top sticks campaign: Safety culture.* Retrieved from http://www.cdc.gov/niosh/stopsticks/safetyculture.html

Centers for Disease Control and Prevention. (2012). *Injection safety: Information for providers.* Retrieved from http://www.cdc.gov/injectionsafety/providers.html

Lavery, I. (2011). Intravenous therapy: Preparation and administration of IV medicines. *British Journal of Nursing, 20*, S28–S34.

Pugliese, G., Gosnell, C., Bartley, J. M., & Robinson, S. (2010). Injection practices among clinicians in United States health care settings. *American Journal of Infection Control, 38*, 789–798. doi:10.1016/j.ajic.2010.09.003

Walsh, L., & Brophy, K. (2010). Staff nurses' sites of choice for administering intramuscular injections to adult patients in the acute care setting. *Journal of Advanced Nursing, 67*, 1034–1040. doi:10.1111/j.1365-2648.2010.05527.x

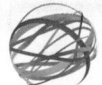

18 Administering Intravenous Therapy

LEARNING OUTCOMES

At the completion of this chapter, the student will be able to:

1. Define the key terms used in the skills of intravenous therapy.
2. Identify common types of intravenous infusion equipment.
3. Identify potential venipuncture sites.
4. Identify indications and contraindications for intravenous therapy and central venous lines.
5. Recognize when it is appropriate to delegate aspects of intravenous therapy to unlicensed assistive personnel.
6. Verbalize the steps used in:
   a. Performing venipuncture.
   b. Starting an intravenous infusion.
   c. Using an electronic infusion device.
   d. Maintaining infusions.
   e. Maintaining intermittent infusion devices.
   f. Discontinuing infusion devices.
   g. Administering blood transfusions.
   h. Managing central venous access devices.
   i. Performing central venous access device dressing changes.
   j. Working with implanted vascular access devices.
7. Calculate and regulate intravenous flow rates.
8. Identify interventions that prevent complications associated with intravenous therapy and central venous access devices.
9. Demonstrate appropriate documentation and reporting of intravenous therapy.

SKILLS

KEY TERMS

Many clients require administration of fluids or medications directly into the vascular system through **intravenous (IV)** (within or into the vein) devices. Nurses provide a significant amount of this type of therapy in the hospital and in ambulatory settings and must have substantial knowledge and skill to practice according to safety standards. Changes in principles and practice of intravenous therapy are always occurring and, therefore, continuing education regarding IV therapy is an ongoing nursing responsibility.

INTRAVENOUS INFUSIONS

An IV **infusion** is the instillation of fluid, electrolytes, medications, blood, or nutrient substances into a vein by means of venipuncture. A physician or other primary care provider is responsible for ordering the type of solution to be administered, the amount to be given, and the rate at which it is to be infused.

IV therapy can be prescribed for these reasons:

- To supply supplemental or complete fluid, electrolytes, or nutrition.
- To provide vitamins and medications.
- To establish a lifeline for rapidly needed medications.

Common Types of Solutions

IV solutions can be classified as isotonic, hypotonic, or hypertonic. Most IV solutions are *isotonic*, having the same concentration of solutes as blood plasma. Isotonic solutions are often used to restore vascular volume. *Hypertonic solutions* have a greater concentration of solutes than plasma; *hypotonic solutions* have a lesser concentration of solutes. Table 18–1 provides examples of IV solutions and nursing implications.

TABLE 18–1	Selected Intravenous Solutions
Type/Examples	**Comments/Nursing Implications**
ISOTONIC SOLUTIONS 0.9% NaCl (normal saline) Lactated Ringer's (a balanced electrolyte solution) 5% dextrose in water (D₅W)	Isotonic solutions such as normal saline and lactated Ringer's initially remain in the vascular compartment, expanding vascular volume. Assess clients carefully for signs of hypervolemia such as bounding pulse and shortness of breath. D₅W is isotonic on initial administration but provides free water when dextrose is metabolized, expanding intracellular and extracellular fluid volumes. D₅W is avoided in clients at risk for increased intracranial pressure (IICP) because it can increase cerebral edema.
HYPERTONIC SOLUTIONS 5% dextrose in normal saline (D₅NS) 5% dextrose in 0.45% NaCl (D₅ ½NS) 5% dextrose in lactated Ringer's (D₅LR)	Hypertonic solutions draw fluid out of the intracellular and interstitial compartments into the vascular compartment, expanding vascular volume. Do not administer to clients with kidney or heart disease or clients who are dehydrated. Watch for signs of hypervolemia.
HYPOTONIC SOLUTIONS 0.45% NaCl (half normal saline) 0.33% NaCl (one-third normal saline)	Hypotonic solutions are used to provide free water and treat cellular dehydration. These solutions promote waste elimination by the kidneys. Do not administer to clients at risk for IICP or third-space fluid shift.

IV solutions can also be categorized according to their purpose. *Nutrient solutions* contain some form of carbohydrate (e.g., dextrose, glucose, or levulose) and water. Water is supplied for fluid requirements, and carbohydrate is supplied for calories and energy. For example, 1 L of 5% dextrose provides 170 calories. Nutrient solutions are useful in preventing dehydration and ketosis but do not provide sufficient calories to promote wound healing, weight gain, or normal growth in children. Common nutrient solutions are 5% dextrose in water (D₅W) and 5% dextrose in 0.45% sodium chloride (dextrose in half normal saline).

Electrolyte solutions contain varying amounts of cations and anions. Commonly used solutions are normal saline (0.9% sodium chloride solution) and lactated Ringer's solution (which contains sodium, chloride, potassium, calcium, and lactate). Lactate is metabolized in the liver to form bicarbonate. Saline and electrolyte solutions are commonly used to restore vascular volume, particularly after trauma or surgery. They also may be used to replace fluid and electrolytes for clients with continuing losses, for example, those experiencing gastric suction or wound drainage. Lactated Ringer's solution is an alkalizing solution that may be given to treat metabolic acidosis. Acidifying solutions, in contrast, are administered to counteract metabolic alkalosis. Examples of acidifying solutions are 5% dextrose in 0.45% sodium chloride and 0.9% sodium chloride solution.

Volume expanders are used to increase the blood volume following severe loss of blood (e.g., from hemorrhage) or loss of plasma (e.g., from severe burns, which draw large amounts of plasma from the bloodstream to the burn site). Examples of expanders are dextran, plasma, albumin, and Hespan (a synthetic plasma expander).

Peripheral Venipuncture Sites

The site chosen for venipuncture varies with the client's age, length of time an infusion is to run, the type of solution used, and the condition of veins. For adults, veins in the arm are commonly used; for infants, veins in the scalp and dorsal foot veins are often used. The larger veins of the adult's forearm are preferred over the metacarpal veins of the hand for infusions that need to be given rapidly and for solutions that are hypertonic, are highly acidic or alkaline, or contain irritating medications. The loss of subcutaneous tissue, thinning of the skin, and fragile veins in the older adult can be a challenge for the nurse when performing a venipuncture. It is common practice for the initial venipuncture to be in the most distal portion of the arm because this allows for subsequent venipunctures to move upward. The veins of the hands of the older adult, however, are not the best initial sites for venipuncture because of the loss of subcutaneous tissue and thinning of the skin (Phillips & Gorski, 2014).

The metacarpal, basilic, and cephalic veins are common venipuncture sites (Figure 18–1 ■). The ulna and radius act as natural splints at these sites, and the client has greater freedom of arm movements for activities such as eating. Although the antecubital basilic and median cubital veins are convenient, they are usually kept for blood draws, bolus injections of medication, and insertion sites for a peripherally inserted central catheter (PICC) line (see Figure 18–1A).

Historically, nurses used their eyes and hands to locate a suitable vein for a venipuncture. This could be especially challenging in some clients such as older adults, dark-skinned clients whose veins may not be visible, or clients who are obese, because their veins may not be visible or palpable. The *Infusion Nursing Standards of Practice* (Infusion Nurses Society [INS], 2011a) state that nurses should "consider using visualization technologies to aid in vein identification and selection" (p. S41). Currently transillumination devices are available that use light to allow for the location and identification of blood vessels. The client's skin color does not affect the ability to highlight veins. One type of device is applied to the client's skin. Focusing bright visible light onto and under the skin helps the nurse locate superficial veins. Another device is used by holding it about 18 cm (7 in.) above the skin. The veins are displayed on the surface of the skin.

Intravenous Infusion Equipment

Because equipment varies according to the manufacturer, the nurse must become familiar with the equipment used in each particular agency. IV equipment consists of IV catheters, catheter stabilization devices, solution containers, infusion administration sets, IV filters, and IV poles.

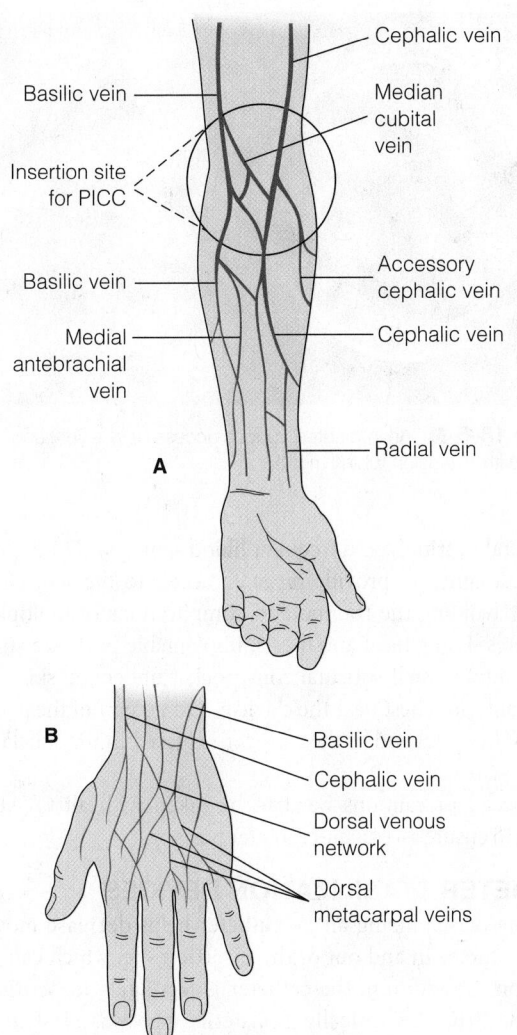

A

B

Figure 18–1 ■ Commonly used venipuncture sites of the *A,* arm, and *B,* hand. *A* also shows the site used for a peripherally inserted central catheter (PICC).

INTRAVENOUS CATHETERS

The *Infusion NursingStandards of Practice* (INS, 2011a) state that the type of IV catheter to be used depends on the client's vascular access needs, which are based on the prescribed therapy, length of treatment, vascular integrity, client preference, and ability and resources available to care for the device (p. S37). All catheters must be radiopaque.

A *peripheral-short catheter* is used for usually less than 1 week. It comes in a variety of gauge sizes (i.e., #14 to #27) and types (e.g., winged or nonwinged, and over-the-needle), and the tip ends in a peripheral vein (INS, 2011a). Over-the-needle catheters (ONCs), also known as **angiocatheters**, are commonly used for adult clients. The plastic catheter fits over a needle (stylet) used to pierce the skin and vein wall (Figure 18–2 ■). Once inserted into the vein, the needle (stylet) is withdrawn and discarded, leaving the catheter in place. The nurse should use peripheral-short catheters equipped with a passive or active safety mechanism to prevent sharps injury. The active safety device requires activation by the nurse, and the passive safety device automatically activates after the stylet is removed from the catheter.

CLINICAL ALERT!

A peripheral-short catheter placed in an emergency situation where aseptic technique has been compromised must be replaced as soon as possible and no longer than 48 hours later (INS, 2011b).

A **butterfly** or **wing-tipped needle** with plastic flaps attached to the shaft is sometimes used (Figure 18–3 ■). The flaps are held tightly together to hold the needle securely during insertion; after insertion, they are flattened against the skin and secured with tape. The butterfly needle is most frequently used for short-term therapy (e.g., less than 24 hours) such as with single-dose therapy, IV push medications, or blood sample retrieval (Phillips & Gorski, 2014).

A *peripheral-midline catheter* is 7.6 to 20.3 cm (3 to 8 in.) in length and inserted near the antecubital area into the basilic, cephalic, or brachial veins, with the preference being the basilica vein because of its larger diameter. The tip is advanced no farther than the distal axillary vein in the upper arm. Although the INS classifies the midline catheter as a peripheral catheter, the midline catheter is managed differently than the peripheral-short catheter. For example, an angiocatheter may stay in a vein for up to 72 hours maximum; a midline catheter can last from 1 to 4 weeks.

A **peripherally inserted central catheter (PICC)** is inserted in the basilic or cephalic vein just above or below the antecubital space of the right arm. The tip of the catheter rests in the superior vena cava. These catheters frequently are used for long-term IV access when the client will be managing IV therapy at home.

When long-term IV therapy or parenteral nutrition is anticipated, or a client is receiving IV medications that are damaging to vessels (e.g., chemotherapy), a **central venous access device (CVAD)** may be inserted. A CVAD is defined by the location of the

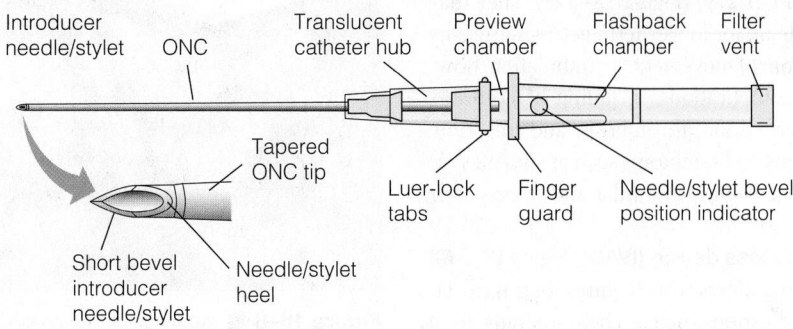

Figure 18–2 ■ Schematic of an over-the-needle angiocatheter.

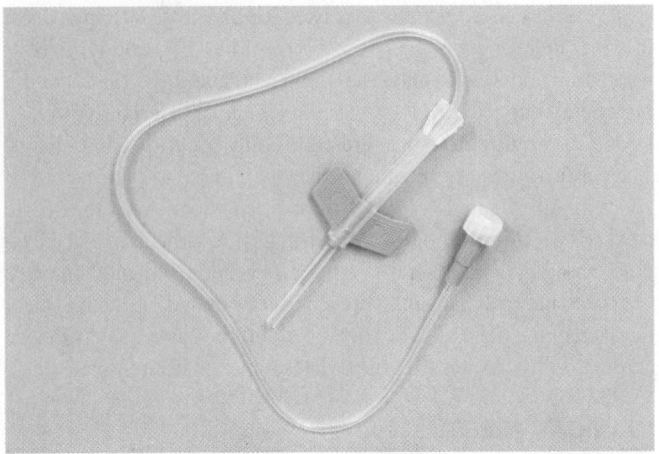

Figure 18–3 ■ A butterfly IV needle.

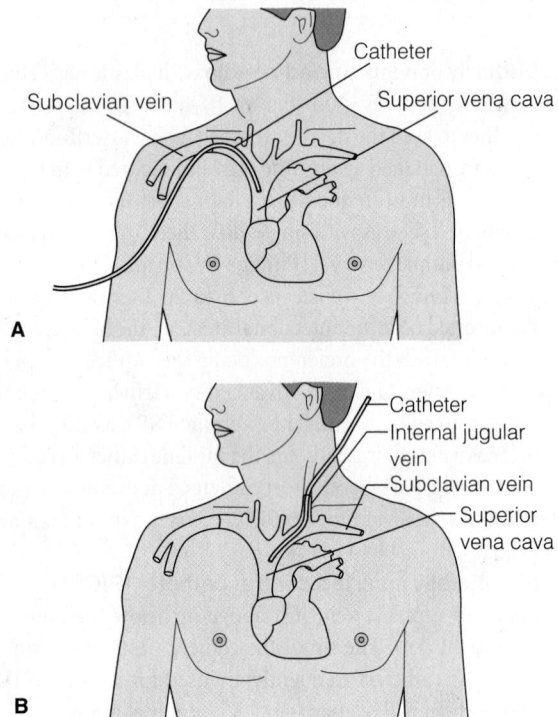

Figure 18–4 ■ Central venous access devices with *A*, subclavian insertion, and *B*, left jugular vein insertion.

catheter tip in a central vein. The CVAD catheter tip should reside in the lower one third of the superior vena cava, above the right atrium (Phillips & Gorski, 2014, p. 279) (Figure 18–4 ■). They may be inserted at a client's bedside or, for longer term access, surgically inserted. CVADs permit freedom of movement for ambulation; however, there is greater risk of complications, including hemothorax or pneumothorax, cardiac perforation, thrombosis, and infection. Assess the client closely for signs and symptoms such as shortness of breath, chest pain, cough, hypotension, tachycardia, and anxiety after the insertion procedure.

An **implanted venous access device (IVAD)** (Figure 18–5 ■) is used for a client with chronic illness who requires long-term IV therapy (e.g., intermittent medications such as chemotherapy, total

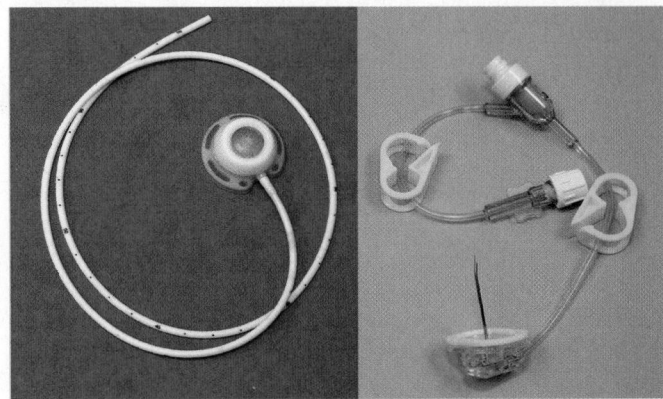

Figure 18–5 ■ An implanted venous access device (left) and a Huber needle with extension tubing (right).

parenteral nutrition, and frequent blood samples). This type of device is designed to provide repeated access to the central venous system, avoiding the trauma and complications of multiple venipunctures. Using local anesthesia, implantable ports are surgically placed into a small subcutaneous pocket under the skin, usually on the anterior chest near the clavicle, and no part of the port is exposed. The distal end of the catheter is placed in the subclavian or jugular vein.

Special precautions need to be taken with all CVADs and IVADs to ensure asepsis and catheter patency.

CATHETER STABILIZATION DEVICES

Securing or stabilizing an IV catheter helps decrease movement of the catheter in and out of the insertion site, which can lead to infection. In addition, the catheter is less likely to be dislodged (Gorski, 2010). Historically, nonsterile tape was used to secure peripheral IV catheters. The INS standards now recommend the use of manufactured catheter stabilization devices (Figure 18–6 ■) as preferred over other methods such as sterile tapes and surgical strips (INS, 2011a).

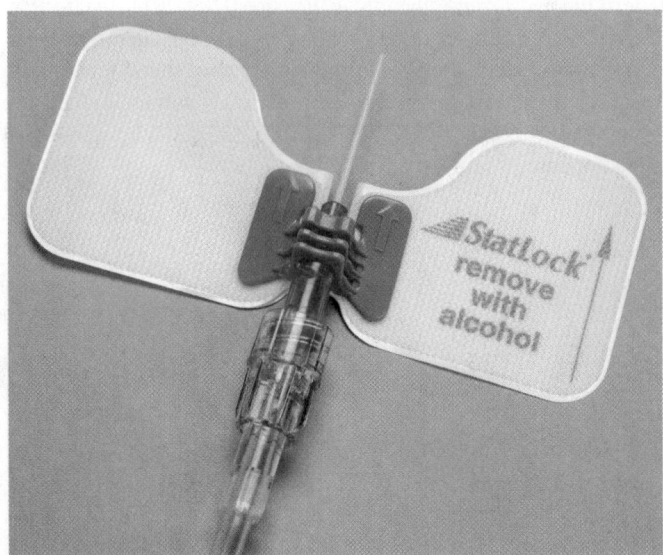

Figure 18–6 ■ Manufactured catheter stabilization device.

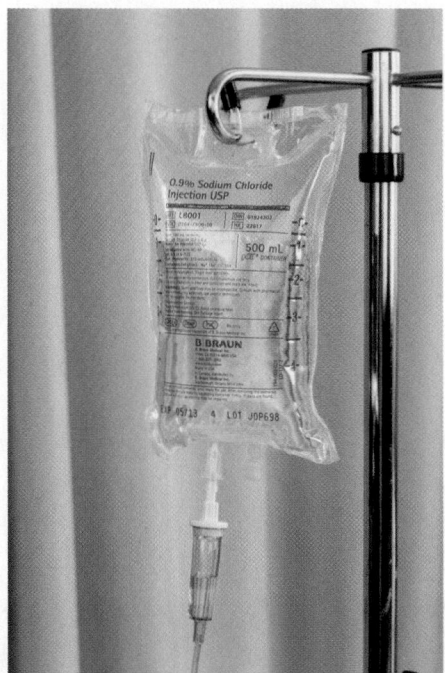

Figure 18–7 ■ A plastic intravenous fluid container.

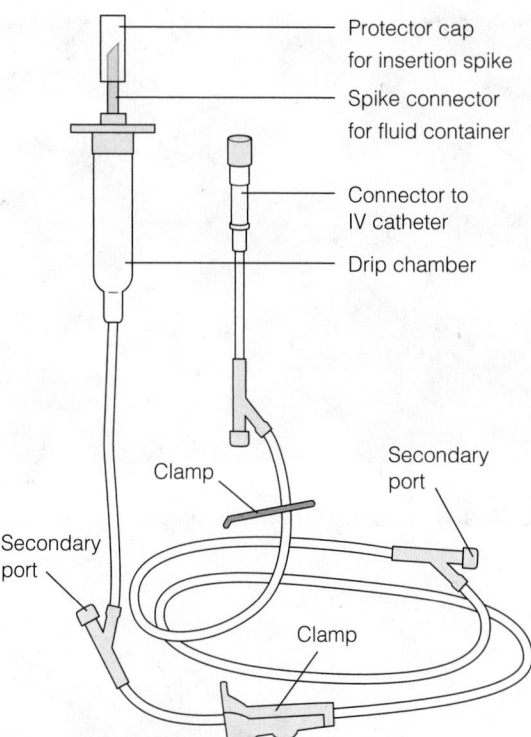

Protector cap
for insertion spike

Spike connector
for fluid container

Connector to
IV catheter

Drip chamber

Secondary
port

Clamp

Secondary
port

Clamp

Figure 18–8 ■ A standard IV administration set.

SOLUTION CONTAINERS

Solution containers are available in various sizes (50, 100, 250, 500, or 1,000 mL); the smaller containers are often used to administer medications. Most solutions are currently dispensed in plastic bags (Figure 18–7 ■). However, glass bottles may need to be used if the administered medications are incompatible with plastic. Glass bottles require an air vent so that air can enter the bottle and replace the fluid that enters the client's vein. Some bottles contain a tube that serves as a vent; other containers require a vent on the administration set. Air vents usually have filters to prevent contamination from the air that enters the container. Air vents are not required for plastic solution bags, because the bags collapse under atmospheric pressure when the solution enters the vein.

It is essential for the solution to be sterile and in good condition, that is, clear. Cloudiness, evidence that the container has been opened previously, or leaks indicate possible contamination. Always check the expiration date on the label. Return any questionable or contaminated solutions to the pharmacy or IV therapy department.

CLINICAL ALERT!

Do not write directly on a plastic IV bag with a ballpoint pen (may puncture the bag) or indelible marker (may absorb through the bag into the solution).

INFUSION ADMINISTRATION SETS

Infusion administration sets (also called administration infusion sets) consist of an insertion spike, a drip chamber, a roller valve or screw clamp, tubing with secondary ports, and a protective cap over the connecter to the IV catheter (Figure 18–8 ■). The insertion spike is kept sterile and inserted into the solution container when the equipment is set up and ready to start. The drip chamber permits a predictable amount of fluid to be delivered. A **macrodrip** drip chamber delivers between 10 and 20 drops (abbreviated **gtts**) per milliliter of solution. The specific amount is written on the package. **Microdrip** sets deliver 60 drops per milliliter of solution (Figure 18–9 ■). A special infusion set is required if the IV flow rate will be regulated by an infusion pump.

Most infusion sets include one or more injection ports for administering IV medications or secondary infusions. Needleless systems are used because they reduce the risk of needlestick injury and contamination of the IV line. The needleless ports can be accessed with either a syringe that has a blunt cannula or a Luer-Lok to administer medications, or an adapter can be added to the IV tubing for administration of secondary infusions (Figure 18–10 ■). When more than one solution needs to be infused at the same time, *secondary sets* such as the tandem and the piggyback IV setups are used. Another variation is a *volume-control set*, which is used if the volume of fluid or medication administered is to be carefully controlled (see Skill 17–8 in Chapter 17 ∞).

Rather than using a continuous infusion, an intermittent infusion lock may be created by attaching a sterile injection cap or device to an existing IV catheter. This keeps the venous access available for the administration of intermittent or emergency medications. The device is commonly referred to as a **saline lock** because periodic injection with saline is used to keep blood from coagulating within the tubing.

INTRAVENOUS FILTERS IV filters are used to remove air and particulate matter from IV infusions and to reduce the risk of complications (e.g., infusion-related phlebitis) associated with

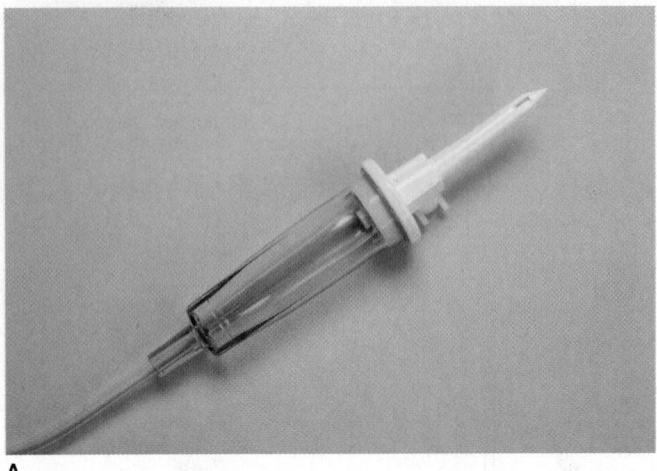

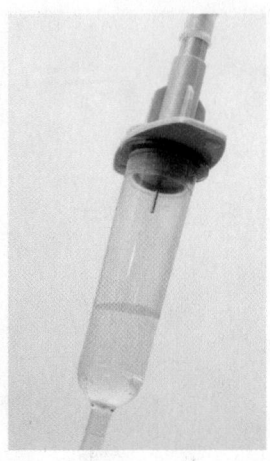

A

B

Figure 18–9 ■ Infusion set spikes and drip chambers: *A*, nonvented macrodrip; *B*, nonvented microdrip.

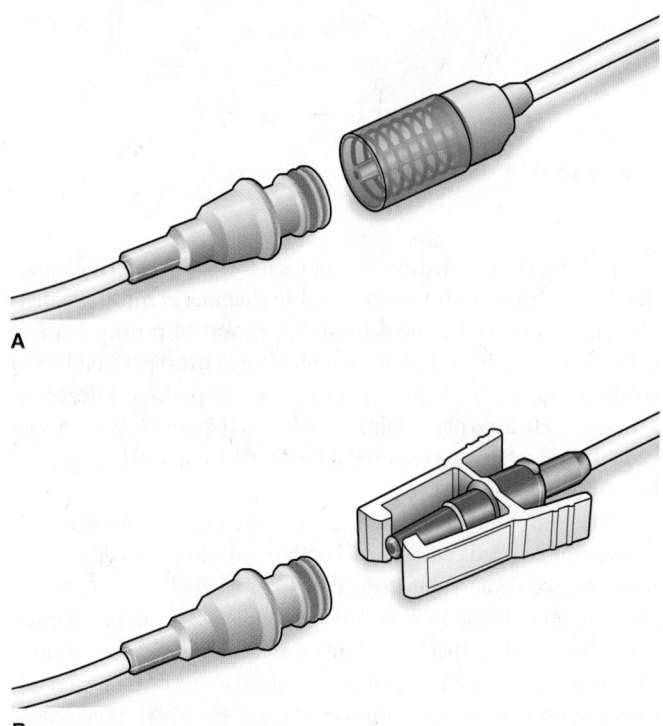

A

B

Figure 18–10 ■ Cannulae used to connect the tubing of secondary sets to primary tubing: *A*, threaded cannula; *B,* lever-lock cannula.

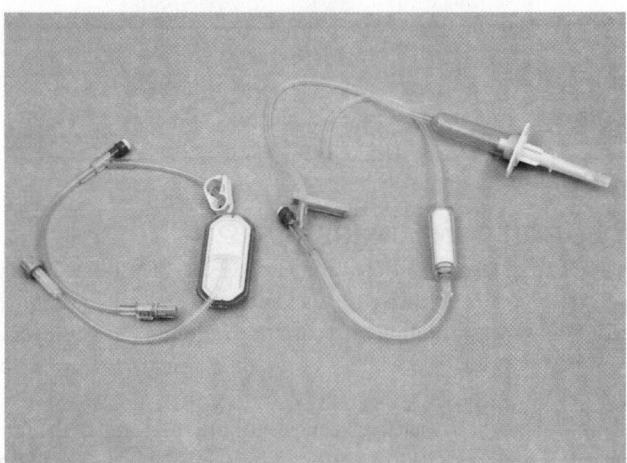

Figure 18–11 ■ Two types of IV filters.

routine IV therapies (Figure 18–11 ■). Most IV filters in current use consist of a membrane (pore size of 0.22 micron, although sizes vary). Some problems associated with filters include (a) clogging of the filter surface, which may stop or slow the flow rate when debris accumulates; and (b) binding of some drugs (e.g., insulin and amphotericin B) to the surface of the filter. When using filters, the nurse must remember that the filter should never be considered a substitute for quality care and meticulous technique.

INTRAVENOUS POLES   IV poles (rods) are used to hang the solution container. Some poles are attached to hospital beds; others are floor models with casters that can be pushed along when a client is up and walking. In the home, plant hangers or robe hooks (even kitchen cabinet knobs or an S-hook over the top of a door) may be used to hang solution containers. The height of most poles is adjustable. The higher the solution container, the greater the force of the solution as it enters the client and the faster the rate of flow.

PERFORMING VENIPUNCTURE

Although the primary care provider is responsible for ordering IV therapy for clients, nurses initiate, monitor, and maintain the prescribed IV infusion. This is true not only in hospitals and long-term care facilities but increasingly in community-based settings such as clinics and clients' homes.

●○● NURSING PROCESS: PERFORMING VENIPUNCTURE

Performing Venipuncture

ASSESSMENT

Before performing venipuncture, the nurse must determine:

- The exact order requiring venipuncture. Generally, the primary care provider will order the fluids, medications, diagnostic study, or transfusion that requires an IV rather than the venipuncture itself. The order to perform the venipuncture is implied. **Rationale:** *The specific aspects of the order assist the nurse with selection of appropriate IV catheter size, type, and placement.*
- Whether the client has any allergies, especially to tape, povidone-iodine, and latex.
- The agency policy about clipping hair in the area before a venipuncture. Shaving is not recommended because of the possibility of nicking the skin and subsequent infection.

- Available arms and hands for a possible insertion site (see Practice Guidelines on page 453). Avoid diseased or injured extremities. Avoid sites that have been used recently. **Rationale:** *Recently used sites will be more prone to complications and discomfort.* Determine if the client is right- or left-handed. **Rationale:** *Leave the dominant hand free if possible.*
- Vital signs for baseline data (pulse, respiratory rate, and blood pressure).
- Bleeding tendencies.

PLANNING

Prior to venipuncture, consider how long the client is likely to have the IV, what kind of fluids will be infused, and what medications the client will be receiving or is likely to receive. These factors may affect choice of vein and catheter size. Review the client record regarding previous venipuncture. Note any difficulties encountered and how they were managed.

DELEGATION

Due to the need for knowledge of anatomy and use of sterile technique, IV infusion therapy is not delegated to unlicensed assistive personnel (UAP). UAP may care for clients receiving IV therapy, and the nurse must ensure that the UAP knows how to perform routine tasks such as bathing and positioning without disturbing the IV. The UAP should also know what complications or adverse signs, such as leakage, should be reported to the nurse.

In many states, a licensed practical nurse or licensed vocational nurse (LPN/LVN) with special IV therapy training may start IV infusions. Check the applicable state's nurse practice act.

Equipment

Substitute appropriate supplies if the client has tape, antiseptic, or latex allergies.

- Nonallergenic tape
- Clean gloves
- Tourniquet
- Antiseptic swabs such as 10% povidone-iodine or 2% chlorhexidine gluconate (CHG) with alcohol or 70% isopropyl alcohol. Chlorhexidine is becoming the standard of practice and is the antiseptic preferred by the INS (Phillips & Gorski, 2014, p. 338).
- IV catheter (Choose an IV catheter of the appropriate type and size based on the size of the vein and the purpose of the IV. A #20- to #22-gauge catheter is indicated for most adults. Always have an extra catheter and ones of different sizes available.)
- Sterile gauze dressing or transparent semipermeable membrane (TSM) dressing (preferred)
- Stabilization device
- Splint, if required
- Towel or bed protector
- Local anesthetic (optional and per agency policy)

IMPLEMENTATION

Preparation

- If possible, select a time to perform the venipuncture that is convenient for the client. Unless initiating IV therapy is urgent, provide any scheduled care before insertion to minimize excessive movement of the affected limb. **Rationale:** *Moving the limb after insertion could dislodge the catheter.*
- Make sure the client's clothing or gown can be removed over the IV apparatus if necessary. Some agencies provide special gowns that open over the shoulder and down the sleeve for easy removal.
- Visitors or family members may be asked to leave the room if desired by the nurse or the client.

Performance

1. Prior to performing the procedure, introduce self and verify the client's identity using agency protocol. Explain to the client what you are going to do, why it is necessary, and how he or she can participate. Venipuncture can cause discomfort for a few seconds, but there should be no ongoing pain after insertion. If possible, explain how long the IV will need to remain in place and how it will be used.
2. Perform hand hygiene and observe other appropriate infection prevention procedures.

3. Prepare the client.
   - Assist the client to a comfortable position, either sitting or lying. Expose the limb to be used but provide for client privacy.
4. Select the venipuncture site.
   - Use the client's nondominant arm, unless contraindicated (e.g., mastectomy, fistula for dialysis). Identify possible venipuncture sites by looking for veins that are relatively straight, not sclerotic or tortuous, and avoid venous valves. The vein should be palpable, but may not be visible, especially in clients with dark skin. Consider the catheter length; look for a site sufficiently distal to the wrist or elbow where the tip of the catheter will not be at a point of flexion. **Rationale:** *Sclerotic veins may make initiating and maintaining the IV difficult. Joint flexion increases the risk of irritation of vein walls by the catheter.*
   - Check agency protocol about shaving if the site is very hairy. Shaving is not recommended. **Rationale:** *Shaving can cause microabrasions, which can increase the risk of infection.*
   - Place a towel or bed protector under the extremity to protect linens (or furniture if in the home).

Continued on page 450

Performing Venipuncture—*continued*

5. Dilate the vein.
- Place the extremity in a dependent position (lower than the client's heart). **Rationale:** *Gravity slows venous return and distends the veins. Distending the veins makes it easier to insert the IV catheter properly.*
- Apply a tourniquet firmly 15 to 20 cm (6 to 8 in.) above the venipuncture site. ❶ Explain that the tourniquet will feel tight. **Rationale:** *The tourniquet must be tight enough to obstruct venous flow but not so tight that it occludes arterial flow. Obstructing arterial flow inhibits venous filling.* If a radial pulse can be palpated, the arterial flow is not obstructed.
- Use the tourniquet on only one client. This avoids cross contamination to other clients. Be sure to ask if the client has a latex allergy.
- For older adults with fragile skin, instead of applying a tourniquet, place the arm in a dependent position to allow the veins to engorge. **Rationale:** *The tourniquet can cause tissue damage and may not be needed to allow the vein to dilate.*
- If the vein is not sufficiently dilated:
  a. Massage or stroke the vein distal to the site and in the direction of venous flow toward the heart. **Rationale:** *This action helps fill the vein.*
  b. Encourage the client to clench and unclench the fist. **Rationale:** *Contracting the muscles compresses the distal veins, forcing blood along the veins and distending them.*
  c. Lightly tap the vein with your fingertips. **Rationale:** *Tapping may distend the vein.*
- If the preceding steps fail to distend the vein so that it is palpable, remove the tourniquet and wrap the extremity in a warm towel for 10 to 15 minutes. **Rationale:** *Heat dilates*

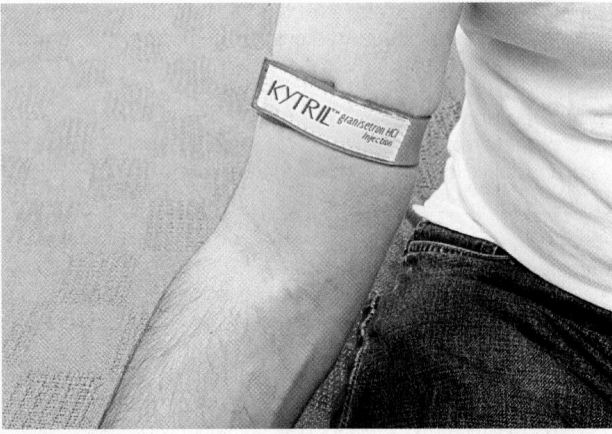

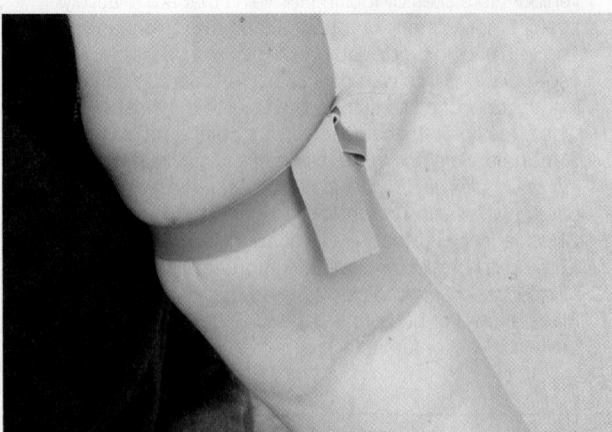

❶ Two types of tourniquets.

superficial blood vessels, causing them to fill. Then repeat the steps to dilate the vein.

6. Minimize insertion pain as much as possible.
- Although the pain of insertion should be brief, prevention can and should be offered. Transdermal analgesic creams (e.g., EMLA, Synera) may also be used, depending on policy. Allow at least 30 to 60 minutes for the topical analgesic to take effect (Phillips & Gorski, 2014).
- If desired and permitted by policy, inject 0.3 mL of 1% lidocaine (without epinephrine) intradermally over the site where you plan to insert the IV catheter. (Be sure to first apply gloves and clean the skin site as described in step 7 below.) Allow 5 to 10 seconds for the anesthetic to take effect (Phillips & Gorski, 2014).

7. Apply clean gloves and clean the venipuncture site. **Rationale:** *Gloves protect the nurse from contamination by the client's blood.*
- Clean the skin at the site of entry with a topical antiseptic swab (e.g., 2% CHG, or alcohol). Some institutions may use an anti-infective solution such as povidone-iodine (check agency protocol). Check for allergies to iodine or shellfish before cleansing skin with Betadine or iodine products.
- When using chlorhexidine solution (preferred), use a back-and-forth motion for a minimum of 30 seconds to scrub the insertion site and surrounding area (Phillips & Gorski, 2014). Allow the site to completely air dry before inserting the catheter. Do *not* fan, blow on, or wipe the skin.
- When using povidone-iodine, apply using swabsticks in a concentric circle beginning at the catheter insertion site and moving outward. The iodine should be in contact with the skin for 2 minutes or longer to completely dry for adequate antisepsis (INS, 2011b, p. 66).

8. Insert the catheter and initiate the infusion.
- Remove the catheter assembly from its sterile packaging. Review instructions for using the catheter because a variety of needle-safety devices are manufactured. Remove the cover of the needle (stylet).
- Use the nondominant hand to pull the skin taut below the entry site. **Rationale:** *This stabilizes the vein and makes the skin taut for needle (stylet) entry. It can also make initial tissue penetration less painful.*
- Holding the ONC at a 15° to 30° angle with needle (stylet) bevel up, insert the catheter through the skin and into the vein. A sudden lack of resistance is felt as the needle (stylet) enters the vein. Use a slow steady insertion technique and avoid jabbing or stabbing motions.
- Once blood appears in the lumen or clear "flashback" chamber of the needle, lower the angle of the catheter until it is almost parallel with the skin, and advance the needle (stylet) and catheter approximately 0.5 to 1 cm (about ¼ in.) farther. ❷ Holding the assembly steady, advance the catheter until the hub is at the venipuncture site. The exact technique depends on the type of device used. **Rationale:** *The catheter is advanced to ensure that it, and not just the stylet, is in the vein.*
- If there is no blood return, try redirecting the catheter assembly again toward the vein. If the stylet has been withdrawn from the catheter even a small distance, or the catheter tip has been pulled out of the skin, the catheter must be discarded and a new one used. **Rationale:** *Reinserting the stylet into the catheter can result in damage or slicing of the catheter. A catheter that has been removed from the skin is considered contaminated and cannot be reused.*
- If blood begins to flow out of the vein into the tissues as the catheter is inserted, creating a hematoma, the insertion has not been successful. This is sometimes referred to as a blown vein. Immediately release the tourniquet and remove

Performing Venipuncture—*continued*

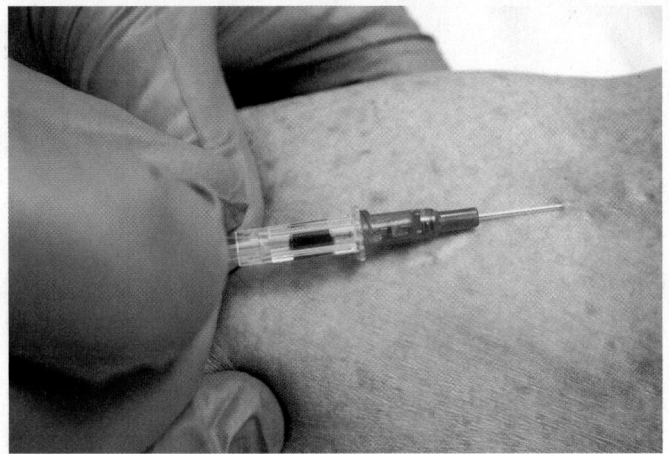

❷ Blood is noted in the flashback chamber once the stylet has entered the vein.

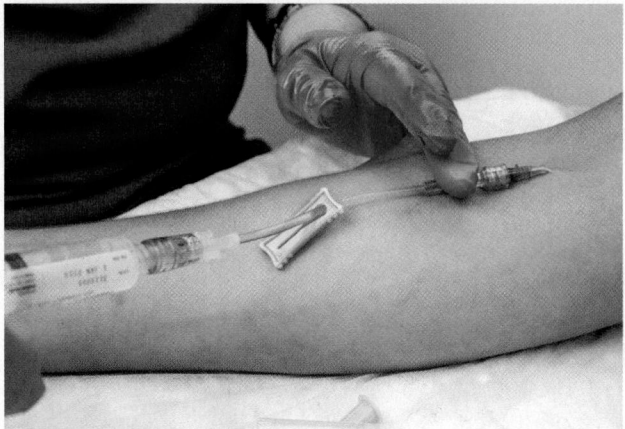

❹ The catheter is stabilized while gently flushing it to determine patency.

the catheter, applying pressure over the insertion site with dry gauze. Attempt the venipuncture in another site, in the opposite arm if possible. **Rationale:** *Placing the tourniquet back on the same arm above the unsuccessful site may cause it to bleed. Placing the IV below the unsuccessful site could result in infusing fluid into the already punctured vein, causing it to leak.*

- Release the tourniquet.
- Put pressure on the vein proximal to the catheter to eliminate or reduce blood oozing out of the catheter. Stabilize the hub with thumb and index finger of the nondominant hand.
- Remove the protective cap from the distal end of the tubing and hold it ready to attach to the catheter, maintaining the sterility of the end.
- Stabilize the catheter hub and apply pressure distal to the catheter with your finger(s). ❸ **Rationale:** *This prevents excessive blood flow through the catheter.*
- Carefully remove the stylet, engage the needle safety device (if it does not engage automatically), and attach the end of the infusion tubing to the catheter hub. Place the stylet directly into a sharps container. If this is not within reach, place the stylet into its original package and dispose in a sharps container as soon as possible.
- Initiate the infusion or flush the catheter with sterile normal saline. ❹ **Rationale:** *Blood must be removed from*

the catheter lumen and tubing immediately. Otherwise, the blood will clot inside the lumen. Watch closely for any signs that the catheter is infiltrated. Infiltration occurs when the tip of the IV is outside the vein and the fluid is entering the tissues instead. It is manifested by localized swelling, coolness, pallor, and discomfort at the IV site. **Rationale:** *Inflammation or infiltration necessitates removal of the IV catheter to avoid further trauma to the tissue.*

9. Stabilize the catheter and apply a dressing.
- Secure the catheter according to the manufacturer's instructions and agency policy. Several methods are used to stabilize the catheter, including the use of a dressing and securement device. If tape is used, it must be sterile tape or surgical strips and they should be applied only to the catheter adapter and not placed directly on the catheter–skin junction site. Using a manufactured stabilization device is preferred (INS, 2011a).
- Apply a dressing. Two methods are used for applying a dressing: a sterile gauze dressing secured with tape and a TSM dressing. ❺ Most common is the TSM because it allows for continuous assessment of the site and it is more comfortable than gauze and tape (Phillips & Gorski, 2014, p. 345). Do not use ointment of any kind under a TSM dressing. Additional tape may be used to secure the IV catheter below the TSM, if necessary. Do not place tape on the TSM dressing.
- Label the dressing with the date and time of insertion, type, gauge and length of catheter used, and your initials. ❻

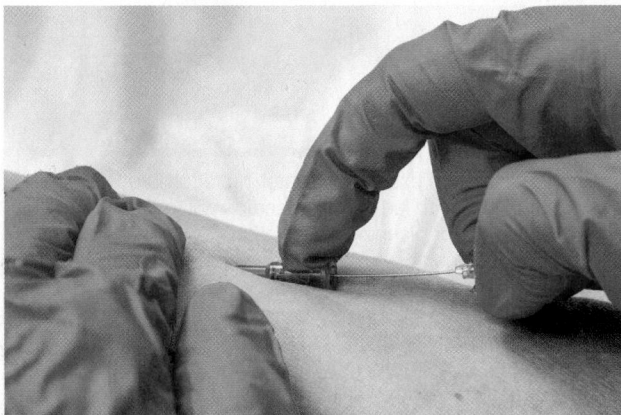

❸ Stabilize the catheter hub and occlude the vein with finger(s) while removing the stylet.

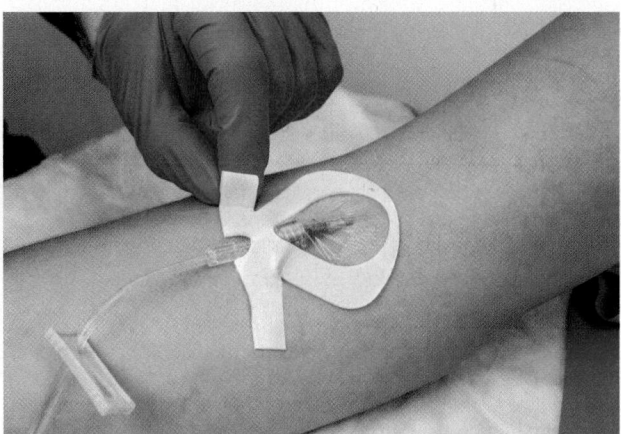

❺ Applying a sterile one-piece IV stabilization and TSM dressing device.

Continued on page 452

Performing Venipuncture—*continued*

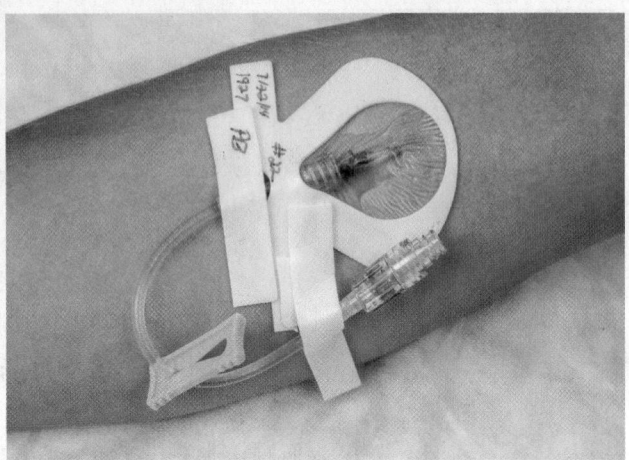

6 IV site labeled with date, time, size of catheter, and initials.

- Apply an IV site protector, if available. Protective devices are available that help prevent dislodgment of the IV catheter and still provide easy assessment of the IV site. **7**
- Loop the tubing and secure it with tape. **Rationale:** *Looping and securing the tubing prevent the weight of the tubing or any movement from pulling on the IV catheter.*

10. Discard the tourniquet.
    - Remove and discard gloves.
    - Perform hand hygiene.
11. Discard all used disposable supplies in appropriate receptacles. Cleanse any blood spills according to agency policy. Clean any reusable supplies.
12. Document relevant data, including assessments.
    - Record the venipuncture on the client's chart. Some agencies provide a special form for this purpose. Include the date and time of the venipuncture; type, length, and gauge of the IV catheter; venipuncture site; how many attempts were made and the location of each attempt; the type of dressing applied; if IV therapy was initiated, also include amount and

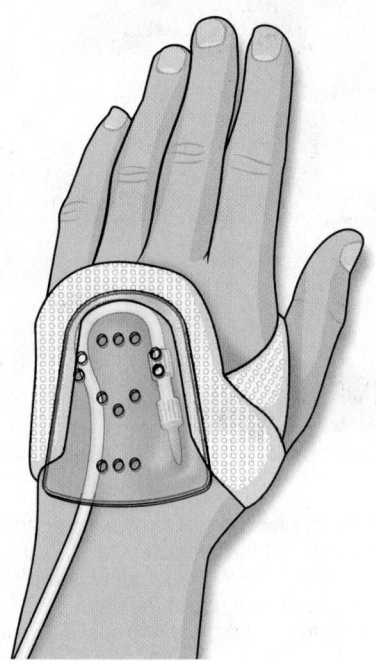

7 IV site protective device.

type of solution used, including any additives, and the flow rate; and the client's general response.

SAMPLE DOCUMENTATION

1/15/2015 0600 Inserted 20-gauge, 1-inch angiocath in the right cephalic vein 4 inches above the (L) wrist on first attempt. StatLock used to stabilize catheter and Tegaderm dressing applied. IV infusing at 125 mL/h. Explained reason for IV. Verbalized understanding. ————————————————— A. Luis, RN

EVALUATION
- Perform follow-up based on findings or outcomes that deviated from expected or normal for the client. Relate findings to previous data if available.
- At least every 4 hours, check the skin status at the IV site (warm temperature and absence of pain, redness, or swelling); status

of the dressing; the client's ability to perform self-care activities; and the client's understanding of any mobility limitations.
- Report significant deviations from normal to the primary care provider.

LIFESPAN CONSIDERATIONS   Venipuncture

INFANTS/CHILDREN
- For infants, veins in the scalp are used for venipuncture.
- Because infants do not have large veins in the antecubital fossa, blood specimens for examination are usually taken from the external jugular and femoral veins.
- Use a doll to demonstrate venipuncture for children and explain the procedure to the parents.
- Explain the procedure to the young client, encourage questions, and be alert for nonverbal cues. Children may not understand things that seem obvious to adults. For example, a child may think the IV therapy is a punishment.

- Venipuncture can be extremely frightening for children. Simply numbing the skin with ice prior to insertion will reduce the discomfort. When prior planning is an option, EMLA cream (lidocaine and prilocaine) topical anesthetic can be applied ahead of time with an occlusive dressing to cover. Remove all of the cream and clean the site prior to insertion.
- Even with analgesia, many children will resist, cry, or become combative. Parents, in turn, may become upset. Offering distractions and rewards may help. Helping the child to take deep, slow breaths can also trigger some degree of relaxation. Sometimes it is necessary to restrain the child

LIFESPAN CONSIDERATIONS   Venipuncture (*continued*)

(see Chapter 12 ∞). Most pediatric professionals believe that it is best if a person other than the child's parent holds the child, so the child doesn't associate the parent with the fear and pain. It is important for the parent to remain with the child, soothing the child with voice, closeness, and touch. Some parents are not able to do this, and they need support and understanding from nursing staff. A calm demeanor on the nurse's part (and relaxation breathing) will help ease this potentially upsetting situation for all concerned.

- A #24-gauge catheter or needle is commonly indicated for use with children.
- Apply age-appropriate restraints, arm boards, or other devices to protect the IV site.

OLDER ADULTS

- The skin of older adults is often fragile and bruises easily. Select an IV site with adequate healthy tissue to support the IV catheter.
- To distend the vein, tap only lightly to prevent trauma.
- Consider not using a tourniquet. The older adult's superficial veins are often large enough to insert the stylet without further distention. Using a tourniquet can cause the vein to burst when the stylet enters.
- Minimize the use of tape to avoid irritating sensitive skin.

PRACTICE GUIDELINES

Vein Selection

- Use distal veins of the arm first; subsequent IV starts should be proximal to the previous site.
- Use the client's nondominant arm whenever possible. **Rationale:** *This minimizes the client's restricted mobility and function.*
- Select a vein that is:
  a. Easily palpated and feels soft and full.
  b. Naturally splinted by bone.
  c. Large enough to allow adequate circulation around the catheter.
- Avoid using veins that are:
  a. In areas of flexion (e.g., the antecubital fossa).
  b. Highly visible. **Rationale:** *These veins tend to roll away from the needle/stylet.*

  c. Damaged by previous use, phlebitis, infiltration, or sclerosis.
  d. Continually distended with blood, knotted, or tortuous.
  e. In a surgically compromised or injured extremity (e.g., following a mastectomy). **Rationale:** *These sites may have impaired circulation and cause discomfort for the client.*
  f. In the foot or legs unless arm veins are inaccessible, and with a primary care provider's order. **Rationale:** *Lower extremity sites are more prone to thrombus formation and subsequent emboli.*

PRACTICE GUIDELINES

General Tips for Easier IV Starts

- Review the client's medical history. Avoid using an arm affected by hemiplegia or with a dialysis access, or on the same side as a mastectomy. Also avoid sites near infections, sites below previous infiltrations or extravasations, and veins affected by phlebitis.
- Dilate the vein. Ways to do this include dangling the client's arm over the side of the bed to encourage dependent vein filling, asking the client to open and close his or her fist, stroking the vein downward or lightly tapping the vein, and applying warm compresses to the site for 10 minutes.
- Make sure the client is positioned comfortably and has been medicated for pain if appropriate. Pain and anxiety stimulate the sympathetic nervous system and trigger vasoconstriction.
- Because of the risk of nerve injuries, as well as discomfort and restriction of movement, hand veins should be a last choice.
- If the ordered IV medication is irritating to veins and therapy is expected to last more than a few days, consult with the IV

nurse or medical team to determine whether the client is a candidate for a midline catheter, a peripherally inserted central catheter, or another type of central venous access device.
- Use the smallest gauge catheter that will accommodate the therapy and allow good venous flow around the catheter tip. For routine hydration or intermittent therapy, use #22- to #27-gauge catheters; for transfusion therapy, use #20- to #24-gauge catheters; and for therapy for neonates or clients with very small, fragile veins, use #24- to #27-gauge catheters.
- Raise the bed or stretcher to a comfortable working height, and keep all equipment within reach. Stabilize the client's hand or arm with your nondominant arm, tucking it under your forearm if necessary to prevent movement.
- Limit your attempts to two. If you are not successful after two tries, ask another nurse to try.

ESTABLISHING INTRAVENOUS INFUSIONS

An IV infusion may be set up before venipuncture so that the infusion can be attached to the IV catheter immediately after it is inserted.

●○○● NURSING PROCESS: ESTABLISHING INTRAVENOUS INFUSIONS

Starting an Intravenous Infusion

SKILL 18–2

ASSESSMENT

- Before preparing the infusion, verify the IV order indicating the type of solution, the amount to be administered, the rate of flow or time over which the infusion is to be completed, and any client allergies (e.g., tape, iodine).
- Assess the IV site:
  - If the IV catheter has already been inserted and is not currently attached to an infusion, ensure that it is patent by aspirating for blood or irrigating with normal saline.

- Inspect the IV site for the presence of infiltration or inflammation. **Rationale:** *Inflammation or infiltration necessitates removal of the IV catheter to avoid further trauma to the tissues.* Discontinue and relocate the IV site if indicated (see Skills 18–1, 18–5, and 18–6).

PLANNING

Prior to initiating the IV infusion, consider how long the client is likely to have the IV, what kinds of fluids will be infused, and what medications the client will be receiving or is likely to receive. These factors may affect the choice of vein and catheter size. Review the client record regarding previous infusions. Note any complications and how they were managed.

Equipment

- Infusion set
- Sterile parenteral solution
- Labels for IV tubing and container
- IV pole
- Nonallergenic tape
- Electronic infusion device or pump, as determined by the nurse
- Clean gloves

DELEGATION

Due to the use of sterile technique, IV infusion therapy is not delegated to UAP. UAP may care for clients receiving IV therapy, and the nurse must ensure that the UAP knows how to perform routine tasks such as bathing and positioning without disturbing the IV. The UAP should also know what complications or adverse signs, such as leakage, should be reported to the nurse.

In many states, an LPN/LVN with special IV therapy training may start IV infusions. Check the state's nurse practice act.

IMPLEMENTATION

Preparation

- If possible, select a time to establish the infusion that is convenient for the client. Unless initiating IV therapy is urgent, provide any scheduled care before initiation to minimize excessive movement of the affected limb.
- Make sure that the client's clothing or gown can be removed over the IV apparatus if necessary. Many agencies provide special gowns that open over the shoulder and down the sleeve for easy removal.

Performance

1. Prior to performing the procedure, introduce self and verify the client's identity using agency protocol. Explain to the client what you are going to do, why it is necessary, and how he or she can participate. If possible, explain how long the infusion will need to remain in place.
2. Perform hand hygiene and observe other appropriate infection prevention procedures.
3. Apply a medication label to the solution container if a medication is added.

    In many agencies, medications and labels are applied in the pharmacy; if they are not, apply the label upside down on the container. **Rationale:** *The label is applied upside down so it can be read easily when the container is hanging up.*
4. Open and prepare the infusion set.
   - Remove tubing from the container and straighten it out.
   - Slide the tubing clamp along the tubing until it is just below the drip chamber to facilitate its access.
   - Close the clamp.
   - Leave the ends of the tubing covered with the plastic caps until the infusion is started. **Rationale:** *This will maintain the sterility of the ends of the tubing.*

5. Spike the solution container.
   - Expose the insertion site of the bag or bottle by removing the protective cover.
   - Remove the cap from the spike and insert the spike into the insertion site of the bag or bottle. ❶
6. Hang the solution container on the pole.
   - Adjust the pole so that the container is suspended about 1 m (3 ft) above the client's head. **Rationale:** *This height is needed to enable gravity to overcome venous pressure and facilitate flow of the solution into the vein.*

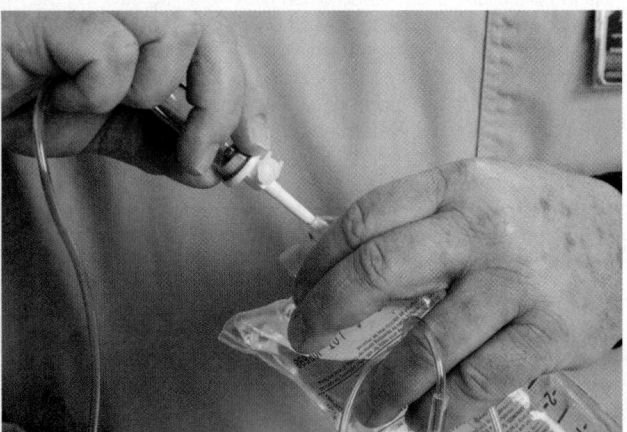

❶ Inserting the spike.

Starting an Intravenous Infusion—*continued*

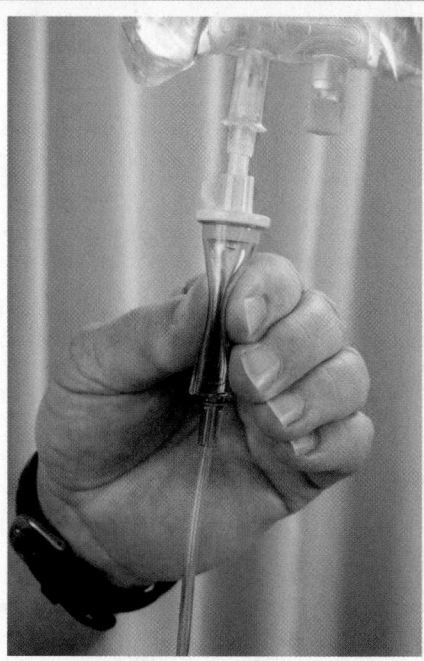

❷ Squeezing the drip chamber.

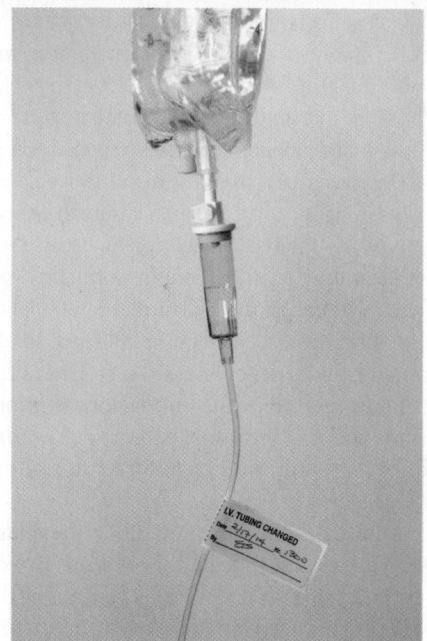

❸ Tubing labeled with date, time, and nurse's initials.

7. Partially fill the drip chamber with solution.
   * Squeeze the chamber gently until it is half full of solution. ❷ **Rationale:** *The drip chamber is partly filled with solution to prevent air from moving down the tubing.*
8. Prime the tubing as described below. The term *prime* means "to make ready" but in common use refers to flushing the tubing to remove air.
   * Remove the protective cap and hold the tubing over a container. Maintain the sterility of the end of the tubing and the cap.
   * Release the clamp and let the fluid run through the tubing until all bubbles are removed. Tap the tubing if necessary with your fingers to help the bubbles move. **Rationale:** *The tubing is primed to prevent the introduction of air into the client. Air bubbles smaller than 0.5 mL usually do not cause problems in peripheral lines.*
   * Reclamp the tubing and replace the tubing cap, maintaining sterile technique.
   * If an infusion control pump, electronic device, or a controller is being used, follow the manufacturer's directions for inserting the tubing and setting the infusion rate (see Skill 18–3).
9. Disconnect the used tubing or remove the cap on an intermittent device.
   * Apply clean gloves.
   * Place a sterile swab under the hub of the catheter. **Rationale:** *This absorbs any leakage that might occur when the tubing is disconnected.*
   * Clamp the tubing. With the fourth or fifth finger of the nondominant hand, apply pressure to the vein above the end of the catheter. **Rationale:** *This helps prevent blood from coming out of the IV catheter during the change of tubing.*
   * Holding the hub of the catheter with the nondominant hand, remove the tubing or cap with the dominant hand, using a

twisting and pulling motion. **Rationale:** *Holding the catheter firmly but gently maintains its position in the vein.*
   * Place the end of the used tubing or cap in a basin or other receptacle.
10. Connect the new tubing, and establish the infusion.
    * Continue to hold the catheter and grasp the new tubing with the dominant hand.
    * Remove the protective tubing cap and, maintaining sterility, insert the tubing end securely into the IV catheter hub.
    * Open the clamp to start the solution flowing.
11. Ensure appropriate infusion flow.
    * Remove and discard gloves.
    * Perform hand hygiene.
    * Apply a padded arm board to splint the joint as needed.
    * Adjust the infusion rate of flow according to the order.
12. Label the IV tubing.
    * Label the tubing with the date and time of attachment and your initials. ❸ This labeling may also be done when the container is set up. **Rationale:** *The tubing is labeled to ensure that it is changed at regular intervals (i.e., according to agency policy).*
13. Loop the tubing and secure it with tape to the client's skin. **Rationale:** *Looping and securing the tubing prevent the weight of the tubing or any movement from pulling on the IV catheter.*
14. Document all assessments and interventions.
    * Record the infusion in the client's chart. Some agencies provide a special form for this purpose. Include the date and time of beginning the infusion; amount and type of solution used, including any additives (e.g., kind and amount of medications); container number; flow rate; and the client's general response.

EVALUATION
* Regularly check the client for intended and adverse effects of the infusion.
* Examine the IV site at regular intervals.

* Perform follow-up based on findings or outcomes that deviated from expected or normal for the client. Relate findings to previous data if available.
* Report significant deviations from normal to the primary care provider.

REGULATING INTRAVENOUS FLOW RATES

An important nursing function is to regulate the flow rate of an IV infusion. Orders for IV infusions may take several forms, for example: "3,000 mL over 24 hours"; "1,000 mL every 8 hours"; "125 mL/h until oral intake is adequate." The nurse initiating the IV calculates the correct flow rate, regulates the infusion, and monitors the client's responses. Unless an infusion control device is being used, the nurse manually regulates the drops per minute of flow using the roller clamp to ensure that the prescribed amount of solution will be infused in the correct time span. Problems that can result from incorrectly regulated infusions include hypervolemia, hypovolemia, electrolyte imbalances, and medication complications.

The number of drops delivered per milliliter of solution varies with different brands and types of infusion sets. This rate, called the **drop factor** (sometimes called the drip factor), is printed on the package of the infusion set. Macrodrips commonly have drop factors of 10, 12, 15, or 20 drops/mL; the drop factor for microdrip is always 60 drops/mL (see Figure 18–9 on page 448).

To calculate flow rates, the nurse must know the volume of fluid to be infused and the specific time for the infusion. Two commonly used methods of indicating flow rates are (1) designating the number of milliliters to be administered in 1 hour (mL/h) and (2) designating the number of drops to be given in 1 minute (gtts/min).

Occasionally, the IV rate order will read "keep vein open" (KVO) or "to keep open" (TKO). This order does not provide adequate direction for the nurse unless agency policy specifies the milliliters per hour equivalent for this order. Generally, the KVO rate is less than 50 mL/h (e.g., 10 to 20 mL/h). Some IV pumps have a keep open rate choice built in. If the IV is not on this type of pump and no policy exists, contact the primary care provider for clarification.

Milliliters per Hour

Hourly rates of infusion can be calculated by dividing the total infusion volume by the total infusion time in hours. For example, if 3,000 mL is infused in 24 hours, the number of milliliters per hour is:

$$\frac{3{,}000 \text{ mL (total infusion volume)}}{24 \text{ h (total infusion time)}} = 125 \text{ mL/h}$$

Nurses need to check infusions at least every hour to ensure that the indicated milliliters per hour have infused and to assess the IV site.

Drops per Minute

The nurse who begins an infusion must regulate the drops per minute to ensure that the prescribed amount of solution will infuse. Drops per minute are calculated by the following formula:

$$\text{Drops per minute} = \frac{\text{Total infusion volume} \times \text{drop factor}}{\text{Total time of infusion in } minutes}$$

If the requirements are 1,000 mL in 8 hours and the drop factor is 20 drops/mL, the drops per minute should be

$$\frac{1{,}000 \text{ mL} \times 20}{8 \times 60 \text{ min (480 min)}} = 42 \text{ drops/min}$$

The nurse regulates the drops per minute by tightening or releasing the IV tubing clamp and counting the drops for 15 seconds, then multiplying that number by 4.

BOX 18–1   Factors Influencing Flow Rates

- *The position of the forearm.* Sometimes a change in the position of the client's arm decreases flow. Slight pronation, supination, extension, or elevation of the forearm on a pillow can increase the flow.
- *The position and patency of the tubing.* Tubing can be obstructed by the client's weight, a kink, or a clamp closed too tightly. The flow rate also diminishes when part of the tubing dangles below the puncture site.
- *The height of the infusion container.* Elevating the height of the infusion bottle a few inches can speed the flow by creating more pressure.
- *Possible infiltration or fluid leakage.* Swelling, a feeling of coldness, and tenderness at the venipuncture site may indicate infiltration.
- *Relationship of the size of the angiocatheter to the vein.* A catheter that is too small may impede the infusion flow.

A number of factors influence flow rates (Box 18–1).

CLINICAL ALERT!

A flow rate control device should be used when administering IV fluid to older adults or pediatric clients. Both of these age groups are especially at risk for complications of fluid overload, which can occur with rapid infusion of IV fluids.

DEVICES TO CONTROL INFUSIONS

Historically, the nurse manually regulated the IV rate with the roller clamp on the administration set. Although the roller clamp can still be used, a number of other devices are currently available to control the rate of an infusion. The term *flow-control device* refers to any manual, mechanical, or electronic infusion device used to regulate the IV flow rate (INS, 2011a, p. S104). The *Infusion Nursing Standards of Practice* (INS, 2011a) state that the choice of a flow-control device (e.g., manual flow regulator, elastomeric balloon pump, electronic infusion pump) should consider the age and mobility of the client, severity of illness, type of therapy, and health care setting (p. S34).

In the acute health care setting, electronic infusion devices (EIDs) are predominantly used to regulate the infusion rate at preset limits. EIDs are powered by electricity or battery and are programmed to regulate the IV flow rate in either drops per minute or milliliters per hour (Phillips & Gorski, 2014, p. 288). They use positive pressure to deliver the IV solution and provide an accurate flow rate, are easy to use, and have alarms that signal problems with the infusion (e.g., when the solution in the IV bag is low, when there is air in the tubing, or when flow is impeded by an occlusion). The alarms are helpful; however, the nurse must still conduct regular assessment and evaluation of the IV site to ensure safe infusion.

CLINICAL ALERT!

Many EIDs use low infusion pressures, often lower than the pressure of a gravity delivery. As a result, they do not detect infiltration. When an infiltration occurs, the inline pressure may even drop and not trigger an alarm. Thus, it is important for the nurse to assess for infiltration in clients with EIDs (Phillips & Gorski, 2014, p. 296).

Another type of flow-control device is the multichannel pump. This type of pump can deliver several medications and fluids at the same time at multiple rates from bags, bottles, or syringes (Phillips & Gorski, 2014, p. 292). The multichannel pump usually has two to four channels with each channel being programmed independently (Figure 18–12 ■). Newer systems, called smart pumps, are EIDs with a computer system. They are programmable and include drug libraries with dose rate calculators, automatic flushing between medications, dual or triple simultaneous line control, memory, multiple alarm settings, air in line, pressure/resistance, battery, schedule reminders, volume settings down to 0.1 mL, panel locks, and digital displays.

Mechanical flow-control devices are often used to regulate infusion rates in home care and/or ambulatory settings. Examples of these nonelectric methods include use of a Dial-A-Flo in-line device and the elastomeric pump. The Dial-A-Flo in-line device (Figure 18–13 ■) is a manual regulator that controls the amount of fluid to be administered. The Dial-A-Flo may be used in situations where a pump is not available or required, but prevention of fluid overload is important. The nurse presets the volume to be infused by rotating the dial to the desired rate. It is important for the nurse to remember that flow rate needs to be verified by counting the drops.

The elastomeric infusion pump (Figure 18–14 ■), a nonelectric portable disposable pump, is prefilled with a medication and connects to the client's needleless connector. It is a lightweight, disposable pump that delivers medications at a controlled rate. The medication is held in a reservoir (balloon) that is inside a rigid, transparent container. The balloon exerts positive pressure, which releases the

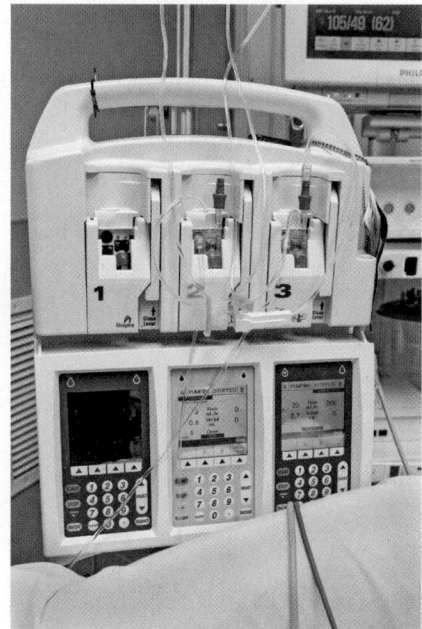

Figure 18–12 ■ Programmable multichannel infusion pumps.

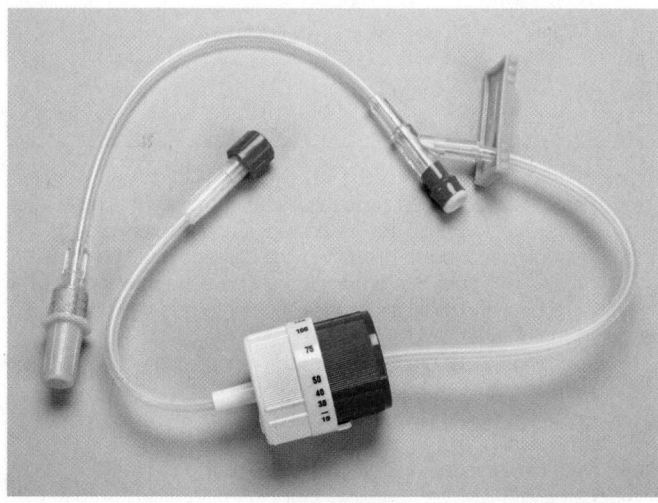

A

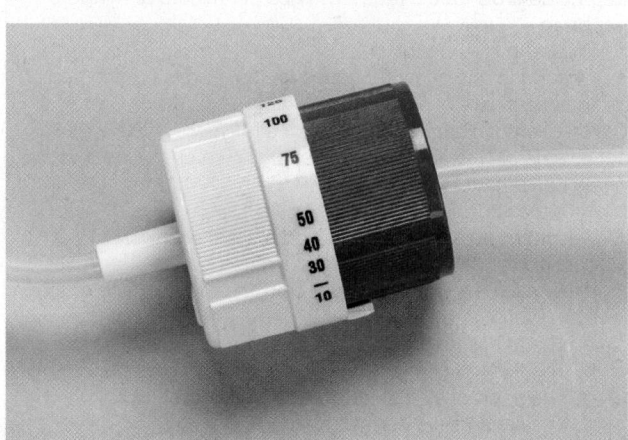

B

Figure 18–13 ■ *A*, The Dial-A-Flo in-line gravity control device; *B*, the manual rate-flow regulator.

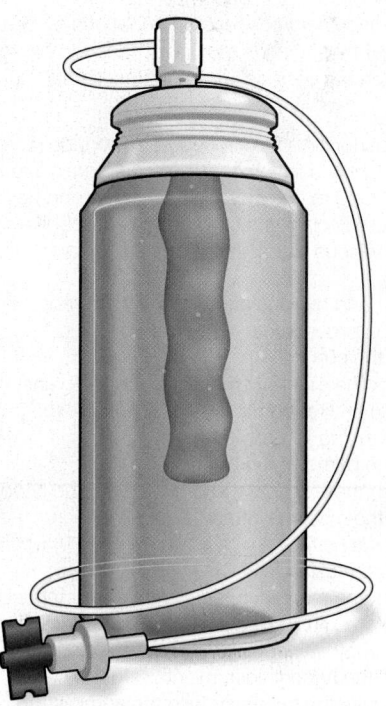

Figure 18–14 ■ An elastomeric infusion pump showing medication in the reservoir and protected by an exterior shell.

solution into the tubing that is attached to the client's vascular access device (Broadhurst, 2012, p. 144). An integrated flow restrictor controls the flow rate, which can be set from 0.5 to 500 mL/h (Phillips & Gorski, 2014, p. 287). The elastomeric infusion pump is portable and can be put in a loose pocket or bag while infusing, allowing the client to be mobile. When the infusion is finished, the entire device is discarded. The elastomeric pump provides ease of use in the home care setting.

●○● NURSING PROCESS: USING AN ELECTRONIC INFUSION DEVICE (EID)

Using an Electronic Infusion Device (EID)

SKILL 18-3

ASSESSMENT
Before preparing the EID, the nurse first verifies the order indicating the type of solution, the amount to be administered, and the rate of flow of the infusion. The appearance of the infusion site and patency of the system should also be assessed.

Planning
Review the client record regarding previous infusions and use of infusion devices. Note any complications and how they were managed.

DELEGATION

Due to the need for sterile technique and technical complexity, use of infusion devices is not delegated to UAP. UAP may care for clients with such devices, and the nurse must ensure that the UAP knows how to perform routine tasks such as positioning and changing gowns when a device is in place. The UAP should also know what complications or adverse signs, such as alarms, should be reported to the nurse. In many states, an LPN/LVN with special IV therapy training may manage infusions. Check the state's nurse practice act.

Equipment
- EID
- IV solution or medication
- IV pole
- IV administration set with EID compatible IV tubing
- Alcohol swabs and tape
- Label for tubing

IMPLEMENTATION
Preparation
- Review the use of the EID outside the client's room. Read all appropriate materials and confirm how to set the device. **Rationale:** *Many types of pumps are available. It is important to read the manufacturer's recommendations for setup.*
- Ensure that the tubing is the correct one for the device. Each manufacturer and model may require different tubing.

Performance
1. Prior to performing the procedure, introduce self and verify the client's identity using agency protocol. Explain to the client what you are going to do, why it is necessary, and how he or she can participate. Explain what the device sounds like during normal use, the various alarms, and to notify the nurse if an alarm sounds.
2. Perform hand hygiene and observe other appropriate infection prevention procedures.
3. Prepare the client.
   - Check the client's identification band against the IV fluid container. **Rationale:** *This ensures that the correct client receives the infusion.*
4. Attach the pump to the IV pole.
   - Attach the EID below and in line with the IV container.
   - Plug the machine into an electric outlet, unless battery power is used.
5. Set up the infusion.
   - Check the manufacturer's directions before using an IV filter or before infusing blood. **Rationale:** *Infusion pump pressures may damage filters or cause rate inaccuracies.*
   - Open the IV container, maintaining the sterility of the port, and spike the container with the administration set.
   - Place the IV container on the IV pole above the pump.
   - Fill the drip chamber.

- Prime the tubing, and close the clamp. Some pumps have a cassette that must also be primed. Manufacturers provide instructions for doing this. Often, the cassette must be tilted to be filled with fluid. Some pumps must have the power on and the tubing and cassette in place in order to perform priming.
6. Insert the IV tubing into the pump.
   - Load the machine according to the manufacturer's instructions.
   - Press the power button to the on position.
7. Initiate the infusion.
   - Perform venipuncture or connect the tubing to the IV catheter.
8. Set the controls for the required drops per minute or milliliters per hour.
   - Press the start button.
   - Check the drip chamber to ensure that fluid is flowing from the container.
9. Set the alarms. **Rationale:** *The alarms notify the nurse when a set volume of fluid has been infused or indicates malfunctioning of the equipment.*
10. Monitor the infusion.
    - Check the volume of fluid infused at least every hour to confirm the actual volume of fluid infused.
    - If the volume infused does not coincide with the time or the alarm sounds, begin at the client level and check that:
      a. The IV has not infiltrated or clotted at the insertion site.
      b. The tubing is not pinched, kinked, or disconnected.
      c. The appropriate tubing clamps are fully open.
      d. The sensors are correctly placed.
      e. The rate/volume settings are accurate.
      f. The drip chamber is correctly filled.
      g. The container still has solution.
      h. The IV container is correctly placed.

Using an Electronic Infusion Device (EID)—*continued*

11. Document relevant information.
  - Record the date and time of starting the infusion, the type and amount of fluid being infused, the rate at which it is

being infused, the infusion device used, the status of the IV insertion site, and any adverse responses of the client.

EVALUATION
- Regularly check the client for intended and adverse effects of the infusion.
- Examine the IV site at regular intervals according to agency policy.

- Perform follow-up based on findings or outcomes that deviated from expected or normal for the client. Relate findings to previous data if available.
- Report significant deviations from normal to the primary care provider.

SKILL 18-3

LIFESPAN CONSIDERATIONS **Regulating Intravenous Flow Rates**

INFANTS/CHILDREN
- Emphasize to children that the EID is not a toy and should not be touched unless an adult is present. Children are naturally curious and will want to examine the equipment.
- Use a volume-control infusion set (Buretrol, Soluset, Volutrol, or Pediatrol) with the pump/controller for pediatric clients (see Figure 17–33 on page 434).
- Explain the procedure to the young client, encourage questions, and be alert for nonverbal cues. Children may not understand

things that seem obvious to adults. For example, a child may think the IV therapy is a punishment.

OLDER ADULTS
- Check the IV flow rate frequently for older clients. Older adults are at increased risk to develop fluid overload if IV fluid is infused too rapidly.
- Check the IV site often for signs of infiltration. Veins become more fragile with aging.

MAINTAINING INFUSIONS

Once an IV infusion has been established, it is the nurse's responsibility to maintain the prescribed flow rate and to prevent complications associated with IV therapy. IV solution containers are changed when only a small amount of fluid remains in the neck of the container and fluid still remains in the drip chamber. However, all IV bags should be changed every 24 hours, regardless of how much solution remains, to minimize the risk of contamination. Change primary administration sets and secondary tubing that remains continuously attached to them "no more frequently than every 96 hours" (INS, 2011b). Change intermittent infusion sets without a primary infusion every 24 hours or whenever their sterility is in question (INS, 2011b). Add-on devices (e.g., extension sets, filters, stopcocks) should be changed at the same time the administration set is changed (INS, 2011b). The *Infusion NursingStandards of Practice* (INS, 2011a) state "routine site care and dressing changes are not performed on short peripheral catheters unless the dressing is soiled or no longer intact" (p. S63).

●○● NURSING PROCESS: MAINTAINING INFUSIONS

Maintaining Infusions

ASSESSMENT
In maintaining the infusion, the nurse will examine the appearance of the infusion site, patency of the system, type of fluid being infused and rate of flow, and the response of the client.

PLANNING
Review the client record regarding previous infusions and use of infusion devices. Note any complications and how they were managed. Gather the pertinent data:
- From the order, determine the type and sequence of solutions to be infused.
- Determine the rate of flow and infusion schedule.

DELEGATION

Due to the need for sterile technique and technical complexity, inspection of IV sites and regulation of IV rates are not delegated to UAP. UAP may care for clients with such devices, and the nurse must ensure that the UAP knows what complications or adverse signs should be reported to the nurse. In many states, an LPN/LVN with special IV therapy training may manage infusions. Check the state's nurse practice act.

Equipment
None

SKILL 18-4

Continued on page 460

Maintaining Infusions—*continued*

IMPLEMENTATION
Performance

1. Prior to performing the procedure, introduce self and verify the client's identity using agency protocol. Explain to the client what you are going to do, why it is necessary, and how he or she can participate.
2. Perform hand hygiene and observe other appropriate infection prevention procedures.
3. Position the client appropriately.
   - Assist the client to a comfortable position, either sitting or lying.
   - Expose the IV site but provide for client privacy.
4. Ensure that the correct solution is being infused.
   - Compare the label on the container (including added medications) to the order. If the solution is incorrect, slow the rate of flow to a minimum to maintain the patency of the catheter. If the infusing solution is contraindicated for the client, stop the infusion and saline-lock the catheter. **Rationale:** *Just stopping the infusion may allow a thrombus to form in the IV catheter. If this occurs, the catheter must be removed and another venipuncture performed before the infusion can be resumed. Because IV tubing contains approximately 12 to 15 mL, it may be desirable to prevent even this much additional incorrect solution to infuse when the correct IV solution container is hung on existing tubing. In this case, all tubing should be removed until new tubing, primed with the correct solution, can be started.*
   - Change the solution to the correct one, using new tubing if indicated.
   - Document and report the error according to agency protocol.
5. Observe the rate of flow every hour.
   - Compare the rate of flow regularly, for example, every hour, against the infusion schedule. **Rationale:** *Infusions that are off schedule can be harmful to a client.* To read the volume in an IV bag, pull the edges of the bag apart at the level of the fluid and read the volume remaining. **Rationale:** *Stretching the bag allows the fluid meniscus to fall to the proper level.*
   - Observe the position of the solution container. If it is less than 1 m (3 ft) above the IV site, readjust it to the correct height of the pole. **Rationale:** *If the container is too low with a gravity IV infusion, the solution may not flow into the vein because there is insufficient gravitational pressure to overcome the pressure of the blood within the vein.*
   - If too much fluid has infused in the time interval, check agency policy. The primary care provider may need to be notified.
   - In some agencies, you will slow the infusion to less than the ordered rate so that it will be completed at the planned time. **Rationale:** *Solution administered too quickly may cause a significant increase in circulating blood volume (which is about 6 L in an adult). Hypervolemia may result in pulmonary edema and cardiac failure.* Assess the client for manifestations of hypervolemia and its complications, including dyspnea; rapid, labored breathing; cough; crackles; tachycardia; and bounding pulses.
   - In other agencies, if the order is for a specified amount of fluid per hour, the IV may be adjusted to the correct rate and the client monitored for signs of fluid overload.
   - If the rate is too slow, check agency practice. Some agencies permit nursing personnel to adjust a rate of flow by a specified amount. Adjustments above this amount may require a primary care provider's order. **Rationale:** *Solution that is administered too slowly can supply insufficient fluid, electrolytes, or medication for a client's needs.*
   - If the prescribed rate of flow is 150 mL/h or more, check the rate of flow more frequently, for example, every 15 to 30 minutes.
6. Inspect the patency of the IV tubing and catheter.
   - Observe the drip chamber. If it is less than half full, squeeze the chamber to allow the correct amount of fluid to flow in.
   - Inspect the tubing for pinches, kinks, or obstructions to flow. Arrange the tubing so that it is lightly coiled and under no pressure. Sometimes the tubing becomes caught under the client's body and the weight blocks the flow.
   - Observe the position of the tubing. If it is dangling below the venipuncture site, coil it carefully on the surface of the bed. **Rationale:** *The solution may not flow upward into the vein against the force of gravity.*
   - Determine catheter position. Some methods include:
     a. Aspirate the catheter for a blood return. Do this slowly and gently.
     b. Lower the solution container below the level of the infusion site and observe for a return flow of blood from the vein. **Rationale:** *A return flow of blood indicates that the IV catheter is patent and in the vein. Blood returns in this instance because venous pressure is greater than the fluid pressure in the IV tubing. Absence of blood return may indicate that the IV catheter is no longer in the vein or that the tip of the catheter is partially obstructed by a thrombus, the vein wall, or a valve in the vein.* (Note: With some catheters, no blood may appear even with patency because the soft catheter walls collapse during siphoning.)
   - If there is leakage, locate the source. If the leak is at the catheter connection, tighten the tubing into the catheter. If the leak is elsewhere in the tubing, slow the infusion and replace the tubing. Estimate the amount of solution lost, if it was substantial. If the IV insertion site is leaking, the catheter will have to be removed and IV access reestablished at a new site.
7. Inspect the insertion site for fluid infiltration. **Infiltration** is the unintentional administration of a nonvesicant solution or medication into the tissue surrounding the IV catheter (Martin, 2013, p. 392).
   - If infiltration is present, stop the infusion and remove the catheter. Restart the infusion at another site.
   - Start supportive treatment (e.g., elevate extremity or apply heat to the site) (INS, 2011b). **Rationale:** *Warmth promotes comfort and vasodilation, facilitating absorption of the fluid from interstitial tissue.*
   - If the infiltration involves a **vesicant** (a medication or fluid that causes blisters, severe tissue injury, or necrosis if it escapes from the vein [Vacca, 2013]), it is called **extravasation** and other measures are indicated. The extravasation of a vesicant drug should be considered an emergency. Usually, vesicants are administered only through central venous infusions and by specially certified nurses. Most nurses relate vesicants to chemotherapy medications, such as paclitaxel; however, a number of nonchemotherapeutic medications are vesicants (e.g., vancomycin, domapine, diazepam, digoxin) (Martin, 2013; Vacca, 2013).
   - For an extravasation:
     a. Stop the infusion immediately.
     b. For a peripheral-short catheter, disconnect the tubing from the catheter hub and attach a 3- or 5-mL syringe. Aspirate any fluid remaining in the hub and catheter.
     c. Remove the catheter. Use a dry gauze pad to control bleeding.

Maintaining Infusions—*continued*

d. Apply a new dry dressing. Do not apply pressure to the area.

e. For a central venous catheter (CVC), do not remove the catheter. Clamp and cap the catheter hub. Follow agency procedure for flushing when extravasation is suspected.

f. Assess motion, sensation, and capillary refill distal to the injury. Measure the circumference of the extremity and compare it with the opposite extremity.

g. Notify the primary care provider.

h. Photograph the site if that is agency policy.

i. The affected arm should be elevated and, depending on the drug, heat or cold therapy should be implemented.

j. Pharmacologic treatment may be instituted depending on the type of vesicant that has caused the damage. Two appropriate medications are hyaluronidase and phentolamine, which are used to lessen tissue injury. The best results occur when administered immediately after an extravasation (Martin, 2013).

k. The lack of recommendations and guidelines for the treatment of extravasation requires health care facilities to develop their own policies and procedures.

8. Inspect the insertion site for **phlebitis** (inflammation of a vein).
   • Inspect and palpate the site at least every 8 hours. Phlebitis can occur as a result of injury to a vein, for example, because of mechanical trauma or chemical irritation. Chemical injury to a vein can occur from IV electrolytes (especially potassium and magnesium) and medications. The clinical signs are redness, warmth, and swelling at the IV site and burning pain along the course of a vein.

• If phlebitis is detected, discontinue the infusion, and apply warm or cold compresses to the venipuncture site. Do not use this injured vein for further infusions.

9. Inspect the IV site for bleeding.
   • Oozing or bleeding into the surrounding tissues can occur while the infusion is freely flowing but is more likely to occur after the catheter has been removed from the vein.
   • Observation of the venipuncture site is extremely important for clients who bleed readily, such as those receiving anticoagulants.

10. Teach the client ways to maintain the infusion system; for example:
    • Inform of any limitations on movement or mobility.
    • Explain alarms if an electronic control device is used.
    • Instruct to notify a nurse if:
      a. The flow rate suddenly changes or the solution stops dripping.
      b. The solution container is nearly empty.
      c. There is blood in the IV tubing.
      d. Discomfort or swelling is experienced at the IV site.
    • Inform that the nurse will be checking the venipuncture site.

11. Document relevant information (often on a specified form).
    • Record the status of the IV insertion site and any adverse responses of the client.
    • Document the client's IV fluid intake at least every 8 hours according to agency policy. Include the date and time, amount and type of solution used, container number, flow rate, and the client's general response. In most agencies, the amount remaining in each IV container is also recorded at the end of the shift.

EVALUATION

• Perform follow-up based on findings or outcomes that deviated from expected or normal for the client. Consider urinary output compared to intake, tissue turgor, specific gravity of urine, vital signs, and lung sounds compared to baseline data.

• Regularly check the client for intended and adverse effects of the infusion. Report significant deviations from normal to the primary care provider.

CLIENT TEACHING CONSIDERATIONS

Intravenous Infusions

Teach the client ways to help maintain the infusion system, for example:

• Avoid sudden twisting or turning movements of the arm with the catheter.
• Avoid stretching or placing tension on the tubing.
• Try to keep the tubing from dangling below the level of the IV catheter.

• Notify a nurse if:
  a. The flow rate suddenly changes or the solution stops dripping.
  b. The client notices the solution container is nearly empty.
  c. There is blood in the IV tubing.
  d. Discomfort or swelling is experienced at the IV site.
  e. The pump or controller alarm sounds.

Ambulatory and Community Settings   Intravenous Infusions   PATIENT-CENTERED CARE

• In the home, plant hangers, robe hooks, or over-the-door S hooks may be used to hang an IV container.
• Evaluate the client's or caregiver's ability to operate the infusion device at home.
• Emphasize the need for hand hygiene and clean technique when handling IV equipment. Set aside a clean area in the home to store the IV equipment.

• Demonstrate the device, and ask for a return demonstration from the client or caregiver.
• Discuss complications, such as infiltration, power failure, or equipment problems, and the measures to take when they arise.
• Make certain the client knows how and where to obtain supplies.

SKILL 18–5

INTERMITTENT INFUSION DEVICES

The purpose of intermittent infusion devices is to provide venous access when IV administration of medications or fluids is needed only on an intermittent basis. The nurse may establish the IV catheter initially as an intermittent device (see Skill 18–1) or convert a continuous IV to intermittent.

●○● NURSING PROCESS: INTERMITTENT INFUSION DEVICES

Maintaining Intermittent Infusion Devices

ASSESSMENT
Gather the pertinent data:
- Assess the patency of the IV catheter and the appearance of the site (evidence of inflammation or infiltration).

PLANNING
Review the primary care provider's order.
- A specific order may be written to insert or convert IV access to a saline lock. The order also may be implied. For example, IV fluids are to be discontinued but the client has orders for an IV antibiotic every 6 hours or is receiving analgesics intravenously.
- From the primary care provider's order, determine the type and sequence of intermittent infusions.
- Review the client record regarding previous infusions and use of infusion devices. Note any complications and how they were managed.

DELEGATION

Due to the need for sterile technique and technical complexity, this procedure is not delegated to UAP. UAP may care for clients with such devices, and the nurse must ensure that the UAP knows what complications or adverse signs should be reported to the nurse. In many states, an LPN/LVN with special IV therapy training may manage intermittent infusion devices. Check the state's nurse practice act.

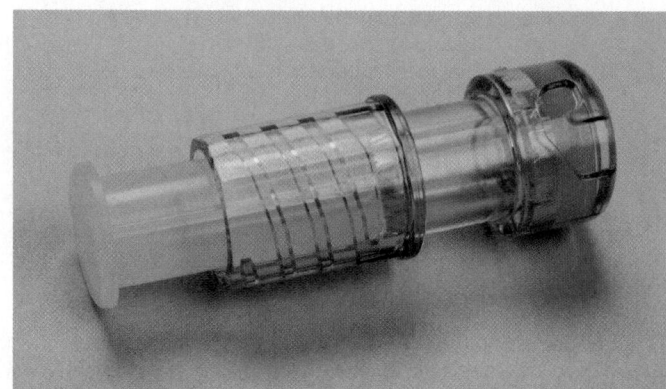

❶ Intermittent infusion device with injection port.

- Sterile 2×2 or 4×4 gauze
- Sterile saline for injection (without preservative) in a prefilled syringe, a 3-mL syringe with a needleless infusion device
- Alcohol wipes
- Tape
- Clean emesis basin

Equipment
- Intermittent infusion cap or device ❶
- Clean gloves
- TSM dressing

IMPLEMENTATION
Performance
1. Prior to performing the procedure, introduce self and verify the client's identity using agency protocol. Explain to the client what you are going to do, why it is necessary, and how he or she can participate. Explain the reason for the intermittent device and that changing an IV to a saline lock should cause no discomfort other than that associated with removing tape from the IV tubing.
2. Perform hand hygiene and observe other appropriate infection prevention procedures.
3. Assist the client to a comfortable position, either sitting or lying. Expose the IV site but provide for client privacy.
4. Assess the IV site and determine the patency of the catheter (see Skill 18–4). If the catheter is not fully patent or there is evidence of phlebitis or infiltration, discontinue the catheter and establish a new IV site.
   - Expose the IV catheter hub and loosen any tape that is holding the IV tubing in place or that will interfere with insertion of the intermittent infusion plug into the catheter.
   - Clamp the IV tubing to stop the flow of IV fluid (see Chapter 17 ∞).

- Open the gauze pad and place it under the IV catheter hub. **Rationale:** *This absorbs any leakage that might occur when the tubing is disconnected.*
- Open the alcohol wipe and intermittent infusion cap, leaving the plug in its sterile package.
5. Remove the IV tubing and insert the intermittent infusion plug into the IV catheter.
   - Apply clean gloves.
   - Stabilize the IV catheter with your nondominant hand and use the little finger to place slight pressure on the vein above the end of the catheter. Twist the IV tubing adapter to loosen it from the IV catheter and remove it, placing the end of the tubing into a clean emesis basin. ❷
   - Pick up the intermittent infusion plug from its package and remove the protective sleeve from the male adapter (see ❶), maintaining its sterility. Insert the plug into the IV catheter, twisting it to seat it firmly, or engage the Luer-Lok.
6. Instill saline solution per agency policy. **Rationale:** *Saline is used to maintain patency of the IV catheter when fluids are not infusing through the catheter.*

Maintaining Intermittent Infusion Devices—*continued*

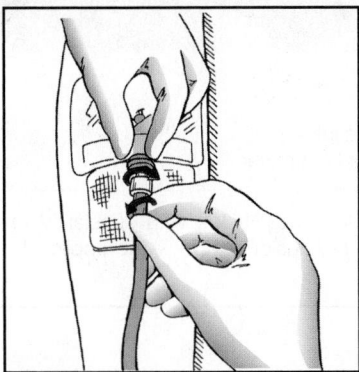

❷ Separating the IV catheter from the infusion tubing.

7. Cover the site with a TSM dressing. **Rationale:** *The TSM dressing provides protection from infection, allows for ease of assessment of the venipuncture site, and also promotes comfort, preventing the plug from catching on clothing or bedding.*

8. Access the device to infuse fluids or medication:
* Cleanse the cap with povidone-iodine or alcohol according to agency policy.
* Use a threaded-lock needleless connector for infusions Figure 18–10 *A*.

9. Flush the device with prescribed solution after each use or every 8 to 12 hours if not in use, according to agency policy. Some recommend flushing the lock by injecting saline using the push–pause method (a rapid succession of push–pause–push–pause movements exerted on the plunger of the syringe barrel) with the rationale that this creates a turbulence within the catheter lumen that causes a swirling effect to remove any debris (e.g., blood or medication) attached to the catheter lumen. However, no research supports this method of flushing. There are differences of opinion and practice regarding this type of flushing versus a smooth injection of the flush solution. Research is needed to provide evidence of which is the most effective (Phillips & Gorski, 2014, p. 359).

10. Remove and discard gloves.
* Perform hand hygiene.

11. Teach the client how to maintain the lock.
* Notify the nurse or primary care provider if the plug or catheter comes out; if the site becomes red, inflamed, or painful; or if any drainage or bleeding occurs at the site.

12. Document relevant information.
* Record the date and time of converting the infusion device, the status of the IV insertion site, and any adverse responses of the client.

EVALUATION

* Perform follow-up based on findings or outcomes that deviated from expected or normal for the client. Relate findings to previous data if available.

* Examine the IV site at regular intervals. Note patency and ease of flushing.
* Report significant deviations from normal to the primary care provider.

CLIENT TEACHING CONSIDERATIONS

Intermittent Infusion Devices

Teach the client how to maintain the lock:

* Avoid manipulating the catheter or infusion plug and protect it from catching on clothing or bedding. A gauze bandage such as Kerlix or Kling may be wrapped over the plug to protect it when it is not in use.

* Cover the site with an occlusive dressing when showering; avoid immersing the site.
* Flush the catheter with saline solution as directed.
* Notify the care provider if the plug or catheter comes out; if the site becomes red, inflamed, or painful; or if any drainage or bleeding occurs at the site.

DISCONTINUING INFUSIONS

When the IV access is no longer required, the nurse removes the IV catheter. A specific order may be written to discontinue IV therapy. Ensure that it is not necessary to maintain an intermittent device.

SKILL 18–6

●○○● NURSING PROCESS: DISCONTINUING INFUSIONS

Discontinuing Infusion Devices

ASSESSMENT
Assess:
* Appearance of the venipuncture site.
* Any bleeding from the infusion site.
* Amount of fluid infused.
* Appearance of IV catheter.

PLANNING
Review the client record regarding the primary care provider's orders. Note if there were any previous infusions and if there were any complications and how they were managed.

In many states, an LPN/LVN with special IV therapy training may discontinue IV infusions. Check the applicable state's nurse practice act.

DELEGATION

In some states and agencies, removal of a peripheral IV catheter may be delegated to UAP. In others, removal of IV infusions or devices is not delegated to UAP. In any case, the nurse must ensure that the UAP knows what complications or adverse signs following removal should be reported to the nurse.

Equipment
* Clean gloves
* Linen-saver pad
* Small sterile dressing and tape

IMPLEMENTATION
Performance
1. Prior to performing the procedure, introduce self and verify the client's identity using agency protocol. Explain to the client what you are going to do, why it is necessary, and how he or she can participate. Explain the reason for discontinuing the IV and that the procedure should cause no discomfort other than that associated with removing the tape.
2. Perform hand hygiene and observe other appropriate infection prevention procedures.
3. Assist the client to a comfortable position, either sitting or lying. Expose the IV site but provide for client privacy. Place a linen-saver pad under the extremity that has the IV.
4. Prepare the equipment.
   * Clamp the infusion tubing. **Rationale:** *Clamping the tubing prevents the fluid from flowing out of the IV catheter onto the client or bed.*
   * Apply clean gloves.
   * Remove the dressing, stabilization device, and tape at the venipuncture site while holding the IV catheter firmly and applying countertraction to the skin. ❶ **Rationale:** *Movement of the IV catheter can injure the vein and cause discomfort to the client. Countertraction prevents pulling the skin and causing discomfort.*
   * Assess the venipuncture site. **Rationale:** *Assess for signs of infection or phlebitis.*
   * Apply the sterile gauze above the venipuncture site. Only touch the upper (top) portion of the gauze pad and maintain sterility of the lower (bottom) portion that is in contact with the venipuncture site.
5. Withdraw the catheter from the vein.
   * Withdraw the catheter by pulling it out along the line of the vein. ❷ **Rationale:** *Pulling it out in line with the vein avoids pain and injury to the vein.* Do not press down on the sterile gauze pad while removing the catheter.
   * Immediately apply firm pressure to the site, using sterile gauze, for 2 to 3 minutes. **Rationale:** *Pressure helps stop the bleeding and prevents hematoma formation.*
   * Hold the client's arm above heart level if any bleeding persists. **Rationale:** *Raising the limb decreases blood flow to the area.*
   * Teach the client to inform the nurse if the site begins to bleed at any time or the client notes any other abnormalities in the area.

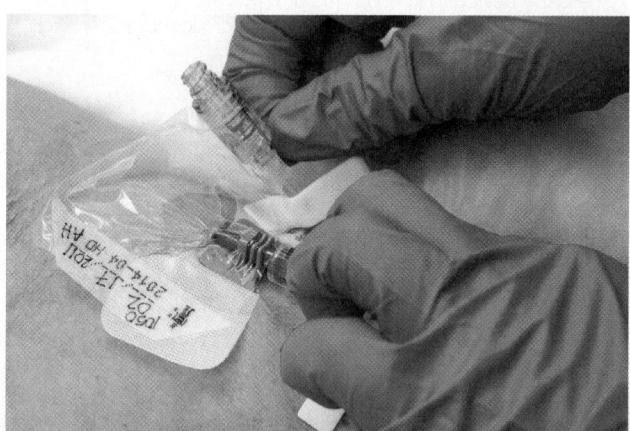

❶ Remove the dressing, stabilization device, and tape while holding the IV catheter firmly.

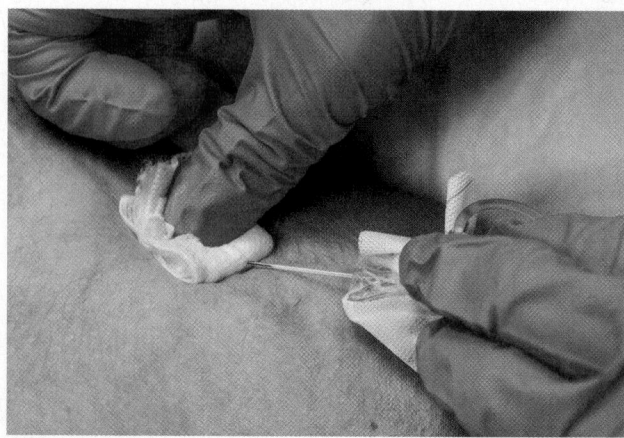

❷ Withdraw the IV catheter from the vein. Do not apply pressure on the sterile gauze pad until the catheter is completely removed.

Discontinuing Infusion Devices—*continued*

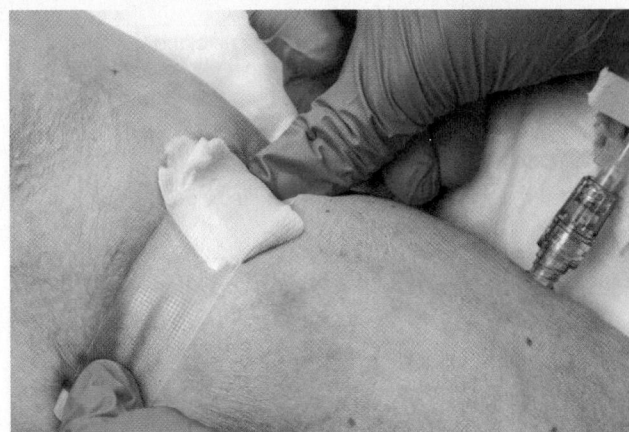

❸ Apply new sterile dressing to the site with tape.

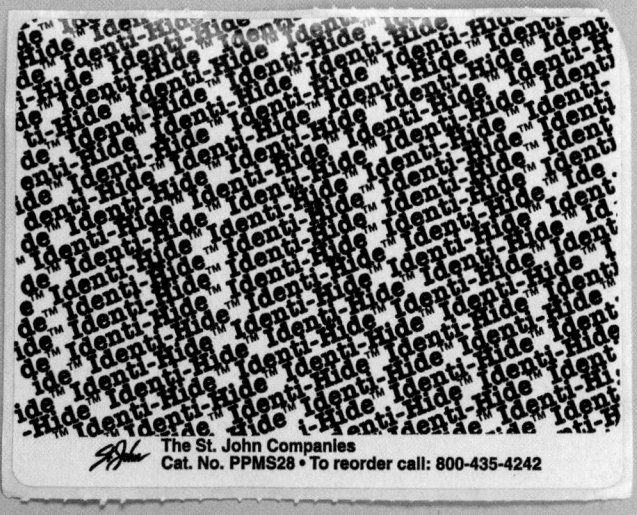

A

6. Examine the catheter removed from the client.
   - Check the catheter to make sure it is intact. **Rationale:** *If a piece of tubing remains in the client's vein, it could move centrally (toward the heart or lungs).*
   - Report a broken catheter to the nurse in charge or primary care provider immediately.
   - If the broken piece can be palpated, apply a tourniquet above the insertion site. **Rationale:** *Application of a tourniquet decreases the possibility of the piece moving until a primary care provider is notified.*
7. Cover the venipuncture site.
   - Apply a new sterile dressing to the site with tape. ❸ **Rationale:** *The dressing maintains the pressure and covers the open area in the skin, preventing infection.*
   - Discard used supplies appropriately.
   - Remove and discard gloves.
   - Perform hand hygiene.
8. Read the amount remaining in the IV solution container prior to discarding the IV solution.
9. Apply a black-out label ❹, *A,* over the existing IV solution label prior to discarding the IV solution into a biohazard container ❹, *B.* **Rationale:** *The existing IV label contains client information. The black-out label conceals client information and ensures client confidentiality. These labels are called IV HIPAA-compliant labels.*
10. Document all relevant information.
    - Record the amount of fluid infused on the intake and output record and in the record, according to agency policy. Include the container number, type of solution used, time of discontinuing the infusion, and the client's response.

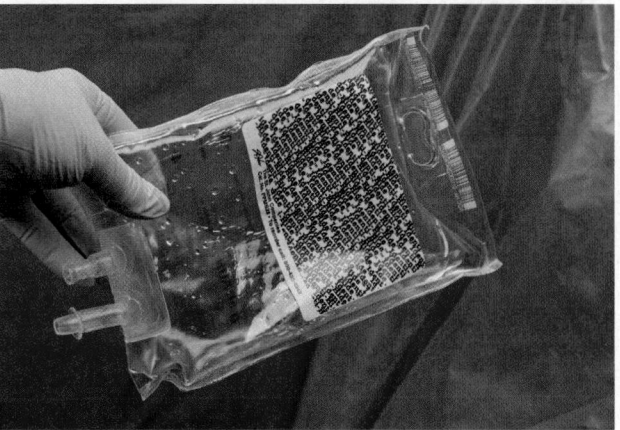

B

❹ *A,* An IV black-out label; *B,* discarding an IV bag into a biohazard container after applying a black-out label to ensure client confidentiality.

EVALUATION
- Perform follow-up based on findings or outcomes that deviated from expected or normal for the client. Relate findings to previous data if available.
- Report significant deviations from normal to the primary care provider.

TABLE 18–2	Blood Products for Transfusion
Product	**Use**
Whole blood	Not commonly used except for extreme cases of acute hemorrhage. Replaces blood volume and all blood products: RBCs, plasma, plasma proteins, fresh platelets, and other clotting factors.
Packed red blood cells (PRBCs)	Used to increase the oxygen-carrying capacity of blood in anemias, surgery, and disorders with slow bleeding. One unit of PRBCs has the same amount of oxygen-carrying RBCs as a unit of whole blood. One unit raises hematocrit by approximately 2% to 3%.
Autologous red blood cells	Used for blood replacement following planned elective surgery. Client donates blood for autologous (to self) transfusion 4 to 5 weeks prior to surgery.
Platelets	Used to replace platelets in clients with bleeding disorders or platelet deficiency. Fresh platelets most effective. Each unit should increase the average adult client's platelet count by about 5,000 platelets/microliter.
Fresh frozen plasma	Provides clotting factors. Does not need to be typed and crossmatched (contains no RBCs).
Albumin and plasma protein fraction	Blood volume expander; provides plasma proteins.
Clotting factors and cryoprecipitate	Used for clients with clotting factor deficiencies. Each provides different factors involved in the clotting pathway; cryoprecipitate contains fibrinogen.

BLOOD TRANSFUSIONS

A blood **transfusion** is the introduction of whole blood or components of the blood (e.g., plasma or erythrocytes) into the venous circulation (Table 18–2). Human blood is commonly classified into four main groups: A, B, AB, and O. The surfaces of an individual's red blood cells (RBCs) contain a number of proteins known as antigens that are unique for each person. These antigens can cause antibody reactions when in contact with mismatched blood. Blood transfusions must be matched to the client's blood type in terms of compatible antigens. Mismatched blood results in destruction (hemolysis) of RBCs.

The **Rh factor** antigen is present on the RBCs of approximately 85% of the people in the United States. Blood that contains the Rh factor is known as Rh positive (Rh^+); blood that does not contain the Rh factor is known as Rh negative (Rh^-). In contrast to the ABO blood groups, Rh^- blood does not naturally contain Rh antibodies. However, after exposure to blood containing Rh factor (e.g., an Rh^- mother carrying a fetus with Rh^+ blood, or transfusion of Rh^+ blood into a client who is Rh^-), Rh antibodies develop. Subsequent exposure to Rh^+ blood places the client at risk for an antigen–antibody reaction and hemolysis of RBCs.

Transfusion Reactions

To avoid transfusing incompatible red blood cells, both blood and recipient are typed and their blood is crossmatched for compatibility. This is referred to as a *type and crossmatch*. Other forms of transfusion reactions may also occur, including febrile or allergic reactions, circulatory overload, and sepsis. Because the risk of an adverse reaction is high when blood is transfused, clients must be frequently and carefully assessed before and during transfusion. Many reactions become evident within 5 to 15 minutes of initiating the transfusion, but reactions can develop any time during a transfusion; for this reason clients are most closely monitored during the initial period of the transfusion. Stop the transfusion immediately if signs of a reaction develop. Keep the line open with normal saline. Do not use the saline attached to the Y-set tubing because the filter contains blood, and you do not want to give the client who is experiencing an acute transfusion reaction one more drop of blood. Instead, use new IV tubing. Disconnect the infusion tubing from the hub of the IV catheter and replace with the new IV tubing. Do not piggyback the new tubing into the access port of the transfusion tubing because it is possible that some of the blood product could be administered to the client. Hydrate the client with normal saline and notify the primary care provider. Continue to monitor vital signs (Phillips & Gorski, 2014). Possible transfusion reactions, their clinical signs and symptoms, and nursing interventions are listed in Table 18–3. The hospital must have a protocol relating to transfusion reactions. Common measures include:

- Notify the blood bank.
- Examine the label on the blood container to check for errors in identifying the client, blood, or blood component.
- Obtain lab specimens (e.g., blood work, urine sample).
- Send the blood container (whether or not it contains any blood), attached infusion set, and IV solution to the blood bank (American Association of Blood Banks [AABB], 2009, p. 79).

Blood Administration

Special precautions are necessary when administering blood. When a transfusion is ordered, the nurse or other personnel obtain blood in plastic bags from the blood bank just before starting the transfusion. One unit of whole blood is 500 mL; a unit of packed RBCs is approximately 300 mL (Phillips & Gorski, 2014). Do not store the blood in the refrigerator on the nursing unit; lack of temperature control may damage the blood. Once blood or a blood product is removed from the blood bank refrigerator, it must be administered within a limited amount of time (e.g., packed RBCs should not hang for more than 4 hours after being removed from the blood bank refrigerator).

TABLE 18–3 Transfusion Reactions

Reaction: Cause	Clinical Signs	Nursing Intervention*
Hemolytic reaction: incompatibility between client's blood and donor's blood	Fever or chills, flank pain, and reddish or brown urine; tachycardia, hypotension	1. Discontinue the transfusion immediately. *Note:* When the transfusion is discontinued, the blood tubing must be removed as well. Use *new* tubing for the normal saline infusion. 2. Maintain vascular access with normal saline, or according to agency protocol. 3. Notify the primary care provider immediately. 4. Monitor vital signs. 5. Monitor fluid intake and output. 6. Send the remaining blood, bag, filter, tubing, a sample of the client's blood, and a urine sample to the laboratory.
Febrile reaction: sensitivity of the client's blood to white blood cells, platelets, or plasma proteins; does not cause hemolysis	Fever; chills; warm, flushed skin; headache; anxiety; nausea	1. Discontinue the transfusion immediately. 2. Keep the vein open with a normal saline infusion. 3. Notify the primary care provider. 4. Give antipyretics as ordered.
Allergic reaction (mild): sensitivity to infused plasma proteins	Flushing, urticaria with or without itching	1. Stop the transfusion immediately. 2. Notify the primary care provider. 3. Administer medication (antihistamines, steroids) as ordered.
Allergic reaction (severe): antibody–antigen reaction	Dyspnea, stridor, decreased oxygen saturation, chest pain, flushing, hypotension	1. Stop the transfusion immediately. 2. Keep the vein open with a normal saline infusion. 3. Notify the primary care provider immediately. 4. Monitor vital signs. Administer cardiopulmonary resuscitation if needed. 5. Administer medications and/or oxygen as ordered.
Circulatory overload: blood administered faster than the circulation can accommodate	Dyspnea, orthopnea, crackles (rales), distended neck veins, tachycardia, hypertension	1. Stop the transfusion immediately. 2. Place the client upright. 3. Notify the primary care provider. 4. Administer diuretics and oxygen as ordered.
Sepsis: contaminated blood administered	High fever, chills, vomiting, diarrhea, hypotension, oliguria	1. Stop the transfusion immediately. 2. Keep the vein open with a normal saline infusion. 3. Notify the primary care provider. 4. Administer IV fluids and antibiotics. 5. Obtain a blood specimen from the client for culture. 6. Send the remaining blood and tubing to the laboratory.

*Nurses should follow the agency's protocol regarding interventions. These may vary among agencies.

Follow agency policies for verifying that the blood is correct for the client. The U.S. Food and Drug Administration (2011) requires blood products to have bar codes to allow for scanning and machine-readable information on blood and blood component container labels to help reduce medication errors.

Traditionally, blood has usually been administered through an #18- to #20-gauge IV needle or catheter with the belief being that using smaller needles may slow the infusion and damage blood cells (hemolysis). However, studies have shown that blood infusing through smaller-gauge catheters can be completed within 4 hours without hemolysis. Current practice guidelines established by the AABB and endorsed by the American Red Cross and the INS recommend that a #14- to #22-gauge IV catheter is acceptable for transfusion of cellular blood components in adults (Makic, Martin, Burns, Philbrick, & Rauen, 2013, p. 36). Large-bore IV catheters are difficult to insert in older adults and oncology clients. Using a smaller gauge catheter (i.e., #22 gauge) is more comfortable for the client, may reduce the number of needlesticks, and avoid complications (e.g., infiltration, hematomas, and phlebitis). Blood administration sets (Y-sets) are used to keep the vein open while starting the transfusion and to flush the line with normal saline before the blood enters the tubing (Figure 18–15 ■). The infusion tubing has a filter inside the drip chamber. A transfusion should be completed within 4 hours of initiation. The maximum time for use of a blood filter is 4 hours (Phillips & Gorski 2014). According to the AABB (2009), "with the exception of 0.9% sodium chloride, no drug or medication should be added to blood or blood components unless they have been approved by the FDA or there is documentation that the addition is safe and does not adversely affect the blood or blood component" (p. 42). If an additional unit needs to be transfused, follow the agency guidelines. A new blood administration set is to be used with each component (Phillips & Gorski, 2014). New IV tubing is used for administering other IV fluids following a transfusion.

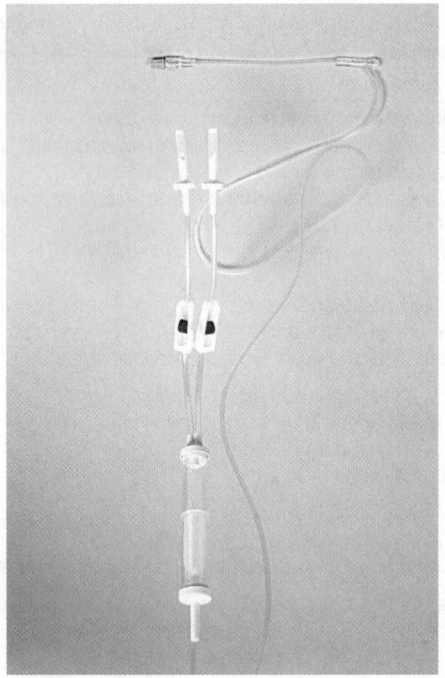

Figure 18–15 ■ Y-set blood tubing.

2014 The Joint Commission National Patient Safety Goals (2013)

GOAL 1: IMPROVE THE ACCURACY OF PATIENT IDENTIFICATION.

Goal 01.03.01: Eliminate transfusion errors related to patient misidentification.
- Before initiating a blood or blood component transfusion:
  - Match the blood or blood component to the order.
  - Match the patient to the blood or blood component.
  - Use a two-person verification process or a one-person verification process accompanied by automated identification technology, such as bar coding.

CLINICAL ALERT!

Normal saline must always be used when giving a blood transfusion. If the client has an infusion of any other IV solution, stop that infusion and flush the line with saline prior to initiating the transfusion, or establish IV access through an additional site. Solutions other than saline can cause damage to the blood components.

●○○● NURSING PROCESS: BLOOD TRANSFUSIONS

SKILL 18–7

Administering Blood Transfusions

ASSESSMENT

Assess:
- Vital signs.
- Physical examination including fluid balance and heart and lung sounds as manifestations of hypo- or hypervolemia.
- Status of infusion site.
- Blood test results such as hemoglobin value or platelet count.
- Any unusual symptoms.

PLANNING
- Review the client record regarding previous transfusions. Note any complications and how they were managed (e.g., allergies or previous adverse reactions to blood).
- Confirm the primary care provider's order for the number and type of units and the desired speed of infusion.
- In some agencies, written consent for transfusion is required. Check policy and obtain as indicated.
- Know the purpose of the transfusion:
  - To restore blood volume after severe hemorrhage.
  - To restore the oxygen-carrying capacity of the blood.
  - To provide plasma factors, such as antihemophilic factor (AHF) or factor VIII, or platelet concentrates, which prevent or treat bleeding.
- Plan to begin the transfusion as soon as the component is ready. A type and crossmatch can take several hours.
- Note any premedications ordered by the primary care provider (e.g., acetaminophen or diphenhydramine). Schedule their administration (usually 30 minutes prior to the transfusion).

DELEGATION

Due to the need for sterile technique and technical complexity, blood transfusion is not delegated to UAP. The nurse must ensure that the UAP knows what complications or adverse signs can occur and should be reported to the nurse. In some states, only RNs can administer blood or blood products.

Equipment
- Unit of whole blood, packed RBCs, or other component
- Blood administration set
- IV pump, if needed
- 250 mL normal saline for infusion
- IV pole
- Venipuncture set containing a #14- to #22-gauge catheter (if one is not already in place).
- Alcohol swabs
- Tape
- Clean gloves

Administering Blood Transfusions—*continued*

IMPLEMENTATION

Preparation

- If the client has an IV solution infusing, check whether the IV catheter and solution are appropriate to administer blood. The IV catheter size can range between #14 to #22 gauge, and the solution *must* be normal saline. Dextrose (which causes lysis of RBCs), Ringer's solution, medications and other additives, and hyperalimentation solutions are incompatible. Refer to step 6 below if the infusing solution is not compatible.
- If the client does not have an IV solution infusing, check agency policies. In some agencies an infusion must be running before the blood is obtained from the blood bank. In this case, you will need to perform a venipuncture on a suitable vein (see Skill 18–1) and start an IV infusion of normal saline.

Performance

1. Prior to performing the procedure, introduce self and verify the client's identity using agency protocol. Explain to the client what you are going to do, why it is necessary, and how he or she can participate. Instruct the client to report promptly any sudden chills, nausea, itching, rash, dyspnea, back pain, or other unusual symptoms.
2. Perform hand hygiene and observe other appropriate infection prevention procedures.
3. Provide for client privacy and prepare the client.
   - Assist the client to a comfortable position, either sitting or lying. Expose the IV site but provide for client privacy.
4. Prepare the infusion equipment.
   - Ensure that the blood filter inside the drip chamber is suitable for the blood components to be transfused. Attach the blood tubing to the blood filter, if necessary. **Rationale:** *Blood filters have a surface area large enough to allow the blood components through easily but are designed to trap clots.*
   - Apply gloves.
   - Close all the clamps on the Y-set: the main flow rate clamp and both Y-line clamps.
   - Insert the piercing pin (spike) into the saline solution.
   - Hang the container on the IV pole about 1 m (3 ft) above the venipuncture site.
5. Prime the tubing.
   - Open the upper clamp on the normal saline tubing, and squeeze the drip chamber until it covers the filter and one third of the drip chamber above the filter.
   - Tap the filter chamber to expel any residual air in the filter.
   - Open the main flow rate clamp, and prime the tubing with saline.
   - Close both clamps.
6. Start the saline solution.
   - If an IV solution incompatible with blood is infusing, stop the infusion and discard the solution and tubing according to agency policy.
   - Attach the blood tubing primed with normal saline to the IV catheter.
   - Open the saline and main flow rate clamps and adjust the flow rate. Use only the main flow rate clamp to adjust the rate.
   - Allow a small amount of solution to infuse to make sure there are no problems with the flow or with the venipuncture site. **Rationale:** *Infusing normal saline before initiating the transfusion also clears the IV catheter of incompatible solutions or medications.*

7. Obtain the correct blood component for the client.
   - Check the primary care provider's order with the requisition.
   - Check the requisition form and the blood bag label with a laboratory technician or according to agency policy. Specifically, check the client's name, identification number, blood type (A, B, AB, or O) and Rh group, the blood donor number, and the expiration date of the blood. Observe the blood for abnormal color, RBC clumping, gas bubbles, and extraneous material. Return outdated or abnormal blood to the blood bank.
   - With another nurse (most agencies require an RN), verify the following before initiating the transfusion (Phillips & Gorski, 2014, p. 731):
     a. *Order:* Check the blood or component against the primary care provider's written order.
     b. *Transfusion consent form:* Ensure the form is completed per facility policy.
     c. *Client identification:* The name and identification number on the client's identification band must be identical to the name and number attached to the unit of blood.
     d. *Unit identification:* The unit identification number on the blood container, the transfusion form, and the tag attached to the unit must agree.
     e. *Blood type:* The ABO group and Rh type on the primary label of the donor unit must agree with those recorded on the transfusion form.
     f. *Expiration:* The expiration date and time of the donor unit should be verified as acceptable.
     g. *Compatibility:* The interpretation of compatibility testing must be recorded on the transfusion form and on the tag attached to the unit.
     h. *Appearance:* There should be no discoloration, foaming, bubbles, cloudiness, clots or clumps, or loss of integrity of the container.

CLINICAL ALERT!

It is safer to have one nurse read the information for verification to the other nurse; this avoids errors that can be made if both nurses look at the tags together.

- If any of the information does not match *exactly*, notify the charge nurse and the blood bank. Do not administer blood until discrepancies are corrected or clarified.
- Sign the appropriate form with the other nurse according to agency policy.
- Make sure that the blood is left at room temperature for no more than 30 minutes before starting the transfusion. Agencies may designate different times at which the blood must be returned to the blood bank if the transfusion has not been started. **Rationale:** *As blood components warm, the risk of bacterial growth also increases.* If the start of the transfusion is unexpectedly delayed, return the blood to the blood bank after 30 minutes. Do **not** store blood in the unit refrigerator. **Rationale:** *The temperature of unit refrigerators is not precisely regulated and the blood may be damaged.*

Continued on page 470

SKILL 18-7

Administering Blood Transfusions—*continued*

8. Prepare the blood bag.
   - Invert the blood bag gently several times to mix the cells with the plasma. **Rationale:** *Rough handling can damage the cells.*
   - Expose the port on the blood bag by pulling back the tabs.
   - Insert the remaining Y-set spike into the blood bag.
   - Suspend the blood bag.
9. Establish the blood transfusion.
   - Close the upper clamp below the IV saline solution container.
   - Open the upper clamp below the blood bag. The blood will run into the saline-filled drip chamber. If necessary, squeeze the drip chamber to reestablish the liquid level with the drip chamber one-third full. (Tap the filter to expel any residual air within the filter.)
   - Readjust the flow rate with the main clamp.
   - Remove and discard gloves.
   - Perform hand hygiene.
10. Observe the client closely for the first 15 minutes.
   - Phillips and Gorski (2014) reported that the AABB recommends that "transfusions of RBCs be started at 1–2 mL/min for the first 15 minutes of the transfusion" (p. 732). **Rationale:** *This small amount is enough to produce a severe reaction but small enough that the reaction could be treated successfully.*
   - Note adverse reactions, such as chills, nausea, vomiting, skin rash, dyspnea, back pain, or tachycardia. **Rationale:** *The earlier a transfusion reaction occurs, the more severe it tends to be. Promptly identifying such reactions helps to minimize the consequences.*
   - Remind the client to call a nurse immediately if any unusual symptoms are felt during the transfusion such as chills, nausea, itching, rash, dyspnea, or back pain.
   - If any of these reactions occur, report these to the nurse in charge, and take appropriate nursing action. See Table 18–3 on page 467.
11. Document relevant data.
   - Record starting the blood, including vital signs, type of blood, blood unit number, sequence number (e.g., #1 of three ordered units), site of the venipuncture, size of the catheter, and drip rate.

SAMPLE DOCUMENTATION

1/21/2015 1400 1 unit of PRBCs (#65234) hung to be infused over 3 hours. IV site in (L) forearm with 22 gauge angiocath. VS taken (see transfusion record). Informed to contact nurse if begins to experience any discomfort during transfusion. Stated he would use the call light.
—————————————————————————————— C. Jones, RN

12. Monitor the client.
   - Fifteen minutes after initiating the transfusion (or according to agency policy), check the vital signs. If there are no signs of a reaction, establish the required flow rate. Most adults can tolerate receiving one unit of blood in 1.5 to 2 hours. Do not transfuse a unit of blood for longer than 4 hours.

   - Assess the client, including vital signs per agency policy. If the client has a reaction and the blood is discontinued, send the blood bag and tubing to the laboratory for investigation of the blood. Check agency policy.
13. Terminate the transfusion.
   - Apply clean gloves.
   - If no infusion is to follow, clamp the blood tubing. Check agency protocol to determine if the blood component bag needs to be returned or if the blood bag and tubing can be disposed of in a biohazard container. The IV line can be discontinued or capped with an adapter, or a new infusion line and solution container may be added. If another transfusion is to follow, clamp the blood tubing and open the saline infusion arm. Check agency protocol. A new blood administration set is to be used with each component (Phillips & Gorski, 2014, p. 733).
   - If the primary IV is to be continued, flush the maintenance line with saline solution. Disconnect the blood tubing system and reestablish the IV infusion using new tubing. Adjust the drip to the desired rate. Often a normal saline or other solution is kept running in case of delayed reaction to the blood.
   - Measure vital signs.
14. Follow agency protocol for appropriate disposition of the used supplies.
   - Discard the administration set according to agency practice.
   - Dispose of blood bags and administration sets.
     a. On the requisition attached to the blood unit, fill in the time the transfusion was completed and the amount transfused.
     b. Attach one copy of the requisition to the client's record and another to the empty blood bag if required by agency policy.
     c. Agency policy generally involves returning the bag to the blood bank for reference in case of subsequent or delayed adverse reaction.
   - Remove and discard gloves.
   - Perform hand hygiene.
15. Document relevant data.
   - Record completion of the transfusion, the amount of blood absorbed, the blood unit number, and the vital signs. If the primary IV infusion was continued, record connecting it. Also record the transfusion on the IV flow sheet and intake and output record.

SAMPLE DOCUMENTATION

4/21/2015 1420 c/o feeling warm, headache, & backache. Skin flushed. T 39.1°C (102.6°F), BP 140/90 mmHg, P 112 beats/min, R 28/min. Approximately 50 mL PRBCs (#65234) infused over past 20 minutes. Infusion stopped. Tubing changed, NS infusing at 15 mL/h. Blood bag and attached tubing sent to blood bank. Dr. Riley notified.
—————————————————————————————— C. Jones, RN

EVALUATION

- Perform follow-up based on findings or outcomes that deviated from expected or normal for the client. Relate findings to previous data if available.

- Report significant deviations from normal to the primary care provider.

WHAT IF   Transfusion Reaction

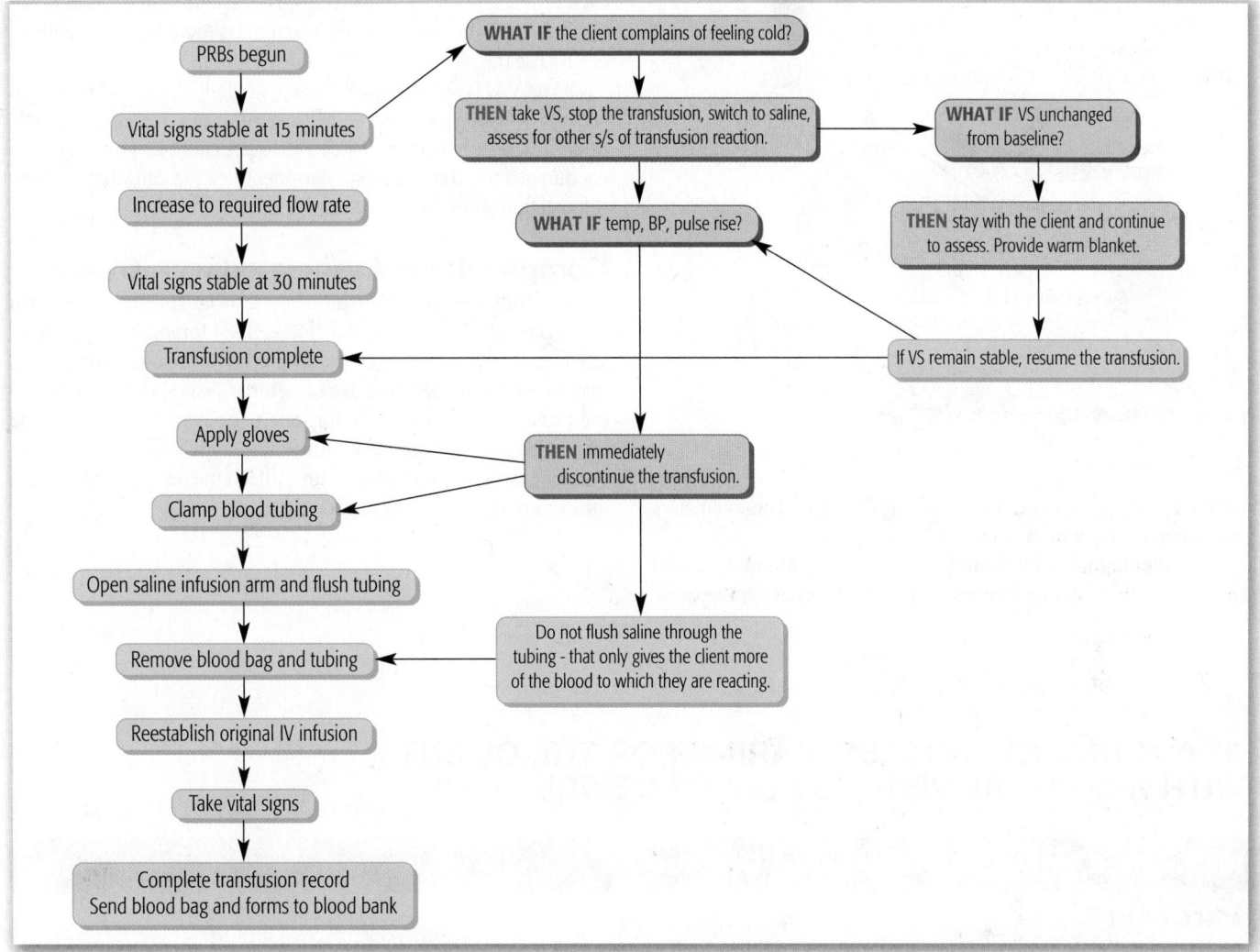

CENTRAL VENOUS ACCESS DEVICES

Sometimes, access to the vascular system through peripheral IV lines is not possible or not desirable. In these cases, central venous access devices (CVADs) may be used. A CVAD is a catheter inserted into a large vein located centrally in the body. The tip of the catheter may terminate in the vein, the superior vena cava, or in the right atrium of the heart. X-ray confirms correct placement of the catheter.

Physicians usually insert CVADs, although nurses who are specially trained may insert certain types. CVADs are inserted primarily to:

- Spare the client numerous venipunctures associated with short-term peripheral IV catheters.
- Administer solutions that are highly irritating to smaller veins (including some types of parenteral nutrition—see Chapter 19 ∞).
- Provide access for frequent blood sampling.
- Monitor central venous pressure (CVP).

Types of CVADs

CVADs are catheters of variable length, usually made of polyurethane or silicone. There are four major types: (1) percutaneous

nontunneled catheters, (2) PICCs, (3) subcutaneously tunneled catheters, and (4) implanted vascular access ports. Percutaneous CVADs are commonly inserted through the chest wall into the subclavian or internal jugular vein and are used primarily in acute care settings (see Figure 18–4 on page 446). A PICC, the most common CVAD used in all settings, is a long venous catheter 45 to 60 cm (18 to 24 in.) in length, inserted in an arm vein and extending into the distal third of the superior vena cava (Figure 18–16 ■). The PICC may be used for short-term needs in the acute care setting and for clients who require longer term infusion needs beyond the acute care setting (Phillips & Gorski, 2014, p. 280). A variation of the PICC, a peripherally inserted midline catheter, is 8 to 20 cm (3 to 8 in.) long and used for therapy lasting 1 to 4 weeks (INS, 2011a, S37). Both catheters are used for inpatient and outpatient settings.

For percutaneous insertion, the practitioner inserts a catheter with needle (stylet) to penetrate the vein. Once the vein is entered and the stylet placed correctly, the catheter is advanced over or through the (stylet) to the desired length and sutured or secured in place. When the catheter is in place, the stylet is withdrawn.

The subcutaneous CVAD is also inserted surgically. Because these catheters are implanted through a subcutaneous tunnel, they are often referred to as subcutaneously tunneled catheters. Examples

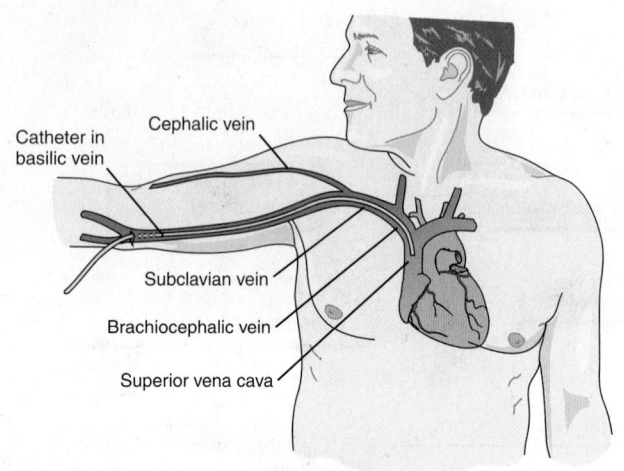

Catheter in basilic vein

Cephalic vein

Subclavian vein

Brachiocephalic vein

Superior vena cava

Figure 18–16 ■ Placement of a PICC line.

are the *Hickman*, *Broviac*, and *Groshong* catheters. These catheters may remain in place for many years.

The nontunneled, PICC, and subcutaneously tunneled CVADs can have from one to four lumens with each lumen having a separate port. These allow simultaneous infusion of total parenteral nutrition therapy, CVP readings, blood transfusions, antibiotics, blood drawing, and any other needed uses. The nurse should be consistent and always use the same port for the same purpose.

An IVAD (see Figure 18–5) is a single-lumen subclavian vein catheter attached to a reservoir that is surgically placed completely under the skin, usually in the client's upper chest. Clients should be encouraged to carry a medical alert identification card that contains information about their implanted port.

Complications Associated with CVADs

Many of the sepsis (infection) problems associated with conventional IV therapy are also associated with CVADs. Moreover, the problems are magnified because (1) clients with CVADs are often critically ill, may be malnourished, and are sometimes immunosuppressed; (2) the catheters are left in place for long periods of time; and (3) the intralipids used in parenteral nutrition therapy support the growth of a wide variety of microorganisms. Infection control is therefore of utmost importance during CVAD therapy.

●○○● NURSING PROCESS: CARING FOR THE CLIENT WITH A CENTRAL VENOUS ACCESS DEVICE

Managing Central Venous Access Devices

SKILL 18–8

ASSESSMENT
In maintaining the CVAD, the nurse examines the appearance of the infusion site, patency of the system, type of fluid being infused and rate of flow, and the response of the client.

Gather the pertinent data:
- From the client record, determine the purpose of the CVAD, how and when it was inserted, and the type of catheter used.
- Determine the type of infusion, rate of flow, and infusion schedule.

PLANNING
Review the client record regarding the insertion of the CVAD and previous infusions. Note any complications and how they were managed.

DELEGATION

Due to the need for sterile technique and technical complexity, the maintaining and monitoring of CVADs are not delegated to UAP. UAP may care for clients with CVADs, and the nurse must ensure that the UAP knows what complications or adverse signs should be reported to the nurse.

Equipment
- Soft-tipped clamp without teeth
- Alcohol, CHG wipes
- TSM dressing
- 10-mL syringe
- Sterile normal saline
- Heparin flush solution (e.g., 10 units heparin per milliliter)

Managing Central Venous Access Devices—*continued*

IMPLEMENTATION
Performance

1. Prior to performing the procedure, introduce self and verify the client's identity using agency protocol. Explain to the client what you are going to do, why it is necessary, and how he or she can participate.
2. Perform hand hygiene and observe other appropriate infection prevention procedures.
3. Position the client appropriately.
   • Assist the client to a comfortable position, either sitting or lying. Expose the IV site but provide for client privacy.
4. Label each lumen of multilumen catheters.
   • Mark each lumen or port of the tubing with a description of its purpose (e.g., the distal lumen for CVP monitoring and infusing blood, the middle lumen for parenteral nutrition, and the proximal lumen for other IV solutions or for blood samples).

   or

   • Use a color code established by the agency to label the proximal, middle, and distal lumens. **Rationale:** *Labeling prevents mixing of incompatible medications or infusions and reserves each lumen for specific therapies.*
5. Monitor tubing connections.
   • Ensure that all tubing connections are secured according to agency protocol.
   • Check the connections every 2 hours.
   • Tape cap ends if agency protocol indicates.
6. Change tubing according to agency policy.
   • See Skill 18–2.
   • Parenteral nutrition tubing should be changed every 24 hours (Phillips & Gorski, 2014).
7. Change the catheter site dressing according to agency policy.
   • Use strict aseptic technique (including the use of sterile gloves and mask) when caring for CVADs.
   • The frequency of dressing changes is dependent on the dressing material. TSM dressings or tape and gauze are acceptable; however, gauze dressings do not allow for visualization of the insertion site and need to be changed every 48 hours or if the site requires visual inspection (Phillips & Gorski, 2014, p. 501). In contrast, TSM dressings allow for visualization and can be left in place for a maximum of 7 days if they remain clean, dry, and intact (INS, 2011a, p. S63). All dressings should be changed when loose or soiled.
   • Assess the site for any redness, swelling, tenderness, or drainage. Compare the length of the external portion of the catheter with its documented length to assess for possible displacement. Report and document any position changes or signs of infection.
   • Follow agency protocol for cleaning solutions and types of dressings. CHG is the preferred agent to clean the insertion site.
   • Clean the skin around the site with CHG solution, using a back-and-forth motion for at least 30 seconds (INS, 2011b). Allow the site to air-dry. A round dressing impregnated with CHG can also be applied to the insertion site to prevent catheter-related bloodstream infections (CRBSIs). ❶
   • Apply a new stabilization device.
   • Apply a sterile dressing.
8. Administer all infusions as ordered.
   • Use an EID for all fluids (see Skill 18–3).
   • Maintain the fluid flow at the prescribed rate.
   • Whenever the line is interrupted for any reason, instruct the client to perform Valsalva's maneuver. If the client is

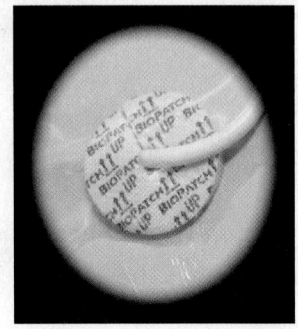

❶ Protective disk with chlorhexidine gluconate (CHG) (BioPatch®).

unable to perform Valsalva's maneuver, place the client in a supine position, and clamp the lumen of the catheter with a soft-tipped clamp. Place a strip of tape over the catheter (about 8 cm [3 in.] from the end) before applying the clamp. **Rationale:** *The clamp is placed over the taped area to prevent damage to the tubing. A clamp without teeth prevents piercing.*

9. Cap lumens without continuous infusions, and flush them regularly.
   • Change the catheter cap as indicated by agency protocol. The catheter hub can be a source of infection. A 15-second scrub of the connection surface of the needleless connector has been shown to prohibit microorganism entry on the surface (Moureau & Dawson, 2010). Also available are commercial single-use Luer access valve disinfection caps. This cap contains isopropyl alcohol, which cleans the needleless connector before access and also protects it from contamination between uses. The cap is twisted onto the needleless connector and left in place until the next access to the connector is needed. The nurse removes and discards the old cap, and the connector is ready for use without further wiping. A study conducted by Wright et al. (2013) concluded that disinfecting caps filled with alcohol-soaked sponges reduced bacterial contamination in catheter hubs and the rate of CRBSIs. See ❷ to ❺.

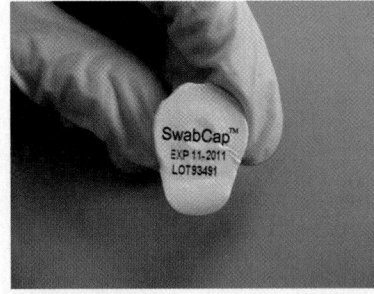

❷ Disinfecting cap (SwabCap™).

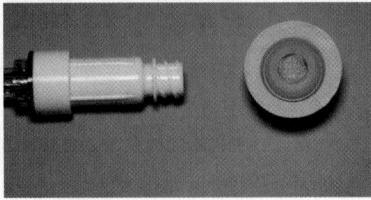

❸ Cap contains disinfecting solution.

Continued on page 474

Managing Central Venous Access Devices—*continued*

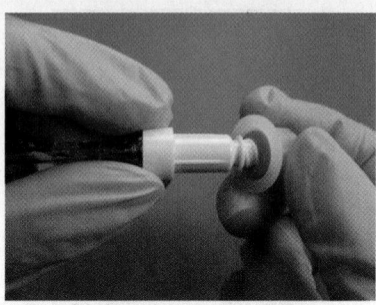

④ Twist cap onto needleless connector.

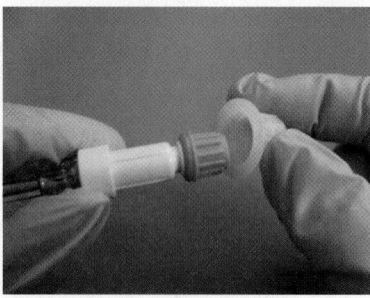

⑤ Remove outer packaging and leave the cap in place.

SAFETY ALERT! | SAFETY

2014 The Joint Commission National Patient Safety Goals (2013)

GOAL 7: REDUCE THE RISK OF HEALTH CARE–ASSOCIATED INFECTIONS.

Goal 7.04.01: Implement evidence-based practices to prevent central line–associated bloodstream infections.

- Perform hand hygiene prior to catheter manipulation.
- Use a standardized protocol to disinfect catheter hubs and injection ports before accessing the ports.

- The solution used and frequency of flushing are determined by agency protocol for the specific type of port being used. Heparin-induced thrombocytopenia (HIT) has been reported with the use of heparin flush solutions. If heparin is used as part of the flushing protocol, the concentration should not be in amounts that cause systemic anticoagulation but in the lowest possible concentration to maintain patency (e.g., 10 units/mL). Many agencies are switching to needleless IV connectors that can be flushed with normal saline solution only.
- Flush the catheter before and after each dose of medication. **Rationale:** *The initial flush is to assess patency of the catheter, and the flush after administration of the medication is to ensure that the complete dose has entered the bloodstream and to prevent contact between incompatible medications.*
- Use a 10-mL syringe to flush the catheter. Never apply force if you feel resistance.
- CVADs need to be locked after the final flush solution to decrease the risk of occlusion (INS, 2011a). Locking a cath-

eter creates a column of fluid inside the lumen to maintain patency (Hadaway, 2012, p. 42). The process for locking a catheter varies depending on the manufacturer of the needleless connector.
- Blood reflux into the catheter lumen after flushing increases the risk of infection. Positive-pressure valve caps on central line catheters can help prevent blood reflux when used with negative-pressure needleless infusion caps (Mathers, 2011, p. 65). Thus, it is important for the nurse to know the type of needleless connector being used: positive-pressure, negative-pressure, or neutral displacement needleless connector.

10. Administer medications as ordered.
   - If a capped lumen used for medication has been flushed with heparin solution, aspirate and discard or flush the line with 5 to 10 mL of normal saline according to agency protocol before giving the medication. **Rationale:** *Many medications are incompatible with heparin.*
   - After the medication is instilled through the lumen, inject normal saline first and then the heparin flush solution if indicated by agency protocol. **Rationale:** *The saline solution flushes the line of the medication. The heparin maintains the patency of the catheter by preventing blood clotting.*

11. Monitor the client for complications.
   - Assess the client's vital signs, skin color, mental alertness, appearance of the catheter site, and presence of adverse symptoms at least every 4 hours.
   - If an air embolism is suspected, give the client 100% oxygen by mask, place the client in a left Trendelenburg position, and notify the primary care provider. **Rationale:** *Lowering the head increases intrathoracic pressure, decreasing the flow of air into the vein during inhalation. A left side-lying position helps prevent the air from moving to the pulmonary artery.*
   - If sepsis is suspected, replace a parenteral nutrition, blood, or other infusion with 5% or 10% dextrose solution, change the IV tubing and dressing, save the remaining solution for lab analysis, record the lot number of the solution and any additives, and notify the primary care provider immediately. When changing the dressing, take a culture of the catheter site as ordered by the primary care provider or according to agency protocol.
   - If a lumen appears to be occluded, the cause could be thrombus, precipitate, or mechanical. An x-ray is done to determine if the catheter is properly located. Fluoroscopy can demonstrate the presence of a thrombus by indicating the fluid path through the catheter. If a thrombus is found, thrombolytic therapy using an enzyme such as recombinant tissue plasminogen activator (t-PA) is indicated. Follow agency guidelines for use of these agents. If drugs infused into the lumen may have created a precipitate, the pharmacist can assist in determining whether an acidic, alkaline, or lipid precipitate is likely and the appropriate solution to dissolve it. If the occlusion is mechanical, consult policy to determine if the nurse may reposition the catheter or if the primary care provider must be notified.

12. Document all relevant information.
   - Record the date and time of any infusion started; type of solution, drip rate, and number of milliliters infusing per hour; dressing or tubing changes; appearance of insertion site; and all other nursing assessments.

EVALUATION
- Perform follow-up based on findings or outcomes that deviated from expected or normal for the client. Relate findings to previous data if available.

- Report significant deviations from normal to the primary care provider.

LIFESPAN CONSIDERATIONS **Managing Central Venous Access Devices**

CHILDREN
- Explain all procedures to the young client beforehand, using play therapy to demonstrate. Encourage questions, and be alert for nonverbal cues. Children may not understand things that seem obvious to adults. For example, a child may think the IV therapy is a punishment.
- Young clients can help with catheter care procedures by holding nonsterile supplies and handing them to the nurse. Participating gives the child a sense of control.
- Tell the young client not to play with the IV tubing, flow clamp, or any other part of the equipment. Encourage the child to decorate the IV tubing with colorful stickers.

Ambulatory and Community Settings **Managing Central Venous Access Devices** | **PATIENT-CENTERED CARE**

- When caring for a central catheter in the home, place equipment on a clean towel or nonsterile drape.
- Assess the home environment and help the client choose a clean, dry place to store the IV supplies.
- Evaluate the client's or caregiver's ability and willingness to perform CVAD care at home. Ask for a return demonstration of all teaching.
- Emphasize the need for hand hygiene and clean technique when working with the CVAD.
- Ensure that the client knows how and where to obtain supplies.
- Discuss possible complications of a CVAD, such as phlebitis, sepsis, or thrombus formation, and explain when to notify the health care provider.

Changing CVAD Dressings

For tunneled catheters that have healed, no dressing is indicated. Options for CVAD dressings include the TSM dressing or the gauze and tape dressing. The INS (2011a) recommends changing TSM dressings when they are damp, loosened, or soiled or at least every 7 days (Phillips & Gorski, 2014, p. 501). Gauze dressings should be changed every 48 hours or if the site requires visual inspection (INS, 2011b). No antibacterial ointment should be applied to the site. If the infusion tubing also requires changing, it may be desirable to do this at the same time as the dressing change (see Skill 18–2).

●○● NURSING PROCESS: CHANGING CENTRAL VENOUS ACCESS DEVICE DRESSINGS

Performing Central Venous Access Device Dressing Changes

ASSESSMENT
Gather the pertinent data. Know the purpose of the central line. Confirm the primary care provider's order for the central line (i.e., whether it is to have an infusion or be capped). Determine:
- Any allergy to tape, iodine, or components of fluids infused.
- Any bleeding tendency. Such clients, especially those receiving anticoagulants, require special observation.
- Client's ability to understand instructions during the procedure and to perform Valsalva's maneuver.

PLANNING
Review the client record regarding previous care of CVADs. Note any complications and how they were managed.

DELEGATION

Due to the need for sterile technique and technical complexity, changing a CVAD dressing is not delegated to UAP. UAP may care for clients with CVADs, and the nurse must ensure that the UAP knows what complications or adverse signs should be reported to the nurse.

Equipment
- Central line (CVAD) dressing set (recommended)
  or
- Two face masks (one for the nurse and one for the client)
- 2% CHG wipes
- Clean gloves
- Sterile gloves
- Catheter securement device (according to agency policy)
- TSM dressing such as Op-Site or Tegaderm
- Nonallergenic 2.5-cm (1-in.) tape
- Dressing label
- Sterile drape

IMPLEMENTATION
Performance
1. Prior to performing the procedure, introduce self and verify the client's identity using agency protocol. Explain to the client what you are going to do, why it is necessary, and how he or she can participate.
2. Perform hand hygiene and observe other appropriate infection prevention procedures.

3. Provide for client privacy and position the client.
   - Assist the client to a comfortable position, either sitting or lying. The client should be supine if the tubing or injection cap is also being changed. **Rationale:** *An upright position during these techniques increases the chances of an air embolism forming.* Expose the CVAD site but provide for client privacy.

Continued on page 476

SKILL 18-9

SKILL 18–9

Performing Central Venous Access Device Dressing Changes—*continued*

4. Prepare the client.
   - Apply a mask, and have the client apply a mask (if tolerated or as agency protocol indicates), and/or ask the client to turn the head away from the insertion site. **Rationale:** *This helps protect the insertion site from the nurse's and client's nasal and oral microorganisms. Turning the client's head also makes the site more accessible.*
5. Prepare the equipment.
   - Establish a sterile field and place the sterile supplies.
6. Remove the old dressing.
   - Apply clean gloves.
   - For a TSM dressing, pull both sides away from the insertion site, stretching it to gently lift off perpendicular to the skin toward the insertion site. ❶ For taped dressings, hold the catheter with one hand and gently pull the tape in the direction of the catheter. **Rationale:** *This prevents catheter displacement and skin irritation.*
   - Remove the stabilization device.
   - Inspect the skin for signs of irritation or infection. Inspect the catheter for signs of drainage. If infection is suspected, take a swab of the drainage for culture, label it, send it to the laboratory, and notify the primary care provider. Measure the length of the external portion of the catheter extending from the skin exit site to the injection cap or infusion tubing. **Rationale:** *This measurement allows comparison with previous measurements to determine if the catheter is migrating in or out.*
   - Remove and discard gloves and dressing.
   - Perform hand hygiene.
7. Cleanse the site.
   - Apply sterile gloves.
   - Clean the catheter insertion site with CHG-based skin prep in a back-and-forth motion, with plenty of friction for a minimum of 30 seconds. ❷ **Rationale:** *The friction allows the solution to get as far as possible into the skin.* The prepped site will be approximately the size of the dressing, 5 to 10 cm (2 to 4 in.). Let the skin dry. If cleansing the skin with povidone-iodine, apply using swabsticks in a concentric circle beginning at the catheter insertion site, moving outward. It must dry completely (e.g., at least 2 minutes) for adequate antisepsis (INS, 2011b, p. 89).
   - If possible, use one hand to lift the catheter so you can clean under it.
   - For additional protection against CRBSI, some agencies use CHG-impregnated sponges at the catheter exit site (see ❶ in Skill 18–8).
8. Apply the new dressing.
   - Apply the stabilization device, surgical strips or sterile tape (INS, 2011b).
   - Apply a new transparent dressing over the exposed catheter, including the hub. **Rationale:** *This type of dressing allows gas exchange but is impermeable to liquids and microorganisms. It also allows visualization of the site.*
   - Remove and discard gloves.
   - Perform hand hygiene.
   - Label the dressing with catheter information, date and time of the dressing change, and your initials.

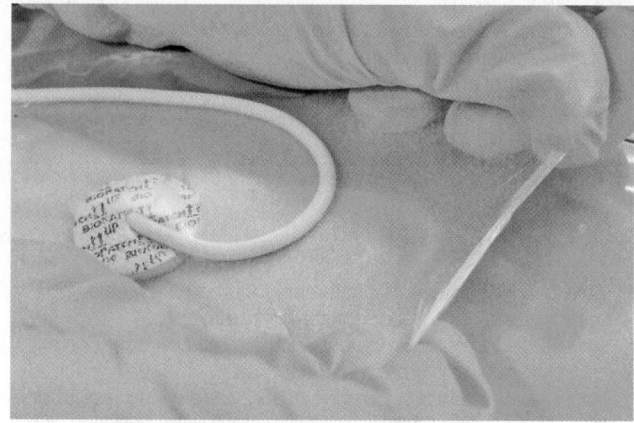

❶ Removing the central line catheter dressing.

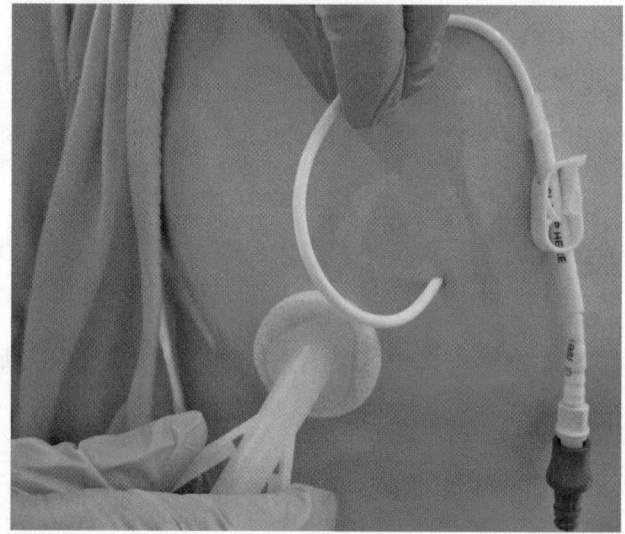

❷ Cleansing the central line insertion site using back-and-forth motions.

9. Document all relevant information.
   - Record the appearance of the catheter insertion site: presence of drainage, the type of dressing applied, client complaints or concerns, and patency of tubing (if evaluated).

SAMPLE DOCUMENTATION

4/13/2015 2030 Dressing changed on Broviac catheter. External portion of 12.7 cm unchanged from previous dressing change. Skin without redness, drainage, or swelling. IV infusing freely. No c/o discomfort. Transparent dressing reapplied using sterile technique. —————————————— J. Valenzuela, RN

EVALUATION

- Perform follow-up based on findings or outcomes that deviated from expected or normal for the client. Relate findings to previous data if available.
- Report significant deviations from normal to the primary care provider.

Implanted Vascular Access Devices

As noted earlier, IVADs or ports are surgically placed completely under the skin. Thus, they have the advantages of not being visible and not requiring dressing changes or other care associated with central lines that have an external component. However, IVADs must be accessed using a needle inserted through the client's skin. This needle must be a noncoring **Huber needle** so that pieces of the port septum are not removed each time the needle is inserted through the septum and into the port reservoir (see Figure 18–5 on page 446 and Figure 18–17 ■).

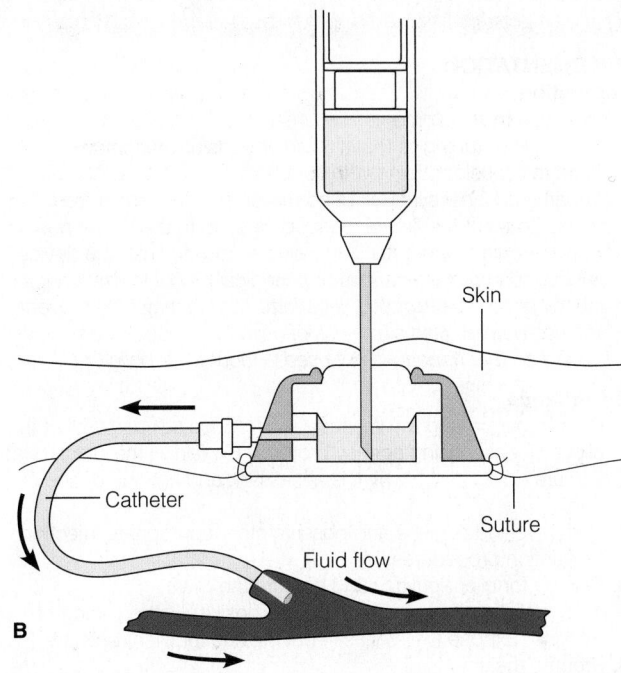

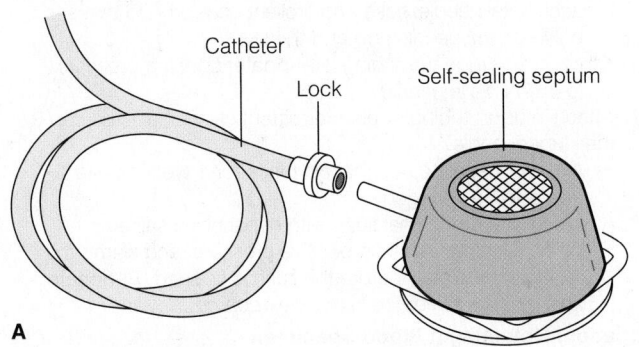

Figure 18–17 ■ An implanted vascular access device: *A,* components; *B,* the device in place.

●○● NURSING PROCESS: IMPLANTED VASCULAR ACCESS DEVICES

Working with Implanted Vascular Access Devices

ASSESSMENT
Gather the pertinent data. Know the purpose of the IVAD. Confirm the primary care provider's order for the IVAD (i.e., whether it is to have an infusion).

PLANNING
Review the client record regarding previous care of the IVAD. Note any complications and how they were managed.

DELEGATION

Due to the need for sterile technique and technical complexity, accessing an IVAD is not delegated to UAP. UAP may care for clients with such devices, and the nurse must ensure that the UAP knows what complications or adverse signs should be reported to the nurse.

Equipment
• IV solution container and administration set
or
• Blood or blood product with transfusion set and priming saline
or
• Blood specimen tubes and syringe and needle
• Sterile gloves
• Mask
• 10-mL syringes of normal saline flush and 5-mL syringes of heparinized saline (10 units/mL of heparin) according to agency policy
• 2% lidocaine with subcutaneous syringe and needle (optional)
• CHG swabs

• Straight or right-angled Huber needle, with attached extension tubing and in-line clamp ❶
• Adhesive or nonallergenic tape
• Dressing materials (e.g., 2×2 gauze, TSM dressing)

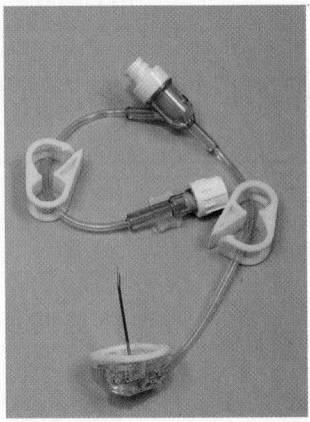

❶ A right angled Huber needle with extension tubing.

Continued on page 478

Working with Implanted Vascular Access Devices—*continued*

IMPLEMENTATION

Preparation

- Assemble the equipment.
- Attach the IV tubing to the infusion or transfusion container.
- Prime the infusion tubing with fluid.
- Prepare and label syringes of normal saline and heparinized saline. Connect the first of these to be used to the Huber needle. Saline followed by heparinized saline is used to flush the device before and after medications or periodically if not in use (check agency policy). **Rationale:** *Heparinized saline may help prevent clotting. There is also some risk of heparin-induced thrombocytopenia so that heparin is not used without clear policy.*

Performance

1. Prior to performing the procedure, introduce self and verify the client's identity using agency protocol. Explain to the client what you are going to do, why it is necessary, and how he or she can participate.
2. Perform hand hygiene and observe other appropriate infection prevention procedures.
3. Provide for client privacy and prepare the client.
   - Assist the client to a comfortable position, either sitting or lying. Expose the IVAD site but provide for client privacy.
4. Prepare the site.
   - Locate the IVAD device and its septum, the disk at the center of the port where the needle will be inserted.
   - Prepare the skin in accordance with agency policy and let the area dry after applying solutions.
   - Apply sterile gloves and mask.
   - *Optional:* Inject 2% lidocaine subcutaneously over the needle insertion site. **Rationale:** *This anesthetizes the area for injection.* It may be ordered during the first few weeks after the implant surgery, when the area is tender and swollen and more pain from the needle puncture is felt. Other topical anesthetics may be used.
   - An ice pack may be placed over the site for several minutes to reduce discomfort from the needle puncture.
5. Insert the Huber needle.
   - Grasp the base of the IVAD device between two fingers of your nondominant hand to stabilize it. IVADs may have top entry or side entry ports, depending on the design.
   - Insert the needle at a 90° angle to the septum, and push it firmly through the skin and septum until it contacts the base of the IVAD chamber.
   - Avoid tilting or moving the needle when the septum is punctured. **Rationale:** *Needle movement can damage the septum and cause fluid leakage.*
   - When the needle contacts the base of the septum, aspirate for blood to determine correct placement. If no blood is obtained, remove the needle and repeat the procedure after having the client move the arms and change position. **Rationale:** *Movement can free the catheter tip from the vessel wall, where it may be lodged.*

- Infuse the saline flush. There should be no discomfort or sign of subcutaneous infiltration with infusion of the flush.
6. Prevent manipulation or dislodgment of the needle.
   - If the needle will remain in place for longer than needed to withdraw a blood sample or flush an unused port, secure the needle.
   - Support the Huber needle with 2×2 dressings and apply an occlusive transparent dressing to the needle site. Some manufacturers' devices include a safety lock to decrease accidental needlesticks and a client comfort pad that sits between the needle hub and the skin.
   - Loop and tape the tubing. **Rationale:** *Looping prevents tension on the needle.*
7. Attach infusion tubing or an intermittent infusion access cap to the Huber needle.
   - A Huber needle can remain in place for 1 week before it needs to be changed.
8. After use, perform a final flush with heparinized saline.
   - When flushing, maintain positive pressure, and clamp the tubing immediately before the flush is finished. **Rationale:** *These actions avoid reflux of the heparnized saline.*

Variation: Obtaining a Blood Specimen

To obtain a blood specimen:

- Withdraw 10 mL of blood (or an amount according to agency policy) and discard it. **Rationale:** *This initial specimen may be diluted with saline and heparin from previous flushes.*
- Draw up the required amount of blood and transfer it to the appropriate containers.
- Slowly instill 10 mL of normal saline, according to agency policy. **Rationale:** *This thoroughly flushes the catheter of blood.*
- Inject 5 mL of heparin flush solution to prevent clotting.
9. Remove and discard gloves.
   - Perform hand hygiene.
10. Document all relevant information.
    - Record the appearance of the IVAD site, any difficulty accessing the port and interventions used, presence of drainage, the type of dressing applied, infusions given, and client complaints or concerns. Note any clinical signs indicating venous thrombosis (pain in the neck, arm, and/or shoulder on the side of the insertion site; neck and/or supraclavicular swelling); infection (redness and swelling at the site); and dislodgment of the needle or catheter (shortness of breath, chest pain, coolness in the chest).

SAMPLE DOCUMENTATION

4/14/2015 0900 Implanted port right chest with skin intact and no swelling. Accessed with #20-gauge 1-inch Huber needle. Prompt blood return, flushed without difficulty. IV infusion begun. No c/o of discomfort. ————————————————— G. Young, RN

EVALUATION

- Perform follow-up based on findings or outcomes that deviated from expected or normal for the client. Relate findings to previous data if available.

- Report significant deviations from normal to the primary care provider.

LIFESPAN CONSIDERATIONS **Working with Implanted Vascular Access Devices**

CHILDREN

- Explain all procedures to the young client beforehand, using play therapy to demonstrate. Encourage questions, and be alert for nonverbal cues. Children may not understand things that seem obvious to adults. For example, a child may think the IV therapy is a punishment.

- IVADs have less impact on self-image than CVTCs because they are not readily visible and require no daily care. As with ports in adults, the IVAD may be used for infusions or for drawing blood.

FOCUSING ON CLINICAL THINKING

Consider This

1. Your client has had surgery on the left arm and now requires IV antibiotics. The client is right-handed. Where would you place the IV and why?

2. You have plugged new IV tubing into the peripheral catheter when you notice that there are several inches of air in the tubing. How would you handle this situation?

3. One hour after starting a new IV on a pump/controller, 125 mL was supposed to have been infused. You check the amount infused but find that slightly less than 100 mL has gone in. What steps would you follow?

4. At shift report, the off-going nurse states that there is 300 mL left in an IV of D_5W with 40 mEq of KCl running at 100 mL/h. When you check the IV about 30 minutes later, it is empty and the client is complaining of stinging at the site. There is redness at the site extending about 5 cm (2 in.) along the vein. What would you do?

5. It is now time to irrigate an intermittent infusion device for patency. The catheter has been in place 48 hours. The transparent membrane dressing shows dried blood. You are unable to aspirate a blood return. What would you do?

6. In discontinuing an IV catheter, you have put pressure on the site after removing the catheter. What other steps should you take?

7. Proper technique for beginning a blood transfusion requires the nurse to close the upper clamp on the priming saline before opening the clamp to the blood. What would happen if the nurse fails to close the saline clamp?

8. Your client will be receiving chemotherapy for cancer for 6 months. The client requests your input on the primary care provider's statement that either an implanted port or a tunneled central catheter would be advisable. How would you respond regarding the advantages and disadvantages of each?

9. Your client with a central IV catheter is unable to perform Valsalva's maneuver. What would you do when disconnecting the tubing to attach a new infusion set?

10. Upon assessing your restless client, you find that the Huber needle has been pulled out of the client's implanted port. What would be your next steps?

See Focusing on Clinical Thinking answers on student resource website.

TEST YOUR KNOWLEDGE

1. The nurse is caring for a client receiving an antineoplastic medication intravenously. The nurse discovers the intravenous site is red, edematous, and painful. Knowing that antineoplastic medications are vesicant medications, the nurse uses which word to document what the client has experienced?
   1. Infiltration
   2. Extravasation
   3. Phlebitis
   4. Thrombophlebitis

2. Which client would the nurse anticipate requires the placement of a central venous catheter?
   1. A client in the same-day surgery unit who might require blood transfusions
   2. A client in the intensive care unit requiring multiple simultaneous intravenous medications
   3. A client in the cardiac care unit diagnosed with possible myocardial infarction
   4. A client on the surgical unit recovering from hernia repair

3. The nurse assigns an unlicensed assistive personnel (UAP) to care for several clients with continuous intravenous (IV) infusions. The UAP can take responsibility for which action?
   1. Changing empty IV solution containers
   2. Confirming the correct IV drip rate
   3. Assessing the client for response to IV therapy
   4. Informing the nurse if they notice anything abnormal

4. The nurse is caring for a client receiving intravenous (IV) therapy. Which would the nurse need to report to the primary care provider?
   1. Completion of each liter of fluid
   2. Initiation of IV fluids
   3. Small infiltration
   4. Extravasation

5. The nurse is caring for a client who has experienced hypovolemia secondary to acute vomiting and diarrhea. What type of fluid does the nurse anticipate will be ordered to administer intravenously?
   1. Hypotonic or isotonic solutions
   2. Hypertonic or isotonic solutions
   3. Hypertonic solutions only
   4. Whole blood

6. The nurse is preparing to initiate IV therapy for a client who is to receive several blood transfusions. Which venipuncture site would the nurse choose?
   1. Metacarpal veins of the hand
   2. Antecubital basilic vein
   3. Cephalic vein
   4. Median cubital vein

7. The nurse is preparing to initiate IV therapy. The primary care provider ordered a continuous infusion of a 0.9% saline solution at a rate of 80 mL per hour. The nurse obtains the solution and tubing that delivers 10 drops per mL. How many drops per minute should the nurse set in order to deliver the prescribed amount? _____

8. The nurse is caring for a client with a continuous intravenous infusion of 5% dextrose in water with 40 mEq of potassium chloride added to each liter. During a routine check of the infusion, the nurse discovers that 4 hours of fluid has infused in the past 1 hour. What would be the nurse's first action?
   1. Notify the primary care provider.
   2. Assess the client.
   3. Reduce the infusion rate.
   4. Notify the charge nurse.

9. The nurse is administering one unit of packed red blood cells as ordered by the primary care provider. While the nurse is measuring vital signs 15 minutes after starting the transfusion, the client complains of chills and back pain. What should the nurse do first?

   1. Stop the blood infusion and keep the vein open by allowing the saline to infuse from the other side of the Y tubing.

   2. Slow the blood transfusion and notify the charge nurse.

   3. Stop the blood transfusion and notify the primary care provider.

   4. Disconnect the blood tubing from the catheter, replacing it with an infusion of normal saline.

10. The nurse is preparing to infuse 1 liter of IV fluid over a 5-hour period using an infusion set that delivers 10 drops per milliliter. How many drops per minute would the nurse deliver? _____

See Answers to Test Your Knowledge in Appendix A.

READINGS AND REFERENCES

References

American Association of Blood Banks. (2009). *Standards for blood banks and transfusion services* (26th ed.). Bethesda, MD: Author.

Broadhurst, D. (2012). Transition to an elastomeric infusion pump in home care: An evidence-based approach. *Journal of Infusion Nursing, 35*, 143–151. doi:10.1097/NAN.0b013e31824d1b7a

Gorski, L. A. (2010). Central venous access device associated infections: Recommendations for best practice in home infusion therapy. *Home Healthcare Nurse, 28*, 221–229. doi:10.1097/NHH.0b013e3181d6c3ad

Hadaway, L. (2012). Needleless connectors for IV catheters. *American Journal of Nursing, 112*(11), 32–44. doi:10.1097/01.NAJ.0000422253.72836.c1

Infusion Nurses Society. (2011a). *Infusion nursing standards of practice.* Norwood, MA: Author.

Infusion Nurses Society. (2011b). *Policies and procedures for infusion nursing* (4th ed.). Norwood, MA: Author.

The Joint Commission. (2013). *Hospital: 2014 National Patient Safety Goals.* Retrieved from http://www.jointcommission.org/hap_2014_npsgs

Makic, M. B. F., Martin, S. A., Burns, S., Philbrick, D., & Rauen, C. (2013). Putting evidence into nursing practice: Four traditional practices not supported by the evidence. *Critical Care Nurse, 33*(2), 28–44. doi:10.4037/ccn2013787

Martin, S. M. (2013). Extravasation management of nonchemotherapeutic medications. *Journal of Infusion Nursing, 36*, 392–396. doi:10.1097/NAN.0000000000000010

Mathers, D. (2011). Evidence-based practice: Improving outcomes for patients with a central venous access device. *Journal of the Association for Vascular Access, 16*, 64–72. doi:10.2309/java.16-2-3

Moureau, N. L., & Dawson, R. B. (2010). Keeping needleless connectors clean, part 2. *Nursing, 40*(6), 61–63.

Phillips, L. D., & Gorski, L. A. (2014). *Manual of I.V. therapeutics. Evidence-based practice for infusion therapy* (6th ed.). Philadelphia, PA: F.A. Davis.

U.S. Food and Drug Administration. (2011). *Bar code label requirements for blood and blood components questions and answers.* Retrieved from http://www.fda.gov/BiologicsBloodVaccines/DevelopmentApprovalProcess/AdvertisingLabelingPromotionalMaterials/BarCodeLabelRequirements/ucm133136.htm

Vacca, V. M. (2013). Vesicant extravasation. *Nursing, 43*(9), 21–22. doi:10.1097/01.NURSE.0000432917.59376.55

Wright, M. O., Tropp, J., Schora, D. M., Dillon-Grant, M., Peterson, K., Boehm, S., . . . Peterson, L. R. (2013). Continuous passive disinfection of catheter hubs prevents contamination and bloodstream infection. *American Journal of Infection Control, 41*, 33–38. doi:10.1016/j.ajic.2012.05.030

Selected Bibliography

Argame, J. (2014). Picking up on PICC lines. *Nursing made Incredibly Easy!, 12*(1), 14–16. doi:10.1097/01.NME.0000432874.05582.bf

Berman, A., Snyder, S., & Frandsen, G. (2016). *Fundamentals of nursing: Concepts, process, and practice* (10th ed.). Upper Saddle River, NJ: Pearson Education.

Dychter, S. S., Gold, D. A., Carson, D., & Haller, M. (2012). Intravenous therapy: A review of complications and economic considerations of peripheral access. *Journal of Infusion Nursing, 35*, 84–91. doi:10.1097/NAN.0b013e31824237ce

Scales, K. (2011). Reducing infection associated with central venous access devices. *Nursing Standard, 25*(36), 49–56. doi:10.7748/ns2011.05.25.36.49.c8517

Tolich, D. J., Blackmur, S., Stahorsky, K., & Wabeke, D. (2013). Blood management: Best practice transfusion strategies. *Nursing, 43*(1), 40–47. doi:10.1097/01.NURSE.0000423955.22755.b1

Weeks, K. (2012). Intermittent IV infusions in acute care: Special considerations. *Nursing, 42*(12), 66–68. doi:10.1097/01.NURSE.0000421393.74230.73

Williams, W. (2013). Fluid management basics. *Nursing made Incredibly Easy!, 11*(4), 48–51. doi:10.1097/01.NME.0000426300.80485.91

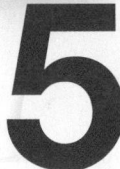

5 Applying the Nursing Process

This unit explores skills of medication administration including administering oral, topical, enteral, parenteral, and intravenous medications. Administering medication requires skill, critical thinking, and knowledge to maintain the client's safety and prevent errors. Medication administration can never be taken lightly. Whether administering a common over-the-counter medication or a prescribed medication, safety is always the highest priority.

CLIENT: Fred   AGE: 52 Years   CURRENT MEDICAL DIAGNOSIS: Anterior Myocardial Infarction

Medical History: Fred was admitted to the coronary care unit (CCU) after being diagnosed with his third myocardial infarction in the emergency department. He used nitroglycerin sublingually for chest pain but the pain did not subside after three pills taken 5 minutes apart, and he called 911. He has now had a device (stent) placed to maintain patency in his left descending coronary artery. He is currently prescribed aspirin 81 mg PO daily, Lipitor 80 mg PO tid, and atenolol 100 mg daily. He has an IV of 5% dextrose in water infusing at 20 mL per hour through which he receives vancomycin 500 mg every 6 hours for an infection that developed at the cardiac catheter insertion site in his left inguinal area. He also has the following prn medications ordered: acetaminophen 650 mg q4hr PO for mild pain,

nitroglycerin 0.4 mg sublingual q5 minutes up to 3 for chest pain, and morphine 10 mg IV q4hr for severe pain.

Personal and Social History: Fred is single, having been divorced 2 years ago. He lives alone and has custody of his 12-year-old son every other weekend and on rotating holidays. He and his ex-wife have a friendly relationship. Fred is a corporate executive and is required to travel extensively. He estimates that he is out of town 3 weeks a month and says he spends a lot of time on airplanes. He has a very sedentary lifestyle and eats in restaurants or has take-out food almost all of the time. He admits he does not have a healthy diet and drinks 1–2 alcoholic beverages per day. He does not smoke and denies using other substances.

Questions

Assessment

1. The nurse is preparing to administer vancomycin at 12 noon using a secondary set. Prior to initiating the medication infusion, what data would the nurse assess?

Analysis

2. List two possible nursing diagnoses that can be identified from the medical/personal history and the assessment data above.

Planning

3. Based on the assessment data and nursing diagnoses, identify one desired outcome.

4. Identify the action verb, measurable criteria, and time line for the outcome.

Implementation

5. Fred receives his medications at 9 AM including Lipitor, aspirin, and atenolol. When and what will the nurse document related to the administration of these medications?

Evaluation

6. Describe the steps to take if the outcome has not been met or has been only partially met.

See *Applying the Nursing Process* suggested answers on student resource website.

6

Nutrition and Elimination

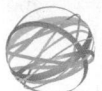

19 Feeding Clients

LEARNING OUTCOMES

At the completion of this chapter, the student will be able to:

1. Define the key terms used in the skills of feeding clients.
2. Describe the characteristics of overnutrition, undernutrition, and protein-calorie malnutrition.
3. Discuss the components and purposes of nutritional assessments and nutritional screenings.
4. State types of and reasons for special or modified diets.
5. Recognize when it is appropriate to delegate feeding of clients to unlicensed assistive personnel.
6. Verbalize the steps used in:
   a. Assisting an adult to eat.
   b. Inserting a nasogastric tube.
   c. Administering a tube feeding.
   d. Removing a nasogastric tube.
   e. Administering a gastrostomy or jejunostomy feeding.
   f. Providing total parenteral nutrition.

7. Identify indications for enteral access devices.
8. Compare and contrast the use of the nasogastric tube, nasoenteric tube, gastrostomy tube, and jejunostomy tube for nutritional support.
9. Compare and contrast the characteristics of intermittent feedings, bolus intermittent feedings, continuous feedings, cyclic feedings, and open and closed systems for enteral feedings.
10. List strategies to help prevent clogged feeding tubes.
11. Compare and contrast total parenteral nutrition and peripheral parenteral nutrition.
12. Demonstrate appropriate documentation and reporting of information related to feeding of clients.

SKILLS

Skill 19–1 Assisting an Adult to Eat
Skill 19–2 Inserting a Nasogastric Tube
Skill 19–3 Administering a Tube Feeding

Skill 19–4 Removing a Nasogastric Tube
Skill 19–5 Administering a Gastrostomy or Jejunostomy Feeding
Skill 19–6 Providing Total Parenteral Nutrition

KEY TERMS

anorexia, 485
bolus intermittent feedings, 499
clear liquid diet, 489
closed systems, 500
continuous feedings, 499
cyclic feedings, 500
diet as tolerated (DAT), 489
dysphagia, 485
emesis, 485
enteral, 494
full liquid diet, 489

gastrostomy, 495
hyperalimentation, 507
intermittent feedings, 499
jejunostomy, 495
light diet, 489
macronutrients, 483
malnutrition, 485
micronutrients, 484
nasogastric tube, 494
nothing by mouth (NPO), 492

nutrients, 483
nutrition, 483
nutritive value, 483
open systems, 500
overnutrition, 485
percutaneous endoscopic gastrostomy (PEG), 495
percutaneous endoscopic jejunostomy (PEJ), 495
peripheral parenteral nutrition (PPN), 507

protein-calorie malnutrition (PCM), 485
pureed diet, 489
regular (standard or house) diet, 489
Salem sump tube, 494
small-bore feeding tube (SBFT), 494
soft diet, 489
total parenteral nutrition (TPN), 507
undernutrition, 485

INTRODUCTION

Nutrition is the sum of all interactions between an organism and the food it consumes. In other words, nutrition is what a person eats and how the body uses it. **Nutrients** are organic, inorganic, and energy-producing substances found in foods and required for body functioning. People require the essential nutrients in foods for the growth and maintenance of all body tissues and the normal functioning of all body processes.

NUTRITION

Adequate food intake consists of a balance of nutrients: water, carbohydrates, proteins, fats, fiber, vitamins, and minerals. Foods differ greatly in their **nutritive value** (the nutrient content of a specified amount of food). Nutrients have three major functions: providing energy for body processes and movement, providing structural material for body tissues, and regulating body processes.

The body's most basic nutrient need is water. Because every cell requires a continuous supply of fuel, the most urgent nutritional need, after water, is for nutrients that provide fuel or energy. The energy-providing nutrients are carbohydrates, fats, and proteins. Hunger impels people to eat enough energy-providing nutrients to satisfy their energy needs.

Carbohydrates, fats, and protein are referred to as **macronutrients**, because they are needed in large amounts (e.g., hundreds of grams) to provide energy. **Micronutrients**, vitamins and minerals, are those required in small amounts (e.g., milligrams or micrograms) to metabolize the energy-providing nutrients.

Although the nutritional content of food is an important consideration when planning a diet, an individual's food preferences and habits are often a major factor affecting actual food intake. Habits about eating are influenced by many factors, as described in Table 19–1.

TABLE 19–1   Factors Affecting Nutrition

Factor	Comments
Development	People in rapid periods of growth (i.e., infancy and adolescence) have increased needs for nutrients. Older adults, on the other hand, need fewer calories and often need to make dietary changes in view of the risk of coronary heart disease, osteoporosis, and hypertension.
Sex	Nutrient requirements are different for men and women because of body composition and reproductive functions. The larger muscle mass of men means a greater need for calories and proteins. Because of menstruation, women require more iron than men prior to menopause. Women who are pregnant or lactating have increased caloric and fluid needs.
Ethnicity and culture	Ethnicity often determines food preferences. Traditional foods (e.g., rice for Asians, pasta for Italians, curry for Indians) are eaten long after other customs are abandoned. Food preferences, however, probably differ as much among individuals of the same cultural background as they do generally between cultures. See Culturally Responsive Care. Between 30 million and 50 million Americans have lactose intolerance (also called lactose maldigestion), a shortage of the enzyme lactase, which is needed to break down the sugar in cow's milk. Certain populations are more widely affected especially African Americans, Ashkenazi Jews, Asians, Native Americans, and Latinos (DeBruyne & Pinna, 2014).
Beliefs about food	Beliefs about effects of foods on health and well-being can affect food choices. Many people acquire their beliefs about food from television, magazines, and other media.
Personal preferences	Some adults are very adventuresome and eager to try new foods. Others prefer to eat the same foods over and over again. Preferences in the tastes, smells, flavors (blends of taste and smell), temperatures, colors, shapes, and sizes of food influence a person's food choices.
Religious practices	Some Roman Catholics avoid meat on certain days, and some Protestant faiths prohibit meat, tea, coffee, or alcohol. Both Orthodox Judaism and Islam prohibit pork. Orthodox Jews observe kosher customs, eating certain foods only if they are inspected by a rabbi and prepared according to dietary laws.
Lifestyle	Certain lifestyles are linked to food-related behaviors. People who are always in a hurry often buy convenience grocery items or eat restaurant meals. Individual differences also influence lifestyle patterns (e.g., cooking skills, concern about health). Some people work at different times, such as evening or night shifts. They might need to adapt their eating habits as a result.
Economics	What, how much, and how often a person eats are frequently affected by socioeconomic status. People with limited incomes, including some older adults, may not be able to afford meat and fresh vegetables. In contrast, people with higher incomes may purchase more proteins and fats and fewer complex carbohydrates. Not all individuals have the financial resources for extensive food preparation and storage.
Medications and therapy	The effects of drugs on nutrition vary considerably. Drugs may alter appetite, disturb taste perception, or interfere with nutrient absorption or excretion. Conversely, nutrients can affect drug utilization. Some nutrients can decrease drug absorption; others enhance absorption.
	Therapies prescribed for certain diseases (e.g., chemotherapy and radiation for cancer) may also adversely affect eating patterns and nutrition. For example, oral ulcers, intestinal bleeding, or diarrhea resulting from the toxicity of antineoplastic agents used in chemotherapy can seriously diminish a person's nutritional status. The effects of radiotherapy depend on the area that is treated. For example, radiotherapy of the head and neck may cause decreased salivation, taste distortions, and swallowing difficulties.
Health	An individual's health status greatly affects eating habits and nutritional status. The lack of teeth, ill-fitting teeth, or a sore mouth makes chewing food difficult. Difficulty swallowing (dysphagia) due to a painfully inflamed throat or a stricture of the esophagus can prevent a person from obtaining adequate nourishment. Disease processes and surgery of the gastrointestinal tract can affect digestion, absorption, metabolism, and excretion of essential nutrients. Autoimmune and genetic disorders such as celiac disease and irritable bowel syndrome may be worsened when eating foods containing wheat or gluten.
Alcohol consumption	The calories consumed in alcoholic drinks include both those of the alcohol itself and of the other beverages added to the drink. Drinking alcohol can lead to weight gain through the addition of these calories to the regular diet plus the effect of alcohol on fat metabolism. Excessive alcohol use can contribute to nutritional deficiencies. Alcohol may replace food in a person's diet, and it can depress the appetite. Excessive alcohol can have a toxic effect on the intestinal mucosa, thereby decreasing the absorption of nutrients.
Advertising	Food producers try to persuade people to change from the product they currently use to the brand of the producer.
Psychological factors	Although some people overeat when stressed, depressed, or lonely, others eat very little under the same conditions. Anorexia and weight loss can indicate severe stress or depression.

Selected Variations in Nutritional Practices and Preferences Among Different Cultures

AFRICAN AMERICAN HERITAGE
- Gifts of food are common and should never be rejected.
- Diets are often high in fat, cholesterol, and sodium.
- Being overweight may be viewed as positive.
- Popular vegetables include black-eyed peas, okra, sweet potatoes, peanuts, corn, hot and sweet peppers, green and lima beans, and collard, turnip, and mustard greens.

ARAB HERITAGE
- Many spices and herbs are used such as cinnamon, allspice, cloves, mint, ginger, and garlic.
- Meats are often skewer roasted or slow simmered; most common are lamb and chicken.
- Bread is served at every meal.
- Muslims do not eat pork, and all meats must be cooked well done.
- Food is eaten (and clients fed) with the right hand.
- Beverages are drunk after the meal, not during.
- Muslims fast during daylight hours during the month of Ramadan (falls on different days of the Gregorian calendar each year because Ramadan is based on the lunar calendar).

CHINESE HERITAGE
- Foods are served at meals in a specific order.
- Each region in China has its own traditional diet.
- Traditional Chinese may not want ice in their drinks.
- Foods are chosen to balance *yin* and *yang* in order to avoid indigestion.
- Soy sauce is used instead of salt

JEWISH HERITAGE
- Dietary laws govern the killing, preparation, and eating of foods.
- Meat and animal milk are not eaten at the same time; dairy substitutes (e.g., margarine) are permitted.
- Pork is one meat that is forbidden to eat.
- All blood must be drained from meats.
- Always wash hands before eating.

MEXICAN HERITAGE
- Rice, beans, and tortillas are core, essential foods.
- Being overweight may be viewed as positive.
- Sweet fruit drinks, including adding sugar to juice, are popular.
- The main meal of the day is at noontime.
- Foods are chosen according to *hot* and *cold* theory.

NAVAJO HERITAGE
- Rites of passage and ceremonies are celebrated with food.
- Herbs are used to treat many illnesses.
- Sheep are the major source of meat.
- Squash and corn are major vegetables.

Altered Nutrition

Malnutrition is commonly defined as the lack of necessary or appropriate food substances but in practice includes both undernutrition and overnutrition (obesity). **Overnutrition** refers to a caloric intake in excess of daily energy requirements, resulting in storage of energy in the form of increased adipose (fat) tissue. As the amount of stored fat increases, the individual becomes overweight or obese.

Undernutrition refers to an intake of nutrients insufficient to meet daily energy requirements as a result of inadequate food intake or improper digestion and absorption of food. An inadequate food intake may be caused by the inability to acquire and prepare food, inadequate knowledge about essential nutrients and a balanced diet, discomfort during or after eating, **dysphagia** (difficulty swallowing), **anorexia** (loss of appetite), nausea or vomiting (**emesis**), and so on. Improper digestion and absorption of nutrients may be caused by food allergies, inadequate production of hormones or enzymes, or by medical conditions resulting in inflammation or obstruction of the gastrointestinal (GI) tract.

Inadequate nutrition is associated with marked weight loss, generalized weakness, altered functional abilities, delayed wound healing, increased susceptibility to infection, decreased immunocompetence, impaired pulmonary function, and prolonged length of hospitalization. Examples of individuals at great risk include the older client who is cognitively impaired or the client with significant dementia who exhibits agitated behaviors at mealtime because of the overwhelming stimuli. Many clients in skilled nursing facilities are dependent on staff assistance for feeding, ranging from verbal direction to total assistance (Table 19–2).

Protein-calorie malnutrition (PCM), historically seen in starving children of underdeveloped countries, is now also recognized as a significant problem of clients with long-term deficiencies in caloric intake (e.g., those with cancer and chronic disease). PCM is an imbalance between protein intake and the body's protein requirements. Characteristics of PCM are depressed visceral proteins (e.g., albumin), weight loss, and visible muscle and fat wasting. Clients with PCM take longer to recover from injuries, have more complications, and tend to stay in the hospital longer.

Nurses must not underestimate the role of nutrition in its importance not only to optimal physical and cognitive function of clients but also to quality of life. Therefore, assessing and promoting adequate nutrition for clients is an important and vital aspect of nursing care.

Nutritional Assessment

The purpose of a nutritional assessment is to identify clients at risk for malnutrition and those with poor nutritional status. In most health care facilities, the responsibility for nutritional assessment and support is shared by the primary care provider, the dietitian, and the nurse. Because a comprehensive nutritional assessment is time consuming and expensive, various levels and types of assessment are available. Generally, nurses perform a nutritional screen. A comprehensive nutritional assessment is often performed by a nutritionist or a dietitian, and the primary care provider. Components of a nutritional assessment are shown in Table 19–3 and may be remembered as ABCD data: anthropometric, biochemical, clinical, and dietary.

NUTRITIONAL SCREENING

A nutritional screen is an assessment performed to identify clients at risk for malnutrition or those who are malnourished (Box 19–1). Clients who are found to be at moderate or high risk are followed

TABLE 19–2 | **Problems Associated with Nutrition in Older Adults**

Problems	Nursing Interventions
Difficulty chewing	Encourage regular visits to the dentist to have dentures repaired, refitted, or replaced. Chop fruits and vegetables finely; shred green, leafy vegetables; select ground meat, poultry, or fish.
Lowered glucose tolerance	Eat more complex carbohydrates (e.g., breads, cereals, rice, pasta, potatoes, and legumes) rather than sugar-rich foods.
Decreased social interaction, loneliness	Promote appropriate social interaction at meals, when possible. Encourage the client and spouse to take an interest in food preparation and serving, perhaps as an activity they can do together. Encourage family or caregivers to present the food at a dining table with place mats, tablecloths, and napkins to trigger eating associations for the older adult. If food preparation is not possible, suggest community resources, such as Meals-on-Wheels.
Loss of appetite and senses of smell and taste	Eat essential, nutrient-dense foods first; follow with desserts and low-nutrient-density foods. Review dietary restrictions, and find ways to make meals appealing within these guidelines. Eat small meals frequently instead of three large meals a day.
Limited income	Suggest using generic brands and coupons. Substitute milk, dairy products, and beans for meat. Avoid convenience foods if able to cook. Buy foods that are on sale and freeze for future use. Suggest community resources and nutrition programs.
Difficulty sleeping at night	Have the major meal at noon instead of in the evening. Avoid tea, coffee, or other stimulants in the evening.

TABLE 19–3 | **Components of a Nutritional Assessment**

	Screening Data	Additional In-Depth Data
Anthropometric Data	• Height • Weight • Ideal body weight • Usual body weight • Body mass index	• Triceps skinfold (TSF) • Mid-arm circumference (MAC) • Mid-arm muscle area (MAMA)
Biochemical Data	• Hemoglobin • Serum albumin • Total lymphocyte count • Skin	• Serum transferrin level • Urinary urea nitrogen • Urinary creatinine excretion • Hair analysis • Neurologic testing
Clinical Data	• Hair and nails • Mucous membranes • Activity level	
Dietary Data	• 24-hour food recall • Food frequency record	• Selective food frequency record • Food diary • Diet history

up with a comprehensive assessment by a dietitian. Medicare standards for nursing homes require that any resident who experiences unplanned or undesired weight loss of 5% or more in 1 month, 7.5% or more in 3 months, or 10% or more in 6 months receive a full nutritional assessment by a nurse.

Nurses carry out nutritional screens through routine nursing histories and physical examinations. Custom-designed screens for a particular population (e.g., older adults and pregnant women) and specific disorders (e.g., cardiac disease) are available.

Screening tools such as the Patient-Generated Subjective Global Assessment (PG-SGA) and the Nutrition Screening Initiative

(NSI) can be incorporated into the nursing history. The PG-SGA (Figure 19–1 ■) is a method of classifying clients as either well nourished, moderately malnourished, or severely malnourished based on a dietary history and physical examination. The PG-SGA was established primarily for use with clients who have cancer, but it has been widely tested and is appropriate for both inpatient and outpatient clients with various diagnoses.

The NSI is an ongoing project of the American Academy of Family Physicians, the American Dietetic Association, the National Council on Aging, and other organizations to promote nutrition screening and improved nutritional care for older adults.

Scored Patient-Generated Subjective
Global Assessment (PG-SGA)

History Boxes 1-4 are designed to be completed by the patient.
[Boxes 1-4 are referred to as the PG-SGA Short Form (SF)]

---

1. Weight *(See Worksheet 1)*

In summary of my current and recent weight:

I currently weigh about_____pounds
I am about_____feet_____tall

One month ago I weighed about_____pounds
Six months ago I weighed about_____pounds

During the past two weeks my weight has:

☐ decreased (1)   ☐ not changed (0)   ☐ increased (0)   Box 1 ☐

---

2. Food Intake: As compared to my normal intake, I would rate my food intake during the past month as:

☐ unchanged (0)
☐ more than usual (0)
☐ less than usual (1)
  I am now taking:
  ☐ *normal food* but less than normal amount (1)
  ☐ little solid food (2)
  ☐ only liquids (3)
  ☐ only nutritional supplements (3)
  ☐ very little of anything (4)
  ☐ only tube feedings or only nutrition by vein (0) Box 2 ☐

---

3. Symptoms: I have had the following problems that have kept me from eating enough during the past two weeks (check all that apply):

☐ no problems eating (0)
☐ no appetite, just did not feel like eating
☐ nausea (1)   ☐ vomiting (3)
☐ constipation (1)   ☐ diarrhea (3)
☐ mouth sores (2)   ☐ dry mouth (1)
☐ things taste funny or have no taste (1) ☐ smells bother me (1)
☐ problems swallowing (2)   ☐ feel full quickly (1)
☐ pain; where?_____ (3)   ☐ fatigue (1)
☐ other**_____ (1)

** Examples: depression, money, or dental problems   Box 3 ☐

©FD Ottery, 2005, 2006, 2014
email: faithotterymdphd@aol.com or info@pt-global.org

---

4. Activities and Function:
Over the past month, I would generally rate my activity as:

☐ normal with no limitations (0)
☐ not my normal self, but able to be up and about with fairly normal activities (1)
☐ not feeling up to most things, but in bed or chair less than half the day (2)
☐ able to do little activity and spend most of the day in bed or chair (3)
  pretty much bedridden, rarely out of bed (3)

Box 4 ☐

Additive Score of the Boxes 1-4 ☐ A

The remainder of this form is to be completed by your doctor, nurse, dietitian, or therapist. Thank you.

Scored Patient-Generated Subjective Global Assessment (PG-SGA)

Worksheet 1 - Scoring Weight (Wt) Loss
To determine score, use 1 month weight data if available. Use 6 month data only if there is no 1 month weight data. Use points below to score weight change and add one extra point if patient has lost weight during the past 2 weeks. Enter total point

Wt loss in 1 month	Points	Wt loss in 6 months
10% or greater	4	20% or greater
5-9.9%	3	10 -19.9%
3-4.9%	2	6 - 9.9%
2-2.9%	1	2 - 5.9%
0-1.9%	0	0 - 1.9%

Numerical score from Worksheet 1 ☐

Additive Score of the Boxes 1-4 (See Side 1) ☐ A

5. Worksheet 2 - Disease and its relation to nutritional requirements

All relevant diagnoses (specify) _____
Primary disease stage (circle if known or appropriate) I II III IV Other _____
One point each:
☐ Cancer ☐ AIDS ☐ Pulmonary or cardiac cachexia ☐ Presence of decubitus, open wound, or fistula
☐ Presence of trauma ☐ Age greater than 65 years ☐ Chronic renal insufficiency

Numerical score from Worksheet 2 ☐ B

---

6. Work Sheet 3 - Metabolic Demand
Score for metabolic stress is determined by a number of variables known to increase protein & calorie needs. The score is additive so that a patient who has a fever of > 102 degrees (3 points) and is on 10 mg of prednisone chronically (2 points) would have an additive score for this section of 5 points.

Stress	none (0)	low (1)	moderate (2)	high (3)	
Fever	no fever	>99 and <101	≥101 and <102	≥102	**Numerical score from Worksheet 3** ☐ C
Fever duration	no fever	<72 hrs	72 hrs	> 72 hrs	
Corticosteroids	no corticosteroids	low dose (<10mg prednisone equivalents/day)	moderate dose (≥10 and <30mg prednisone equivalents/day)	high dose steroid (≥ 30mg prednisone equivalents/day)	

---

7. Worksheet 4 - Physical Exam
Physical exam includes a subjective evaluation of 3 aspects of body composition: fat, muscle, & fluid status. Since this is subjective, each aspect of the exam is rated for degree of deficit. Muscle deficit impacts point score more than fat deficit. Definition of categories: 0 = no deficit, 1+ = mild deficit, 2+ = moderate 3+ = severe

Muscle Status:				
clavicles (pectoralis & deltoids)	0	1+	2+	3+
interosseous muscles	0	1+	2+	3+
thigh (quadriceps)	0	1+	2+	3+
Global muscle status rating	**0**	**1+**	**2+**	**3+**
orbital fat pads	0	1+	2+	3+
triceps skin fold	0	1+	2+	3+
Global fat deficit rating	**0**	**1+**	**2**	**3+**

Fluid Status:				
sacral edema	0	1+	2+	3+
Global fluid status rating	**0**	**1+**	**2+**	**3+**

Numerical score from Worksheet 4 ☐ D

Total PG-SGA score ☐
(Total numerical score of A+B+C+D above)
(See triage recommendations below)

Global PG-SGA rating (A, B, or C) = ☐

Clinician Signature_____ RD RN PA MD DO Other____ Date_____

Worksheet 5 - PG-SGA Global Assessment Categories

Category	Stage A Well nourished	Stage B Moderately malnourished	Stage C Severely malnourished
Weight	No wt loss OR Recent wt gain	≤5% wt loss in 1 month (or 10% in 6 mos) OR Progressive wt loss	>5% wt loss in 1 month (or >10% in 6 mos) OR Progressive wt loss
Nutrient intake	No deficit OR Significant recent improvement	Definite decrease in intake	Severe deficit in intake
Nutrition Impact Symptoms	None OR Significant recent improvement allowing adequate intake	Present of nutrition impact symptoms (PG-SGA Box 3)	Present of nutrition impact symptoms (PG-SGA Box 3)
Functioning	No deficit OR Recent improvement	Moderate functional deficit OR Recent deterioration	Severe functional deficit OR recent significant deterioration
Physical Exam	No deficit OR Chronic deficient but tissue, recent improvement	Evidence of mild to moderate loss of muscle mass / SQ fat / muscle tone on palpation	Obvious signs of malnutrition (e.g., severe loss muscle, SQ possible edema)

Nutritional Triage Recommendations: Additive score is used to define specific nutritional interventions including patient & family education, symptom management including pharmacologic intervention, and appropriate nutrient intervention (food, nutritional supplements, enteral, or parenteral triage).
First line nutrition intervention includes optimal symptom management.

Triage based on PG-SGA point score
0-1 No intervention required at this time. Re-assessment on routine and regular basis during treatment.
2-3 Patient & family education by dietitian, nurse, or other clinician with pharmacologic intervention as indicated by symptom survey (Box 3) and lab values as appropriate.
4-8 Requires intervention by dietitian, in conjunction with nurse or physician as indicated by symptoms (Box 3).
≥ 9 Indicates a critical need for improved symptom management and/or nutrient intervention options.

©FD Ottery, 2005, 2006, 2014 email: faithotterymdphd@aol.com or info@pt-global.org

---

Figure 19–1 ■ Scored Patient-Generated Subjective Global Assessment (PG-SGA).
From © Faith D. Ottery, 2005, 2006, 2014 email: faithotterymdphd@aol.com or http://www.pt-global.org. Reprinted with permission.

BOX 19–1 | **Summary of Risk Factors for Nutritional Problems**

DIET HISTORY
- Chewing or swallowing difficulties (including ill-fitting dentures, dental caries, and missing teeth)
- Inadequate food budget
- Inadequate food intake
- Inadequate food preparation facilities
- Inadequate food storage facilities
- IV fluids (other than total parenteral nutrition) for 10 or more days
- Living and eating alone
- No intake for 10 or more days
- Physical disabilities
- Restricted or fad diets

MEDICAL HISTORY
- Adolescent pregnancy or closely spaced pregnancies
- Alcohol or substance abuse
- Catabolic or hypermetabolic condition: burns, trauma
- Chronic illness: end-stage renal disease, liver disease, HIV, chronic obstructive pulmonary disease (COPD), cancer

- Fluid and electrolyte imbalance
- Gastrointestinal problems: anorexia, dysphagia, nausea, vomiting, diarrhea, constipation
- Neurologic or cognitive impairment
- Oral and gastrointestinal surgery
- Unintentional weight loss or gain of 10% within 6 months

MEDICATION HISTORY
- Antacids
- Antidepressants
- Antihypertensives
- Anti-inflammatory agents
- Antineoplastic agents
- Aspirin
- Digitalis
- Diuretics (thiazides)
- Laxatives
- Potassium chloride

The NSI estimates that approximately half of older adults in hospitals, nursing homes, and home care are malnourished. The NSI screens older adults using a nutrition checklist that contains nine warning signs of conditions that can interfere with good nutrition (Box 19–2).

Nursing interventions to promote optimal nutrition for hospitalized clients are often provided in collaboration with the primary care provider, who writes the diet orders, and the dietitian, who informs clients about special diets. The nurse reinforces this instruction and, in addition, creates an atmosphere that encourages eating, provides assistance with eating, monitors the client's appetite and food intake, administers enteral and parenteral feedings, and consults with the primary care provider and dietitian about nutritional problems that arise.

BOX 19–2 | **Nutritional Screening Tool**

Read the statement. Circle the number in the Yes column for those that apply to you. Total your nutritional assessment.

Nutritional Assessment Statements	Yes
I have an illness or condition that made me change the kind or amount of food I eat.	2
I eat fewer than two meals per day.	3
I eat few fruits, vegetables, or milk products.	2
I have three or more drinks of beer, liquor, or wine almost every day.	2
I have tooth or mouth problems that make it hard for me to eat.	2
I do not always have enough money to buy the food I need.	4
I eat alone most of the time.	1
I take three or more different prescribed or over-the-counter drugs a day.	1
Without wanting to, I have lost or gained 10 pounds in the last 6 months.	2
I am not always physically able to shop, cook, or feed myself.	2
Total	_____

If you scored 0–2: Good! Recheck your nutritional score in 6 months.
If you scored 3–5: You are at moderate nutritional risk. See what can be done to improve your eating habits and lifestyle. Recheck your score in 3 months.
If you scored 6 or above: You are at high nutritional risk. Take this checklist to your doctor, nurse practitioner, or home health nurse. Ask for help to improve your nutritional health.

From *Determine Your Nutritional Health*, by the Nutrition Screening Initiative, 2008, Washington, DC: National Council On Aging. Reprinted with permission by the Nutrition Screening Initiative, a project of the American Dietetic Association, funded in part by a grant from Ross Products Division, Abbott Laboratories, Inc.

BOX 19–3	Examples of Foods for Clear Liquid, Full Liquid, and Soft Diets

Clear Liquid	Full Liquid	Soft
Coffee, regular and decaffeinated Tea Carbonated beverages Bouillon, fat-free broth Clear fruit juices (apple, cranberry, grape) Other fruit juices, strained Popsicles Gelatin Sugar, honey Hard candy	All foods on clear liquid diet plus: Milk and milk drinks Puddings, custards Ice cream, sherbet Vegetable juices Refined or strained cereals (e.g., cream of rice) Cream, butter, margarine Eggs (in custard and pudding) Smooth peanut butter Yogurt	All foods on full and clear liquid diets, plus: Meat: all lean, tender meat, fish, or poultry (chopped, shredded); spaghetti sauce with ground meat over pasta Meat alternatives: scrambled eggs, omelet, poached eggs; cottage cheese and other mild cheese Vegetables: mashed potatoes, sweet potatoes, or squash; vegetables in cream or cheese sauce; other cooked vegetables as tolerated (e.g., spinach, cauliflower, asparagus tips), chopped and mashed as needed; avocado Fruits: cooked or canned fruits; bananas, grapefruit and orange sections without membranes, applesauce Breads and cereals: enriched rice, barley, pasta; all breads; cooked cereals (e.g., oatmeal) Desserts: soft cake, bread pudding

Assisting Clients with Special Diets

Alterations in the client's diet are often needed to treat a disease process such as diabetes mellitus, to prepare for a special examination or surgery, to increase or decrease weight, to restore nutritional deficits, or to allow an organ to rest and promote healing. Diets are modified in one or more of the following aspects: texture, kilocalories, food sources, specific nutrients, seasonings, or consistency.

Hospitalized clients who do not have special needs eat the **regular (standard or house) diet**, a balanced diet that supplies the metabolic requirements of a sedentary person (about 2,000 kilocalories [Kcal]). Most agencies offer clients a daily menu from which to select their meals for the next day; others provide standard meals to each client on the general diet.

A variation of the regular diet is the **light diet**, designed for postoperative and other clients who are not ready for the regular diet. Foods in the light diet are plainly cooked and fat is usually minimized, as are bran and foods containing a great deal of fiber.

Diets modified in consistency are often given to clients before and after surgery or procedures or to promote healing in clients with GI distress. These diets include clear liquid, full liquid, soft, and diet as tolerated. In some agencies, clients who have had GI surgery are not permitted red-colored liquids or candy because, if vomited, the color may be confused with blood.

CLEAR LIQUID DIET

The **clear liquid diet** is limited to water, tea, coffee, clear broths, ginger ale or other carbonated beverages, strained and clear juices, and plain gelatin. Note that "clear" does not necessarily mean "colorless." This diet provides the client with fluid and carbohydrates (in the form of sugar) but does not supply adequate protein, fat, vitamins, minerals, or calories. It is a short-term diet (24 to 36 hours) provided for clients after certain surgeries or in the acute stages of infection, particularly of the GI tract. The major objectives of this diet are to relieve thirst, prevent dehydration, and minimize stimulation of the GI tract. Examples of foods allowed in clear liquid diets are shown in Box 19–3.

FULL LIQUID DIET

The **full liquid diet** contains only liquids or foods that turn to liquid at body temperature, such as ice cream (see Box 19–3). Full liquid diets are often eaten by clients who have GI disturbances or are otherwise unable to tolerate solid or semisolid foods. This diet is not recommended for long-term use because it is low in iron, protein, and calories. In addition, its cholesterol content may be high because of the amount of cow's milk offered. Clients who must receive only liquids for long periods are usually given a nutritionally balanced oral supplement, such as Ensure or Sustacal. The full liquid diet is monotonous and difficult for clients to accept. Planning six or more feedings per day may encourage a more adequate intake.

SOFT DIET

The **soft diet** is easily chewed and digested. It is often ordered for clients who have difficulty chewing and swallowing. It is a low-residue (low-fiber) diet containing very few uncooked foods; however, restrictions vary among agencies and according to individual tolerance. Examples of foods that can be included in a soft or semisoft diet are shown in Box 19–3. The **pureed diet** is a modification of the soft diet. Liquid may be added to the food, which is then blended to a semisolid consistency.

DIET AS TOLERATED

Diet as tolerated (DAT) is ordered when the client's appetite, ability to eat, and tolerance for certain foods may change. For example, on the first postoperative day a client may be given a clear liquid diet. If no nausea occurs, normal intestinal motility has returned as evidenced by active bowel sounds and client reports of passing gas, and the client feels like eating, the diet may be advanced to a full liquid, light, or regular diet.

MODIFICATION FOR DISEASE

Many special diets may be prescribed to meet requirements that take into account disease processes or altered metabolism. For example, a client with diabetes mellitus may need a diet recommended by the

American Diabetes Association, an obese client may need a calorie-restricted diet, a client with cardiac problems may need sodium and cholesterol restrictions, and a client with allergies will need a hypoallergenic diet.

Some clients must follow certain diets (e.g., the diabetic diet) for a lifetime. If the diet is long term, the client must understand the diet and also develop a healthy, positive attitude toward it. Assisting clients and support persons with special diets is a function shared by the dietitian or nutritionist and the nurse. The dietitian informs the client and support persons about the specific foods allowed and not allowed and assists the client with meal planning. The nurse reinforces this instruction, assists the client to make changes, and evaluates the client's responses.

DYSPHAGIA

Some clients may have no difficulty with choosing a healthy diet, but be at risk for nutritional problems due to dysphagia. These clients may have inadequate solid or fluid intake, be unable to swallow their medications, or aspirate food or fluids into the lungs—causing pneumonia. Clients at risk for dysphagia include older adults, those who have experienced a stroke, individuals with cancer who have had radiation therapy to the head and neck, and others with cranial nerve dysfunction. Consider dysphagia if the client exhibits the following behaviors: coughs, chokes, or gags while eating; complains of pain when swallowing; has a gurgling voice; requires frequent oral suctioning. Nurses may be the first persons to detect dysphagia and are in an excellent position to recommend further evaluation; implement specialized feeding techniques and diets; and work with clients, family members, and other health care professionals to develop a plan to assist the client with difficulties (Box 19–4). If the client condition suggests dysphagia, the nurse should review the history in detail; interview the client or family; assess the mouth, throat, and chest; and observe the client swallowing. Although absence of or a reduced gag reflex indicates the client will have difficulty swallowing, presence of the gag reflex should not be interpreted as indicating that swallowing will not be impaired.

A gag reflex can be elicited by very light touching of the back of the tongue or posterior wall of the oropharynx with a tongue blade. The client should have immediate elevation of the palate, the muscles of the pharynx should constrict, and the client may begin making gagging sounds indicating a normal gag reflex. If none of this happens the gag reflex is not present.

A multidisciplinary group developed the National Dysphagia Diet (NDD), which delineates standards of food textures (American Dietetic Association, 2002). The four levels of liquid foods are thin, nectar-like, honey-like, and spoon-thick liquids. The four levels of semisolid/solid foods are pureed, mechanically altered, advanced/mechanically soft, and regular/general. If a client has dysphagia, the dietitian, occupational therapist, swallowing specialist, speech-language pathologist, and/or primary care provider can use these levels to determine a consistent approach to a particular client's dysphagia. For example, a mechanically soft diet may result in lower pneumonia rates than a pureed diet in stroke clients with a history of aspiration pneumonia. Or, clients who cannot tolerate thin liquids can be taught to add fluid-thickening agents. Early detection and intervention can prevent the adverse outcomes of dysphagia in most clients.

All dietary instructions must be individually designed to meet the client's intellectual ability, motivation level, lifestyle, culture, language, and economic status. Both nutritionists and dietitians help to adapt a diet to suit the client. Simple verbal instructions need to be given and reinforced with written material. Family and support persons must be included in the dietary instruction.

Stimulating the Appetite

Physical illness, unfamiliar or unpalatable food, environmental and psychological factors, and physical discomfort or pain may depress the appetites of many clients. A short-term decrease in food intake usually is not a problem for adults; over time, however, it leads to weight loss, decreased strength and stamina, and other nutritional problems. A decreased food intake is often accompanied by a decrease in fluid intake, which may cause fluid and electrolyte problems. Stimulating a person's appetite requires the nurse to determine the reason for the lack of appetite and then deal with the problem. Some general interventions for improving the client's appetite are summarized in Box 19–5.

BOX 19–4 | Promoting Safety for the Client with Dysphagia

- Assess level of alertness and orientation.
- Provide a quiet, relaxed, distraction-free environment. Avoid rushing.
- Sit the client up as high as possible in bed or in a chair.
- Encourage to eat only a small amount at a time.
- Place food toward the back of the tongue.
- Remind the client to chew thoroughly.
- Position the head in a neutral position or slightly flexed.
- Ensure that the client swallows an entire bite of food before taking another bite.
- Remove food if the client begins to cough or choke.
- Check the mouth for unswallowed food after completion of a meal. Remove unswallowed food.
- Ask the client to remain in an upright position for 20 to 30 minutes after eating.

BOX 19–5 | Improving Appetite

- Provide familiar food that the person likes. Often the relatives of clients are pleased to bring food from home but may need some guidance about special diet requirements.
- Select small portions so as not to discourage the client.
- Avoid unpleasant or uncomfortable treatments immediately before or after a meal.
- Provide a tidy, clean environment that is free of unpleasant sights and odors. A soiled dressing, a used bedpan, an uncovered irrigation set, or even used dishes can negatively affect the appetite.
- Encourage or provide oral hygiene before mealtime. This improves the client's ability to taste.
- Relieve illness symptoms that depress appetite before mealtime; for example, give an analgesic for pain or an antipyretic for a fever or allow rest for fatigue.
- Reduce psychological stress. A lack of understanding of therapy, the anticipation of an operation, and fear of the unknown can cause anorexia. Often, the nurse can help by discussing feelings with the client, giving information and assistance, and allaying fears.

Assisting Clients with Meals

Because clients in health care agencies are frequently confined to their beds, meals are brought to the client. The client receives a tray that has been assembled in a central kitchen. Nursing personnel may be responsible for giving out and collecting the trays; however, in most settings this is done by dietary personnel. Long-term care facilities and some hospitals serve meals to mobile clients in a special group dining area.

Individuals who frequently require help with their meals include older adults who are weakened, individuals with disabilities such as visual impairments, those who must remain in a back-lying position, or those who cannot use their hands. The client's nursing care plan will indicate that assistance is required with meals.

The nurse must be sensitive to clients' potential feelings of embarrassment, resentment, and loss of autonomy. Whenever possible, the nurse should help clients feed themselves rather than feed them. Some clients become depressed because they require help and because they believe they are burdensome to busy nursing personnel. Although feeding a client is time consuming, nurses should try to appear unhurried and convey that they have ample time. Sitting at the bedside is one way to convey this impression. If the client is to be fed by unlicensed assistive personnel (UAP), the nurse must ensure that the same standards are met.

When feeding a client, ask in which order the client would like to eat the food. If the client cannot see, tell the client which food is being offered. Always allow ample time for the client to chew and swallow the food before offering more. Also, provide fluids as requested or, if the client is unable to communicate, offer fluids after every three or four mouthfuls of solid food. It is important to make the time a pleasant one, choosing topics of conversation that are of interest to clients who want to talk.

Although normal utensils should be used whenever possible, special utensils may be needed to assist a client to eat. For clients who have difficulty drinking from a cup or glass, a straw often permits them to obtain liquids with less effort and less spillage. Special drinking cups are also available. One model has a spout; another is specially designed to permit drinking with less tipping of the cup than is normally required.

Many adaptive feeding aids are available to help clients maintain independence. Figures 19–2 ■ and 19–3 ■ show some of these aids. A standard eating utensil with a built-up or widened handle helps clients who cannot grasp objects easily. Utensils with wide handles can be purchased, or a regular eating utensil can be modified by taping foam around the handle. The foam increases friction and thus steadies the client's grasp. Handles may be bent or angled to compensate for limited motion. Collars or bands that prevent the utensil from being dropped can be attached to the end of the handle and fit over the client's hand. Plates with rims and plastic or metal plate guards enable the client to pick up the food by first pushing it against this raised edge. A suction cup or damp sponge or cloth may be placed under the dish to keep it from moving while the client is eating. No-spill mugs and two-handled drinking cups are especially useful for individuals with impaired hand coordination. Stretch terry cloth and knitted or crocheted glass covers enable the client to keep a secure grasp on a glass. Lidded tip-proof glasses are also available. In the hospital or long-term care setting, these aids are usually provided for clients by occupational therapists.

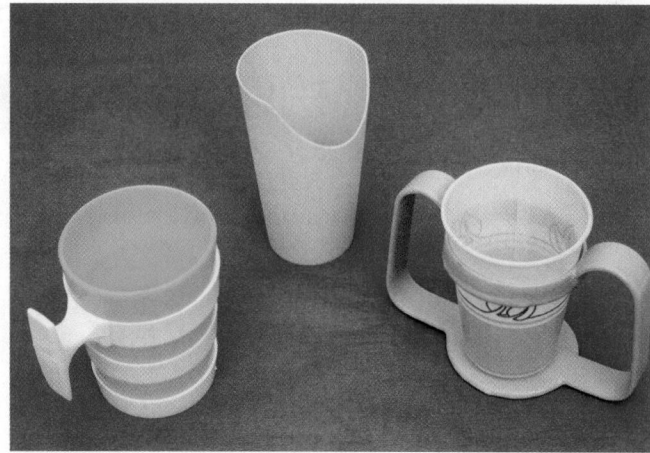

Figure 19–2 ■ *Left to right:* glass holder, cup with hole for nose, two-handled cup holder.

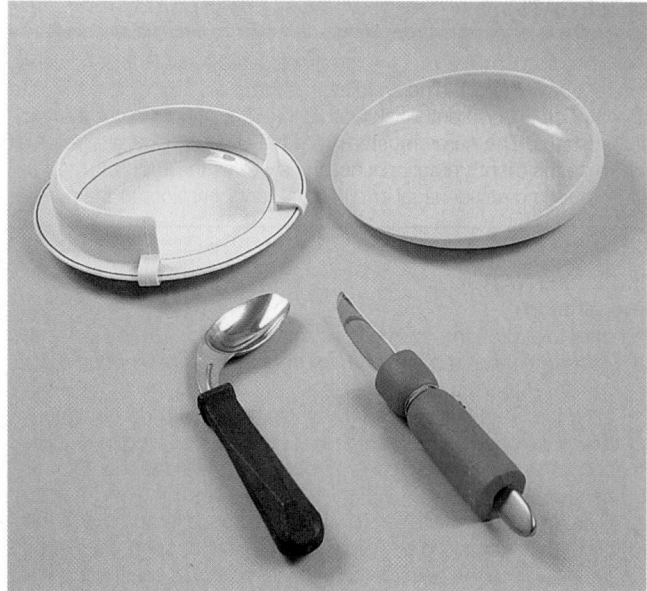

Figure 19–3 ■ Dinner plate with guard attached and lipped plate facilitate scooping; wide-handled spoon and knife facilitate grip.

Special mealtime care is required for clients with dementia, cognitive impairment, or medical disorders that put them at risk for aspiration. Often, feeding a client is delegated to UAP. If possible, assigning the same person to feed an individual client each time can be beneficial in a number of ways. The UAP develops a rapport and relationship with the client that may promote better eating through cuing and guidance. The UAP, by knowing the client, would be able to determine if any changes are occurring such as improved appetite, changes in mental status, or signs of swallowing problems such as coughing and choking. For clients with cognitive impairments, a helpful strategy is to provide one course at a time and give only those eating utensils that the person can use. By reducing the distractions, the client can focus on eating the meal. Skill 19–1 explains the steps involved in assisting adult clients to eat.

●○○● NURSING PROCESS: ASSISTING CLIENTS WITH MEALS

Assisting an Adult to Eat

ASSESSMENT

Assess the client's:
- Self-care abilities for eating and assistance required (note hand coordination, level of consciousness, and visual acuity).
- Appetite for and tolerance of food and fluid.
- Need for a special diet.
- Food allergies and food likes and dislikes.

PLANNING

Confirm the client's diet order:
- Check the client's chart or plan of care for the diet order and to determine whether the client is fasting for laboratory tests or surgery or whether the primary care provider has ordered **nothing by mouth (NPO)**. For clients who are fasting or NPO, ensure that the appropriate signs are placed on either the room door or the client's bed, according to agency practice.
- If there is a change in the type of food the client is to receive, notify the dietary staff.

DELEGATION

Assisting or feeding a client is often delegated to UAP. It is, however, the responsibility of the nurse to assess the client's ability to eat and to identify actual or potential risk factors that may affect the client's nutritional status. The nurse must instruct the UAP about strategies that promote the client's nutritional health as well as the importance of the UAP reporting any unusual or different client behaviors to the nurse.

INTERPROFESSIONAL PRACTICE

Assisting the client with meals may be within the scope of practice for other health care providers. For example, occupational therapists may work with clients who need to develop modified feeding or swallowing techniques. Although the therapists may verbally communicate their findings and plan to the health care team members, the nurse must also know where to locate their documentation in the client's medical record.

Equipment
- Meal tray with the correct food and fluids
- Extra napkin or small towel
- Straw, special drinking cup, weighted glass, or other adaptive feeding aid as required

IMPLEMENTATION

Preparation

Prepare the client and overbed table.
- Assist the client to the bathroom or onto a bedpan or commode if the client needs to urinate.
- Offer the client assistance in washing the hands prior to a meal. If the client has problems with oral hygiene, brushing the teeth or using a mouthwash can improve the taste in the mouth and hence the appetite.
- Clear the overbed table so that there is space for the tray. If the client must remain in a lying position in bed, arrange the overbed table close to the bedside so that the client can see the food.

Performance

1. Prior to feeding the client, introduce self and verify the client's identity using agency protocol. Explain to the client what you are going to do, why it is necessary, and how he or she can participate.
2. Perform hand hygiene and observe other appropriate infection prevention procedures.
3. Provide for client privacy if appropriate.
4. Position the client and yourself appropriately.
   - Assist the client to a comfortable position for eating. Most people sit during a meal; if it is permitted, assist the client to sit in bed ❶ or in a chair.
   - If the client is unable to sit, assist the client to a lateral position. **Rationale:** *It is easier to swallow in a lateral position than in a back-lying position.*
   - If the client requires assistance with feeding, assume a sitting position, if possible, beside the client. ❷ **Rationale:** *This conveys a more relaxed presence and encourages the client to eat an adequate meal.*
5. Assist the client as required.
   - Check the tray for the client's name, the type of diet, and completeness. If the diet does not seem to be correct,

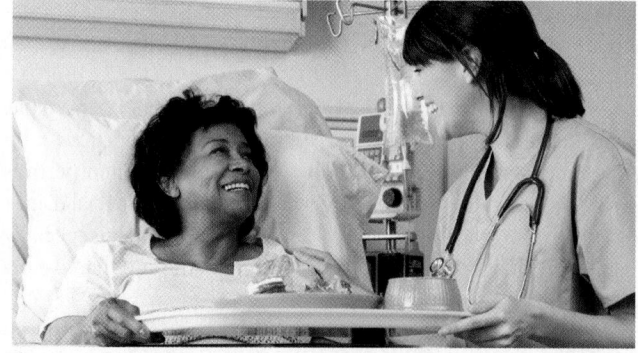

❶ A supported sitting position contributes to a client's comfort while eating.
Monkey Business Images/Shutterstock.

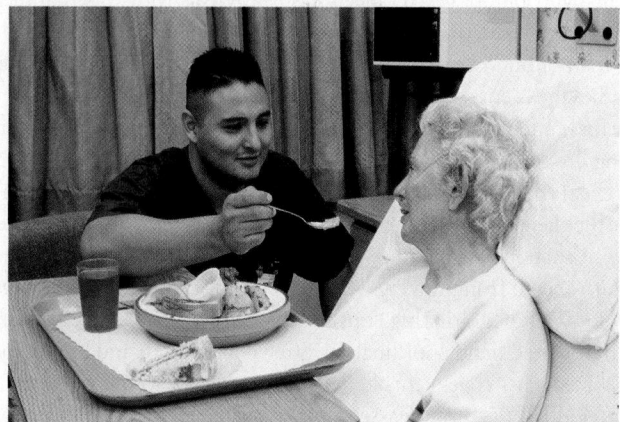

❷ Sitting at the same level as the client facilitates comfort and communication.

Assisting an Adult to Eat—*continued*

check it against the client's health record. Do not leave an incorrect diet for a client to eat.

- Encourage the client to eat independently, assisting as needed. Do not take over the feeding process. **Rationale:** *Participation by the client enhances feelings of independence.*
- Remove the food covers, butter the bread, pour the drink, and cut the meat, if needed.
- For a client with a visual impairment, identify the placement of the food as you would describe the time on a clock. For instance, say "The potatoes are at 8 o'clock, the chicken at 12 o'clock, and the green beans at 4 o'clock." ❸
- If the client needs assistance with feeding:
  a. Ask in which order the client desires to eat the food.

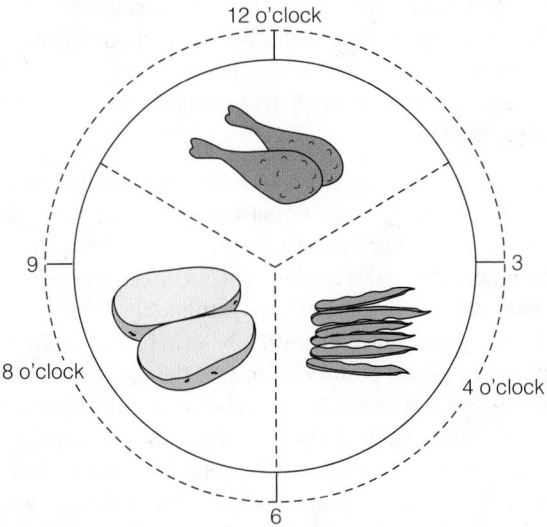

❸ For a client who is visually impaired, the nurse can use the clock system to describe the location of food on the plate.

  b. Use normal utensils whenever possible. **Rationale:** *Using ordinary utensils enhances self-esteem.*
  c. If the client is visually impaired, tell which food you are giving.
  d. Warn the client if the food is hot or cold.
  e. Allow ample time for the client to chew and swallow the food before offering more.
  f. Provide fluids as requested or, if the client is unable to ask, offer fluids after every three or four mouthfuls of solid food.
  g. Use a straw or special drinking cup for fluids that would spill from normal containers.
  h. Make the time a pleasant one, choosing topics of conversation that are of interest to the client, if the person wants to talk.

6. After the meal, ensure client comfort.
   - Assist the client to clean the mouth and hands.
   - Reposition the client.
   - Replace the food covers and remove the food tray from the bedside.
7. Document all relevant information.
   - Note how much and what the client has eaten and the amount of fluid taken. In many agencies, nurses record the percentage of the meal consumed, but describing the amount and size of individual items eaten provides greater accuracy.
   - Record fluid intake and calorie count as required. In a hospital or subacute inpatient setting, a calorie count is usually calculated by the dietary department. It is based on a detailed list of foods and fluids consumed that has been recorded by nursing personnel.
   - If the client is on a special diet or is having problems eating, record the amount of food eaten and any pain, fatigue, or nausea experienced.
   - If the client is not eating, notify the nurse in charge so that the diet can be changed or other nursing measures can be taken (e.g., rescheduling the meals, providing small, more frequent meals, or obtaining special self-feeding aids).

EVALUATION
- Note the client's appetite, tolerance of food and fluids taken, amount of fluid intake, calorie count, if required, any chewing or swallowing difficulties, and the need for any adjustments in food consistency (e.g., minced or pureed foods, need for special feeding aids).
- Relate these findings to previous assessment data if available.
- Report significant deviations from usual to the primary care provider.

LIFESPAN CONSIDERATIONS | Assisting an Adult to Eat

OLDER ADULTS
- Offer fluids frequently to prevent dry mouth. Initially avoid dry foods such as crackers and sticky foods such as bananas. **Rationale:** *Saliva production decreases with age.*
- Allow the older client time to eat and offer to rewarm the food if needed. **Rationale:** *Hand tremors and arthritic joint changes may slow the eating process for older clients.*

- Observe for dysphagia and adapt the older client's diet accordingly. **Rationale:** *Esophageal nerve degeneration, which often occurs with aging, can affect the ability to swallow.*
- Older clients may need extra seasoning on food. **Rationale:** *Aging decreases the ability to taste, especially sweet and salty foods.*

- Assess the home for adequate facilities to prepare and store food such as a working refrigerator and stove.
- Assess the client's and caregiver's ability to obtain food and prepare meals.
- Evaluate problems that can interfere with eating such as ill-fitting dentures, sore gums, constipation, diarrhea, or a special diet.

- Instruct the caregiver about the importance of regular, nutritious meals and allowing the client to remain independent when possible.
- Provide written guidelines for the client's diet and any special feeding techniques.

ENTERAL NUTRITION

An alternative method to ensure adequate nutrition includes **enteral** (through the GI system) methods. Enteral nutrition (EN), also referred to as total enteral nutrition (TEN), is provided when the client is unable to ingest foods or the upper GI tract is impaired but the remainder of the intestinal tract is functional. Enteral feedings are administered through nasogastric and small-bore feeding tubes, or through gastrostomy or jejunostomy tubes.

Enteral Access Devices

Enteral access is achieved by means of nasogastric or nasointestinal (nasoenteric) tubes, or gastrostomy or jejunostomy tubes.

A **nasogastric tube** is inserted through one of the nostrils, down the nasopharynx, and into the alimentary tract. In some instances, the tube is passed through the mouth and pharynx (orogastric), although this route may be more uncomfortable for the conscious adult client and cause gagging. This approach, however, is used for infants, who are nose breathers; for premature infants, who have no gag reflex; and for adults in critical care units.

Traditional firm, nasogastric tubes are placed into the stomach. Examples are the Levin tube, a flexible rubber or plastic, single-lumen tube with holes near the tip, and the **Salem sump tube**, with a double lumen (Figure 19–4 ■). The larger lumen of the Salem sump tube allows delivery of liquids to the stomach or removal of gastric contents. When the Salem tube is used for suction of gastric contents, the smaller vent lumen (the proximal port is often referred to as the *blue pigtail*) allows for an inflow of atmospheric air, which prevents a vacuum if the gastric tube adheres to the wall of the stomach. Irritation of the gastric mucosa is thereby avoided.

Nasogastric tubes are used for feeding clients who have adequate gastric emptying, bowel motility, and intact cough and gag reflexes,

and for clients who require short-term feedings. Skill 19–2 provides guidelines for inserting a nasogastric tube. Skill 19–4 outlines the steps for removing a nasogastric tube.

Nasogastric tubes may be inserted for reasons other than providing a route for feeding the client, including:

- To prevent nausea, vomiting, and gastric distention following surgery. In this case, the tube is attached to a suction source.
- To remove stomach contents for laboratory analysis.
- To lavage (wash) the stomach in cases of poisoning or overdose of oral medications.

Another tube often used for feeding that is softer, more flexible, and less irritating is the **small-bore feeding tube (SBFT)**. This tube comes in different sizes (i.e., 8, 10, and 12 Fr). The smaller sizes are more comfortable for the client but do clog easier. The SBFT, sometimes called a nasoenteric (or nasointestinal) tube, is longer than the nasogastric tube (often 101 cm [40 in.] for an adult) because the tip may be placed postpyloric or into the upper small intestine (Figures 19–5 ■ and 19–6A ■). It can be inserted nasally or orally. If the client is intubated, sedated, or comatose, the oral insertion route is preferable. But, if the client is awake and has no other oral tubes, the nasal insertion route is more comfortable and better tolerated. Some agencies may allow only specially trained nurses or primary care providers to insert this type of tube. Postpyloric feeding tubes are most beneficial for clients with the following characteristics (Sekino, Yoshitomi, Nakamura, Makita, & Sumikawa, 2012):

- Cannot tolerate gastric feedings.
- Must be kept flat in bed.

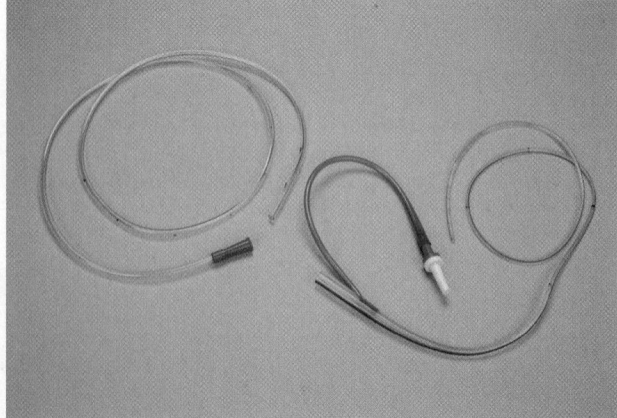

Figure 19–4 ■ *Left,* Single-lumen Levin tube; *Right,* double-lumen Salem sump tube with filter on air vent port.

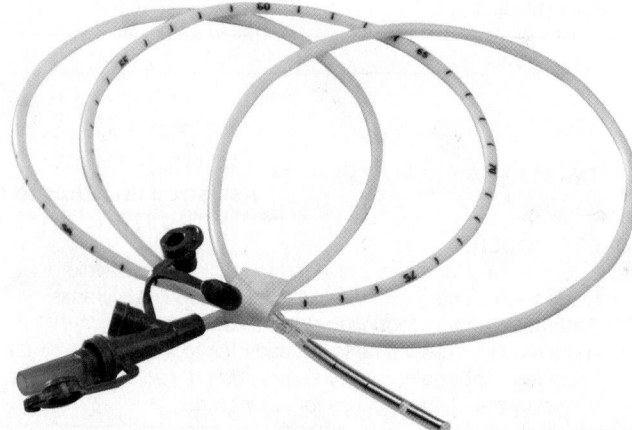

Figure 19–5 ■ A polyurethane feeding tube designed for nasogastric and nasoduodenal feeding with a weighted tip for easier insertion. The feeding port is incompatible with luer lock or IV connections, reducing the risk of accidental connection or infusion. Tubes can be 8Fr-12Fr and 36"-55" long.
Courtesy Covidien.

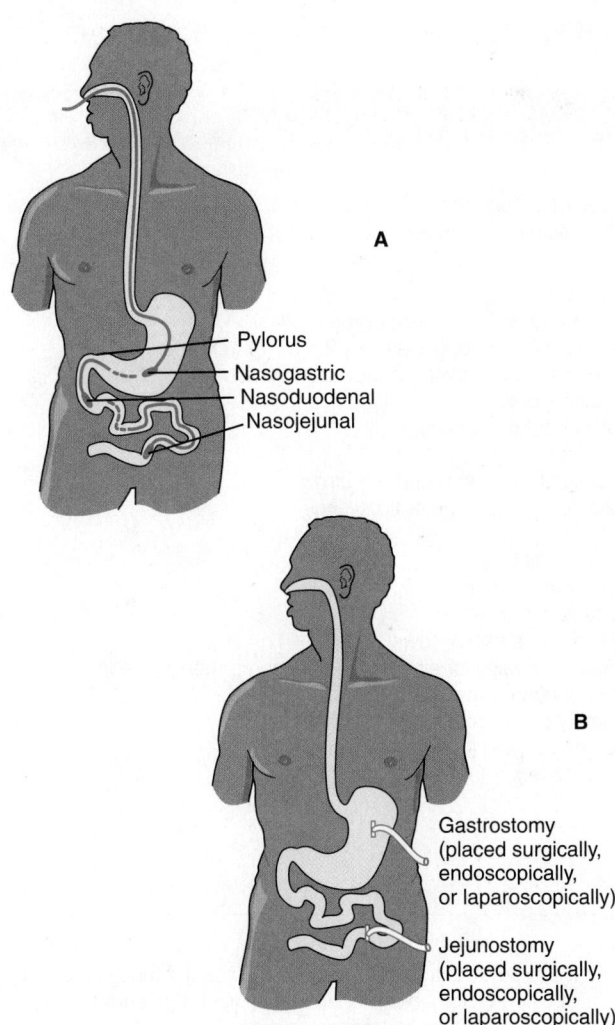

Figure 19–6 ■ Placements for enteral access: *A,* for nasoenteric/nasointestinal tubes; *B,* for gastrostomy and jejunostomy tubes.

• Require positive pressure ventilation.
• Have impaired gastric motility.
• Require continuous gastric decompression.
• Are high risk for aspiration.

   Gastrostomy and **jejunostomy** devices are used for long-term nutritional support, generally more than 6 to 8 weeks. Tubes are placed surgically or by laparoscopy through the abdominal wall into the stomach (gastrostomy; see Figure 19–6*B*) or into the jejunum (jejunostomy; see Figure 19–6*B*). A **percutaneous endoscopic gastrostomy (PEG)** (Figure 19–7 ■) or **percutaneous endoscopic jejunostomy (PEJ)** (Figure 19–8 ■) is created by using an endoscope to visualize the inside of the stomach, making a puncture through the skin and subcutaneous tissues of the abdomen into the stomach, and inserting the PEG or PEJ catheter through the puncture.

   The surgical opening is sutured tightly around the tube or catheter to prevent leakage. Care of this opening before it heals requires surgical asepsis. The catheter has an external bumper and an internal inflatable retention balloon to maintain placement. When the tract is established (about 1 month), the tube or catheter can be removed and reinserted for each feeding. Alternatively, a skin-level tube can be used that remains in place (Figure 19–9 ■). A feeding set is attached when needed.

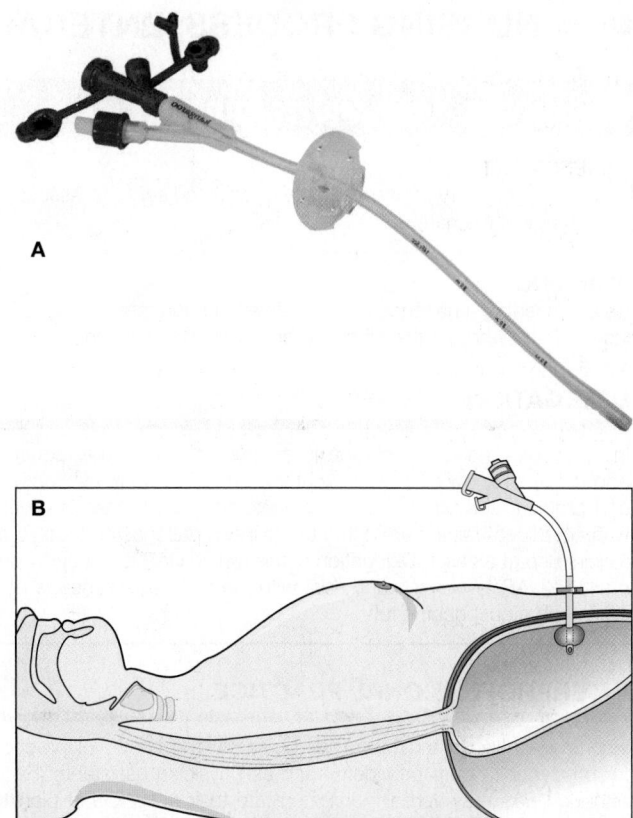

Figure 19–7 ■ Percutaneous endoscopic gastrostomy (PEG) tube: *A,* Courtesy Covidien.

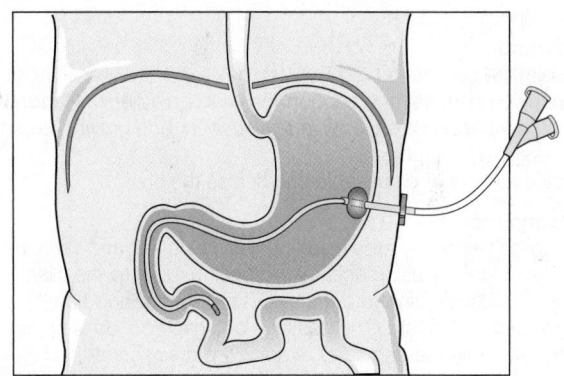

Figure 19–8 ■ Percutaneous endoscopic jejunostomy (PEJ) tube.

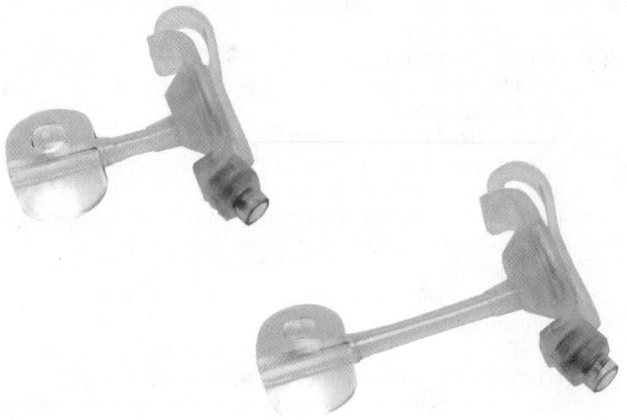

Figure 19–9 ■ Low-profile gastrostomy feeding tubes. Courtesy Covidien.

● ○ ○ ● **NURSING PROCESS: ENTERAL NUTRITION**

Inserting a Nasogastric Tube

ASSESSMENT
- Check for history of nasal surgery or deviated septum. Assess patency of the nares.
- Determine presence of the gag reflex.
- Assess mental status or ability to cooperate with the procedure.

PLANNING
Before inserting a nasogastric tube, determine the size of tube to be inserted and whether the tube is to be attached to suction.

DELEGATION

Insertion of a nasogastric tube is an invasive procedure requiring application of knowledge (e.g., anatomy and physiology, risk factors) and problem solving. In some agencies, only health care providers with advanced training are permitted to insert nasogastric tubes that require use of a stylet. Delegation of this skill to UAP is not appropriate. The UAP, however, can assist with the oral hygiene needs of a client with a nasogastric tube.

INTERPROFESSIONAL PRACTICE

Inserting a nasogastric tube may be within the scope of practice for other health care providers such as physician assistants (PAs). Although PAs may verbally communicate their actions and plan to the health care team members, the nurse must also know where to locate their documentation in the client's medical record.

Equipment
- Large- or SBFT (nonlatex preferred)
- Nonallergenic adhesive tape, 2.5 cm (1 in.) wide
- Commercial securement device, if available
- Clean gloves
- Water-soluble lubricant
- Facial tissues
- Glass of water and drinking straw
- 20- to 50-mL catheter tip syringe
- Basin
- pH test strip or meter
- Bilirubin dipstick
- Stethoscope
- Disposable pad or towel
- Antireflux valve for air vent if Salem sump tube is used
- Suction apparatus
- Safety pin and elastic band
- Clamp or plug (optional)
- CO_2 detector (optional)

IMPLEMENTATION
Preparation
- Assist the client to a high-Fowler's position if the client's health condition permits, and support the head on a pillow. **Rationale:** *It is often easier to swallow in this position, and gravity helps the passage of the tube.*
- Place a towel or disposable pad across the chest.

Performance
1. Prior to performing the insertion, introduce self and verify the client's identity using agency protocol. Explain to the client what you are going to do, why it is necessary, and how he or she can participate. The passage of a gastric tube is unpleasant because the gag reflex is activated during insertion. Establish a method for the client to indicate distress and a desire for you to pause the insertion. Raising a finger or hand is often used for this.
2. Perform hand hygiene and observe other appropriate infection prevention procedures.
3. Provide for client privacy.
4. Assess the client's nares.
   - Apply clean gloves.
   - Ask the client to hyperextend the head and, using a flashlight, observe the intactness of the tissues of the nostrils, including any irritations or abrasions.
   - Examine the nares for any obstructions or deformities by asking the client to breathe through one nostril while occluding the other.
   - Select the nostril that has the greater airflow.
5. Prepare the tube.
   - If a SBFT is being used, ensure the stylet or guidewire is secured in position. **Rationale:** *An improperly positioned stylet or guidewire can traumatize the nasopharynx, esophagus, and stomach.*
   - If a large-bore tube is being used, place the tube in a basin of warm water while preparing the client. **Rationale:** *This allows the tubing to become more pliable and flexible. However, if the softened tube becomes difficult to control, it may be helpful to place the distal end in a basin of ice water to help it hold its shape.*
6. Determine how far to insert the tube.
   - Use the tube to mark off the distance from the tip of the client's nose to the tip of the earlobe and then from the tip of the earlobe to the tip of the xiphoid. ❶ **Rationale:** *This length approximates the distance from the nares to the stomach. This distance varies among individuals.*
   - Mark this length with adhesive tape if the tube does not have markings.
7. Insert the tube.
   - Lubricate the tip of the tube well with water-soluble lubricant or water to ease insertion. In some agencies, topical lidocaine anesthetic is used on the tube or in the client's nose to numb the area (Uri, Yosefov, Haim, Behrbalk, & Halpern, 2011). **Rationale:** *A water-soluble lubricant dissolves if the tube accidentally enters the lungs. An oil-based lubricant, such as petroleum jelly, will not dissolve and could cause respiratory complications if it enters the lungs.*
   - Insert the tube, with its natural curve downward, into the selected nostril. Ask the client to hyperextend the neck, and gently advance the tube toward the nasopharynx. **Rationale:** *Hyperextension of the neck reduces the curvature of the nasopharyngeal junction.*
   - Direct the tube along the floor of the nostril and toward the midline. **Rationale:** *Directing the tube along the floor avoids the projections (turbinates) along the lateral wall.*

Inserting a Nasogastric Tube—*continued*

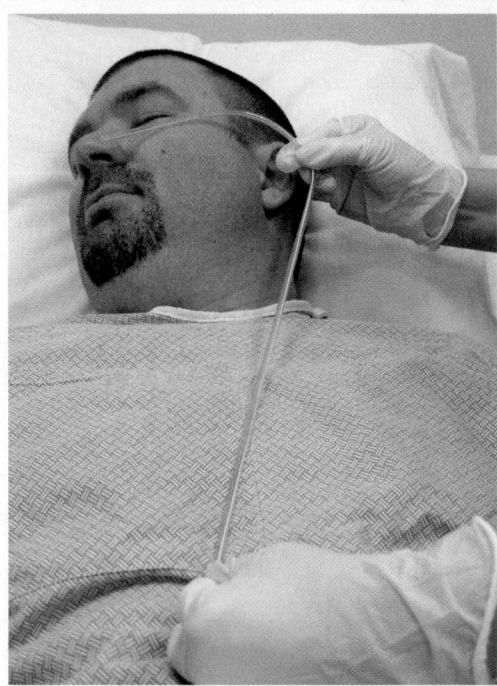

❶ Measuring the appropriate length to insert a nasogastric tube.

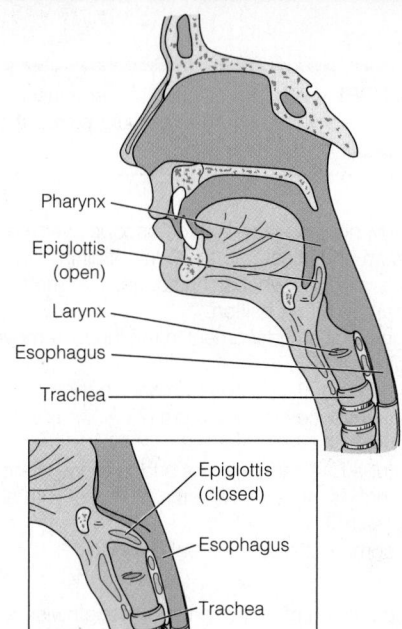

❷ Swallowing closes the epiglottis.

- Slight pressure and a twisting motion are sometimes required to pass the tube into the nasopharynx, and the client's eyes may water at this point. **Rationale:** *Tears are a natural body response. Provide the client with tissues as needed.*
- If the tube meets resistance, withdraw it, relubricate it, and insert it in the other nostril. **Rationale:** *The tube should never be forced against resistance because of the danger of injury.*
- Once the tube reaches the oropharynx (throat), the client will feel the tube in the throat and may gag and retch. Ask the client to tilt the head forward, and encourage the client to drink and swallow. **Rationale:** *Tilting the head forward facilitates passage of the tube into the posterior pharynx and esophagus rather than into the larynx; swallowing moves the epiglottis over the opening to the larynx.* ❷
- If the client gags, stop passing the tube momentarily. Have the client rest, take a few breaths, and take sips of water to calm the gag reflex.
- In cooperation with the client, pass the tube 5 to 10 cm (2 to 4 in.) with each swallow, until the indicated length is inserted.
- If the client continues to gag and the tube does not advance with each swallow, withdraw it slightly, and inspect the throat by looking through the mouth. **Rationale:** The tube may be coiled in the throat. If so, withdraw it until it is straight, and try again to insert it.
- If a CO_2 detector is used, after the tube has been advanced approximately 30 cm (12 in.), draw air through the detector. ❸ Any change in color of the detector indicates placement of the tube in the respiratory tract. Immediately withdraw the tube and reinsert.
8. Ascertain correct placement of the tube.
- Nasogastric tubes are radiopaque, and position can be confirmed by x-ray. If a SBFT is used, leave the stylet or guidewire in place until correct position is verified by x-ray.

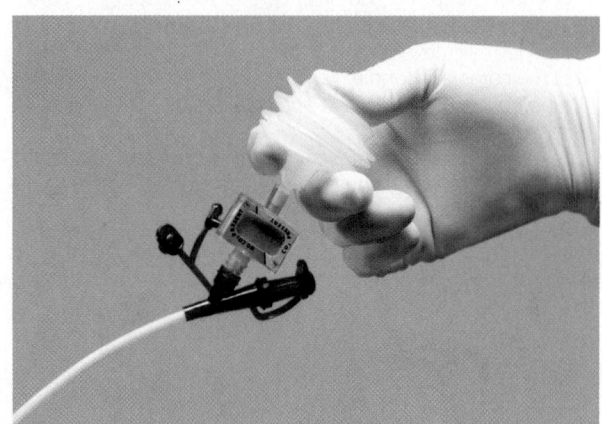

❸ After drawing air into the tube using a syringe or attached bellows, match the sensor color to the legend on the detector. This example shows purple—no CO_2 present.
Courtesy Covidien.

This is the only definitive method of verifying feeding tube tip placement. If an x-ray is not feasible, at least two of the following methods should be used.
- Aspirate stomach contents, and check the pH, which should be acidic. **Rationale:** *Testing pH is one way to determine location of a feeding tube. Gastric contents are commonly pH 1 to 5; pH of 6 or greater would indicate the contents are from lower in the intestinal tract or in the respiratory tract. However, pH may not discriminate between gastric and esophageal placement (Stepter, 2012).*
- Aspirate can also be tested for bilirubin. Bilirubin levels in the lungs should be almost zero, while levels in the stomach will be approximately 1.5 mg/dL and in the intestine over 10 mg/dL.

Continued on page 498

Inserting a Nasogastric Tube—*continued*

SAFETY ALERT! | SAFETY

If the stylet of a SBFT has been removed, never reinsert it while the tube is in place. The stylet is sharp and could pierce the tube and injure the client or cut off the tube end.

- Historically, nurses placed a stethoscope over the client's epigastrium and injected 5 to 20 mL of air into the tube while listening for a whooshing sound. This method does not guarantee tube position.
- If the signs indicate placement in the lungs, remove the tube and begin again.
- If the signs do not indicate placement in the lungs or stomach, advance the tube 5 cm (2 in.), and repeat the tests.

9. Secure the tube by taping it to the bridge of the client's nose.
   - If the client has oily skin, wipe the nose first with alcohol to defat the skin.
   - Apply a commercial securement device

   or

   - Cut 7.5 cm (3 in.) of tape, and split it lengthwise at one end, leaving a 2.5-cm (1-in.) tab at the end.
   - Place the tape over the bridge of the client's nose, and bring the split ends either under and around the tubing, or under the tubing and back up over the nose. ❹ Ensure that the tube is centrally located prior to securing with tape to maximize airflow and prevent irritation to the side of the nares. **Rationale:** *Taping in this manner prevents the tube from pressing against and irritating the edge of the nostril.*

10. Once correct position has been determined, attach the tube to a suction source or feeding apparatus as ordered, or clamp the end of the tubing.

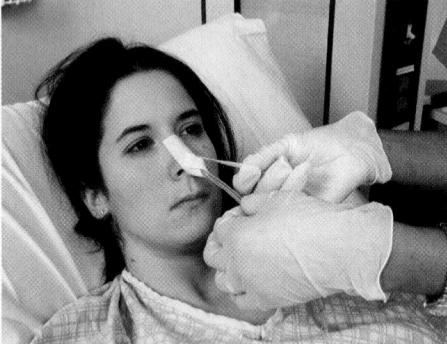

❹ Taping a nasogastric tube to the bridge of the nose.

11. Secure the tube to the client's gown.
    - Loop an elastic band around the end of the tubing, and attach the elastic band to the gown with a safety pin.

    or

    - Attach a piece of adhesive tape to the tube, and pin the tape to the gown. **Rationale:** *The tube is attached to prevent it from dangling and pulling.* If a Salem sump tube is used, attach the antireflux valve to the vent port (if used) and position the port above the client's waist. **Rationale:** *This prevents gastric contents from flowing into the vent lumen.*
    - Remove and discard gloves.
    - Perform hand hygiene.

12. Document relevant information: the insertion of the tube, the means by which correct placement was determined, and client responses (e.g., discomfort or abdominal distention).

13. Establish a plan for providing daily nasogastric tube care.
    - Inspect the nostril for discharge and irritation.
    - Clean the nostril and tube with moistened, cotton-tipped applicators.
    - Apply water-soluble lubricant to the nostril if it appears dry or encrusted.
    - Change the adhesive as required to secure the tube and prevent skin trauma from either tape or pressure of the tube against the nares.
    - Give frequent mouth care. Due to the presence of the tube, the client may breathe through the mouth.

14. If suction is applied, ensure that the patency of both the nasogastric and suction tubes is maintained.
    - Irrigation of the tube may be required at regular intervals. In some agencies, irrigation must be ordered by the primary care provider. Prior to irrigation, always recheck placement.
    - If a Salem sump tube is used, follow agency policies for irrigating the vent lumen with air to maintain patency of the suctioning lumen. Often, a sucking sound can be heard from the vent port if it is patent.
    - Keep accurate records of the client's fluid intake and output, and record the amount and characteristics of the drainage.

15. Document the type of tube inserted, date and time of tube insertion, type of suction used, color and amount of gastric contents, and the client's tolerance of the procedure.

SAMPLE DOCUMENTATION

11/5/2015 1030 Feeding tube (#8 Fr) inserted without difficulty through (R) nare with stylet in place. To x-ray to check placement. Radiologist reports tube tip in stomach. Stylet removed. Aspirate pH 4. Tube secured to nose. Verbalizes understanding of need to not pull on tube. ———————————————————— L. Traynor, RN

EVALUATION

Conduct appropriate follow-up, such as degree of client comfort, client tolerance of the nasogastric tube, correct placement of the nasogastric tube in the stomach, client understanding of restrictions, color and amount of gastric contents if attached to suction, or stomach contents aspirated.

LIFESPAN CONSIDERATIONS Inserting a Nasogastric Tube

INFANTS AND YOUNG CHILDREN
- Restraints may be necessary during tube insertion and throughout therapy. **Rationale:** *Restraints will prevent accidental dislodging of the tube.*
- Place the infant in an infant seat or position the infant with a rolled towel or pillow under the head and shoulders.
- When assessing the nares, obstruct one of the infant's nares and feel for air passage from the other. If the nasal passageway is very small or is obstructed, an orogastric tube may be more appropriate.

- Measure appropriate nasogastric tube length from the nose to the tip of the earlobe and then to the point midway between the umbilicus and the xiphoid process.
- If an orogastric tube is used, measure from the tip of the earlobe to the corner of the mouth to the xiphoid process.
- Do not hyperextend or hyperflex an infant's neck. **Rationale:** *Hyperextension or hyperflexion of the neck could occlude the airway.*
- Tape the tube to the area between the end of the nares and the upper lip as well as to the cheek.

Testing Feeding Tube Placement

Tube placement is confirmed by radiography, particularly when a SBFT has been inserted or when the client is at risk for aspiration. After placement is confirmed, the nurse marks the tube with indelible ink or tape at its exit point from the nose and documents the length of visible tubing for baseline data. The nurse is responsible, however, for verifying tube placement (i.e., GI placement versus respiratory placement) before each intermittent feeding and at regular intervals (e.g., at least once per shift) when continuous feedings are being administered.

Methods nurses use to check tube placement include the following:

1. Aspirate GI secretions. Because SBFTs offer more resistance during aspirations than large-bore tubes and are more likely to collapse when negative pressure is applied, it may not be possible to obtain an aspirate. If obtained, gastric secretions tend to be a grassy-green, off-white, or tan color; intestinal fluid is stained with bile and has a golden yellow or brownish green color.
2. Measure the pH of aspirated fluid. Testing the pH of aspirates can help distinguish gastric from respiratory and intestinal placement (see Skill 19–2, step 8).
3. Confirm the length of tube insertion with the insertion mark. If more of the tube is now exposed, the position of the tip should be questioned.

Currently, the most effective method is radiographic verification of tube placement. Repeated x-ray studies, however, are not feasible in terms of cost and radiation exposure. More research is required to devise effective alternatives, especially for placement of SBFTs. In the meantime, nurses should (a) ensure initial radiographic verification of SBFTs, (b) aspirate contents when possible and check their acidity, (c) closely observe the client for signs of obvious distress, and (d) consider tube dislodgment after episodes of coughing, sneezing, and vomiting.

Enteral Feedings

The type and frequency of feedings and amounts to be administered are ordered by the primary care provider. Liquid feeding mixtures are available commercially or may be prepared by the dietary department in accordance with the primary care provider's orders. A standard formula provides 1 Kcal per milliliter of solution with protein, fat, carbohydrate, minerals, fiber, and vitamins in specified proportions.

Enteral feedings can be given intermittently or continuously. **Intermittent feedings** are the administration of 300 to 500 mL of enteral formula several times per day. The stomach is the preferred site for these feedings, which are usually administered over at least

30 minutes. Initial intermittent feedings should be no more than 120 mL. If tolerated, increase by 120 mL each feeding until the goal is reached (DeBruyne & Pinna, 2014). **Bolus intermittent feedings** are those that use a syringe to deliver the formula into the stomach. Because the formula is delivered rapidly by this method (e.g., over 5 minutes), it is not usually recommended but may be used in long-term situations if the client tolerates it. These feedings must be given only into the stomach; the client must be monitored closely for distention and aspiration.

Continuous feedings are generally administered over a 24-hour period using an infusion pump (often referred to as a kangaroo pump) that guarantees a constant flow rate (Figure 19–10 ■).

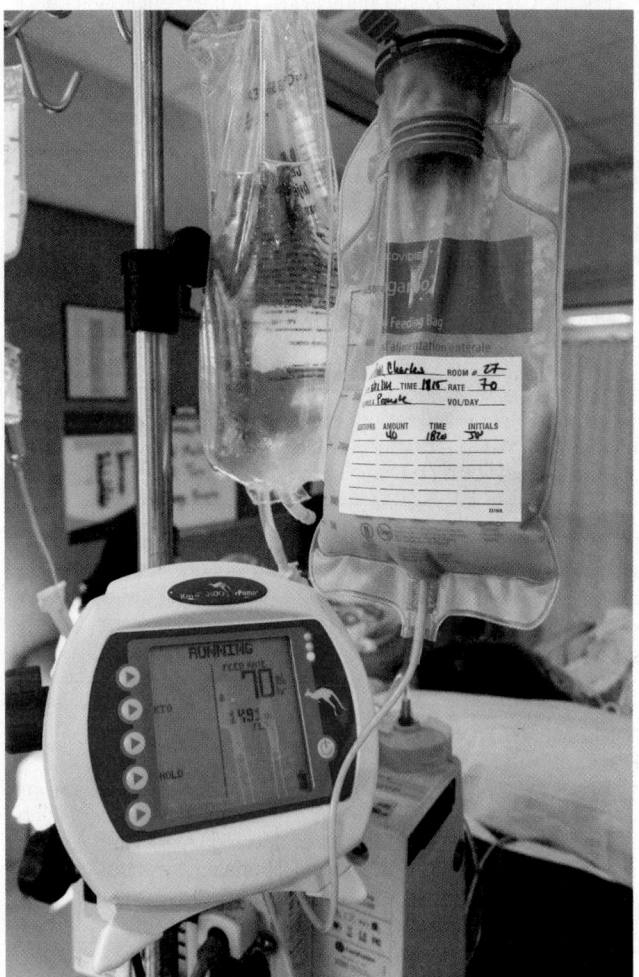

Figure 19–10 ■ An enteric feeding pump.

Initial intermittent feedings should be no more than 60 mL per hour. If tolerated, increase by 20 mL each feeding until the goal is reached (DeBruyne & Pinna, 2014). Continuous feedings are essential when feedings are administered in the small bowel.

Cyclic feedings are continuous feedings that are administered in less than 24 hours (e.g., 12 to 16 hours). These feedings, often administered at night, allow the client to attempt to eat regular meals throughout the day. Because nocturnal feedings may use higher nutrient densities and higher infusion rates than the standard continuous feeding, particular attention needs to be given to monitoring fluid status.

Enteral feedings are administered to clients through open or closed systems. **Open systems** use an open-top container or a syringe for administration. Enteral feedings for use with open systems are provided in flip-top cans or powdered formulas that are reconstituted with sterile water. Sterile water, rather than tap water, reduces the risk of microbial contamination. Open systems should have no more than 8 to 12 hours of formula poured at one time (DeBruyne & Pinna, 2014). At the completion of this time, remaining formula should be discarded and the container rinsed before new formula is poured. The bag and tubing should be replaced every 24 hours. **Closed systems** consist of a prefilled container that is spiked with enteral tubing and attached to the enteral access device. Prefilled containers can hang safely for as long as 48 hours if sterile technique is used. Closed systems materials are more expensive than open systems but if nursing care costs are included, closed systems are less expensive (Phillips, Roman, & Glassman, 2013).

Skill 19–3 provides the essential steps involved in administering a tube feeding, and Skill 19–5 indicates the steps involved in administering a gastrostomy or jejunostomy tube feeding.

●○● NURSING PROCESS: TUBE FEEDING

Administering a Tube Feeding

SKILL 19–3

ASSESSMENT
Assess:
- For any clinical signs of malnutrition or dehydration.
- For allergies to any food in the feeding. If the client is lactose intolerant, check the tube feeding formula. Notify the primary care provider if any incompatibilities exist.
- For the presence of bowel sounds.
- For any problems that suggest lack of tolerance of previous feedings (e.g., delayed gastric emptying, abdominal distention, diarrhea, cramping, or constipation).

PLANNING
Before commencing a tube feeding, determine the type, amount, and frequency of feedings and tolerance of previous feedings.

DELEGATION

Administering a tube feeding requires application of knowledge and problem solving and it is not usually delegated to UAP. Some agencies, however, may allow a trained UAP to administer a feeding. In this case, it is the responsibility of the nurse to assess tube placement and determine that the tube is patent. The nurse should reinforce major points, such as making sure the client is sitting upright, and instruct the UAP to report any difficulty administering the feeding or any complaints voiced by the client.

INTERPROFESSIONAL PRACTICE

Administering a tube feeding is generally not performed by other health care providers, although it may not be prohibited by their scope of practice.

Equipment
- Correct type and amount of feeding solution
- 60-mL catheter-tip syringe
- Emesis basin
- Clean gloves
- pH test strip or meter
- Large syringe or calibrated plastic feeding bag with label and tubing that can be attached to the feeding tube or prefilled bottle with a drip chamber, tubing, and a flow-regulator clamp
- Measuring container from which to pour the feeding (if using open system)
- Water (60 mL unless otherwise specified) at room temperature
- Feeding pump as required

SAFETY ALERT! | SAFETY

Do not add colored food dye to tube feedings. Previously, blue dye was often added to assist in recognition of aspiration. However, the U.S. Food and Drug Administration reports cases of many adverse reactions to the dye, including toxicity and death.

IMPLEMENTATION
Preparation
- Assist the client to a Fowler's position (at least 30° elevation) in bed or a sitting position in a chair, the normal position for eating. If a sitting position is contraindicated, a slightly elevated right side-lying position is acceptable. **Rationale:** *These positions enhance the gravitational flow of the solution and prevent aspiration of fluid into the lungs.*

Performance
1. Prior to performing the feeding, introduce self and verify the client's identity using agency protocol. Explain to the client what you are going to do, why it is necessary, and how he or she can participate. Inform the client that the feeding should not cause any discomfort but may cause a feeling of fullness.
2. Perform hand hygiene and observe other appropriate infection prevention procedures.

Administering a Tube Feeding—*continued*

3. Provide privacy for this procedure if the client desires it. Tube feedings are embarrassing to some people.

4. Assess tube placement prior to initiating a feeding or three times per day for continuous feedings.
- Apply clean gloves.
- Examine the placement mark on the tube to determine if it has advanced or slipped out.
- Attach the syringe to the open end of the tube and aspirate. Check the pH.
- Allow 1 hour to elapse before testing the pH if the client has received a medication.
- Use a pH meter rather than pH paper if the client is receiving a continuous feeding. Follow agency policy if the pH is 6 or greater.

5. Assess residual feeding contents.
- If the tube is placed in the stomach, aspirate all contents and measure the amount before administering the feeding. **Rationale:** *This is done to evaluate absorption of the last feeding; that is, whether undigested formula from a previous feeding remains. If the tube is in the small intestine, residual contents cannot be aspirated.*
- If 100 mL (or more than half of the last feeding) is withdrawn, check with the nurse in charge or refer to agency policy before proceeding. The precise amount of residual requiring intervention is usually determined by the primary care provider's order or by agency policy. **Rationale:** *At some agencies, a feeding is delayed when the specified amount or more of formula remains in the stomach.*

or

- Reinstill the gastric contents into the stomach if this is the agency policy or primary care provider's order. **Rationale:** *Removal of the contents could disturb the client's electrolyte balance.*
- If the client is on a continuous feeding, check the gastric residual every 4 to 6 hours or according to agency protocol.

6. Administer the feeding.
- Before administering feeding:
  a. Check the expiration date of the feeding.
  b. Warm the feeding to room temperature. **Rationale:** *An excessively cold feeding may cause abdominal cramps.*
  c. When an open system is used, clean the top of the feeding container with alcohol before opening it. **Rationale:** *This minimizes the risk of contaminants entering the feeding syringe or feeding bag.*

Feeding Bag (Open System)
- Hang the labeled bag from an infusion pole about 30 cm (12 in.) above the tube's point of insertion into the client.
- Clamp the tubing and add the formula to the bag.
  a. Apply a label that indicates the date, time of starting the feeding, and nurse's initials on the feeding bag.
- Open the clamp, run the formula through the tubing, and reclamp the tube. **Rationale:** *The formula will displace the air in the tubing, thus preventing the instillation of excess air into the client's stomach or intestine.*
- Attach the bag to the feeding tube ❶ and regulate the drip by adjusting the clamp to the drop factor on the bag (e.g., 20 drops/mL) if not placed on a pump.

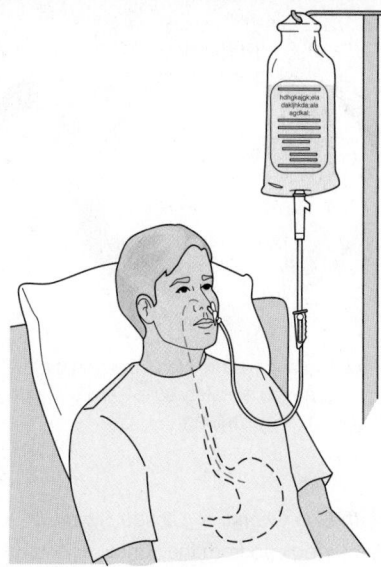

❶ Using a calibrated plastic bag to administer a tube feeding.

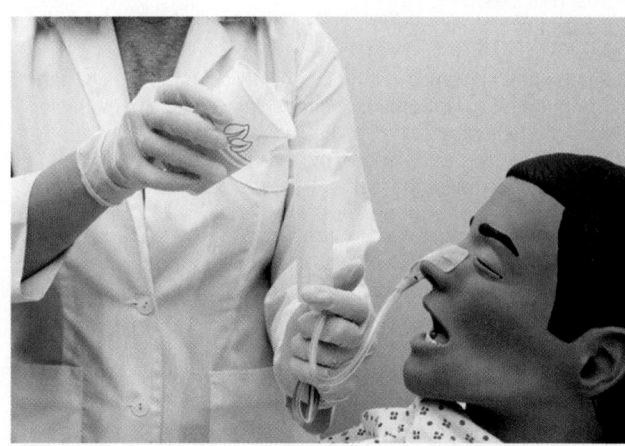

❷ Using the barrel of a syringe to administer a tube feeding.

Syringe (Open System)
- Remove the plunger from the syringe and connect the syringe to a pinched or clamped nasogastric tube. **Rationale:** *Pinching or clamping the tube prevents excess air from entering the stomach and causing distention.*
- Add the feeding to the syringe barrel. ❷
- Permit the feeding to flow in slowly at the prescribed rate. Raise or lower the syringe to adjust the flow as needed. Pinch or clamp the tubing to stop the flow for a minute if the client experiences discomfort. **Rationale:** *Quickly administered feedings can cause flatus, cramps, and/or vomiting.*

Continued on page 502

Administering a Tube Feeding—*continued*

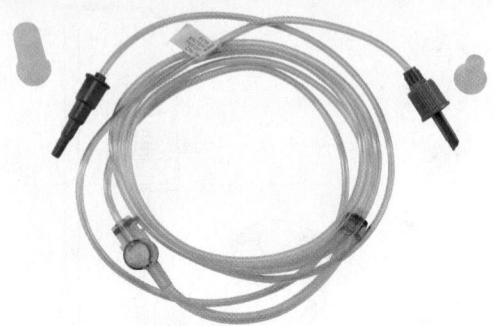

❸ Feeding set with spike and tubing. Note, the port on the cap can only be accessed using a special safety screw spike to prevent accidental connection using intravenous tubing.

Courtesy Covidien.

Prefilled Bottle with Drip Chamber (Closed System)

- Remove the screw-on cap from the container and attach the administration set with tubing. ❸
- Close the clamp on the tubing.
- Hang the container on an intravenous (IV) pole about 30 cm (12 in.) above the tube's insertion point into the client. **Rationale:** *At this height, the formula should run at a safe rate into the stomach or intestine.*
- Squeeze the drip chamber to fill it to one third to one half of its capacity.
- Open the tubing clamp, run the formula through the tubing, and reclamp the tube. **Rationale:** *The formula will displace the air in the tubing, thus preventing the instillation of excess air.*
- Attach the feeding set tubing to the feeding tube and regulate the drip rate to deliver the feeding over the desired length of time or attach to a feeding pump.

7. If another bottle is not to be immediately hung, flush the feeding tube before all of the formula has run through the tubing.
   - Instill 50 to 100 mL of water through the feeding tube or medication port. **Rationale:** *Water flushes the lumen of the tube, preventing future blockage by sticky formula.*
   - Be sure to add the water before the feeding solution has drained from the neck of a syringe or from the tubing of an administration set. **Rationale:** *Adding the water before the syringe or tubing is empty prevents the instillation of air into the stomach or intestine and thus prevents unnecessary distention.*

8. Clamp the feeding tube.
   - Clamp the feeding tube before all of the water is instilled. **Rationale:** *Clamping prevents leakage and air from entering the tube if done before water is instilled.*

9. Ensure client comfort and safety.
   - Secure the tubing to the client's gown. **Rationale:** *This minimizes pulling of the tube, thus preventing discomfort and dislodgment.*
   - Ask the client to remain sitting upright in Fowler's position or in a slightly elevated right lateral position for at least 30 minutes. **Rationale:** *These positions facilitate digestion*

and movement of the feeding from the stomach along the alimentary tract, and prevent the potential aspiration of the feeding into the lungs.
   - Check the agency's policy on the frequency of changing the nasogastric tube and the use of smaller lumen tubes if a large-bore tube is in place. **Rationale:** *These measures prevent irritation and erosion of the pharyngeal and esophageal mucous membranes.*
   - Remove and discard gloves.
   - Perform hand hygiene.

10. Dispose of equipment appropriately.
    - If the equipment is to be reused, wash it thoroughly with soap and water so that it is ready for reuse.
    - Change the equipment every 24 hours or according to agency policy.

11. Document all relevant information.
    - Document the feeding, including amount and kind of solution taken, duration of the feeding, and assessments of the client.
    - Record the volume of the feeding and water administered on the client's intake and output record.

SAMPLE DOCUMENTATION

11/5/2015 1330 Aspirated 20 mL pale yellow fluid from NG tube, pH 5. Returned residual. Placed in Fowler's position. 1 liter room-temperature ordered formula begun @ 60 mL/hour on pump. No nausea reported. ──────────── L. Traynor, RN

12. Monitor the client for possible problems.
    - Carefully assess the client receiving tube feedings for problems.
    - To prevent dehydration, give the client supplemental water in addition to the prescribed tube feeding as ordered.

Variation: Continuous-Drip Feeding

- Interrupt the feeding at least every 4 to 6 hours, or as indicated by agency protocol or the manufacturer, and aspirate and measure the gastric contents. **Rationale:** *This determines adequate absorption and verifies correct placement of the tube. If placement of a SBFT is questionable, a repeat x-ray should be done.*
- Determine agency protocol regarding withholding a feeding. Many agencies withhold the feeding if more than 75 to 100 mL of feeding is aspirated. If the feeding is withheld, flush the tubing with water to prevent formula from clogging the tube.
- To prevent spoilage or bacterial contamination, do not allow the feeding solution to hang longer than 12 hours for an open system and 48 hours for a closed system. Check agency policy or the manufacturer's recommendations regarding time limits.
- Follow agency policy regarding how frequently to change the feeding bag and tubing. Changing the feeding bag and tubing every 24 hours reduces the risk of contamination.

Administering a Tube Feeding—*continued*

EVALUATION

Perform a follow-up examination of the following:

- Tolerance of feeding (e.g., nausea, cramping)
- Bowel sounds
- Regurgitation and feelings of fullness after feedings
- Weight gain or loss

- Fecal elimination pattern (e.g., diarrhea, flatulence, constipation)
- Skin turgor
- Urine output and specific gravity.

Relate findings to previous assessment data if available. Report significant deviations from normal to the primary care provider.

LIFESPAN CONSIDERATIONS   Administering a Tube Feeding

INFANTS AND YOUNG CHILDREN

- Feeding tubes may be removed after each feeding and reinserted at the next feeding to prevent irritation of the mucous membrane, nasal airway obstruction, and stomach perforation that may occur if the tube is left in place continuously. Check agency practice.
- Formula should not be allowed to hang more than 4 hours (DeBruyne & Pinna, 2014).
- Position a small child or infant in your lap, provide a pacifier, and hold and cuddle the child during feedings. This promotes comfort, supports the normal sucking instinct of the infant, and facilitates digestion.

OLDER ADULTS

- Physiological changes associated with aging may make the older adult more vulnerable to complications associated with enteral feedings. Decreased gastric emptying may necessitate checking frequently for gastric residual. Diarrhea from administering the feeding too fast or at too high a concentration may cause dehydration. If the feeding has a high concentration of glucose, assess for hyperglycemia because with aging, the body has a decreased ability to handle increased glucose levels.
- Conditions such as hiatal hernia and diabetes mellitus may cause the stomach to empty more slowly. This increases the risk of aspiration in a client receiving a tube feeding. Checking for gastric residual more frequently can help document this if it is an ongoing problem. Changing the formula or the rate of administration, repositioning the client, or obtaining a primary care provider's order for a medication to increase stomach emptying may resolve this problem.

CLIENT TEACHING CONSIDERATIONS

Tube Feedings

Clients and caregivers need the following instructions to manage these feedings:

- Teach and provide the client or caregiver the rationale for how to assess for tube placement using pH measurement before administering the feeding. Instruct regarding actions to take if the pH is greater than 5.
- Preparation of the formula. Include the name of the formula and how much and how often it is to be given; the need to inspect the formula for the expiration date and leaks and cracks in bags or cans; how to mix or prepare the formula, if needed; and aseptic techniques such as cleansing the container's top with alcohol before opening it, and changing the syringe administration set and reservoir every 24 hours.
- Proper storage of the formula. Include the need to refrigerate diluted or reconstituted formula and formula that contains additives.
- Administration of the feeding. Include proper hand cleansing technique, how to fill and hang the feeding bag, operation of an infusion pump if indicated, the feeding rate, and client positioning during and after the feeding.
- Discuss strategies for hanging formula containers if an IV pole is unavailable or inconvenient.
- Management of the enteral access device. Include site care; aseptic precautions; dressing change, as indicated; how the site should look normally; and flushing protocols (e.g., type of irrigant and schedule).
- Daily monitoring needs. Include temperature, weight, and intake and output.
- Signs and symptoms of complications to report. Include fever, increased respiratory rate, decrease in urine output, increased stool frequency or diarrhea, and altered level of consciousness.
- Whom to contact about questions or problems. Include emergency telephone numbers of the home care agency, nursing clinician, and/or primary care provider, or other 24-hour on-call emergency service.
- Plan for optimal timing of feedings to allow for daily activities. Many clients can tolerate having the majority of their feedings run during sleep so they are free from the equipment during the day.

●○○● NURSING PROCESS: REMOVING A NASOGASTRIC TUBE

SKILL 19–4

Removing a Nasogastric Tube

ASSESSMENT
Assess:
- For the presence of bowel sounds.
- For the absence of nausea or vomiting when the tube is clamped.

PLANNING
DELEGATION

Due to the need for assessment of client status, the skill of removing a nasogastric tube is not delegated to UAP.

INTERPROFESSIONAL PRACTICE

Removing a nasogastric tube may be within the scope of practice for other health care providers such as PAs. Although PAs may verbally communicate their actions and plan to the health care team members, the nurse must also know where to locate their documentation in the client's medical record.

Equipment
- Disposable pad or towel
- Tissues
- Clean gloves
- 50-mL syringe (optional)
- Moisture-proof trash bag

IMPLEMENTATION
Preparation
- Confirm the primary care provider's order to remove the tube.
- Assist the client to a sitting position if health permits.
- Place the disposable pad or towel across the client's chest to collect any spillage of secretions from the tube.
- Provide tissues to the client to wipe the nose and mouth after tube removal.

Performance
1. Prior to performing the removal, introduce self and verify the client's identity using agency protocol. Explain to the client what you are going to do, why it is necessary, and how he or she can participate.
2. Perform hand hygiene and observe other appropriate infection prevention procedures.
3. Provide for client privacy.
4. Detach the tube.
   - Apply clean gloves.
   - Disconnect the nasogastric tube from the suction apparatus, if present.
   - Unpin the tube from the client's gown.
   - Remove the adhesive securing the tube to the nose.
5. Remove the nasogastric tube.
   - *Optional:* Instill 50 mL of air into the tube. **Rationale:** *This clears the tube of any contents such as feeding or gastric drainage and decreases the chances of dragging any drainage through the esophagus and nasopharynx.*
   - Ask the client to take a deep breath and to hold it. **Rationale:** *This closes the glottis, thereby preventing accidental aspiration of any gastric contents.*

- Pinch the tube with the gloved hand. **Rationale:** *Pinching the tube prevents any contents inside the tube from draining into the client's throat.*
- Smoothly withdraw the tube.
- Place the tube in the trash bag. **Rationale:** *Placing the tube immediately into the bag prevents the transference of microorganisms from the tube to other articles or people.*
- Observe the intactness of the tube.
6. Ensure client comfort.
   - Provide mouth care if desired.
   - Assist the client as required to blow the nose. **Rationale:** *Excessive secretions may have accumulated in the nasal passages.*
7. Dispose of the equipment appropriately.
   - Place the pad, bag with tube, and gloves in the receptacle designated by the agency. **Rationale:** *Correct disposal prevents the transmission of microorganisms.*
   - Remove and discard gloves.
   - Perform hand hygiene.
8. Document all relevant information.
   - Record the removal of the tube, the amount and appearance of any drainage if connected to suction, and any relevant assessments of the client.

SAMPLE DOCUMENTATION

11/8/2015 1500 NG tube removed intact without difficulty. Oral & nasal care given. No bleeding or excoriation noted. States is hungry & thirsty. 60 mL apple juice given. No c/o nausea. — L. Traynor, RN

EVALUATION
- Perform a follow-up examination, such as presence of bowel sounds, absence of nausea or vomiting when tube is removed, and intactness of tissues of the nares.

- Relate findings to previous assessment data if available.
- Report significant deviations from normal to the primary care provider.

●○● NURSING PROCESS: GASTROSTOMY OR JEJUNOSTOMY FEEDING

Administering a Gastrostomy or Jejunostomy Feeding

ASSESSMENT
See Skill 19–3.

PLANNING
Before beginning a gastrostomy or jejunostomy feeding, determine the type and amount of feeding to be instilled, frequency of feedings, and any pertinent information about previous feedings (e.g., the positioning in which the client best tolerates the feeding).

DELEGATION

See Skill 19–3.

INTERPROFESSIONAL PRACTICE

See Skill 19–3.

Equipment
- Correct amount of feeding solution
- Graduated container and tubing with clamp to hold the feeding
- 60-mL catheter-tip syringe

For a Tube That Remains in Place
- Mild soap and water
- Clean gloves
- Petrolatum, zinc oxide ointment, or other skin protectant
- Precut 4×4 gauze squares
- Uncut 4×4 gauze squares
- Paper tape

For Tube Insertion
- Clean gloves
- Moisture-proof bag
- Water-soluble lubricant
- Feeding tube (if needed)

IMPLEMENTATION
Preparation
See Skill 19–3.

Performance
1. Prior to performing the feeding, introduce self and verify the client's identity using agency protocol. Explain to the client what you are going to do, why it is necessary, and how he or she can participate.
2. Perform hand hygiene and observe other appropriate infection prevention procedures.
3. Provide for client privacy.
4. Insert a feeding tube, if one is not already in place.
   - Wearing gloves, remove the dressing. Then discard the dressing and gloves in the moisture-proof bag.
   - Perform hand hygiene.
   - Apply new clean gloves.
   - Lubricate the end of the tube, and insert it into the ostomy opening 10 to 15 cm (4 to 6 in.).
5. Check the location and patency of the tube.
   - Determine correct placement of the tube by aspirating and checking the pH of the return.
   - Follow agency policy related to amount of residual formula. This may include withholding the feeding, rechecking in 3 to 4 hours, or notifying the primary care provider if a large residual remains.
   - For continuous feedings, check the residual every 4 to 6 hours and hold feedings according to agency policy.
   - Remove the syringe plunger. Pour 15 to 30 mL of water into the syringe, remove the tube clamp, and allow the water to flow into the tube. **Rationale:** *This determines the patency of the tube. If water flows freely, the tube is patent.*
   - If the water does not flow freely, notify the nurse in charge and/or the primary care provider.
6. Administer the feeding.
   - Hold the barrel of the syringe 7 to 15 cm (3 to 6 in.) above the ostomy opening.
   - Slowly pour the solution into the syringe and allow it to flow through the tube by gravity.
   - Just before the syringe is empty, add 30 mL of water. **Rationale:** *Water flushes the tube and preserves its patency.*

- If the tube is to remain in place, hold it upright, remove the syringe, and then clamp or plug the tube to prevent leakage.
- If a tube was inserted for the feeding, remove it.
- Remove and discard gloves.
- Perform hand hygiene.
7. Ensure client comfort and safety.
   - After the feeding, ask the client to remain in the sitting position or a slightly elevated right lateral position for at least 30 minutes. **Rationale:** *This minimizes the risk of aspiration.*
   - Assess status of peristomal skin. **Rationale:** *Gastric or jejunal drainage contains digestive enzymes that can irritate the skin.* Document any redness and broken skin areas.
   - Check orders about cleaning the peristomal skin, applying a skin protectant, and applying appropriate dressings. Generally, the peristomal skin is washed with mild soap and water at least once daily. The tube may be rotated between thumb and forefinger to release any sticking and promote tract formation. Petrolatum, zinc oxide ointment, or other skin protectant may be applied around the stoma, and precut 4×4 gauze squares may be placed around the tube. The precut squares are then covered with regular 4×4 gauze squares, and the tube is coiled and taped over them.
   - Observe for common complications of enteral feedings: aspiration, hyperglycemia, abdominal distention, diarrhea, and fecal impaction. Report findings to the primary care provider. Often, a change in formula or rate of administration can correct problems.
   - When appropriate, teach the client how to administer feedings and when to notify the primary care provider concerning problems.
8. Document all assessments and interventions.

SAMPLE DOCUMENTATION

6/24/2015 2045 No fluid aspirated from gastrostomy tube. Placed in Fowler's position. 30 mL water flowed freely by gravity through tube. 250 mL room-temperature Ensure formula given over 20 minutes. No complaints of discomfort. ——————————— L. Traynor, RN

EVALUATION
See Skill 19–3.

WHAT IF   Administering a Gastrostomy Feeding Using an Open System

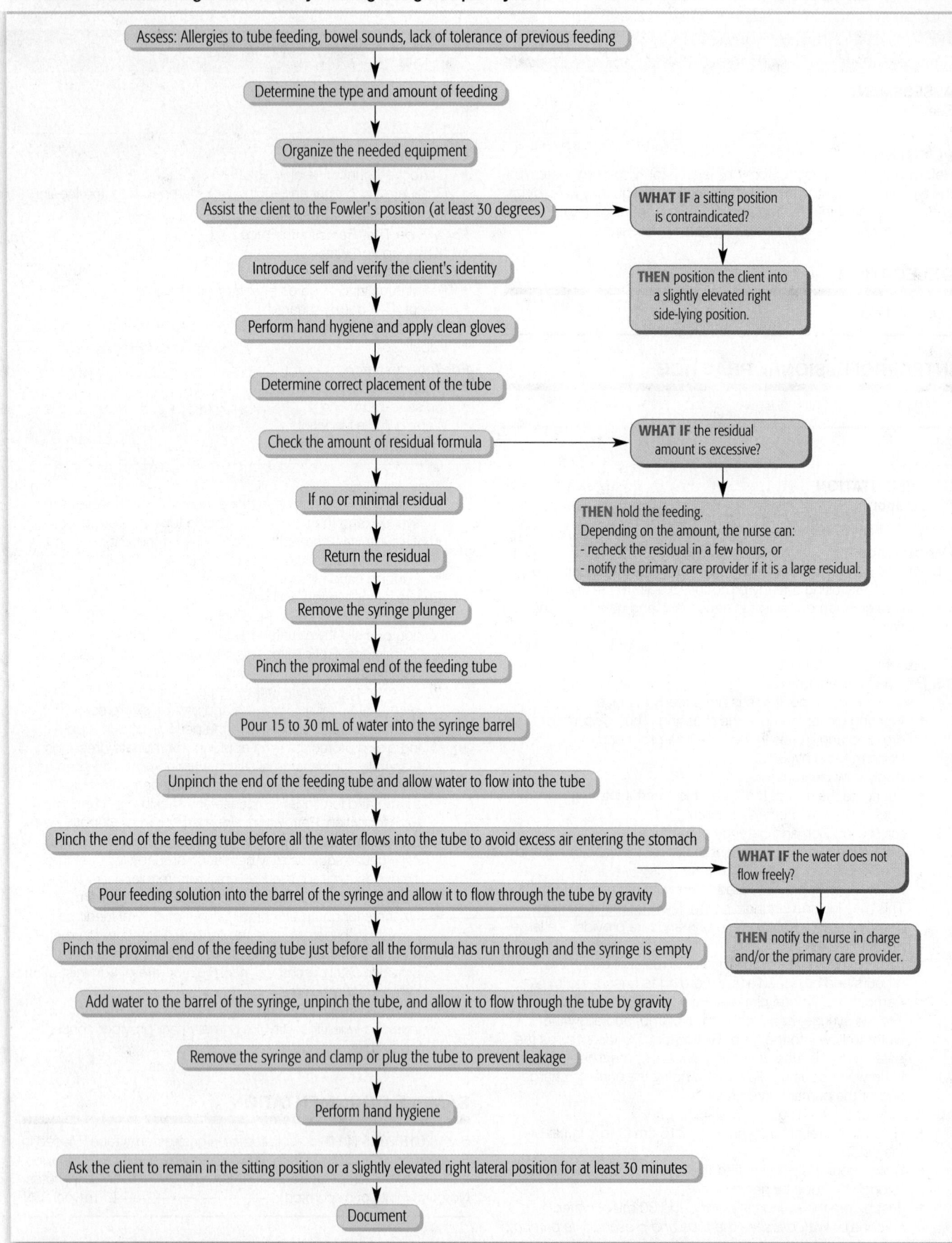

Managing Clogged Feeding Tubes

Even if feeding tubes are flushed with water before and after feedings and medications, they still become clogged—especially SBFTs. This can occur when the feeding container runs dry, solid medication is not adequately crushed, or medications are mixed with formula. Even the important practice of aspirating to check residual volume increases the incidence of clogging. To avoid the necessity of removing the tube and reinserting a new tube, both prevention and intervention strategies must be used.

To prevent clogged feeding tubes, flush liberally (at least 30 mL water) before, between, and after each separate medication is instilled, using a 60-mL piston syringe. Too great a pressure can rupture the tube—especially SBFTs. Do not add medications to formula or to each other since the combination could create a precipitate that clogs the tube.

Many strategies have been used to try to unclog feeding tubes. The first strategy that should be tried is to reposition the client, which may allow a kink to straighten. Alternately flush and aspirate the tube with water. Strategies that have shown inconsistent effectiveness include instilling meat tenderizer, carbonated beverages, or cranberry juice (Stepter, 2012), or flushing with small-barrel syringes. Until 2013, only enteric-coated and extended-release pancreatic enzymes were available as unclogging agents in the United States. However, an effective uncoated enzyme product, used in combination with sodium bicarbonate, is now available (Klang, Gandhi, & Mironova, 2013). Commercial unclogging kits containing a combination of acids, buffers, antibacterial agents, enzymes, and metal inhibitors are available.

PARENTERAL NUTRITION

Parenteral nutrition has two forms: total and peripheral. **Total parenteral nutrition (TPN)**, also referred to as **hyperalimentation**, is the IV infusion of water, protein, carbohydrates, electrolytes, minerals, and vitamins. Because TPN solutions are hypertonic (highly concentrated in comparison to the solute concentration of blood), they are administered only into high-flow central veins, where they are diluted by the client's blood. Access to these veins is through a central venous catheter or a peripherally inserted central catheter (PICC). See Chapter 18 ∞. TPN is used when enteral access is not possible or the client is unable to tolerate the enteral feedings.

TPN formulas provide all of the known essential nutrients in quantities that promote weight maintenance or gain and wound healing. Between 10% and 50% dextrose in water, plus a mixture of amino acids and special additives, such as vitamins (e.g., B complex, C, D, K), minerals (e.g., potassium, sodium, chloride, calcium, phosphate, magnesium), and trace elements (e.g., zinc, manganese), are mixed together in one container and infused as the primary TPN solution. Lipid emulsions containing primarily essential fatty acids are administered from a separate container through a Y-connector into the TPN intravenous line or are combined with the TPN solution.

The proportion of nutrients and total calories delivered varies with the individual's nutritional needs. Thus, a thorough nutritional assessment is required to determine the appropriate TPN regimen. Examples of clients who may receive TPN include those with severe malnutrition, burns, bowel disease disorders, cancer, or major surgeries where nothing may be taken by mouth for more than 5 days. A description of the components of parenteral nutrition is provided in Table 19–4.

TPN is not risk-free. Infection control is of utmost importance. The nurse must always observe surgical aseptic technique when changing solutions, tubing, dressings, and filters. Because TPN solutions are high in dextrose, infusions are started gradually to prevent hyperglycemia. Levels are monitored during the infusion. When TPN therapy is to be discontinued, the TPN infusion rates are decreased slowly to prevent hypoglycemia.

Clients are also at increased risk of fluid and electrolyte imbalances and require frequent evaluation and modification of the TPN mixture. In addition, clients on long-term TPN are at high risk for developing liver, gallbladder, and metabolic bone conditions (DeBruyne & Pinna, 2014).

Peripheral parenteral nutrition (PPN), delivered into the smaller peripheral veins, cannot handle as concentrated a solution as central lines but can accommodate lipids. For example, a 20% lipid emulsion can provide nearly 2,000 Kcal per day through a peripheral vein. PPN is considered to be a safe and convenient form of therapy. One major disadvantage, however, is the frequent incidence of phlebitis associated with PPN. Substituting glycerol for dextrose may reduce vein irritation (Julian, 2013). Peripheral parenteral nutrition is administered to clients whose needs for IV nutrition will last only a short time or in whom placement of a central venous catheter is contraindicated. It is a form of therapy used more frequently to *prevent* nutritional deficits than to correct them.

TABLE 19–4	Components of Parenteral Nutrition
Component	**Description**
Protein	Supplied as crystalline synthetic amino acids; contains essential and nonessential amino acids (4 calories/gram of protein; 1 gram nitrogen/6 grams protein)
Carbohydrate	Supplied as dextrose at 3.4 calories/gram (DeBruyne & Pinna, 2014). Peripheral administration 0% to 10% dextrose; central administration up to 50%, although usual is 20% to 25%
Electrolytes	Added to formula; can include sodium, potassium, chloride, acetate, calcium, phosphorus, magnesium; administered according to need
Minerals	Added to formula; can include zinc, chromium, manganese, and copper; administered according to need
Vitamins	Recommended allowances of vitamins A, thiamine, riboflavin, B_6, B_{12}, C, D, E, folic acid, niacin, biotin, and pantothenic acid
Fat/lipids	Contains primarily essential fatty acids; 9 calories/gram

SKILL 19–6

●○○● NURSING PROCESS: PARENTERAL NUTRITION

Providing Total Parenteral Nutrition

ASSESSMENT
- Gather the pertinent data. Know the purpose of the TPN.
- Confirm the order for the TPN.
- Obtain the client's vital signs, including recent body temperature, weight, fluid balance, and any allergy to ingredients in the TPN solution.
- Know the client's recent lab values.

PLANNING
Review the client record regarding previous TPN. Note any complications and how they were managed.

DELEGATION

Due to the need for sterile technique and technical complexity, administration of TPN is not delegated to UAP. UAP may care for clients receiving TPN, and the nurse must ensure that the UAP knows what complications or adverse signs should be reported to the nurse.

INTERPROFESSIONAL PRACTICE

Providing ongoing TPN is generally not in the scope of practice for other health care providers. However, other qualified professionals such as PAs may insert the IV access device.

Equipment
- TPN solution
- Timing tape
- Infusion pump
- Tubing with filter

IMPLEMENTATION
Preparation
- Inspect and prepare the solution.
- Remove the ordered TPN solution from the refrigerator 1 hour before use, and check each ingredient and the proposed rate against the order on the chart. **Rationale:** *Infusion of a cold solution can cause pain, hypothermia, and venous spasm and constriction.*
- Inspect the solution for cloudiness or presence of particles, and ensure that the container is free from cracks or tears. For lipids, examine the bag for separation of emulsion, fat globules, or froth.
- Before administering any TPN solution:
  - Check its expiration date. Most solutions must be used within 24 hours of preparation, unless they are refrigerated.
  - Two licensed nurses need to check the nutrients in the bag with the order written by the primary care provider. **Rationale:** *This is another check that ensures the solution was properly prepared by the pharmacist.*
  - Apply a timing tape on the solution container.

PERFORMANCE
1. Prior to performing the procedure, introduce self and verify the client's identity using agency protocol. Explain to the client what you are going to do, why it is necessary, and how he or she can participate.
2. Perform hand hygiene and observe other appropriate infection prevention procedures.
3. Provide for client privacy and prepare the client.
   - Assist the client to a comfortable position, either sitting or lying. If necessary, expose the central line site but provide for client privacy.
4. Change the solution container to the TPN solution ordered.
   - Ensure that correct placement of the central line catheter has been confirmed by x-ray examination.
   - Ensure that the tubing has an in-line filter connected at the end of the TPN tubing. For plain TPN, use a 0.22-micron filter. ❶, *A.* For TPN with lipids, the filter must be 1.2 microns. ❶, *B.* Plain lipids are infused without a filter. **Rationale:** *The filter traps bacteria and particles that can form in the TPN solution.*
   - Attach and connect the tubing to an infusion pump, if not present. See Skill 18–3 on pages 458–459. **Rationale:** *A pump eliminates the changes in flow rate that occur with alterations in the client's activity and position.*

❶ *A,* A 0.22-micron filter used for TPN; *B,* a 1.2-micron filter for use with TPN containing lipids.

- Attach the TPN solution to the IV administration tubing. If a multiple-lumen tube is in place, attach the infusion to the appropriate lumen. If possible, a lumen should be dedicated to TPN use only.
- If lipids are being infused separately from the TPN, connect the lipid tubing to the injection port closest to the client (below the TPN filter).
5. Regulate and monitor the flow rate.
   - Establish the prescribed rate of flow and monitor the infusion at least every 30 minutes.
   - Never accelerate an infusion that has fallen behind schedule. **Rationale:** *Wide fluctuations in blood glucose can occur if the rate of TPN infusion is irregular.*
   - Never interrupt or discontinue the infusion abruptly. If TPN solution is temporarily unavailable, infuse a solution containing at least 5% to 10% dextrose. **Rationale:** *This prevents rebound hypoglycemia.*
   - During the initial stage of a lipid infusion (i.e., the first hour), closely monitor vital signs and signs of any side effects (e.g., fever, flushing, diaphoresis, dyspnea, cyanosis, headache, nausea, or vomiting).

Providing Total Parenteral Nutrition—*continued*

- Start lipid infusions very slowly according to the primary care provider's orders, the manufacturer's directions, and agency policy. For a 10% emulsion, start at 1 mL/min for the first 5 minutes, then up to 4 mL/min for the next 25 minutes. If well tolerated, set the ordered rate thereafter.
6. Monitor the client for complications.
   - Change the administration set and filter every 24 hours.
   - Monitor the vital signs every 4 hours. If fever or abnormal vital signs occur, notify the primary care provider. **Rationale:** *An elevated temperature is one of the earliest indications of catheter-related sepsis.*
   - Collect double-voided urine specimens in accordance with agency policy, and test the urine for specific gravity. If the specific gravity is abnormal, notify the primary care provider, who may alter the constituents of the TPN solution.
   - Assess capillary (finger-stick) blood glucose levels every 6 hours or according to agency protocol (see Skill 4–1 in Chapter 4 ∞). **Rationale:** *Blood glucose is tested to make certain the infusion is not running too rapidly for the body to metabolize glucose or too slowly for caloric needs to be met.* Notify the primary care provider of abnormal glucose

levels. For hyperglycemia, supplementary insulin may be ordered subcutaneously or added directly to the TPN solution. For hypoglycemia, the infusion rate may need to be increased.
   - Measure the daily fluid intake and output and calorie intake. **Rationale:** *Precise replacement for fluid and electrolyte deficits can then be more readily determined.*
   - Monitor the results of laboratory tests (e.g., serum electrolytes and blood urea nitrogen) and report abnormal findings to the primary care provider.
7. Assess weight and anthropometric measurements.
   - Weigh the client daily, at the same time and in the same garments. A gain of more than 0.5 kg (1.1 lb) per day indicates fluid excess and should be reported.
   - Measure arm circumference and triceps skinfold thickness weekly or in accordance with agency protocol to assess the physical changes.
8. Document all relevant information.
   - Record the type and amount of infusion, rate of infusion, vital signs q4h, finger-stick blood glucose levels as ordered, client's weight daily, and anthropometric measurements.

EVALUATION

- Perform follow-up based on findings or outcomes that deviated from expected or normal for the client. Relate findings to previous data if available.

- Report significant deviations from normal to the primary care provider.

Chapter **19** Review

FOCUSING ON CLINICAL THINKING

Consider This

1. A 75-year-old female client has recently been diagnosed with chronic lung cancer that has left her susceptible to pneumonia. As a result, her primary care provider has ordered three different oral medications that have resulted in her losing her appetite and a 22-pound weight loss. Once overweight, the client is now within the weight parameters for her height and age. The client tells her home health nurse that "nothing sounds good and nothing tastes good." The client lives alone and is responsible for her own meal preparation.
   a. Do you have any concerns regarding this client's nutritional needs?
   b. What information would be helpful to you as the nurse in order to meet or maintain the client's nutritional needs?
   c. What suggestions do you have for ways to enhance the client's intake during this period of decreased appetite?
   d. Do you think the client is a good candidate for a feeding tube? Why or why not?

2. It is time for the next tube feeding. You have just checked feeding tube placement and obtained the pH of the aspirated fluid for the following three clients. What actions would you take for each client?
   Client A: pH 3
   Client B: pH 6
   Client C: pH 7

3. Contaminated enteral feeding formula can put the client at risk for many problems. How can you minimize or avoid the risk of contamination for both the open and closed feedings systems?

4. How must TPN be infused differently if it has lipids combined in the same infusion bag?

See Focusing on Clinical Thinking answers on student resource website.

TEST YOUR KNOWLEDGE

1. The nurse is assessing a client's intake of micronutrients. The nurse would consider the intake of which of the following?
   1. Carbohydrates, proteins, and fats
   2. Fat-soluble vitamins and protein
   3. Vitamins and minerals
   4. Minerals and carbohydrates

2. While caring for a client with a medical diagnosis of anorexia and malnutrition, the nurse needs to assess for which of the following? Select all that apply.
   1. Reduced cardiac output
   2. Impaired pulmonary function
   3. An incompetent immune response
   4. Altered functional abilities
   5. Dysphagia

3. The nurse is preparing to assess the nutritional status of an older adult client in a long-term care facility. What screening tool would best suit this purpose?
   1. A comprehensive nutritional assessment
   2. The Nutrition Screening Initiative (NSI)
   3. The Patient-Generated Subjective Global Assessment (PG-SGA)
   4. A daily nutrition intake log

4. The nurse is caring for a client who is 48 hours post–bowel resection with creation of a colostomy. This morning the nurse assessed the return of bowel sounds. In what order would this client's diet progress?
   1. Full liquid diet
   2. Regular diet
   3. Clear liquid diet
   4. NPO
   5. Soft diet

5. The nurse would anticipate the need for an enteral access device in which client?
   1. A client who has severe acute dysphagia
   2. A client whose bowel sounds have not yet returned after abdominal surgery
   3. A client who dislikes the taste of facility meals
   4. A client who recently had a cerebrovascular accident

6. The nurse is caring for a client in a chronic vegetative state with inadequate gastric emptying. What type of enteral access device would the nurse anticipate finding in this client?
   1. Nasogastric tube
   2. Nasoenteric tube
   3. Gastrostomy tube
   4. Jejunostomy tube

7. If the nurse is administering bolus intermittent feedings, the enteral access device must be what type?
   1. Nasojejunal
   2. Percutaneous jejunostomy
   3. Gastrostomy
   4. Nasointestinal

8. The nurse is caring for a client with a nasogastric feeding tube in place. What interventions would the nurse perform to reduce the risk of clogging the tube when administering feedings or medications? Select all that apply.
   1. Administer the feeding and medication as fast as possible so they cannot solidify in the tube.
   2. Mix medication with feeding to dilute the medication thoroughly.
   3. Flush the tube liberally with water before, between, and after each medication instillation.
   4. Use the largest barrel syringe possible to reduce the pressure in the tube.
   5. Crush solid medications thoroughly and mix in water before instillation.

9. The nurse has just inserted a nasogastric tube. All of the following methods are acceptable means of assessing placement *except:*
   1. Aspirate the tube to determine if gastric contents are obtained.
   2. Test contents aspirated from the tube for pH.
   3. Perform a radiologic examination.
   4. Auscultate the epigastrium while instilling 60 mL of air.

10. The nurse is caring for a client who requires assistance with eating. The client repeatedly apologizes to the nurse, saying "I'm such a burden. I can't even feed myself. I'm like a little baby. I'm so sorry." What strategy is the most appropriate for the nurse to use?
    1. Feed the client quickly so as not to make the client feel like it is taking a great deal of time out of the nurse's day.
    2. Appear unhurried, sit at the bedside, and encourage the client to feed himself/herself as much as possible.
    3. Feed all of the solid foods first, and then offer liquids.
    4. Minimize conversation so that the client can eat faster.

See Answers to Test Your Knowledge in Appendix A.

READINGS AND REFERENCES

References

American Dietetic Association. (2002). *National dysphagia diet: Standardization for optimal care.* Chicago, IL: Author.

DeBruyne, L. K., & Pinna, K. (2014). *Nutrition for health and healthcare* (5th ed.). Belmont, CA: Wadsworth/Cengage.

Julian, M. K. (2013). Caring for your patient receiving TPN. *Nursing Made Incredibly Easy, 11*(1), 8–11. doi:10.1097/01.NME.0000423373.68269.52

Klang, M. G., Gandhi, U. D., & Mironova, O. (2013). Dissolving a nutrition clog with a new pancreatic enzyme

formulation. *Nutrition in Clinical Practice, 28,* 410–412. doi:10.1177/0884533613481477

Nutrition Screening Initiative. (2008). *Determine your nutritional health.* Washington, DC: National Council on Aging.

Phillips, W., Roman, B., & Glassman, K. (2013). Economic impact of switching from an open to a closed enteral nutrition feeding system in an acute care setting. *Nutrition in Clinical Practice, 28,* 510–514. doi:10.1177/0884533613489712

Sekino, M., Yoshitomi, O., Nakamura, T., Makita, T., & Sumikawa, K. (2012). A new technique for post-pyloric

feeding tube placement by palpation in lean critically ill patients. *Anaesthesia & Intensive Care, 40*(1), 154–158.

Stepter, C. R. (2012). Maintaining placement of temporary enteral feeding tubes in adults: A critical appraisal of the evidence. *Medsurg Nursing, 21*(2), 61–68, 102.

Uri, O., Yosefov, L., Haim, A., Behrbalk, E., & Halpern, P. (2011). Lidocaine gel as an anesthetic protocol for nasogastric tube insertion in the ED. *American Journal of Emergency Medicine, 29,* 386–390. doi:10.1016/j.ajem.2009.10.011

Selected Bibliography

Akhtar, S. R. (2011). TPN? And when? *Critical Care Alert*, *19*(8), 57–58.

Berman, A., Snyder, S., & Frandsen, G. (2016). *Kozier & Erb's fundamentals of nursing: Concepts, process, and practice* (10th ed.). Upper Saddle River, NJ: Pearson.

Chan, E., Ng, I., Tan, S., Jabin, K., Lee, L., & Ang, C. (2012). Nasogastric feeding practices: A survey using clinical scenarios. *International Journal of Nursing Studies*, *49*, 310–319. doi:10.1016/j.ijnurstu.2011.09.014

Chasen, M., & Bhargava, R. (2012). Gastrointestinal symptoms, electrogastrography, inflammatory markers, and PG-SGA in patients with advanced cancer. *Supportive Care in Cancer*, *20*, 1283–1290. doi:10.1007/s00520-011-1215-8

Dandeles, L. M., & Lodolce, A. E. (2011). Efficacy of agents to prevent and treat enteral feeding tube clogs. *Annals of Pharmacotherapeutics*, *45*, 676–680. doi:10.1345/aph.1P487

Di Sabatino, A., & Corazza, G. (2012). Nonceliac gluten sensitivity: Sense or sensibility? *Annals of Internal Medicine*, *156*, 309–311. doi:10.7326/0003-4819-156-4-201202210-00010

Fletcher, J. (2013). Parenteral nutrition: Indications, risks and nursing care. *Nursing Standard*, *27*(46), 50–57. doi:10.7748/ns2013.07.27.46.50.e7508

Gabrielson, D. K., Scaffidi, D., Leung, E., Stoyanoff, L., Robinson, J., Nisenbaum, R., . . . Darling, P. B. (2013). Use of an abridged scored Patient-Generated Subjective Global Assessment (abPG-SGA) as a nutritional screening tool for cancer patients in an outpatient setting. *Nutrition & Cancer*, *65*, 234–239. doi:10.1080/01635581.2013.755554

Gomes Jr., C., Lustosa, S., Matos, D., Andriolo, R., Waisberg, D., & Waisberg, J. (2012). Percutaneous endoscopic gastrostomy versus nasogastric tube feeding for adults with swallowing disturbances. *Cochrane Database of Systematic Reviews*, Issue 3, Art. No.: CD008096. doi:10.1002/14651858.CD008096.pub3

Hanson, L. C., Carey, T. S., Caprio, A. J., Lee, T., Ersek, M., Garrett, J., . . . Mitchell, S. L. (2011). Improving decision-making for feeding options in advanced dementia: A randomized, controlled trial. *Journal of the American Geriatrics Society*, *59*, 2009–2016. doi:10.1111/j.1532-5415.2011.03629.x

Karon, B. S. (2011). Tips from the clinical experts. Blood specimens from patients receiving TPN. *Medical Laboratory Observer*, *43*(10), 38–39.

Kirkland, L., Kashiwagi, D., Brantley, S., Scheurer, D., & Varkey, P. (2013). Nutrition in the hospitalized patient. *Journal of Hospital Medicine*, *8*(1), 52–58. doi:10.1002/jhm.1969

Longo, M. (2011). Best evidence: Nasogastric tube placement verification. *Journal of Pediatric Nursing*, *26*, 373–376. doi:10.1016/j.pedn.2011.04.030

Lundin, K., & Alaedini, A. (2012). Non-celiac gluten sensitivity. *Gastrointestinal Endoscopy Clinics of North America*, *22*, 723–734. doi:10.1016/j.giec.2012.07.006

Pan, H., Cai, S., Ji, J., Jiang, Z., Liang, H., Lin, F., & Liu, X. (2013). The impact of nutritional status, nutritional risk, and nutritional treatment on clinical outcome of 2248 hospitalized cancer patients: A multi-center, prospective cohort study in Chinese teaching hospitals. *Nutrition and Cancer*, *65*(1), 62–70. doi:10.1080/01635581.2013.741752

Payne, C., Methven, L., Fairfield, C., & Bell, A. (2011). Consistently inconsistent: Commercially available starch-based dysphagia products. *Dysphagia*, *26*(1), 27–33. doi:10.1007/s00455-009-9263-7

Peate, I., & Gault, C. (2013). Clinical skills series/4: Nasogastric tube insertion. *British Journal of Healthcare Assistants*, *6*, 272–277.

Pietzak, M. (2012). Celiac disease, wheat allergy, and gluten sensitivity: When gluten free is not a fad. *Journal of Parenteral & Enteral Nutrition*, *36*(1 Suppl.), 68S–75S. doi:10.1177/0148607111426276

Roth, R. A. (2014). *Nutrition and diet therapy* (11th ed.). Clifton Park, NY: Delmar/Cengage.

Shah, Z. M., Suraiya, H. S., Poi, P. J., Tan, K. S., Lai, P. S., Ramakrishnan, K., & Mahadeva, S. (2012). Long-term nasogastric tube feeding in elderly stroke patients—An assessment of nutritional adequacy and attitudes to gastrostomy feeding in Asians. *Journal of Nutrition, Health & Aging*, *16*, 701–706. doi:10.1007/s12603-012-0027-y

Son, Y., & Song, E. (2013). High nutritional risk is associated with worse health-related quality of life in patients with heart failure beyond sodium intake. *European Journal of Cardiovascular Nursing*, *12*, 184–192. doi:10.1177/1474515112443439

Upile, T., Stimpson, P., Christie, M., Mahil, J., Tailor, H., & Jerjes, W. (2011). Use of gel caps to aid endoscopic insertion of nasogastric feeding tubes: A comparative audit. *Head & Neck Oncology*, *3* doi:10.1186/1758-3284-3-24

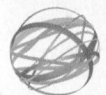 **20** Assisting with Urinary Elimination

LEARNING OUTCOMES

At the completion of this chapter, the student will be able to:

1. Define the key terms used in urinary elimination.
2. Identify essential components of a urinary elimination history.
3. Recognize when it is appropriate to delegate urinary care to unlicensed assistive personnel.
4. Verbalize the steps used in:
   a. Assisting clients with the use of a urinal.
   b. Applying an external urinary device.
   c. Performing urinary catheterization.
   d. Performing catheter care and removal.
   e. Performing bladder irrigation.
   f. Performing urinary ostomy care.
5. Identify indications and contraindications for urinary catheterization.
6. Identify reasons for using various types of urinary catheters or drainage systems.
7. Identify essential interventions for:
   a. Clients requiring catheterization.
   b. Clients requiring bladder irrigation.
   c. Clients with urinary diversion ostomies.
8. Demonstrate appropriate documentation and reporting of urinary elimination skills.

SKILLS

Skill 20–1 Assisting with a Urinal
Skill 20–2 Applying an External Urinary Device
Skill 20–3 Performing Urinary Catheterization

Skill 20–4 Performing Catheter Care and Removal
Skill 20–5 Performing Bladder Irrigation
Skill 20–6 Performing Urinary Ostomy Care

KEY TERMS

catheter, *518*
CAUTI, *518*
condom catheter, *516*
external catheter, *516*
Foley catheter, *519*

ileal conduit, *531*
ileal loop, *531*
irrigation, *529*
meatus, *512*
micturition, *513*

Robinson catheter, *519*
suprapubic catheter, *527*
urinary incontinence (UI), *514*
urinary retention, *513*

urinary sheath, *516*
urination, *513*
voiding, *513*

Elimination from the urinary tract is usually taken for granted. Only when a problem arises do most people become aware of their urinary habits and any associated symptoms. The nurse's role in urinary elimination may be to (a) assist the client with urinary control, (b) obtain a urine specimen (voided or catheterized), (c) assess for urine retention using a bladder scanner, or (d) establish bladder emptiness through catheterization.

THE URINARY SYSTEM

Urine is formed in the kidneys and then carried into the kidney pelvis and the ureter. The ureters extend from the kidneys to the urinary bladder. The urinary bladder lies behind the symphysis pubis. In the male, it lies in front of the rectum and above the prostate gland (Figure 20–1 ■); in the female, it lies in front of the uterus and vagina (Figure 20–2 ■).

The urethra of the adult female is approximately 4 cm (1.5 in.) in length. In the adult male, it is about 20 cm (8 in.) long. The urethra extends from the bladder to the external surface of the body. This external opening is called the urinary **meatus** or the urethral orifice.

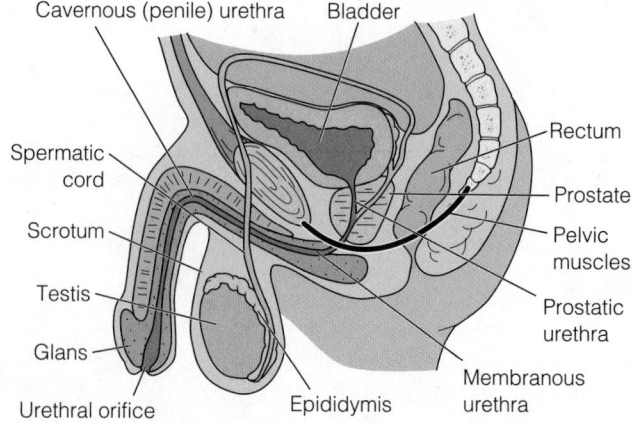

Figure 20–1 ■ The male urogenital system.

In the female, it is located between the labia minora, in front of the vagina and below the clitoris (Figure 20–3 ■); in the male, it is located at the distal end of the penis (see Figure 20–1).

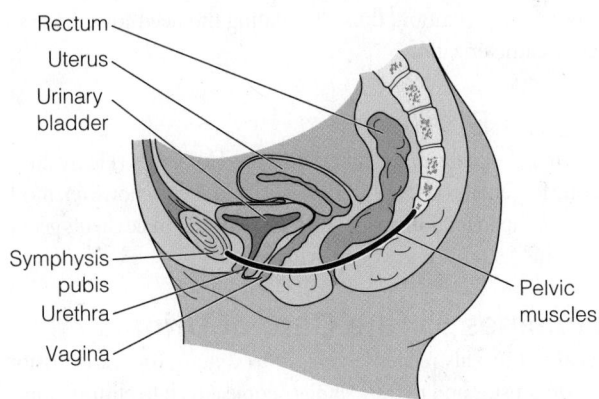

Figure 20–2 ■ The female urogenital system.

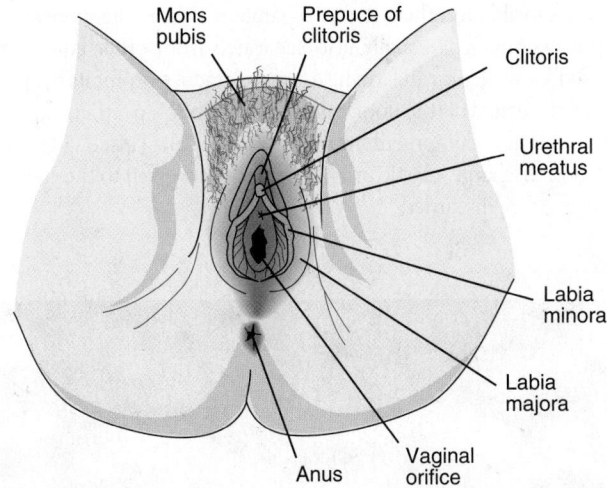

Figure 20–3 ■ Location of the female urinary meatus in relation to surrounding structures.

The urethra, in both males and females, has a continuous mucous membrane lining with the bladder and the ureters. Thus, an infection of the urethra can readily extend through the urinary tract to the kidneys.

Micturition, **voiding**, and **urination** all refer to the process of emptying the urinary bladder. Urine collects in the bladder until pressure stimulates special sensory nerve endings in the bladder wall called *stretch receptors*. This occurs when the adult bladder contains between 250 and 450 mL of urine. Messages sent from these nerves to the brain result in (a) contraction of the detrusor muscle and (b) relaxation of the internal sphincter muscle. As a result, urine can be released from the bladder, but it is still held back by the external urinary sphincter. In the female, the external urethral sphincter is situated at about the midpoint of the urethra; in the male, it is distal to the prostatic portion of the urethra.

If the time and place are appropriate for urination, the conscious portion of the brain relaxes the external urethral sphincter muscle, and urination takes place. If the time and place are inappropriate, the micturition reflex usually subsides until the bladder becomes more filled and the reflex is stimulated again. Table 20–1 shows variations in urinary elimination among different age groups.

URINARY CONTROL

Urinary control problems fall into two major categories: retention and incontinence.

Urinary retention is the accumulation of urine in the bladder and inability of the bladder to empty itself. Because urine production continues, retention results in distention of the bladder. With urinary retention, some adult bladders may distend to hold 3,000 to 4,000 mL of urine. Acute urinary retention is the most common complication in the first 2 to 4 hours postoperatively (Palese, Buchini, Deroma, & Barbone, 2010). Causes of chronic urinary retention can include paraplegia, quadriplegia, multiple sclerosis, and urethral or perineal trauma (Bullman, 2011, p. 259).

TABLE 20–1	Variations in Urinary Elimination by Age	
Age	**Average Daily Urine Output**	**Other Variations**
1–2 days	15–60 mL	Ability to concentrate urine is minimal; therefore, urine appears light yellow in color. Voluntary urinary control absent.
3–10 days	100–300 mL	
10 days–2 months	250–450 mL	
2 months–1 year	400–500 mL	
1–3 years	500–600 mL	Urine effectively concentrated, normal amber color; voluntary control begins.
3–5 years	600–700 mL	Full urinary control.
5–8 years	700–1,000 mL	
8–14 years	800–1,400 mL	
Adult	1,200–1,500 mL	Kidneys continue to grow until about age 40; begin to diminish in size and function after age 50.
Older adult	1,500 mL or less	Ability to concentrate urine declines.

Occasionally, a person will have urinary retention with overflow. In this situation, the bladder is holding urine, and only the overflow urine is excreted when the pressure of the urine overwhelms sphincter control. The client then voids small amounts of urine frequently or dribbles urine, while the bladder remains distended.

Urinary incontinence (UI) is a temporary or permanent inability of the external sphincter muscles to control the flow of urine from the bladder. It is the opposite of retention. The severity of urinary incontinence ranges from occasionally leaking urine during coughing or sneezing to having an urge to void that is so strong that a person cannot make it to the bathroom in time. UI is a health symptom, not a disease. It has been estimated that 20 million women and 6 million men experience some type of UI in their lifetime (Scemons, 2013, p. 53). Shultz (2012) found that 30% of homebound older adults are incontinent, and UI contributed significantly to their being homebound. More than half of all residents in long-term care (LTC) facilities are incontinent and UI is the second leading cause of institutionalization (p. 32). In spite of the high numbers of adults with UI, it is underreported and undertreated, and can lead to a decreased qualify of life (Keyock & Newman, 2011). It is important to remember that UI is *not* a normal part of aging and often is treatable.

Bladder Scanning

Historically, it was difficult for the nurse to truly assess the presence and amount of urine in the client's bladder without the invasive procedure of catheterization, which increases the risk of urinary tract infection. Current technology using sound waves (ultrasound) permits quick, noninvasive, and accurate determination of bladder volume through bladder scanning. A handheld, cordless scanner requires less than 5 seconds to display the bladder volume on its liquid crystal screen (Figure 20–4 ■).

Use of a bladder scan enables the nurse to determine if the client is retaining urine after voiding (also called postvoid residual [PVR]), or has urinary retention, thus eliminating the need for unnecessary, invasive catheterization.

URINALS

Two urinal designs are available: One is used for males (Figure 20–5 ■) and one for females (Figure 20–6 ■). Female clients, however, most often use a bedpan for both urine and feces, whereas male clients generally use a urinal for urine and a bedpan for feces.

Guidelines for the Care of Urinals

The care of urinals relates largely to preventing the transmission of microorganisms and to the feelings people attach to elimination.

- To maintain medical asepsis, each hospitalized client is provided with a separate urinal.
- Urinals are stored in an appropriate place out of sight. Bedside units are often designed to provide a specific place for urinals that is not visible to others and is separate from the client's personal possessions. It is usually also separated from other equipment used for hygienic care. Medical aseptic practice prohibits the placing of a urinal on the floor, under the bed, or on overbed tables.
- Elimination equipment must be thoroughly rinsed after use. Upon discharge, plastic urinals are generally given to the client to keep or are discarded.

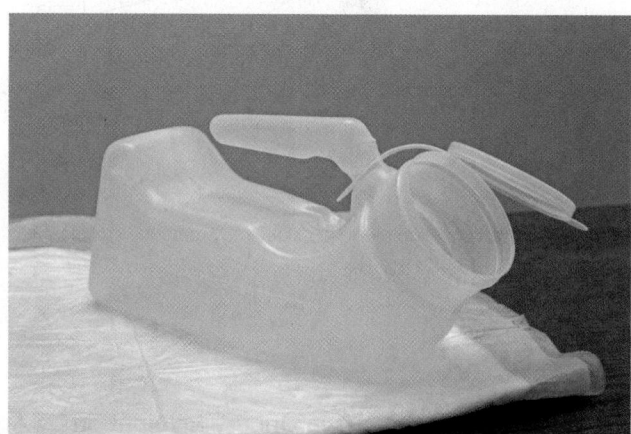

Figure 20–5 ■ Male urinal.

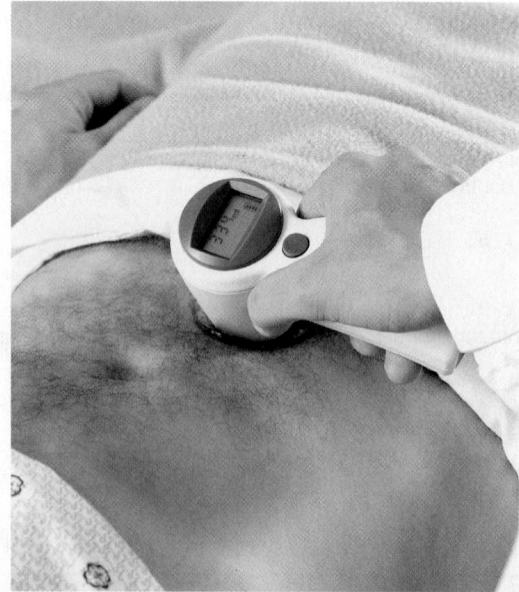

Figure 20–4 ■ A handheld, portable ultrasound device can measure bladder urine volume noninvasively.

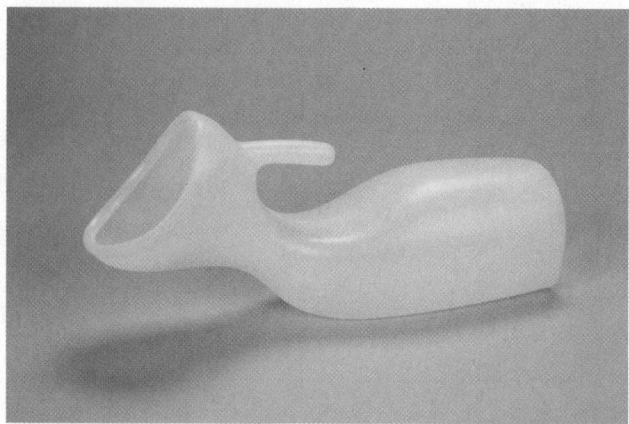

Figure 20–6 ■ Female urinal.

●○● NURSING PROCESS: URINARY ELIMINATION AND USING A URINAL

Assisting with a Urinal

ASSESSMENT

The following assessment items relate to various aspects of urinary elimination. The nurse selects items appropriate to the particular skill being performed. Determine the client's usual patterns and frequency of urination. Ask the client the approximate number of times that voiding occurs each day. Determine any recent alterations in voiding with regard to:

- Passage of unusually large or small amounts of urine.
- Voiding at more frequent intervals than usual for the client.
- Trouble getting to the bathroom in time or feeling an urgency to void.
- Painful voiding.
- Difficulty starting urine stream.
- Frequent dribbling of urine or feeling of bladder fullness associated with voiding small amounts of urine.
- Reduced force of stream.
- Accidental leakage of urine and when this occurs (e.g., when coughing, laughing, or sneezing; at night; during the day).

Obtain the medical history of urinary elimination problems, urinary tract disease or surgery, and other diseases that may affect urinary elimination, including:

- Infections of the kidney, bladder, or urethra.
- Urinary calculi (stones).
- Kidney surgery, bladder surgery, prostate removal, or other surgical procedures that alter urinary routes (e.g., ureterostomy).
- Cardiovascular disease, such as hypertension or heart disease.
- Chronic diseases that alter urinary characteristics or impair urinary function, such as diabetes mellitus, neurologic disease (e.g., multiple sclerosis), and cancer.

Assess the volume and characteristics of the client's urine, including:

- When the client last voided and the amount. (Unanticipated volumes of less than 30 mL or more than 500 mL per hour must be reported immediately.)
- Dark, cloudy, or discolored urine.

- Presence of mucous plugs.
- Offensive odor.

Determine any factors influencing urinary elimination:

- *Medications:* Any medications that could increase urinary output (e.g., diuretic), cause retention of urine (e.g., anticholinergic–antispasmodic, antidepressant–antipsychotic, antiparkinsonism drugs, antihistamines, antihypertensives), or discolor urine (e.g., multivitamins, chemotherapy).
- *Fluid intake:* Amount and kind of fluid taken each day (e.g., six glasses of water, five cups of coffee, three cola drinks with or without caffeine; rate of IV fluids).
- *Environmental factors:* Any problems with toileting (mobility, dexterity with clothing, toilet seat too low, facility without grab bar).
- *Diagnostic procedures:* Recent procedures such as a cystoscopy or spinal anesthetic.

Determine the presence of pain:

- *Bladder pain:* Pain over the suprapubic region.
- *Kidney or flank pain:* Pain between the ribs and ileum that may spread to the abdomen and be associated with nausea and vomiting or pain at the costovertebral angle, which may radiate to the umbilicus.
- *Ureteral pain:* Pain in the back, which may radiate to the abdomen, upper thigh, testes, or labia.

Review data from diagnostic tests and examinations, including:

- Urine pH under 4.5 or over 8.
- Specific gravity under 1.010 or over 1.025.
- Presence of glucose or acetone in the urine.
- Presence of occult or visible blood in the urine.
- Presence of protein, urobilinogen, or nitrite in the urine.
- Presence of microorganisms in the urine.
- Blood serum: blood urea nitrogen (BUN), creatinine, sodium, potassium.

PLANNING

In preparing to assist the client with use of a urinal, determine if there are any restrictions in positioning the client. Inquire whether the client has used a urinal previously. If so, determine if the client has any unique needs related to the use of the urinal. Locate the client's urinal.

DELEGATION

Assisting the client with a urinal is often delegated to unlicensed assistive personnel (UAP). Ensure that UAP are aware of any specimens that need to be collected. The nurse must validate and interpret abnormal findings.

Equipment

- Clean urinal
- Toilet tissue
- Equipment for a specimen if required (see Skills 4–3 through 4–5 in Chapter 4 ∞)
- Clean gloves

IMPLEMENTATION

Preparation

- Assist the client to an appropriate position.
  - Both males and females confined to bed may prefer a semi-Fowler's position, or the male may prefer a standing position at the side of the bed if health permits.

Performance

1. Prior to performing the procedure, introduce self and verify the client's identity using agency protocol. Explain to the client what you are going to do, why it is necessary, and how he or she can participate. Discuss how the results will be used in planning further care or treatments.

2. Perform hand hygiene and observe other appropriate infection prevention procedures.
3. Provide for client privacy.
4. Assist the client with using the urinal.
   - Offer the urinal so that the client can position it independently.

   or

   - Place the urinal between the client's legs with the handle uppermost so that urine will flow into it.
   - Leave the signal cord within reach of the person. **Rationale:** *The client can then call for assistance if required.*

Continued on page 516

SKILL 20-1

Assisting with a Urinal—*continued*

- Leave for 2 to 3 minutes or until the client signals.

or

- Remain if the client needs support to stand at the bedside or other assistance.

5. Assist the client with removing the urinal as needed.
   - Apply clean gloves.
   - Remove the urinal.
   - If wet, wipe the area around the urethral orifice with a tissue. Dry the perineum.
   - Change the linens or pad under the client if it is wet.
   - Provide the client with hand wipes, a dampened washcloth, or water, soap, and a towel to wash and dry hands.

6. Attend to the urine as required.
   - Measure the urine if the client is on monitored intake and output, and transfer a specimen to the appropriate container if required.

- Empty and rinse out the urinal, and return it to the bedside unit. If the male client prefers, the urinal may be hung on the side rail by its handle for easy access.
- Remove and discard gloves.
- Perform hand hygiene.

7. Document findings in the client record using forms or checklists supplemented by narrative notes when appropriate. Record the amount of urine, if it was measured, and all assessment data (e.g., cloudy urine, reddened perineum).

SAMPLE DOCUMENTATION

4/22/2015 1320 Assisted with use of urinal due to arm in cast. Voided 450 mL dark yellow, clear, odorless urine. Specimen to lab for UA. Encouraged to drink more fluids; ice water and juice placed at bedside. Client verbalizes agreement to increase fluid intake. ————

———— K. Clark, RN

EVALUATION

- Perform a detailed follow-up based on findings that deviated from expected or normal for the client. Relate findings to previous assessment data if available.

- Report significant deviations from normal to the primary care provider.

LIFESPAN CONSIDERATIONS   Voiding

INFANTS
- Babies have no conscious control, and the urine is released after a small amount accumulates in the bladder.

CHILDREN
- In children, 50 to 200 mL stimulates stretch receptors in the bladder.
- Urinary control normally takes place between 2 and 4 1/2 years of age. Boys are usually slower than girls in developing this control.
- Teaching proper perineal hygiene can reduce infection. Girls should learn to wipe from front to back and wear cotton underwear. **Rationale:** *Wiping from front to back prevents stool or vaginal secretions from contaminating the urethral meatus. Wearing cotton underwear is recommended instead of nylon because it "breathes" and is less likely to support bacterial growth.*
- Teach children and parents that they should go to the bathroom as soon as the sensation to void is felt and not try to hold the urine in.

OLDER ADULTS
- Bladder capacity decreases, as does ability to completely empty the bladder.
- Decreased muscle tone may lead to nocturia, frequency, and increased residual.
- Altered cognition may lead to incontinence since it prevents the person from understanding the need to urinate and the actions needed to perform the activity.
- Many older men have enlarged prostate glands, which can inhibit complete emptying of the bladder. This often results in urinary retention and urgency, which sometimes causes incontinence.
- Women past menopause have decreased estrogen, which results in a decrease in perineal tone and support of bladder, vagina, and pelvic tissues. This often results in urgency and stress incontinence and can even increase the incidence of urinary tract infections (UTIs).
- Increased stiffness and pain in joints, previous joint surgery, and neuromuscular problems can impair mobility and often make it difficult to get to the bathroom.

APPLYING AN EXTERNAL URINARY DEVICE

To prevent the complications and inconveniences associated with incontinence in males, a **condom catheter**, also referred to as a **urinary sheath** or **external catheter**, attached to a urinary drainage system may be used. A condom appliance is preferable to an internal retention catheter because it avoids entrance into the urethra and bladder, thus minimizing the risk of urinary tract or bladder infection. Methods of applying condom appliances vary. The nurse needs to follow the manufacturer's instructions when applying a condom catheter. First, the nurse determines when the client experiences incontinence. Some clients may require a condom appliance at night only, others continuously.

●○○● NURSING PROCESS: APPLYING AN EXTERNAL URINARY DEVICE

Applying an External Urinary Device

ASSESSMENT
- Review the client record to determine a pattern to voiding and other pertinent data, such as latex sensitivity/allergy.

PLANNING
- Discuss the use of external urinary devices with the client and/or family. Research has shown that condom catheters may be more comfortable and cause fewer UTIs than indwelling catheters (Kyle, 2011).
- Determine if the client has had an external catheter previously and any difficulties with it.
- Perform any procedures that are best completed without the catheter in place; for example, weighing the client would be easier without the tubing and bag.

DELEGATION

Applying a condom catheter may be delegated to UAP. However, the nurse must determine if the specific client has unique needs such as impaired circulation or latex allergy that would require special training of the UAP in the use of the condom catheter. Abnormal findings must be validated and interpreted by the nurse.

Equipment
- Condom sheath of appropriate size: small, medium, large, extra large (Use the manufacturer's size guide as indicated. Use latex-free silicone for clients with latex allergies. Use self-adhering condoms or those with Velcro or some other external securing device.) ❶

IMPLEMENTATION
Preparation
- Assemble the leg drainage bag or urinary drainage bag for attachment to the condom sheath.
- If the condom supplied is not rolled onto itself, roll the condom outward onto itself to facilitate easier application.

Performance
1. Prior to performing the procedure, introduce self and verify the client's identity using agency protocol. Explain to the client what you are going to do, why it is necessary, and how he can participate.
2. Perform hand hygiene and observe other appropriate infection prevention procedures.
3. Position the client in either a supine or a sitting position. Provide for client privacy.
   - Drape the client appropriately with the bath blanket, exposing only the penis.
4. Apply clean gloves.
5. Inspect and clean the penis.
   - Clean the genital area and dry it thoroughly. **Rationale:** *This minimizes skin irritation and excoriation after the condom is applied.*
6. Apply and secure the condom.
   - Roll the condom smoothly over the penis, leaving 2.5 cm (1 in.) between the end of the penis and the rubber or plastic connecting tube. ❷ **Rationale:** *This space prevents irritation of the tip of the penis and provides for full drainage of urine.*

- Apply clean gloves and examine the client's penis for swelling or excoriation that would contraindicate use of the condom catheter.

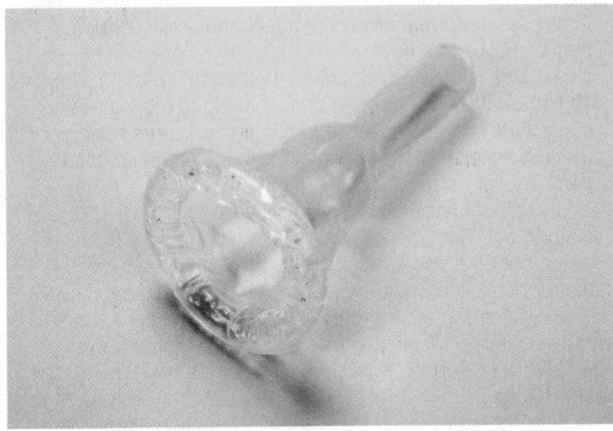

❶ An external or condom catheter.

- Leg drainage bag if ambulatory or urinary drainage bag with tubing
- Clean gloves
- Basin of warm water and soap
- Washcloth and towel
- External fixation device (e.g., flexible, self-adhesive tape or Velcro strap, if needed)

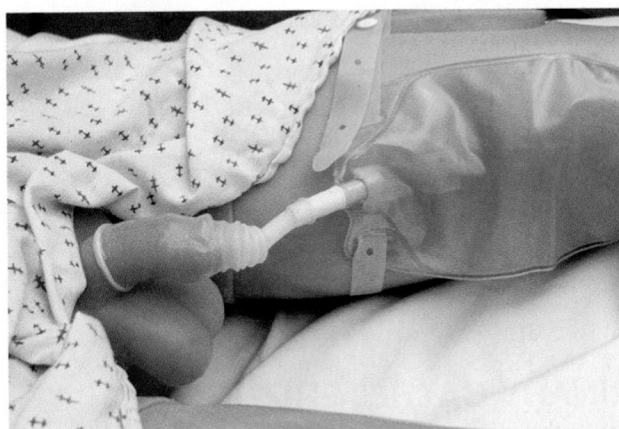

❷ The self-adhering condom rolled over the penis.

- Secure the condom firmly, but not too tightly, to the penis. Avoid catching pubic hair if possible. Some condoms have an adhesive inside the proximal end that adheres to the skin of the base of the penis. Many condoms are packaged with special fixation material. If neither is present, use a strip of flexible self-adhesive tape or Velcro around the base of the penis over the condom. Ordinary tape is *contraindicated* because it is not flexible and can stop blood flow.

Continued on page 518

SKILL 20–2

Applying an External Urinary Device—*continued*

7. Securely attach the urinary drainage system.
   - Make sure that the tip of the penis is not touching the condom and that the condom is not twisted. **Rationale:** *A twisted condom could obstruct the flow of urine.*
   - Attach the urinary drainage system to the condom.
   - Remove and discard gloves.
   - Perform hand hygiene.
   - If the client is to remain in bed, attach the urinary drainage bag to the bed frame.
   - If the client is ambulatory, attach the bag to the client's leg. ❸ **Rationale:** *Attaching the drainage bag to the leg helps control the movement of the tubing and prevents twisting of the thin material of the condom appliance at the tip of the penis.*

8. Teach the client about the drainage system.
   - Instruct the client to keep the drainage bag below the level of the condom and to avoid loops or kinks in the tubing. Instruct the client to report pain, irritation, swelling, or wetness/leaking around the penis to health care personnel.

9. Inspect the penis 30 minutes following the condom application and at least every 4 hours. Check for urine flow. Document these findings.
   - Assess the penis for swelling and discoloration. **Rationale:** *This indicates that the condom is too tight.*
   - Assess urine flow if the client has voided. Normally, some urine is present in the tube if the flow is not obstructed.
   - Assess for redness and/or skin blistering the first few days. **Rationale:** *This could indicate a latex allergy.*

10. Change the condom as indicated and provide skin care. In most settings, the condom is changed daily.
    - Remove the elastic or Velcro strip, apply clean gloves, and roll off the condom.
    - Wash the penis with soapy water, rinse, and dry it thoroughly.
    - Assess the foreskin for signs of irritation, swelling, and discoloration.

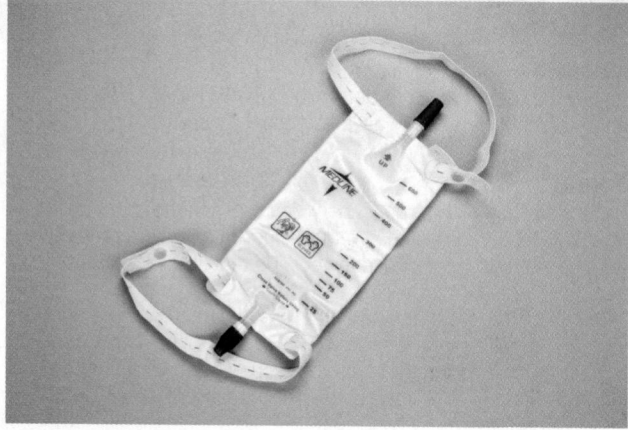

❸ Urinary drainage leg bag.

   - Reapply a new condom.
   - Remove and discard gloves.
   - Perform hand hygiene.

11. Document in the client record using forms or checklists supplemented by narrative notes when appropriate. Record the application of the condom, the time, and pertinent observations, such as irritated areas on the penis.

SAMPLE DOCUMENTATION

4/22/2015 2245 Condom catheter applied for the night per client request. Glans clean, skin intact. Catheter attached to bedside collection bag. Instructed to notify staff if pain, irritation, swelling, or wetness/leaking occurs. Verbalized that he would. —————————
——————————————————————————— L. Chan, RN

EVALUATION
- Perform a detailed follow-up based on findings that deviated from expected or normal for the client. Relate findings to previous assessment data if available.

- Report significant deviations from normal to the primary care provider.

URINARY CATHETERIZATION

Urinary catheterization is the introduction of a hollow, flexible tube or **catheter** through the urethra into the urinary bladder. This is usually performed only when absolutely necessary, because the danger exists of introducing microorganisms into the bladder. The most frequent health care–associated infection in hospitals is a urinary tract infection (UTI), and indwelling urethral catheters cause 80% of these UTIs (Institute for Healthcare Improvement, 2011). A catheter-associated urinary tract infection (**CAUTI**) is a "urinary tract infection that occurs while an indwelling catheter is in place or within 48 hours of its removal" (Seckel, 2013, p. 63). Clients with a CAUTI remain in the hospital longer and need to be placed on antibiotic therapy, which increases health care costs. The high incidence and high costs related to CAUTI, in addition to the fact that most are preventable, resulted in the Centers for Medicare and Medicaid Services (CMS) not reimbursing hospitals unless the CAUTI was documented as present on admission (Magers, 2013). It is well documented that the risk to the client of developing a CAUTI correlates to the duration of the catheter being in place. According to the Centers for Disease Control and Prevention (CDC), the risk of infection increases by 5% for each day that a catheter remains in place (Lee & Carter, 2013, p. 53). Oman et al. (2012) reported that urinary catheters are often "retained for days because of convenience, misunderstanding of their necessity/appropriateness, or lack of clear orders for removal" (p. 548). Best practice is to remove a urinary catheter that is not necessary. Box 20–1 provides evidence-based guidelines for preventing CAUTIs.

BOX 20-1   Preventing or Reducing the Risk of CAUTIs

AVOID UNNECESSARY USE OF URINARY CATHETERS
- Develop criteria for appropriate catheter insertion.
- Consider alternatives to an indwelling catheter such as an external condom catheter.
- Use a bladder scanner to assess for urinary retention.

INSERT URINARY CATHETERS USING ASEPTIC TECHNIQUE
- Catheters should only be inserted by trained individuals.
- Use aseptic technique and sterile equipment.
- Ensure that the catheter kit includes all necessary items in one place.
- Use the smallest catheter possible that allows for proper drainage and decreases urethral trauma.

URINARY CATHETER MAINTENANCE
- Use hand hygiene and standard precautions during any manipulation of the catheter or collecting system.
- Maintain a sterile, closed drainage system.
- Maintain unobstructed urine flow; keep catheter and tubing from kinking.
- Keep the collection bag below the level of the bladder at all times. Do not rest the bag on the floor.
- Empty the collection bag regularly with a separate, clean collecting container for each client; and prevent contact of the drainage spigot with the nonsterile collecting container.

PRACTICES TO AVOID
- Irrigation of catheters, except in cases of catheter obstruction.
- Disconnecting the catheter from the drainage tubing.
- Replacing catheters routinely.
- Cleaning the periurethral area with antiseptics. Routine hygiene (cleaning the meatus during daily bathing) is appropriate.

REVIEW URINARY CATHETER NECESSITY DAILY AND REMOVE PROMPTLY
- Assess the need for a catheter in daily nursing assessments; contact the primary care provider if criteria for continued use are not met.
- Develop nursing protocols that allow nurses to remove urinary catheters if criteria for necessity are not met and there are no contraindications for removal
- Implement automatic stop orders for 48 to 72 hours after catheter insertion. Continue catheter use only with a documented order from the primary care provider.
- Use alerts in the chart or computerized charting system to inform the primary care provider of the presence of a catheter and require an order for continued use.

From *How-to-Guide: Prevent Catheter-Associated Urinary Tract Infections*, by Institute for Healthcare Improvement, 2011, Cambridge, MA: Author; "Using Evidence-Based Practice to Reduce Catheter-Associated Urinary Tract Infections," by T. L. Magers, 2013, *American Journal of Nursing, 113*(6), pp. 34–42; and "Maintaining Urinary Catheters: What Does the Evidence Say?" by M. A. Seckel, 2013, *Nursing, 43*(2), pp. 63–65.

SAFETY ALERT! | SAFETY

2014 The Joint Commission National Patient Safety Goals (2013)

GOAL 7: REDUCE THE RISK OF HEALTH CARE–ASSOCIATED INFECTIONS.
- Implement evidence-based practices to prevent indwelling catheter-associated urinary tract infections (CAUTIs).
  - Insert indwelling urinary catheters according to established evidence-based guidelines.
  - Manage indwelling urinary catheters according to established evidence-based guidelines.
  - Measure and monitor CAUTI prevention processes and outcomes in high-volume areas.

Another hazard is trauma with urethral catheterization, particularly in the male client, whose urethra is longer and more tortuous than that of a female client. It is important to insert a catheter along the normal contour of the urethra. Damage to the urethra can occur if the catheter is forced through strictures or at an incorrect angle. In males, the urethra is normally curved, but it can be straightened by elevating the penis to a position perpendicular to the body.

Catheters are commonly made of rubber or plastics although they may be made from latex, silicone, or polyvinyl chloride (PVC). They are sized by the diameter of the lumen using the French (Fr) scale: the larger the number, the larger the lumen of the catheter. Sizes 14 (4.7 mm), 16 (5.3 mm), and 18 (6 mm) are commonly used for adults. The lumen of a silicone catheter is slightly larger than that of a same-sized latex catheter.

The straight catheter, or **Robinson catheter**, is a single-lumen tube with a small eye or opening about 1.25 cm (0.5 in.) from the insertion tip (Figure 20–7 ■).

The retention catheter, or **Foley catheter**, is a double-lumen catheter. The larger lumen drains urine from the bladder. A second, smaller lumen is used to inflate a balloon near the tip of the catheter to hold the catheter in place within the bladder (Figure 20–8 ■). Some catheter manufacturers apply an antimicrobial coating to their catheters to reduce CAUTIs. The outside end of this two-way retention catheter is bifurcated; that is, it has two openings, one to drain the urine, the other to inflate the balloon (see Figure 20–8).

A variation of the indwelling catheter is the coudé (elbowed) catheter, which has a curved tip (Figure 20–9 ■). This is sometimes used for men who have a hypertrophied prostate, because its tip is somewhat stiffer than the tip of a regular catheter and thus it can be better controlled during insertion, and passage is often less traumatic.

Clients who require continuous or periodic bladder irrigations may have a three-way Foley catheter (Figure 20–10 ■). It is similar to the two-way Foley catheter described earlier, except that it has a third lumen (channel) through which sterile fluid can flow into the urinary bladder. The fluid then exits the bladder through the drainage lumen, along with the urine.

The balloons of retention catheters are sized by the volume of fluid used to inflate them. The size of the retention catheter balloon is indicated on the catheter along with the diameter, for example, "#16 Fr—5 mL balloon." The purpose of the catheter balloon is to secure the catheter in the bladder. Historically, nurses pretested the catheter balloon to prevent insertion of a defective catheter. Some

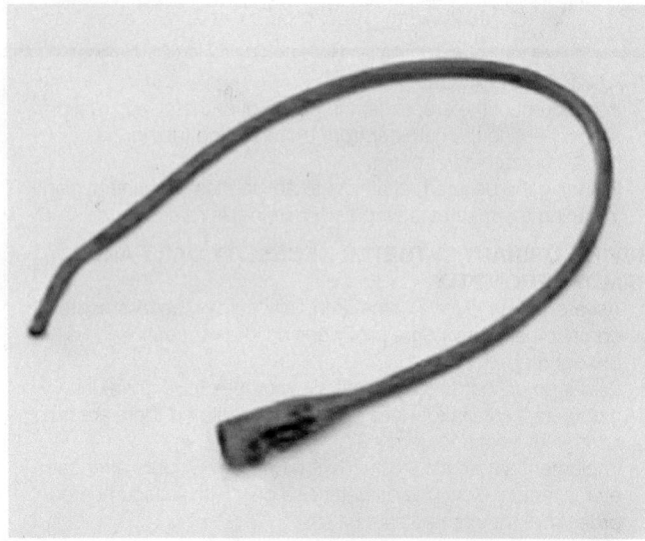

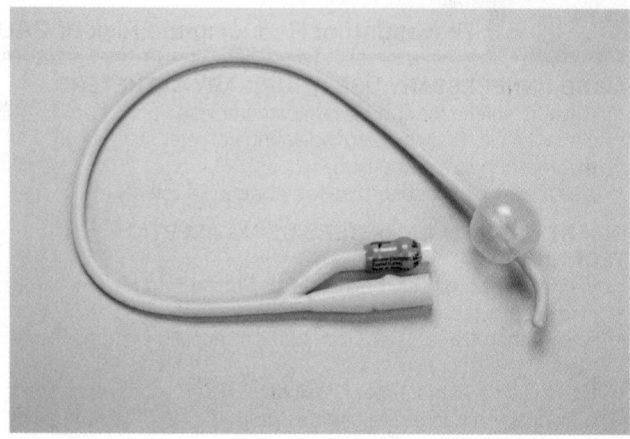

Figure 20–9 ■ Coudé catheter.

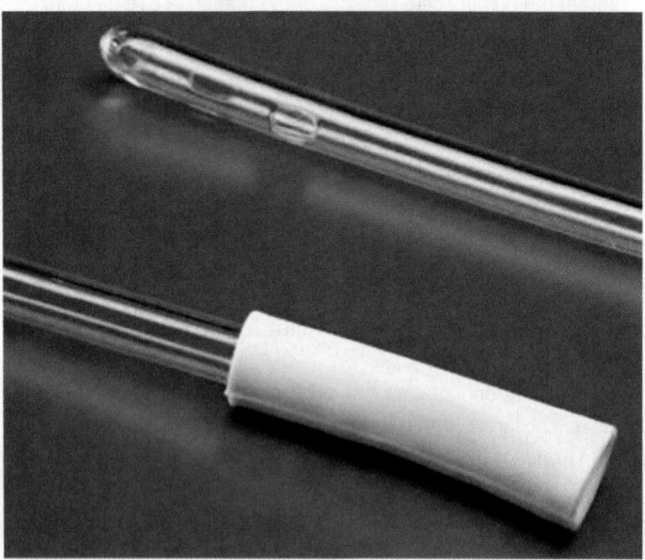

Figure 20–7 ■ Red rubber or plastic Robinson straight catheters.
Courtesy Covidien.

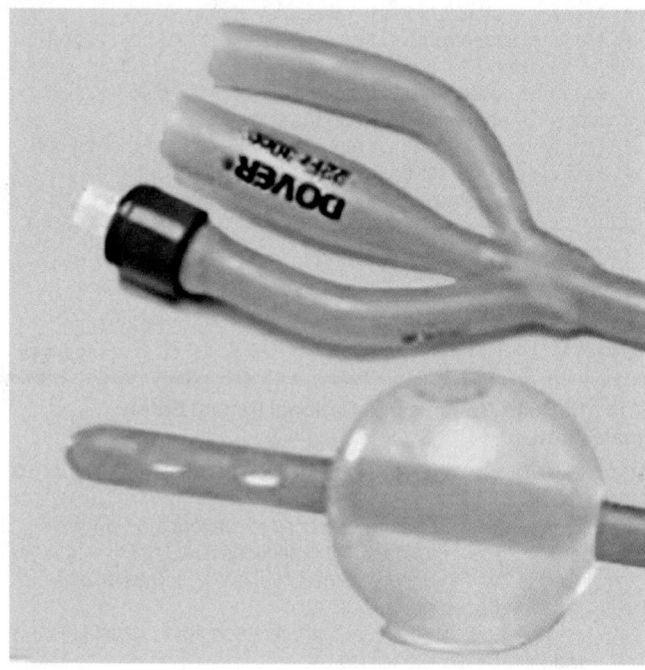

Figure 20–10 ■ A three-way Foley catheter, often used for continuous bladder irrigation.
Courtesy Covidien.

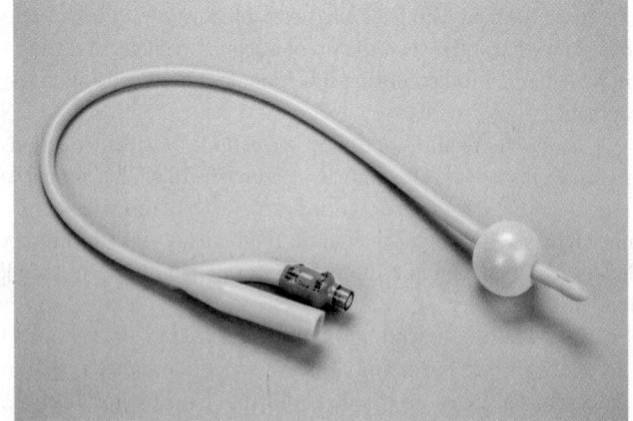

Figure 20–8 ■ A retention (Foley) catheter with the balloon inflated.

catheter manufacturers (e.g., Bard) test the balloon as part of their quality assurance process and do not recommend pretesting of the balloon by the nurse. Pretesting of *silicone* balloons in particular is *not* recommended because the silicone can form a cuff or crease at the balloon area that can cause trauma to the urethra during catheter insertion. It is important to follow the manufacturer's instructions for the proper volume to use for balloon inflation. Improperly inflated catheter balloons may cause drainage and deflation difficulties. See Box 20–2 for guidelines in selecting an appropriate catheter.

BOX 20–2	Selecting a Urinary Catheter

- Determine appropriate catheter length by the client's gender. For adult female clients, use a 22-cm catheter; for adult male clients, use a 40-cm catheter.
- Determine appropriate catheter size by the size of the urethral canal. Use sizes such as #8 or #10 for children, #14 or #16 for adults. Men frequently require a larger size than women, for example, #18.
- Select the appropriate balloon size. For adults, use a 5-mL balloon to facilitate optimal urine drainage. The smaller balloons allow more complete bladder emptying because the catheter tip is closer to the urethral opening in the bladder. However, a 30-mL balloon is commonly used to achieve hemostasis of the prostatic area following a prostatectomy. Use 3-mL balloons for children.

Retention catheters are usually connected to a closed gravity drainage system. This system consists of the catheter, drainage tubing, and a collecting bag for the urine. A closed system cannot be opened anywhere along the system, from catheter to collecting bag. Some health facilities, however, may use an open system, which consists of separate packages for the catheter and the drainage tubing and collecting bag. The open system requires the nurse to be especially vigilant to ensure sterile technique is maintained when connecting the catheter and drainage tubing. The closed system is preferred because it reduces the risk of microorganisms entering the system and infecting the urinary tract. Urinary drainage systems typically depend on the force of gravity to drain urine from the bladder to the collecting bag.

●○● NURSING PROCESS: URINARY CATHETERIZATION

Performing Urinary Catheterization

SKILL 20-3

ASSESSMENT
- Determine the most appropriate method of catheterization based on the purpose and any criteria specified in the order such as total amount of urine to be removed or size of catheter to be used.
- Use a straight catheter if only a one-time urine specimen is needed, if the amount of residual urine is being measured, or if temporary decompression/emptying of the bladder is required.
- Use an indwelling/retention catheter if the bladder must remain empty, intermittent catheterization is contraindicated, or continuous urine measurement/collection is needed.
- Assess the client's overall condition. Determine if the client is able to participate and hold still during the procedure and if the

client can be positioned supine with the head relatively flat. For a female client, determine if she can have knees bent and hips externally rotated.
- Determine when the client last voided or was last catheterized.
- If catheterization is being performed because the client has been unable to void, when possible, complete a bladder scan to assess the amount of urine present in the bladder. **Rationale:** *This prevents catheterizing the bladder when insufficient urine is present. Often, a minimum of 500 to 800 mL of urine indicates urinary retention and the client should be reassessed until that amount is present.*

PLANNING
- Allow adequate time to perform the catheterization. Although the entire procedure can require as little as 15 minutes, several sources of difficulty could result in a much longer time period. If possible, it should not be performed just prior to or after the client eats.
- Some clients may feel uncomfortable being catheterized by nurses of the opposite gender. If this is the case, obtain the client's permission. Also consider whether agency policy requires or encourages having a person of the client's same gender present for the procedure.

DELEGATION

Due to the need for sterile technique and detailed knowledge of anatomy, insertion of a urinary catheter is not delegated to UAP.

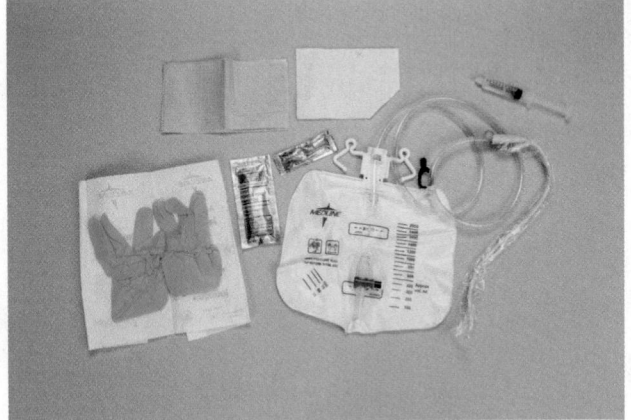

❶ A closed indwelling catheter insertion kit.

Equipment
- Sterile catheter of appropriate size (An extra catheter should also be at hand.)
- Catheterization kit ❶ or individual sterile items:
  - Sterile gloves
  - Waterproof drape(s)
  - Antiseptic solution
  - Cleansing balls
  - Forceps
  - Water-soluble lubricant
  - Urine receptacle
  - Specimen container

- For an indwelling catheter:
  - Syringe prefilled with sterile water in amount specified by catheter manufacturer
  - Collection bag and tubing
- 5 to 10 mL 2% Xylocaine gel or water-soluble lubricant for urethral injection (if agency permits)
- Clean gloves
- Supplies for performing perineal cleansing
- Bath blanket or sheet for draping the client
- Adequate lighting (Obtain a flashlight or lamp if necessary.)

Continued on page 522

Performing Urinary Catheterization—*continued*

IMPLEMENTATION
Preparation

- If using a catheterization kit, read the label carefully to ensure that all necessary items are included.
- Apply clean gloves and perform routine perineal care to cleanse the meatus from gross contamination. For women, use this time to locate the urinary meatus relative to surrounding structures. ❷
- Remove and discard gloves.
- Perform hand hygiene.

Performance

1. Prior to performing the procedure, introduce self and verify the client's identity using agency protocol. Explain to the client what you are going to do, why it is necessary, and how he or she can participate.
2. Perform hand hygiene and observe other appropriate infection prevention procedures.
3. Provide for client privacy.
4. Place the client in the appropriate position and drape all areas except the perineum.
   - *Female:* supine with knees flexed, feet about 2 feet apart, and hips slightly externally rotated, if possible
   - *Male:* supine, thighs slightly abducted or apart.
5. Establish adequate lighting. Stand on the client's right if you are right-handed, on the client's left if you are left-handed.
6. If using a collecting bag and it is not contained within the catheterization kit, open the drainage package and place the end of the tubing within reach. **Rationale:** *Because one hand is needed to hold the catheter once it is in place, open the package while two hands are still available.*
7. If agency policy permits, apply clean gloves and inject 10 to 15 mL Xylocaine gel or water-soluble lubricant into the urethra of the male client. Wipe the underside of the penile shaft to distribute the gel up the urethra. Wait at least 5 minutes for the gel to take effect before inserting the catheter.
   - Remove and discard gloves.
   - Perform hand hygiene.

8. Open the catheterization kit. Place a waterproof drape under the buttocks (female) or penis without contaminating the center of the drape with your hands.
9. Apply sterile gloves.
10. Organize the remaining supplies:
    - Saturate the cleansing balls with the antiseptic solution.
    - Open the lubricant package.
    - Remove the specimen container and place it nearby with the lid loosely on top.
11. Attach the prefilled syringe to the indwelling catheter inflation hub. Apply agency policy regarding pretesting of the balloon. **Rationale:** *There is little research regarding pretesting of the balloon; however, some balloons (e.g., silicone) may form a cuff on deflation, which can irritate the urethra on insertion.*
12. Lubricate the catheter 2.5 to 5 cm (1 to 2 in.) for females, 15 to 17.5 cm (6 to 7 in.) for males, and place it with the drainage end inside the collection container.
13. If desired, place the fenestrated drape over the perineum, exposing the urinary meatus.
14. Cleanse the meatus. *Note:* The nondominant hand is considered contaminated once it touches the client's skin.
    - *Females:* Use your nondominant hand to spread the labia so the meatus is visible. Establish firm but gentle pressure on the labia. The antiseptic may make the tissues slippery but the labia must not be allowed to return over the cleaned meatus. *Note:* Location of the urethral meatus is best identified during the cleansing process. Pick up a cleansing ball with the forceps in your dominant hand and wipe one side of the labia majora in an anteroposterior direction. ❸ Use great care that wiping the client does not contaminate this sterile hand. Use a new ball for the opposite side. Repeat for the labia minora. Use the last ball to cleanse directly over the meatus.

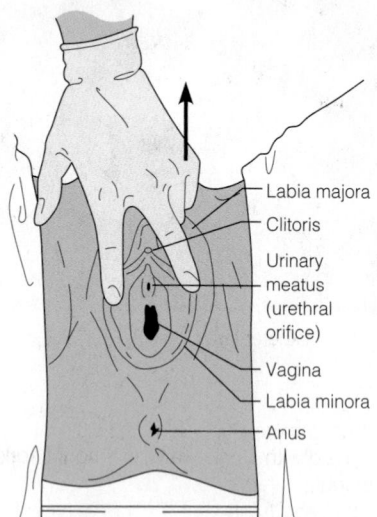

Labia majora
Clitoris
Urinary meatus (urethral orifice)
Vagina
Labia minora
Anus

❷ To expose the urinary meatus, separate the labia minora and retract the tissue upward.

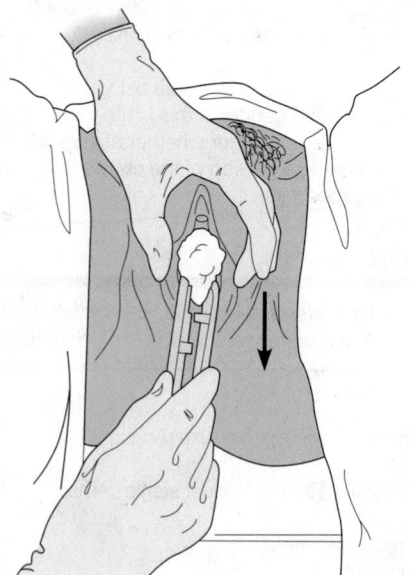

❸ When cleaning the labia minora, move the swab downward.

Performing Urinary Catheterization—*continued*

- *Males:* Use your nondominant hand to grasp the penis just below the glans. If necessary, retract the foreskin. Hold the penis firmly upright, with slight tension. **Rationale:** *Lifting the penis in this manner helps straighten the urethra.* Pick up a cleansing ball with the forceps in your dominant hand and wipe from the center of the meatus in a circular motion around the glans to the base. Use great care that wiping the client does not contaminate this sterile hand. Use a new ball and repeat three more times. The antiseptic may make the tissues slippery, but the foreskin must not be allowed to return over the cleaned meatus and the penis must not be dropped.

15. Insert the catheter.
    - Grasp the catheter firmly 5 to 7.5 cm (2 to 3 in.) from the tip. Ask the client to take a slow deep breath and insert the catheter as the client exhales. Slight resistance is expected as the catheter passes through the sphincter. If necessary, twist the catheter or hold pressure on the catheter until the sphincter relaxes.
    - Advance the catheter 5 cm (2 in.) farther after the urine begins to flow through it. **Rationale:** *This is to be sure it is fully in the bladder, will not easily fall out, and the balloon is into the bladder completely.* For male clients, some experts recommend advancing the catheter to the "Y" bifurcation of the catheter. Check your agency's policy.
    - If the catheter accidentally contacts the labia or slips into the vagina, it is considered contaminated and a new, sterile catheter must be used. The contaminated catheter may be left in the vagina until the new catheter is inserted to help avoid mistaking the vaginal opening for the urinary meatus.

16. Hold the catheter with the nondominant hand.

17. For an indwelling catheter, inflate the retention balloon with the designated volume.
    - Without releasing the catheter (and, for females, without releasing the labia), hold the inflation valve between two fingers of your nondominant hand while you attach the syringe (if not left attached earlier when testing the balloon) and inflate with your dominant hand. If the client complains of discomfort, immediately withdraw the instilled fluid, advance the catheter farther, and attempt to inflate the balloon again.
    - Pull gently on the catheter until resistance is felt to ensure that the balloon has inflated and to place it in the trigone of the bladder. ❹

18. Collect a urine specimen if needed. For a straight catheter, allow 20 to 30 mL to flow into the bottle without touching the catheter to the bottle. For an indwelling catheter preattached to a drainage bag, a specimen may be taken from the bag this initial time only.

19. Allow the straight catheter to continue draining into the urine receptacle. If necessary (e.g., an open system), attach the drainage end of an indwelling catheter to the collecting tubing and bag.

20. Examine and measure the urine. In some cases, only 750 to 1,000 mL of urine are to be drained from the bladder at one time. Check agency policy for further instructions if this should occur.

21. Remove the straight catheter when urine flow stops. For an indwelling catheter, secure the catheter tubing to the thigh for

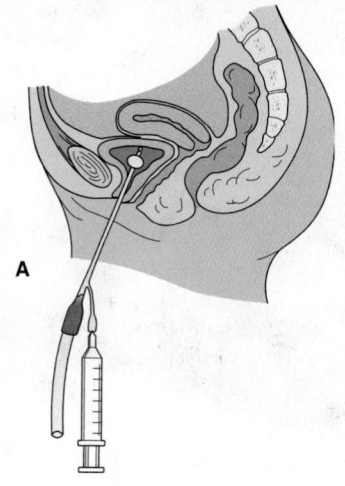

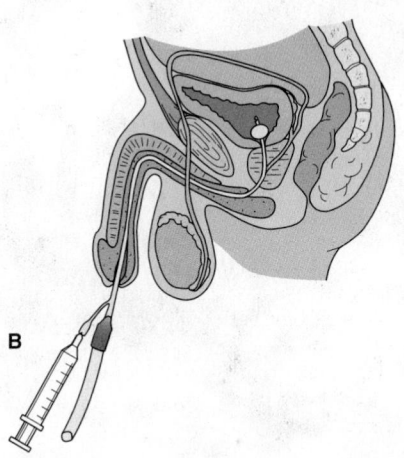

❹ Placement of catheter and inflated balloon of a closed system in *A,* female client; *B,* male client.

female clients or the upper thigh or lower abdomen for male clients to prevent movement on the urethra or excessive tension or pulling on the retention balloon (Fisher, 2010; Herter & Kazer, 2010). Adhesive and nonadhesive catheter-securing devices are available and should be used to secure the catheter tubing to the client. ❺ **Rationale:** *This prevents unnecessary trauma to the urethra.* Next, hang the bag below the level of the bladder. No tubing should fall below the top of the bag. ❻

22. Wipe any remaining antiseptic or lubricant from the perineal area. Replace the foreskin if retracted earlier. Return the client to a comfortable position. Instruct the client on positioning and moving with the catheter in place.

23. Discard all used supplies in appropriate receptacles.

24. Remove and discard gloves.
    - Perform hand hygiene.

Continued on page 524

Performing Urinary Catheterization—*continued*

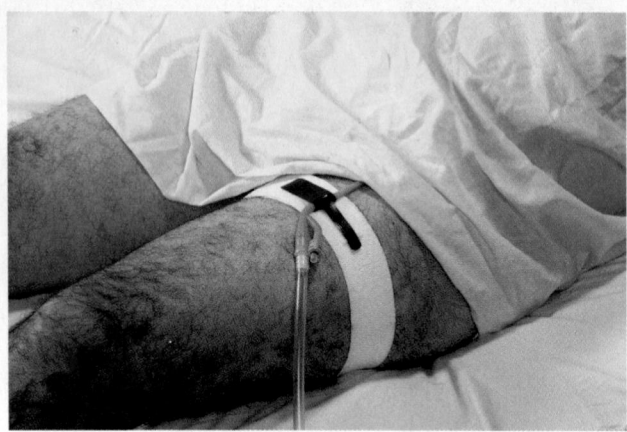

A

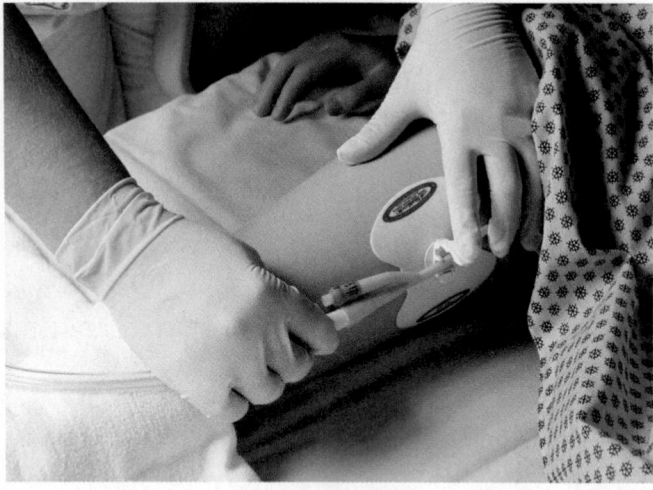

B

❺ Catheter securement devices: *A,* nonadhesive device (Velcro strap); *B,* adhesive device.

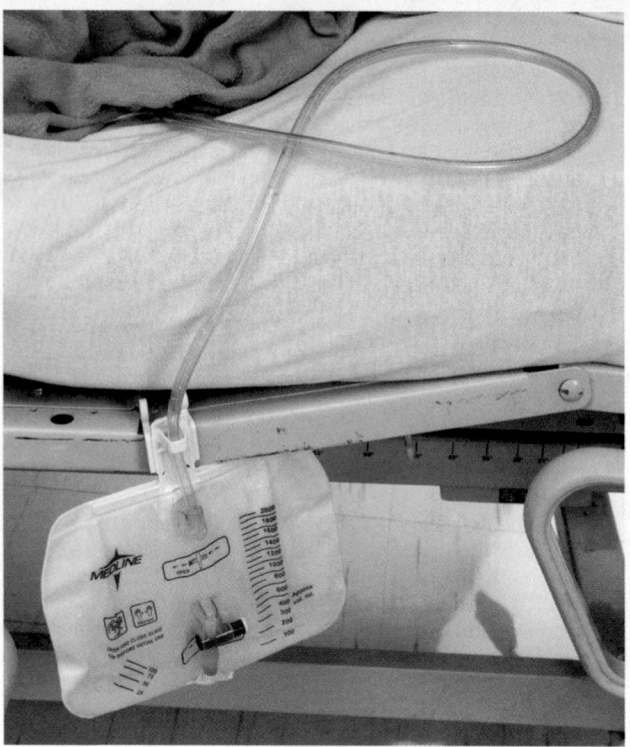

❻ Correct position for a urine drainage bag and tubing.

25. Document the catheterization procedure, including catheter size and results, in the client record using forms or checklists supplemented by narrative notes when appropriate.

SAMPLE DOCUMENTATION

2/24/2015 0530 Client agreed to insertion of pre-op indwelling catheter as per order. #16 Foley with 5-mL balloon inserted without difficulty, secured to thigh, connected to straight drainage. Immediate return of 300 mL pale, clear yellow urine. ——————— G. Hampton, RN

EVALUATION
- Notify the primary care provider of the catheterization results.
- Perform a detailed follow-up based on findings that deviated from expected or normal for the client. Relate findings to previous assessment data if available.

- Teach the client how to care for the indwelling catheter, to drink more fluids, and other appropriate instructions.

LIFESPAN CONSIDERATIONS Urinary Catheterization

INFANTS/CHILDREN
- Adapt the size of the catheter for pediatric clients.
- Ask a family member to assist in holding the child during catheterization, if appropriate.

OLDER ADULTS
- Obtaining consent and cooperation may take longer than with younger clients.
- When catheterizing older adults, be very attentive to problems of limited movement, especially in the hips. Arthritis, or previous hip or knee surgery, may limit movement and cause discomfort. Modify the position (e.g., side-lying) as needed to perform the procedure safely and comfortably. For women, obtain the assistance of another nurse to flex and hold the client's knees and hips as necessary or place her in a modified Sims' position.
- If the female meatus cannot be visualized, insert a gloved finger into the vagina and press gently upward. **Rationale:** *This action may straighten the urethra and make the meatus visible.*

CLIENT TEACHING CONSIDERATIONS

Urinary Catheterization

For indwelling catheters, instruct the client to:

- Never pull on the catheter.
- Keep the catheter tubing attached to the leg using a catheter-securing device.
- Ensure that there are no kinks or twists in the tubing.
- Keep the urine drainage bag below the level of the bladder.
- Report signs and symptoms of UTI including burning, urgency, abdominal pain, and cloudy urine; in older adults, confusion may be an early sign.
- Maintain adequate oral intake of fluids.

Ambulatory and Community Settings   Urinary Catheterization

PATIENT-CENTERED CARE

- Clients with spinal cord injuries who are unable to stimulate voiding may use intermittent straight catheterization every few hours. The client or another caregiver can perform this procedure once taught by a nurse. Often, the client will use clean rather than sterile technique and reuse equipment since the microorganisms to which the client is exposed are his or her own.
- For intermittent self-catheterization, instruct the client to:
  - Follow instructions for clean technique.
  - Wash hands well with warm water and soap prior to handling equipment or performing catheterization.
  - Monitor for signs and symptoms of UTI including burning, urgency, abdominal pain, and cloudy urine; in older adults, confusion may be an early sign.
  - Ensure adequate oral intake of fluids.
  - After each catheterization, assess the urine for color, odor, clarity, and the presence of blood.
  - Wash reusable catheters thoroughly with soap and water after use, dry, and store in a clean place.
- For ambulatory clients, those in the home, or those using wheelchairs who have indwelling catheters, modifications are needed in securing the catheter and maintaining the collection bag below bladder level. A leg bag may substitute for a hanging bag for those who are upright.
- Discuss with the client and family ways to minimize UTIs in those requiring frequent catheterization. Increased fluid intake and urine acidification through drinking cranberry juice are two examples. Also discuss modifications in hygiene and sexual intercourse that may be indicated for individuals with indwelling catheters.
- Teach the client and family when and how to empty the collection bag and to assess the urine for signs of infection, bleeding, or other complications.
- Clients with an indwelling catheter should take a shower rather than a tub bath. **Rationale:** *Sitting in a tub allows bacteria easier access into the urinary tract.*

WHAT IF   Urinary Catheterization Using an Indwelling Catheter

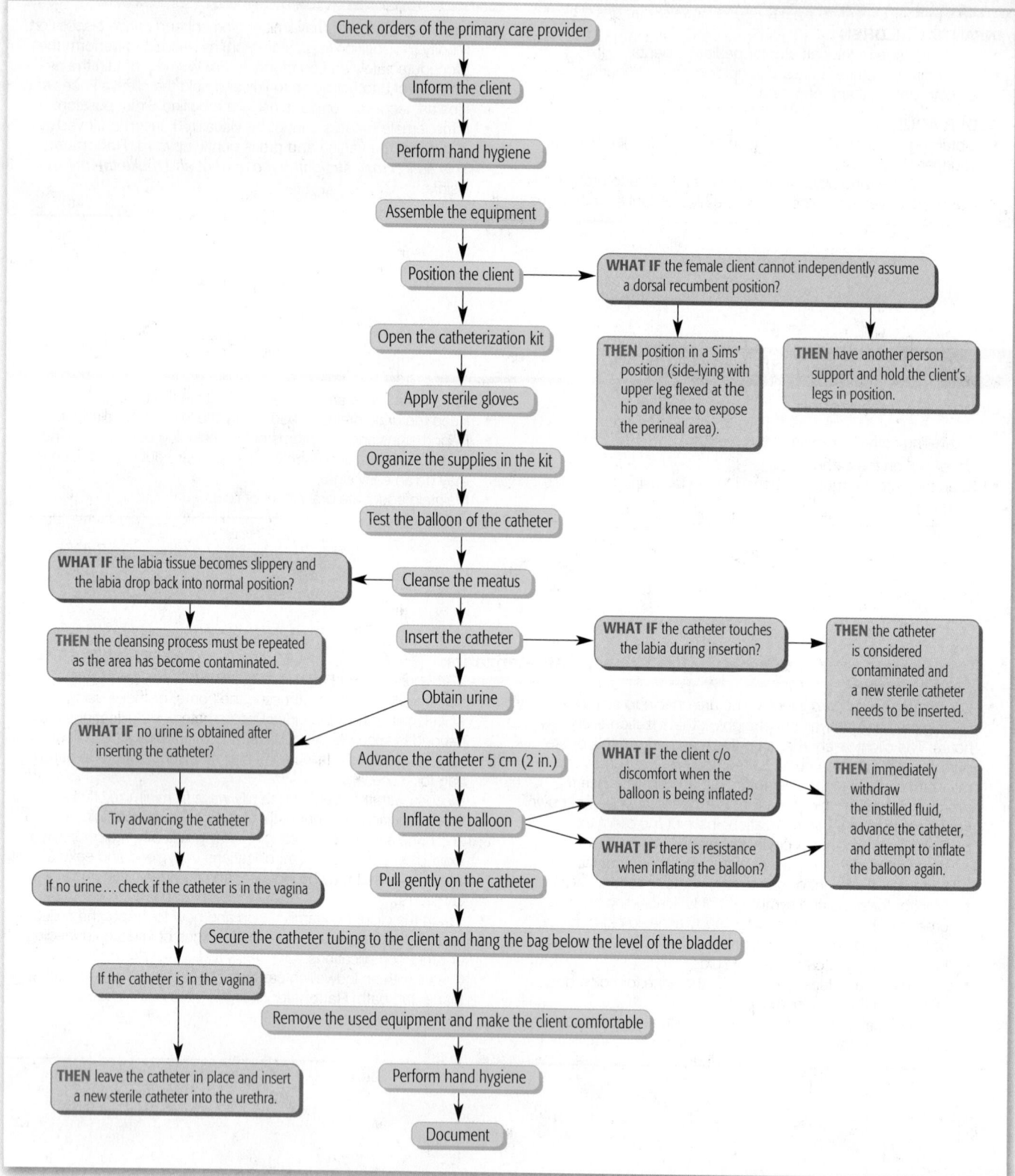

Catheter Care and Removal

Nursing care for a client with an indwelling catheter consists primarily of steps to reduce the chance of developing a UTI. It includes performing steps and client and family teaching about maintaining adequate fluid intake (3 L/day if possible), emptying and recording urine output, and maintaining the patency and cleanliness of the drainage system.

Perineal care practices for clients with indwelling catheters vary significantly according to agency policy. In general, routine perineal care involving washing with soap and water and removing discharge or crusts that may form around the catheter is considered sufficient.

Indwelling catheters are removed after their purpose has been achieved, usually on the order of the primary care provider. Unfortunately, not all primary care providers know which of their clients has an indwelling catheter. As a result, some facilities have incorporated an alert system that requires the provider to take an action after a specified time frame. Also, some health care facilities allow the nurse to remove an indwelling catheter through the use of a protocol with specific criteria (Wenger, 2010).

Some clients may have a **suprapubic catheter**, an indwelling catheter that has been inserted surgically through the abdominal wall above the symphysis pubis into the urinary bladder. The suprapubic catheter may have a pigtail or balloon that holds it in the bladder depending on the manufacturer (Figure 20–11 ■). The physician inserts the catheter using local anesthesia or during bladder or vaginal surgery. The catheter may be secured in place with sutures to reinforce the security of the catheter and is then attached to a closed drainage system. The suprapubic catheter may be placed for temporary bladder drainage until the client is able to resume normal voiding (e.g., after urethral, bladder, or vaginal surgery) or it may become a permanent device (e.g., urethral or pelvic trauma).

Care of the catheter insertion site involves sterile technique. Dressings around the newly placed suprapubic catheter are changed whenever they are soiled with drainage to prevent bacterial growth around the insertion site and reduce the potential for infection. Cleanse with 4×4s with chlorhexidine gluconate and warm water. The area is dressed with a 4×4 and taped in an occlusive fashion (Bullman, 2011). Securing the catheter tube to the abdomen helps to reduce tension at the insertion site. For catheters that have been in place for an extended period, no dressing may be needed and the healed insertion tract enables removal and replacement of the catheter as needed. Formation, however, of a healed insertion tract takes approximately 6 weeks to 6 months to develop. Before that time, the catheter needs to be replaced within 30 minutes if it falls out to avoid the opening closing over (Bullman, 2011; Winder, 2012). The nurse

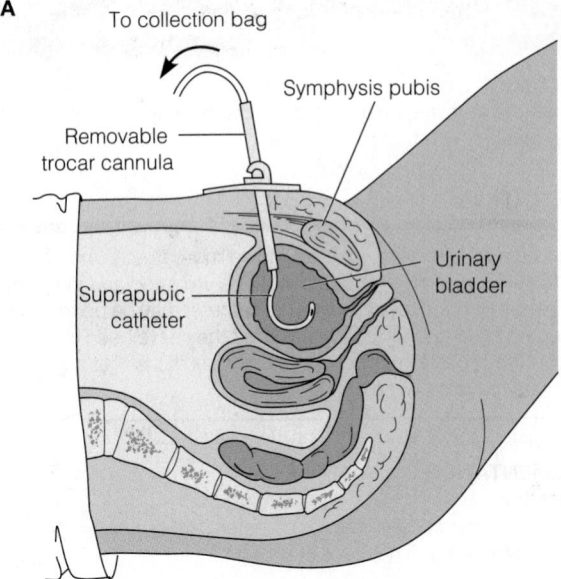

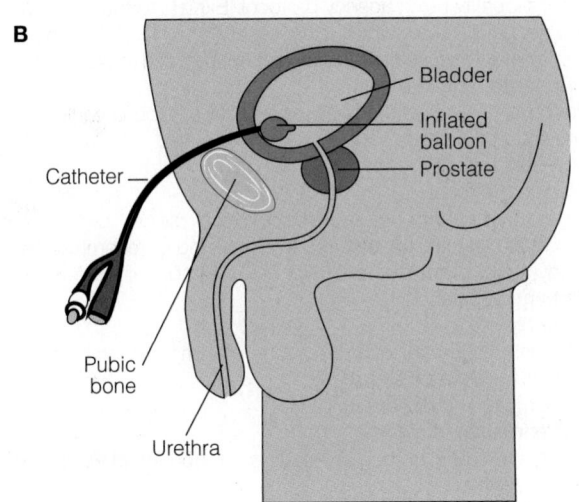

Figure 20–11 ■ A suprapubic catheter in place: *A,* using a pigtail loop; *B,* using a balloon to keep catheter in place.

assesses the insertion area at regular intervals. If pubic hair invades the insertion site, it may be carefully trimmed with scissors. Any redness or discharge at the skin around the insertion site must be reported.

●○● NURSING PROCESS: CATHETER CARE AND REMOVAL

Performing Catheter Care and Removal

ASSESSMENT
- Review the client record to determine the length of time the catheter has been in place and any difficulties reported with the system. Routine changing of the catheter and tubing is not recommended. If there are significant sediment, blood, or mucous threads in the tubing or the system is not draining adequately, the tubing and/or catheter may need to be replaced using aseptic technique.

- Assess the client for any complaints of discomfort from the catheter. The initial sensation of the need to void is common after insertion and should have diminished within a few minutes.
- Examine the perineal area for redness, discharge, or lesions.

SKILL 20-4

Continued on page 528

Performing Catheter Care and Removal—*continued*

PLANNING

If the catheter requires changing, an entire new system with collecting bag must be used.

DELEGATION

Routine care of the client with an indwelling catheter may be delegated to UAP. Abnormal findings must be validated and interpreted by the nurse. Removal of an indwelling catheter may be performed by UAP according to agency policy, provided they have been thoroughly trained in the procedure and is aware of conditions that could arise that require the assistance of a nurse.

Equipment

- Clean gloves (three pairs)
- Washcloth, soap, and towels

For catheter removal:

- Paper towel or waste receptacle
- Luer-Lok or slip tip syringe at least as large as the size of the retention balloon (printed on the inflation port)

IMPLEMENTATION

Preparation

Determine an appropriate time for catheter care or removal, and the client's knowledge and need for teaching.

Performance

1. Prior to performing the procedure, introduce self and verify the client's identity using agency protocol. Explain to the client what you are going to do, why it is necessary, and how he or she can participate. Discuss how the results will be used in planning further care or treatments.

2. Perform hand hygiene and observe other appropriate infection prevention procedures.

3. Provide for client privacy.

4. Prepare the client.
   - Ask the client to assume a back-lying position.
   - Obtain a sterile urine specimen if ordered or recommended by agency protocol. See Skill 4–5 in Chapter 4 ∞.

5. Perform catheter care.
   - Apply clean gloves.
   - Wash the urinary meatus and the proximal catheter with soap and water. Dry gently.
   - Remove and discard gloves.
   - Perform hand hygiene.

6. Empty the collection bag at least every 8 hours and whenever close to half full.
   - Apply clean gloves.
   - Obtain the graduated container used for measuring urine for that client.
   - Place a paper towel on the floor below the bag.
   - Remove the end of the drainage tube from its protective housing on the collection bag without touching the end.
   - Point the tube into the container and release the clamp. Do not let the tube touch the container to avoid contamination.
   - After the bag is completely emptied, cleanse the end of the tube according to agency policy (e.g., with an alcohol swab), clamp the tube, and replace it into the protective housing.
   - Note the volume and characteristics of the urine. Empty the container into the toilet if the urine does not need to be saved.
   - Rinse the container and return it to its storage location.
   - Remove and discard gloves.
   - Perform hand hygiene.

7. To remove the catheter:
   - Place a towel or receptacle between the client's legs.
   - Remove the catheter-securing device from where it has been secured to the client.
   - Apply clean gloves.
   - Insert the syringe into the injection port of the catheter, and withdraw the fluid from the balloon. After the fluid has been aspirated, the walls of the balloon do not deflate to their original shape but collapse into uneven ridges, forming a "cuff" around the catheter. This cuff is more pronounced with a silicone catheter (Wilson, 2012). This cuff can cause discomfort to the client as the catheter is removed. There is minimal research about balloon cuffing that occurs following deflation of a catheter balloon. One recent research study by Chung and So (2012) specifically tested four balloon deflation methods. They found that active deflation (rapid deflation of balloon within 5 seconds) caused the greatest degree of catheter balloon cuffing, followed by passive deflation (very slow active deflation over 30 seconds). Passive auto-deflation (attaching an empty syringe to the balloon inflow channel to allow for gentle autodeflation) and excision of the balloon inflow channel caused the least cuffing (p. 176).
   - Do not pull the catheter while the balloon is inflated; doing so will injure the urethra.
   - After all of the fluid is removed from the balloon, gently withdraw the catheter and place it in the waste receptacle.
   - Dry the perineal area with a towel.
   - Measure the urine in the drainage bag.

8. Measure the urine in the drainage bag (see step 6 above).

9. Discard all used supplies in appropriate receptacles.
   - Remove and discard gloves.
   - Perform hand hygiene.

10. Document the procedure and assessment data.
    - Record the time the catheter was removed; the intactness of the catheter; and the amount, color, and clarity of the urine.

11. Determine the time of first voiding and the amount voided over the first 8 hours. Compare this with the fluid intake. **Rationale:** *When the fluid output is considerably less than the fluid intake, the bladder may be retaining urine.* If urine retention is suspected, scan or palpate the bladder for fullness. Use non-invasive methods to encourage voiding such as allowing the client to hear running water or placing the client's hand in water. Notify the primary care provider if the client has not voided in 8 hours (or another interval specified by policy) because the client may need to be recatheterized. Record the voiding or other action taken.

Performing Catheter Care and Removal—*continued*

SAMPLE DOCUMENTATION

7/3/2015 1015 Foley removed intact after aspirating balloon for 10 mL fluid without difficulty. Moderate amount white sediment noted around catheter tip. Peri care provided. Skin intact and without lesions. Taught to continue goal intake of fluids of 150 mL/hour. Verbalized agreement. ————————— S. Brown, RN

7/3/2015 1645 Up to BR. Voided 600 mL amber urine. c/o slight burning at start of urination. States will continue fluid intake. Dr. Wertz notified of burning on urination. ————— S. Brown, RN

EVALUATION
- Perform detailed follow-up based on findings that deviated from expected or normal for the client. Relate findings to previous assessment data if available.
- Report significant deviations from normal to the primary care provider.

URINARY IRRIGATIONS

An **irrigation** is a flushing or washing out with a specified solution. Bladder irrigation is carried out on a primary care provider's order, usually to wash out the bladder and sometimes to apply medication to the bladder lining. Catheter irrigations may also be performed to maintain or restore the patency of a catheter, for example, to remove blood clots blocking the catheter. Sterile technique is used.

There are three ways of irrigating a catheter or bladder for a client with an indwelling catheter: (1) Closed intermittent irrigation maintains the closed system by injecting the solution through an aspiration port, (2) closed intermittent or continuous irrigation irrigates through a three-way catheter (see Figure 20–10), and (3) an open intermittent system irrigates through a catheter after separating the catheter and tubing. The closed method is the preferred technique for catheter or bladder irrigation because it is associated with a lower risk of UTI. This method is most often used for clients who have had genitourinary surgery. The continuous irrigation helps prevent blood clots from occluding the catheter. Occasionally an open irrigation may be necessary to restore catheter patency. The risk of injecting microorganisms into the urinary tract is greater with open irrigations because the connection between the indwelling catheter and the drainage tubing is broken. Strict precautions must be taken to maintain the sterility of both the drainage tubing connector and the interior of the indwelling catheter. The open method of catheter or bladder irrigation is performed with double-lumen indwelling catheters. It may be necessary for clients who develop blood clots and mucous fragments that occlude the catheter, or when it is undesirable to change the catheter. To continuously irrigate an adult bladder, 1,000 mL is commonly used; for open catheter irrigation, 200 mL is normally required.

●○● NURSING PROCESS: URINARY IRRIGATIONS

Performing Bladder Irrigation

ASSESSMENT
- Determine the client's current urinary drainage system. Review the client record for recent intake and output and any difficulties the client has been experiencing with the system. Review the results of previous irrigations.
- Assess the client for any discomfort, bladder spasms, or distended bladder.

PLANNING
Before irrigating a catheter or bladder, check (a) the reason for the irrigation; (b) the order authorizing the continuous or intermittent irrigation (in most agencies, a primary care provider's order is required); (c) the type of sterile solution, the amount, and strength to be used, and the rate (if continuous); and (d) the type of catheter in place. If these are not specified on the client's chart, check agency protocol.

DELEGATION

Due to the need for sterile technique, urinary irrigation is generally not delegated to UAP. If the client has continuous irrigation, the UAP may care for the client and note abnormal findings. These must be validated and interpreted by the nurse.

Equipment
- Clean gloves (2 pairs)
- Retention catheter in place
- Drainage tubing and bag (if not in place)
- Drainage tubing clamp
- Antiseptic swabs
- Sterile receptacle
- Sterile irrigating solution warmed or at room temperature (Label the irrigant clearly with the words "Bladder Irrigation," including the information about any medications that have been added to the original solution, and the date, time, and nurse's initials.)
- Infusion tubing
- IV pole

Continued on page 530

Performing Bladder Irrigation—*continued*

IMPLEMENTATION
Performance

1. Prior to performing the procedure, introduce self and verify the client's identity using agency protocol. Explain to the client what you are going to do, why it is necessary, and how he or she can participate. The irrigation should not be painful or uncomfortable. Discuss how the results will be used in planning further care or treatments.
2. Perform hand hygiene and observe other appropriate infection prevention procedures.
3. Provide for client privacy.
4. Apply clean gloves.
5. Empty, measure, and record the amount and appearance of urine present in the drainage bag. Discard urine and gloves. **Rationale:** *Emptying the drainage bag allows more accurate measurement of urinary output after the irrigation is in place or completed. Assessing the character of the urine provides baseline data for later comparison.*
6. Prepare the equipment.
   • Perform hand hygiene.
   • Connect the irrigation infusion tubing to the irrigating solution and flush the tubing with solution, keeping the tip sterile. **Rationale:** *Flushing the tubing removes air and prevents it from being instilled into the bladder.*
   • Apply clean gloves and cleanse the port with antiseptic swabs.
   • Connect the irrigation tubing to the input port of the three-way catheter.
   • Connect the drainage bag and tubing to the urinary drainage port if not already in place.
   • Remove and discard gloves.
   • Perform hand hygiene.
7. Irrigate the bladder.
   • For closed continuous bladder irrigation using a three-way catheter, open the clamp on the urinary drainage tubing (if present). ❶ **Rationale:** *This allows the irrigating solution to flow out of the bladder continuously.*
     a. Apply clean gloves.
     b. Open the regulating clamp on the irrigating fluid infusion tubing, and adjust the flow rate as prescribed by the

primary care provider or to 40 to 60 drops per minute if not specified.
   c. Assess the drainage for amount, color, and clarity. The amount of drainage should equal the amount of irrigant entering the bladder plus expected urine output. Empty the bag frequently so that it does not exceed half full.
• For closed intermittent irrigation, determine whether the solution is to remain in the bladder for a specified time.
   a. If the solution is to remain in the bladder (a bladder irrigation or instillation), close the clamp to the urinary drainage tubing. **Rationale:** *Closing the flow clamp allows the solution to be retained in the bladder and in contact with the bladder walls.*
   b. If the solution is being instilled to irrigate the catheter, open the flow clamp on the urinary drainage tubing. **Rationale:** *Irrigating solution will flow through the urinary drainage port and tubing, removing mucous shreds or clots.*
   c. If a three-way catheter is used, open the flow clamp to the irrigating fluid infusion tubing, allowing the specified amount of solution to infuse. Then close the clamp on the infusion tubing.

or

   d. If a two-way catheter is used, connect an irrigating syringe with a needleless adapter to the injection port on the drainage tubing and instill the solution.
   e. After the specified period that the solution is to be retained has passed, open the drainage tubing flow clamp and allow the bladder to empty.
   f. Assess the drainage for amount, color, and clarity. The amount of drainage should equal the amount of irrigant entering the bladder plus expected urine output.
• Remove and discard gloves.
• Perform hand hygiene.
8. Assess the client and the urinary output.
   • Assess the client's comfort.
   • Apply clean gloves.
   • Empty the drainage bag and measure the contents. Subtract the amount of irrigant instilled from the total volume of drainage to obtain the volume of urine output.
   • Remove and discard gloves.
   • Perform hand hygiene.
9. Document findings in the client record using forms or checklists supplemented by narrative notes when appropriate.
   • Note any abnormal constituents such as blood clots, pus, or mucous shreds.

Variation: Open Irrigation Using a Two-Way Indwelling Catheter

1. Assemble the equipment. Use an irrigation set ❷ or assemble individual items as follows:
   • Clean gloves
   • Disposable water-resistant towel
   • Sterile irrigating solution
   • Sterile basin
   • Sterile 30- to 50-mL irrigating syringe
   • Antiseptic swabs
   • Sterile protective cap for drainage tubing.
2. Prepare the client (see steps 1 through 5 of main procedure for catheter irrigation).
3. Prepare the equipment.
   • Perform hand hygiene.
   • Using aseptic technique, open supplies and pour the irrigating solution into the sterile basin or receptacle. **Rationale:** *Aseptic technique is vital to reduce the risk of instilling microorganisms into the urinary tract during the irrigation.*

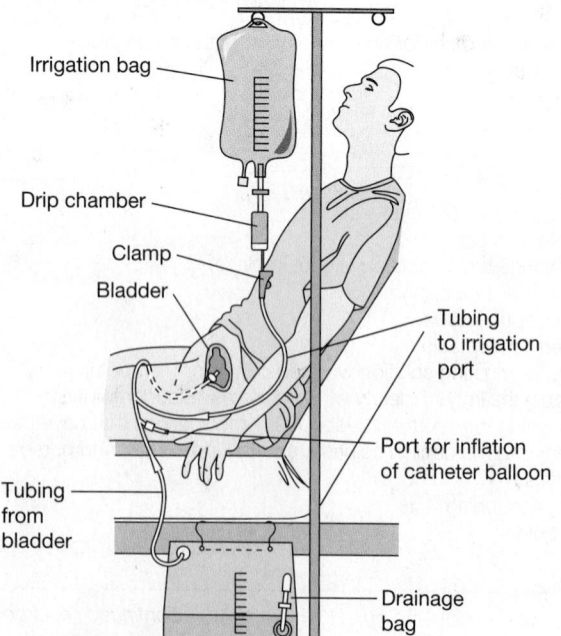

Irrigation bag

Drip chamber

Clamp

Bladder

Tubing to irrigation port

Port for inflation of catheter balloon

Tubing from bladder

Drainage bag

❶ A continuous bladder irrigation (CBI) setup.

Performing Bladder Irrigation—*continued*

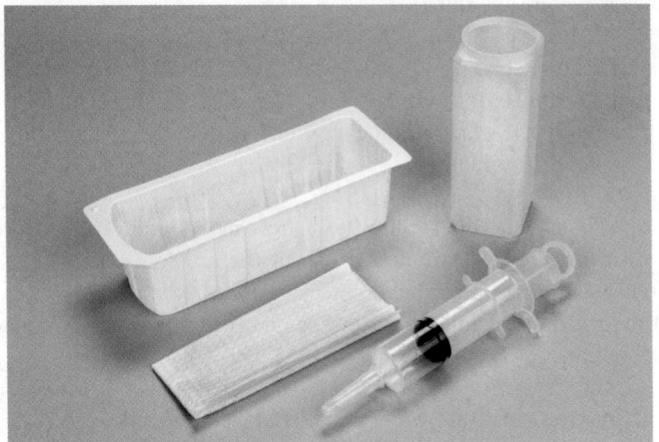

2 An irrigation set.

- Place the disposable water-resistant towel under the catheter.
- Apply clean gloves.
- Disconnect the catheter from the drainage tubing and place the catheter end in the sterile basin. Place the sterile protective cap over the end of the drainage tubing. **Rationale:** *The end of the drainage tubing will be considered contaminated if it touches bed linens or skin surfaces.*

- Draw the prescribed amount of irrigating solution into the syringe, maintaining the sterility of the syringe and solution.
4. Irrigate the bladder.
   - Insert the tip of the syringe into the catheter opening.
   - Gently and slowly inject the solution into the catheter at approximately 3 mL per second. In adults, about 30 to 40 mL generally is instilled for catheter irrigations; 100 to 200 mL may be instilled for bladder irrigation or instillation. **Rationale:** *Gentle instillation reduces the risks of injury to bladder mucosa and of bladder spasms.*
   - Remove the syringe and allow the solution to drain back into the basin.
   - Continue to irrigate the client's bladder until the total amount to be instilled has been injected or when fluid returns are clear and/or clots are removed.
   - Remove the protective cap from the drainage tube and wipe with an antiseptic swab.
   - Reconnect the catheter to the drainage tubing.
   - Remove and discard gloves.
   - Perform hand hygiene.
   - Assess the drainage for amount, color, and clarity. The amount of drainage should equal at least the amount of irrigant entering the bladder plus any urine that may have been dwelling in the bladder. Determine the amount of fluid used for the irrigation and subtract it from the total output on the client's input and output record.
5. Assess the client and the urinary output and document the procedure as in steps 8 and 9 above.

EVALUATION
- Perform detailed follow-up based on findings that deviated from expected or normal for the client. Relate findings to previous assessment data if available.

- Report significant deviations from normal to the primary care provider.

URINARY DIVERSION

A urinary diversion is the surgical rerouting of urine from the kidneys to a site other than the bladder. Permanent urinary diversions are indicated for any condition that requires removal of the bladder (cystectomy). There are two categories of diversions: incontinent and continent.

With incontinent diversions clients have no control over the passage of urine and require the use of an external ostomy appliance to contain the urine. The most common type of incontinent urinary diversion is the **ileal conduit** or **ileal loop** (Figure 20–12 ■). The client must wear an external pouch over the stoma to collect the continuous flow of urine. Continent diversion entails creation of a mechanism that allows the client to control the passage of urine, such as intermittent catheterization of the internal reservoir (e.g., Kock pouch). The person with a Kock pouch has had a reservoir for urine created from a piece of bowel (Figure 20–13 ■). This continent diversion also has valves that close as the reservoir fills, preventing urine leakage. In this case, the client inserts a clean catheter into the valve approximately every 4 hours to empty the urine. Between catheterizations, a small dressing is worn to protect the stoma and clothing.

Application of a urinary diversion ostomy appliance is similar to application of a bowel diversion ostomy (see Skill 21–4 in Chapter 21 ∞). Essential interventions include peristomal care, application of a clean

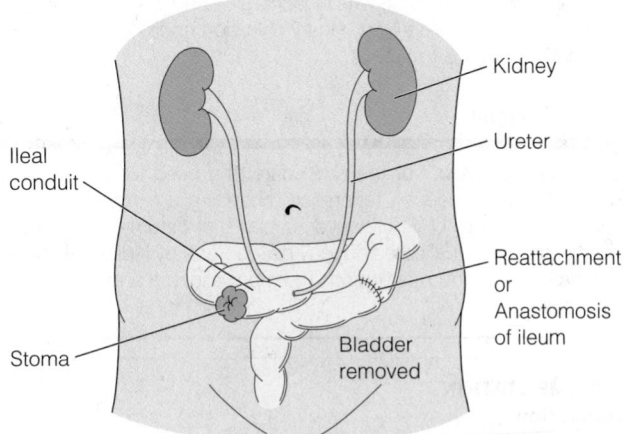

Figure 20–12 ■ An incontinent urinary diversion (ileal conduit).

appliance when required, and teaching self-care to the client and support people.

Temporary disposable urinary diversion appliances are often attached to a urinary drainage system, especially during the night, to prevent accumulation and stagnation of urine in the appliance. Empty these bags at least every 8 hours or when about one-third full.

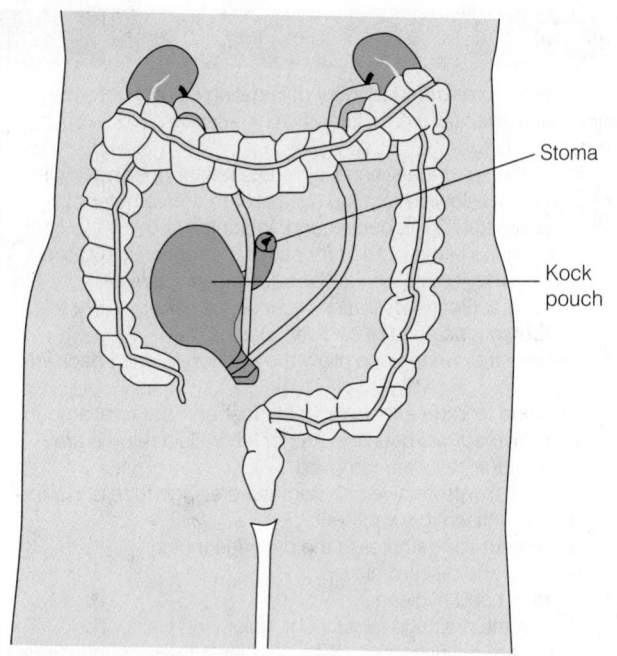

Figure 20–13 ■ The Kock pouch – a continent urinary diversion.

To avoid separation of the appliance from the skin, pouches that are not attached to a drainage system must be emptied several times a day when they are one-third full.

Peristomal skin barriers such as Skin-Prep liquid or wipes or a similar product, or ready-made wafer-type or disk-type barriers, are used according to the manufacturer's directions. The Karaya ring seal, although effective in protecting the skin, is less effective with urinary ostomies than with bowel ostomies because urine tends to melt the product.

The client will also need to learn ways to reduce the odor of urine. Use of deodorant drops in the appliance, soaking a reusable pouch in a diluted vinegar solution, a diet that makes the urine more acidic, and drinking plenty of fluids all help control odor.

Information about ostomy clubs and other applicable community services should also be included. The hole in the abdominal wall, the stoma, and the presence of a bag and fluid can trigger body image issues, feelings of loss, and shame. Refer the client for formal counseling support as needed.

●○● NURSING PROCESS: URINARY DIVERSION

SKILL 20–6

Performing Urinary Ostomy Care

ASSESSMENT
Assess the amount and character of urine drainage; stoma size, shape, and color; status of the peristomal skin; allergies to tape; and the learning needs of the client and support people.

PLANNING
Review the client's record to determine the type of urinary diversion. Determine when the device was last changed and any pertinent findings at that time. Generally, a urinary diversion appliance adheres to the client's skin for 3 to 5 days.

DELEGATION

Due to the complexity of the procedure, the need for assessment skills, and use of aseptic technique, changing a urostomy device is not delegated to UAP. However, aspects of ostomy function are observed during usual care and may be recorded by individuals other than the nurse. Abnormal findings must be validated and interpreted by the nurse.

Equipment
* One- or two-piece urinary pouch
* Tail closure clamp
* Clean gloves
* Cleaning materials, including tissues, warm water, mild soap (optional), cotton balls, washcloth or gauze pads, towel
* Skin barrier/prep (gel, liquid, powder, or film)
* Stoma measuring guide
* Pen or pencil and scissors
* Deodorant liquid drops (optional)
* Bedpan or graduated cylinder

IMPLEMENTATION
Preparation
* Determine the need for an appliance change.
  * Assess the used appliance for leakage of urine. **Rationale:** *Urine irritates the peristomal skin.*
  * Ask the client about any discomfort at or around the stoma. **Rationale:** *A burning sensation may indicate breakdown beneath the faceplate of the pouch.*
  * Assess the fullness of the pouch. **Rationale:** *The weight of an overly full bag may loosen the faceplate and separate it from the skin, causing the urine to leak and irritate the peristomal skin.*
* If there is pouch leakage or discomfort at or around the stoma, change the appliance.

* Select an appropriate time to change the appliance.
  * Avoid times close to meals or visiting hours. **Rationale:** *Ostomy odor may reduce appetite or embarrass the client.*

Performance
1. Prior to performing the procedure, introduce self and verify the client's identity using agency protocol. Explain to the client what you are going to do, why it is necessary, and how he or she can participate. Discuss how the results will be used in planning further care or treatments. Changing an ostomy appliance should not cause discomfort, but it may be distasteful to the client. Communicate acceptance and support to the client.

Performing Urinary Ostomy Care—*continued*

It is important to change the appliance competently and quickly. Include support people as appropriate.

2. Perform hand hygiene and observe other appropriate infection prevention procedures.

3. Provide for client privacy.

4. Assist the client to a comfortable sitting or lying position in bed or a sitting or standing position in the bathroom. **Rationale:** *Lying or standing positions may facilitate smoother pouch application.*

5. Empty and remove the ostomy appliance. *Note:* Because urine flows continuously, if the stoma can be measured for the new appliance with the appliance in place, perform step 8 first. This can usually be accomplished if the pouch is thin or transparent enough to fit the measuring guide snugly over the stoma while it is in place.
   • Apply clean gloves.
   • Empty the pouch through the bottom opening into a bedpan or graduated cylinder. **Rationale:** *Emptying before removing the pouch prevents spillage of urine onto the client's skin.*
   • Peel the bag off slowly while holding the client's skin taut. **Rationale:** *Holding the skin taut minimizes client discomfort and prevents abrasion of the skin.*
   • Place gauze pads over the stoma, and change as needed. **Rationale:** *This absorbs urine seepage from the stoma. Incontinent urinary diversions drain continually. As a result, some type of wicking material (e.g., rolled dry gauze pad or tampon) can be placed over the stoma to absorb the urine and keep the skin dry throughout the measurement and change of the ostomy appliance (Avent, 2012).*

6. *Clean* and dry the peristomal skin and stoma.
   • Use warm water, mild soap (optional), and damp cotton balls, gauze, or a washcloth and towel to clean the skin and stoma. Check agency practice on the use of soap. **Rationale:** *Soap is sometimes not advised because it can be irritating to the skin.*
   • Dry the area thoroughly by patting with a towel or cotton balls. **Rationale:** *Excess rubbing can abrade the skin.*

7. *Assess* the stoma and peristomal skin.
   • Inspect the stoma for color, size, shape, and bleeding.
   • Inspect the peristomal skin for any redness, ulceration, or irritation. Transient redness after removal of adhesive is normal.

8. Prepare and apply the new pouch.
   • Use the guide to measure the size of the stoma.
   • On the backing of the skin barrier, trace a circle the same size as the stomal opening.
   • Cut out the traced stoma pattern to make an opening in the skin barrier. Make the opening no more than 0.3 cm (1/8 in.) larger than the stoma. **Rationale:** *This allows space for the stoma to expand slightly when functioning and minimizes the risk of urine contacting peristomal skin.*
   • Remove the backing to expose the sticky adhesive side of the barrier. The backing can be saved and used as a pattern when making an opening for future skin barriers.
   • Apply the peristomal skin barrier to the faceplate of the ostomy appliance or around the stoma depending on the manufacturer's recommendations. Skin barrier powder may be used on irritated skin, but Skin-Prep liquid may not be applied to irritated skin.
   • Center the faceplate over the stoma, and gently press it onto the client's skin, smoothing out any wrinkles or bubbles. Hold in place for about 30 seconds. **Rationale:** *The heat and pressure help activate the adhesives in the skin barrier.*
   • Remove the air from the pouch. **Rationale:** *Removing the air helps the pouch lie flat against the abdomen.*
   • *Optional:* Place approximately 10 drops of deodorant in the pouch.
   • Close the pouch by turning up the bottom a few times, fan-folding its end lengthwise, and securing it with a tail closure clamp or replacing the drainage outlet cap.
   • Discard all used supplies in appropriate receptacles.
   • Remove and discard gloves.
   • Perform hand hygiene.

9. Document findings in the client record using forms or checklists supplemented by narrative notes when appropriate.

SAMPLE DOCUMENTATION

8/31/2015 0900 Urostomy bag changed due to slight leakage. Had been in place for 3 days. No redness or irritation around stoma. Stoma pink, bled a few drops when washed. Client states home care RN changes the appliance when home. ————————— M. Earl, RN

EVALUATION

• Perform detailed follow-up based on findings that deviated from expected or normal for the client. Relate findings to previous assessment data if available.

• Report significant deviations from normal to the primary care provider.

FOCUSING ON CLINICAL THINKING

Consider This

1. An older male client requests that the urinal be left in place between his legs at all times. How would you respond, and why?

2. Needing to use the urinal every 30 to 60 minutes around the clock has exhausted an 85-year-old man. However, he voids only 15 to 30 mL each time. Is a condom catheter an appropriate solution?

3. While removing an indwelling catheter, only about 75% of the amount of balloon fluid indicated on the catheter is retrieved. How would you proceed?

4. Following a transurethral resection of the prostate gland (TURP), significant bleeding may occur. The primary care provider may order "irrigate catheter prn." How would you determine if the catheter requires irrigating?

5. The hospitalized client's urostomy bag was last emptied 4 hours ago at 4 AM. It now contains 100 mL. Is this acceptable? If not, what steps would you take?

See Focusing on Clinical Thinking answers on student resource website.

TEST YOUR KNOWLEDGE

1. Which terms are acceptable for use in documenting the process of emptying the urinary bladder? Select all that apply.
   1. Urination
   2. Voiding
   3. Maturation
   4. Micturition
   5. Incontinence

2. The nurse is obtaining a urinary elimination history. Which should be emphasized due to likely influence on urinary elimination?
   1. Cardiovascular system disease
   2. Integumentary system disease
   3. Immune system disease
   4. Respiratory system disease

3. The nurse is preparing to assist a male client with using a urinal. In what order would the nurse perform this procedure? Place the following steps of the procedure in the proper order.
   1. Place the urinal between the client's legs.
   2. Pull the curtain around the bed or close the door to the room.
   3. Apply clean gloves.
   4. Rinse the urinal and return it to the client's bedside.
   5. Remove the urinal.

4. The nurse is caring for a client with prostatic hypertrophy and urinary retention. Which catheter would be the *best* choice for this client?
   1. Foley catheter
   2. Robinson catheter
   3. Condom catheter
   4. Coudé catheter

5. While preparing a client for thoracic surgery, the nurse prepares to insert a retention catheter. Which is the *least* appropriate indication for inserting a retention catheter?
   1. Accurate measurement of intake and output
   2. Avoidance of soiling of the surgical incision and dressing
   3. Avoidance of urine retention and bladder distention
   4. Client's inability to void normally postoperatively secondary to anesthesia

6. When inserting a Foley catheter as opposed to a straight catheter, the nurse must complete which action?
   1. Perform hand hygiene.
   2. Obtain a collection bag and tubing.
   3. Apply sterile gloves.
   4. Lubricate the tip of the catheter prior to insertion.

7. The nurse is caring for a client with a retention catheter in place. What is the nurse's primary concern when caring for this client?
   1. Maintain the client on bed rest to prevent backflow of urine from the drainage bag back into the bladder.
   2. Encourage fluid to produce urine output.
   3. Reduce the risk of infection.
   4. Reduce the risk of skin breakdown.

8. The nurse is teaching a client with a urinary diversion how to reduce the odor of urine. The nurse recognizes that the client needs further teaching when the client says:
   1. "I will soak my reusable pouch in diluted vinegar solution to reduce the smell of urine."
   2. "If I drink plenty of fluids, that will help to reduce the urine smell."
   3. "I can put some baking soda in the pouch to make my urine less acidic."
   4. "I can buy deodorant drops to put in the pouch and that will lessen the smell of urine."

9. The nurse can delegate which action to an unlicensed assistive personnel (UAP)?
   1. Inserting a straight catheter
   2. Obtaining a urinary elimination history
   3. Performing bladder irrigation
   4. Emptying a urinary drainage bag for a client with a retention catheter

10. The nurse will notify the primary care provider for which client with a retention catheter?
    1. Client A: 25 mL of urine during hour 1; 35 mL of urine during hour 2; and 27 mL of urine during hour 3
    2. Client B: 25 mL of urine during hour 1; 30 mL of urine during hour 2; and 35 mL of urine during hour 3
    3. Client C: 35 mL of urine during hour 1; 30 mL of urine during hour 2; and 35 mL of urine during hour 3
    4. Client D: 45 mL of urine during hour 1; 50 mL of urine during hour 2; and 35 mL of urine during hour 3

See Answers to Test Your Knowledge in Appendix A.

READINGS AND REFERENCES

References

Avent, Y. (2012). Understanding urinary diversions. *Nursing made Incredibly Easy!, 10*(4), 47–52. doi:10.1097/01 .NME.0000415018.34438.86

Bullman, S. (2011). Ins and outs of suprapubic catheters—A clinician's experience. *Urologic Nursing, 31*(5), 259e–264e.

Chung, E., & So, K. (2012). In vitro analysis of balloon cuffing phenomenon: Inherent biophysical properties of catheter material or mechanics of catheter balloon deflation? *Surgical Innovation, 19,* 175–180. doi:10.1177/1553350611399589

Fisher, J. (2010). The importance of effective catheter securement. *British Journal of Nursing, 19*(Suppl. 8), S14–S18.

Herter, R., & Kazer, M. W. (2010). Best practices in urinary catheter care. *Home Healthcare Nurse, 28,* 342–349. doi:10.1097/NHH.0b013e3181df5d79

Institute for Healthcare Improvement. (2011). *How-to-guide: Prevent catheter-associated urinary tract infections.* Cambridge, MA: Author.

The Joint Commission. (2013). *Hospital: 2014 National Patient Safety Goals.* Retrieved from http://www.jointcommission .org/standards_information/npsgs.aspx

Keyock, K. L., & Newman, D. K. (2011). Understanding stress urinary incontinence. *The Nurse Practitioner, 36*(10), 24–36. doi:10.1097/01.NPR.0000405281.55881.7a

Kyle, G. (2011). The use of urinary sheaths in male incontinence. *British Journal of Nursing, 20,* 338.

Lee, F. M., & Carter, J. R. (2013). Reducing CAUTIs with a bladder retraining program. *Nursing made Incredibly Easy!, 11*(6), 53–54.

Magers, T. L. (2013). Using evidence-based practice to reduce catheter-associated urinary tract infections. *American Journal of Nursing, 113*(6), 34–42. doi:10.1097/ 01.NAJ.0000430923.07539.a7

Oman, K. S., Makic, M. B., Fink, R., Schraeder, N., Hulett, T., Keech, T., & Wald, H. (2012). Nurse-directed interventions to reduce catheter-associated urinary tract infections. *American Journal of Infection Control, 40,* 548–553. doi:10.1016/j.ajic.2011.07.018

Palese, A., Buchini, S., Deroma, L., & Barbone, F. (2010). The effectiveness of the ultrasound bladder scanner in reducing urinary tract infections: A meta-analysis. *Journal of Clinical Nursing, 19,* 2970–2979. doi:10.1111/j.1365-2702.2010.03281.x

Scemons, D. (2013). Urinary incontinence in adults. *Nursing, 43*(11), 52–60. doi:10.1097/ 01.NURSE.0000435202.96023.d6

Schultz, J. (2012). Rethink urinary incontinence in older women. *Nursing, 42*(11), 32–40. doi:10.1097/ 01.NURSE.0000421371.52320.aa

Seckel, M. A. (2013). Maintaining urinary catheters: What does the evidence say? *Nursing, 43*(2), 63–65. doi:10.1097/ 01.NURSE.0000425872.18314.db

Wenger, J. E. (2010). Cultivating quality: Reducing rates of catheter-associated urinary tract infection. *American Journal of Nursing, 110*(8), 40–45. doi:10.1097/ 01.NAJ.0000387691.47746.b5

Wilson, M. (2012). Addressing the problems of long-term urethral catheterization: Part 2. *British Journal of Nursing, 21*(1), 16–25.

Winder, A. (2012). Good practice in catheter care. *Journal of Community Nursing, 26*(6), 15–20.

Selected Bibliography

Berman, A., Snyder, S., & Frandsen, G. (2016). *Kozier & Erb's fundamentals of nursing: Concepts, process, and practice* (10th ed.). Upper Saddle River, NJ: Pearson.

Davis, C., Chrisman, J., & Walden, P. (2012). To scan or not to scan? Detecting urinary retention. *Nursing made Incredibly Easy!, 10*(4), 53–54. doi:10.1097/ 01.NME.0000415016.88696.9d

Dumont, C., & Wakeman, J. (2010). Preventing catheter-associated UTIs: Survey report. *Nursing, 40*(12), 24–30. doi:10.1097/01.NURSE.0000390665.67826.56

Jindal, T., Kamal, M. R., Mandal, S. N., & Karmakar, D. (2012). Catheter-induced urethral erosion. *Urologic Nursing, 32*(2), 100–101.

Mangnall, J. (2012). OptiLube active. The role of lubricants in urinary catheterization. *British Journal of Community Nursing, 17*(9), 414–420.

Nazarko, L. (2012). Catheter-associated urinary tract infection. *Nursing & Residential Care, 14*(11), 578–583.

Uberoi, V., Calixte, N., Coronel, V. R., Furlong, D. J., Orlando, R. P., & Lerner, L. B. (2013). Reducing urinary catheter days. *Nursing, 43*(1), 26–20. doi:10.1097/01.NURSE .0000423971.46518.4d

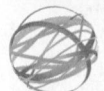

21 Assisting with Fecal Elimination

LEARNING OUTCOMES

At the completion of this chapter, the student will be able to:

1. Define the key terms used in the skills of fecal elimination.
2. Describe factors that affect fecal elimination.
3. Describe guidelines for the care of bedpans.
4. List:
   a. Types of ostomy appliances.
   b. The various pieces of equipment involved with an ostomy appliance.
5. Recognize when it is appropriate to delegate assistance with fecal elimination to unlicensed assistive personnel.

6. Verbalize the steps used in:
   a. Assisting with a bedpan.
   b. Administering an enema.
   c. Removing a fecal impaction.
   d. Changing a bowel diversion ostomy appliance.
7. Demonstrate appropriate documentation and reporting related to fecal elimination.

SKILLS

Skill 21–1 Assisting with a Bedpan
Skill 21–2 Administering an Enema

Skill 21–3 Removing a Fecal Impaction
Skill 21–4 Changing a Bowel Diversion Ostomy Appliance

KEY TERMS

bedpan, *539*
carminative enema, *542*
chyme, *538*
cleansing enema, *542*
colostomy, *548*
commode, *539*
constipation, *542*

defecation, *536*
divided colostomy, *548*
double-barreled colostomy, *549*
enema, *542*
feces, *536*
gastrocolic reflex, *538*
ileostomy, *548*

impaction, *546*
incontinence, *539*
loop colostomy, *548*
meconium, *537*
ostomy, *548*
ostomy appliance, *549*
retention enema, *542*

return-flow enema, *542*
single (end)
   colostomy, *548*
stoma, *548*
stool, *536*

DEFECATION

Elimination of the waste products of digestion from the body is essential to health. The excreted waste products are referred to as **feces** or **stool**. **Defecation** is the expulsion of feces from the anus and rectum. It is also called a bowel movement. The frequency of defecation is highly individual, varying from several times per day to two or three times per week. The amount defecated also varies from person to person. When peristaltic waves move the feces into the sigmoid colon and the rectum, the sensory nerves in the rectum are stimulated and the individual becomes aware of the need to defecate.

CLINICAL ALERT!

Individuals (especially children) may use very different terms for a bowel movement. The nurse may need to try several different common words before finding one the client understands.

When the internal anal sphincter relaxes, feces move into the anal canal. After the individual is seated on a toilet or bedpan, the external anal sphincter is relaxed voluntarily. Expulsion of the feces is assisted by contraction of the abdominal muscles and the diaphragm, which increases abdominal pressure, and by contraction of the muscles of the pelvic floor, which moves the feces through the anal canal. Normal defecation is facilitated by (a) thigh flexion, which increases the pressure within the abdomen, and (b) a sitting position, which increases the downward pressure on the rectum.

If the defecation reflex is ignored, or if defecation is consciously inhibited by contracting the external sphincter muscle, the urge to defecate normally disappears for a few hours before occurring again. Repeated inhibition of the urge to defecate can result in expansion of the rectum to accommodate accumulated feces and eventual loss of sensitivity to the need to defecate. Constipation can be the ultimate result.

Feces

Normal feces are made of about 75% water and 25% solid materials. They are soft but formed. Normal feces require a normal fluid intake; feces that contain less water may be hard and difficult to expel. Feces are normally brown, chiefly due to the presence of stercobilin and urobilin, which are derived from bilirubin (a red pigment in bile). Another factor that affects fecal color is the action of bacteria such as *Escherichia coli*, which are normally present in the large intestine.

| TABLE 21–1 | Characteristics of Normal and Abnormal Feces | | |

Characteristic	Normal	Abnormal	Possible Cause of Abnormal Feces
Color	Adult: brown	Clay or white	Absence of bile pigment (bile obstruction); diagnostic study using barium
	Infant: yellow	Black or tarry	Drug (e.g., iron); bleeding from upper gastrointestinal tract (e.g., stomach, small intestine); diet high in red meat and dark green vegetables (e.g., spinach)
		Red	Bleeding from lower gastrointestinal tract (e.g., rectum); some foods (e.g., beets)
		Pale	Malabsorption of fats; diet high in milk and milk products and low in meat
		Orange or green	Intestinal infection
Consistency	Formed, soft, semisolid, moist	Hard, dry	Dehydration; decreased intestinal motility resulting from lack of fiber in diet, lack of exercise, emotional upset, laxative abuse
		Diarrhea	Increased intestinal motility (e.g., due to irritation of the colon by bacteria)
Shape	Cylindrical (contour of rectum) about 2.5 cm (1 in.) in diameter in adults	Narrow, pencil-shaped, or stringlike stool	Obstructive condition of the rectum
Amount	Varies with diet (about 100–400 g/day)		
Odor	Aromatic: affected by ingested food and person's own bacterial flora	Pungent	Infection, blood
Constituents	Small amounts of undigested roughage, sloughed dead bacteria and epithelial cells, fat, protein, dried constituents of digestive juices (e.g., bile pigments, inorganic matter)	Pus Mucus Parasites Blood Large quantities of fat Foreign objects	Bacterial infection Inflammatory condition Gastrointestinal bleeding Malabsorption Accidental ingestion of foreign object

The amount of gas produced a day varies among individuals; passing gas around 13 to 21 times a day is normal (National Digestive Diseases Information Clearinghouse, 2013). The gases include carbon dioxide, methane, hydrogen, oxygen, and nitrogen. Some are swallowed with food and fluids taken by mouth, others are formed through the action of bacteria in the large intestine, and other gas diffuses from the blood into the gastrointestinal tract. The action of microorganisms is also responsible for the odor of feces and flatus. Table 21–1 lists the characteristics of normal and abnormal feces.

Factors That Affect Defecation

Defecation patterns vary at different stages of life. Circumstances of diet, fluid intake and output, activity, psychological factors, lifestyle, medications and medical procedures, disease, pain, and positioning also affect defecation.

DEVELOPMENT

Newborns and infants, toddlers, children, and older adults are groups within which members have similarities in elimination patterns.

NEWBORNS AND INFANTS **Meconium** is the first fecal material passed by the newborn, normally up to 24 hours after birth. It is black, tarry, odorless, and sticky. Transitional stools, which follow for about a week, are generally greenish yellow; they contain mucus and are loose.

Infants pass stool frequently, often after each feeding. Because the intestine is immature, water is not well absorbed and the stool is soft, liquid, and frequent. When the intestine matures bacterial flora increase. After solid foods are introduced, the stool becomes less frequent and firmer.

Infants who are breast-fed have light yellow to golden feces that are loose in texture. Infants who are taking formula will have dark yellow or tan stool that is more formed.

TODDLERS Some control of defecation starts at 1½ to 2 years of age. By this time, children have learned to walk, and the nervous and muscular systems are sufficiently well developed to permit bowel control. A desire to control daytime bowel movements and to use the toilet generally starts when the child becomes aware of (a) the discomfort caused by a soiled diaper and (b) the sensation that indicates the need for a bowel movement. Daytime control is typically attained by age 2½, after a process of toilet training.

SCHOOL-AGE CHILDREN AND ADOLESCENTS School-age children and adolescents have bowel habits similar to those of adults. Patterns of defecation vary in frequency, quantity, and consistency. Some school-age children may delay defecation because of an activity such as play.

OLDER ADULTS Toner and Claros (2012) state that "up to half of all older adults suffer from constipation" (p. 32) This is due, in part, to reduced activity levels, inadequate amounts of fluid and fiber intake, and muscle weakness. Many older people believe that "regularity" means a bowel movement every day. Those who do not meet this criterion often seek over-the-counter preparations to relieve what they believe to be constipation. Older adults should be advised that normal patterns of bowel elimination vary considerably. For some, a normal pattern may be every other day; for others, twice a day. Constipation can be relieved by increasing the fiber intake to 20 to 35 grams per day, unless contraindicated (Tabloski & Connell, 2014). Adequate roughage in the diet, adequate exercise, and 6 to 8 glasses of fluid daily are essential preventive measures for constipation. A cup of hot water or tea at a regular time in the morning is helpful for some. The **gastrocolic reflex** (increased peristalsis of the colon after food has entered the stomach) is an important consideration. For example, toileting is recommended 30 minutes after meals, especially after breakfast when the gastrocolic reflex is strongest (Toner & Claros, 2012).

DIET

Sufficient bulk (cellulose, fiber) in the diet is necessary to provide fecal volume. Bland diets and low-fiber diets are lacking in bulk and therefore create insufficient residue of waste products to stimulate the reflex for defecation. Low-residue foods, such as rice, eggs, and lean meats, move more slowly through the intestinal tract. Increasing fluid intake with such foods increases their rate of movement.

Certain foods are difficult or impossible for some people to digest. This inability results in digestive upsets and, in some instances, the passage of watery stools. Irregular eating can also impair regular defecation. Individuals who eat at the same times every day usually have a regularly timed, physiological response to the food intake and a regular pattern of peristaltic activity in the colon.

FLUID

Even when fluid intake is inadequate or output (urine or vomitus, for example) is excessive for some reason, the body continues to reabsorb fluid from the **chyme** (contents of the colon). The chyme becomes drier than normal, resulting in hard feces. In addition, reduced fluid intake slows the chyme's passage along the intestines, further increasing the reabsorption of fluid from the chyme. Healthy fecal elimination usually requires a daily fluid intake of 2,000 to 3,000 mL. If chyme moves abnormally quickly through the large intestine, however, there is less time for fluid to be absorbed into the blood; as a result, the feces are soft or even watery.

ACTIVITY

Activity stimulates peristalsis, thus facilitating the movement of chyme along the colon. Weak abdominal and pelvic muscles are often ineffective in increasing the intra-abdominal pressure during defecation or in controlling defecation. Weak muscles can result from lack of exercise, immobility, or impaired neurologic functioning. Confinement in bed or long periods of impaired mobility can often result in constipation.

PSYCHOLOGICAL FACTORS

Some people who are anxious or angry experience increased peristaltic activity and subsequent nausea or diarrhea. In contrast, people who are depressed may experience slowed intestinal motility, resulting in constipation. How a person responds to these emotional states is the result of individual differences in the response of the enteric nervous system to vagal stimulation from the brain.

DEFECATION HABITS

Early bowel training may establish the habit of defecating at a regular time. Many people defecate after breakfast, when the gastrocolic reflex causes mass peristaltic waves in the large intestine. If a person ignores this urge to defecate, water continues to be reabsorbed, making the feces hard and difficult to expel. When the normal defecation reflexes are inhibited or ignored, these conditioned reflexes tend to be progressively weakened. When habitually ignored, the urge to defecate is ultimately lost. Adults may ignore these reflexes because of the pressures of time or work. Clients who are hospitalized may suppress the urge because of embarrassment about using a bedpan, because of lack of privacy, or because defecation is too uncomfortable.

MEDICATIONS

Some medications can have side effects that interfere with normal elimination. Some cause diarrhea as a side effect or adverse reaction; others, such as large doses of certain tranquilizers and repeated administration of morphine and codeine, cause constipation because they decrease gastrointestinal activity through their action on the central nervous system. Iron supplements act more locally on the bowel mucosa and can cause constipation or diarrhea.

Some medications directly affect elimination. Laxatives are medications that stimulate bowel activity and so assist fecal elimination. Other medications soften stool, facilitating defecation. Certain medications suppress peristaltic activity and may be used to treat diarrhea.

Medications can also affect the appearance of the feces. Any drug that can cause gastrointestinal bleeding (e.g., aspirin products) has the potential to produce red or black stool. Iron salts lead to black stool because of the oxidation of the iron, antibiotics may cause a gray-green discoloration, and antacids can cause a whitish discoloration or white specks in the stool. Pepto-Bismol, a common over-the-counter drug, causes stools to be black.

DIAGNOSTIC PROCEDURES

Before certain diagnostic procedures, such as visualization of the colon (colonoscopy or sigmoidoscopy), the client is restricted from ingesting food or fluid. The client may also be given a cleansing enema prior to the examination. In these instances normal defecation usually will not occur until eating resumes.

ANESTHESIA AND SURGERY

General anesthetics cause the normal colonic movements to cease or slow by blocking parasympathetic stimulation to the muscles of the colon. Clients who have regional or spinal anesthesia are less likely to experience this problem.

Surgery that involves direct handling of the intestines can cause temporary cessation of intestinal movement. This condition, called ileus, usually lasts 24 to 48 hours. Listening for bowel sounds that reflect intestinal motility is an important nursing assessment following surgery.

PATHOLOGIC CONDITIONS

Spinal cord injuries and head injuries can decrease the sensory stimulation for defecation. Impaired mobility may limit the client's ability to respond to the urge to defecate, and the client may experience constipation. Or, a client may experience fecal **incontinence** (loss of control of expulsion of feces) because of poorly functioning anal sphincters.

PAIN

Clients who experience discomfort when defecating (e.g., hemorrhoids, following rectal surgery) often suppress the urge to defecate to avoid the pain. Such clients can experience constipation as a result. Clients taking narcotic analgesics for pain may also experience constipation as a side effect of the medication.

POSITIONING

Although the squatting position best facilitates defecation, on a toilet seat the best position for most people seems to be leaning forward.

For clients who have difficulty sitting down and getting up from the toilet, an elevated toilet seat can be attached to a regular toilet. Clients then do not have to lower themselves as far onto the seat and do not have to lift as far off the seat. Elevated toilet seats can be purchased from a medical supply store for use in the home.

A bedside **commode** is a portable chair with a toilet seat and a removable collection receptacle beneath the seat. It is often used for the adult client who can get out of bed but is unable to walk to the bathroom. Some commodes have wheels and can slide over the base of a regular toilet when the waste receptacle is removed, thus providing clients the privacy of a bathroom. Some commodes have a seat and can be used as a chair (Figure 21–1 ■). Potty chairs are available for children.

Clients restricted to bed may need to use a **bedpan**, a receptacle for urine and feces. Female clients use a bedpan for both urine and feces; male clients use a bedpan for feces and a urinal for urine.

BEDPANS

There are two main types of bedpans: the regular, or high-back, pan; and the slipper, or fracture, pan (Figure 21–2 ■). The slipper pan has a low back and is used for people who are unable to elevate their buttocks because of physical problems or therapy that contraindicates such movement. Many people confined to bed are able to use a bedpan independently, provided the equipment is placed within safe and easy reach. Some, however, require varying degrees of assistance from a nurse. The nurse has to determine the individual's needs and provide the appropriate assistance. Using a bedpan can be embarrassing to many people. For the older client or clients who are physically impaired or critically ill, it can also be a tiring procedure.

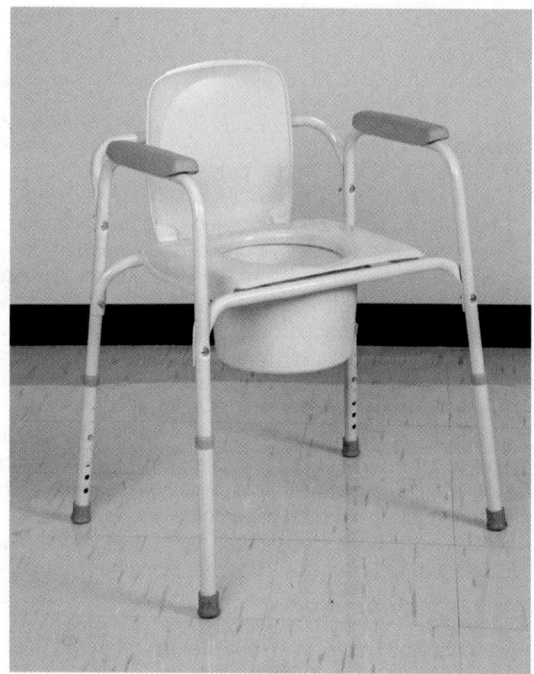

Figure 21–1 ■ A commode with an overlying seat.

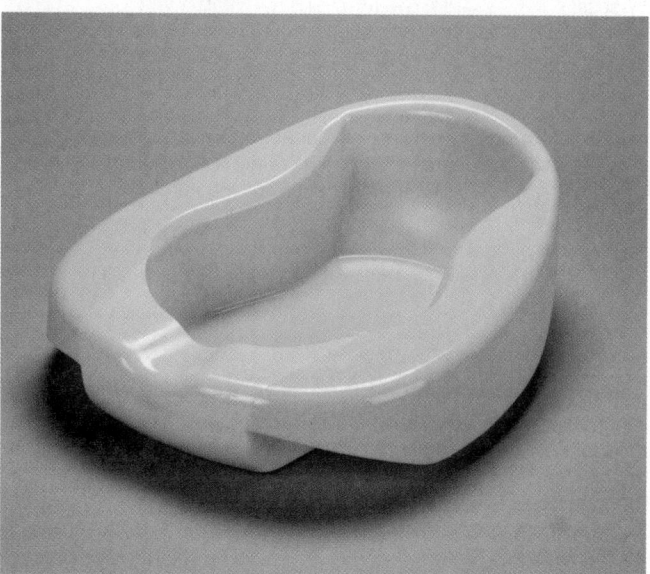
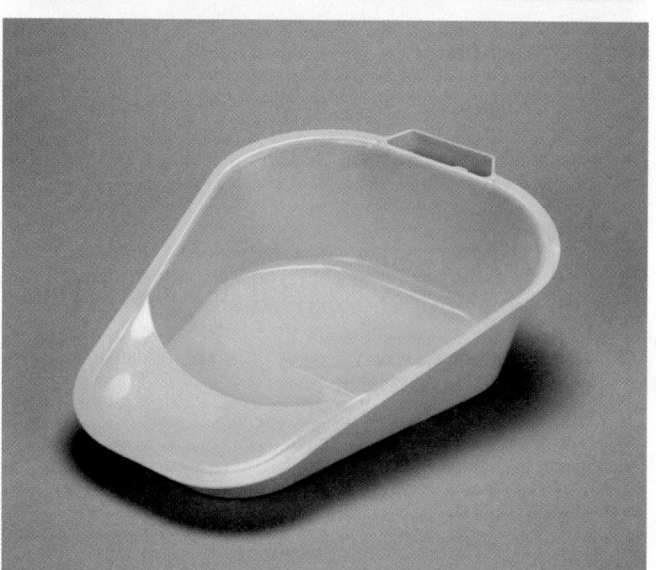

Figure 21–2 ■ *Top,* The high-back or regular bedpan; *Bottom,* the slipper or fracture pan.

Guidelines for the Care of Bedpans

The care of bedpans relates largely to preventing the transmission of microorganisms and to the feelings people attach to elimination.

- To maintain medical asepsis, each client in a hospital is provided with a separate bedpan.
- Bedpans are stored in an appropriate place out of sight. Bedside units are often designed to provide a specific place for bedpans that is not visible to others and is separate from the client's personal possessions. It is usually also separated from other equipment used for hygienic care. Medical aseptic practice prohibits placing a bedpan on the floor, under the bed, or on bedside tables.
- Bedpans should always be handled from the outside while wearing gloves. Slipper (fracture) pans have handles that the nurse can use to carry them. The high-back bedpan needs to be supported with both hands on its base for transport.
- Elimination equipment is thoroughly cleaned after use. Rinsing devices are generally located in the client bathrooms or the dirty utility room.

●○●● NURSING PROCESS: BEDPANS

SKILL 21–1

Assisting with a Bedpan

ASSESSMENT

Assess:
- Defecation pattern: The frequency and time of day of the client's defecation. Has this pattern changed recently? Does it ever change? If so, does the client know what factors affect it?
- Abdominal distention.
- Bowel sounds: Auscultate all four abdominal quadrants to determine the degree of activity or frequency of sounds. See Skill 3–15, Assessing the Abdomen, in Chapter 3 ∞.
- Perianal region and anus: Inspect these areas for discolorations, inflammations, scars, lesions, fissures, fistulas, or hemorrhoids.
- Presence of abdominal or rectal pain.
- Level of mobility and amount of assistance needed.
- Need for a stool specimen.

PLANNING

Inquire whether the client has used a bedpan previously. Locate the client's bedpan.

DELEGATION

Unlicensed assistive personnel (UAP) commonly assist clients with bedpans. The nurse must determine if the specific client has unique needs that would require special training of the UAP in the use of the bedpan. Ensure that personnel are aware of any specimens that need to be collected. Abnormal findings must be validated and interpreted by the nurse.

Equipment
- Clean bedpan and cover
- Toilet tissue
- Basin of water, soap, washcloth, and towel
- Equipment for a specimen if required (see Skill 4–2 in Chapter 4 ∞)
- Clean gloves
- Disposable absorbent pad

IMPLEMENTATION

Preparation
- Adjust the bed to a height appropriate to prevent back strain.
- Elevate the rail on the opposite side of the bed. **Rationale:** *This prevents the client from falling and provides a hand grasp for the client if needed.*

Performance
1. Prior to performing the procedure, introduce self to the client and verify the client's identity using agency protocol. Explain to the client what you are going to do, why it is necessary, and how he or she can participate.
2. Perform hand hygiene and observe other appropriate infection prevention procedures.
3. Apply clean gloves.
4. Provide for client privacy.
5. Prepare the client.
   - For clients who can assist by raising their buttocks, fold down the top bed linen on the near side to expose the hip, and adjust the gown so that it will not fall into the bedpan. **Rationale:** *A pie fold of the top bed linens exposes the client minimally and facilitates placement of the bedpan.*
   - For clients who cannot raise their buttocks onto and off a bedpan, fold the top bed linens down to the hips.

6. Place the client on the bedpan.
   - For clients who can lift their buttocks:
     a. Ask the client to flex the knees, rest his or her weight on the back and the heels, and then raise the buttocks. The client can use a trapeze, if present, or grasp the side rail for support. Assist the client to lift the buttocks by placing the hand nearest the person's head palm up under the lower back, resting the elbow on the mattress, and using the forearm as a lever. **Rationale:** *Use of appropriate body mechanics by both the client and nurse prevents unnecessary muscle strain and exertion.*
     b. Place the absorbent pad on the bed where the bedpan will be located. Position a regular bedpan under the buttocks with the narrow end toward the foot of the bed and the buttocks resting on the smooth, rounded rim. Place a slipper (fracture) pan with the flat end under the client's buttocks. ❶ **Rationale:** *Improper placement of the bedpan can cause skin abrasion to the sacral area and spillage of the bedpan's contents.*
   - For clients who cannot lift their buttocks:
     a. Assist the client to a side-lying position.

Assisting with a Bedpan—*continued*

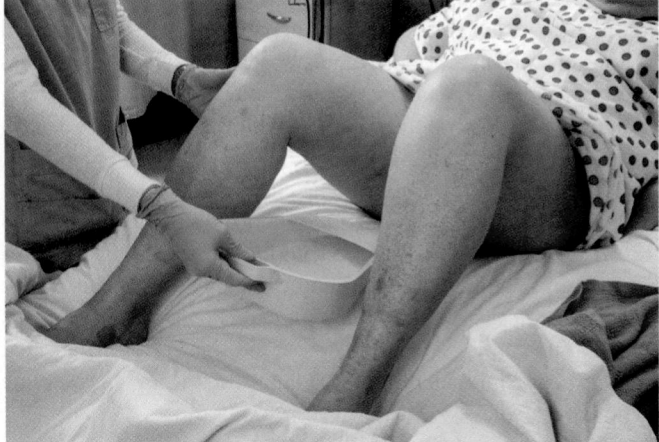

❶ Placing a slipper (fracture) bedpan under the buttocks.

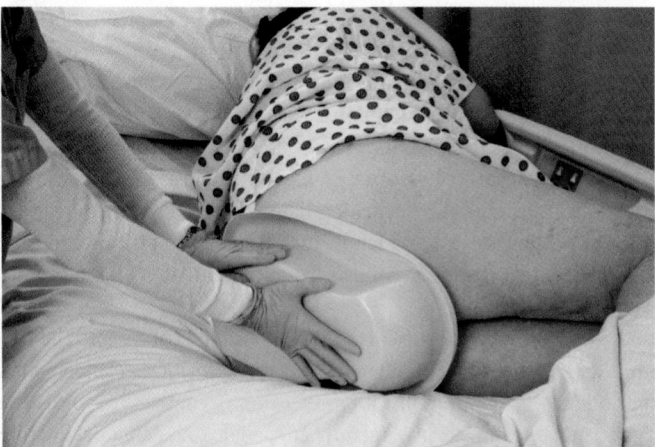

❷ Placing a regular bedpan against the client's buttocks.

b. Place the bedpan against the buttocks with the open rim toward the foot of the bed.
c. Smoothly roll the client onto the bedpan while holding the bedpan against the buttocks. ❷

7. Elevate the head of the bed to a semi-Fowler's position. **Rationale:** *This position relieves strain on the client's back and permits a more normal position for elimination.* Recheck the position of the bedpan because it may have been repositioned while the head of the bed was being raised.
   • If the person is unable to assume a semi-Fowler's position, place a small pillow under the back, or help the client to another comfortable position.

8. Replace the top bed linen.
9. Provide the client with toilet tissue, raise the side rail, lower the bed height, and ensure that the call light is readily accessible. Ask the client to signal when finished. Leave only when, in your judgment, it is safe to do so. **Rationale:** *Having necessary items within reach prevents falls.*

Do not leave anyone on a bedpan longer than 15 minutes unless the individual is able to remove the pan without assistance. **Rationale:** *Lengthy stays on a bedpan can cause skin breakdown.*

Removing a Bedpan

10. Return the bed to the position used when giving the bedpan.
    • Hold the bedpan steady to prevent spillage of its contents.
    • Cover the bedpan, and place it on an adjacent chair with a pad or towel under it. **Rationale:** *Covering the bedpan reduces offensive odors and reduces the client's embarrassment.*

11. Assist the client with any needed hygienic measures.
    • Wrap toilet tissue several times around the gloved hand, and wipe the person from the pubic area to the anal area, using one stroke for each piece of tissue. **Rationale:** *Cleaning in this direction—from the less soiled area to the more soiled area—helps prevent the spread of microorganisms.*
    • Place the soiled tissue in the bedpan.
    • Wash the anal area with soap and water as indicated, and thoroughly dry the area. **Rationale:** *Adequate washing and drying prevents skin abrasion and excessive accumulation of microorganisms.*
    • Remove the disposable absorbent pad or replace the draw-sheet if it is soiled.
    • Offer the client materials to wash and dry the hands. **Rationale:** *Hand washing following elimination is a practice that helps prevent the spread of microorganisms.*

12. Attend to any unpleasant odors in the environment.
    • Spray the air with an air freshener as needed unless contraindicated because of respiratory problems or allergies, or because it is offensive. **Rationale:** *Elimination odor can be embarrassing to clients and visitors alike. However, sprays may be harmful to people with respiratory problems, and some perfume sprays are offensive to some people.*

13. Attend to the used bedpan.
    • Acquire a specimen if required. Place it in the appropriately labeled container.
    • Empty and clean the bedpan. Provide a clean bedpan cover, if necessary, before returning it to the client's unit.
    • Remove and discard gloves.
    • Perform hand hygiene.

14. Document findings (e.g., color, odor, amount, and consistency of feces) in the client record using forms or checklists supplemented by narrative notes when appropriate.

EVALUATION
• Perform follow-up treatment or client teaching based on findings that deviated from expected or normal for the client. Relate findings to previous data if available.

• Report significant deviations from normal to the primary care provider.

ENEMAS

An **enema** is a solution introduced into the rectum and large intestine and can be used as a treatment for constipation. **Constipation** refers to the passage of small, dry, hard stool or the passage of no stool for a period of time. It is important to define constipation in relation to the person's regular elimination pattern, but it may be defined as fewer than three bowel movements per week. It occurs when the movement of feces through the large intestine is slow, thus allowing time for additional reabsorption of fluid from the large intestine.

The action of an enema varies depending on the type of enema. Enemas are classified into four types or groups: cleansing, carminative, retention, and return-flow.

A **cleansing enema** is intended to remove feces. It is given chiefly to:

- Prevent the escape of feces during surgery.
- Prepare the intestine for certain diagnostic tests such as x-ray or visualization tests (e.g., colonoscopy).
- Remove feces in instances of constipation or impaction.

Cleansing enemas use a variety of solutions. Table 21–2 lists commonly used solutions.

Hypertonic solutions exert osmotic pressure, which draws fluid from the interstitial space into the colon. The increased volume in the colon stimulates peristalsis and therefore defecation. A commonly used hypertonic enema is the commercially prepared Fleet phosphate enema. Hypotonic solutions (e.g., tap water) exert a lower osmotic pressure than the surrounding interstitial fluid, causing water to move from the colon into the interstitial space. Before the water moves from the colon, it stimulates peristalsis and defecation. Because the water moves out of the colon, the tap water enema should not be repeated because of danger of circulatory overload when the water moves from the interstitial space into the circulatory system.

SAFETY ALERT! | SAFETY

Special precautions must be used to alert nurses to possible contraindications when Fleet enemas are prescribed for clients with renal failure. The label on a Fleet enema warns that using more than one enema every 24 hours can be harmful. Clients and family may underestimate the risks for a client with decreased renal function because a Fleet enema can be obtained over the counter in stores (Cohen, 2012).

Isotonic solutions, such as physiological (normal) saline, are considered the safest enema solutions to use. They exert the same osmotic pressure as the interstitial fluid surrounding the colon. Therefore, there is no fluid movement into or out of the colon. The instilled volume of saline in the colon stimulates peristalsis. Soapsuds enemas stimulate peristalsis by increasing the volume in the colon and irritating the mucosa. Only pure soap (i.e., castile soap) should be used in order to minimize mucosa irritation.

As shown in Table 21–2, some enemas are large volume (i.e., 500 to 1,000 mL) for an adult and others are small volume (90 to 120 mL), including hypertonic solutions. The amount of solution administered for a high-volume enema will depend on the age and medical condition of the individual. For example, clients with certain cardiac or renal diseases would be adversely affected by significant fluid retention that might result from large-volume hypotonic enemas.

Cleansing enemas may also be described as high or low depending on how much of the colon needs to be cleansed. A high enema is given to cleanse as much of the colon as possible. The client changes from the left lateral position to the dorsal recumbent position and then to the right lateral position during administration so that the solution can follow the large intestine. The low enema is used to clean the rectum and sigmoid colon only. The client maintains a left lateral position during administration.

A **carminative enema** is given primarily to help relieve abdominal distention by expelling flatus. The solution instilled into the rectum releases gas, which in turn distends the rectum and the colon, thus stimulating peristalsis. For an adult, 60 to 80 mL of fluid is instilled.

A **retention enema** introduces oil or medication into the rectum and sigmoid colon. The liquid is retained for a relatively long period (e.g., 1 to 3 hours). An oil retention enema acts to soften the feces and to lubricate the rectum and anal canal, thus facilitating passage of the feces. Antibiotic enemas are used to treat infections locally, anthelmintic enemas to kill helminths such as worms and intestinal parasites, and nutritive enemas to administer fluids and nutrients to the rectum.

A **return-flow enema** is used occasionally to expel flatus. Alternating flow of 100 to 200 mL of fluid into and out of the rectum and sigmoid colon stimulates peristalsis. This process is repeated five or six times until the flatus is expelled and abdominal distention is relieved.

TABLE 21–2 | Commonly Used Enema Solutions

Solution	Constituents	Action	Time to Take Effect	Adverse Effects
Hypertonic	90–120 mL of solution (e.g., sodium phosphate [Fleet's])	Draws water into the colon	5–10 min	Retention of sodium
Hypotonic	500–1,000 mL of tap water	Distends colon, stimulates peristalsis, and softens feces	15–20 min	Fluid and electrolyte imbalance; water intoxication
Isotonic	500–1,000 mL of normal saline	Distends colon, stimulates peristalsis, and softens feces	15–20 min	Possible sodium retention
Soapsuds	500–1,000 mL (3–5 mL soap to 1,000 mL water)	Irritates mucosa, distends colon	10–15 min	Irritates and may damage mucosa
Oil (mineral, olive, cottonseed)	90–120 mL	Lubricates the feces and the colon mucosa	0.5–3 h	

Some clients may wish to administer their own enemas. If this is appropriate, the nurse validates the client's knowledge of correct technique and assists as needed.

From a holistic perspective, it is important for the nurse to remember that clients may perceive this type of procedure as a significant violation of personal space. Cultural sensitivity pertaining to personal space, gender of the caregiver, and the potential meaning of the structures and fluids found in this private area of the body needs to be considered. Keep in mind the client's potential discomfort with the gender of the caregiver and try to accommodate the client's preferences whenever possible. When it is not possible to honor the client's wishes, respectfully explain the circumstances. A gentle, matter-of-fact approach is often most helpful. Also, insertion of anything foreign into an orifice of a client's body may trigger memories of past abuse for some clients. Monitor the client for emotional responses to the procedure (both subtle and extreme) because this could indicate a history of trauma and require appropriate referral for counseling. Simply asking the client to describe the experience will give the nurse more information for possible referral.

The following are guidelines for administering enemas:

- Enemas for adults are usually given at 37°C to 42°C (99°F to 106°F), unless otherwise specified. High temperatures can be injurious to the bowel mucosa; cold temperatures are uncomfortable for the client and may trigger a spasm of the sphincter muscles.
- The force of flow of the solution is governed by (a) the height of the solution container, (b) size of the tubing, (c) viscosity of the fluid, and (d) resistance of the rectum. The higher the solution container is held above the rectum, the faster the flow and the greater the force (pressure) in the rectum. During most adult enemas, the solution container should be no higher than 30 cm (12 in.) above the rectum. During a high cleansing enema, the solution container is usually held 30 to 44 cm (12 to 18 in.) above the rectum because the fluid is instilled farther to clean the entire bowel.
- The time it takes to administer an enema largely depends on the amount of fluid to be instilled and the client's tolerance. Large volumes, such as 1,000 mL, may take 10 to 15 minutes to instill; small volumes require less time.
- The amount of time the client retains the enema solution depends on the purpose of the enema and the client's ability to contract the external sphincter to retain the solution. Oil retention enemas are usually retained 1 to 3 hours. Other enemas are normally retained 5 to 10 minutes.

●○○● NURSING PROCESS: ENEMAS

Administering an Enema

ASSESSMENT

Assess:
- When the client last had a bowel movement and the amount, color, and consistency of the feces.
- Presence of abdominal distention.
- Whether the client has sphincter control.
- Whether the client can use a toilet or commode or must remain in bed and use a bedpan.

PLANNING

Before administering an enema, determine that there is a primary care provider's order. At some agencies, a primary care provider must order the kind of enema and the time to give it, for example, the morning of an examination. At other agencies, enemas are given at the nurses' discretion (i.e., as necessary on a prn order). In addition, determine the presence of kidney or cardiac disease that contraindicates the use of a hypotonic or hypertonic solution.

DELEGATION

Administration of some enemas may be delegated to UAP. However, the nurse must ensure the personnel are competent in the use of standard precautions. Abnormal findings such as inability to insert the rectal tip, client inability to retain the solution, or unusual return from the enema must be validated and interpreted by the nurse.

Equipment
- Disposable linen-saver pad
- Bath blanket
- Bedpan or commode
- Clean gloves
- Water-soluble lubricant if tubing is not prelubricated
- Paper towel

Large-Volume Enema
- Solution container with tubing of correct size and tubing clamp
- Correct solution, amount, and temperature

Small-Volume Enema
- Prepackaged container of enema solution with lubricated tip

IMPLEMENTATION

Preparation
- Lubricate about 5 cm (2 in.) of the rectal tube (some commercially prepared enema sets already have lubricated nozzles). **Rationale:** *Lubrication facilitates insertion through the sphincter and minimizes trauma.*
- Run some solution through the connecting tubing of a large-volume enema set and the rectal tube to expel any air in the tubing, then close the clamp. **Rationale:** *Air instilled into the rectum, although not harmful, causes unnecessary distention.*

Continued on page 544

SKILL 21-2

SKILL 21-2

Administering an Enema—*continued*

Performance

1. Prior to performing the procedure, introduce self and verify the client's identity using agency protocol. Explain to the client what you are going to do, why it is necessary, and how he or she can participate. Discuss how the results will be used in planning further care or treatments. Indicate that the client may experience a feeling of fullness while the solution is being administered. Explain the need to hold the solution as long as possible.

2. Perform hand hygiene and observe other appropriate infection prevention procedures.

3. Apply clean gloves.

4. Provide for client privacy.

5. Assist the adult client to a left lateral position, with the right leg as acutely flexed as possible ❶ and the linen-saver pad under the buttocks. **Rationale:** *This position facilitates the flow of solution by gravity into the sigmoid and descending colon, which are on the left side. Having the right leg acutely flexed provides for adequate exposure of the anus.*

6. Insert the enema tube.
   - For clients in the left lateral position, lift the upper buttock. ❷ **Rationale:** *This ensures good visualization of the anus.*
   - Insert the tube smoothly and slowly into the rectum, directing it toward the umbilicus. ❸ **Rationale:** *The angle follows the normal contour of the rectum. Slow insertion prevents spasm of the sphincter.*
   - Insert the tube 7 to 10 cm (3 to 4 in.). **Rationale:** *Because the anal canal is about 2.5 to 5 cm (1 to 2 in.) long in the adult, insertion to this point places the tip of the tube beyond the anal sphincter into the rectum.*
   - If resistance is encountered at the internal sphincter, ask the client to take a deep breath, then run a small amount of solution through the tube. **Rationale:** *This relaxes the internal anal sphincter.*
   - Never force tube or solution entry. If instilling a small amount of solution does not permit the tube to be advanced or the solution to freely flow, withdraw the tube. Check for any stool that may have blocked the tube during insertion. If present, flush it and retry the procedure. You may also perform a digital rectal examination to determine if there is an impaction or other mechanical blockage. If resistance persists, end the procedure and report the resistance to the primary care provider and nurse in charge.

7. Slowly administer the enema solution.
   - Raise the solution container, and open the clamp to allow fluid flow.

   or

   - Compress a pliable container by hand.
   - During most low enemas, hold or hang the solution container no higher than 30 cm (12 in.) above the rectum. **Rationale:** *The higher the solution container is held above the rectum, the faster the flow and the greater the force (pressure) in the rectum.* During a high enema, hang the solution container between 30 to 45 cm (12 to 18 in.). **Rationale:** *The fluid must be instilled farther to clean the entire bowel.* See agency protocol.
   - Administer the fluid slowly. If the client complains of fullness or pain, lower the container or use the clamp to stop the flow for 30 seconds, and then restart the flow at a slower rate. **Rationale:** *Administering the enema slowly and stopping the flow momentarily decreases the likelihood of intestinal spasm and premature ejection of the solution.*

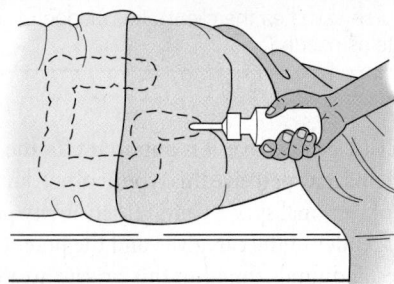

❶ Assuming a left lateral position for an enema. Note the commercially prepared enema.

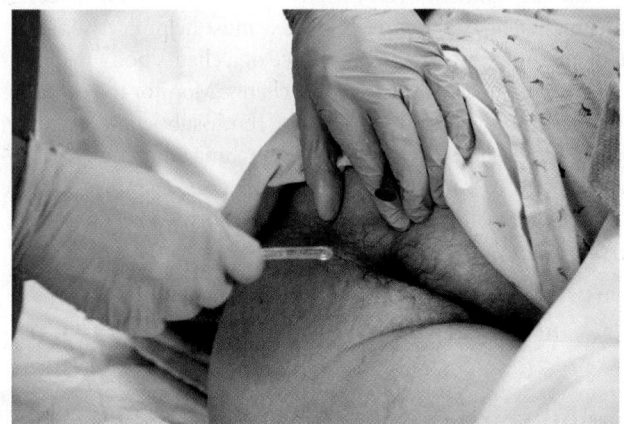

❷ Inserting the enema tube.

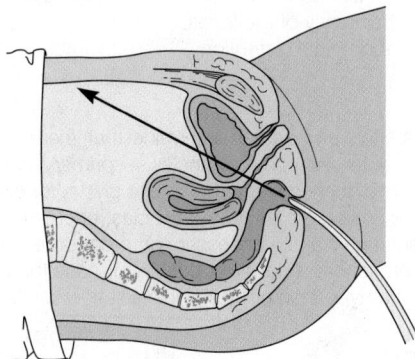

❸ Inserting the enema tube following the direction of the rectum.

   - If you are using a plastic commercial container, roll it up as the fluid is instilled. This prevents subsequent suctioning of the solution. ❹ After all the solution has been instilled or when the client cannot hold any more and feels the desire to defecate (the urge to defecate usually indicates that sufficient fluid has been administered), close the clamp and remove the enema tube from the anus.
   - Place the enema tube in a disposable towel as you withdraw it.

Administering an Enema—*continued*

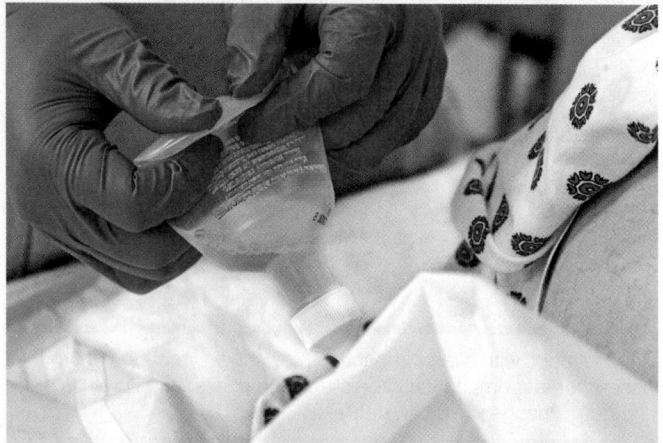

④ Rolling up a commercial enema container.

8. Encourage the client to retain the enema.
   - Ask the client to remain lying down. **Rationale:** *It is easier for the client to retain the enema when lying down than when sitting or standing, because gravity promotes drainage and peristalsis.*
   - Request that the client retain the solution for the appropriate amount of time, for example, 5 to 10 minutes for a cleansing enema or at least 30 minutes for a retention enema.
9. Assist the client to defecate.
   - Assist the client to a sitting position on the bedpan, commode, or toilet. A sitting position facilitates the act of defecation.
   - Ask the client who is using the toilet not to flush it. The nurse needs to observe the feces.
   - If a specimen of feces is required, ask the client to use a bedpan or commode.

- Remove and discard gloves.
- Perform hand hygiene.
10. Document the type and volume, if appropriate, of enema given. Describe the results.

SAMPLE DOCUMENTATION

8/2/2015 1000. States last BM five days ago. Abdomen distended and firm. Bowel sounds hypoactive. Fleet enema given per order resulting in large amount of firm brown stool. States he "feels better."
———— M. Lopez, RN

Variation: Administering an Enema to a Client Who Is Incontinent
Occasionally a nurse needs to administer an enema to a client who is unable to control the external sphincter muscle and thus cannot retain the enema solution for even a few minutes. In that case, after the rectal tube is inserted, the client assumes a supine position on a bedpan. The head of the bed can be elevated slightly, to 30° if necessary for easier breathing, and pillows support the client's head and back.

Variation: Administering a Return-Flow Enema
For a return-flow enema, the solution (100 to 200 mL for an adult) is instilled into the client's rectum and sigmoid colon. Then the solution container is lowered so that the fluid flows back out through the rectal tube into the container, pulling the flatus with it. The inflow–outflow process is repeated five or six times (to stimulate peristalsis and the expulsion of flatus), and the solution is replaced several times during the procedure if it becomes thick with feces.

Document type of solution; length of time solution was retained; the amount, color, and consistency of the returns; and the relief of flatus and abdominal distention in the client record using forms or checklists supplemented by narrative notes when appropriate.

EVALUATION
- Perform a detailed follow-up based on findings that deviated from expected or normal for the client. Relate findings to previous assessment data if available. Report significant deviations from expected to the primary care provider.

LIFESPAN CONSIDERATIONS | Administering an Enema

INFANTS/CHILDREN
- Provide a careful explanation to the parents and the child before the procedure. An enema is an intrusive procedure and therefore threatening.
- The enema solution should be isotonic (usually normal saline). Some hypertonic commercial solutions (e.g., Fleet phosphate enema) can lead to hypovolemia and electrolyte imbalances. In addition, the osmotic effect of the enema may produce diarrhea and subsequent metabolic acidosis.
- Infants and small children do not exhibit sphincter control and need to be assisted in retaining the enema. The nurse administers the enema while the infant or child is lying with the buttocks over the bedpan, and the nurse firmly presses the buttocks together to prevent the immediate expulsion of the solution. Older children can usually hold the solution if they understand what to do and are not required to hold it for too long a period. It may be necessary to ensure that the bathroom is available for an ambulatory child before starting the procedure or to have a bedpan ready.
- Enema temperature should be 37.7°C (100°F) unless otherwise ordered.
- Large-volume enemas consist of 50 to 200 mL in children less than 18 months old, 200 to 300 mL in children 18 months to 5 years, and 300 to 500 mL in children 5 to 12 years old.

- Careful explanation is especially important for the preschool child.
- For infants and small children, the dorsal recumbent position is frequently used. Position them on a small padded bedpan with support for the back and head. Secure the legs by placing a diaper under the bedpan and then over and around the thighs. Place the underpad under the client's buttocks to protect the bed linen, and drape the client with the bath blanket.
- Insert the tube 5 to 7.5 cm (2 to 3 in.) in the child and only 2.5 cm (1 in.) in the infant.
- For children, lower the height of the solution container appropriately for the age of the child. See agency protocol.
- To assist a small child in retaining the solution, apply firm pressure over the anus with tissue wipes, or firmly press the buttocks together.

OLDER ADULTS
- Older adults may fatigue easily.
- Older adults may be more susceptible to fluid and electrolyte imbalances. Use tap water enemas with great caution.
- Monitor the client's tolerance during the procedure, watching for vagal episodes (e.g., slow pulse) and dysrhythmias.
- Protect older adults' skin from prolonged exposure to moisture.
- Assist older clients with perineal care as indicated.

Teach the caregiver or client the following:
- To make an isotonic saline solution, mix 1 teaspoon of table salt with 500 mL of tap water.
- Use enemas only as directed. Do not rely on them for regular bowel evacuation.

- Prior to administration, make sure a bedpan, commode, or toilet is nearby.

FECAL IMPACTION

Fecal **impaction** is a mass or collection of hardened feces in the rectum. Impaction results from prolonged retention and accumulation of fecal material. A client who has a fecal impaction will experience the passage of liquid fecal seepage (diarrhea) and no normal stool. The liquid portion of the feces seeps out around the impacted mass (Figure 21–3 ■). Impaction can also be assessed by digital examination of the rectum, during which the hardened mass can often be palpated. Although fecal impaction can generally be prevented, digital removal of impacted feces is sometimes necessary. When fecal impaction is suspected, the client is often given an oil retention enema, a cleansing enema 2 to 4 hours later, and daily additional cleansing enemas (see Skill 21–2), suppositories, or stool softeners. If these measures fail, manual removal is often necessary.

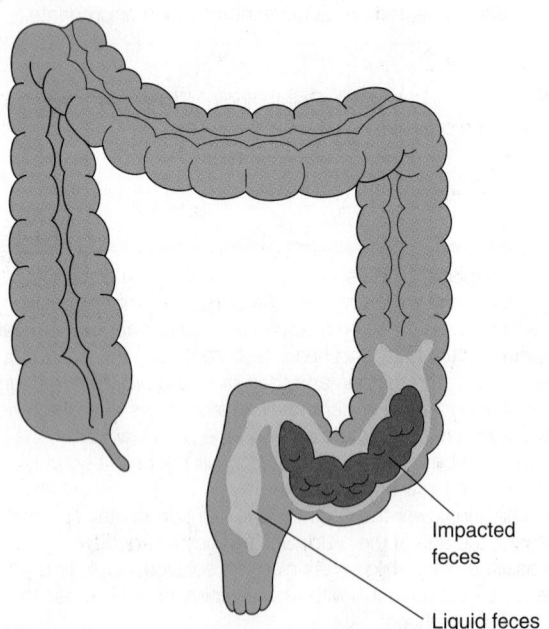

Figure 21–3 ■ Fecal impaction with liquid feces leaking around the impaction.

Impacted feces

Liquid feces

CLINICAL ALERT!

An older adult with a fecal impaction may show symptoms of delirium. Assess for fecal impaction if the client with constipation problems has a sudden change in mental status.

Removing a Fecal Impaction Digitally

Digital removal involves breaking up the fecal mass digitally and removing it in portions. Because the bowel mucosa can be injured during this procedure, some agencies restrict and specify the personnel permitted to conduct digital disimpactions. Rectal stimulation is also contraindicated for some people because it may cause an excessive vagal response, resulting in cardiac arrhythmia (e.g., slowing of the heart rate). Before disimpaction it is suggested an oil retention enema be given and held for 30 minutes. After a disimpaction, the nurse can use various interventions to remove remaining feces, such as a cleansing enema or the insertion of a suppository.

CLINICAL ALERT!

Clients with a history of cardiac disease and/or dysrhythmias may be at risk with digital stimulation to remove an impaction. If in doubt, the nurse should check with the primary care provider before performing the procedure.

Because manual removal of an impaction can be painful, the nurse may use, if the agency permits, 1 to 2 mL of lidocaine (Xylocaine) gel on a gloved finger inserted into the anal canal as far as the nurse can reach. The lidocaine will anesthetize the anal canal and rectum and should be inserted 5 minutes before the disimpaction procedure.

Disimpacting the client requires great sensitivity and a caring, yet matter-of-fact, approach. Be aware of personal facial expressions or anything that may convey distaste or disgust to the client. When dealing with fecal matter, many clients feel a sense of shame that relates to childhood experiences that may have been traumatic in some way. Control issues may also be triggered, and can manifest in many ways. Confusion and negative feelings are easily triggered in both client and nurse. Awareness and an ability to discuss these issues with a client, when appropriate, are important to providing sensitive care. Self-awareness will help the nurse be more therapeutically present to the client.

●○○● NURSING PROCESS: FECAL IMPACTION

Removing a Fecal Impaction

ASSESSMENT
Assess:
- Presence of an impaction by digital examination; presence of nausea, headache, abdominal pain, malaise, abdominal distention, or sudden change in mental status.
- Baseline pulse rate and rhythm.

PLANNING
DELEGATION

Due to the potential results of stimulation of the vagus nerve during the procedure, digital removal of an impaction is generally not delegated to UAP.

Equipment
- Bath blanket
- Disposable absorbent pad
- Bedpan and cover
- Toilet tissue
- Clean gloves
- Lubricant
- Soap, water, and towel
- Topical lidocaine (if agency permits)

IMPLEMENTATION
Preparation
- Check agency policy to determine if a primary care provider's order is required. **Rationale:** *Rectal manipulation can cause stimulation of the vagus nerve, resulting in a slowing of the heart rate.*
- If the agency permits the use of the topical anesthetic lidocaine, 1 to 2 mL should be inserted into the anal canal 5 minutes prior to the procedure. **Rationale:** *This will numb the anal and rectal areas, reducing the pain of the procedure.*

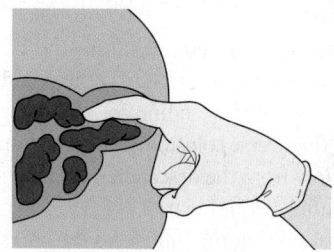

❶ Digital removal of fecal impaction.

Performance
1. Prior to performing the procedure, introduce self and verify the client's identity using agency protocol. Explain to the client what you are going to do, why it is necessary, and how he or she can participate. Discuss how the results will be used in planning further care or treatments. This procedure is distressing, tiring, and uncomfortable, so the person may desire the presence of another nurse or support person.
2. Perform hand hygiene and observe other appropriate infection prevention procedures.
3. Apply clean gloves.
4. Provide for client privacy.
5. Assist the client to a right or left lateral or Sims' position with the back toward you. **Rationale:** *When the person lies on the right side, the sigmoid colon is uppermost; thus, gravity can aid removal of the feces. Positioning on the left side allows easier access to the sigmoid colon.*
6. Place the disposable absorbent pad under the client's hips, and arrange the top bed linen to ensure that it falls obliquely over the hips, exposing only the buttocks.
7. Place the bedpan and toilet tissue nearby on the bed or a bedside chair.
8. Lubricate the gloved index finger. **Rationale:** *Lubricant reduces resistance by the anal sphincter as the finger is inserted.*
9. Remove the impaction. Have the client take slow, deep breaths during the procedure. Ensure the client does not hold their breath. **Rationale:** *Holding the breath can stimulate a vagal response.*
   - Gently insert the index finger into the rectum, moving the finger along the length of the rectum toward the umbilicus.

- Gently massage around the stool to loosen and dislodge the stool. **Rationale:** *Gentle action prevents damage to the rectal mucosa. A circular motion around the rectum dislodges the stool, stimulates peristalsis, and relaxes the anal sphincter.*
- Work the finger into the hardened mass of stool to break it up. ❶ If you cannot break up the impaction with one finger, insert two fingers and try to break up the impaction scissor style.
- Work the stool down to the anus, remove it in small pieces, and place them in the bedpan.
- Carefully continue to remove as much fecal material as possible; at the same time, assess for bleeding or signs of pallor, feelings of faintness, shortness of breath, perspiration, or changes in pulse rate. Terminate the procedure if these occur. Manual stimulation should be minimal. **Rationale:** *Manual stimulation could result in mucosal damage, excessive vagal nerve stimulation, and subsequent cardiac arrhythmia.*
- Assist the client to a position on a clean bedpan, commode, or toilet. **Rationale:** *Digital stimulation of the rectum may induce the urge to defecate.*
10. Assist the client with hygienic measures as needed.
    - Wash the rectal area with soap and water and dry gently.
    - Remove and discard gloves.
    - Perform hand hygiene.
11. Document the results of the procedure in the client record using forms or checklists supplemented by narrative notes when appropriate.

EVALUATION
- Perform a detailed follow-up based on findings that deviated from expected or normal for the client.
- Report significant deviations from normal (such as extensive bleeding) to the primary care provider.
- Perform client teaching to help prevent the formation of an impaction in the future.

BOWEL DIVERSION OSTOMIES

An **ostomy** is an opening on the abdominal wall for the elimination of feces or urine. A **colostomy** is an opening into the colon (large bowel). The purpose of bowel ostomies is to divert and drain fecal material. Bowel diversion ostomies are often classified according to (a) their status as permanent or temporary, (b) their anatomic location, and (c) the construction of the **stoma**, the opening created in the abdominal wall by an ostomy. A stoma is generally pink or red in color and moist. Initially, slight bleeding may occur when the stoma is touched and this is considered normal. A person does not feel the stoma because there are no nerve endings in the stoma.

Colostomies can be either temporary or permanent. Temporary colostomies are generally performed for traumatic injuries or inflammatory conditions of the bowel. They allow the distal diseased portion of the bowel to rest and heal. Permanent colostomies are performed to provide a means of elimination when the rectum or anus is nonfunctional as a result of a birth defect or removed for a disease such as cancer of the bowel.

An **ileostomy** generally empties from the distal end of the small intestine. A cecostomy empties from the cecum (the first part of the ascending colon). An ascending colostomy empties from the ascending colon, a transverse colostomy from the transverse colon, a descending colostomy from the descending colon, and a sigmoidostomy from the sigmoid colon (Figure 21–4 ■).

The location of the ostomy influences the character and management of the fecal drainage. The farther along the bowel, the more formed the stool (because the large bowel reabsorbs water from the fecal mass) and the more control over the frequency of stomal discharge can be established. For example:

- An ileostomy produces liquid fecal drainage. Drainage is constant and cannot be regulated. Ileostomy drainage contains some digestive enzymes, which are damaging to the skin. For this reason, a client with an ileostomy must wear an appliance continuously and take special precautions to prevent skin breakdown. Compared to colostomies, however, odor is minimal because fewer bacteria are present.

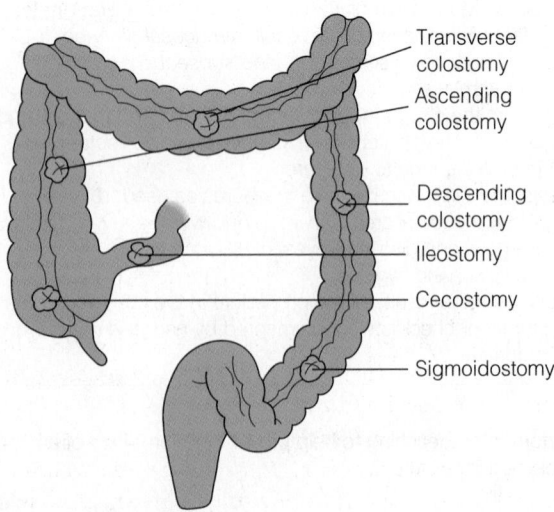

Figure 21–4 ■ The locations of bowel diversion ostomies.

Transverse colostomy
Ascending colostomy
Descending colostomy
Ileostomy
Cecostomy
Sigmoidostomy

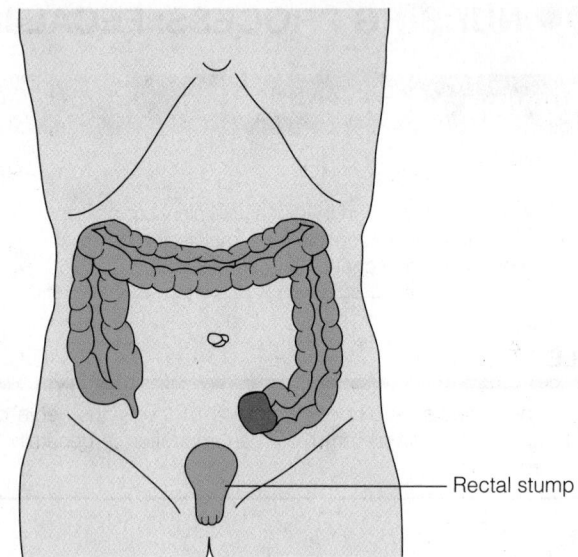

Rectal stump

Figure 21–5 ■ End colostomy: the diseased portion of bowel is removed and a rectal pouch remains.

- An ascending colostomy is similar to an ileostomy in that the drainage is liquid and cannot be regulated, and digestive enzymes are present. Odor, however, is a problem requiring control.
- A transverse colostomy produces a malodorous, mushy drainage because some of the liquid has been reabsorbed. There is usually no control.
- A descending colostomy produces increasingly solid fecal drainage. Stools from a sigmoidostomy are of normal or formed consistency, and the frequency of discharge can be regulated. People with a sigmoidostomy may not have to wear an appliance at all times, and odors can usually be controlled.

The length of time that an ostomy is in place also helps to determine the consistency of the stool, particularly with transverse and descending colostomies. Over time, the stool becomes more formed because the remaining functioning portions of the colon tend to compensate by increasing water reabsorption.

There are four major types of stoma constructions: the single, loop, divided, and double-barreled colostomies. A **single (end) colostomy** has only one stoma. The single stoma is created when one end of bowel is brought out through an opening onto the anterior abdominal wall. This is referred to as an end or terminal colostomy; the stoma is permanent (Figure 21–5 ■).

In the **loop colostomy**, a loop of bowel is brought out onto the abdominal wall and supported by a plastic bridge or a piece of rubber tubing (Figure 21–6 ■). A loop stoma has two openings: the proximal or afferent end, which is active, and the distal or efferent end, which is inactive. The loop colostomy is usually performed in an emergency procedure and is often situated on the right transverse colon. It is a bulky stoma that is more difficult to manage than a single stoma.

The **divided colostomy** consists of two edges of bowel brought out onto the abdomen but separated from each other (Figure 21–7 ■). The opening from the digestive or proximal end is the colostomy. The distal end in this situation is often referred to as a mucous fistula, since this section of bowel continues to secrete mucus. The divided colostomy is often used in situations

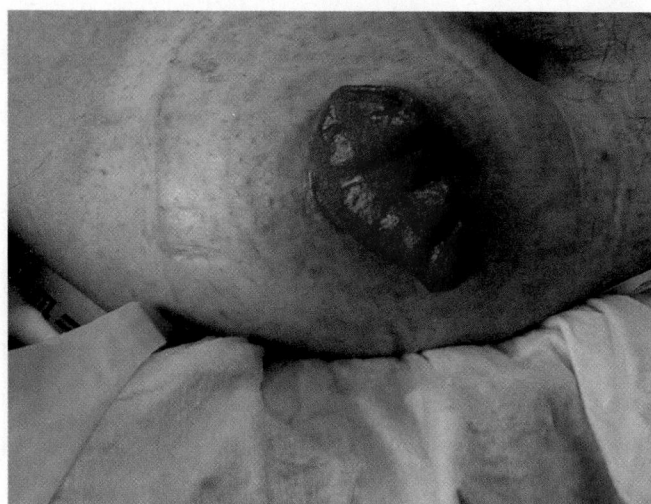

Figure 21–6 ■ Loop colostomy.
Courtesy of Cory Patrick Hartley, RN.

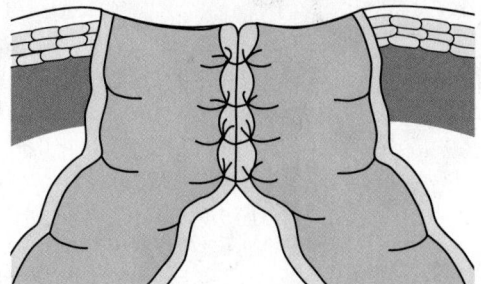

Figure 21–8 ■ Double-barreled colostomy.

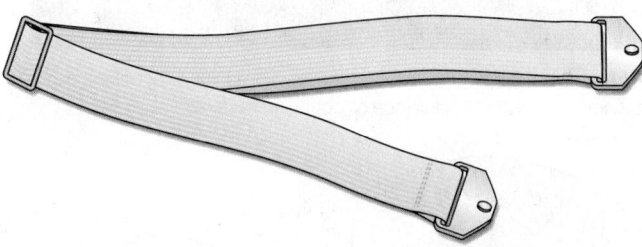

Figure 21–9 ■ Adjustable ostomy belt.

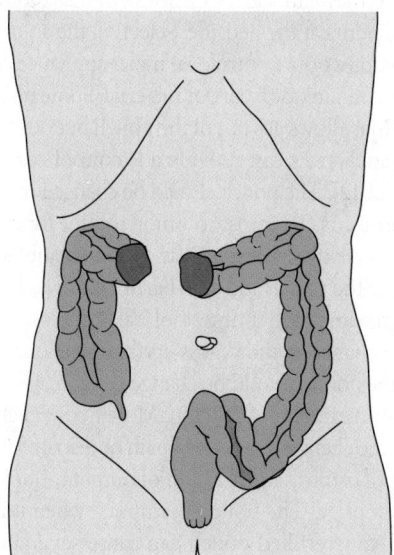

Figure 21–7 ■ Divided colostomy with two separated stomas.

Members of local chapters of such an organization have been known to meet and visit with a person who has a new ostomy. It is common for a client with a new ostomy to feel frightened and alone. Talking with another person who has experienced the surgery may help the client realize that he or she is not alone and others are willing to listen and help.

Stoma and Skin Care

Care of the stoma and skin is important for all clients who have ostomies. The fecal material from a colostomy or ileostomy is irritating to the peristomal skin. This is particularly true of stool from an ileostomy, which contains digestive enzymes. It is important to assess the peristomal skin for irritation each time the appliance is changed. Any irritation or skin breakdown needs to be treated immediately. The skin is kept clean by washing off any excretion and drying thoroughly.

An **ostomy appliance** consists of a skin barrier and a pouch and should protect the skin, collect stool, and control odor. Some clients may prefer to also wear an adjustable ostomy belt, which attaches to an ostomy pouch to hold the pouch firmly in place (Figure 21–9 ■). Appliances can be one piece with the skin barrier attached by the manufacturer to the pouch (Figure 21–10*A* ■), or an appliance can consist of two pieces: a separate pouch with a flange and a separate skin barrier with a flange where the pouch fastens to the barrier at the flange (Figure 21–10*B*). The pouch can be removed without removing the skin barrier when using a two-piece appliance. Pouches can be closed or drainable (Figure 21–11 ■). A drainable pouch usually has a clip where the end of the pouch is folded over the clamp and clipped (Figure 21–12 ■). Newer drainable pouches have an integrated closure system instead of a clamp. The client folds up the end of the pouch three times and presses firmly to seal the pouch.

where spillage of feces into the distal end of the bowel needs to be avoided.

The **double-barreled colostomy** (Figure 21–8 ■) resembles a double-barreled shotgun. In this type of colostomy, the proximal and distal loops of bowel are sutured together for about 10 cm (4 in.) and both ends are brought up onto the abdominal wall.

The stoma and the presence of a bag and fluid can trigger negative body image issues, feelings of loss, and shame. Clients with fecal diversions need considerable psychological support, instruction, and physical care. Many agencies have access to a wound ostomy continence nurse (WOCN) to assist these clients. If possible, clients should meet with the WOCN prior to the surgery to assist in the placement of the colostomy. National organizations (e.g., United Ostomy Associations of America) have support groups whose mission is to improve the quality of life of people who have, or will have, an ostomy.

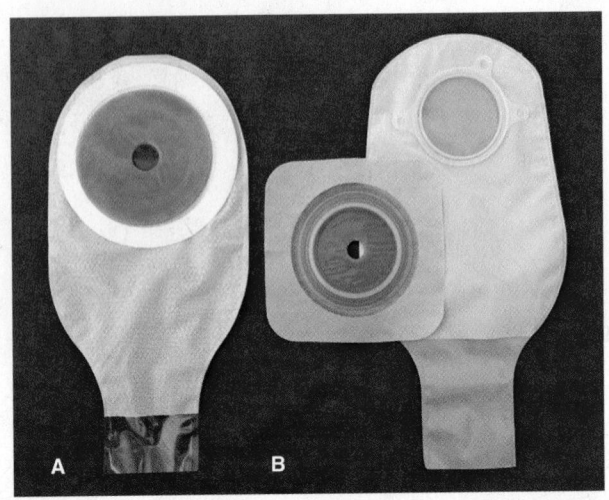

Figure 21–10 ■ *A,* One-piece ostomy appliance or pouching system; *B,* two-piece ostomy appliance or pouching system.

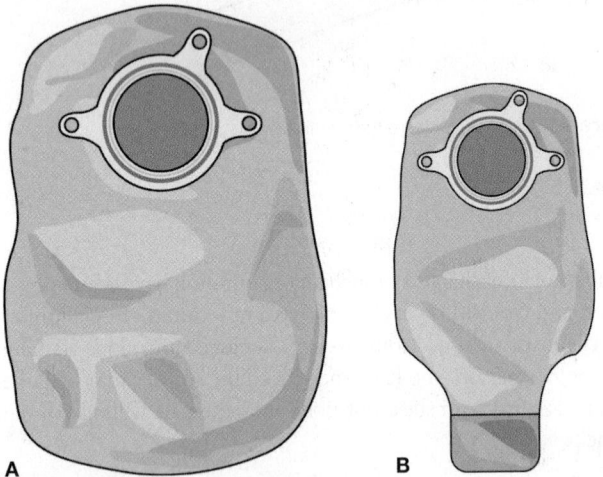

Figure 21–11 ■ *A,* Closed pouch; *B,* drainable pouch.

Drainable pouches are usually used by people who need to empty the pouch more than twice a day.

Closed pouches are often used by people who have a regular stoma discharge (e.g., sigmoid colostomy) and only have to empty the pouch one or two times a day. Some people find it easier to change a

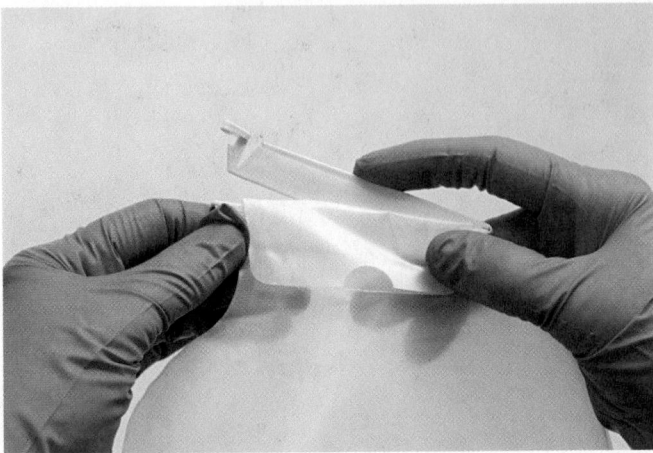

Figure 21–12 ■ Applying a pouch clamp.

closed pouch than to empty a drainable pouch, which requires some dexterity.

Odor control is essential to clients' self-esteem. As soon as clients are ambulatory, they can learn to work with the ostomy in the bathroom to avoid odors at the bedside. Selecting the appropriate kind of appliance promotes odor control. An intact appliance contains odors. Most pouches contain odor-barrier material. Some pouches also have a pouch filter that allows gas out of the pouch but not the odor.

Ostomy appliances can provide a leakproof seal for about 3 to 7 days (Avent, 2012). The pouch should be changed on a routine basis, before leakage occurs. The most common routine for changing the appliance is twice weekly (Hollister, 2011). Some manufacturers recommend removing the pouch and skin barrier twice a week to clean and inspect the peristomal skin unless stool leaks onto the peristomal skin, necessitating a change. If the skin is erythematous, eroded, denuded, or ulcerated, the pouch should be changed every 24 to 48 hours to allow appropriate treatment of the skin. More frequent changes are recommended if the client complains of pain or discomfort.

The type of ostomy and amount of output influences how often the pouch is emptied. The pouch is emptied when it is one-third to one-half full. An overfilled pouch can cause separation of the skin barrier from the skin, resulting in stool coming in contact with the skin. This results in the entire appliance needing to be removed and a new one applied.

●○○ NURSING PROCESS: BOWEL DIVERSION OSTOMIES

Changing a Bowel Diversion Ostomy Appliance

SKILL 21–4

ASSESSMENT
Determine:
- The type of ostomy and its placement on the abdomen. Surgeons often draw diagrams when there are two stomas. If there is more than one stoma, it is important to confirm which is the functioning stoma.
- The type and size of appliance currently used and the special barrier substance applied to the skin, according to the nursing care plan.

Assess:
- Stoma color: The stoma should appear pink or red, similar in color to the mucosal lining of the inner cheek and slightly moist.

Very pale or darker-colored stomas with a dusky bluish or purplish hue indicate impaired blood circulation to the area. Notify the surgeon immediately.
- Stoma size and shape: Most stomas protrude slightly from the abdomen. New stomas normally appear swollen, but swelling generally decreases over 2 or 3 weeks or for as long as 6 weeks. Failure of swelling to recede may indicate a complication (e.g., blockage) in need of follow-up by the surgeon.
- Stomal bleeding: Bleeding initially when the stoma is touched is normal, but other bleeding should be reported.

Changing a Bowel Diversion Ostomy Appliance—*continued*

- Status of peristomal skin: Any redness and irritation of the peristomal skin—the 5 to 13 cm (2 to 5 in.) of skin surrounding the stoma—should be noted. Transient redness after removal of adhesive is normal.
- Amount and type of feces: Assess the amount, color, odor, and consistency. Inspect for abnormalities, such as pus or blood.

- Complaints: Complaints of burning sensation under the skin barrier may indicate skin breakdown. The presence of abdominal discomfort and/or distention also needs to be determined.
- The client's and family members' learning needs regarding the ostomy and self-care.
- The client's emotional status, especially strategies used to cope with body image changes and the ostomy.

PLANNING
Review features of the appliance to ensure that all parts are present and functioning correctly.

DELEGATION

Care of a *new* ostomy is not delegated to UAP. However, aspects of ostomy function are observed during usual care and may be recorded by a WOCN in addition to the unit nurse. Abnormal findings must be validated and interpreted by the nurse. In some agencies, UAP may remove and replace well-established ostomy appliances.

Equipment
- Clean gloves
- Bedpan
- Moisture-proof bag (for disposable pouches)
- Cleaning materials, including warm water, mild soap (optional), washcloth, towel
- Tissue or gauze pad
- Skin barrier (optional)
- Stoma measuring guide
- Pen or pencil and scissors
- New ostomy pouch with optional belt
- Tail closure clamp
- Deodorant for pouch (optional)

IMPLEMENTATION
Preparation
- Determine the need for an appliance change.
  - Assess the used appliance for leakage of stool. **Rationale:** *Stool can irritate the peristomal skin.*
  - Ask the client about any discomfort at or around the stoma. **Rationale:** *A burning sensation may indicate breakdown beneath the faceplate of the pouch.*
  - Assess the fullness of the pouch. **Rationale:** *The weight of an overly full bag may loosen the skin barrier and separate it from the skin, causing the stool to leak and irritate the peristomal skin.*
- If there is pouch leakage or discomfort at or around the stoma, change the appliance.
- Select an appropriate time to change the appliance.
  - Avoid times close to meal or visiting hours. **Rationale:** *Ostomy odor and stool may reduce appetite or embarrass the client.*
  - Avoid times immediately after meals or the administration of any medications that may stimulate bowel evacuation. **Rationale:** *It is best to change the pouch when drainage is least likely to occur.*
  - The best time to change a pouching system is first thing in the morning or 2 to 4 hours after meals, when the bowel is least active (Scemons, 2013, p. 37).

Performance
1. Prior to performing the procedure, introduce self and verify the client's identity using agency protocol. Explain to the client what you are going to do, why it is necessary, and how he or she can participate. Discuss how the results will be used in planning further care or treatments. Changing an ostomy appliance should not cause discomfort, but it may be distasteful to the client. Communicate acceptance and support to the client. It is important to change the appliance competently and quickly. Include support people as appropriate.
2. Perform hand hygiene and observe other appropriate infection prevention procedures.
3. Apply clean gloves.
4. Provide for client privacy, preferably in the bathroom, where clients can learn to deal with the ostomy as they would at home.
5. Assist the client to a comfortable sitting or lying position in bed or preferably a sitting or standing position in the bathroom.

Rationale: *Lying or standing positions may facilitate smoother pouch application, that is, avoid wrinkles.*
6. Unfasten the belt if the client is wearing one.
7. Empty the pouch and remove the ostomy skin barrier.
   - Empty the contents of a drainable pouch through the bottom opening into a bedpan or toilet. **Rationale:** *Emptying before removing the pouch prevents spillage of stool onto the client's skin.*
   - If the pouch uses a clamp, do not throw it away because it can be reused.
   - Assess the consistency, color, and amount of stool.
   - Peel the skin barrier off slowly, beginning at the top and working downward, while holding the client's skin taut. **Rationale:** *Holding the skin taut minimizes client discomfort and prevents abrasion of the skin.*
   - Discard the disposable pouch in a moisture-proof bag.
8. Clean and dry the peristomal skin and stoma.
   - Use toilet tissue to remove excess stool.
   - Use warm water, mild soap (optional), and a washcloth to clean the skin and stoma. ❶ Check agency practice on the use of soap. **Rationale:** *Soap is sometimes not advised*

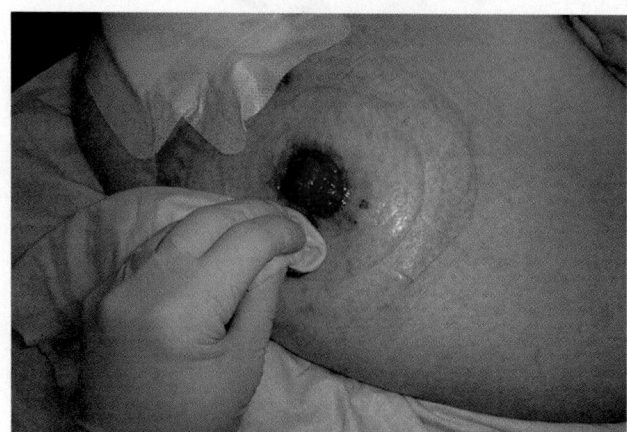

❶ Cleaning the skin.
Courtesy of Cory Patrick Hartley, RN.

Continued on page 552

Changing a Bowel Diversion Ostomy Appliance—*continued*

because it can be irritating to the skin. If soap is allowed, do not use deodorant or moisturizing soaps. **Rationale:** *They may interfere with the adhesives in the skin barrier.*

- Dry the area thoroughly by patting with a towel. **Rationale:** *Excess rubbing can abrade the skin.*

9. Assess the stoma and peristomal skin.
   - Inspect the stoma for color, size, shape, and bleeding.
   - Inspect the peristomal skin for any redness, ulceration, or irritation. Transient redness after the removal of adhesive is normal.

10. Place a piece of tissue or gauze over the stoma, and change it as needed. **Rationale:** *This absorbs any seepage from the stoma while the ostomy appliance is being changed.*

11. Prepare and apply the skin barrier (peristomal seal).
    - Use the guide to measure the size of the stoma. ❷
    - On the backing of the skin barrier, trace a circle the same size as the stomal opening.
    - Cut out the traced stoma pattern to make an opening in the skin barrier. ❸ Make the opening no more than 0.3 cm (1/8 in.) larger than the stoma (Piras & Hurley, 2011).

Rationale: *This allows space for the stoma to expand slightly when functioning and minimizes the risk of stool contacting peristomal skin.*

- Remove the backing to expose the sticky adhesive side. The backing can be saved and used as a pattern when making an opening for future skin barriers.

For a One-Piece Pouching System
- Center the one-piece skin barrier and pouch over the stoma and gently press it onto the client's skin for 30 seconds. ❹ and ❺
  Rationale: *The heat and pressure help activate the adhesives in the skin barrier.*

For a Two-Piece Pouching System
- Center the skin barrier over the stoma and gently press it onto the client's skin for 30 seconds.
- Remove the tissue over the stoma before applying the pouch.
- Snap the pouch onto the flange or skin barrier wafer.
- For drainable pouches, close the pouch according to the manufacturer's directions.
- Remove and discard gloves.
- Perform hand hygiene.

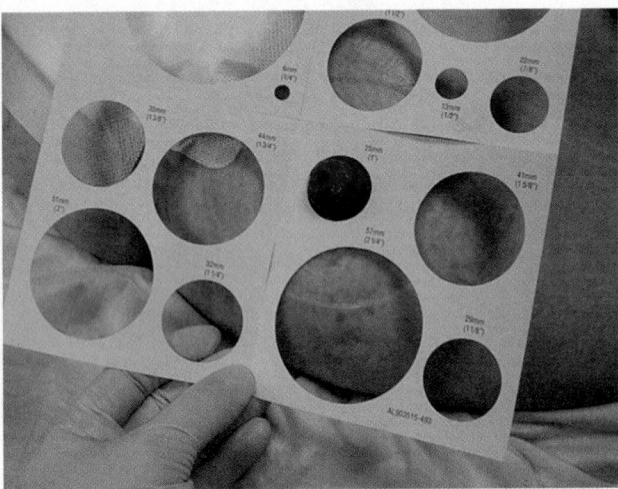

❷ A guide for measuring the stoma.
Courtesy of Cory Patrick Hartley, RN.

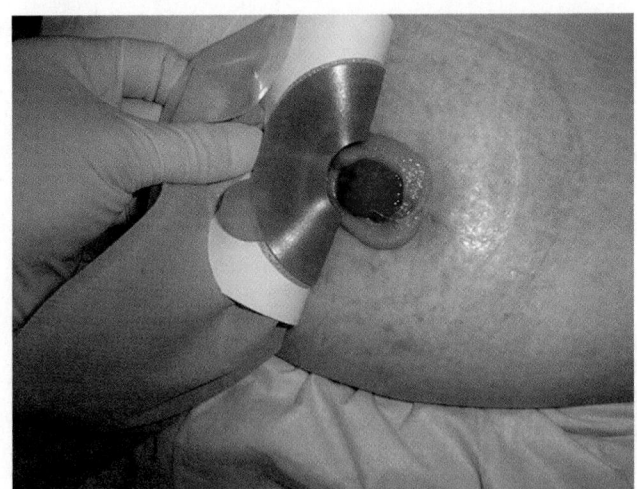

❹ Centering the skin barrier over the stoma.
Courtesy of Cory Patrick Hartley, RN.

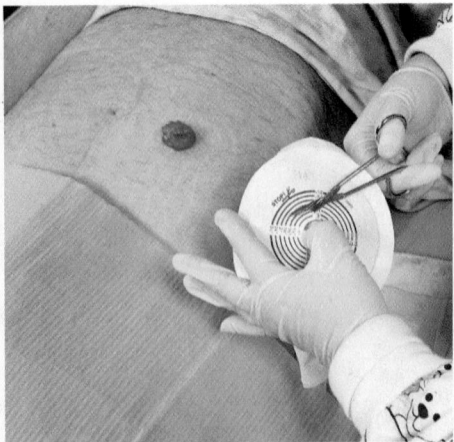

❸ The nurse is making a stoma opening on a disposable one-piece pouch.

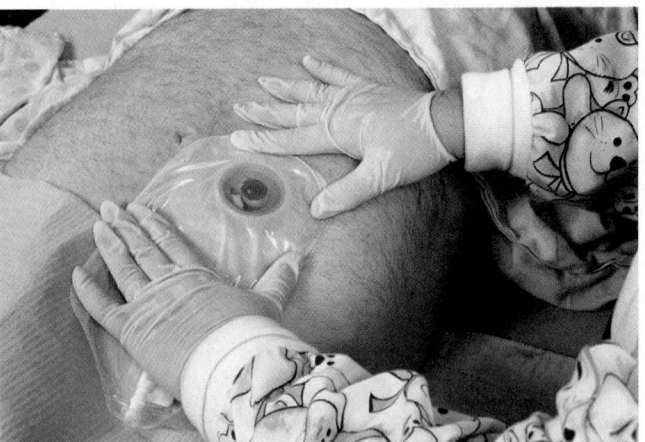

❺ Pressing the skin barrier of a disposable one-piece pouch for 30 seconds to activate the adhesives in the skin barrier.

Changing a Bowel Diversion Ostomy Appliance—*continued*

12. Document the procedure in the client record using forms or checklists supplemented by narrative notes when appropriate. Record pertinent assessments and interventions. Report any increase in stoma size, change in color indicative of circulatory impairment, and presence of skin irritation or erosion. Record on the client's chart discoloration of the stoma, the appearance of the peristomal skin, the amount and type of drainage, the client's reaction to the procedure, the client's experience with the ostomy, and skills learned by the client.

SAMPLE DOCUMENTATION

8/3/2015 0900 Colostomy bag changed. Moderate to large amount of semiformed brown stool. Stoma reddish color. No redness or irritation around stoma. Client looked at stoma today and started asking questions about how she will be able to change the pouch when she is home. Asked if she would like to do the next changing of the pouch. Stated "yes."——————————— G. Hsu, RN

EVALUATION

- Relate findings to previous data if available. Adjust the teaching plan and nursing care plan as needed. Reinforce the teaching each time the care is performed. Encourage and support self-care as soon as possible because clients should be able to perform self-care by discharge. **Rationale:** *Client learning is facilitated by consistent nursing interventions.*

Variation: Emptying a Drainable Pouch
- Empty the pouch when it is one-third to one-half full of stool or gas. **Rationale:** *Emptying before it is overfull helps avoid breaking the seal with the skin and stool then coming in contact with the skin.*
- While wearing gloves, hold the pouch outlet over a bedpan or toilet. Lift the lower edge up.
- Unclamp or unseal the pouch.
- Drain the pouch. Loosen feces from the sides by moving fingers down the pouch.
- Clean the inside of the tail of the pouch with a tissue or a premoistened towelette.
- Apply the clamp or seal the pouch.
- Dispose of used supplies.
- Remove and discard gloves.
- Perform hand hygiene.
- Document the amount, consistency, and color of stool.

- Perform detailed follow-up based on findings that deviated from expected or normal for the client. Report significant deviations from normal to the primary care provider.

Ambulatory and Community Settings   **Changing an Ostomy Appliance** | PATIENT-CENTERED CARE |

- Provide the client with the names and phone numbers of a WOCN, supply vendor, and other resource people to contact when needed. Provide pertinent Internet resources for information and support.
- Inform the client of signs to report to a health care provider (e.g., peristomal redness, skin breakdown, and changes in stomal color).
- Provide client and family education regarding care of the ostomy and appliance when traveling.

- Educate the client and family regarding infection control precautions, including proper disposal of used pouches since these cannot be flushed down a toilet.
- Younger clients may have special concerns about odor and appearance. Provide information about ostomy care and community support groups. A visit from someone who has had an ostomy under similar circumstances may be helpful.

Colostomy Irrigation

A colostomy irrigation, similar to an enema, is a form of stoma management used only for clients who have a sigmoid or descending colostomy. The purpose of irrigation is to distend the bowel sufficiently to stimulate peristalsis, which stimulates evacuation. When a regular evacuation pattern is achieved, the wearing of a colostomy pouch is unnecessary. Currently, colostomy irrigations are not routinely taught to clients. Routine daily irrigations for control of the time of elimination ultimately become the client's decision. Some clients prefer to control the time of elimination through rigid dietary regulation and not be bothered with irrigations, which can take up to an hour to complete. When regulation by irrigation is chosen, it should be done at the same time each day. Control by irrigations also necessitates

some control of the diet. For example, laxative foods that might cause an unexpected evacuation need to be avoided.

For some clients, a relatively small amount of fluid (300 to 500 mL) stimulates evacuation. For others, up to 1,000 mL may be needed because a colostomy has no sphincter and the fluid tends to return as it is instilled. This problem is reduced by the use of a cone on the irrigating catheter. The cone helps to hold the fluid within the bowel during the irrigation. Clients who choose to practice colostomy irrigation need to be motivated to master the procedure. In addition, good manual dexterity and eyesight, along with uninterrupted time (approximately 60 minutes), is needed (Williams, 2011). These requirements may deter clients from using this alternative method of regaining bowel control. See Practice Guidelines for the technique of irrigating a colostomy.

PRACTICE GUIDELINES

Irrigating a Colostomy

- Fill the solution bag with 500 mL of warm (body temperature) tap water or other solution as ordered.
- Hang the solution bag on an IV pole so that the bottom of the container is at the level of the client's shoulder or 30 to 45 cm (12 to 18 in.) above the stoma.
- Attach the colon catheter securely to the tubing.
- Open the regulator clamp, and run fluid through the tubing to expel air from it. Close the clamp until ready for the irrigation.
- Provide privacy.
- Perform hand hygiene.
- Apply clean gloves.
- Assist the client who must remain in bed to a side-lying position. Place a disposable pad on the bed in front of the client, and place the bedpan on top of the disposable pad, beneath the stoma. Assist an ambulatory client to sit on the toilet or on a commode in the bathroom.
- Remove the colostomy bag and dispose of the used pouch in a plastic bag.
- Center the irrigation drainage sleeve over the stoma and attach it snugly. Direct the lower, open end of the drainage sleeve into the bedpan or between the client's legs into the toilet.

- Lubricate the tip of the stoma cone or colon catheter with a water-soluble lubricant.
- Using a rotating motion, insert the catheter or stoma cone through the opening in the top of the irrigation drainage sleeve and gently through the stoma. Insert a catheter only 7 cm (3 in.); insert a stoma cone just until it fits snugly. Use of a stoma cone avoids the risk of perforating the bowel.
- Open the tubing clamp, and allow the fluid to flow into the bowel. If cramping occurs, stop the flow until the cramps subside and then resume the flow.
- After all the fluid is instilled, remove the catheter or cone and allow the colon to empty, usually 10 to 15 minutes.
- Cleanse the base of the irrigation drainage sleeve, and seal the bottom with a drainage clamp, following the manufacturer's instructions.
- Encourage an ambulatory client to move around for about 30 minutes to completely empty the colon.
- Empty and remove the irrigation sleeve.
- Clean the area around the stoma, and dry it thoroughly.
- Apply a skin barrier and colostomy appliance as needed.

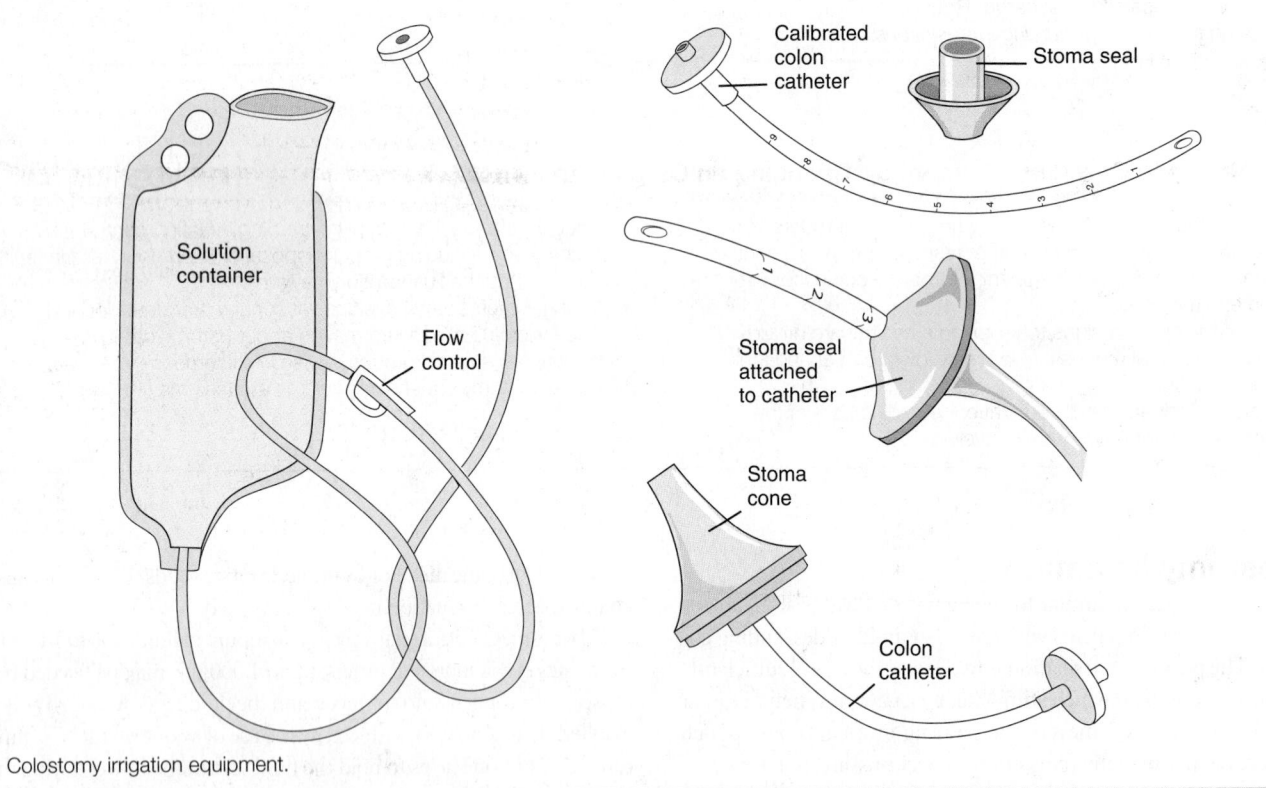

Colostomy irrigation equipment.

FOCUSING ON CLINICAL THINKING

Consider This

1. An extremely heavy male client has requested the bedpan for a bowel movement. How would you assist him in getting onto the bedpan?

2. After you have administered about 150 mL of a soapsuds enema to the client, fluid begins to leak back out of the anus and the client complains of rectal discomfort. What would you do?

3. During a home visit, a young client shares that her grandmother taught her to use digital stimulation to remove hard stool every week or so. What advice would you provide to this client?

4. When beginning to assist a client in changing a colostomy bag, you notice that the client is not using a skin barrier. When you ask about this, the client states that the barriers are too expensive since the bag is changed every day. The client's skin around the stoma appears in good condition. How would you respond?

See Focusing on Clinical Thinking answers on student resource website.

TEST YOUR KNOWLEDGE

1. While obtaining an admission history, the client tells the nurse that she occasionally suffers from mild constipation and asks how she can change her diet to reduce this problem. The nurse teaches the client to increase which of the following to help reduce constipation? Select all that apply.
   1. Fiber intake
   2. Fat- and carbohydrate-containing foods
   3. Iron-rich foods
   4. Fluid intake
   5. Caffeine intake

2. When questioned about his bowel elimination habits, the client tells the nurse, "My work has kept me so busy that I often ignore the need to have a bowel movement and then I end up constipated." The nurse explains to the client that repeatedly ignoring the need to defecate can result in:
   1. Bowel obstruction.
   2. Rupture of the rectum.
   3. Constipation.
   4. Fecal incontinence.

3. The client has just defecated and called the nurse into the room to remove the bedpan. What is the nurse's first action upon entering the room?
   1. Remove the bedpan.
   2. Apply clean gloves.
   3. Change the linen as necessary.
   4. Clean the client's anal area using toilet paper.

4. The nurse is performing discharge teaching for a client with a newly created ostomy and informs the client that one disadvantage of a one-piece ostomy appliance is that:
   1. It is harder to apply.
   2. The pouch has to be removed in order to empty it.
   3. When the bag needs to be changed, the skin barrier must be replaced as well.
   4. It is more likely to leak.

5. The nurse is ordering supplies for a client with a newly created sigmoidostomy. What are essential supplies? Select all that apply.
   1. A skin barrier
   2. An ostomy pouch
   3. A deodorant
   4. An adjustable ostomy belt
   5. A stoma measuring guide

6. After the client has defecated, the nurse removes the regular bedpan and carries it to be emptied by holding it:
   1. With one hand held flat under the bottom of the bedpan.
   2. Firmly, with fingers of one hand wrapped inside the back edge of the bedpan.
   3. At a 30° angle, using two hands to help to reduce the odor for the nurse.
   4. Flat in two hands away from the body, without touching the inside of the bedpan, to avoid spilling or contaminating the uniform.

7. The nurse is preparing to administer a cleansing enema to a client who is continent and able to participate. The enema will be most effective if the client is placed in which position?
   1. A left lateral position with the right leg flexed
   2. A right lateral position with the left leg flexed
   3. A semi-Fowler's position while sitting on the bedpan
   4. A prone position

8. The nurse has received an order to digitally disimpact a client's fecal mass. Before performing the disimpaction, what should the nurse do to make the procedure more effective *and* less traumatic for the client?
   1. Explain the procedure to the client.
   2. Administer an oil retention enema.
   3. Lubricate the gloved finger.
   4. Administer a cathartic suppository.

9. The nurse is assessing the client's ostomy appliance to determine if it needs to be changed. Which would indicate that the appliance needs to be changed?
   1. The appliance is snugly in place without leakage.
   2. The client denies any discomfort at or around the stoma.
   3. The skin around the stoma was intact and healthy when the appliance was last changed 5 days ago.
   4. The skin around the stoma was erythematous when the appliance was last changed 48 hours ago.

10. The nurse, working on a pediatric unit, is caring for an 18-month-old toddler. The child's mother says, "I have been working so hard to toilet train her but she keeps having accidents. When will she learn to control her bowels?" What is the nurse's best response?
    1. "Have you spoken with her pediatrician about this? She may need to be tested to make sure there are no physical problems contributing to her inability to become toilet trained."
    2. "Children normally attain control of their bowel movements by the age of 2½ so it is normal for a child at 18 months to have accidents."
    3. "There are some wonderful books you can buy that will help you to toilet train your child. You may not be approaching it correctly."
    4. "What are you feeding her? Perhaps it is related to her diet."

See Answers to Test Your Knowledge in Appendix A.

READINGS AND REFERENCES

References

Avent, Y. (2012). Understanding fecal diversions. *Nursing made Incredibly Easy!, 10*(5), 11–16. doi:10.1097/01.NME.0000418044.19439.98

Cohen, M. R. (2012). Fleet enemas: Don't underestimate the risk. *Nursing, 42*(12), 12. doi:10.1097/01.NURSE.0000422652.36748.22

Hollister, Inc. (2011). *Understanding your colostomy.* Retrieved from http://www.hollister.com/us/ostomy/learning/booklets.asp

National Digestive Diseases Information Clearinghouse. (2013). *Gas in the digestive tract.* Retrieved from http://digestive.niddk.nih.gov/ddiseases/pubs/gas

Piras, S. E., & Hurley, S. (2011). Ostomy care: Are you prepared? *Nursing made Incredibly Easy!, 9*(5), 46-48. doi:10.1097/01.NME.0000403198.60545.dd

Scemons, D. (2013). The ins and outs of ostomy management. *Nursing Made Incredibly Easy!, 11*(5), 32–42. doi:10.1097/01.NME.0000432867.93012.55

Tabloski, P. A., & Connell, W. F. (2014). *Gerontological nursing* (3rd ed.). Upper Saddle River, NJ: Pearson.

Toner, F., & Claros, E. (2012). Preventing, assessing, and managing constipation in older adults. *Nursing, 42*(12), 32–39. doi:10.1097/01.NURSE.0000422642.83383.17

Williams, J. (2011). Principles and practices of colostomy irrigation. *Gastrointestinal Nursing, 9*(9), 15–16.

Selected Bibliography

Berman, A., Snyder, S., & Frandsen, G. (2016). *Kozier & Erb's fundamentals of nursing: Concepts, process, and practice* (10th ed.). Upper Saddle River, NJ: Pearson.

Black, P. (2011). Choosing the correct stoma appliance. *Journal of Community Nursing, 25*(6), 44.

Burch, J. (2012). Stoma care and enhanced recovery. *Gastrointestinal Nursing, 10*(7), 26–32. doi:10.12968/gasn.2012.10.7.26

Burch, J. (2013). Choosing the correct accessory for each stoma type: An update. *British Journal of Nursing, 22*(Suppl. 16), S10–S13.

Burch, J. (2013). Stoma complications: An overview. *British Journal of Community Nursing, 18*(8), 375–378.

Chandler, P., & Lowther, C. (2013). Stoma care: Use of the colostomy Conseal plug. *Gastrointestinal Nursing, 11*(2), 15–16. doi:10.12968/gasn.2013.11.2.15

Daniels, G., & Schmelzer, M. (2013). Giving laxatives safely and effectively. *MEDSURG Nursing, 22*(5), 290–302

Gallagher, D. L., & Thompson, D. L. (2012). Identifying and managing fecal incontinence. *Journal of Wound, Ostomy and Continence Nursing, 39*(1), 95–97. doi:10.1097/WON.0b013e31823fe683

Gardiner, A. (2013). Constipation: Causes, assessment and management. *Nursing and Residential Care, 15*(6), 410–415.

Gardiner, A. (2013). Understanding the functions required to maintain continence. *Nursing and Residential Care, 15*(5), 250–257.

Mayo Clinic. (2012). *Dietary fiber: Essential for a healthy diet.* Retrieved from http://www.mayoclinic.com/health/fiber/NU00033

Palmer, S. (2013). Focus on healthy carbs. *Environmental Nutrition, 36*(10), 1–4.

Peate, I., & Gault, C. (2013). Clinical skills series/2: Enemas and suppositories. *British Journal of Healthcare Assistants, 7*(2), 76–81.

Slater, R. (2012). Choosing one- and two-piece appliances. *Nursing and Residential Care, 14*(8), 410–413.

Williams, J. (2012). Inserting suppositories and enemas into a colostomy. *Gastrointestinal Nursing, 10*(1), 13–14.

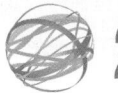

22 Caring for the Client with Peritoneal Dialysis

LEARNING OUTCOMES

At the completion of this chapter, the student will be able to:

1. Define the key terms used in the skills of peritoneal dialysis.
2. Recognize when it is appropriate to delegate aspects of peritoneal dialysis to unlicensed assistive personnel.
3. Identify key elements of assisting the primary care provider with insertion of a peritoneal dialysis catheter.
4. Verbalize the steps used in:
   a. Assisting with peritoneal dialysis catheter insertion.
   b. Conducting peritoneal dialysis procedures.
5. Demonstrate appropriate documentation and reporting of skills related to peritoneal dialysis.

SKILLS

Skill 22–1 Assisting with Peritoneal Dialysis Catheter Insertion

Skill 22–2 Conducting Peritoneal Dialysis Procedures

KEY TERMS

continuous ambulatory peritoneal dialysis (CAPD), *560*

continuous cycling (or cycler-assisted) peritoneal dialysis (CCPD), *560*

dialysate, *557*
dialysis, *557*
dwell, *560*

end-stage renal disease (ESRD), *557*
peritoneal dialysis (PD), *557*

Anuria (lack of urine production), oliguria (inadequate urine production), and both acute and chronic renal failure can occur as a result of kidney disease, severe heart failure, burns, and shock. These conditions can be fatal if some other means is not used to remove the body wastes. **Dialysis** is the technique by which blood is filtered for the removal of these wastes and of excess fluid. When *hemodialysis* is used, intravascular needles or catheters are inserted directly into blood vessels so that the blood can be removed from the body, cycled through machines that filter the blood, and then returned to the body. This chapter describes another type of dialysis: *peritoneal dialysis*.

If the kidneys have permanently failed, clients are diagnosed with **end-stage renal disease (ESRD)**, which, by definition, requires dialysis to provide the functions that the kidneys are no longer able to provide. The impact of the diagnosis is compounded by the significant lifestyle changes required by the ongoing need for dialysis. Some clients use denial as a coping mechanism. Anger, loss, and depression are common reactions in these individuals. Assessing the client's emotional experience and support system is essential to providing holistic care. Research shows that peritoneal dialysis offers clients a sense of control, independence, self-efficacy, and freedom. However, clients also face risks for impaired self-esteem, physical incapacitation, reduced social functioning, and poor sense of self-worth. Strategies that strengthen social support and promote resilience and confidence in clients are integral to achieving positive adjustment, improved psychosocial outcomes, and treatment satisfaction (Tong et al., 2013). Referral to support groups can provide necessary resources for clients with chronic renal disease and their caregivers. Organizations such as the American Association of Kidney Patients (AAKP), the National Kidney Foundation, and the Renal Support Network provide support groups.

PERITONEAL DIALYSIS

Peritoneal dialysis (PD) is the technique of instillation and drainage of a solution (a **dialysate**) into the peritoneal cavity to filter impurities, excess fluid, and electrolytes from the blood that would normally be excreted through the kidneys. In this procedure, the peritoneum is used as the dialyzing surface rather than an artificial membrane such as that used in hemodialysis machines.

PD has some significant advantages over hemodialysis. Peritoneal dialysis is generally cheaper, clients have lower rates of acquiring hepatitis B and hepatitis C, and no anticoagulation is needed. Research comparing the two types of dialysis is complex and often flawed but most research confirms that survival outcomes are similar when the comparisons are scientifically sound (Davies, 2013). Probably the most important advantage of PD is the client's ability to undergo treatment at home and independently. If PD is a medical option, the client need not go to a treatment facility several times each week and can take more responsibility for their own health management.

The dialysate solution commonly contains water, glucose, sodium, calcium, chloride, and magnesium. Lactate and potassium may also be included. When the solution is instilled into the peritoneal cavity, the body's waste products, excess electrolytes, and excess fluids pass by diffusion and osmosis across the semipermeable peritoneal membrane into the dialysate. The dialysate containing these waste products is then drained from the peritoneal cavity, and the cycle is repeated as needed. This process replaces kidney function.

For peritoneal dialysis, the primary care provider inserts a catheter into the peritoneal cavity. Some variations in the catheter include bent (swan neck) or straight (Tenckhoff) subcutaneous portions and coiled or straight intra-abdominal portions. Dacron cuffs along

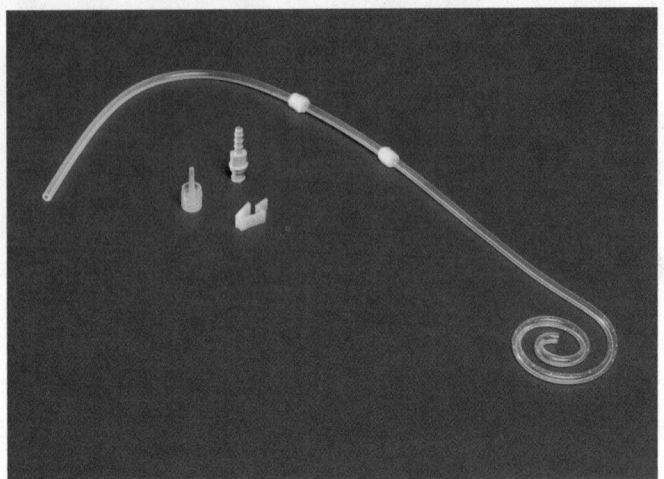

Figure 22–1 ■ An Argyle double-cuff curl catheter. This multiple side-hole catheter has two or three cuffs, a removable hub, and a screw cap. The two cuffs closest to the tip are Dacron and are designed to hold the catheter in place. When present, the third cuff, nearest the hub, is impregnated with an antibacterial agent and intended to reduce tunnel infection and peritonitis.
Courtesy Covidien.

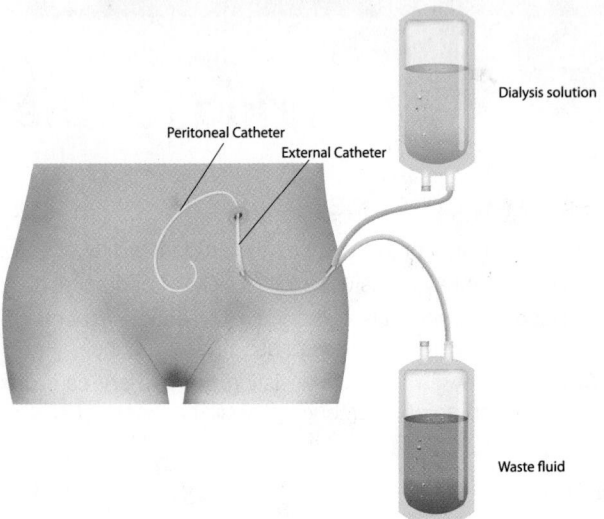

Figure 22–2 ■ Peritoneal dialysis system.
GRei, Shutterstock.

the catheter length promote tissue adhesions that serve as mechanical barriers to catheter movement and to infection (Figure 22–1 ■). Catheters are usually made of silicone elastomer and come in a variety of diameters and lengths. If the abdomen cannot be used for the exit site, the client wants to be able to swim or soak, the client is obese and has difficulty manipulating a catheter at the belt line, or or the client is incontinent, a presternal catheter which has the exit site located on the upper chest wall instead of the abdomen, can be used.

Catheter insertion may be done at the bedside, in the radiology department, or in the operating room using either open or laparoscopic technique. Nurses assist with the insertion of the catheter, change the dressing at the catheter site, perform fluid exchanges, and assist with removal of the catheter. The basic peritoneal dialysis system and its components are shown in Figure 22–2 ■.

Many nurses may not have an active role in assisting with PD procedures, but they should be familiar with the principles. Assisting with PD catheter insertion and performing dialysis procedures should be done only after sufficient training and supervision.

●○● NURSING PROCESS: BEGINNING PERITONEAL DIALYSIS

SKILL 22–1

Assisting with Peritoneal Dialysis Catheter Insertion

ASSESSMENT
Assess:
- Vital signs and weight for baseline data and subsequent comparisons.
- Abdominal girth, respiratory status (rate, character, and breath sounds), and presence of edema. These are indicators of fluid retention.

- Results of blood analyses. Commonly, these include electrolytes, glucose, blood urea nitrogen (BUN), creatinine, albumin, hemoglobin, hematocrit, iron, bicarbonate, and parathyroid hormone.
- Allergies to any products used (e.g., lidocaine, shellfish, latex).

PLANNING
- Confirm the order for PD and determine the type of catheter and insertion equipment preferred by this primary care provider for the client.
- Confirm that the primary care provider has determined the insertion and exit sites. Catheter exit site should avoid the client's usual waistband or belt line and be on the side opposite the client's dominant hand (Frost & Bagul, 2012). The selected position is marked with a surgical skin marker while the client is standing or seated because the site shifts when the client is in a supine position during placement.
- Ensure that consent for this invasive procedure has been obtained.

DELEGATION

Assisting with peritoneal catheter insertion is a sterile procedure and not delegated to unlicensed assistive personnel (UAP).

INTERPROFESSIONAL PRACTICE

Any health care provider for whom sterile technique is within their scope of practice may assist in PD catheter insertion.

Assisting with Peritoneal Dialysis Catheter Insertion—*continued*

Equipment

- Sterile gloves, masks, caps, goggles, and gowns for the primary care provider, nurse, and anyone assisting; mask for the client
- Sterile peritoneal dialysis set containing:
  - Peritoneal catheter
  - Local anesthetic (e.g., lidocaine), #25-gauge 5/8-inch needle, and 3-mL syringe
  - Alcohol sponges
  - Scalpel with a blade
  - Precut gauze to place around the catheter
  - Drape
  - Transfer set
  - Protective transfer set cap
  - Sutures, needles, and needle driver
  - Trocar (the sharp, needle-like instrument used to make a hole in body tissues)
- Connector
- 4×4 gauze square
- Specimen container
- Antiseptic ointment (e.g., mupirocin). Do not use mupirocin with polyurethane catheters because it can damage the catheter (Crabtree, Piraino, Firanek, Abu-Alfa, & Guest, 2012).
- 10-mL syringe and 1.5-inch needle
- Scissors
- Skin preparation/dressing set containing:
  - Chlorhexidine gluconate 2%, povidone-iodine, or other disinfecting solution
  - Razor and blade or scissors
  - Gauze sponges
  - Nonallergenic tape

IMPLEMENTATION

Preparation

Although the primary care provider will have already done initial client and family teaching, the nurse reinforces key elements. Review the technique of peritoneal dialysis and its purpose with the client and family.

- Explain that since the kidneys are not functioning properly, this procedure will rid the blood and body of excess waste and fluid that are normally excreted by the kidneys.
- Explain that inserting the trocar (which is the primary care provider's responsibility) may be uncomfortable. The discomfort can be reduced by the client tensing the abdominal muscles as if for a bowel movement.
- Explain that the purpose of the masks, gowns, gloves, and caps is to reduce the possibility of contaminating the site during insertion. Then explain that the client will also need to wear a mask for the same reason.
- If ordered, administer analgesics.
- Administer prophylactic antibiotic medication as ordered. The medication should be administered 30 to 60 minutes prior to catheter insertion (Frost & Bagul, 2012).

Performance

1. Prior to performing the procedure, introduce self and verify the client's identity using agency protocol. Explain to the client what your role will be, why it is necessary, and how he or she can participate. Remind the client that additional teaching will be done at the time of the actual peritoneal dialysis treatment.
2. Perform hand hygiene and observe other appropriate infection prevention procedures throughout the various phases of the procedure. Assist the client with use of the mask.
3. Provide for client privacy.
4. Prepare the client.
   - Ask the client to urinate before the procedure. In some cases, bowel cleansing is also done prior to catheter insertion. **Rationale:** *Emptying the bladder and bowels moves them away from the peritoneal wall and lessens the danger that they will be punctured by the trocar.*
   - Assist the client to a supine position, and arrange the bedding to expose the area around the umbilicus.

   Rationale: *The insertion site is usually in the midline just below the umbilicus. Note:* The insertion site is not the same as the exit site since the catheter is tunneled from the peritoneal cavity to the skin exit site.
5. Prepare the solution and the tubing (see Skill 22–2).
6. Implement surgical aseptic practices and body fluid precautions according to agency protocol.
   - Apply masks. **Rationale:** *Applying masks prior to breaking the seals on the packages reduces the chance of contamination.*
   - Apply cap, gown, and goggles.
   - Open the dialysis set and any sterile supplies not part of the set (see the skills in Chapter 7 ∞).
   - Apply sterile gloves.
7. Assist the primary care provider as needed during and after the catheter insertion.
   - Ensure that the transfer set that has been connected to the catheter is securely capped.
   - Cover the catheter site with the antiseptic ointment and precut sterile gauze, and tape the occlusive dressing in place.
8. Remove and discard gloves.
   - Perform hand hygiene.
9. Recheck vital signs. Report to the primary care provider if significantly different from baseline.
10. Document findings in the client record using forms or checklists supplemented by narrative notes when appropriate. Record the date and time of the procedure, the client's response, and the appearance of the exit site and dressing.

SAMPLE DOCUMENTATION

5/19/2015 1430 Double-cuff coiled Tenckhoff peritoneal catheter inserted in right lower quadrant by Dr. Novar under local anesthesia using sterile technique throughout. Post-insertion VS consistent with baseline. Catheter taped to abdominal skin. Dry, sterile, occlusive dressing applied to exit site. ———————— U. Schmidt, RN

EVALUATION

Perform detailed follow-up based on any findings that deviated from expected for the client.

PERFORMING PERITONEAL DIALYSIS

Three major types of peritoneal dialysis are currently used: intermittent peritoneal dialysis (IPD), **continuous ambulatory peritoneal dialysis (CAPD)**, and **continuous cycling (or cycler-assisted) peritoneal dialysis (CCPD)**. IPD is performed within the acute care setting and involves the infusion and drainage of one bag of dialysate solution at a time with periods of no dialysis between infusions.

The CAPD technique allows the clients to go home with a peritoneal catheter in place and perform the exchange on themselves. The dialysate is allowed to remain in the abdomen (**dwell**) for 4 to 6 hours, three to four times each day and overnight. The client is ambulatory and free to resume normal activities between exchanges. No machine is needed, although a clean environment and space to store supplies are required. With CAPD, the focus of nursing care is on teaching the client and family to perform the dialysis treatments at home.

CCPD is performed both in the acute care setting and at home by some clients who are capable of maintaining and operating the cyclers.

CCPD (also called automated peritoneal dialysis, or APD) involves the cycling of dialysate infused through a mechanical cycler and warmer. Large bags of dialysate are used so that three to five exchanges can be done over 8 to 10 hours in one night. The cycler has a timer, which controls the clamp that opens to allow dwelled fluid to drain, and a meter that records the amounts of fluid instilled and drained. Sensors trigger alarms and turn the cycler off if there is blockage of either the drainage or instillation tubing. Some clients using CCPD also perform a manual change during the day.

The majority of complications experienced by clients undergoing peritoneal dialysis are catheter related such as occlusion or infection. However, complications can also arise during and after the dialysis that are related to the procedure and the composition of the dialysate. Most of these complications are due to either the absorption or loss of elements in the dialysate. For example, both protein and fluid are removed during the exchange, which can result in hypotension. Hypoproteinemia may cause peripheral edema. The presence of the dialysis fluid may cause low back pain or gastroesophageal reflux.

●○● NURSING PROCESS: PERFORMING PERITONEAL DIALYSIS

Conducting Peritoneal Dialysis Procedures

SKILL 22–2

ASSESSMENT

Assess each time dialysis is begun, and periodically during continuous dialysis:

- Vital signs and weight for baseline data and subsequent comparisons. The term *dry weight* refers to the client's weight without the fluid retention that occurs in clients with ESRD. Clients undergoing peritoneal dialysis should weigh near their dry weight when measured after draining the dialysate.

- Abdominal girth, respiratory status (rate, character, and breath sounds), presence of edema. **Rationale:** *These are indicators of fluid retention.*
- Results of blood analyses. Commonly, these include electrolytes, glucose, BUN, creatinine, albumin, hemoglobin, hematocrit, iron, bicarbonate, and parathyroid hormone.
- Allergies to any products used (e.g., lidocaine, shellfish, latex).

PLANNING

Review the client record for information about previous dialysis procedures. Note any complications and how these were managed and may be prevented. Before initiating dialysis, determine the primary care provider's order specifying the amount and type of solution for each peritoneal exchange, the number of exchanges, the length of time the fluid is to remain in the peritoneal cavity, and whether only a specific amount of fluid is to be withdrawn from the peritoneal cavity.

DELEGATION

Conducting peritoneal dialysis procedures is not delegated to UAP. However, the client's status is observed during usual care and may be recorded by persons other than the nurse. Abnormal findings must be validated and interpreted by the nurse.

INTERPROFESSIONAL PRACTICE

Any health care provider for whom sterile technique is within their scope of practice and who has the appropriate training or experience may perform aspects of PD treatments. Although the providers may verbally communicate their findings and plan to other health care team members, the nurse must also know where to locate their documentation in the client's medical record.

Equipment

For Infusing the Dialysate
- Container of peritoneal solution at body temperature, of the amount and kind ordered by the primary care provider. Bags range in size from 1 to 3 L.
- IV pole

SKILL 22-2

Conducting Peritoneal Dialysis Procedures—*continued*

- Sterile peritoneal dialysis administration set (separate or combined pieces):
  - Y-connector
  - IV-type tubing for dialysate
  - Drainage bag with tubing
- Sterile transfer set cap
- Dialysis log or flow sheet
- Clean gloves
- Mask and goggles
- Povidone-iodine swabs or other antiseptic per agency protocol (Some agencies recommend a sterile bowl and antiseptic for soaking the transfer set tubing.)

For Changing the Catheter Site Dressing
- Sterile gloves and masks (gowns and goggles as needed)

- Sterile cotton-tipped applicators
- Chlorhexidine gluconate, povidone-iodine solution, or soap and water as specified by agency protocol
- Povidone-iodine, mupirocin, gentamicin, or other antimicrobial ointment
- Precut sterile 2×2 gauze or slit transparent occlusive dressing
- Nonallergenic tape

CLINICAL ALERT!

In addition to antimicrobial ointment applied to the catheter exit site, clients may be given intranasal mupirocin for 5 to 7 days every month if they are identified as a nasal *Staphylococcus aureus* carrier.

IMPLEMENTATION
Preparation
Determine when the last dressing change was performed. Following initial catheter insertion, the dressing is not changed for several days to allow for stabilization of the catheter exit site. Subsequently, the dressing should be changed when wet, soiled, or loose, or at intervals specified by agency policy.

Performance
1. Prior to performing the procedure, introduce self and verify the client's identity using agency protocol. Explain to the client what you are going to do, why it is necessary, and how he or she can participate. Discuss how the results will be used in planning further care or treatments.
2. Perform hand hygiene and observe other appropriate infection prevention procedures.
3. Provide for client privacy.
4. Prepare the solution and the tubing.
   - Examine the label on the container and check the expiration date. Examine the dialysate solution. It should be clear and the seals unbroken.
   - Warm the dialysate using an approved warmer (not a microwave oven) to at least body temperature. **Rationale:** *Warmed solution enhances exchange and is more comfortable for the client.*
   - Following agency policy for the required technique, add any prescribed medication to the dialysate solution. For example, this may require soaking the injection port of the bag in antiseptic solution. Heparin is sometimes added. **Rationale:** *This prevents the accumulation of fibrin in the catheter.*
   - Apply the mask and spike the solution container. Close the clamp, and hang the container on the IV pole.
   - Prime the tubing: Remove the protective cap and hold the tubing over a cup or basin. Maintain the sterility of the end of the tubing and the cap. Open the clamp and let the fluid run through the tubing, removing all bubbles. Close the tubing clamp. **Rationale:** *This rids the tubing of air that could enter the peritoneal cavity, causing discomfort and preventing free drainage outflow.*
5. Connect the solution to the catheter.
   - Apply clean gloves and goggles, keeping the mask on.
   - Free the catheter end from the dressing if necessary.
   - Cleanse or soak the end of the transfer set that connects to the Y-connector with povidone-iodine or other specified disinfectant for the time listed in the agency protocol (usually 5 minutes). If tubing is not already attached, remove the cap from the transfer set and attach the Y-connector and end of the tubing from the solution to the catheter.
   - Connect the drainage receptacle to the outflow tubing if not preattached. Close the outflow tubing clamp.

- If necessary, cover the catheter site with the precut sterile gauze, and tape the dressing in place. Minimize handling of the catheter.
6. Remove and discard gloves, goggles, and mask.
   - Perform hand hygiene.
7. Infuse the peritoneal dialysate.
   - Open the clamp on the inflow tubing so that the dialysate can flow into the peritoneal cavity for the time specified by the order. If no rate is specified, the client can usually tolerate a steady open flow.
   - Observe the client for any signs of discomfort, particularly respiratory distress or abdominal pain.
   - After the fluid has infused, clamp the inflow tubing. **Rationale:** *With the tubing clamped, air will not enter the peritoneal cavity.*
   - Leave the fluid in the cavity for the designated time.
8. Ensure client comfort and safety.
   - Assist the client into a comfortable position.
   - Monitor the client's vital signs.
   - Periodically assess the client's comfort during the dwell time.
9. Remove the fluid.
   - Unclamp the outflow tubing, and permit the fluid to drain into the drainage bag by gravity for about 30 minutes.
   - If the fluid does not drain freely, assist the client to change position, or raise the head of the bed. If specified, drain only the amount ordered.
10. Assess the outflow fluid.
    - Observe the appearance of the outflow fluid. **Rationale:** *A cloudy, pink-tinged, or blood-tinged return may indicate peritonitis (infection/inflammation of the peritoneal cavity).* During the first two to four exchanges following insertion of the peritoneal dialysis catheter, the return may be blood tinged but should quickly progress to a straw-color return.
    - Apply clean gloves.
    - Measure the amount of outflow fluid, and discard the fluid and used supplies in an appropriate area.
11. Calculate the fluid balance for each exchange.
    - Compare the amount of outflow fluid with the amount of solution infused for each exchange.
    - If more fluid was infused than removed, the client's fluid balance is positive (+); if more fluid was removed than infused, the fluid balance is negative (–).
    Example:

    $$\begin{array}{r} + \ 2{,}000 \text{ mL dialysate solution infused} \\ - \ 1{,}500 \text{ mL fluid returned in drainage bag} \\ \hline = \ \ \ 500 \text{ mL balance for this exchange} \end{array}$$

    - Repeat steps for each exchange.

Continued on page 562

Conducting Peritoneal Dialysis Procedures—*continued*

CLINICAL ALERT!

The longest time interval in the peritoneal dialysis sequence is the dwell. Often, the nurse begins the exchange by draining the abdomen and then instilling the new bag of dialysate, initiating the next dwell. In this case, the nurse proceeds after step 3 to step 9 and then after step 13 back to step 4 to infuse the new bag. The Y-connector and IV tubing are usually removed during the dwell.

12. Calculate the cumulative fluid balance at least every 24 hours. The cumulative fluid balance should be negative.
    • Add the balance from each exchange (from step 10) to the total exchange balance:
    Example:

Previous cumulative exchange balance	+ 500 mL
Present exchange balance	– 700 mL
Cumulative exchange balance	– 200 mL

13. Check the dressing at the catheter exit site if present.
    • Assess the dryness of the dressing. **Rationale:** *The dressing should remain dry during dialysis.*
    • To change the catheter exit site dressing, use the equipment listed on page 561. See Skills 31–2 and 31–3 in Chapter 31 ∞ for dressing change technique. Do not forcibly remove crusts or scabs (Hain & Chan, 2013). **Rationale:** *This may irritate skin and increase the risk of exit site infection.* Dressings may not be necessary for well-healed insertion sites.

EVALUATION
• Perform detailed follow-up based on findings that deviated from expected or normal for the client. Relate findings to previous assessment data if available.

14. If another bag is not to be infused at this time, or after the infusion of the new bag, disconnect the catheter from the tubing, and cover the end of the catheter with a new sterile cap. **Rationale:** *This allows the catheter to remain in place between each of the exchanges without contamination of the catheter.*
15. Remove and discard gloves.
    • Perform hand hygiene.
16. Document findings in the client record using forms or checklists supplemented by narrative notes when appropriate. Include the time during which the fluid infused, the exchange number, dialysate and additives used, details of the exchange balance, color of outflow solution from the client, the client's response, appearance of the catheter exit site and dressing, and the client's weight before and after the set of exchanges (daily). These may be written in the nurse's notes or on a flowchart.

SAMPLE DOCUMENTATION

5/20/2015 0830 First 1L dialysate infused over 20 minutes thru PD catheter. VS unchanged, no complaints of discomfort. Insertion site dressing clean & dry. ———————————————— S. Everley, RN

5/20/2015 1330 VS stable, dressing & intact. 950 mL pink-tinged fluid returned from PD catheter by gravity flow over 20 minutes. PD bag #2, 1L, infused in 15 minutes. Ambulated in hall independently. ———————————————— S. Everley, RN

• Report significant deviations from normal to the primary care provider.

Ambulatory and Community Settings **Peritoneal Dialysis** **PATIENT-CENTERED CARE**

Most clients undergoing peritoneal dialysis perform these procedures themselves at home. The nurse performs initial teaching and documents that the client and family are knowledgeable and able to demonstrate the techniques involved. In addition, the nurse assists with arrangements for all equipment and supplies that the client requires for home care.

For clients using CAPD, the double bag system of a dialysate solution bag and a drainage bag is used. A special belt that stabilizes the catheter is available.

Teach the client and family:
• Store supplies in a clean, cool, dry place.
• Examine the solution for any signs of contamination before using it.
• Warm the dialysate using a heating pad that has been checked for appropriate temperature, for about 1 hour.
• Hang the dialysate bag at approximately shoulder height for infusion. Assist the client with obtaining an IV pole or other hanging device.

• Perform thorough hand washing and wear a surgical mask when changing tubing.
• Drain the dialysate from the abdomen into the empty bag. A one-way valve prevents used dialysate from backing up into the new dialysate bag.
• Record weight and dialysis fluid balance daily or as ordered. Weight should be measured after draining the dialysate, and on the same scale, at the same time of day, and wearing similar clothing each time.
• Instill the new dialysate.
• Disconnect the tubing with the two bags attached. Discard the drained dialysate, bags, and tubing while using appropriate infection prevention techniques, as advised by the health care provider.
• Report any signs of peritonitis:
    • Fever
    • Nausea or vomiting
• Redness or pain around the exit site.

Chapter 22 Review

FOCUSING ON CLINICAL THINKING

Consider This

1. As you prepare to assist with the procedure of insertion of a peritoneal dialysis catheter, the client expresses relief that the catheter will be in place for only 24 hours. How would you respond?

2. The client on continuous ambulatory peritoneal dialysis is to have daily weights taken. When would be an appropriate time to record the weight?

See Focusing on Clinical Thinking Answers on student resource website.

TEST YOUR KNOWLEDGE

1. The nurse is caring for a client undergoing peritoneal dialysis. The primary care provider specifies the components of the _____ solution used in the procedure.
   1. Dialysis
   2. Dialysate
   3. Dialyzer
   4. Instillation

2. The nurse is caring for a client who produces 50 to 60 mL of urine per day as a result of kidney failure. How would the nurse document this quantity of urine?
   1. Anuria
   2. Oliguria
   3. Polyuria
   4. Hydruria

3. The nurse is caring for a client requiring peritoneal dialysis. The nurse can safely delegate what aspect of care for this client to unlicensed assistive personnel (UAP)?
   1. Assisting with peritoneal catheter insertion
   2. Conducting the peritoneal dialysis procedure
   3. Observing the status of the client while assisting with activities of daily living (ADLs)
   4. Assessing the outflow fluid

4. The nurse is caring for a client receiving peritoneal dialysis and can safely ask the UAP to do which of the following (with proper instructions)? Select all that apply.
   1. Change the peritoneal catheter dressing.
   2. Measure vital signs.
   3. Obtain a daily weight.
   4. Instill dialysate.
   5. Assist the client to eat breakfast.

5. The nurse is preparing to assist the primary care provider with the insertion of a peritoneal dialysis catheter. The nurse's role in ensuring that the client is prepared for the procedure is which of the following? Select all that apply.
   1. Initial client and family teaching
   2. Reinforcing key elements of client and family teaching
   3. Initial explanation of the client's diagnosis and need for peritoneal dialysis
   4. Providing information for the informed consent
   5. Reviewing the technique of peritoneal dialysis and its purpose with the client and family

6. The nurse is assisting the primary care provider with the insertion of a peritoneal dialysis catheter. As the primary care provider prepares to insert the trocar, which action would the nurse instruct the client to perform?
   1. Tense the abdominal muscles to reduce discomfort.
   2. Take a deep breath to distend the abdomen.
   3. Hold the breath to avoid abdominal movement.
   4. Drink fluids to distend the stomach.

7. The nurse is preparing the dialysate for a client requiring peritoneal dialysis. After warming the solution, the nurse adds substances commonly ordered to reduce complications. Which substance is commonly added?
   1. Sodium
   2. Chloride
   3. Calcium
   4. Heparin

8. The nurse has performed peritoneal dialysis throughout the shift and exchanged fluid three times. Each infusion consisted of 500 mL. On the first exchange 600 mL of fluid was returned, on the second exchange 550 mL was returned, and on the third exchange 475 mL was returned. What is the client's cumulative fluid balance? _____

9. The nurse is assigned a client who has been receiving peritoneal dialysis for the past year. On initial rounds the nurse sees that the peritoneal outflow is cloudy and pink tinged. What would be the best nursing action at this time?
   1. Inform the primary care provider because this could indicate peritonitis.
   2. Do nothing because this is normal-appearing fluid.
   3. Make the client NPO because this could indicate bowel perforation.
   4. Partially clamp the outflow because this indicates that too much dialysate is being removed at one time.

10. The nurse, caring for a client receiving peritoneal dialysis, recognizes that which of the following is a normal condition?
    1. Pulse rate of 76 beats/min that increases to 88 beats/min while peritoneal fluid is indwelling
    2. Temperature of 38.1°C (100.6°F) oral
    3. Serum potassium of 3.1 mEq/L
    4. Weight gain of 5 pounds in 24 hours

See Answers to Test Your Knowledge in Appendix A.

READINGS AND REFERENCES

References

Crabtree, J. H., Piraino, B., Firanek, C. A., Abu-Alfa, A. K., & Guest, S. (2012). *Access care and complications management: Care of the adult patient on peritoneal dialysis.* Retrieved from http://www.qxmd.com/references/access-care-guide

Davies, S. (2013). Peritoneal dialysis-current status and future challenges. *Nature Reviews Nephrology, 9,* 399–408. doi:10.1038/nrneph.2013.100

Frost, J. H., & Bagul, A. (2012). A brief recap of tips and surgical manoeuvres to enhance optimal outcome of surgically placed peritoneal dialysis catheters. *International Journal of Nephrology, 2012,* pp. 1–7. doi:10.1155/2012/251584

Hain, D. J., & Chan, J. (2013). Best available evidence for peritoneal dialysis catheter exit-site care. *Nephrology Nursing Journal, 40*(1), 63–69.

Tong, A., Lesmana, B., Johnson, D., Wong, G., Campbell, D., & Craig, J. (2013). The perspectives of adults living with peritoneal dialysis: Thematic synthesis of qualitative studies. *American Journal of Kidney Diseases, 61,* 873–888. doi:10.1053/j.ajkd.2012.08.045

Selected Bibliography

Agarwal, A. K., Salman, L., & Asif, A. (2013). *Peritoneal dialysis: Types, procedures and risks factors.* Hauppauge, NY: Nova Science.

Chui, B., Manns, B., Pannu, N., Dong, J., Wiebe, N., Jindal, K., & Klarenbach, S. (2013). Health care costs of peritoneal dialysis technique failure and dialysis modality switching. *American Journal of Kidney Diseases, 61,* 104–111. doi:10.1053/j.ajkd.2012.07.010

Flythe, J., & Brunelli, S. (2013). Racial disparities in survival on peritoneal dialysis. *American Journal of Kidney Diseases, 62,* 10–11. doi:10.1053/j.ajkd.2013.04.001

Gultekin, F., Cakmak, G., Karakaya, K., Emre, A., Tascilar, O., Oner, M., . . . Kulah, E. (2013). Our long-term results of Tenckhoff peritoneal dialysis catheters placement via laparoscopic preperitoneal tunneling technique. *Seminars in Dialysis, 26,* 349–354. doi:10.1111/sdi.12003

Hagen, S. M., van Alphen, A. M., IJzermans, J. N. M., & Dor, F. J. M. F. (2011). Laparoscopic versus open peritoneal dialysis catheter insertion, the LOCI-trial: A study protocol. *BMC Surgery, 11,* 35. doi:10.1186/1471-2482-11-35

Hall, R. K., O'Hare, A. M., Anderson, R. A., & Colón-Emeric, C. S. (2013). End-stage renal disease in nursing homes: A systematic review. *Journal of the American Medical Directors Association, 14,* 242–247. doi:10.1016/j.jamda.2013.01.004

Krediet, R., & Struijk, D. (2013). Peritoneal changes in patients on long-term peritoneal dialysis. *Nature Reviews Nephrology, 9,* 419–429. doi:10.1038/nrneph.2013.99

Lecouf, A., Ryckelynck, J., Ficheux, M., Henri, P., & Lobbedez, T. (2013). A new paradigm: Home therapy for patients who start dialysis in an unplanned way. *Journal of Renal Care, 39*(S1), 50–55. doi:10.1111/j.1755-6686.2013,00336.x

Lomas, C. (2012). Do-it-yourself dialysis. *Nursing Standard, 27*(11), 16–17.

McQuillan, R. F., Chiu, E., Nessim, S., Lok, C. E., Roscoe, J. M., Tam, P., & Jassal, S. V. (2012). A randomized controlled trial comparing mupirocin and Polysporin triple ointments in peritoneal dialysis patients: The MP3 study.

Clinical Journal of the American Society of Nephrology, 7, 297–303. doi:10.2215/CJN.07970811

Mehrotra, R. (2013). Nutritional issues in peritoneal dialysis patients: How do they differ from that of patients undergoing hemodialysis? *Journal of Renal Nutrition, 23,* 237–240. doi:10.1053/j.jrn.2013.01.031

Mehrotra, R., & Singh, H. (2013). Peritoneal dialysis–associated peritonitis with simultaneous exit-site infection. *Clinical Journal of the American Society of Nephrology, 8,* 126–130. doi:10.2215/CJN.06910712

Noordzij, M., & Jager, K. J. (2012). Survival comparisons between haemodialysis and peritoneal dialysis. *Nephrology Dialysis Transplantation, 27,* 3385–3387. doi:10.1093/ndt/gfs031

Segal, J., & Messana, J. (2013). Prevention of peritonitis in peritoneal dialysis. *Seminars in Dialysis, 26,* 494–502. doi:10.1111/sdi.12114

Shahbazi, N., & McCormick, B. (2011). Peritoneal dialysis catheter insertion strategies and maintenance of catheter function. *Seminars in Nephrology, 31,* 138–151. doi:10.1016/j.semnephrol.2011.01.003

Xie, J., Kiryluk, K., Ren, H., Zhu, P., Huang, X., Shen, P., . . . Chen, N. (2011). Coiled versus straight peritoneal dialysis catheters: A randomized controlled trial and meta-analysis. *American Journal of Kidney Diseases, 58,* 946–955.

Yngman-Uhlin, P., Fernström, A., Börjeson, S., & Edéll-Gustafsson, U. (2012). Evaluation of an individual sleep intervention programme in people undergoing peritoneal dialysis treatment. *Journal of Clinical Nursing, 21,* 3402–3417. doi:10.1111/j.1365-2702.2012.04282.x

6 Applying the Nursing Process

This unit explores skills related to nutrition and elimination. Meeting the client's nutritional needs is essential to promoting health, preventing illness, and enhancing recovery from injury and disease. Urinary and bowel elimination are basic human needs that can be affected by illness, injury, medications, and treatments. The nurse plays an important role in assessing and maintaining nutrition and elimination when providing client care in any setting.

Client: Michael   AGE: 78 Years   CURRENT MEDICAL DIAGNOSIS: Cerebrovascular Accident, Hypertension, Chronic Renal Failure

Medical History: Michael, 78 years old, is an African American who emigrated from Sierra Leone 12 years ago. He was diagnosed with hypertension at age 35 and was intermittently compliant with his treatment plan, often choosing to stop taking his antihypertensive medication because he "felt fine" and didn't think he needed it. He was diagnosed with chronic renal failure 10 years ago, and his kidney function has steadily declined. Two weeks ago while playing cards at home he suddenly lost sensation and function on the left side of his body. He was rushed to the emergency department where he was diagnosed with a cerebrovascular accident (stroke). When his condition stabilized he was transferred to a rehabilitation facility where he receives occupational and physical therapy as well as assistance with meeting his self-care needs. He takes hydrochlorothiazide 50 mg and atenolol 100 mg PO daily to control his hypertension, and furosemide 40 mg PO daily to improve urine output. Michael has developed dysphagia, constipation, and occasional urinary incontinence.

Personal and Social History: Michael is married and has four grown children and 10 grandchildren. Two of his children live nearby. His wife is anxious for him to recover enough to return home. They live in a two-story detached home.

Questions

Assessment

1. What assessment data will the nurse collect related to the client's nutritional and elimination status?

Analysis

2. List two possible nursing diagnoses that can be identified from the medical/personal history and assessment data above related to nutrition and/or elimination.

Planning

3. Based on the assessment data and nursing diagnoses, identify one desired outcome.
4. Identify the action verb, measurable criteria, and time line for the outcome.

Implementation

5. What interventions can the nurse provide to improve Michael's ability to meet nutritional requirements?
6. What interventions can the nurse provide to treat Michael's constipation?
7. Suggest interventions to reduce urinary incontinence.

Evaluation

8. What data might the nurse collect to indicate the desired outcome has been met?

See Applying the Nursing Process suggested answers on student resource website.

UNIT

7

Circulatory and Ventilatory Support

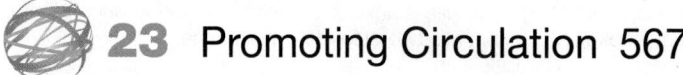

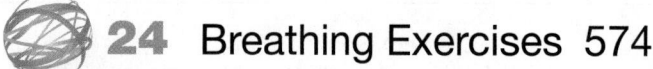
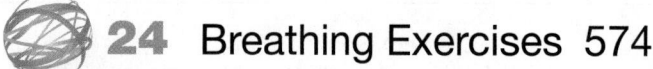
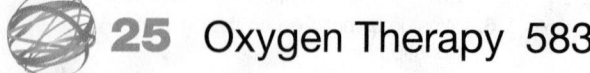

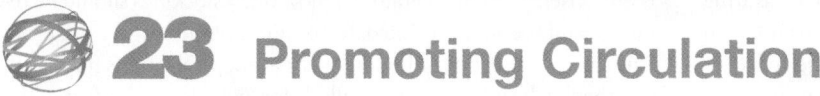

23 Promoting Circulation

LEARNING OUTCOMES

At the completion of this chapter, the student will be able to:

1. Define the key terms used in the skills of promoting circulation.
2. Describe two measures to help prevent venous stasis.
3. Identify indications and contraindications for applying anti-emboli stockings and sequential compression devices.
4. Recognize when it is appropriate to delegate circulatory support to unlicensed assistive personnel.

5. Verbalize the steps used in:
   a. Applying antiemboli stockings.
   b. Applying a sequential compression device.
6. Demonstrate appropriate documentation and recording of skills used to promote circulation.

SKILLS

Skill 23–1 Applying Antiemboli Stockings

Skill 23–2 Applying a Sequential Compression Device

KEY TERMS

antiemboli (elastic) stockings, *567*
deep venous thrombosis (DVT), *567*
Homans' sign, *568*

intermittent pneumatic
   compression devices
   (IPCDs), *570*

pulmonary embolism (PE), *567*
sequential compression devices
   (SCDs), *570*

venous thromboembolism
   (VTE), *567*

Most people in good health give little thought to their cardiovascular function. Changing position frequently, ambulating, and exercising usually maintain adequate cardiovascular functioning. Immobility, however, is highly detrimental to cardiovascular function.

PREVENTING VENOUS STASIS

When clients have limited mobility or are confined to bed, venous return to the heart is impaired and the risk of venous stasis (decreased blood movement) increases. Immobility is a problem not only for clients who are ill or debilitated but also for some travelers who sit with legs dependent for long periods in a motor vehicle or an airplane.

Venous stasis may allow clots (venous thrombosis) to develop in a deep vein, often in the thigh or calf. This is called **deep venous thrombosis (DVT)** or deep vein thrombosis. If the thrombus breaks free, it can travel and become a **pulmonary embolism (PE)** where it blocks a pulmonary artery or one of its branches. Blood flow and gas exchange in the lungs are then impaired. If the clot is large enough, sudden death can occur. DVT is associated with the development of about 90% of all PEs (Larkin, Mitchell, & Petrie, 2012). The term **venous thromboembolism (VTE)** incorporates both DVT and PE. VTE is one of the most common preventable causes of hospital-related death, especially among older adults, because advancing age is a major risk for VTE (McNamara, 2014; Pollak & McBane, 2014).

Preventing venous stasis is an important nursing intervention to reduce the risk of complications following surgery, trauma, or major medical problems. Positioning and leg exercises are discussed in Chapters 10 ∞ and 13 ∞, respectively. Antiemboli stockings and

sequential compression devices are additional measures to help prevent venous stasis.

Antiemboli Stockings

Antiemboli (elastic) stockings are firm elastic hosiery. They exert external pressure on the leg and compress the veins which decrease the pooling of venous blood in the extremities and thereby facilitate the return of venous blood to the heart. Elastic stockings are frequently used for clients with limited mobility because of restricted activities or prolonged standing (e.g., supermarket checkers, surgeons, and nurses). These stockings also are often used postoperatively to avoid complications such as DVT and PE.

The nurse needs to remember that not all clients will benefit from elastic stockings. Clients with peripheral arterial disease, massive leg edema, gangrene of the foot or leg, current diagnosis of DVT, recent bypass graft, dermatitis, cellulitis, or thigh or calf circumference that exceeds the size specified in the fitting instructions are not appropriate candidates for compression stockings. Stockings that are too small can impair subcutaneous tissue oxygenation or create a tourniquet effect, resulting in skin damage and impaired venous return. It is important for a nurse to thoroughly assess the client for contraindications before applying elastic stockings.

Several types of stockings are available. One type extends from the foot to the knee, and another from the foot to midthigh. These stockings usually have a partial foot that exposes the heel or toes so that the extremity circulation can be assessed. Elastic stockings usually come in a variety of sizes (i.e., small, medium and large), but some clients may require custom-made stockings.

When obtaining antiemboli stockings for a client, it is important to follow the manufacturer's recommendations for measuring and fitting the stockings to ensure the stockings are applied and worn correctly. Ill-fitting thigh-length stockings should not be rolled or folded down the leg to make them fit. Rolling and folding are incorrect procedures and should be corrected, because they can cause the stockings to have a tourniquet effect and decrease circulation. There is no consensus in the literature of how often stockings should be removed and the skin inspected. Recommendations range from every 8 hours to once every 24 hours. Check agency policy. It is important that the skin be inspected, particularly for high-risk clients (e.g., older adults). See Skill 23–1 on applying antiemboli stockings.

●○● NURSING PROCESS: APPLYING ANTIEMBOLI STOCKINGS

SKILL 23–1

Applying Antiemboli Stockings

ASSESSMENT
Assess and compare both lower extremities for:
- Presence and force (e.g., strong, faint, easily obliterated) of posterior tibial and dorsalis pedis pulses.
- Skin color (note pallor, cyanosis, or other pigmentation).
- Skin temperature (e.g., warm, cool).

- Presence of edema.
- Skin condition (e.g., thickened, shiny, taut).
- **Homans' sign** (pain in calf with passive dorsiflexion of the foot). A positive Homans' sign should be reported because it *could* indicate DVT; it is not a conclusive sign of DVT.

PLANNING
Before applying antiemboli stockings, determine the presence of actual or potential circulatory problems, and determine if an order for the stockings has been written by the primary care provider.

Equipment
- Single-use (disposable) tape measure (to prevent cross-infection)
- Clean knee-high or thigh-high antiemboli stockings of appropriate size

DELEGATION

Unlicensed assistive personnel (UAP) frequently remove and apply antiemboli stockings as part of hygiene care. The nurse should stress the importance of removing and reapplying the stockings and reporting any changes in the client's skin to the nurse. The nurse is responsible for assessment of the skin.

IMPLEMENTATION
Preparation
Take measurements as needed to obtain the appropriate size stockings.
- Measure the length of both legs from the heel to the gluteal fold (for thigh-length stockings) or from the heel to the popliteal space or bend of the knee (for knee-length stockings).
- Measure the circumference of each calf and each thigh at the widest point.
- Compare the measurements to the size chart on the back of the manufacturer's package to obtain stockings of the correct size. Obtain two sizes if there is a significant difference. **Rationale:** *Stockings that are too large for the client do not place adequate pressure on the legs to facilitate venous return. They may bunch, increasing the risk of pressure and skin irritation. Stockings that are too small may impede blood flow to the feet and cause skin breakdown.*

Performance
1. Prior to performing the procedure, introduce self and verify the client's identity using agency protocol. Explain to the client what you are going to do, why it is necessary, and how he or she can participate.
2. Perform hand hygiene and observe other appropriate infection prevention procedures.
3. Provide for client privacy.
4. Select an appropriate time to apply the stockings.
   - Apply stockings in the morning, if possible, before the client gets out of bed. **Rationale:** *In sitting and standing positions,* the veins can become distended so that edema occurs; the stockings should be applied before this happens.
   - Assist the client who has been ambulating to lie down and elevate the legs for 15 to 30 minutes before applying the stockings. **Rationale:** *This facilitates venous return, reduces swelling, and simplifies application of the stockings.*
5. Prepare the client.
   - Assist the client to a lying position in bed.
   - Wash and dry the legs as needed.
6. Apply the stockings.
   - Reach inside the stocking from the top, and grasping the heel, turn the upper portion of the stocking inside out so the foot portion is inside the stocking leg. **Rationale:** *Firm elastic stockings are easier to fit over the foot and calf when inverted in this manner rather than bunching up the stocking.*
   - Ask the client to point the toes, and then position the stocking on the client's foot. With the heel of the stocking down and stretching each side of the stocking, ease the stocking over the toes, taking care to place the toe and heel portions of the stocking appropriately. ❶ **Rationale:** *Pointing the toes makes application easier.*
   - Grasp the loose portion of the stocking at the ankle and gently pull the stocking over the leg, turning it right side out in the process. ❷ and ❸ If applying thigh-length stockings, stretch them over the knee until the top is below the gluteal fold.

Applying Antiemboli Stockings—*continued*

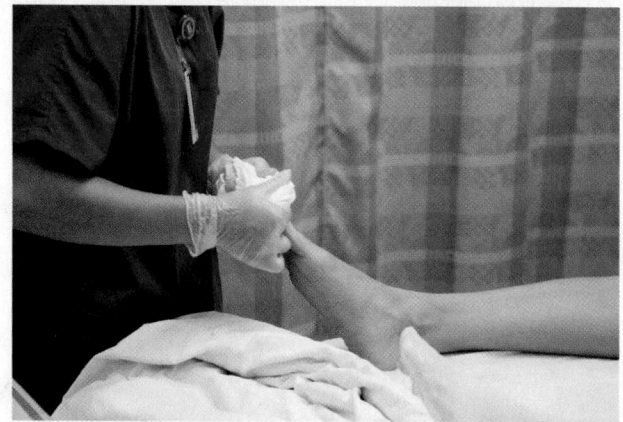

❶ Applying the stocking over the toes.

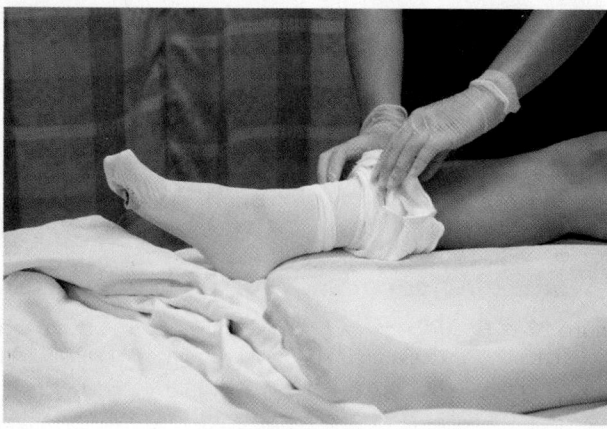

❷ Pulling the stocking snugly over the leg.

- Inspect the client's leg and stocking, smoothing any folds or creases. Ensure that the stocking is not rolled down or bunched at the top or ankle. Ensure that the stocking is distributed evenly and that the heel is properly centered in the heel pocket. **Rationale:** *Folds and creases can cause skin irritation under the stocking; bunching of the stocking can further impair venous return.*
- Remove the stockings per agency policy, inspecting the legs and skin while the stockings are off.
- Soiled stockings may be laundered by hand with warm water and mild soap. Hang to dry.

7. Document the procedure. Record the procedure, your assessment data, and the time when stockings are removed and reapplied.

SKILL 23-1

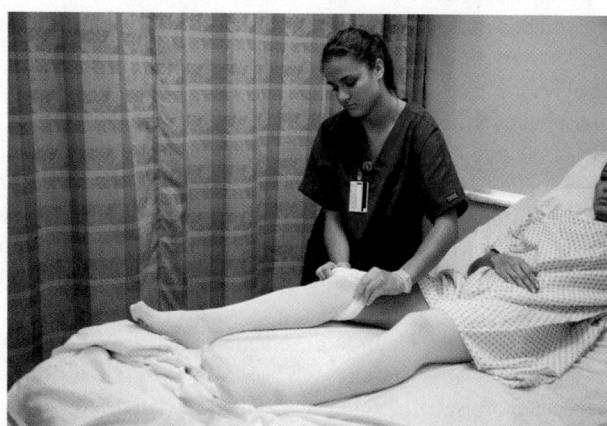

❸ For thigh-length stockings, stretch the stocking over the knee until the top is below the gluteal fold.

EVALUATION

- Remove antiembolism stockings per agency policy for skin care and inspection.
- Note the appearance of the legs and skin integrity, presence of edema, peripheral pulses, and skin color and temperature. Compare to previous assessment data.

- If complications occur, remove the stockings and report findings to the primary care provider.

LIFESPAN CONSIDERATIONS   Antiemboli Stockings

CHILDREN
- Antiemboli stockings are infrequently used on children.

OLDER ADULTS
- Because the elastic is quite strong in antiemboli stockings, older adults may need assistance with putting on the stockings. Clients with arthritis may need to have another person put the stockings on for them.
- Many older adults have circulation problems and wear antiemboli stockings. It is important to check for wrinkles in the stockings and to see if the stocking has rolled down or twisted.

If so, correct immediately. **Rationale:** *The stockings must be evenly distributed over the limb to promote rather than hinder circulation.*
- Stockings should be removed at least once a day (check agency policy) so that a thorough assessment can be made of the legs and feet. **Rationale:** *Redness and skin breakdown on the heels can occur quickly and go undetected if not thoroughly assessed on a regular basis.*
- Provide information about the importance of wearing the elastic stockings, how to wear them correctly, and how to take care of them.

- Teach the client or caregiver how to apply the antiemboli stockings.
- Stress the importance of no wrinkles or rolling down of the stockings and the rationale.
- Instruct the client or caregiver to remove the stockings daily and inspect the skin on the legs.
- Provide instructions about:
  - Laundering the stockings. They should be air-dried because putting them in a dryer can affect the elasticity of the stockings.

- The need for two pairs of stockings to allow for one pair to be worn while the other is being laundered.
- Replacing the stockings when they lose their elasticity.
- The slipperiness of stockings if worn without slippers or shoes. If the client is ambulatory, emphasize the need for footwear to prevent falling.

Sequential Compression Devices

Clients who are undergoing surgery or are immobilized due to illness or injury or are in a critical care unit may benefit from **sequential compression devices (SCDs)** to promote venous return from the legs. Another term used in the literature is **intermittent pneumatic compression devices (IPCDs)**, but because there are different types of IPCDs, they are often collectively referred to as SCDs. SCDs are useful in preventing thrombi and edema, which may result from venous stasis, but they are not used for clients who have arterial insufficiency, cellulitis, infection of the extremity, active DVT, or preexisting venous thrombosis. SCDs inflate and deflate disposable sleeves to promote venous flow. The plastic sleeves are attached by tubing to an air pump that alternately inflates and deflates portions of the sleeve to a specified pressure.

The SCD is available in foot (sometimes called a foot pump), knee-length, or thigh-length sleeves. The foot pump artificially stimulates the venous plantar plexus (a large vein located in the foot) to increase blood circulation in the foot. The inflation and deflation of the pump simulate the blood flow that results from walking. For the knee-length or thigh-length SCDs, the ankle area inflates first, followed by the calf region and then the thigh area. This sequential inflation and deflation counteracts blood stasis in the lower extremities and increases venous blood flow toward the heart (Figure 23–1 ■). Larkin et al. (2012) indicate that "another benefit of mechanical compression devices is that they contribute to increasing the fibrinolytic activity within the vasculature and thus to preventing fibrin clot formation" (p. 517).

Both knee-high and thigh-high SCDs are equally effective against VTE if they are worn 90% of the day or for more than 21 of each 24 hours (Stone & Chamberlin, 2011). Clients may not wear them because of discomfort, warmth, or soiling, particularly for the thigh-high SCDs. Stone and Chamberlin (2011) conducted a study and found that using only the knee-high SCDs as the standard for the intensive care units (ICUs) in their hospital resulted in increased

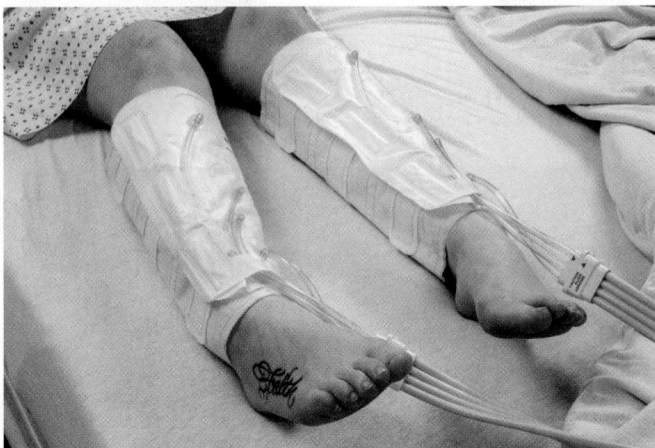

Figure 23–1 ■ The sequential venous compression device enhances venous return. SCDs are available in foot, knee-high, or thigh-high length.

client compliance with wearing SCDs and no newly diagnosed DVTs in the ICU a year after the change was implemented.

The SCD is removed for ambulation and usually discontinued when the client resumes activities. To avoid falls, remind the client that the SCD needs to be removed before ambulating, particularly when the client needs to use the bathroom during the night.

Sequential compression therapy often complements other preventive measures. The client's risk level for VTE often determines the preventive measures used. For example, clients at low risk may require only antiemboli stockings. Clients at moderate risk may have both antiemboli stockings and sequential therapy as part of their treatment. The primary care provider may order antiemboli stockings, sequential therapy, and anticoagulation therapy for a client who is high risk.

Skill 23–2 outlines how to apply a sequential compression device.

●○● NURSING PROCESS: APPLYING A SEQUENTIAL COMPRESSION DEVICE

Applying a Sequential Compression Device

ASSESSMENT

Assess for baseline data:

- Cardiovascular and peripheral vascular status, including heart rate and rhythm, peripheral pulses, and capillary refill

- Color and temperature of extremities
- Movement and sensation of feet and lower extremities and Homans' sign

Applying a Sequential Compression Device—*continued*

SKILL 23-2

PLANNING

- Check the primary care provider's order for type of SCD sleeve. **Rationale:** *Foot, knee-length, and thigh-length sleeves are available.*
- Read the manufacturer's directions for connecting and operating the compression controller.

DELEGATION

UAP often remove and reapply the SCD when performing hygiene care. The nurse should check that the UAP knows the correct application process for the SCD. Reinforce the importance of not allowing the SCD to be removed for long periods of time because the purpose of the SCD is to promote circulation. Remind UAP to inspect the SCD sleeve and tubing each time prior to applying the sleeves.

Equipment

- Measuring tape
- SCD, including disposable sleeves, air pump, and tubing

IMPLEMENTATION
Performance

1. Prior to performing the procedure, introduce self and verify the client's identity using agency protocol. Explain to the client what you are going to do, why it is necessary, and the procedure for applying the sequential compression device. **Rationale:** *The client's participation and comfort will be increased by understanding the rationale for applying the SCD.*
2. Perform hand hygiene and observe other appropriate infection prevention procedures.
3. Provide for client privacy and drape the client appropriately.
4. Prepare the client.
   - Place the client in a dorsal recumbent or semi-Fowler's position.
   - Measure the client's legs as recommended by the manufacturer if a thigh-length sleeve is required. **Rationale:** *Foot and knee-length sleeves come in just one size; the thigh circumference determines the size needed for a thigh-length sleeve.*
5. Apply the sequential compression sleeves.
   - Place a sleeve under each leg with the opening at the knee.
   - Wrap the sleeve securely around the leg, securing the Velcro tabs. ❶ Allow two fingers to fit between the leg and the sleeve. **Rationale:** *This amount of space ensures that the sleeve does not impair circulation when inflated.* Ensure that there is no overlapping or creases in the SCD. **Rationale:** *This prevents skin breakdown.*
6. Connect the sleeves to the control unit and adjust the pressure as needed.
   - Connect the tubing to the sleeves and control unit, ensuring that arrows on the plug and the connector are in alignment and that the tubing is not kinked or twisted. **Rationale:** *Improper alignment or obstruction of the tubing by kinks or twists will interfere with operation of the SCD.*
   - Turn on the control unit and adjust the alarms and pressures as needed. The sleeve cooling control and alarm should be on; ankle pressure is usually set at 35 to 55 mmHg.

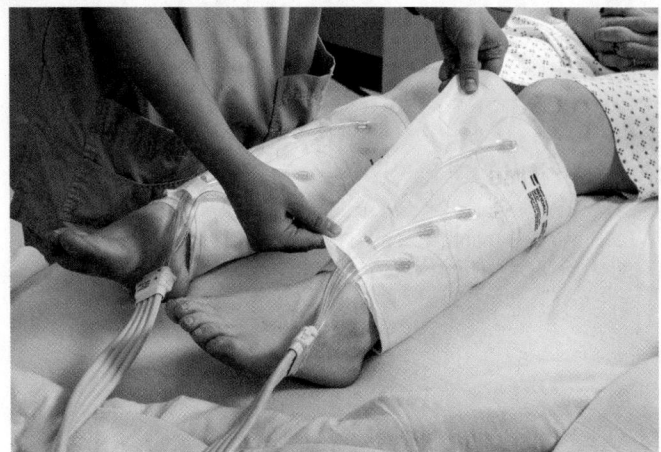

❶ Applying a sequential compression device to the leg.

Rationale: *It is important to have the sleeve cooling control on for comfort and to reduce the risk of skin irritation from moisture under the sleeve. Proper pressure settings prevent injury to the client. Alarms warn of possible control unit malfunctions.*

7. Document the procedure.
   - Record baseline assessment data and application of the SCD. Note control unit settings.
   - Assess and document skin integrity and neurovascular and peripheral vascular status per agency policy while the SCD is in place. Remove the unit and notify the primary care provider if the client complains of numbness and tingling or leg pain. These may be symptoms of nerve compression.

EVALUATION

- Perform appropriate follow-up assessments, such as peripheral vascular status including pedal pulses, skin color and temperature, skin integrity, and neurovascular status, including movement and sensation.
- Compare to the baseline data, if available.
- Report significant deviations from normal to the primary care provider.

LIFESPAN CONSIDERATIONS | Sequential Compression Devices

CHILDREN
- Because young children tend to be more active, the SCD is rarely necessary unless the child is immobile (e.g., comatose or in the critical care setting).

OLDER ADULTS
- The SCD sleeves may become loose as clients move around in bed. Check that the sleeves are secure and properly positioned.

Ambulatory and Community Settings | Sequential Compression Devices | PATIENT-CENTERED CARE

- An SCD may be used in the home. Inform the client or caregiver how to apply the device correctly and how to operate the system, including how to respond to the alarm.

Chapter 23 Review

FOCUSING ON CLINICAL THINKING

Consider This

1. The client brought her own antiemboli stockings from home. The UAP tells you that the client's stockings are loose and do not stay up. What will you do?

2. The client is on a sequential compression device, and the nurse is monitoring neurovascular checks every 2 hours. During this last check, the client states that his leg is starting to feel numb. What action, if any, would you take?

See Focusing on Clinical Thinking answers on student resource website.

TEST YOUR KNOWLEDGE

1. When the nurse dorsiflexes the client's foot, the client complains of pain in the calf of that leg. The nurse documents this using which terminology?
   1. Positive Babinski
   2. Positive Homans' sign
   3. Negative Babinski
   4. Negative Homans' sign

2. The nurse is caring for a client diagnosed with deep venous thrombosis (DVT). This means the client has:
   1. An inflamed vein.
   2. A blood clot in the vein.
   3. A clot that is traveling through the circulatory system.
   4. A blood clot in the vein causing inflammation.

3. The nurse knows that which client is at greatest risk for venous stasis?
   1. A client with atrial fibrillation (irregular heart rate)
   2. A client in the same-day surgery center
   3. A pregnant client required to maintain bed rest due to premature labor
   4. A client with diabetes

4. A nurse is working at a primary care provider's office and is collecting an admission history from a client who is planning a long plane trip. To prevent venous stasis, the nurse educates the client on the importance of which topic?
   1. Drinking extra fluids
   2. Elevating the legs
   3. Getting up and walking at least once an hour
   4. Eating a low-sodium diet

5. The nurse is preparing to apply antiemboli stockings on a postoperative client at risk for venous stasis. What should the nurse determine before applying the stockings?
   1. Potential or current circulatory problems
   2. Intake and output
   3. Alteration in vital signs
   4. Risk for respiratory distress

6. The nurse is preparing to apply antiemboli stockings on a client. Put the steps the nurse will follow in the proper order when performing this procedure.
   1. Compare the client's measurements to the size chart.
   2. Ask the client to point the toes.
   3. Obtain measurements of the leg.
   4. Pull the stocking over the ankle and then up the leg.
   5. Turn the upper portion of the stocking inside out so the foot portion is inside the stocking's leg.

7. The nurse has received a primary care provider's order to apply antiemboli stockings on a postoperative client. What is the best time for the nurse to apply the stockings?
   1. While the client is sitting in the chair after lunch
   2. Prior to the client going to sleep at night
   3. Midafternoon
   4. In the morning before the client gets out of bed

8. The nurse is caring for a client at moderate risk for deep venous thrombosis (DVT) or pulmonary emboli (PE) and anticipates that the primary care provider will order which treatment for the client?
   1. Antiemboli stockings
   2. A sequential compression device
   3. Antiemboli stockings and a sequential compression device
   4. Antiemboli stockings, a sequential compression device, and anticoagulant therapy

9. The nurse would not apply a sequential compression device (SCD) in clients with which condition? Select all that apply.
   1. Cellulitis of the leg
   2. Deep venous thrombosis in the thigh
   3. Hypertension
   4. Arterial insufficiency
   5. Infected wound on the leg

10. When preparing to apply a sequential compression device, the nurse should place the client in what position?
    1. Dorsal lithotomy
    2. High-Fowler's
    3. Prone
    4. Semi-Fowler's

See Answers to Test Your Knowledge in Appendix A.

READINGS AND REFERENCES

References

Larkin, B., Mitchell, K., & Petrie, K. (2012). Translating evidence to practice for mechanical venous thromboembolism prophylaxis. *AORN Journal, 96*, 513–527. doi:10.1016/j.aorn.2012.07.011

McNamara, S. A. (2014). Prevention of venous thromboembolism. *AORN Journal, 99*, 642–647. doi:10.1016/j.aorn.2014.02.001

Pollak, A. W., & McBane, R. D. (2014). Succinct review of the new VTE prevention and management guidelines. *Mayo Clinic Proceedings,89*, 394–408. doi:10.1016/j.mayocp.2013.11.015

Stone, A., & Chamberlin, L. (2011). Out with the thigh-high, in with the knee-high sequential compression devices. *Critical Care Nurse, 31*(2), e37.

Selected Bibliography

Berman, A., Snyder, S., & Frandsen, G. (2016). *Kozier & Erb's fundamentals of nursing: Concepts, process, and practice* (10th ed.). Upper Saddle River, NJ: Pearson.

Blakemore, S. (2012). Drive to screen all adult inpatients for risk of blood clots will save lives. *Nursing Older People, 24*(9), 7. doi:10.7748/nop2012.11.24.9.7.p9734

Choi, M., & Hector, M. (2012). Management of venous thromboembolism for older adults in long-term care facilities. *Journal of the American Academy of Nurse Practitioners, 24*, 335–344. doi:10.1111/j.1745-7599.2012.00733.x

Elpern, E., Killeen, K., Patel, G., & Senecal, P. A. (2013). The application of intermittent pneumatic compression devices for thromboprophylaxis. *American Journal of Nursing, 113*(4), 30–36. doi:10.1097/01.NAJ.0000428736.48428.10

Meetoo, D. (2013). Understanding and managing deep vein thrombosis. *Nurse Prescribing, 11*, 390–395.

Warren, E. (2013). Ten things the practice nurse can do about peripheral arterial disease. *Practice Nurse, 43*(12), 14–18.

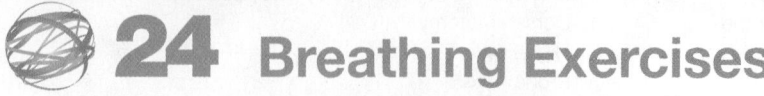

24 Breathing Exercises

LEARNING OUTCOMES

At the completion of this chapter, the student will be able to:

1. Define the key terms used in the skills of breathing exercises.
2. State nursing interventions to maintain the normal respirations of a client.
3. Describe abnormal breathing patterns and sounds.
4. Recognize when it is appropriate to delegate the performance of breathing exercises and use of the incentive spirometer to unlicensed assistive personnel.

5. Verbalize the steps used in:
   a. Teaching abdominal (diaphragmatic) breathing.
   b. Using an incentive spirometer.
6. Demonstrate appropriate documentation and reporting of use of an incentive spirometer.

SKILLS

Skill 24–1 Teaching Abdominal (Diaphragmatic) Breathing

Skill 24–2 Using an Incentive Spirometer

KEY TERMS

abdominal (diaphragmatic) breathing, 575
atelectasis, 580
chronic obstructive pulmonary disease (COPD), 575
expectorate, 575
flow-oriented SMI, 578
huff coughing, 575
incentive spirometer, 578
mucus clearance device (MCD), 576
orthopneic position, 574
pursed-lip breathing, 575
sustained maximal inspiration devices (SMIs), 578
tripod position, 574
volume-oriented SMI, 578

Most people in good health give little thought to their respiratory function. Changing position frequently, ambulating, and exercising usually maintain adequate ventilation and gas exchange. Client Teaching Considerations lists other ways to promote healthy breathing. Many people tend to breathe in a shallow fashion and do not draw air into the lowest regions of the lungs, thus limiting potential gas exchange.

Mounting evidence supports the use of slow, abdominal breathing to facilitate pain relief (see Chapter 9 ∞) and to decrease blood pressure in clients with essential hypertension (Jones, Sangthong, & Pachirat, 2010). Deep, slow breathing also facilitates the beneficial "relaxation response" identified by Dr. Herbert Benson (1996).

PROMOTING OXYGENATION

When people become ill, their respiratory function may be inhibited because of pain and immobility. Shallow respirations inhibit both diaphragmatic excursion and lung distensibility. The result of inadequate chest expansion is pooling of respiratory secretions, which ultimately harbor microorganisms and promote infection. Additionally, shallow respirations may potentiate alveolar collapse, which may cause decreased diffusion of gases and subsequent hypoxemia. This situation is often compounded when opioids are given for pain, because they further depress the rate and depth of respiration.

Interventions by the nurse to maintain the normal respirations of clients include:

- Positioning the client to allow for maximum chest expansion
- Encouraging or providing frequent changes in position
- Encouraging deep breathing and coughing
- Encouraging ambulation.

The semi-Fowler's or high-Fowler's position allows maximum chest expansion and encourages deeper breaths in clients who are confined to bed, particularly those with dyspnea. The nurse also encourages clients to turn from side to side frequently, so that alternate sides of the chest are permitted maximum expansion. Sitting in a chair and ambulating also increases lung capacity and encourages deeper breaths.

Clients in respiratory distress cannot lie flat in bed. They must sit up to relieve their dyspnea or labored breathing. This is called the **orthopneic position**, which is an adaptation of the high-Fowler's position. Some clients also sit upright and lean on their arms or elbows. This is called the **tripod position** (Figure 24–1 ■). Clients with dyspnea often sit in bed and lean over their overbed tables (which are raised to a suitable height), sometimes with a pillow for support. A client in this position can also press the lower part of the chest against

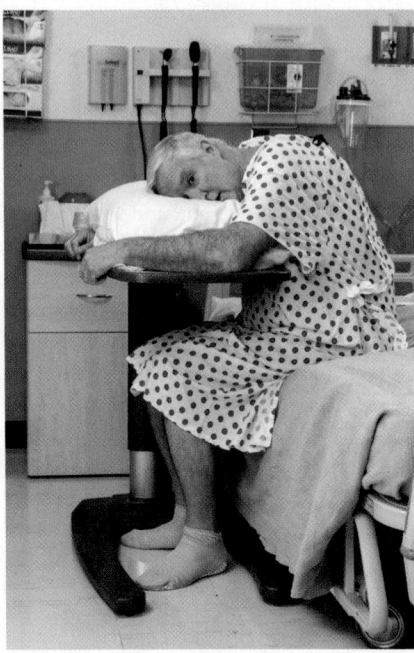

Figure 24–2 ■ A client using the overbed table to assist with breathing.

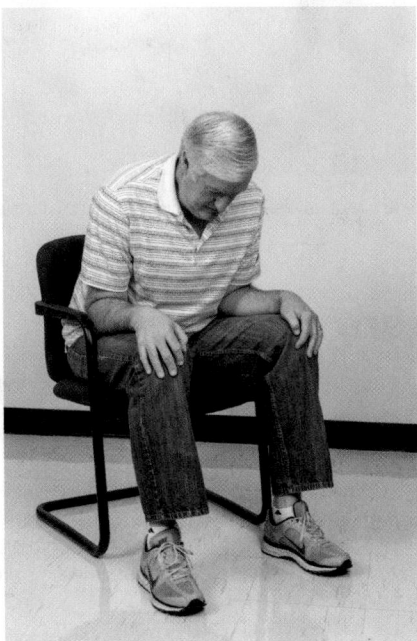

Figure 24–1 ■ Tripod position to assist breathing.

the table to help in exhaling (Figure 24–2 ■). The advantage of these positions is that the position forces the diaphragm down and forward and stabilizes the chest, which reduces the work of breathing.

DEEP BREATHING AND COUGHING

The nurse can facilitate respiratory functioning by encouraging deep-breathing exercises and coughing to remove secretions from the airways. When coughing raises secretions high enough, the client may either **expectorate** (cough up) or swallow them. Swallowing the secretions is not harmful, but it does not allow the nurse to view the secretions for documentation purposes or to obtain a specimen for testing.

Breathing exercises are frequently indicated for clients with restricted chest expansion, such as people with **chronic obstructive pulmonary disease (COPD)** or clients recovering from thoracic or abdominal surgery. COPD is a disease process that decreases the ability of the lungs to perform ventilation. Instructing and encouraging the client to take deep, sustained breaths is among the safest, most effective, and least expensive strategies for keeping the lungs expanded.

Commonly employed breathing exercises are abdominal (diaphragmatic) and pursed-lip breathing. **Abdominal (diaphragmatic) breathing** permits deep, full breaths with little effort. **Pursed-lip breathing** helps the client develop control over breathing and helps alleviate dyspnea (Facchiano, Snyder, & Núñez, 2011). The pursed lips create a resistance to the air flowing out of the lungs, thereby prolonging exhalation and preventing airway collapse by maintaining positive airway pressure. The client is taught to inhale normally through the nose and exhale through pursed lips as if about to whistle and blow slowly and purposefully, tightening the abdominal muscles to assist with exhalation. Clients may practice by slowly blowing a ping-pong ball across a table or visualizing that they are trying to make a candle flame waver.

Forceful, repeated coughing is often ineffective and can cause pain for a postsurgical client. Some clients may lack the strength or ability to cough normally. Normal forceful coughing involves the client inhaling deeply and then coughing twice while exhaling. Another cough technique such as forced expiratory technique, or **huff coughing**, may be taught as an alternative for those clients who are unable to perform a normal forceful cough. A client with a pulmonary condition (e.g., COPD) is instructed to exhale through pursed lips and to exhale with a "huff" sound in mid-exhalation. The huff cough helps prevent high expiratory pressures that collapse diseased airways and helps keep the airways open while moving secretions up and out of the lungs (Hess, MacIntyre, Mishoe, Galvin, & Adams, 2012). Skill 24–1 explains how to teach clients to perform abdominal (diaphragmatic) breathing exercises and provides instructions for coughing techniques.

A **mucus clearance device (MCD)** is used for clients with excessive secretions caused by disorders such as cystic fibrosis, COPD, and bronchiectasis. The Flutter mucus clearance device is an example of one of these devices. It is a small, handheld device with a hard plastic mouthpiece at one end and a perforated cover at the other end. Inside the device is a steel ball that sits in a circular cone shape (Figure 24–3 ■). The client inhales slowly and then, keeping the cheeks firm, exhales quickly through the device. This causes the steel ball to move up and down, resulting in vibrations that loosen mucus and assist its movement up the airways to be expectorated (Hess et al., 2012).

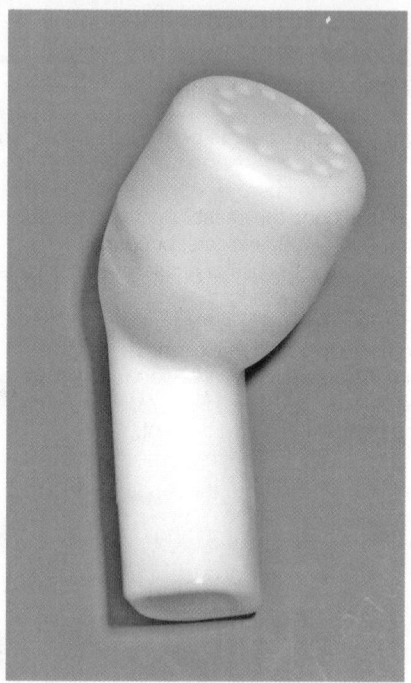

Figure 24–3 ■ Mucus clearance device, also known as a "Flutter."

●○○● NURSING PROCESS: DEEP BREATHING AND COUGHING

Teaching Abdominal (Diaphragmatic) Breathing

ASSESSMENT

The following items relate to various aspects of the history and assessment of clients relative to respiratory techniques. Also see Skill 3–11, Assessing the Thorax and Lungs, in Chapter 3 ∞.

Assess:

- *Current respiratory problems:* What recent changes has the client experienced in breathing pattern (e.g., shortness of breath; difficulty breathing; need to be in an upright position to breathe; use of accessory neck, shoulder, intercostal, or abdominal muscles during respirations; or rapid and shallow breathing)? Which activities might cause the preceding symptom(s) to occur? What pollutants has the client been exposed to?
- *History of respiratory disease:* Has the client had colds, allergies, asthma, tuberculosis, bronchitis, pneumonia, or emphysema? How frequently have these occurred? How long did they last? How were they treated?
- *Presence of a cough:* Is it productive or nonproductive? If a cough is productive, when is sputum produced? What are the amount, color, thickness, and odor (e.g., thick, frothy, pink, rusty, or blood tinged)?
- *Lifestyle:* Does the client smoke? If so, how much? Do any members of the client's family smoke? Are there any occupational hazards (e.g., inhaling fumes) to the respiratory system?
- *Pain:* Does the client experience any pain associated with breathing or activity? Where is the pain located? What words does the client use to describe the pain? How long does it last, and how does it affect breathing? What activities precede the pain? Does anything make the pain better or worse?
- *Medication history:* Has the client taken or does the client take any over-the-counter or prescription medications for breathing? Which ones? What are the dosages, times taken, and effects on the client, including side effects?

Observe (see Box 24–1 for definitions and description of terms):

- Breathing pattern (rate, rhythm, depth, and quality). Note any signs of hyperventilation, hypoventilation, tachypnea, or bradypnea.
- Ease or effort of breathing and posture assumed for breathing (e.g., orthopneic).
- Breath sounds audible without amplification (e.g., stridor, wheezes).
- Chest movements (e.g., retractions, flail chest, or paradoxical breathing). Note the specific location of retractions: intercostals, substernal, suprasternal, or supraclavicular.
- Clinical signs of hypoxia (e.g., increased pulse rate, rapid or deep respirations, cyanosis of the skin and nail beds, restlessness, anxiety, dizziness [vertigo], or faintness [syncope]).
- The location of any surgical incision in relation to the muscles needed for breathing. An incision can impede appropriate lung expansion.

Palpate for:

- Respiratory excursion (see Chapter 3 ∞).
- Vocal (tactile) fremitus (see Chapter 3 ∞).

Percuss the chest for:

- Diaphragmatic excursion (see Chapter 3 ∞).
- Chest sounds (flatness, dullness, resonance, hyperresonance, or tympany).

Auscultate the lungs for:

- Breath sounds (normal, adventitious, or absent). (See Tables 3–5 and 3–6 in Chapter 3 ∞.)

Check the results of:

- Sputum analysis.
- Venous blood samples (e.g., complete blood count).
- Arterial blood samples (blood gases).
- Pulmonary function tests.
- Pulse oximetry.

Teaching Abdominal (Diaphragmatic) Breathing—*continued*

PLANNING
DELEGATION

Unlicensed assistive personnel (UAP) can reinforce and assist clients in performing breathing exercises. However, it is the responsibility of the nurse to teach the client the breathing exercises, to evaluate the effectiveness of the teaching, and to assess the outcomes of the breathing exercises (e.g., ease of breathing, effectiveness of cough, and breath sounds).

INTERPROFESSIONAL PRACTICE

Teaching deep breathing and coughing may be within the scope of practice for specific health care providers. For example, in addition to nurses, respiratory therapists may teach and reinforce this skill. Although these therapists may verbally communicate their findings and plan to the health care team members, the nurse must also know where to locate their documentation in the client's medical record.

Equipment
None (although a pillow is optional for splinting an abdominal or thoracic incision).

IMPLEMENTATION
Preparation
- Before starting to teach breathing exercises, determine if the location of a surgical incision prevents deep breathing because of pain. If so, administer analgesic medication 30 minutes prior to implementing deep-breathing exercises.

Performance
1. Prior to performing the procedure, introduce self and verify the client's identity using agency protocol. Explain to the client what you are going to do, why it is necessary, and how he or she can participate. Discuss how deep breathing and coughing will help keep the lungs expanded and clear of secretions, thus preventing respiratory complications.
2. Perform hand hygiene and observe other appropriate infection prevention procedures.
3. Provide for client privacy.
4. Prepare the client.
   - Assist the client to assume a comfortable semi-Fowler's or sitting position in bed or on a chair, or a lying position in bed with one pillow. **Rationale:** *This increases lung capacity and allows for deeper breathing.*
   - Have the client flex the knees. **Rationale:** *This relaxes the muscles of the abdomen.*
   - Have the client place one or both hands on the abdomen just below the ribs. **Rationale:** *This will help the client to evaluate depth of inspiration through movement of the abdomen.*
5. Perform abdominal breathing. Instruct the client to:
   - Breathe in deeply through the nose with the mouth closed, to stay relaxed, not to arch the back, and to concentrate on feeling the abdomen rise as far as possible. **Rationale:** *When a person breathes in, the diaphragm contracts (drops), the lungs fill with air, and the abdomen rises or protrudes.*
   - Hold the breath for 3 to 5 seconds. **Rationale:** *This helps keep the alveoli open.*
   - Breathe out slowly.
   - Perform relaxed diaphragmatic breathing as needed for respiratory status.
6. Perform forced expiratory technique (huff coughing) as the next step, if needed (e.g., if coughing is going to be beneficial to maintain or improve oxygenation).
   - Instruct clients who have had thoracic or abdominal surgery to place their hands or a pillow over the incisional site and to apply gentle pressure while deep breathing or coughing. **Rationale:** *This helps decrease incisional strain and discomfort and facilitates effective coughing.*
   - Instruct the client to take three to four slow deep breaths, inhaling through the nose and exhaling through pursed lips as if gently blowing out a candle. **Rationale:** *Increasing lung volume increases airflow through the small airways, expands the lungs, and helps mobilize secretions on expiration.* Limit the active deep breaths. **Rationale:** *This helps avoid fatigue and hyperventilation.*
   - Ask the client to inhale deeply and hold his or her breath for a few seconds.
   - Instruct the client to cough twice while exhaling. **Rationale:** *The first cough loosens the mucus; the second expels the secretions.*
   - For huff coughing, the client leans forward and exhales sharply with a "huff" sound mid-exhalation. **Rationale:** *This helps keep the airways open while moving secretions up and out of the lungs.*
   - Inhale by taking rapid short breaths in succession ("sniffing"). **Rationale:** *This prevents mucus from moving back into smaller airways.*
   - Allow the client to rest and breathe slowly between coughs. Try to avoid prolonged episodes of coughing. **Rationale:** *Prolonged episodes may cause fatigue and hypoxia.*
   - Instruct the client to perform several relaxed diaphragmatic breaths before the next cough effort.
7. Document the teaching and assessments for the exercises performed and the client's response.

Variation: Pursed-Lip Breathing
- Teach the client to inhale through the nose and then, pursing lips as if about to whistle, breathe out slowly and gently, making a slow "whooshing" sound without puffing out the cheeks. **Rationale:** *This pursed-lip breathing creates a resistance to air flowing out of the lungs, increases pressure within the bronchi (main air passages), and minimizes collapse of smaller airways, a common problem for people with COPD.*
- Instruct the client to inhale deeply through the nose and count to 3.
- Have the client concentrate on tightening the abdominal muscles while breathing out slowly and evenly through pursed lips while counting to 7 or until the client cannot exhale any more. **Rationale:** *Tightening the abdominal muscles and leaning forward help compress the lungs and enhance effective exhalation.*
- Teach the client how to perform pursed-lip breathing while walking: Inhale while taking two steps, then exhale through pursed lips while taking the next four steps.
- Instruct the client to use this exercise whenever feeling short of breath and to increase gradually to 5 to 10 minutes four times a day. **Rationale:** *Regular practice will help the client do this type of breathing without conscious effort.*

EVALUATION
- Determine the client's ability to perform the breathing exercises and to comply with the instructions.
- Compare current assessment data (e.g., ease of breathing, cough, secretions) to prior assessment data gathered before starting the breathing exercises.
- Report significant deviations from normal to the primary care provider.

BOX 24–1   Abnormal Breathing Patterns and Sounds

BREATHING PATTERNS
Rate
- *Tachypnea*—rapid respiration marked by quick, shallow breaths
- *Bradypnea*—abnormally slow breathing
- *Apnea*—cessation of breathing

Volume/Depth
- *Hyperventilation*—an increase in the amount of air in the lungs; characterized by prolonged and deep breaths
- *Hypoventilation*—reduction in the amount of air in the lungs; characterized by shallow respirations

Rhythm
- *Cheyne-Stokes breathing*—rhythmic waxing and waning of respirations, from very deep to very shallow breathing and temporary apnea

Ease or Effort
- *Dyspnea*—difficult and labored breathing during which the individual has a persistent, unsatisfied need for air and feels distressed
- *Orthopnea*—ability to breathe only in upright sitting or standing positions

BREATH SOUNDS
Audible Without Amplification
- *Stridor*—a shrill, harsh sound heard during inspiration with laryngeal obstruction
- *Stertor*—snoring or sonorous respiration, usually due to a partial obstruction of the upper airway
- *Wheeze*—continuous, high-pitched musical squeak or whistling sound occurring on expiration and sometimes on inspiration when air moves through a narrowed or partially obstructed airway
- *Bubbling*—gurgling sounds heard as air passes through moist secretions in the respiratory tract

Audible by Stethoscope
- *Crackles (rales)*—dry or wet crackling sounds simulated by rolling a lock of hair near the ear; generally heard on inspiration as air moves through accumulated moist secretions (Fine to medium crackles occur when air passes through moisture in small air passages and alveoli; medium to coarse crackles occur when air passes through moisture in the bronchioles, bronchi, and trachea.)
- *Gurgles (rhonchi)*—continuous, coarse, low-pitched, harsh, moaning or snoring sound more audible during expiration as the air moves through tenacious mucus or narrowed bronchi
- *Wheeze*—continuous, high-pitched musical squeak or whistling sound occurring on expiration and sometimes on inspiration when air moves through a narrowed or partially obstructed airway
- *Pleural friction rub*—coarse, leathery, or grating sound produced by the rubbing together of inflamed pleura

CHEST MOVEMENTS
- *Intercostal retraction*—indrawing between the ribs
- *Substernal retraction*—indrawing beneath the breastbone
- *Suprasternal retraction*—indrawing above the breastbone
- *Supraclavicular retraction*—indrawing above the clavicles
- *Tracheal tug*—indrawing and downward pull of the trachea during inspiration
- *Flail chest*—the ballooning out of the chest wall through injured rib spaces; results in paradoxical breathing, during which the chest wall balloons on expiration but is depressed or sucked inward on inspiration

SECRETIONS AND COUGHING
- *Hemoptysis*—the presence of blood in the sputum
- *Productive cough*—a cough accompanied by expectorated secretions
- *Nonproductive cough*—a dry, harsh cough without secretions

INCENTIVE SPIROMETRY

Incentive spirometers, also referred to as **sustained maximal inspiration devices (SMIs)**, measure the flow of air inhaled through the mouthpiece and are used to:

- Improve pulmonary ventilation.
- Counteract the effects of anesthesia or hypoventilation.
- Loosen respiratory secretions.
- Facilitate respiratory gaseous exchange.

Incentive spirometry is designed to mimic natural sighing or yawning by encouraging the client to take long, slow, deep breaths. It is a commonly used device because it is simple and cost effective. Two general types are the flow-oriented spirometer and the volume-oriented spirometer.

The **flow-oriented SMI** consists of one or more clear plastic chambers containing freely movable colored balls or disks. The balls or disks are elevated as the client inhales. The client is asked to keep them elevated as long as possible with a maximal sustained inhalation (Figure 24–4 ■). The longer the inspiratory flow is maintained, the larger the volume, so the client is encouraged to take slow, deep breaths. Unfortunately, a client can generate a high flow (with low volume) by taking a quick, forceful inhalation. When doing this, the client does not meet the therapeutic volume or deep-breathing objectives. Therefore, effective client education is necessary. Flow-oriented SMIs are low-cost devices, are often disposable, and can be used independently by

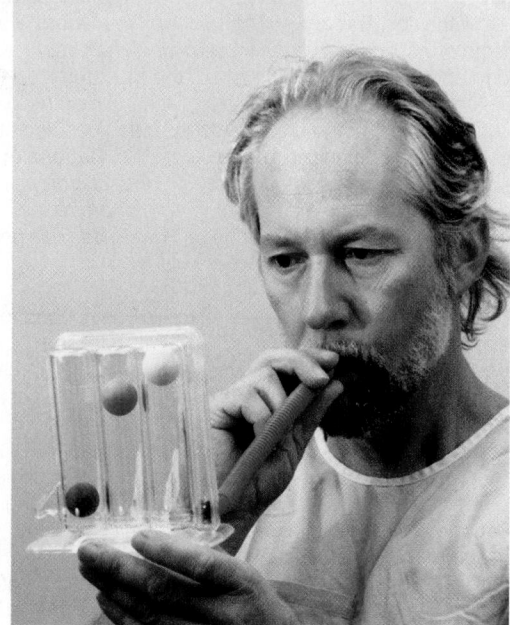

Figure 24–4 ■ Flow-oriented SMI or incentive spirometer.

clients. They do not, however, measure the specific volume of air inhaled.

The **volume-oriented SMI**, in contrast, measures the inhalation volume maintained by the client. A plastic disposable device is shown in Figure 24–5 ■. When the client inhales, a piston-like plate or accordion-pleated cylinder rises as the client inspires, and markings on the side indicate the volume of inspiration achieved by the client.

When using an incentive spirometer, the client should be assisted into, preferably, an upright sitting position in bed or on a chair. This position facilitates maximum ventilation. Skill 24–2 describes how to assist a client with an incentive spirometer or SMI.

A number of recent studies (Davis, 2012; Wren, Martin, Yoon, & Bech, 2010) compared clients who received deep-breathing exercises alone with clients who received deep-breathing exercises and incentive spirometry. The results were positive, with some studies stating that the addition of incentive spirometry improved lung function, reduced pulmonary complications, and shortened hospital stay. Other studies, however, stated there was no evidence of benefit from the use of incentive spirometry (Lamar, 2012). The studies often recommended the need for additional research to determine the role of incentive spirometry. Given the changing health care environment and increasing economic constraints in health care, it is possible that incentive spirometers may not be prescribed on a routine basis, but will be reserved primarily for clients who are at high risk for pulmonary complications, such as postoperative clients.

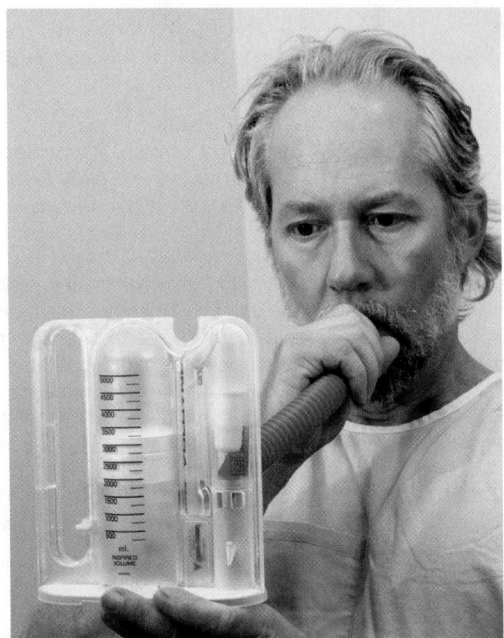

Figure 24–5 ■ Plastic disposable volume-oriented SMI.

●○● NURSING PROCESS: INCENTIVE SPIROMETRY

Using an Incentive Spirometer

ASSESSMENT
- Auscultate the client's lungs before use of the incentive spirometer.
- Note the location of a surgical incision that could impede lung expansion. If present, assess pain level and determine if an analgesic may facilitate use of the SMI device.
- Determine the client's knowledge level pertaining to correct use of the device.
- Ensure that the incentive spirometer is not contraindicated (e.g., clients with tachypnea).

PLANNING
Before assisting a client to use an SMI device, determine the "target" inspiratory volume level as an incentive for the client. This can be based on the preoperative assessment, if done, or use the guide included in the manufacturer's literature.

DELEGATION

It is the responsibility of the nurse to teach the client how to use the incentive spirometer, assess the client's performance, and evaluate the outcomes of the therapy. UAP, however, can reinforce and assist clients in using the incentive spirometer. The nurse should inform the UAP of the key points to using the incentive spirometer correctly.

INTERPROFESSIONAL PRACTICE

Teaching how to use an incentive spirometer may be within the scope of practice for specific health care providers. For example, in addition to nurses, respiratory therapists may teach and reinforce this skill. Although these therapist may verbally communicate their findings and plan to the health care team members, the nurse must also know where to locate their documentation in the client's medical record.

Equipment
- Flow-oriented or volume-oriented SMI
- Mouthpiece or breathing tube
- Label for mouthpiece
- Progress chart
- Nose clip (optional)

IMPLEMENTATION
Preparation
- Determine if the client has a disposable SMI at the bedside.
- This skill should not be performed immediately after a meal or other physically stressful activity.

Performance
1. Prior to performing the skill, introduce self and verify the client's identity using agency protocol. Explain to the client what you are going to do, why it is necessary, and how he or she can participate. Discuss how the results will be used in planning further care or treatments.

2. Perform hand hygiene and observe other appropriate infection prevention procedures.
3. Provide for client privacy.
4. Prepare the client.
   - Assist the client to an upright position in bed or on a chair. If the person is unable to assume a sitting position for a flow spirometer, have the person assume any position. **Rationale:** *A sitting position facilitates maximum ventilation of the lungs.*

SKILL 24–2

Continued on page 580

Using an Incentive Spirometer—*continued*

For a Flow-Oriented SMI

* Instruct the client to use the spirometer as follows:
    a. Hold the spirometer in the upright position. **Rationale:** *A tilted flow-oriented spirometer requires less effort to raise the balls or disks; a volume-oriented device will not function correctly unless upright.*
    b. Exhale normally.
    c. Seal the lips tightly around the mouthpiece, take in a slow deep breath to elevate the balls, and then hold the breath for 2 seconds initially, increasing to 6 seconds (optimum) to keep the balls elevated if possible. Instruct the client to *avoid* brisk low-volume breaths that snap the balls to the top of the chamber. The client may use a nose clip if the person has difficulty breathing only through the mouth. **Rationale:** *A slow, deep breath ensures maximal ventilation. Greater lung expansion is achieved with a very slow inspiration than with a brisk shallow breath. Sustained elevation of the balls ensures adequate ventilation of the alveoli (lung air sacs).*
    d. Remove the mouthpiece and exhale normally.
    e. Cough productively, as needed, after using the spirometer. **Rationale:** *Deep ventilation may loosen secretions and stimulate coughing. Effective coughing can facilitate the removal of the loose secretions.*
    f. Relax and take several normal breaths before using the spirometer again.
    g. Repeat the procedure to a total of 10 breaths, encouraging the client to take progressively deeper breaths up to the maximal goal.
    h. Repeat the series of breaths once each hour while awake. **Rationale:** *Practice increases inspiratory volume, maintains alveolar ventilation, and prevents* **atelectasis** *(collapse of the air sacs).*

For a Volume-Oriented SMI

* Set the spirometer to a "target" volume. **Rationale:** *This provides an incentive and motivation for the client. The nurse can start low and increase the "target" after client success.*
* Instruct the client to use the spirometer as follows:
    a. Exhale normally.
    b. Seal the lips tightly around the mouthpiece and take in a slow, deep breath until the piston is elevated to the predetermined level. The piston level may be visible to the client to identify the volume obtained.
    c. Hold the breath for 6 seconds to ensure maximal alveolar ventilation.
    d. Remove the mouthpiece and exhale normally.
    e. Cough productively, as needed, after using the spirometer. **Rationale:** *Deep ventilation may loosen secretions and stimulate coughing. Effective coughing can facilitate the removal of the loose secretions.*
    f. Relax and take several normal breaths before using the spirometer again.
    g. Repeat the procedure to a total of 10 breaths, encouraging the client to take progressively deeper breaths up to the maximal goal.
    h. Repeat the series of breaths once each hour while awake. **Rationale:** *Practice increases inspiratory volume, maintains alveolar ventilation, and prevents atelectasis.*
    i. Encourage the client to record the top volume achieved at each hour he or she performed the technique. **Rationale:** *This facilitates cooperation of the client and assists in evaluating outcomes of the skill.*

For All Devices

5. Clean the equipment.
    * Clean the mouthpiece with water and shake it dry. Label the mouthpiece and a disposable SMI with the client's name. A disposable SMI may be left at the bedside for the client to use as prescribed.
6. Document all relevant information.
    * Record the skill, including type of spirometer, number of breaths taken, volume or flow levels achieved, client response, and results of auscultation. Also include, when appropriate, client education and the ability of the client to perform the procedure without prompting.

SAMPLE DOCUMENTATION

6/12/2015 1030 Coarse rales in RLL. Instructed on use of incentive spirometer. Able to use correctly and raise one ball for 3 seconds. Use of IS stimulated cough resulting in production of small amount light-colored thick mucus. Encouraged to continue using IS each hour. —————————————————————— S. Lee, RN

EVALUATION

* Conduct appropriate follow-up:
    * Auscultate lung sounds and compare to sounds heard before the procedure.
    * Assess the client's color, heart rate, and respiratory rate.
    * Assess the degree of dyspnea before, during, and after use of the incentive spirometer. Watch for fatigue or dizziness in the client.
* Compare current findings with previous inspiratory volume levels and note the trend of the data.
* Report significant deviations from normal to the primary care provider.

LIFESPAN CONSIDERATIONS Incentive Spirometers

CHILDREN

* Consider the developmental level of the child when choosing a method to promote breathing exercises. Examples include an incentive spirometer, pinwheels, or other blow toys.
* The SMI device can be a game for young clients. Demonstrate the procedure beforehand and show the child how to take slow, deep breaths.
* Nasal clips may be needed if the younger client does not understand how to prevent breathing through the nose.

OLDER ADULTS

* Older adults may have trouble sealing their lips around the mouthpiece of a spirometer because of dentures or a dry mouth.

- Show the client how to use and clean the SMI device.
- Make certain the client understands how often to use the SMI.
- Ask the client to demonstrate use of the SMI.
- Evaluate the client's ability to use the SMI.

- Provide client with a time schedule for SMI use and instruct client to record use and results.
- Offer written material to reinforce verbal instructions.

Chapter 24 Review

FOCUSING ON CLINICAL THINKING

Consider This

1. Your assigned client, a 45-year-old male, had emergency abdominal surgery last night. He smoked one pack of cigarettes a day prior to surgery. Because of the emergency nature of the surgery, he received no preoperative teaching about deep breathing, coughing, or the incentive spirometer that is sitting at his bedside. He refuses to perform any breathing exercises or to use the incentive spirometer. What will you do?

2. At your next visit after observing the client using the flow-oriented SMI correctly, you ask the client how it is working. The client reports that he stopped using it because coughing after its use was nonproductive. What would you say to the client?

See Focusing on Clinical Thinking answers on student resource website.

TEST YOUR KNOWLEDGE

1. The nurse is telling a client with chronic obstructive pulmonary disease (COPD) to breathe out slowly and gently, like blowing out a candle, to prolong exhalation. The nurse is teaching the client what type of breathing? _____

2. The nurse is caring for a client who is 36 hours postoperative following chest surgery. On entering the client's room, the nurse finds the client leaning forward and coughing while exhaling. The nurse recognizes that the client:
   1. Is not working effectively to clear the airways.
   2. Is properly performing huff coughing.
   3. Is in respiratory distress.
   4. Needs further teaching on how to cough and deep breathe.

3. A postoperative surgical client has a respiratory rate of 22 per minute, audible rhonchi in the lower lobes, and an oxygen saturation of 90%. The nurse uses which strategies to improve gas exchange? Select all that apply.
   1. Position the client in the orthopneic position.
   2. Position the client in a supine or prone position.
   3. Encourage bed rest.
   4. Encourage ambulation.
   5. Encourage fluids.

4. The nurse assesses the postoperative client's respirations and finds that the client is breathing shallowly. When encouraged to take deep breaths the client says, "It hurts when I take a deep breath." To assist the client to breathe deeply, the nurse would use which strategy?
   1. Teach the client to use a pillow to splint the incision site while deep breathing.
   2. Apply a binder to the chest to splint the incision.
   3. Encourage the client to reduce fluid intake to prevent production of secretions.
   4. Position the client in a high-Fowler's position.

5. When assessing the client's breath sounds, the nurse auscultates a continuous high-pitched musical squeak/whistle on expiration. The nurse recognizes this is the result of:
   1. Laryngeal obstruction.
   2. Fluid in the air passages and alveoli.
   3. Pleural friction rub.
   4. Narrowed or partially obstructed airway.

6. The nurse assesses the client's respiratory effort and notes indrawing of muscles beneath the breastbone with inspiration. How would the nurse document this assessment?
   1. Intercostal retractions
   2. Substernal retractions
   3. Suprasternal retractions
   4. Supraclavicular retractions

7. The client is providing a return demonstration of abdominal breathing. Which action by the client determines that the nurse's teaching has been effective?
   1. Breathes quickly in and out through the mouth
   2. Arches the back while breathing
   3. Takes a deep breath through the nose
   4. Places the hands behind the head

8. After teaching the client how to use abdominal breathing, the nurse goes on to teach the client how to huff cough. The nurse has the client do which action prior to coughing?
   1. Exhale through the mouth.
   2. Exhale through the nose.
   3. Inhale deeply and hold the breath for a few seconds.
   4. Inhale deeply.

9. The nurse is caring for a client who is 36 hours postoperative following chest surgery. After teaching the client how to use an incentive spirometer, the nurse recognizes that further teaching is needed when the client does which action?

    1. Uses the SMI immediately after eating.

    2. Takes slow deep breaths.

    3. Assumes an upright sitting position.

    4. Exceeds the set volume level.

10. The nurse is choosing an incentive spirometer for the postoperative client and knows that a disadvantage of flow-oriented sustained maximal inspiration devices (SMIs) is:

    1. The client can generate a high flow with low volume by taking quick forceful inhalation and not meet the goal of therapy.

    2. They are expensive.

    3. They are difficult for a client to use.

    4. The client is unable to determine effectiveness without the nurse's evaluation.

See Answers to Test Your Knowledge in Appendix A.

READINGS AND REFERENCES

References

Benson, H. (1996). *Timeless healing: The power and biology of belief.* New York, NY: Scribner.

Davis, S. P. (2012). Incentive spirometry after abdominal surgery. *Nursing Times, 108,* 22–23.

Facchiano, L., Snyder, C., & Núñez, D. E. (2011). A literature review on breathing retraining as a self-management strategy operationalized through Rosswurm and Larrabee's evidence-based practice model. *Journal of the American Academy of Nurse Practitioners, 23,* 421–426. doi:10.1111/j.1745-7599.2011.00623.x

Hess, D. R., MacIntyre, N. R., Mishoe, S. C., Galvin, W. F., & Adams, A. B. (2012). *Respiratory care: Principles and practice* (2nd ed.). Sudbury, MA: Jones & Bartlett.

Jones, C. U., Sangthong, B., & Pachirat, O. (2010). An inspiratory load enhances the antihypertensive effects of home-based training with slow deep breathing: A randomized trial. *Journal of Physiotherapy, 56,* 179–186.

Lamar, J. (2012). Relationship of respiratory care bundle with incentive spirometry to reduce pulmonary complications in a medical general practice unit. *MEDSURG Nursing, 21*(1), 33–37.

Wren, S. M., Martin, M., Yoon, J. K., & Bech, F. (2010). Postoperative pneumonia-prevention program for the inpatient surgical ward. *Journal of American College of Surgeons, 210,* 491–495. doi:10.1016/j.jamcollsurg.2010.01.009

Selected Bibliography

Berman, A., Snyder, S., & Frandsen, G. (2016). *Kozier & Erb's fundamentals of nursing: Concepts, process, and practice* (10th ed.). Upper Saddle River, NJ: Pearson.

Lange, B., Flynn, S., Chang, C., Rizzo, A., & Bolas, M. (2011). Breathe: A game to motivate the adherence of breathing exercises. *Journal of Physical Therapy Education, 25*(1), 30–35.

Wang, Q., Zhang, X., & Li, Q. (2010). Effects of a flutter mucus-clearance device on pulmonary function test results in healthy people 85 years and older in China. *Respiratory Care, 55*(11), 1449–1452.

Yamaguti, W., Sakamoto, E., Panazzolo, D., Peixoto, C., Cerri, G., & Albuquerque, A. (2010). Diaphragmatic mobility in healthy subjects during incentive spirometry with a flow-oriented device and with a volume-oriented device. *Jornal Brasileiro de Pneumologia, 36*(6), 738–745.

25 Oxygen Therapy

LEARNING OUTCOMES

At the completion of this chapter, the student will be able to:

1. Define the key terms used in the skills of oxygen delivery.
2. Identify indications and contraindications for oxygen therapy.
3. Describe oxygen delivery systems.
4. Recognize when it is appropriate to delegate oxygen therapy or measurement of peak expiratory flow to unlicensed assistive personnel.
5. Discuss the care of clients requiring noninvasive continuous positive pressure ventilation.

6. Verbalize the steps used in:
   a. Administering oxygen by cannula, mask, and face tent.
   b. Measuring peak expiratory flow.
7. Demonstrate appropriate documentation and reporting of oxygen therapy.

SKILLS

Skill 25–1 Administering Oxygen by Cannula, Face Mask, or Face Tent

Skill 25–2 Measuring Peak Expiratory Flow

KEY TERMS

bilevel positive airway pressure (BiPAP), *592*
continuous positive airway pressure (CPAP), *592*
face mask, *585*
face tents, *587*

fraction of inspired oxygen (FiO_2), *585*
humidifier, *584*
hypercapnia, *588*
hypercarbia, *588*
hypoxemia, *583*

nasal cannula, *585*
noninvasive positive pressure ventilation (NPPV), *592*
nonrebreather mask, *586*
obstructive sleep apnea (OSA), *592*
oxygen concentrators, *590*

partial rebreather mask, *586*
peak expiratory flow rate (PEFR), *591*
regulator, *583*
transtracheal catheter, *587*
Venturi mask, *586*

Clients who have difficulty ventilating all areas of their lungs, those whose gas exchange is impaired, or people with heart failure may benefit from supplemental oxygen therapy. Although oxygen is, of course, naturally occurring in our air, the medical administration of oxygen is considered to be a process similar to that of administering medications and requires comparable nursing actions. Determining the effectiveness of oxygen therapy involves several measures, including checking vital signs and peripheral blood oxygen saturation (pulse oximetry).

OXYGEN THERAPY

Supplemental oxygen is indicated for clients who have **hypoxemia** (decreased oxygen concentration of arterial blood), for example, people who have reduced ability for diffusion of oxygen through the respiratory membrane (e.g., as a result of pneumonia or cystic fibrosis), hyperventilation, or substantial loss of lung tissue due to tumors or surgery. Others who may require oxygen are those with severe anemia or blood loss, or similar conditions in which there are inadequate numbers of red blood cells or hemoglobin to carry the oxygen.

Oxygen therapy is prescribed by the primary care provider, who specifies the specific concentration, method of delivery, and depending on the method, liter flow per minute (L/min). The order may also call for the nurse to titrate the oxygen to achieve a desired saturation

level as measured by pulse oximetry (see Skill 2–7 in Chapter 2 ∞). When administering oxygen as an *emergency measure*, the nurse may initiate the therapy and then contact the primary care provider for an order.

Oxygen is supplied in two ways in health care facilities: by portable systems—cylinders or tanks—and from wall outlets. Generally, oxygen cylinders are encased in metal carriers equipped with wheels for transport and a broad flat base on which the cylinder stands at the bedside to prevent it from falling. When not in use, a cap on the top protects the valves and outlets. Accidentally opened outlets can turn a tank into a dangerous projectile. Tanks should be placed away from traffic areas, anywhere they can be knocked or fall over, and heat sources. Long-term care or assisted living facilities may use similar oxygen supplies or those used more commonly in the home.

A **regulator** that releases oxygen at a safe level and at a desirable rate must be attached before the oxygen supply is used. On a cylinder, the content gauge indicates the pressure or amount of oxygen remaining in the tank, and the flow meter or flow indicator indicates the gas flow in L/min (Figure 25–1 ■). A flow meter is also required for wall-outlet systems. Flow is only indicated when the cylinder or wall-outlet system valve is open.

Oxygen administered from a cylinder or wall-outlet system is dry. Dry gases dehydrate the respiratory mucous membranes.

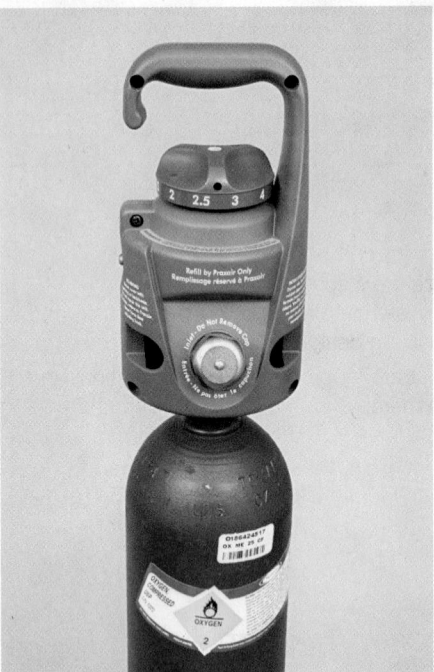

Figure 25–1 ■ An oxygen tank with regulator and flow indicator.

Humidifying devices such as a **humidifier** that add water vapor to inspired air are thus an essential adjunct of oxygen therapy, particularly for liter flows over 4 L/min. These devices provide 20% to 40% humidity. A humidifier bottle is one such device. It is attached below the flow meter gauge so that the oxygen passes through water and then through the specific oxygen tubing and equipment prescribed for the client (e.g., nasal cannula or mask) (Figure 25–2 ■).

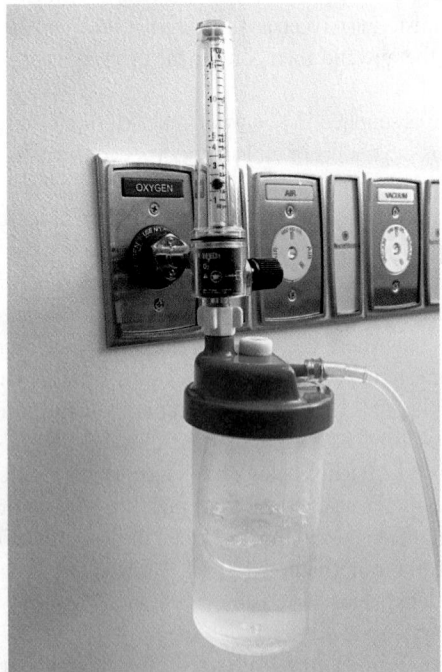

Figure 25–2 ■ An oxygen humidifier attatched to a wall-outlet oxygen flow meter.

Humidifiers prevent mucous membranes from drying and becoming irritated, and they loosen secretions for easier expectoration. Oxygen passing through water picks up water vapor before it reaches the client. The more bubbles created during this process, the more water vapor is produced. Very low liter flows (e.g., 1 to 2 L/min by nasal cannula) do not require humidification. When a client is breathing very low flow oxygen, enough atmospheric air is inhaled (which naturally has water vapor in it) to prevent mucosal drying.

Safety Precautions for Oxygen Therapy

Safety precautions are essential during oxygen therapy (Box 25–1). Although oxygen by itself will not burn or explode, it does facilitate combustion. For example, a bed sheet ordinarily burns slowly when ignited in the atmosphere; however, if saturated with free-flowing oxygen and ignited by a spark, it will burn rapidly and explosively. The greater the concentration of oxygen, the more rapidly fires start and burn, and such fires are difficult to extinguish. Because oxygen is colorless, odorless, and tasteless, people are often unaware of its presence. It is important to teach clients about this aspect of oxygen therapy.

Like any medication, oxygen is not completely harmless to the client. Clients can receive an inadequate amount or an excessive amount of oxygen, and both can lead to a decline in the client's condition. An inadequate amount of oxygen (hypoxia) will lead to cell death, and if left untreated, can ultimately lead to death. Excessive amounts of oxygen can lead to pulmonary tissue damage and increased duration of mechanical ventilation, ICU stays, and hospital lengths of stay (Blakeman, 2013; Kallet, 2012; Martin & Grocott, 2013). Oxygen toxicity can develop from breathing greater than 50% oxygen for 12 hours (Kallet, 2012). The lowest concentration needed to achieve the desired blood oxygen saturation (e.g., greater than 90% or a level prescribed by the primary care provider) should be used.

BOX 25–1 **Oxygen Therapy Safety Precautions**

- For home oxygen use or when the facility permits smoking, teach family members and visitors to smoke only outside or in provided smoking rooms away from the client and oxygen equipment.
- Place cautionary signs reading "No Smoking: Oxygen in Use" on the client's door, at the foot or head of the bed, and on the oxygen equipment.
- Instruct the client and visitors about the hazard of smoking when oxygen is in use.
- Make sure that electric devices (such as razors, hearing aids, radios, televisions, and heating pads) are in good working order to prevent the occurrence of short-circuit sparks.
- Avoid materials that generate static electricity, such as woolen blankets and synthetic fabrics. Cotton blankets should be used, and clients and caregivers should be advised to wear cotton fabrics.
- Avoid the use of volatile, flammable materials, such as oils, greases, alcohol, ether, and acetone (e.g., nail polish remover), near clients receiving oxygen.
- Be sure that electric monitoring equipment, suction machines, and portable diagnostic machines are all electrically grounded.
- Make known the location of fire extinguishers, and make sure personnel are trained in their use.

OXYGEN DELIVERY EQUIPMENT

Low-flow or high-flow systems are available to deliver oxygen to the client. The choice of system depends on the client's oxygen needs, comfort, and developmental considerations. Low-flow systems deliver oxygen via small-bore tubing. Low-flow administration devices include nasal cannulas, face masks, oxygen tents, and transtracheal catheters. Because room air is also inhaled along with the supplemental oxygen with these types of devices, the total concentration of oxygen in the inspired air, called **fraction of inspired oxygen (FiO$_2$)**, will vary depending on the respiratory rate, tidal volume, and L/min flow.

High-flow systems supply all of the oxygen required during ventilation in precise amounts, regardless of the client's respirations and effort. The high-flow system used to deliver a precise and consistent method for controlling the FiO$_2$ is a Venturi device with large-bore tubing.

Cannula

The **nasal cannula**, also called nasal prongs, is the most common inexpensive low-flow device used to administer oxygen. It is easy to apply and does not interfere with the client's ability to eat or talk. It also is relatively comfortable, permits some freedom of movement, and is well tolerated by both children and adults. It consists of a tube with short curved prongs that fit into the nostrils. One end of the tube connects to the oxygen supply. The cannula is often held in place by an elastic band that fits around the client's head or under the chin (Figure 25–3A ■). As long as the nasal airway is open, the cannula will deliver adequate oxygen, even to clients who breathe primarily through the mouth.

Cannulas deliver a relatively low concentration of oxygen (24% to 44%) at flow rates of 2 to 6 L/min. Each liter per minute adds approximately 4% more oxygen, and humidification may be recommended for flow rates greater than 4 L/min. Above 6 L/min, however, there is a tendency for the client to swallow air and the FiO$_2$ is not increased. When greater than 6 L/min is required to ensure adequate oxygenation, the client will require a mask, a rebreather mask, or possibly intubation and artificial ventilation. Limitations of the plain nasal cannula include the inability to deliver higher concentrations of oxygen and that it can be drying and irritating to mucous membranes.

A reservoir nasal cannula is an oxygen-conserving device (also referred to as an Oxymizer). It is used primarily in the home setting. It stores oxygen in the reservoir while the client breathes out and then delivers a 100% oxygen bolus when the client breathes in. As a result, it delivers a higher oxygen concentration at a lower flow rate than a plain nasal cannula, because it conserves oxygen. It can deliver FiO$_2$ of 0.5 or greater while providing the same benefits of a plain nasal cannula. The two styles of reservoir nasal cannulas (Oxymizers) are the mustache and pendant styles (See Figure 25–3B and C). Humidification is not necessary with the reservoir nasal cannula, because it collects the water vapor while the client breathes out, and returns it when the client breathes in.

Face Mask

A **face mask** that covers the client's nose and mouth may be used for oxygen inhalation. Most masks are made of clear, pliable plastic that can be molded to fit the face. They are held to the client's head with elastic bands. Some have a metal clip that can be bent over the bridge of the nose for a snug fit. There are several holes in the sides of the mask (exhalation ports) to allow the escape of exhaled carbon dioxide and intake of room air. To avoid rebreathing of carbon dioxide by the client while wearing a mask, a minimum 5 L/min oxygen flow rate is required.

Some masks have reservoir bags, which provide higher oxygen concentrations to the client. A portion of the client's expired air is directed into the bag. Because this air comes from the upper respiratory passages (e.g., the trachea and bronchi), where it does not take part in gaseous exchange, its oxygen concentration remains the same as that of inspired air.

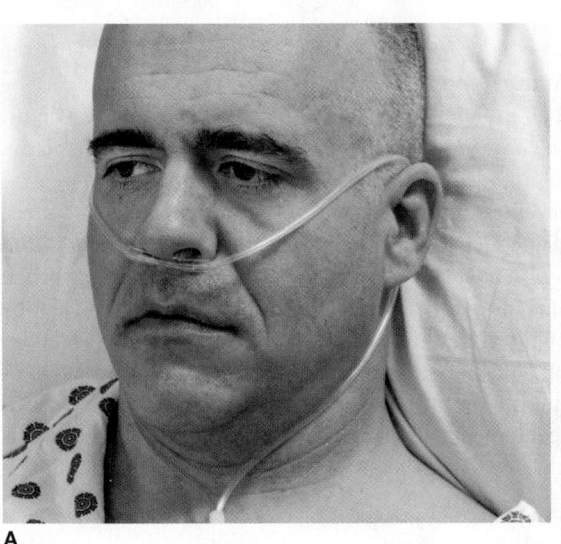
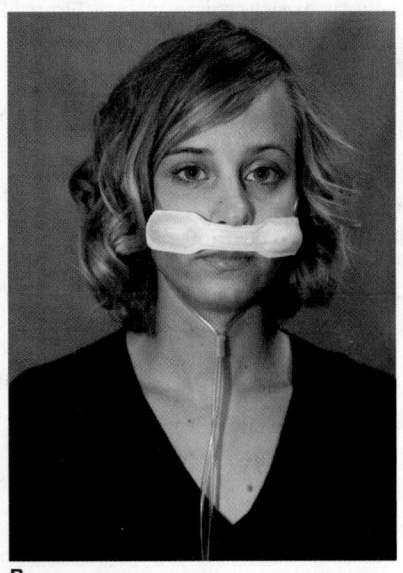
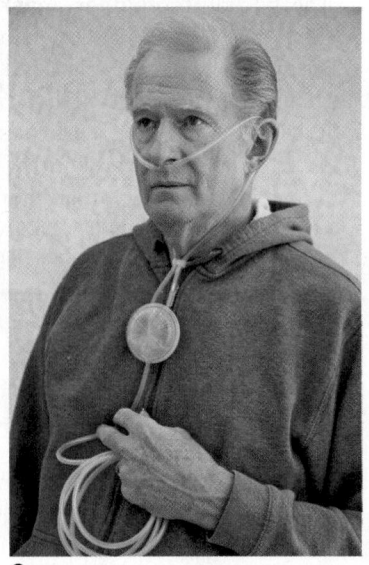

A   B   C

Figure 25–3 ■ *A,* A nasal cannula; *B,* mustache-style reservoir nasal cannula; *C,* pendant-style reservoir nasal cannula.

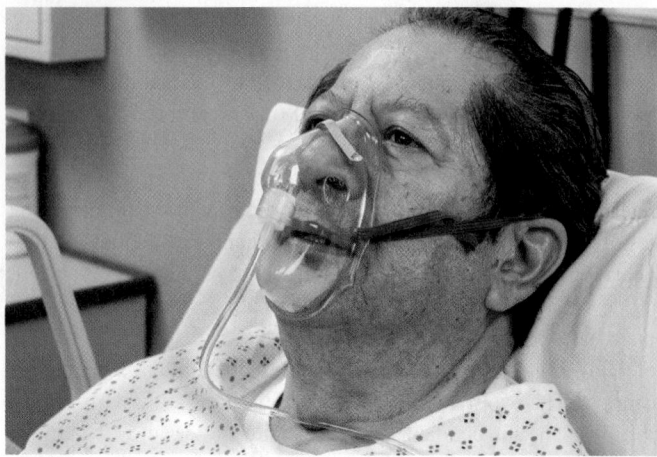

Figure 25–4 ■ A simple face mask.

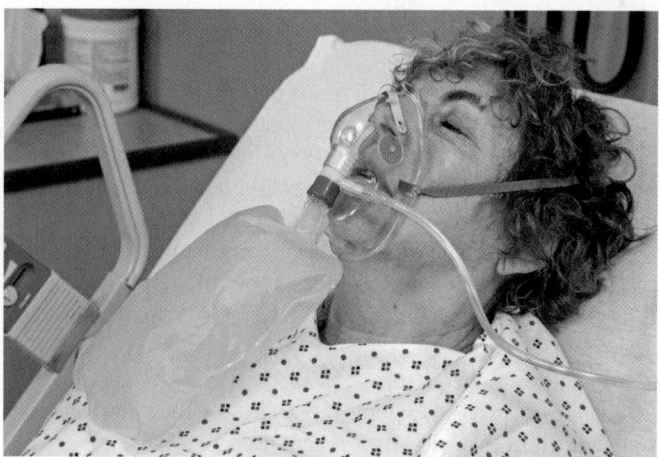

Figure 25–6 ■ A nonrebreather mask.

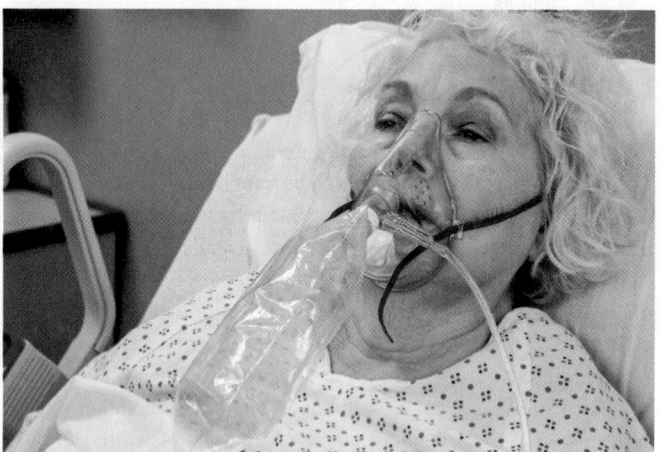

Figure 25–5 ■ A partial rebreather mask.

A variety of oxygen masks are marketed:

- The simple face mask delivers oxygen concentrations from 40% to 60% at liter flows of 5 to 8 L/min (Figure 25–4 ■).
- The **partial rebreather mask** delivers oxygen concentrations of 40% to 60% at liter flows of 6 to 10 L/min. The oxygen reservoir bag that is attached allows the client to rebreathe about the first third of the exhaled air in conjunction with oxygen (Figure 25–5 ■). Thus, it increases the FiO_2 by recycling expired oxygen. The partial rebreather bag must not totally deflate during inspiration to avoid carbon dioxide buildup. If this problem occurs, the liter flow of oxygen needs to be increased so that the bag remains one-third to one-half full.
- The **nonrebreather mask** delivers the highest oxygen concentration possible—95% to 100%—by means other than intubation or mechanical ventilation, at liter flows of 10 to 15 L/min. One-way valves on the mask and between the reservoir bag and the mask prevent the room air and the client's exhaled air from entering the bag so only the oxygen in the bag is inspired (Figure 25–6 ■). In some cases, one of the side valves is removed so that the client can still inhale room air if the oxygen supply is accidentally cut off. To prevent carbon dioxide buildup, the nonrebreather bag must not totally deflate during inspiration. If it does, the nurse can correct this problem by increasing the liter flow of oxygen.

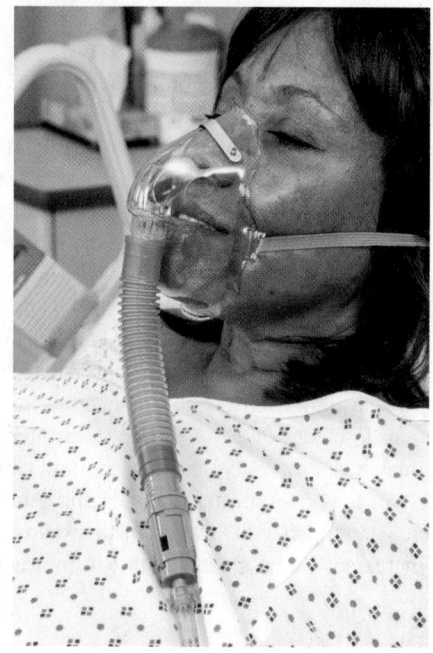

Figure 25–7 ■ A Venturi mask.

- The **Venturi mask** delivers oxygen concentrations varying from 24% to 50% at liter flows of 4 to 10 L/min. The Venturi mask (Figure 25–7 ■) has a section of wide-bore tubing and can have color-coded jet adapters that correspond to a precise oxygen concentration and liter flow. For example, in some cases, a blue adapter delivers a 24% concentration of oxygen at 4 L/min and a green adapter delivers a 35% concentration of oxygen at 8 L/min. However, colors and concentrations may vary by manufacturers so the equipment must be examined carefully. Other manufacturers use a dial for setting the desired concentration. Turning the oxygen source flow rate higher than specified by the equipment manufacturer will not increase the concentration delivered to the client.

Initiating oxygen by mask is much the same as initiating oxygen by cannula, except that the nurse must find a mask of appropriate size. Smaller sizes are available for children. Administering oxygen by mask or face tent is detailed in Skill 25–1. Limitations of masks

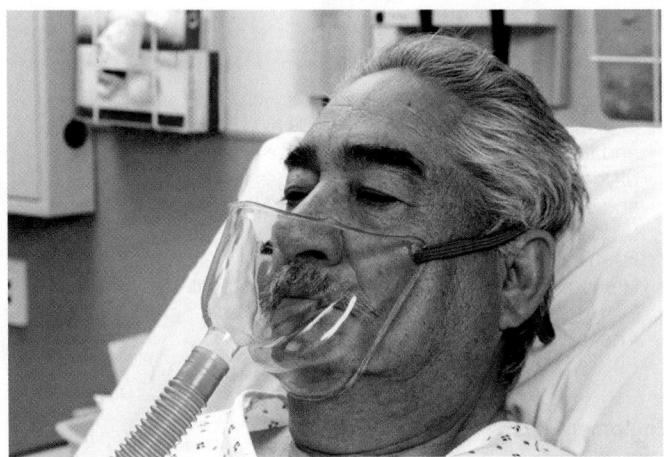

Figure 25–8 ■ An oxygen face tent.

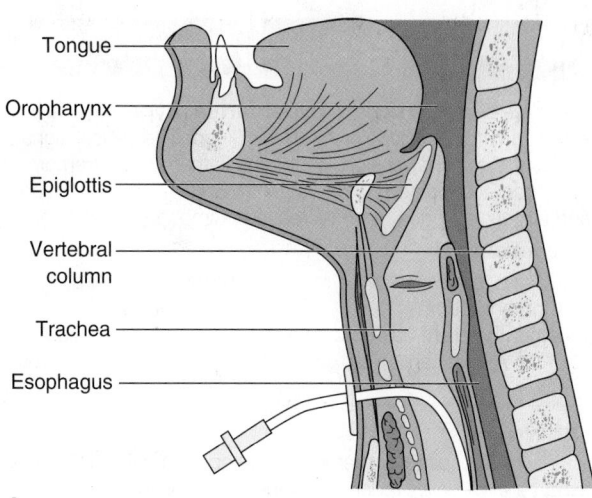

A

include difficulty in achieving a proper fit and poor tolerance by some clients who may complain of feeling hot or "smothering."

Face Tent

Face tents (Figure 25–8 ■) can replace oxygen masks when masks are poorly tolerated by clients. Face tents provide varying concentrations of oxygen (e.g., 30% to 50% concentration of oxygen at 4 to 8 L/min). Frequently inspect the client's facial skin for dampness or chafing, and dry and treat as needed. As with face masks, the client's facial skin must be kept dry.

Transtracheal Catheter

A **transtracheal catheter** is placed through a surgically created tract in the lower neck directly into the trachea (Figure 25–9 ■). Once the tract has matured (healed), the client removes and cleans the catheter two to four times per day. Oxygen applied to the catheter at greater than 1 L/min should be humidified, and high flow rates, as much as 15 to 20 L/min, can be administered.

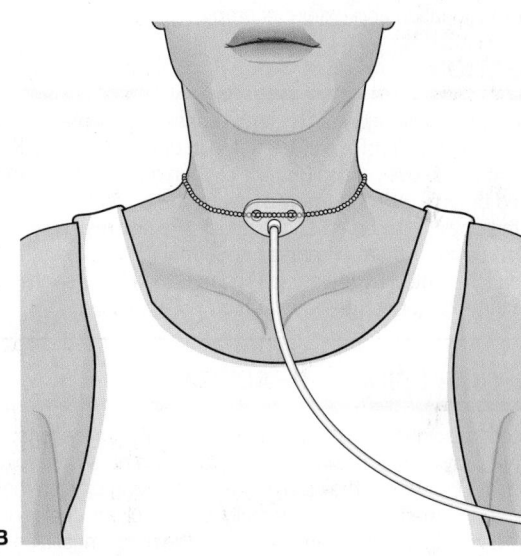

B

Figure 25–9 ■ *A,* Schematic of a transtracheal catheter; *B,* transtracheal catheter in place.

●○● NURSING PROCESS: OXYGEN DELIVERY

Administering Oxygen by Cannula, Face Mask, or Face Tent

Before administering oxygen, check (a) the order for oxygen, including the administering device and the liter flow rate (L/min) or the percentage of oxygen; (b) the levels of oxygen (PaO_2) and carbon dioxide ($PaCO_2$) in the client's arterial blood (PaO_2 is normally 80 to 100 mmHg; $PaCO_2$ is normally 35 to 45 mmHg); and (c) whether the client has COPD. *Note:* If the client has not had arterial blood gases ordered, oxygen saturation should be checked using a noninvasive oximeter.

ASSESSMENT
See also Skill 3–11, Assessing the Thorax and Lungs, in Chapter 3 ∞.
    Assess:
* *Skin and mucous membrane color:* Note whether cyanosis is present, presence of mucus, sputum production, and impedance of airflow.

* *Breathing patterns:* Note depth of respirations and presence of tachypnea, bradypnea, or orthopnea.
* *Chest movements:* Note whether there are any intercostal, substernal, suprasternal, supraclavicular, or tracheal retractions during inspiration or expiration.
* *Chest wall configuration* (e.g., kyphosis, unequal chest expansion, barrel chest).
* *Lung sounds:* audible by auscultating the chest and by ear.
* *Presence of clinical signs of hypoxemia:* tachycardia, tachypnea, restlessness, dyspnea, cyanosis. Tachycardia and tachypnea are often early signs of respiratory distress.
* *Level of consciousness:* Cerebral hypoxia may appear as drowsiness, poor concentration, and confusion. Confusion is a later sign of severe oxygen deprivation.

SKILL 25-1

Continued on page 588

Administering Oxygen by Cannula, Face Mask, or Face Tent—*continued*

- *Presence of clinical signs of* **hypercarbia** (**hypercapnia**): elevated carbon dioxide levels in the blood. The clinical signs are restlessness, hypertension, headache, lethargy, and tremor.
- *Presence of clinical signs of oxygen toxicity:* tracheal irritation and cough, dyspnea, and decreased pulmonary ventilation.

  Determine:
- Vital signs, especially pulse rate and quality, and respiratory rate, rhythm, and depth.
- Whether the client has chronic obstructive pulmonary disease (COPD). A high carbon dioxide level in the blood is the normal stimulus to breathe. However, people with COPD and other lung diseases may have a chronically high carbon dioxide level, and their stimulus to breathe is hypoxemia. During continuous oxygen administration, arterial blood gas levels of oxygen (PO_2) and carbon dioxide (PCO_2) are measured periodically to monitor hypoxemia.
- Results of diagnostic studies such as chest x-ray.
- Hemoglobin, hematocrit, and complete blood count.
- Oxygen saturation level.
- Arterial blood gases, if available.
- Pulmonary function tests, if available.

PLANNING

Consult with a respiratory therapist as needed in the beginning and ongoing care of clients receiving oxygen therapy. In many agencies, the therapist establishes the initial equipment and client teaching. However, it is important for the nurse to continually assess the client's need for oxygenation and oxygen therapy.

DELEGATION

Initiating the administration of oxygen is considered similar to administering a medication and is not delegated to unlicensed assistive personnel (UAP). However, reapplying the oxygen delivery device may be performed by the UAP, and many aspects of the client's response to oxygen therapy are observed during usual care and may be recorded by individuals other than the nurse. Abnormal findings must be validated and interpreted by the nurse. The nurse is also responsible for ensuring that the correct delivery method is being used.

INTERPROFESSIONAL PRACTICE

Administering oxygen may be within the scope of practice for specific health care providers. For example, in addition to nurses, respiratory therapists are involved in the care of clients receiving oxygen therapy. Although these therapists may verbally communicate their findings and plan to the health care team members, the nurse must also know where to locate their documentation in the client's medical record.

Equipment
Cannula
- Oxygen supply with a flow meter and adapter
- Humidifier with distilled water or tap water according to agency protocol
- Nasal cannula and tubing
- Tape (optional)
- Padding for the elastic band (optional)

Face Mask
- Oxygen supply with a flow meter and adapter
- Humidifier with distilled water or tap water according to agency protocol
- Prescribed face mask of the appropriate size
- Padding for the elastic band

Face Tent
- Oxygen supply with a flow meter and adapter
- Humidifier with distilled water or tap water according to agency protocol
- Face tent of the appropriate size

IMPLEMENTATION
Preparation
- Determine the need for oxygen therapy, and verify the order for the therapy.
  - Perform a respiratory assessment to develop baseline data if not already available.
- Prepare the client and support people.
  - Assist the client to a semi-Fowler's position if possible. **Rationale:** *This position permits easier chest expansion and hence easier breathing.*
  - Explain that oxygen is not dangerous when safety precautions are observed. Inform the client and support people about the safety precautions connected with oxygen use.

Performance
1. Prior to performing the procedure, introduce self and verify the client's identity using agency protocol. Explain to the client what you are going to do, why it is necessary, and how he or she can participate. Discuss how the effects of the oxygen therapy will be used in planning further care or treatments.
2. Perform hand hygiene and observe other appropriate infection prevention procedures.
3. Provide for client privacy, if appropriate.
4. Set up the oxygen equipment and the humidifier according to standards and protocols.
   - Attach the flow meter to the wall outlet or tank. ❶ The flow meter should be in the OFF position.

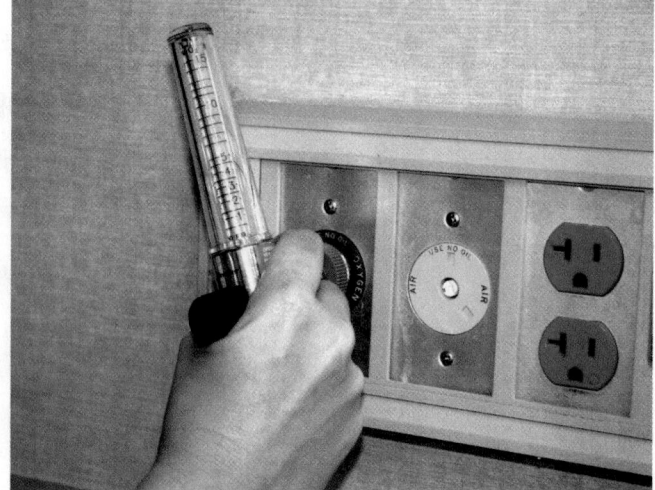

❶ Attach the flow meter to the wall outlet.

- If needed, fill the humidifier bottle with tap or distilled water, or normal saline, per agency policy. (This can be done before coming to the bedside.)
- Attach the humidifier bottle to the base of the flow meter.

Administering Oxygen by Cannula, Face Mask, or Face Tent—*continued*

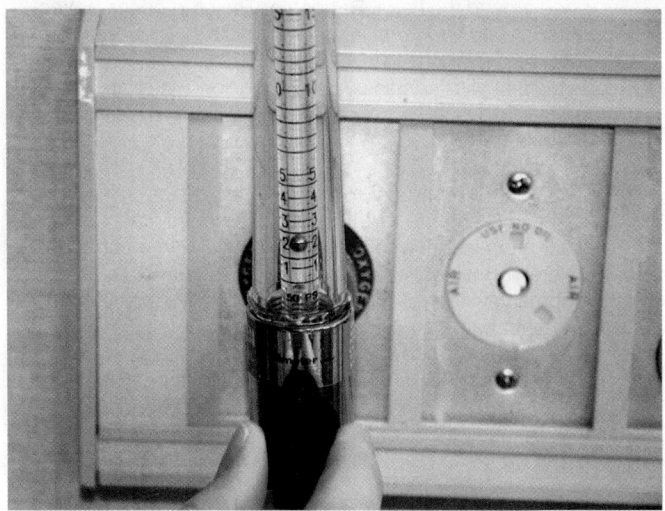

2 This flow meter is set to deliver 2 L/min.

- Attach the prescribed oxygen tubing and delivery device to the humidifier.
5. Turn on the oxygen at the prescribed rate, and ensure proper functioning.
   - Check that the oxygen is flowing freely through the tubing. There should be no kinks in the tubing, and the connections should be airtight. There should be bubbles in the humidifier as the oxygen flows through. You should feel the oxygen at the outlets of the cannula, mask, or tent.
   - Set the oxygen at the flow rate ordered. **2**
6. Apply the appropriate oxygen delivery device.
   Cannula
   - Put the cannula over the client's face, with the outlet prongs curved downward, fitting into the nares, and the elastic band around the head or the tubing over the ears and under the chin (see Figure 25–3). Some models have a strap to adjust under the chin.
   - If the cannula will not stay in place, tape it at the sides of the face.
   - Pad the tubing and band over the ears and cheekbones as needed.
   Face Mask
   - Guide the mask toward the client's face, and apply it from the nose downward.
   - Fit the mask and metal nose bracket to the contours of the client's face (see Figure 25–4). **Rationale:** *The mask should*

mold to the face, so that very little oxygen escapes into the eyes or around the cheeks and chin.
   - Secure the elastic band around the client's head so that the mask is comfortable but snug.
   - Pad the band behind the ears and over bony prominences. **Rationale:** *Padding will prevent irritation from the mask.*
   Face Tent
   - Place the tent over the client's face, and secure the ties around the head (see Figure 25–8).
7. Assess the client regularly.
   - Assess the client's vital signs (including oxygen saturation), level of anxiety, color, and ease of respirations. Provide support while the client adjusts to the device. Some clients may complain of claustrophobia.
   - Assess the client in 15 to 30 minutes, depending on the client's condition, and regularly thereafter.
   - Assess the client regularly for clinical signs of hypoxia, tachycardia, confusion, dyspnea, restlessness, and cyanosis. Review arterial blood gas results if they are available.
   Nasal Cannula
   - Assess the client's nares for encrustations and irritation. Apply a water-soluble lubricant as required to soothe the mucous membranes.
   - Assess the top of the client's ears for any signs of irritation from the cannula strap. If present, padding with a gauze pad may help relieve the discomfort.
   Face Mask or Tent
   - Inspect the facial skin frequently for dampness or chafing, and dry and treat it as needed.
8. Inspect the equipment on a regular basis.
   - Check the liter flow and the level of water in the humidifier in 30 minutes and whenever providing care to the client.
   - Be sure that water is not collecting in dependent loops of the tubing.
   - Make sure that safety precautions are being followed.
9. Document findings in the client record using forms or checklists supplemented by narrative notes when appropriate.

SAMPLE DOCUMENTATION

9/16/2015 0930 Returned from physical therapy with c/o dyspnea. Resp. 26/min, shallow. P 92 beats/min, BP 160/98 mmHg, SpO_2 92%. Skin warm, no cyanosis. Lung sounds clear, no retractions. O_2 per nasal cannula applied @ 2 L/min. ———— P. Isola, RN
9/16/2015 1000 No further c/o dyspnea. Resp. 20/min, P 88 beats/min, BP 152/92 mmHg, SpO_2 96%. O_2 per nasal cannula continues @ 2 L/min. ———— P. Isola, RN

EVALUATION
- Perform follow-up based on findings that deviated from expected or normal for the client. Relate findings to previous data if available.
- Check oxygen saturation (pulse oximetry) and repeat assessment skills to evaluate adequacy of oxygenation.
- Report significant deviations from normal to the primary care provider.

LIFESPAN CONSIDERATIONS   Oxygen Delivery

INFANTS
Oxygen Hood
- An oxygen hood is a rigid plastic dome that encloses an infant's head. It provides precise oxygen levels and high humidity.
- The gas should not be allowed to blow directly into the infant's face, and the hood should not rub against the infant's neck, chin, or shoulder.

CHILDREN
Oxygen Tent
- The tent consists of a rectangular, clear, plastic canopy with outlets that connect to an oxygen or compressed air source and to a humidifier that moisturizes the air or oxygen.
- Because the enclosed tent becomes very warm, some type of cooling mechanism is provided to maintain the temperature at 20°C to 21°C (68°F to 70°F).
- Cover the child with a gown or a cotton blanket. Some agencies provide gowns with hoods, or a small towel may be wrapped around the head. **Rationale:** *The child needs protection from chilling and from the dampness and condensation in the tent.*
- Flood the tent with oxygen by setting the flow meter at 15 L/min for about 5 minutes. Then, adjust the flow meter according to orders (e.g., 10 to 15 L/min). **Rationale:** *Flooding the tent quickly increases the oxygen to the desired level.*
- The tent can deliver approximately 30% oxygen.
- Children may fight having a mask placed on their faces. They are often fearful when placed in oxygen tents or hoods. These are normal responses that vary based on experience, developmental stage, degree of threat to body image, and attachment/abandonment issues. Providing safe toys and a beloved blanket or pillow to hold can help, as can fostering the parent–child bond even though separated by the plastic. Encourage parents to interact with their child around and through the tubing and tent.

Ambulatory and Community Settings   Home Oxygen Delivery   PATIENT-CENTERED CARE

Three major oxygen systems for home care use are available in most communities: cylinders or tanks of compressed gas, liquid (cryogenic) oxygen, and oxygen concentrators.

1. *Cylinders ("green tanks"):* These are the system of choice for clients who need oxygen episodically (e.g., on a prn basis). Advantages are that cylinders deliver all liter flows (1 to 15 L/min), and oxygen evaporation does not occur during storage. Disadvantages are that the cylinders are heavy and awkward to move, the supply company must be notified when a refill is needed, and they are costly for the high-use client. A size "D" tank weighs about 8 pounds and stores 425 L of oxygen. An "E" tank holds 680 L and is transported on wheels. The large "H" tank weighs 150 pounds. The gauge on a full tank reads a pressure of at least 2,000 pounds per square inch (psi), and a tank is considered empty when it reads less than 500 psi.

2. *Liquid oxygen:* Liquid systems have two parts—a large stationary container and a portable unit with a small lightweight tank, refilled from the stationary unit. Liquid reservoirs store oxygen at –212°C (–350°F) in a smaller amount of space than compressed gas. Advantages are that these reservoirs are lighter in weight and cleaner in appearance than cylinders and they are not as difficult to operate. Disadvantages of liquid oxygen are that not all home care medical supply and service companies carry it, oxygen evaporation occurs when the unit is not used, only low flows (1 to 4 L/min) can be used or freezing occurs, and the portable unit designed to be carried over the shoulder weighs 4 to 10 pounds, a possible burden to the typical client with COPD. A wheeled cart can be used to carry the unit but may be awkward.

3. **Oxygen concentrators:** Concentrators are electrically powered systems that manufacture oxygen from room air. At 1 L/min, such a system can deliver a concentration of about 95% oxygen, but the concentration drops when the flow rate increases (e.g., 75% concentration at 4 L/min). Advantages are that they are more attractive in appearance, resembling furniture rather than medical equipment; they eliminate the need for regular delivery of oxygen or refilling of cylinders; because the supply of oxygen is constant, they alleviate the client's anxiety about running out of oxygen; and they are the most economical system when continuous use is required. Major disadvantages of a concentrator are that it is expensive, lacks real portability (small units weigh 28 pounds), tends to be noisy, and is powered by electricity; an emergency backup unit (e.g., an oxygen tank) must be provided for clients for whom a power failure could be life threatening; and heat produced by the concentrator motor is a problem for those who live in trailers, small houses, or warm climates where air conditioners are required. The oxygen concentrator must also be checked periodically with an O_2 analyzer to ensure that it is adequately delivering oxygen.

Another type of oxygen concentrator is the *oxygen enricher*. It uses a plastic membrane that allows water vapor to pass through with the oxygen, thus eliminating the need for a humidifying device. It is also thought to filter out bacteria present in the air. The enricher provides an O_2 concentration of 40% at all flow rates, it tends to be quieter than the concentrator, there is less chance of combustion (because the gas is only 40% oxygen), it has only two moving parts (thus decreasing the risk of something going wrong), and a nebulizer can be operated off the enricher because of the high flow rate.

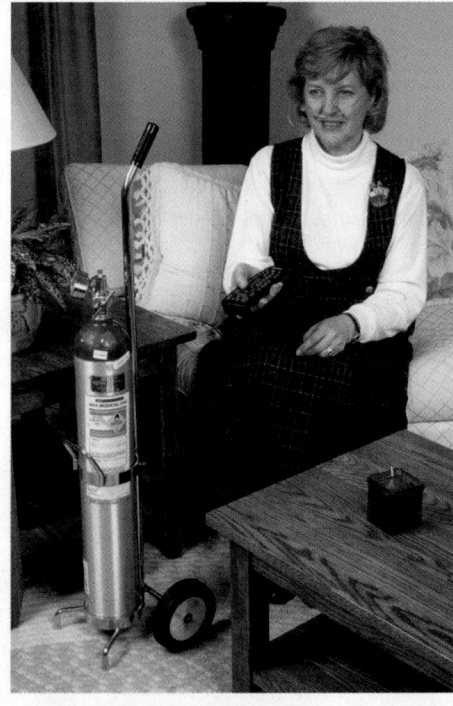

Using a portable oxygen system in the home.
Aaron Haupt/Getty Images.

Social services or the case manager needs to ensure that the client has appropriate help in choosing a reputable home oxygen vendor. Services furnished should include:

- A 24-hour emergency service.
- Trained personnel to make the initial delivery and instruct the client in safe, appropriate use of the oxygen and maintenance of the equipment.
- At least monthly follow-up visits to check the equipment and reinstruct the client as necessary.

- A regular cost review to ensure that the system is the most cost-effective one for that client, with routine notification of the primary care provider or home care professional if it seems that another system is more appropriate.

The nurse also needs to ensure that the client knows about the financial reimbursements available from Medicare and Medicaid or other insurance agencies.

PEAK EXPIRATORY FLOW

Some clients have acute or chronic respiratory disorders, such as asthma or COPD, that affect the amount of air that can be expired from the lungs. In these situations, the measurement of the maximum amount the client can expire may be helpful in directing therapy. This measurement is the **peak expiratory flow rate (PEFR)**. Measuring PEFR before and after a breathing treatment, for example,

can assist the health care team in determining whether additional respiratory therapy is needed.

Note: PEFR evaluates the volume the client can *exhale*. This is not the same as evaluating the volume the client can *inhale*. The client's inspiratory volume is often measured through incentive spirometry (see Skill 24–2 on page 579).

●○● NURSING PROCESS: PEAK EXPIRATORY FLOW

Measuring Peak Expiratory Flow

ASSESSMENT

Perform a thorough respiratory and chest assessment (see Skill 3–11, Assessing the Thorax and Lungs, in Chapter 3 ∞). Examine vital signs, blood gas results, and other relevant laboratory values (e.g., hemoglobin).

PLANNING

Review the client record for previous assessments, PEFR measurements, and resultant changes in therapy.

DELEGATION

PEFR measurement may be delegated to trained UAP. The nurse should double-check any values found to be abnormal or significantly different from previous results and must interpret the findings. Modifications in the treatment regimen may not be initiated by UAP.

INTERPROFESSIONAL PRACTICE

PEFR measurement may be within the scope of practice for specific health care providers. For example, in addition to nurses, respiratory therapists are involved in the care of clients with acute or chronic respiratory disorders. Although these therapists may verbally communicate their findings and plan to the health care team members, the nurse must also know where to locate their documentation in the client's medical record.

Equipment
- Peak flow meter

IMPLEMENTATION

Performance

1. Prior to performing the procedure, introduce self and verify the client's identity using agency protocol. Explain to the client what you are going to do, why it is necessary, and how he or she can participate. Discuss how the results will be used in planning further care or treatments.
2. Perform hand hygiene and observe other appropriate infection prevention procedures.
3. Provide for client privacy.
4. Position the client.
   - If possible, the client should be sitting with the chest free from contact with the bed or chair. If not possible, place the client in semi-Fowler's or high-Fowler's position.
5. Reset the marker on the flow meter to the zero position. ❶
6. Assist the client to use the flow meter.
   - Ask the client to take a deep breath in. ❷
   - The client places the mouthpiece in the mouth with the teeth around the opening and the lips forming a tight seal.
   - Have the client exhale as quickly and forcefully as possible. If you suspect the client is exhaling a significant amount of air through the nose, apply a nose clip.

7. Perform step 6 two more times, allowing the client to rest for 5 to 10 seconds in between. Record the highest level achieved.
8. Document findings in the client record using forms or checklists supplemented by narrative notes when appropriate.
9. Normal or expected PEFR is established based on age and size, and a reference chart is included with each peak flow meter. Percentage of predicted PEFR differs for each individual and the primary care provider helps determine that for the client. There are three peak flow zones, which are based on the traffic light concept: red meaning danger, yellow meaning caution, and green meaning safe. The green or safe zone is from 80% to 100%. The yellow or caution zone is from 50% to 80%. This means that the large airways are beginning to narrow. The red or danger zone is less than 50%, which means severe narrowing of the large airways has occurred (Johns Hopkins, n.d.). Clients are taught to use their individual peak flow meter to anticipate early changes in their condition as part of their self-care plan.

Continued on page 592

Measuring Peak Expiratory Flow—*continued*

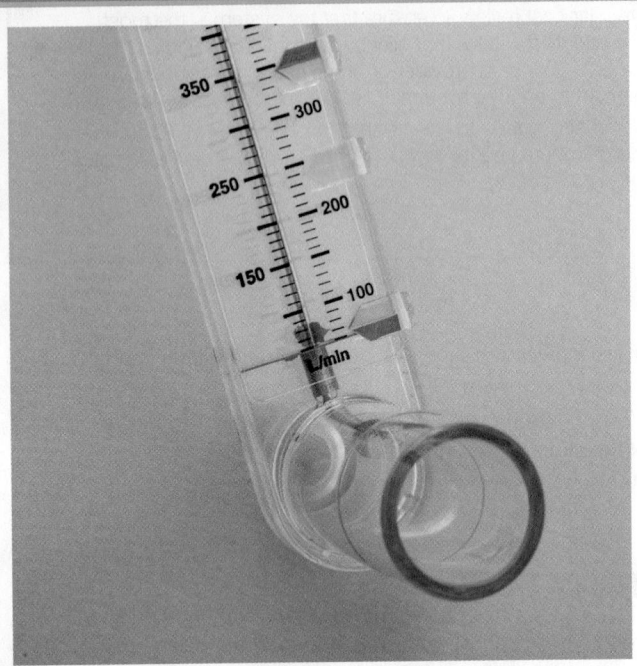

❶ Peak flow meter with marker in the zero position.

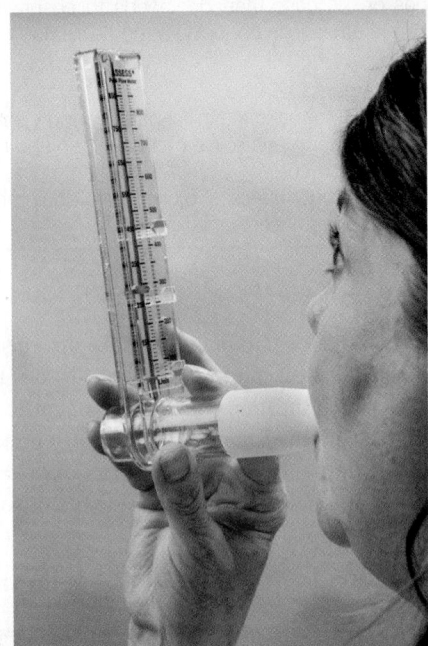

❷ PEFR measurement.

EVALUATION
- Perform follow-up based on findings that deviated from expected or normal for the client. Relate findings to previous assessment data if available.

- Report significant deviations from normal or expected to the primary care provider.

NONINVASIVE POSITIVE PRESSURE VENTILATION

Some clients require mechanical assistance to maintain adequate breathing. When the condition is not life threatening, the assistance may be accomplished by the use of **noninvasive positive pressure ventilation (NPPV)**, that is, delivery of air or oxygen under pressure without the need for an invasive tube such as an endotracheal or tracheostomy tube. Conditions requiring noninvasive ventilation include acute and chronic respiratory failure, pulmonary edema, COPD, and obstructive sleep apnea.

This discussion focuses on the use of noninvasive ventilation devices in the treatment of sleep apnea due to the prevalence of this condition. Sleep apnea affects 12 million Americans. When breathing stops (apnea), the person's carbon dioxide level rises, breathing is stimulated, and then it resumes. There are varying types of sleep apnea, but **obstructive sleep apnea (OSA)** is the most common. Risk factors include male gender, obesity, and age over 40; however, it can affect anyone at any age, including children. OSA can lead to a number of health problems including hypertension, fatigue, memory problems, other cardiovascular disease, and headaches. If an underlying cause can be treated, OSA may be reduced or eliminated. The most common and least invasive treatment for OSA is positive pressure ventilation. A mask fitted over the client's nose during sleep provides air under pressure during inhalation and exhalation so that the airway is kept open and cannot collapse. This mask and pump system is called **continuous positive airway pressure (CPAP)**. A variation of CPAP is **bilevel positive airway pressure (BiPAP)**

in which the pressure delivered during exhalation is less than the pressure delivered during inhalation (Figure 25–10 ■).

The nurse's primary role in caring for clients using CPAP or BiPAP devices is to ensure optimal functioning and use of the device since it may need to be used nightly for the remainder of their lives (see Practice Guidelines). Clients may experience significant issues with adherence to CPAP therapy due to discomfort or other barriers, so the nurse should provide client education and support as well as collaborating with the respiratory therapist and other involved health care providers.

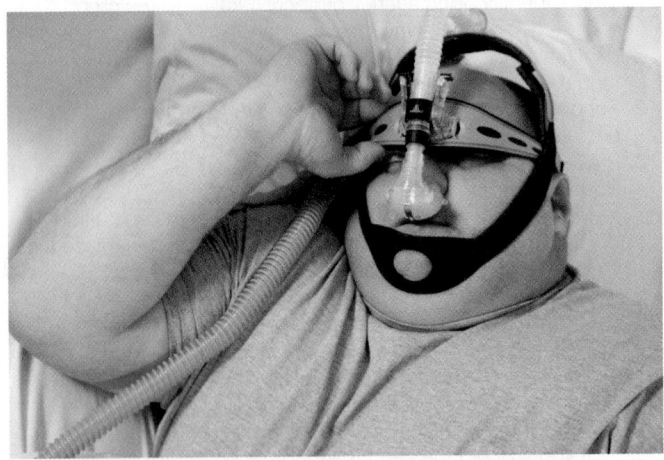

Figure 25–10 ■ A CPAP machine in use in a client's home.
Custom Medical Stock Photo, Inc.

PRACTICE GUIDELINES

Continuous Positive Airway Pressure Device Use in Obstructive Sleep Apnea

- Encourage clients to try other treatment measures that could reduce OSA such as weight loss or oral appliances that advance the lower jaw and base of the tongue, which can block the airway.
- Recommend clients join a community support group for others with OSA using CPAP/BiPAP.
- Review proper use of the equipment, including the pressure setting prescribed by the primary care provider.
- Assess proper fit of the mask. The mask may need to be replaced if the client gains or loses significant weight.
- If the client complains that the air being forced in is bothersome, use a pump that allows for gradual increase in pressure over 15 minutes (ramping) and heated humidification of the air. If humidification is used, the water chamber must be routinely cleaned to prevent fungal growth.
- Instruct the client to wash the mask daily with warm, soapy water.
- In order for full CPAP/BiPAP effectiveness, the client must sleep with the mouth closed so that exhalation is done against the positive pressure. Problems with a dry mouth can occur due to mouth breathing. This may be prevented by using a chin strap or a full face mask.

Chapter 25 Review

FOCUSING ON CLINICAL THINKING

Consider This

1. The client has a primary care provider's order for "oxygen by mask at 6 L/min." However, the client complains of feeling as though not enough air is being delivered and frequently removes the mask. What alternatives might the nurse suggest?

2. The hospitalized client's PEFR is markedly lower in the morning than it was the previous evening. What might explain this finding, and how would the nurse respond?

See Focusing on Clinical Thinking answers on student resource website.

TEST YOUR KNOWLEDGE

1. The nurse is caring for a client with obstructive sleep apnea. The nurse anticipates an order for which type of equipment?
   1. Oxygen by face mask
   2. Room air by Venturi mask
   3. Room air by CPAP
   4. Oxygen by nasal cannula

2. A client with a medical diagnosis of chronic obstructive pulmonary disease (COPD) has an oxygen saturation of 82%. Delivering oxygen by what method and concentration would be safest for this client?
   1. Nasal cannula at 6 L/min
   2. Nonrebreather mask at 100% oxygen concentration
   3. Nasal cannula at 2 L/min
   4. Venturi mask at 50% oxygen concentration

3. On entering a client's room, the nurse finds the client short of breath, dyspneic, with an oxygen saturation of 75% and fingernails that are cyanotic. What is the nurse's priority action?
   1. Begin oxygen administration.
   2. Call the primary care provider and request an order for oxygen administration.
   3. Call the respiratory therapist.
   4. Return to the room in 15 minutes to reevaluate the client's condition.

4. The client has been receiving high-concentration oxygen therapy. The nurse finds the client complaining of a scratchy throat and displaying a cough and mild dyspnea. The nurse suspects which complication?
   1. Hypercarbia
   2. Hypoxia
   3. Oxygen toxicity
   4. Hypercapnia

5. The nurse administers oxygen to a client via a nasal cannula. What nursing intervention will prevent rhinorrhea or nasal irritation?
   1. Connect a humidifier bottle to the flow meter.
   2. Apply a warming device to the nasal cannula tubing.
   3. Instill normal saline nose drops every 4 hours.
   4. Remove the cannula for 1 hour every 4 hours.

6. The nurse may delegate which responsibility related to oxygen therapy to unlicensed assistive personnel?
   1. Initiating oxygen therapy
   2. Determining the client's response to therapy
   3. Measuring oxygen saturation
   4. Changing the oxygen flow rate based on client response to therapy

7. A client with pneumonia is receiving oxygen therapy because of an oxygen saturation of 85%. The previous nurse reports that after beginning oxygen at 4 L/min, the client's oxygen saturation increased to 94%. The nurse is now assessing the client at the beginning of the shift. Which finding would the nurse need to report to the primary care provider immediately?
   1. Oxygen saturation of 98% and respiratory rate of 22 breaths per minute
   2. Oxygen saturation of 94% and respiratory rate of 20 breaths per minute
   3. Oxygen saturation of 88% and respiratory rate of 26 breaths per minute
   4. Oxygen saturation of 84% and respiratory rate of 28 breaths per minute

8. The nurse is preparing to measure peak expiratory airflow on a client. How will the nurse position the client to optimize the measurement?
   1. Semi-Fowler's position
   2. High-Fowler's position
   3. Supine position
   4. Sitting position with chest not touching the chair or bed

9. A new nurse asks why a client was placed on a noninvasive positive pressure ventilation device instead of being intubated. Which is the best response?
   1. "For short-term assistance, the noninvasive ventilation device has fewer side effects than invasive ventilation."
   2. "When the condition is not life threatening, a noninvasive ventilation device is more comfortable for the client and avoids the complications of invasive ventilation."
   3. "This is a short-term option until intubation for invasive ventilation can be scheduled."
   4. "This method of ventilation is less expensive than invasive ventilation."

10. The nurse is caring for a client diagnosed with sleep apnea who uses face mask CPAP. While the nurse is performing the admission history, the client admits he uses the CPAP machine only occasionally. Which would be the nurse's best response?
   1. "Well, you really should use it all the time."
   2. "It can be very dangerous for you if you don't use the CPAP every night."
   3. "Tell me about the reasons you don't use it every night."
   4. "Why don't you like using the machine every night?"

See Answers to Test Your Knowledge in Appendix A.

READINGS AND REFERENCES

References

Blakeman, T. C. (2013). Evidence for oxygen use in the hospitalized patient: Is more really the enemy of good? *Respiratory Care, 58,* 1679–1693. doi:10.4187/respcare.02677

Johns Hopkins. (n.d.). *Peak flow measurement.* Retrieved from http://www.hopkinsmedicine.org/healthlibrary/printv.aspx?d=92,P07755

Kallet, R. H. (2012). Is pulmonary oxygen toxicity still a clinically relevant issue? *Critical Care Alert, 20*(6), 41–43.

Martin, D. S., & Grocott, M. P. W. (2013). Oxygen therapy in critical illness. *Critical Care Medicine, 41,* 423–432.

Selected Bibliography

Berman, A., Snyder, S., & Frandsen, G. (2016). *Kozier & Erb's fundamentals of nursing: Concepts, process, and practice* (10th ed.). Upper Saddle River, NJ: Pearson.

Cataletto, M. (2011). Fundamentals of oxygen therapy. *Nursing made Incredibly Easy!, 9*(2), 22–24. doi:10.1097/01.NME.0000394045.03830.3d

Eastwood, G. M., Reade, M. C., Peck, L., Baldwin, I., Considine, J., & Bellomo, R. (2012). Critical care nurses' opinion and self-reported practice of oxygen therapy: A survey. *Australian Critical Care, 25,* 23–30. doi:10.1016/j.aucc.2011.05.001

Heffner, J. E. (2013). The story of oxygen. *Respiratory Care, 58*(1), 18–31. doi:10.4187/respcare.01831

Lynes, D., & Kelly, C. (2013). Acute oxygen therapy for patients in the community. *Nursing Standard, 27*(21), 63–68. doi:10.7748/ns2013.01.27.21.63.e7058

Preston, W. (2013). The increasing use of non-invasive ventilation. *Practice Nursing, 24*(3), 114–119.

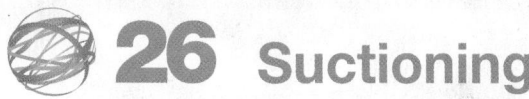

26 Suctioning

LEARNING OUTCOMES

At the completion of this chapter, the student will be able to:

1. Define the key terms used in the skills of suctioning.
2. Describe four types of artificial airways.
3. Differentiate among oropharyngeal, nasopharyngeal, endotracheal, and tracheostomy suctioning.
4. Compare and contrast open and closed airway/tracheal suction systems.
5. List common complications associated with suctioning.
6. Recognize when it is appropriate to delegate suctioning to unlicensed assistive personnel.
7. Verbalize the steps used in:
   a. Oropharyngeal, nasopharyngeal, and nasotracheal suctioning.
   b. Suctioning a tracheostomy or endotracheal tube.
8. Demonstrate appropriate documentation and reporting of suctioning.

SKILLS

Skill 26–1 Oropharyngeal, Nasopharyngeal, and Nasotracheal Suctioning

Skill 26–2 Suctioning a Tracheostomy or Endotracheal Tube

KEY TERMS

artificial airways, *595*
closed suction system, *601*
endotracheal tube (ETT), *596*
hyperinflation, *602*
hyperoxygenation, *602*
hyperventilation, *602*
in-line suctioning, *601*
nares, *595*
naris, *595*
nasopharyngeal airways, *595*
nasopharyngeal suctioning, *597*
open suction system, *601*
open-tipped catheter, *597*
oropharyngeal airways, *595*
oropharyngeal suctioning, *597*
suctioning, *597*
tracheostomy, *597*
whistle-tipped catheter, *597*
Yankauer suction tube, *597*

Artificial airways are inserted to maintain a patent air passage for clients whose airways have become or may become obstructed. A patent airway is necessary so that air can flow into and from the lungs. Four of the more common types of airways are oropharyngeal, nasopharyngeal, endotracheal, and tracheostomy.

OROPHARYNGEAL AND NASOPHARYNGEAL AIRWAYS

Oropharyngeal and nasopharyngeal airways are used to keep the upper air passages open when secretions or the tongue may obstruct them (e.g., in a client who is sedated, is semi-comatose, or has an altered level of consciousness). These airways are easy to insert and have a low risk of complications. Sizes vary and should be appropriate to the size and age of the client. The nasopharyngeal airway should be well lubricated with a water-soluble lubricant prior to insertion. The oropharyngeal airway may be lubricated with water or saline, if necessary.

Oropharyngeal airways (Figure 26–1 ■) stimulate the gag reflex and are only used for clients with altered levels of consciousness (e.g., because of general anesthesia, overdose, or head injury). To insert the airway:

- Place the client in a supine or semi-Fowler's position.
- Apply clean gloves.
- Hold the lubricated airway by the outer flange, with the distal end pointing or curved upward.

- Open the client's mouth and insert the airway along the top of the tongue.
- When the distal end of the airway reaches the soft palate at the back of the mouth, rotate the airway 180° downward and slip it past the uvula into the oral pharynx.
- If not contraindicated, place the client in a side-lying position or with the head turned to the side to allow secretions to drain out of the mouth.
- The oropharynx may be suctioned as needed by inserting the suction catheter alongside the airway.
- Remove and discard gloves.
- Perform hand hygiene.
- Do not tape the airway in place; remove it when the client begins to cough or gag.
- Provide mouth care at least every 2 to 4 hours, keeping suction available at the bedside.
- As appropriate for the client's condition, remove the airway every 8 hours to assess the mouth and provide oral care. Reinsert the airway immediately.

Nasopharyngeal airways are tolerated better by alert clients. They are inserted through the **nares** (nostrils), terminating in the oropharynx (Figure 26–2 ■). When caring for a client with a nasopharyngeal airway, provide frequent oral and nares care, reinserting the airway in the opposite **naris** (nostril) every 8 hours or as ordered to prevent breakdown of the mucosa.

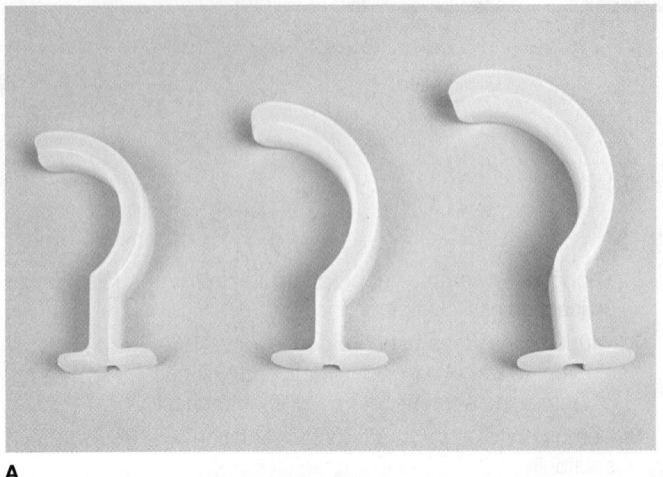

A

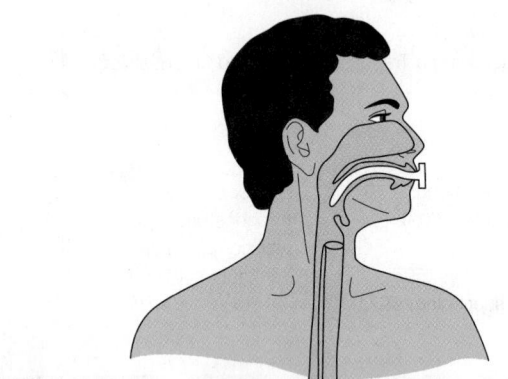

B

Figure 26–1 ■ *A*, Oropharyngeal airways; *B*, an oropharyngeal airway in place.

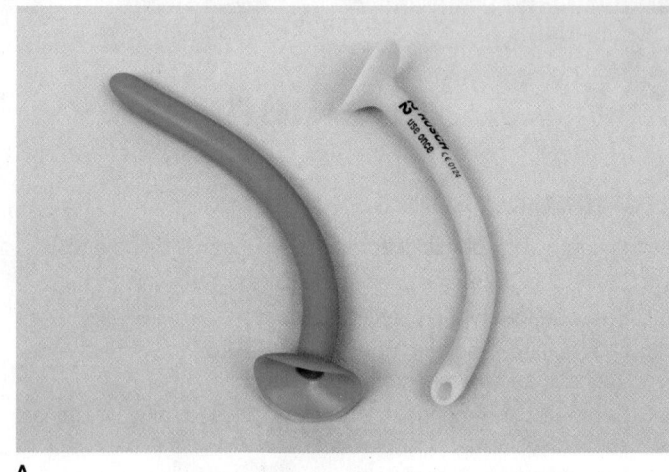

A

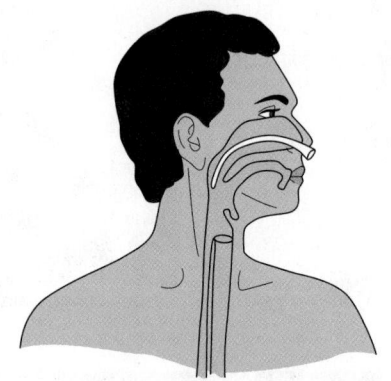

B

Figure 26–2 ■ *A*, Nasopharyngeal airways; *B*, a nasopharyngeal airway in place.

ENDOTRACHEAL TUBES

Endotracheal tubes (ETTs) are most commonly inserted in clients who have had general anesthetics or for those in emergency situations in which mechanical ventilation is required. An ETT is inserted by an anesthesiologist, primary care provider, certified registered nurse anesthetist (CRNA), or respiratory therapist with specialized education. It is inserted through either the mouth or the nose and into the trachea with the guide of a laryngoscope (Figure 26–3 ■). The tube terminates just superior to (above) the bifurcation of the trachea, or carina, into the bronchi. The tube may have an air-filled cuff to prevent air leakage around it. Because an endotracheal tube passes through the epiglottis and glottis, the client is unable to speak

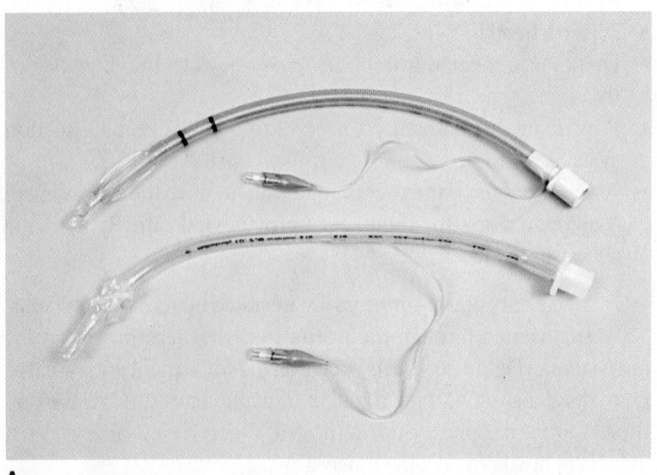

A

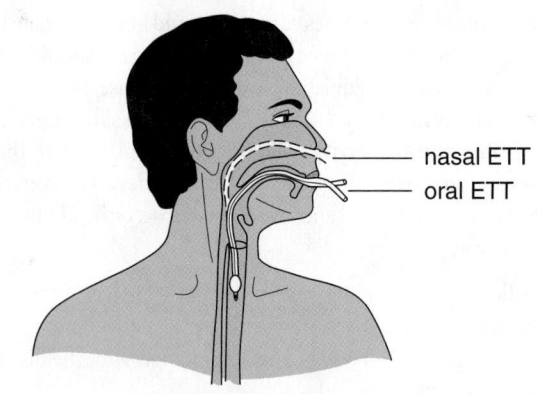

nasal ETT
oral ETT

B

Figure 26–3 ■ *A*, Endotracheal tubes; *B*, an endotracheal tube in place.

BOX 26–1 Nursing Interventions for Clients with Endotracheal Tubes

- Perform hand hygiene before and after contact with the client. Wear gloves when handling respiratory secretions or objects contaminated with respiratory secretions.
- Assess the client's respiratory status at least every 2 hours, or more frequently if indicated. Include in your assessment respiratory rate, rhythm, depth, equality of chest excursion, and lung sounds; level of consciousness; oxygen saturation, percentage of oxygen used and by what means (e.g., ventilator); and skin color.
- Frequently assess nasal and oral mucosa for redness and irritation. Report any abnormal findings to the primary care provider.
- Secure the ETT with tape or a commercially prepared holder to prevent movement of the tube farther into or out of the trachea. Assess the position of the tube frequently. Notify the primary care provider immediately if the tube is dislodged out of the airway. If the tube advances into a main bronchus, it will need to be repositioned to ensure ventilation of both lungs.
- Unless contraindicated, elevate the head of the bed 30° to 45°.
- Using sterile technique, suction the ETT as needed to remove excessive secretions. Perform subglottic suctioning before deflating the cuff of the ETT or before moving the tube. Wear goggles when performing suctioning.

- Closely monitor cuff pressure, maintaining a pressure of 20 to 25 mmHg (or as recommended by the tube manufacturer) to minimize the risk of tracheal tissue necrosis. If recommended, deflate the cuff periodically.
- Provide oral hygiene and nasal care every 2 to 4 hours. Use an oropharyngeal airway or bite block to prevent the client from biting down on an oral ETT. Move oral ETTs to the opposite side of the mouth every 8 hours or per agency protocol, taking care to maintain the position of the tube in the trachea. **Rationale:** *This prevents irritation to the oral mucosa.*
- Provide humidified air or oxygen because the ETT bypasses the upper airways, which normally moisten the air.
- If the client is on mechanical ventilation, ensure that all alarms are enabled at all times because the client cannot call for help should an emergency occur.
- Communicate frequently with the client, providing a note pad or picture board for the client to use in communicating.
- Inform the client and family that an ETT is usually used as a short-term artificial airway. Instruct the client and family not to manipulate the tube and to call for the nurse if the client is uncomfortable.

---

while it is in place. Nursing interventions for clients with endotracheal tubes are shown in Box 26–1.

TRACHEOSTOMY

Clients who need airway support due to a temporary or permanent condition may have a **tracheostomy**, a surgical incision in the trachea just below the larynx. A curved tracheostomy tube is inserted to extend through the stoma into the trachea (Figure 26–4 ■). Tracheostomy tubes are available in different sizes and may be plastic, silicone, or metal, and cuffed, uncuffed, or fenestrated. See Chapter 27 ∞ for more information on the client with a tracheostomy.

UPPER AIRWAY SUCTIONING

When clients have difficulty handling their secretions or an airway is in place, suctioning may be necessary to clear air passages. **Suctioning** is aspirating secretions through a catheter connected to a negative pressure, stand-alone suction machine or wall suction outlet. Even though the upper airways (the oropharynx and nasopharynx) are not sterile, sterile technique is recommended for all suctioning to avoid introducing pathogens into the airways. It is best to check

the agency's policy because some facilities may use clean rather than sterile technique for nasopharyngeal and oropharyngeal suctioning with the rationale that the catheter does not extend down to the lower airway.

Oropharyngeal and **nasopharyngeal suctioning** remove secretions from the upper respiratory tract. In contrast, tracheal suctioning (through an ETT or tracheostomy) is used to remove secretions from the trachea and bronchi or the lower respiratory tract, and sterile technique is always used.

Suction catheters are flexible, plastic, and may be either open tipped or whistle tipped (Figure 26–5 ■). The **whistle-tipped catheter** is less irritating to respiratory tissues, although the **open-tipped catheter** may be more effective for removing thick mucous plugs. An oral suction tube, or **Yankauer suction tube**, is used to suction the oral cavity (Figure 26–6 ■). Alert clients can be taught how to use this method of oral suctioning. Most suction catheters have a thumb port on the side to control the suction. The catheter is connected to suction tubing, which in turn is connected to a collection chamber and suction control gauge (Figure 26–7 ■).

The nurse decides when suctioning is needed by assessing the client for signs of respiratory distress or evidence that the client is unable to cough up and expectorate secretions. Dyspnea, bubbling or

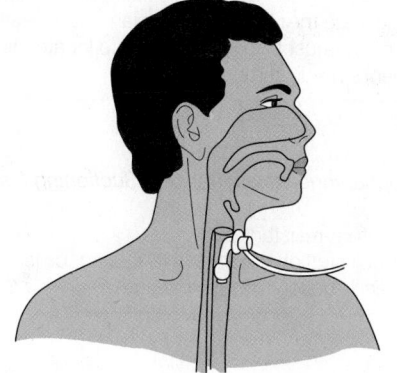

Figure 26–4 ■ A tracheostomy tube in place.

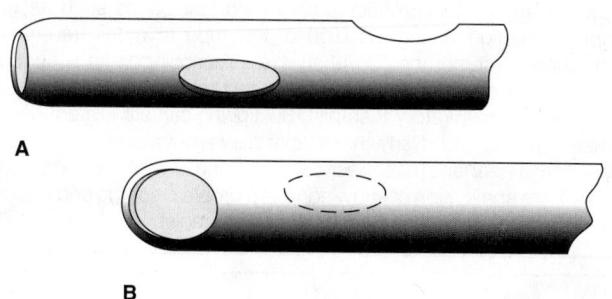

A

B

Figure 26–5 ■ Types of suction catheters: *A*, open tipped; *B*, whistle tipped.

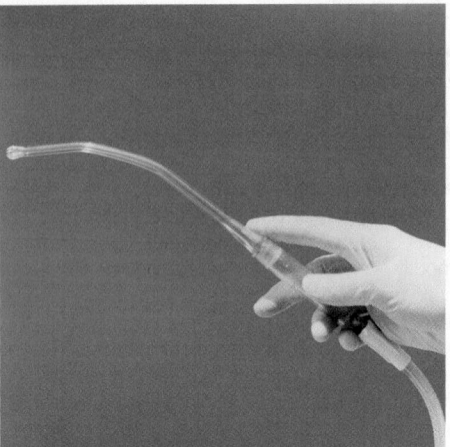

Figure 26–6 ■ Oral (Yankauer) suction tube.

rattling (adventitious) breath sounds, poor skin color (pallor, duskiness, or cyanosis), restlessness, tachycardia, or decreased oxygen saturation (SpO$_2$) levels (also known as O$_2$ sat) may indicate the need for suctioning. Good nursing judgment and critical thinking are necessary, because suctioning irritates mucous membranes, can increase secretions if performed too frequently, and can cause the client's O$_2$ sat to drop further, put the client in bronchospasm, and if the client has a head injury, cause the intracranial pressure to increase. In other words, suctioning is based on clinical need versus a fixed schedule.

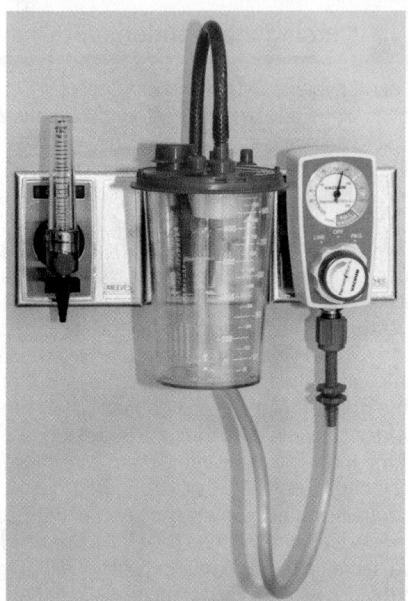

Figure 26–7 ■ A wall suction unit.

In addition to removing secretions that obstruct the airway and facilitating ventilation, suctioning can be performed to obtain secretions for diagnostic purposes and to prevent infection that may result from accumulated secretions. Skill 26–1 outlines oropharyngeal, nasopharyngeal, and nasotracheal suctioning.

●○● NURSING PROCESS: UPPER AIRWAY SUCTIONING

Oropharyngeal, Nasopharyngeal, and Nasotracheal Suctioning

ASSESSMENT

Assess for clinical signs indicating the need for suctioning:
- Restlessness, anxiety, agitation
- Noisy respirations
- Adventitious (abnormal) breath sounds when the chest is auscultated
- Change in mental status

- Skin color
- Rate and pattern of respirations
- Pulse rate and rhythm
- Decreased oxygen saturation

PLANNING
DELEGATION

Oral suctioning using a Yankauer suction tube can be delegated to unlicensed assistive personnel (UAP) and to the client or family, if appropriate, because this is not a sterile procedure. The nurse needs to review the procedure and important points such as not applying suction during insertion of the tube to avoid trauma to the mucous membrane. Oropharyngeal suctioning uses a suction catheter and, although not a sterile procedure, should be performed by a nurse or respiratory therapist. Suctioning can stimulate the gag reflex, hypoxia, and dysrhythmias that may require problem solving. Nasopharyngeal and nasotracheal suctioning use sterile technique and require application of knowledge and problem solving and should be performed by the nurse or respiratory therapist.

INTERPROFESSIONAL PRACTICE

Suctioning a client may be within the scope of practice for specific health care providers. For example, in addition to nurses, respiratory therapists may help suction a client. Although these therapists may verbally communicate their findings and plan to the health care team members, the nurse must also know where to locate their documentation in the client's medical record.

Equipment
Oral and Nasopharyngeal/Nasotracheal Suctioning (using sterile technique)
- Towel or moisture-resistant pad
- Portable or wall suction machine with tubing, collection receptacle, and suction pressure gauge

Oropharyngeal, Nasopharyngeal, and Nasotracheal Suctioning—*continued*

- Sterile disposable container for fluids
- Sterile normal saline or water
- Goggles or face shield, if appropriate
- Moisture-resistant disposal bag
- Sputum trap, if specimen is to be collected

Oral and Oropharyngeal Suctioning (using clean technique)
- Yankauer suction catheter or suction catheter kit
- Clean gloves

Nasopharyngeal or Nasotracheal Suctioning (using sterile technique)
- Sterile gloves
- Sterile suction catheter kit (#12 to #18 Fr for adults, #8 to #10 Fr for children, and #5 to #8 Fr for infants)
- Water-soluble lubricant
- Y-connector

IMPLEMENTATION
Performance
1. Prior to performing the procedure, introduce self and verify the client's identity using agency protocol. Explain to the client what you are going to do, why it is necessary, and how he or she can participate. Inform the client that suctioning will relieve breathing difficulty and, although the procedure is painless, it is noisy and can cause discomfort by stimulating the cough, gag, or sneeze reflex. **Rationale:** *Knowing that the procedure will relieve breathing problems is often reassuring and enlists the client's cooperation.*
2. Perform hand hygiene and observe other appropriate infection prevention procedures.
3. Provide for client privacy.
4. Prepare the client.
   - Position a conscious client who has a functional gag reflex in the semi-Fowler's position with the head turned to one side for oral suctioning or with the neck hyperextended for nasal suctioning. **Rationale:** *These positions facilitate the insertion of the catheter and help prevent aspiration of secretions.*
   - Position an unconscious client in the lateral position, facing you. **Rationale:** *This position allows the tongue to fall forward, so that it will not obstruct the catheter on insertion. The lateral position also facilitates drainage of secretions from the pharynx and prevents the possibility of aspiration.*
   - Place the towel or moisture-resistant pad over the pillow or under the chin.
5. Prepare the equipment.
   - Turn the suction device on and set to appropriate negative pressure on the suction gauge. The amount of negative pressure should be high enough to clear secretions but not too high. **Rationale:** *Too high of a pressure can cause the catheter to adhere to the tracheal wall and cause irritation or trauma. A rule of thumb is to use the lowest amount of suction pressure needed to clear the secretions.*

For Oral and Oropharyngeal Suctioning
- Apply clean gloves.
- Moisten the tip of the Yankauer or suction catheter with water or saline. **Rationale:** *This reduces friction and eases insertion.*
- Pull the tongue forward, if necessary, using gauze.
- Do not apply suction (that is, leave your finger off the port) during insertion. **Rationale:** *Applying suction during insertion causes trauma to the mucous membrane.*
- Advance the catheter about 10 to 15 cm (4 to 6 in.) along one side of the mouth into the oropharynx. **Rationale:** *Directing the catheter along the side prevents gagging.*
- It may be necessary during oropharyngeal suctioning to apply suction to secretions that collect in the mouth and beneath the tongue.
- Remove and discard gloves. Perform hand hygiene.

For Nasopharyngeal and Nasotracheal Suctioning
- Open the lubricant.
- Open the sterile suction package.
  a. Set up the cup or container, touching only the outside.
  b. Pour sterile water or saline into the container.

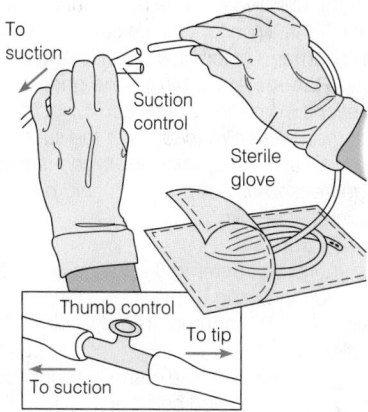

❶ Attaching the catheter to the suction unit.

  c. Apply the sterile gloves, or apply an unsterile glove on the nondominant hand and then a sterile glove on the dominant hand. **Rationale:** *The sterile gloved hand maintains the sterility of the suction catheter, and the unsterile gloved hand holds the suction connecting tubing and prevents transmission of the microorganisms to the nurse.*
- With your sterile gloved hand, pick up the sterile suction catheter and attach it to the suction connecting tubing being held in your nonsterile (nondominant) gloved hand. ❶
- Test the pressure of the suction and the patency of the catheter by applying your sterile gloved finger or thumb to the port or open branch of the Y-connector (the suction control) to create suction.
- If needed, apply or increase supplemental oxygen.
6. Lubricate and introduce the catheter.
   - Lubricate the catheter tip with sterile water, saline, or water-soluble lubricant. **Rationale:** *This reduces friction and eases insertion.*
   - Remove oxygen with the nondominant hand, if appropriate.
   - *Without applying suction*, insert the catheter into either naris and advance it along the floor of the nasal cavity. **Rationale:** *This avoids the nasal turbinates.*
   - Never force the catheter against an obstruction. If one nostril is obstructed, try the other.
7. Perform suctioning.
   - Apply your finger to the suction control port to start suction, and gently rotate the catheter. **Rationale:** *Gentle rotation of the catheter ensures that all surfaces are reached and prevents trauma to any one area of the respiratory mucosa due to prolonged suction.*
   - Apply intermittent suction for 5 to 10 seconds while slowly withdrawing the catheter, then remove your finger from the control and remove the catheter. **Rationale:** *Intermittent suction lessens the occurrence of trauma or irritation to the trachea and nasopharynx.*
   - A suction attempt should last only 10 to 15 seconds. During this time, the catheter is inserted, the suction is applied and discontinued, and the catheter is removed.

Continued on page 600

SKILL 26-1

Oropharyngeal, Nasopharyngeal, and Nasotracheal Suctioning—*continued*

8. Rinse the catheter and repeat suctioning as above.
- Rinse and flush the catheter and tubing with sterile water or saline.
- Relubricate the catheter, and repeat suctioning until the air passage is clear.
- Allow sufficient time between each suction for ventilation and oxygenation. Limit suctioning to 5 minutes total. **Rationale:** *Applying suction for too long may cause secretions to increase or may decrease the client's oxygen supply.*
- Encourage the client to breathe deeply and to cough between suctions. Monitor oxygen saturation and the client's respiration effort and color. Use supplemental oxygen, if appropriate. **Rationale:** *Coughing and deep breathing help carry secretions from the trachea and bronchi into the pharynx, where they can be reached with the suction catheter. Deep breathing and supplemental oxygen replenish oxygen that was decreased during the suctioning process.*

9. Obtain a specimen if required.
- Use a sputum trap. ❷
- Attach the suction catheter to the tubing of the sputum trap.
- Attach the suction tubing to the sputum trap air vent.
- Suction the client. The sputum trap will collect the mucus during suctioning.
- Remove the catheter from the client. Disconnect the sputum trap tubing from the suction catheter. Remove the suction tubing from the trap air vent.

❷ A sputum collection trap.

- Connect the tubing of the sputum trap to the air vent. **Rationale:** *This retains any microorganisms in the sputum trap.*
- Connect the suction catheter to the tubing.
- Flush the catheter to remove secretions from the tubing.

10. Promote client comfort.
- Offer to assist the client with oral or nasal hygiene.
- Assist the client to a position that facilitates breathing.

11. Dispose of equipment and ensure availability for the next suction.
- Dispose of the catheter, gloves, water, and waste container.
  a. Rinse the suction tubing as needed by inserting the end of the tubing into the used water container.
  b. Wrap the catheter around your sterile gloved hand and hold the catheter as the glove is removed over it for disposal.
- Perform hand hygiene.
- Empty and rinse the suction collection container as needed or indicated by protocol. Change the suction tubing and container daily.
- Ensure that supplies are available for the next suctioning (suction kit, gloves, and water or normal saline).

12. Assess the effectiveness of suctioning.
- Auscultate the client's breath sounds to ensure they are clear of secretions. Observe skin color, respiratory rate, heart rate, level of anxiety, and oxygen saturation levels.

13. Document relevant data.
- Record the procedure: the amount, consistency, color, and odor of sputum (e.g., foamy, white mucus; thick, green-tinged mucus; or blood-tinged mucus) and the client's respiratory status before and after the procedure. This may include lung sounds, rate and character of breathing, and oxygen saturation.
- If the procedure is carried out frequently, it may be appropriate to record only once, at the end of the shift; however, the frequency of the suctioning must be recorded.

SAMPLE DOCUMENTATION

11/12/2015 0830 Producing large amounts of thick, tenacious white mucus to back of oral pharynx but unable to expectorate into tissue. Uses Yankauer suction tube as needed. SpO_2 sat increased from 89% before suctioning to 93% after suctioning. RR also decreased from 26 to 18–20 after suctioning. Lungs clear to auscultation throughout all lobes. Continuous O_2 at 2 L/min via n/c. Will continue to reassess.
———— L. Webb, RN

EVALUATION

- Conduct appropriate follow-up, such as appearance of secretions suctioned; breath sounds; respiratory rate, rhythm, and depth; pulse rate and rhythm; oxygen saturation; and skin color.
- Compare findings to previous assessment data if available.
- Report significant deviations from normal to the primary care provider.

LIFESPAN CONSIDERATIONS Suctioning

INFANTS
- A bulb syringe is used to remove secretions from an infant's nose or mouth. Care needs to be taken to avoid stimulating the gag reflex.

CHILDREN
- A catheter is used to remove secretions from an older child's mouth or nose.

OLDER ADULTS
- Older adults often have cardiac and/or pulmonary disease, thus increasing their susceptibility to hypoxemia related to suctioning. Watch closely for signs of hypoxemia. If noted, stop suctioning and hyperoxygenate.

- Teach clients and families that the most important aspect of infection control is frequent hand washing.
- Airway suctioning in the home is considered a clean procedure.
- The catheter or Yankauer should be flushed by suctioning recently boiled or distilled water to rinse away mucus, followed by the suctioning of air through the device to dry the internal surface and, thus, discourage bacterial growth. The outer surface

of the device may be wiped with alcohol or hydrogen peroxide. The suction catheter or Yankauer should be allowed to dry and then be stored in a clean, dry area.
- Suction catheters treated in the manner described above may be reused. It is recommended that catheters be discarded after 24 hours. Yankauer suction tubes may be cleaned, boiled, and reused

TRACHEOSTOMY OR ENDOTRACHEAL TUBE SUCTIONING

Following endotracheal intubation or a tracheostomy, the trachea and surrounding respiratory tissues are irritated and react by producing excessive secretions. Sterile suctioning is necessary to remove these secretions from the trachea and bronchi to maintain a patent airway. The frequency of suctioning depends on the client's health and how recently the intubation was done. Additionally, suctioning may be necessary in clients who have increased secretions because of pneumonia or inability to clear secretions because of altered level of consciousness.

Open Suction System

The traditional method of suctioning an ETT or tracheostomy is sometimes referred to as the *open method*. If a client is connected to a ventilator, the nurse disconnects the client from the ventilator, suctions the airway, reconnects the client to the ventilator, and discards the suction catheter. This is called an open airway suction system.

Suctioning, by itself, causes hypoxemia (low oxygen in the blood). The repeated disconnecting of the client from the ventilator can also contribute to hypoxemia. Other drawbacks to the **open suction system** include the nurse needing to wear personal protective equipment (e.g., goggles or face shield, gown) to avoid exposure

to the client's sputum and the potential cost of one-time catheter use, especially if the client requires frequent suctioning.

Closed Suction System

With the **closed suction system** (sometimes called **in-line suctioning**) (Figure 26–8 ■), the nurse is not exposed to any secretions because the suction catheter is enclosed in a plastic sheath. The suction catheter attaches to the ventilator tubing, and the client does not need to be disconnected from the ventilator. The catheter can be reused as many times as necessary until the system is changed. The nurse needs to inquire about the agency's policy for changing the closed suction system.

Complications of Suctioning

Suctioning is associated with several complications: hypoxemia, trauma to the airway, nosocomial or health care–associated infection, and cardiac dysrhythmia, which is related to the hypoxemia. The following techniques are used to minimize or decrease these complications:

- *Suction only as needed.* Because suctioning the client with an ETT or tracheostomy is uncomfortable for the client and potentially hazardous because of hypoxemia, it should be performed only when indicated and not on a fixed schedule.
- *Sterile technique.* Infection of the lower respiratory tract can occur during tracheal suctioning. The nurse using sterile technique during the suctioning process can prevent this complication.

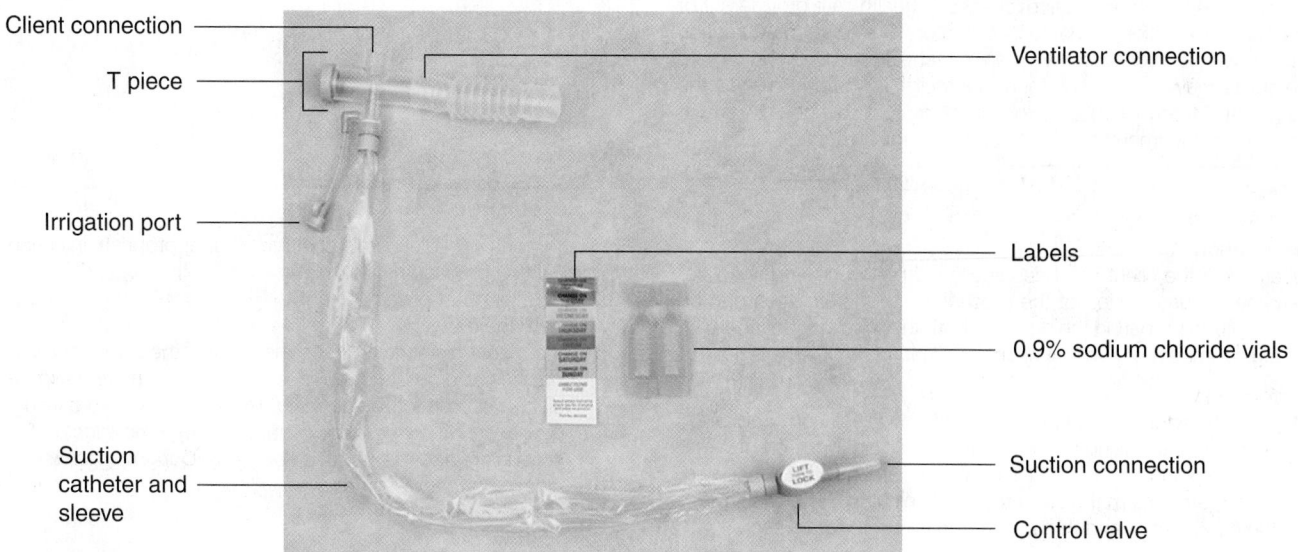

Client connection —
T piece —
Irrigation port —
Suction catheter and sleeve —

Ventilator connection
Labels
0.9% sodium chloride vials
Suction connection
Control valve

Figure 26–8 ■ A closed airway suction (in-line) system.

- **Hyperinflation.** This involves giving the client breaths that are greater than the tidal volume set on the ventilator through the ventilator circuit or via a manual resuscitation bag. Three to five breaths are delivered before and after each pass of the suction catheter.
- **Hyperventilation.** This involves increasing the number of breaths the client is receiving. This can be done through the ventilator or using a manual resuscitation bag. Note that both hyperinflation and hyperventilation help prevent suction hypoxemia; however, they should be used with caution because they can cause injury from overdistention of the lungs (Hess et al., 2012).
- **Hyperoxygenation.** This can be done with a manual resuscitation bag or through the ventilator and is performed by increasing the oxygen flow (usually to 100%) before suctioning and between suction attempts. This is the best technique to avoid suction-related hypoxemia.

- *Safe catheter size.* For tracheostomy and endotracheal suctioning, the outer diameter of the suction catheter should not exceed one half the internal diameter of the tracheostomy or endotracheal tube to allow air to enter around the catheter during suctioning so that hypoxia and trauma to the airway can be prevented (Nance-Floyd, 2011). A rule of thumb to determine suction catheter size is to double the millimeter size of the artificial airway. For example, an artificial airway (e.g., tracheostomy) diameter of 8 mm × 2 = 16. A size 16 French suction catheter would be the largest size catheter that would be safe to use.
- *No saline instillation.* Instilling normal saline into the airway has been a common practice and a routine part of the suctioning procedure. It was thought that the saline would facilitate removal of secretions and improve the client's oxygenation status. Research, however, has shown that saline instillation does *not* facilitate removal of secretions and causes adverse effects such as hypoxemia and increased risk of pneumonia (Ntoumenopoulos, 2013; Pierson, 2013).

●○○● NURSING PROCESS: TRACHEOSTOMY OR ENDOTRACHEAL TUBE SUCTIONING

Suctioning a Tracheostomy or Endotracheal Tube

SKILL 26–2

ASSESSMENT
Assess the client for the presence of adventitious (abnormal) breath sounds. Assess the client's cough reflex and note the client's ability or inability to remove the secretions through coughing.

PLANNING
DELEGATION

Suctioning a tracheostomy or ETT is a sterile, invasive technique requiring application of scientific knowledge and problem solving. This skill is performed by a nurse or respiratory therapist and is not delegated to UAP.

INTERPROFESSIONAL PRACTICE

Suctioning a client with a tracheostomy or endotracheal tube may be within the scope of practice for specific health care providers. For example, in addition to nurses, respiratory therapists may suction a client with a tracheostomy or endotracheal tube. Although these therapists may verbally communicate their findings and plan to the health care team members, the nurse must also know where to locate their documentation in the client's medical record.

Equipment
- Resuscitation bag (bag valve mask) connected to 100% oxygen
- Sterile towel (optional)
- Equipment for suctioning (see Skill 26–1)
- Goggles and mask if necessary
- Gown (if necessary)
- Sterile gloves
- Moisture-resistant bag

IMPLEMENTATION
Preparation
Determine if the client has been suctioned previously and, if so, review the documentation of the procedure. This information can be very helpful in preparing the nurse for both the physiological and psychological impact of suctioning on the client.

Performance
1. Prior to performing the procedure, introduce self and verify the client's identity using agency protocol. Explain to the client what you are going to do, why it is necessary, and how he or she can participate. Inform the client that suctioning usually stimulates the cough reflex and that this assists in removing the secretions.

2. Perform hand hygiene and observe other appropriate infection prevention procedures.
3. Provide for client privacy.
4. Prepare the client.
   - If not contraindicated, place the client in the semi-Fowler's position to promote deep breathing, maximum lung expansion, and productive coughing. **Rationale:** *Deep breathing oxygenates the lungs, counteracts the hypoxic effects of suctioning, and may induce coughing. Coughing helps to loosen and move secretions.*

Suctioning a Tracheostomy or Endotracheal Tube—*continued*

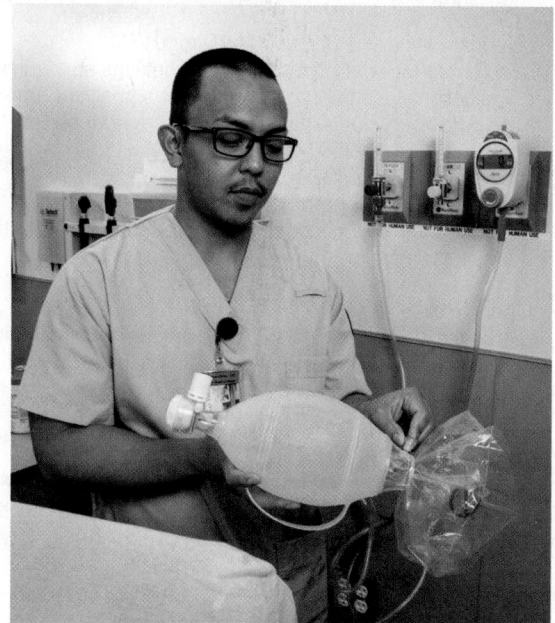

❶ Attaching the resuscitation apparatus to the oxygen source.

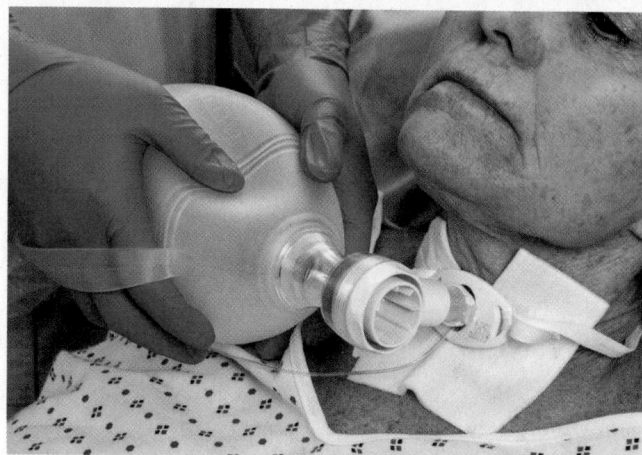

❷ Attaching the resuscitator to the tracheostomy tube.

5. Prepare the equipment (open suction system). See the *Variation* section for a closed suction system.
   * Attach the resuscitation apparatus to the oxygen source. **❶** Adjust the oxygen flow to 100%.
   * Open the sterile supplies:
     a. Suction kit or catheter
     b. Sterile basin/container.
   * Pour sterile normal saline or water in the sterile basin.
   * Place the sterile towel, if used, across the client's chest below the tracheostomy or on a workspace.
   * Turn on the suction, and set the pressure in accordance with agency policy. The suction pressure should be set at what is needed to adequately remove secretions. Hess et al. (2012) states that the suction pressure "should *not exceed* 100 mmHg in infants, 125 mmHg in children and 150 mmHg in adults" (p. 413). Nance-Floyd (2011) recommends using suction pressure of up to 120 mmHg for open system suctioning and up to 160 mmHg for closed system suctioning (p. 15).
   * Apply goggles, mask, and gown if necessary.
   * Apply sterile gloves. Some agencies recommend putting a sterile glove on the dominant hand and an unsterile glove on the nondominant hand. **Rationale:** *The sterile gloved hand maintains the sterility of the suction catheter, and the unsterile glove holds the suction connecting tubing and prevents the transmission of the microorganisms to the nurse.*
   * Holding the catheter in the dominant hand and the connector in the nondominant hand, attach the suction catheter to the suction tubing (see Skill 26–1, Figure **❶**).
6. Flush and lubricate the catheter.
   * Using the dominant hand, place the catheter tip in the sterile saline solution.
   * Using the thumb of the nondominant hand, occlude the thumb control and suction a small amount of the sterile solution through the catheter. **Rationale:** *This determines that the suction equipment is working properly and lubricates the outside and the lumen of the catheter. Lubrication eases insertion and reduces tissue trauma during insertion. Lubricating the lumen also helps prevent secretions from sticking to the inside of the catheter.*

7. If the client does not have copious secretions, hyperventilate the lungs with a resuscitation bag before suctioning.
   * Summon an assistant, if one is available, for this step.
   * Using your nondominant hand, turn on the oxygen to 12 to 15 L/min.
   * If the client is receiving oxygen, disconnect the oxygen source from the tracheostomy tube using your nondominant hand.
   * Attach the resuscitator to the tracheostomy or ETT. **❷**
   * Compress the Ambu bag three to five times, as the client inhales. This is best done by a second person who can use both hands to compress the bag.
   * Observe the rise and fall of the client's chest to assess the adequacy of each ventilation.
   * Remove the resuscitation device and place it on the bed or the client's chest with the connector facing up.

Variation: Using a Ventilator to Provide Hyperventilation
If the client is on a ventilator, use the ventilator for hyperventilation and hyperoxygenation. Newer models have a mode that provides 100% oxygen for 2 minutes and then switches back to the previous oxygen setting as well as a manual breath or sigh button. **Rationale:** *The use of ventilator settings provides more consistent delivery of oxygenation and hyperinflation than a resuscitation device.*

8. If the client has copious secretions, do not hyperventilate with a resuscitator. *Instead:*
   * Keep the regular oxygen delivery device on and increase the liter flow or adjust the FiO_2 to 100% for several breaths before suctioning. **Rationale:** *Hyperventilating a client who has copious secretions can force the secretions deeper into the respiratory tract.*
9. Quickly but gently insert the catheter *without* applying any suction.
   * With your nondominant thumb off the suction port, quickly but gently insert the catheter into the trachea through the tracheostomy tube. **❸ Rationale:** *To prevent tissue trauma and oxygen loss, suction is not applied during insertion of the catheter.*
   * Insert the catheter about 0.5 to 1 cm (0.2 to 0.4 in.) past the distal end of the tube for an open system, and 1 to 2 cm (0.4 to 08. in.) past the distal end for a closed system (Nance-Floyd, 2011) or until the client coughs. If you feel resistance, withdraw the catheter about 1 to 2 cm (0.4 to 0.8 in.) before applying suction. **Rationale:** *Resistance usually means that the catheter tip has reached the bifurcation of the trachea. Withdrawing the catheter prevents damaging the mucous membranes at the bifurcation.*

Continued on page 604

Suctioning a Tracheostomy or Endotracheal Tube—*continued*

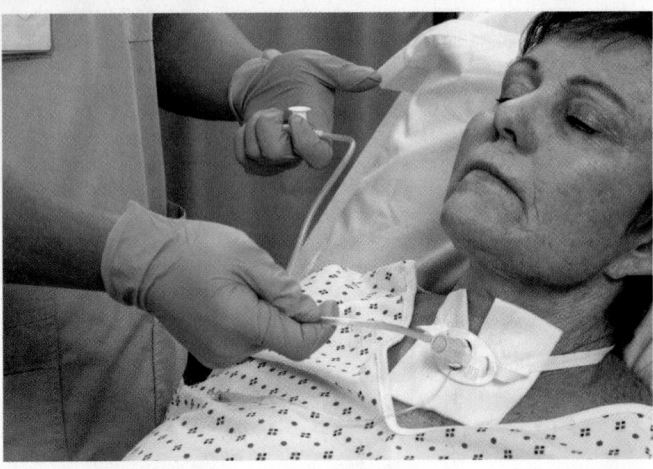

❸ Inserting the catheter into the trachea through the tracheostomy tube. *Note:* Suction is *not* applied while inserting the catheter.

10. Perform suctioning.
    - Apply suction for 5 to 10 seconds by placing the nondominant thumb over the thumb port. **Rationale:** *Suction time is restricted to a maximum of 10 seconds, preferably less to minimize oxygen loss.*
    - Rotate the catheter by rolling it between your thumb and forefinger while slowly withdrawing it. **Rationale:** *This prevents tissue trauma by minimizing the suction time against any part of the trachea.*
    - Withdraw the catheter completely, and release the suction.
    - Hyperventilate the client.
    - Suction again, if needed.
11. Reassess the client's oxygenation status and repeat suctioning.
    - Observe the client's respirations and skin color. Check the client's pulse if necessary, using your nondominant hand. If the client is on a cardiac monitor, assess the rate and rhythm.
    - Encourage the client to breathe deeply and to cough between suctions.
    - Allow 2 to 3 minutes with oxygen, as appropriate, between suctions when possible. **Rationale:** *This provides an opportunity for reoxygenation of the lungs.*
    - Flush the catheter and repeat suctioning until the air passage is clear and the breathing is relatively effortless and quiet.
    - After each suction, pick up the resuscitation bag with your nondominant hand and ventilate the client with no more than three breaths.
12. Dispose of equipment and ensure availability for the next suction.
    - Flush the catheter and suction tubing.
    - Turn off the suction and disconnect the catheter from the suction tubing.
    - Wrap the catheter around your sterile hand and peel the glove off so that it turns inside out over the catheter. Remove the other glove.
    - Discard the gloves and the catheter in the moisture-resistant bag.
    - Perform hand hygiene.
    - Replenish the sterile fluid and supplies so that the suction is ready for use again. **Rationale:** *Clients who require*

suctioning often require it quickly, so it is essential to leave the equipment at the bedside ready for use.*
    - Be sure that the ventilator and oxygen settings are returned to presuctioning settings. **Rationale:** *On some ventilators this is automatic, but always check. It is very dangerous for clients to be left on 100% oxygen.*
13. Provide for client comfort and safety.
    - Assist the client to a comfortable, safe position that aids breathing. If the client is conscious, a semi-Fowler's position is frequently indicated. If the client is unconscious, Sims' position aids in the drainage of secretions from the mouth.
14. Document relevant data.
    - Record the suctioning, including the amount and description of suction returns, how the client tolerated the procedure, and any other relevant assessments.

SAMPLE DOCUMENTATION

11/13/2015 1000 Coarse crackles in RLL and LLL. Requires suctioning about every 1–2 hrs. Obtain large amount of pinkish-tinged white thin mucus via ETT. Breath sounds clearer after suctioning. SpO$_2$ increases from 90% before suctioning to 95% after suctioning. Client signals when he wants to be suctioned. ——————— C. Holmes, RN

Variation: Closed Suction System (In-Line Catheter)
- If a catheter is not attached, apply clean gloves, aseptically open a new closed catheter set, and attach the ventilator connection on the T-piece to the ventilator tubing. Attach the client connection to the ETT or tracheostomy.
- Attach one end of the suction connecting tubing to the suction connection port of the closed system and the other end of the connecting tubing to the suction device.
- Turn suction on, occlude or kink the tubing, and depress the suction control valve (on the closed catheter system) to set suction to the appropriate level. Release the suction control valve.
- Use the ventilator to hyperoxygenate and hyperinflate the client's lungs.
- Unlock the suction control mechanism if required by the manufacturer.
- Advance the suction catheter enclosed in its plastic sheath with the dominant hand. Steady the T-piece with the nondominant hand.
- Depress the suction control valve, apply intermittent suction for no more than 10 seconds, and gently withdraw the catheter.
- Repeat as needed, remembering to provide hyperoxygenation and hyperinflation as needed.
- When completed suctioning, withdraw the catheter into its sleeve and close the access valve, if appropriate. **Rationale:** *If the system does not have an access valve on the client connector, the nurse needs to observe for the potential of the catheter migrating into the airway and partially obstructing the artificial airway.*
- Flush the catheter by instilling normal saline into the irrigation port and applying suction. Repeat until the catheter is clear.
- Close the irrigation port and close the suction valve.
- Remove and discard gloves.
- Perform hand hygiene.

EVALUATION
- Perform a follow-up examination of the client to determine the effectiveness of the suctioning (e.g., respiratory rate, depth, and character; breath sounds; color of skin and nail beds; character and amount of secretions suctioned; and changes in vital signs [e.g., heart rate, oxygen saturation]).
- Relate findings to previous assessment data if available.
- Report significant deviations from normal to the primary care provider.

LIFESPAN CONSIDERATIONS | Suctioning a Tracheostomy or Endotracheal Tube

INFANTS AND CHILDREN
- An assistant or parent may be needed to gently hold the child and to keep hands out of the way. The assistant or parent should maintain the child's head in the midline position.

ADULTS AND OLDER ADULTS
- Health care–associated pneumonia and ventilator-associated pneumonia (VAP) can occur because of infected secretions in the upper airway. Oral antiseptic rinses (e.g., chlorhexidine gluconate) reduce the rate of nosocomial pneumonia in critically ill clients (Booker, Murff, Kitko, & Jablonski, 2013).
- Do a thorough lung assessment before and after suctioning to determine effectiveness of suctioning and to be aware of any special problems.

Ambulatory and Community Settings | Suctioning a Tracheostomy or Endotracheal Tube | **PATIENT-CENTERED CARE**

- Whenever possible, the client should be encouraged to clear the airway by coughing.
- Clients may need to learn to suction their secretions if they cannot cough effectively.
- Clean gloves should be used when endotracheal suctioning is performed in the home environment.

- The nurse needs to instruct the caregiver on how to determine the need for suctioning and the correct process and rationale underlying the practice of suctioning to avoid potential complications.
- Stress the importance of adequate hydration. It thins secretions, which can aid in their removal by coughing or suctioning.

Chapter 26 Review

FOCUSING ON CLINICAL THINKING

Consider This

1. A client who has a history of coronary artery disease (CAD) and chronic pulmonary disease recently had major abdominal surgery and is currently on a ventilator. He has copious amounts of secretions and requires frequent suctioning. The nurses are using the open suction system. Upon suctioning, the client becomes restless and anxious, his heart rate decreases, and the cardiac monitor shows an occasional missed and extra beat. What actions would you take when caring for this client?

2. You have just suctioned and cleared a client's endotracheal tube of secretions. You assessed the client's need for upper airway suctioning and removed a small amount of oral secretions. As you start to remove your gloves and discard the catheter, the client begins coughing and loosens up a moderate amount of secretions from his lower airway. How do you proceed?

3. A client requires nasopharyngeal suctioning. You notice that the client's right naris is reddened and sore, and minimal bleeding occurs after suctioning. What actions would you take to promote both comfort and oxygenation needs for this client?

See Focusing on Clinical Thinking answers on student resource website.

TEST YOUR KNOWLEDGE

1. The unlicensed assistive person (UAP) tells the nurse that the client needs "a new plastic thing—you know, that thing she uses to suction out her mouth." The nurse recognizes that the UAP is talking about which piece of suction equipment?
   1. In-line suction catheter
   2. Yankauer suction tube
   3. Whistle-tipped catheter
   4. Open airway suction system

2. The nurse is caring for a client who just returned from surgery and is still sedated. When stimulated the client breathes normally, but when the client is sleeping deeply the airway becomes intermittently blocked by the tongue. What type of artificial airway might the nurse insert to maintain a patent airway until the sedation level diminishes?
   1. Nasopharyngeal airway
   2. Oropharyngeal airway
   3. Endotracheal airway
   4. Tracheostomy

3. The nurse is caring for a client who has no respiratory effort after experiencing head trauma. It is expected that the client will require long-term airway maintenance. What type of airway would the nurse anticipate would be the best choice for this client?
   1. Nasopharyngeal airway
   2. Oropharyngeal airway
   3. Endotracheal airway
   4. Tracheostomy

4. The nurse is preparing to suction the client. Which form of airway suctioning must be performed using sterile technique?
   1. Oropharyngeal suctioning
   2. Nasopharyngeal suctioning
   3. Oropharyngeal or nasopharyngeal suctioning
   4. Endotracheal suctioning

5. Which represents proper nasopharyngeal/nasotracheal suction technique?
   1. Lubricate the suction catheter with petroleum jelly before and between insertions.
   2. Apply suction intermittently while inserting the suction catheter.
   3. Rotate the catheter while applying suction.
   4. Hyperoxygenate with 100% oxygen for 30 minutes before and after suctioning.

6. The nurse is admitting an adult client who has a tracheostomy and requires suctioning. The nurse will set the suction to which pressure setting?
   1. 60 to 100 mmHg
   2. 100 to 140 mmHg
   3. 80 to 120 mmHg
   4. 160 to 200 mmHg

7. The nurse is preparing to suction a client requiring mechanical ventilation via an endotracheal tube. Which are advantages of a closed airway suctioning system? Select all that apply.
   1. The nurse is not exposed to secretions.
   2. The client does not need to be disconnected from the ventilator.
   3. The catheter can be reused many times until the system is changed.
   4. The nurse does not need to insert the catheter as far into the trachea.
   5. The nurse does not need to wear goggles.

8. The nurse is caring for a client with a tracheostomy in place. The primary care provider has ordered suctioning of the tracheostomy every 4 hours. The nurse knows that scheduled suctioning is contraindicated because (select all that apply):
   1. Suctioning is uncomfortable for the client.
   2. More frequent suctioning may be required at some times.
   3. Less frequent suctioning may be required at some times.
   4. Suctioning increases the risk of nosocomial infections.
   5. Suctioning is time consuming and costly.

9. The nurse is preparing to suction the nasopharynx. Place the following steps in the order in which the nurse would perform them:
   1. Test the pressure of the suction and patency of the catheter.
   2. Lubricate the tip and introduce the catheter.
   3. Rinse and flush the suction catheter.
   4. Attach the catheter to the suction source.
   5. Apply suction for 5 to 10 seconds.

10. The nurse is preparing to suction an adult client's endotracheal tube using an open system. It is important that the nurse do which action prior to inserting the catheter?
   1. Apply suction to the catheter.
   2. Set suction at 60 mmHg.
   3. Reduce the oxygen concentration delivered to the client.
   4. Give breaths greater than the client's usual tidal volume.

See Answers to Test Your Knowledge in Appendix A.

READINGS AND REFERENCES

References

Booker, S., Murff, S., Kitko, L., & Jablonski, R. (2013). Mouth care to reduce ventilator-associated pneumonia. *American Journal of Nursing, 113*(10), 24–30. doi:10.1097/01.NAJ.0000435343.38287.3a

Hess, D. R., MacIntyre, N. R., Mishoe, S. C., Galvin, W. R., & Adams, A. B. (2012). *Respiratory care principles and practice* (2nd ed.). Sudbury, MA: Jones & Bartlett.

Nance-Floyd, B. (2011). Tracheostomy care: An evidence-based guide to suctioning and dressing changes. *American Nurse Today, 6*(7), 14–16.

Ntoumenopoulos, G. (2013). Endotracheal suctioning may or may not have an impact, but it does depend on what you measure! *Respiratory Care, 58,* 1707–1710. doi:10.4187/respcare.02745

Pierson, D. J. (2013). Effects of standardizing procedures on adverse effects of endotracheal suctioning. *Critical Care Alert, 21*(7), 54–55.

Selected Bibliography

Berman, A., Snyder, S., & Frandsen, G. (2016). *Kozier & Erb's fundamentals of nursing: Concepts, process, and practice* (10th ed.). Upper Saddle River, NJ: Pearson.

McClean, E. B. (2012). Tracheal suctioning in children with chronic tracheostomies: A pilot study applying suction both while inserting and removing the catheter. *Journal of Pediatric Nursing, 27,* 50–54. doi:10.1016/j.pedn.2010.11.007

Özden, D., & Görgülü, S. R. (2012). Development of standard practice guidelines for open and closed system suctioning. *Journal of Clinical Nursing, 21,* 1327–1338. doi:10.1111/j.1365-2702.2011.03997.x

Preston, W. (2013). The increasing use of non-invasive ventilation. *Practice Nursing, 24*(3), 114–119.

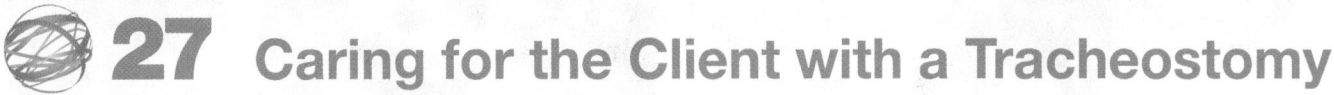

27 Caring for the Client with a Tracheostomy

LEARNING OUTCOMES

At the completion of this chapter, the student will be able to:

1. Define the key terms used in the skills of caring for the client with a tracheostomy.
2. List three types of tracheostomy tubes.
3. Identify parts of a tracheostomy tube and their purposes.
4. Describe methods of facilitating communication for a client with a tracheostomy.
5. Recognize when it is appropriate to delegate tracheostomy care to unlicensed assistive personnel.

6. Verbalize the steps used in:
   a. Providing tracheostomy care.
   b. Capping a tracheostomy tube with a speaking valve.
7. Demonstrate appropriate documentation and reporting of tracheostomy care.

SKILLS

Skill 27–1 Providing Tracheostomy Care

Skill 27–2 Capping a Tracheostomy Tube with a Speaking Valve

KEY TERMS

cuffed tracheostomy tube, *608*
fenestrated tracheostomy
 tube, *608*

flange, *607*
inner cannula, *608*
obturator, *607*

outer cannula, *607*
tracheostomy, *607*

uncuffed tracheostomy tube, *608*
weaned, *608*

Clients who need long-term airway support or who have a need to bypass the upper airway may have a **tracheostomy**, a surgical opening in the trachea just below the larynx. A tube is usually inserted through this opening, and an artificial airway is created. A tracheostomy is created using one of two techniques: the traditional open surgical method or a percutaneous insertion. The percutaneous method can be done at the bedside. The open technique is done in the operating room, and a surgical incision is made in the trachea just below the larynx. A curved tracheostomy tube is inserted to extend through the stoma into the trachea (Figure 27–1 ■).

TRACHEOSTOMY

Advantages of a tracheostomy over endotracheal intubation include improved client comfort and reduced laryngeal, pharyngeal, oral, and nasal damage that can be caused by long-term endotracheal tube placement. The use of nasogastric or nasoenteric tubes for nutrition may not be necessary because a client can swallow effectively with a tracheostomy tube in place. Management of oral secretions is improved, and clients, with the use of adaptive devices, are able to speak with tracheostomy tubes.

Tracheostomy Tubes

Tracheostomy tubes may be either a soft, flexible plastic or silicone, or a rigid metal. They are available in different sizes, and they may

or may not have a cuff. Tracheostomy tubes (Figure 27–2 ■) have an **outer cannula** that is inserted into the trachea, with a **flange** that rests against the neck and allows the tube to be secured in place with tracheostomy twill ties or a Velcro collar. All tubes also have an **obturator** that is used to insert the outer cannula and is then removed. The obturator, along with a spare tracheostomy tube of the same size or smaller, is kept at the client's bedside in case the tube or outer cannula becomes dislodged and needs to be reinserted. Some tracheostomy tubes have an inner cannula that is inserted and locked into place inside the outer cannula. The purpose of the inner cannula is to prevent tube obstruction by allowing regular cleaning or replacement. Many plastic inner cannulas are cleaned with a solution of full or half-strength hydrogen peroxide and sterile water. Some facilities, however, recommend using normal saline only. Morris, Whitmer, and McIntosh (2013) note that it is important to check the manufacturers' instructions for cleaning tracheostomy tubes because silicone tubes and metal tubes can be damaged by using hydrogen peroxide (p. 21). The outer cannula of the tracheostomy tube remains in place to maintain a patent airway.

CLINICAL ALERT!

Some inner cannulas are disposable. These cannulas have a different method of attachment than the nondisposable tubes. Also, the different types of disposable tubes are not interchangeable.

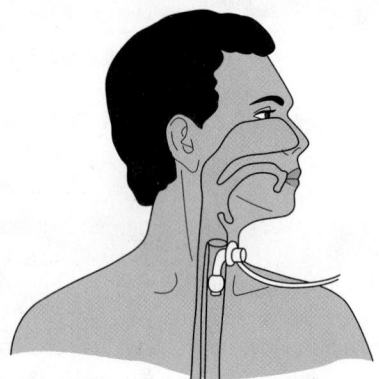

Figure 27–1 ■ A tracheostomy tube in place.

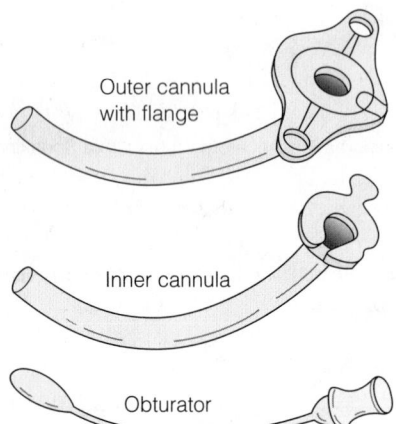

Figure 27–2 ■ Components of a tracheostomy tube.

Outer cannula
with flange

Inner cannula

Obturator

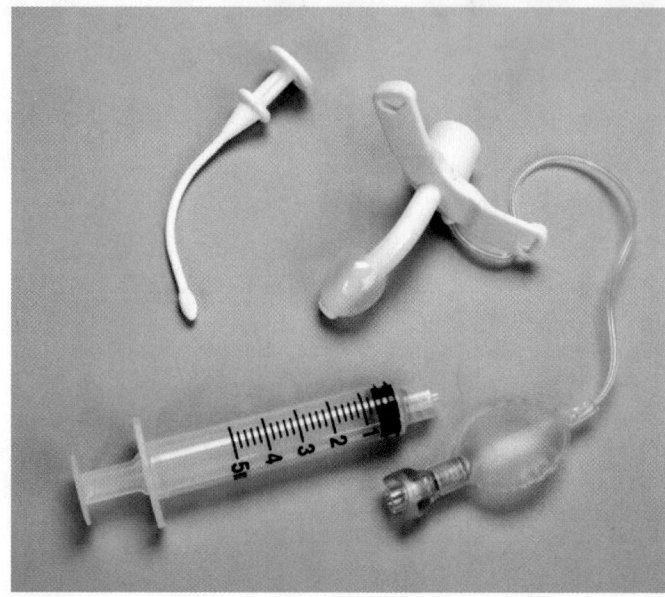

Figure 27–3 ■ A tracheostomy tube with a low-pressure cuff.

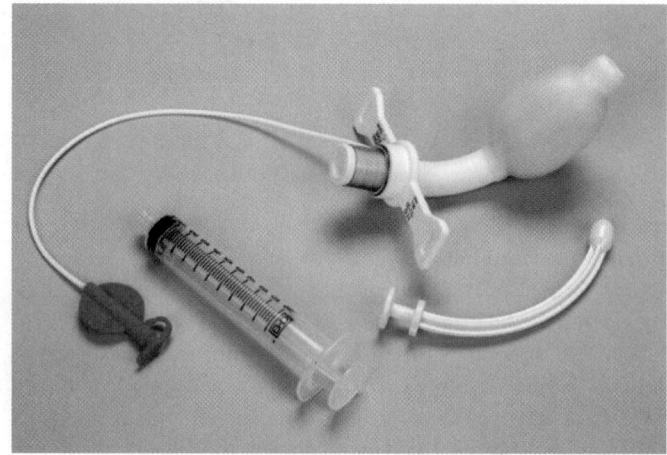

Figure 27–4 ■ A tracheostomy tube with a foam cuff.

Three types of tracheostomy tubes are available: uncuffed, cuffed, and fenestrated. An uncuffed tube may be plastic or metal, which allows for air to flow around the tube. A child with a permanent tracheostomy may use an **uncuffed tracheostomy tube** because a child's trachea is resilient enough to seal the air space around the tube. **Cuffed tracheostomy tubes** (Figure 27–3 ■) are surrounded by an inflatable cuff that produces an airtight seal between the tube and the trachea. This seal prevents aspiration of oropharyngeal secretions, and air leakage between the tube and the trachea. Cuffed tubes are often used immediately after a tracheostomy and are essential when ventilating a tracheostomy client with a mechanical ventilator.

Low-pressure cuffs are commonly used to distribute a low, even pressure against the trachea, thus decreasing the risk of tracheal tissue necrosis. They do not need to be deflated periodically to reduce pressure on the tracheal wall. The foam cuff does not require injected air; instead when the port is opened, ambient air enters the balloon, which then conforms to the client's trachea (Figure 27–4 ■). Air is removed from the cuff prior to insertion or removal of the tube.

If the client has a tracheostomy tube with a cuff that needs to be inflated, the nurse needs to ensure that the air pressure within the cuff is within safe limits (less than 25 cm H_2O). The cuff pressure should be checked at least every 8 hours or once a shift using a cuff manometer (Barnett, 2012; Frace, 2010).

The **fenestrated tracheostomy tube** has holes in the outer cannula (Figure 27–5 ■). The **inner cannula** is in place when the client is on mechanical ventilation. When the client is being **weaned** (gradual discontinuation of mechanical support), the inner cannula is removed, the cuff is deflated, and the external opening of the tracheostomy tube is plugged. The client can then breathe around the tube and through the fenestration and also talk because the tracheostomy tube is plugged. If the client becomes tired and needs to return to using the ventilator, the nurse can easily do this by removing the plug from the tracheostomy tube, inserting the inner cannula (which occludes the fenestration), inflating the cuff, and attaching the ventilator.

TRACHEOSTOMY CARE

The nurse provides tracheostomy care for the client with a new or recent tracheostomy to maintain patency of the tube and reduce the risk of infection. Initially, a tracheostomy may need to be suctioned (see Chapter 26 ∞) and cleaned as often as every 1 to 2 hours. After the initial inflammatory response subsides, tracheostomy care may be required only once or twice a day, depending on the client. For a client with a new tracheostomy, aseptic technique should be used when providing tracheostomy care in order to prevent infection.

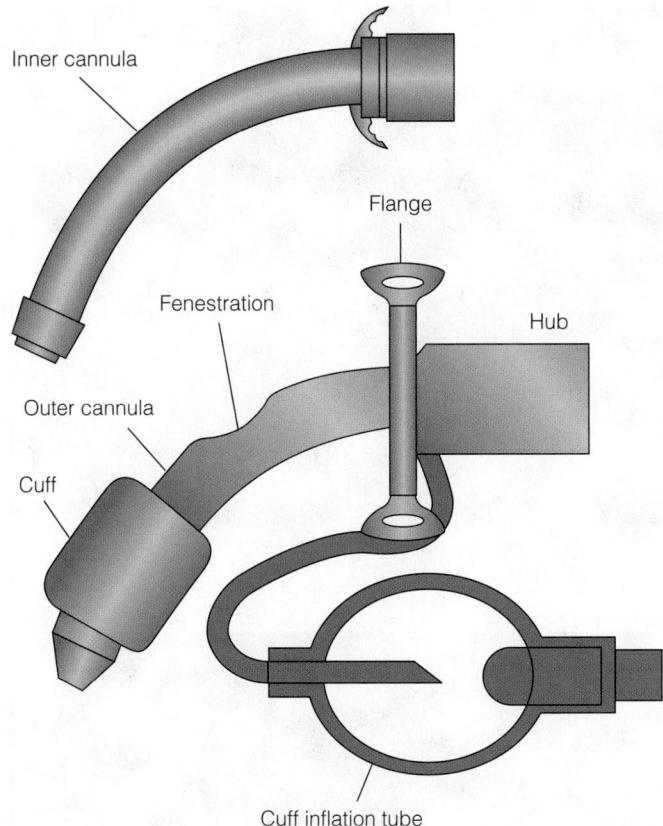

Figure 27–5 ■ A fenestrated tracheostomy tube.

Inner cannula

Flange

Fenestration

Hub

Outer cannula

Cuff

Cuff inflation tube

After the stoma has healed, clean gloves can be used while changing the dressing and tie tapes. Skill 27–1 describes tracheostomy care.

Tracheostomy Dressing and Ties

As part of tracheostomy care, the tracheostomy dressing and the ties need to be changed whenever they become soiled. Soiled dressings harbor microorganisms and can be a potential source of skin excoriation, breakdown, and infection around the tracheostomy incision. Usually, the dressing is changed after the cannula is cleaned, but more frequent dressing changes may be necessary. The dressing technique is described in Skill 27–1.

Before applying a new dressing, the nurse needs to check any special orders or agency protocols regarding application of solutions around the tracheostomy site. Non–cotton-filled 4×4 gauze dressings are used. Do not cut the gauze square because gauze fibers can be aspirated. Precut, nonraveling tracheostomy dressings are commonly available either in separate packages or as part of a tracheostomy cleaning kit. Newer products include a nonadhesive hydrocellular dressing consisting of a cushioned pad that absorbs large amounts of secretions.

Tracheostomy ties should be replaced as needed, according to agency policy. Twill tape and specially manufactured Velcro ties are available. Twill tape is inexpensive and readily available; however, it is easily soiled and can trap moisture that leads to irritation of the skin of the neck. Velcro ties are becoming more commonly used. They are wider, more comfortable, and cause less skin abrasion.

For client safety, the literature recommends a two-person technique when changing the securing device to prevent tube dislodgement. This involves one person holding the tracheostomy tube in place while the other changes the securing device (see Skill 27–1).

●○● NURSING PROCESS: TRACHEOSTOMY

Providing Tracheostomy Care

ASSESSMENT
Assess:
- Respiratory status including ease of breathing, rate, rhythm, depth, lung sounds, and oxygen saturation level.
- Pulse rate.
- Character and amount of secretions from the tracheostomy site.

- Presence of drainage on the tracheostomy dressing or ties.
- Appearance of the incision (note any redness, swelling, purulent discharge, or odor).

PLANNING
DELEGATION

Tracheostomy care involves application of scientific knowledge, sterile technique, and problem solving, and therefore needs to be performed by a nurse or respiratory therapist.

INTERPROFESSIONAL PRACTICE

Providing tracheostomy care may be within the scope of practice for specific health care providers. For example, in addition to nurses, respiratory therapists may help provide tracheostomy care for a client. Although these therapists may verbally communicate their findings and plan to the health care members, the nurse must also know where to locate their documentation in the client's medical record.

Equipment
- Sterile disposable tracheostomy cleaning kit or supplies including sterile containers, sterile nylon brush and/or pipe cleaners, sterile applicators, gauze squares
- Disposable inner cannula if applicable
- Towel or drape to protect bed linens
- Sterile suction catheter kit (suction catheter and sterile container for solution)
- Sterile normal saline (Some agencies may use a mixture of hydrogen peroxide and sterile normal saline. Check agency protocol for soaking solution.)
- Sterile gloves (two pairs—one pair for suctioning if needed)
- Clean gloves
- Moisture-resistant bag
- Commercially prepared sterile tracheostomy dressing or sterile 4×4 gauze dressing
- Cotton twill ties or Velcro collar
- Clean scissors

Continued on page 610

SKILL 27-1

Providing Tracheostomy Care—*continued*

IMPLEMENTATION
Performance

1. Prior to performing the procedure, introduce self and verify the client's identity using agency protocol. Explain to the client what you are going to do, why it is necessary, and how he or she can participate. Provide for a means of communication, such as eye blinking or raising a finger, to indicate pain or distress. Follow through by carefully observing the client throughout the procedure. Offer periodic eye contact, caring touch, and verbal reassurance. Some clients respond well to a sense of efficiency and gentle humor, and nurses must decide when to use this approach.

2. Perform hand hygiene and observe other appropriate infection prevention procedures.

3. Provide for client privacy.

4. Prepare the client and the equipment.
   - Assist the client to a semi-Fowler's or Fowler's position to promote lung expansion.
   - Suction the tracheostomy tube, if needed. (See Skill 26–2 in Chapter 26 ∞.)
   - If suctioning was required, allow the client to rest and restore oxygenation.
   - Open the tracheostomy kit or sterile basins.
   - Establish a sterile field.
   - Open other sterile supplies as needed including sterile applicators, suction kit, tracheostomy dressing, and disposable inner cannula if applicable.
   - Pour the soaking solution and sterile normal saline into separate containers.
   - Apply clean gloves.
   - Remove the oxygen source.
   - Unlock the inner cannula (if present) and remove it by gently pulling it out toward you in line with its curvature. Place the inner cannula in the soaking solution. **Rationale:** *This moistens and loosens dried secretions.*
   - Based on client's respiratory assessments, place the oxygen source over or near the outer cannula. **Rationale:** *This prevents oxygen desaturation by maintaining oxygen to the client.*
   - Remove the soiled tracheostomy dressing. Place the soiled dressing in your gloved hand and peel the glove off so that it turns inside out over the dressing. Remove and discard gloves and the dressing.
   - Perform hand hygiene.
   - Apply sterile gloves. Keep your dominant hand sterile during the procedure.

5. Clean the inner cannula. (See the *Variation* section for using a disposable inner cannula.)
   - Remove the inner cannula from the soaking solution.
   - Clean the lumen and entire inner cannula thoroughly, using the brush or pipe cleaners moistened with sterile normal saline. ❶ Inspect the cannula for cleanliness by holding it at eye level and looking through it into the light.
   - Rinse the inner cannula thoroughly in the sterile normal saline.
   - After rinsing, gently tap the cannula against the inside edge of the sterile saline container. Use a pipe cleaner folded in half to dry only the inside of the cannula; do not dry the outside. **Rationale:** *This removes excess liquid from the cannula and prevents possible aspiration by the client, while leaving a film of moisture on the outer surface to lubricate the cannula for reinsertion.*

6. Replace the inner cannula, securing it in place.
   - Insert the inner cannula by grasping the outer flange and inserting the cannula in the direction of its curvature.

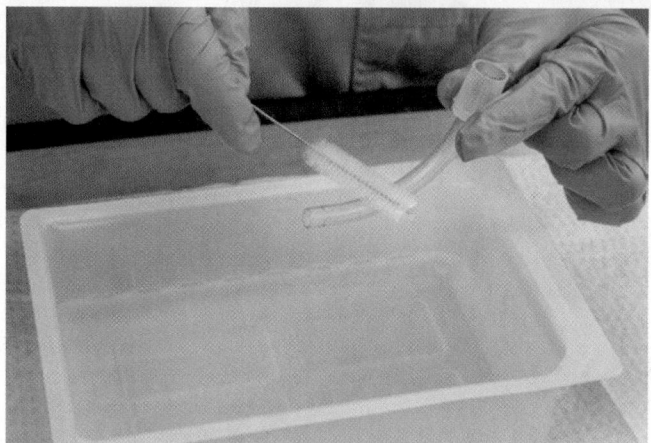
❶ Cleaning the inner cannula with a brush.

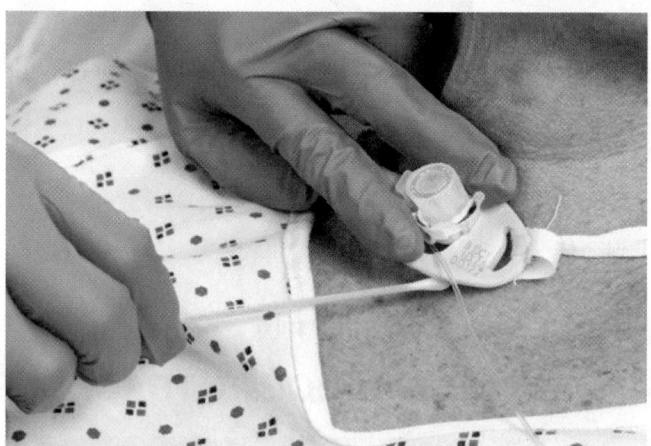
❷ Using an applicator stick to clean the tracheostomy site.

   - Lock the cannula in place by turning the lock (if present) into position to secure the flange of the inner cannula to the outer cannula.

7. Clean the incision site and tube flange.
   - Using sterile applicators or gauze dressings moistened with normal saline, clean the incision site. ❷ Handle the sterile supplies with your dominant hand. Use each applicator or gauze dressing only once and then discard. **Rationale:** *This avoids contaminating a clean area with a soiled gauze dressing or applicator.*
   - Hydrogen peroxide may be used (usually in a half-strength solution mixed with sterile normal saline; use a separate sterile container if this is necessary) to remove crusty secretions around the tracheostomy site. Do not use directly on the site. Check agency policy. Thoroughly rinse the cleaned area using gauze squares moistened with sterile normal saline. **Rationale:** *Hydrogen peroxide can be irritating to the skin and inhibit healing if not thoroughly removed.*
   - Clean the flange of the tube in the same manner.
   - Thoroughly dry the client's skin and tube flanges with dry gauze squares.

8. Apply a sterile dressing.
   - Use a commercially prepared split-gauze ❸ or nonadhesive hydrocellular tracheostomy dressing, which is a cushioned

Providing Tracheostomy Care—*continued*

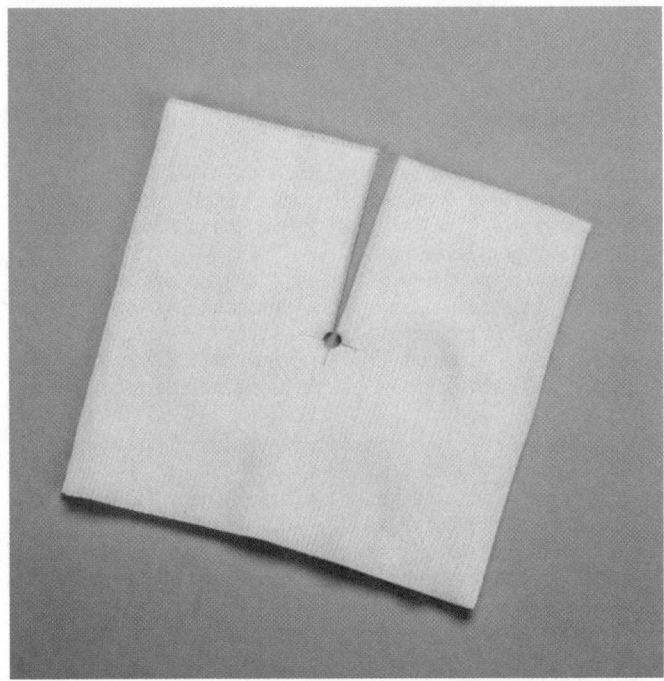

❸ A commercially prepared tracheostomy dressing of nonraveling material.

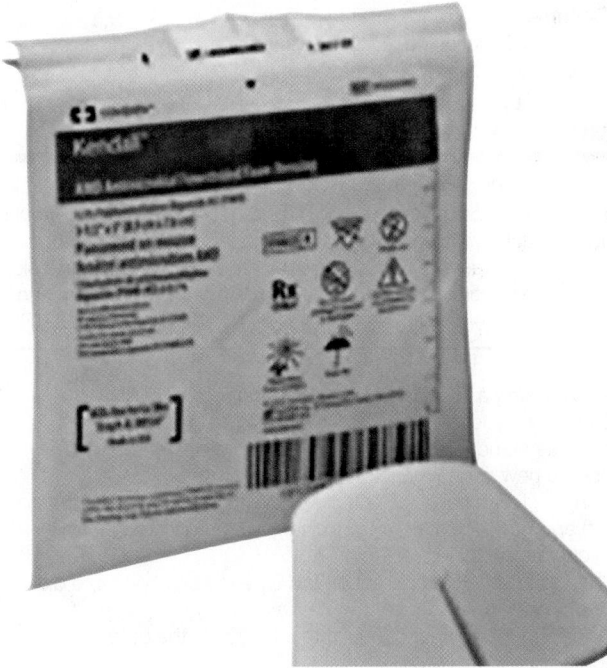

❹ Using a nonadhesive hydrocellular tracheostomy dressing.
Courtesy Covidien.

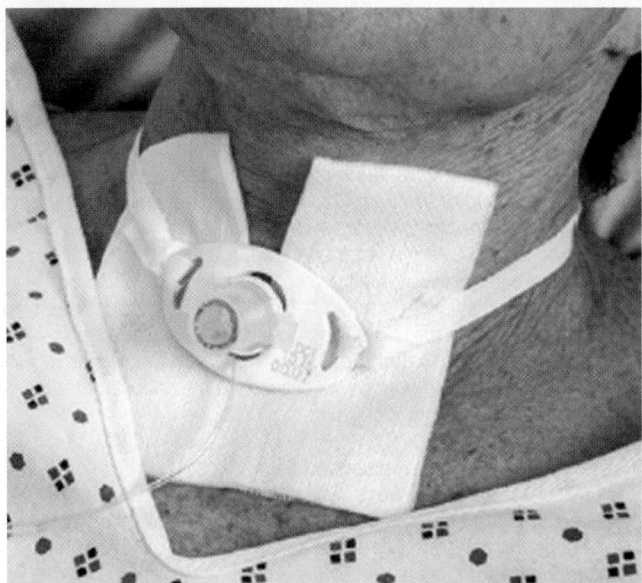

❺ A tracheostomy dressing placed under the flange of the tracheostomy tube.

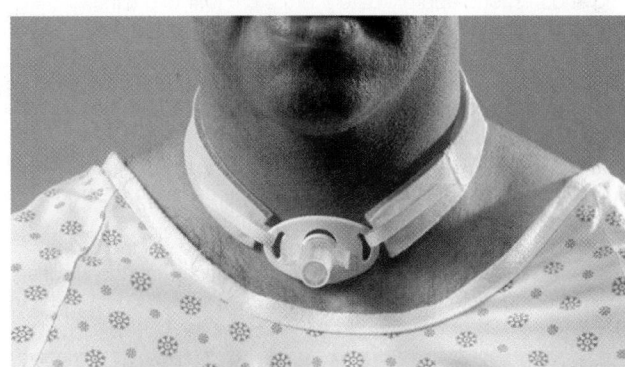

❻ A Velcro tracheostomy collar.

pad that absorbs large amounts of secretions. ❹ Never use cotton-filled gauze squares or cut a 4×4 gauze. **Rationale:** *Cotton lint or gauze fibers can be aspirated by the client, potentially creating a tracheal abscess.*
- Place the dressing under the flange of the tracheostomy tube. ❺
- While applying the dressing, ensure that the tracheostomy tube is securely supported. **Rationale:** *Excessive movement of the tracheostomy tube irritates the trachea.*

9. Change the tracheostomy twill ties or Velcro collar. ❻
- Change as needed to keep the skin clean and dry.
- Twill tape and specially manufactured Velcro ties are available. Twill tape is inexpensive and readily available; however, it is easily soiled and can trap moisture that leads to irritation of the skin of the neck. Velcro ties are becoming more commonly used. They are wider, more comfortable, and cause less skin abrasion.
- For client safety, the literature recommends a two-person technique when changing the securing device to prevent tube dislodgement. This involves one person holding the tracheostomy tube in place while the other changes the securing device.

Two-Strip Method (Twill Tie)
- Cut two unequal strips of twill ties, one approximately 25 cm (10 in.) long and the other about 50 cm (20 in.) long. **Rationale:** *Cutting one tie longer than the other allows them to be fastened at the side of the neck for easy access and to avoid the pressure of a knot on the skin at the back of the neck.*
- Cut a 1-cm (0.4-in.) lengthwise slit approximately 2.5 cm (1 in.) from one end of each tie. To do this, fold the end of the tie back

Continued on page 612

Providing Tracheostomy Care—*continued*

onto itself about 2.5 cm (1 in.), then cut a slit in the middle of the tie from its folded edge.

- Leaving the old ties in place, thread the slit end of one clean tie through the eye of the tracheostomy flange from the bottom side; then thread the long end of the tie through the slit, pulling it tight until it is securely fastened to the flange. **Rationale:** *Leaving the old ties in place while securing the clean ties prevents inadvertent dislodging of the tracheostomy tube. Securing ties in this manner avoids the use of knots in the flange area, which can come untied or cause pressure and irritation.*
- If old ties are very soiled or it is difficult to thread new ties onto the tracheostomy flange with old ties in place, have an assistant apply a sterile glove and hold the tracheostomy in place while you replace the ties. **Rationale:** *This is very important because movement of the tube during this procedure may cause irritation and stimulate coughing. Coughing can dislodge the tube if the ties are undone.*
- Repeat the process for the second tie.
- Ask the client to flex the neck. Slip the longer tie under the client's neck, place a finger between the tie and the client's neck ❼, and tie the ties together at the side of the neck. **Rationale:** *Flexing the neck increases its circumference the way coughing does. Placing a finger under the tie prevents making the tie too tight, which could interfere with coughing or place pressure on the jugular veins.*
- Tie the ends of the ties using square knots. Cut off any long ends, leaving approximately 1 to 2 cm (0.4 to 0.8 in.). **Rationale:** *Square knots prevent slippage and loosening. Adequate ends beyond the knot prevent the knot from inadvertently untying.*
- Once the clean ties are secured, remove the soiled ties and discard.

One-Strip Method (Twill Tie)
- Cut a length of twill tie 2.5 times the length needed to go around the client's neck from one tube flange to the other.
- Thread one end of the tie into the slot on one side of the flange.
- Bring both ends of the tie together. Take them around the client's neck, keeping them flat and untwisted.

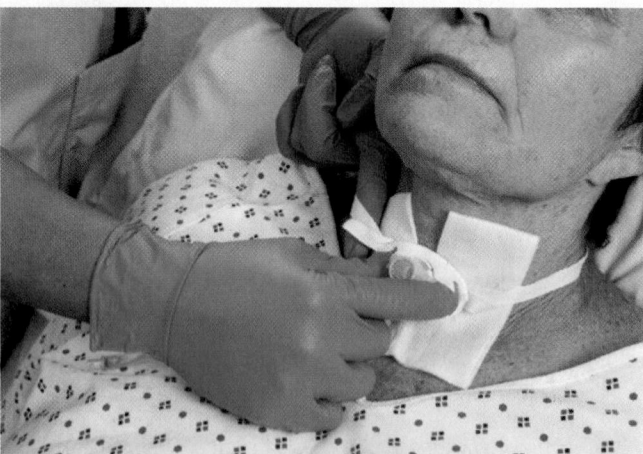

❼ Placing a finger underneath the tie tape before tying it.

- Thread the end of the tie next to the client's neck through the slot from the back to the front.
- Have the client flex the neck. Tie the loose ends with a square knot at the side of the client's neck, allowing for slack by placing one finger under the ties as with the two-strip method. Cut off long ends.
- Tape and pad the tie knot.
- Place a folded 4×4 gauze square under the tie knot, and apply tape over the knot. **Rationale:** *This reduces skin irritation from the knot and prevents confusing the knot with the client's gown ties.*
- Check the tightness of the ties.
- Frequently check the tightness of the tracheostomy ties and position of the tracheostomy tube. **Rationale:** *Swelling of the neck may cause the ties to become too tight, interfering with coughing and circulation. Ties can loosen in restless clients, allowing the tracheostomy tube to extrude from the stoma.*

Velcro Collar Method
- Thread one piece of the collar with the Velcro end on one side of the flange.
- Place the collar around the back of the client's neck, keeping it flat.
- Thread the other piece of the collar with the Velcro end into the slot on the other side of the flange.
- Take the second piece of the collar around the back of the client's neck, keeping it flat.
- Have the client flex the neck, and secure the two pieces of the collar together with the Velcro, allowing space for one to two fingers between the collar and the client's neck.
- Check the tightness of the collar as with the tie method.

10. Remove and discard sterile gloves.
   - Perform hand hygiene.
11. Document all relevant information.
   - Record suctioning, tracheostomy care, and the dressing change, noting your assessments.

SAMPLE DOCUMENTATION

12/11/2015 0900 Respirations 18–20/min. Lung sounds clear. Able to cough up secretions requiring little suctioning. Inner cannula changed. Trach dressing changed. Minimal amount of serosanguineous drainage present. Trach incision area pink to reddish in color 0.2 cm around entire opening. No broken skin noted in the reddened area. ———————————————————— J. Garcia, RN

Variation: Using a Disposable Inner Cannula
- Check policy for frequency of changing the inner cannula because standards vary among institutions.
- Open a new cannula package.
- Using a gloved hand, unlock the current inner cannula (if present) and remove it by gently pulling it out toward you in line with its curvature.
- Check the cannula for amount and type of secretions and discard properly.
- Pick up the new inner cannula, touching only the outer locking portion.
- Insert the new inner cannula into the tracheostomy.
- Lock the cannula in place by turning the lock (if present) or clip in place.

EVALUATION
- Perform appropriate follow-up such as determining character and amount of secretions, drainage from the tracheostomy, appearance of the tracheostomy incision, pulse rate and respiratory status compared to baseline data, and complaints of pain or discomfort at the tracheostomy site.

- Relate findings to previous assessment data if available.
- Report significant deviations from normal to the primary care provider.

INFANTS AND CHILDREN
- An assistant should always be present while tracheostomy care is performed.
- Always keep a sterile, packaged tracheostomy tube taped to the child's bed so that if the tube dislodges, a new one is available for immediate reintubation.

OLDER ADULTS
- Older adult skin is fragile and prone to breakdown. Care of the skin at the tracheostomy stoma is very important.

PATIENT-CENTERED CARE

- For tracheostomies older than 1 month, clean technique (rather than sterile technique) is used for tracheostomy care.
- Stress the importance of good hand hygiene to the caregiver.
- Tap water may be used for rinsing the inner cannula.
- Teach the caregiver the tracheostomy care procedure and observe a return demonstration. Periodically reassess caregiver knowledge and/or tracheostomy care technique.

- Inform the caregiver of the signs and symptoms that may indicate an infection of the stoma site or lower airway.
- Names and telephone numbers of health care personnel who can be reached for emergencies or advice must be available to the client and/or caregiver.
- If the tracheostomy is permanent, provide contact information for available support groups.

Humidification

When the client breathes through a tracheostomy, air is no longer filtered and humidified as it is when passing through the upper airways; therefore, special precautions are necessary. Humidity may be provided with a tracheostomy mist collar (Figure 27–6 ■). Clients with long-term tracheostomies may use a heat moisture exchange device known as a "Swedish nose," which fits onto the connector of the inner cannula (Barnett, 2012) as shown in Figure 27–7 ■. They may also wear a stoma protector such as a 4×4 gauze held in place with a cotton tie over the stoma or a light scarf to filter air as it enters the tracheostomy.

Facilitating Communication

A client with a tracheostomy tube cannot speak because the vocal cords are above the level of the tracheostomy tube. Because air no longer passes over the vocal cords, speech is not possible. Alternative

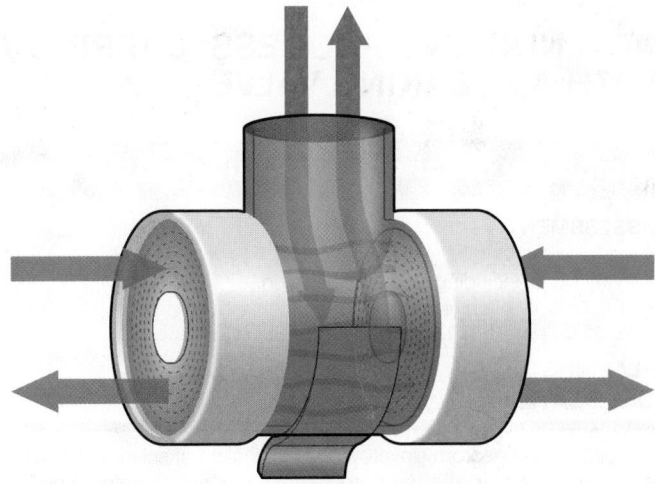

Figure 27–7 ■ A heat moisture exchange device.

methods for communication are necessary to avoid client frustration. Writing materials can be used if the client has the strength and coordination. Some clients may prefer a communication board that allows them to communicate by pointing to a picture or phrase on the board. Some clients may be able to use their finger to occlude the tracheostomy tube to allow them to speak. This method, however, can lead to an infection of the airway.

A more reliable method is to use a commercially available tracheostomy speaking valve. These devices are one-way valves that are connected to the tracheostomy tube opening. The device opens during inspiration but closes during expiration, forcing exhalation to occur around the tube and past the vocal cords, thus permitting speech. One example of a speaking valve is the Shiley™ valve (Figure 27–8 ■).

Clients with a tracheostomy who can use a speaking valve need to be alert and responsive. The speaking valve cannot be used with an endotracheal tube or with a tracheostomy tube that has a foam-filled cuff. The Shiley™ speaking valve can be used on or off a ventilator and is safe for infants and adults. A fenestrated tracheostomy tube

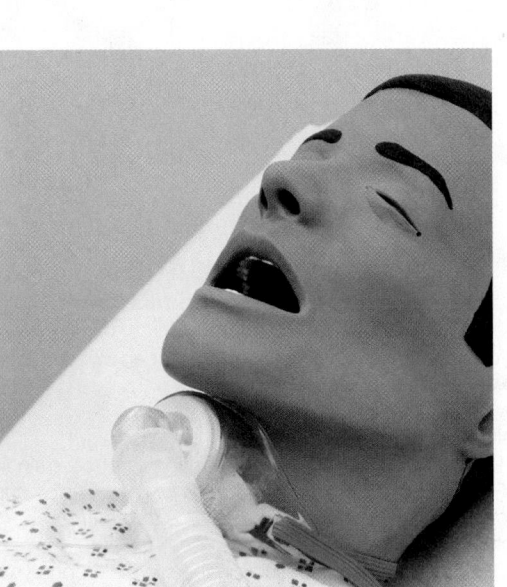

Figure 27–6 ■ A tracheostomy mist collar.

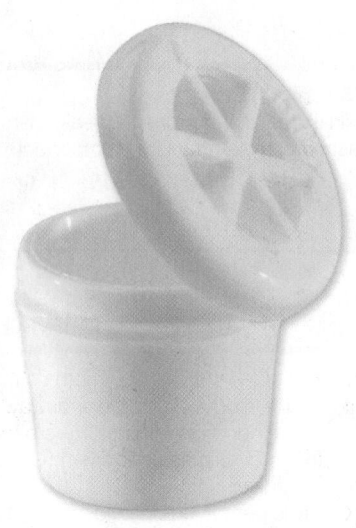

Figure 27–8 ■ A Shiley™ tracheostomy speaking valve.
Dover, Kendall, Monoject, Shiley, Aqua-Seal, Kangaroo and Argyle are trademarks of a Covidien company. Image provided courtesy of Covidien. © 2014 Covidien.

is preferred. Airway patency is a key factor when using a one-way speaking valve. Thus, it is important for the nurse to place signs in appropriate places that state: "A speaking valve is in place. DO NOT inflate cuff of tracheostomy tube." The nurse should explain to clients using a speaking valve that there will be a few changes from normal. For example, their voice will be deeper and hoarser than usual, and they will feel a different air pressure in the upper airway. As they become used to the different air pressure, they will be able to tolerate the speaking valve for longer periods of time. The speaking valve should not be used when a client is drowsy or sleeping. Skill 27–2 describes the process of capping a tracheostomy with a Shiley™ one-way speaking valve.

●○● NURSING PROCESS: CAPPING A TRACHEOSTOMY TUBE WITH A SPEAKING VALVE

Capping a Tracheostomy Tube with a Speaking Valve

SKILL 27-2

ASSESSMENT
Assess:
- Vital signs, including oxygen saturation.
- Respiratory effort (e.g., work of breathing).
- Presence of and amount of secretions.
- Ability to tolerate cuff deflation.

PLANNING
DELEGATION

Capping a tracheostomy involves the application of scientific knowledge, assessment skills, and problem solving, and therefore needs to be performed by a nurse or a respiratory therapist.

Equipment
- Suction apparatus
- Sterile suction catheters
- Sterile 10-mL syringe
- Clean gloves
- Sterile gloves
- Shiley™ speaking valve and storage container

INTERPROFESSIONAL PRACTICE

Capping a tracheostomy tube with a speaking valve may be within the scope of practice for specific health care providers. For example, in addition to nurses, respiratory therapists may help a client to communicate by capping a tracheostomy tube with a speaking valve. Although these therapists may verbally communicate their findings and plan to the health care team members, the nurse must also know where to locate their documentation in the client's medical record.

IMPLEMENTATION
Preparation
Check the primary care provider's orders for speaking valve application. Check for other orders such as special monitoring or changes to ventilator settings, if appropriate. Determine the client's type of tracheostomy. Gather equipment.

Performance
1. Prior to performing the procedure, introduce self and verify the client's identity using agency protocol. Explain to the client what you are going to do, why it is necessary, and how he or she can participate.

2. Perform hand hygiene and observe other appropriate infection prevention procedures.
3. Provide for client privacy.
4. Position the client.
   - Assist the client to a Fowler's position if not contraindicated. **Rationale:** *This position enhances lung expansion and may decrease fears about not being able to breathe.*
5. Suction the airways.
   - Using clean technique, suction the client's oropharynx if there are any secretions present. **Rationale:** *This removes*

Capping a Tracheostomy Tube with a Speaking Valve—*continued*

secretions that may be pooled above the cuff and avoids secretions entering lower airways when the cuff is deflated.
- Ask the client to cough. **Rationale:** *This will help clear secretions and allows the nurse to assess the client's cough reflex.*
- Remove and discard clean gloves and the used suction catheter.
- Perform hand hygiene.
- Using sterile technique, suction the client if indicated. (See Skill 26–2 in Chapter 26 ∞.) Suction the tracheostomy. If the secretions are excessive, report this finding to the nurse in charge or primary care provider to determine whether to proceed with the procedure.
- Remove and discard sterile gloves and the used suction catheter, if appropriate.
- Perform hand hygiene.

6. Prepare the tracheostomy tube.
   - Apply clean gloves.

For a Fenestrated Uncuffed Tracheostomy Tube
- Remove the inner cannula.

For a Cuffed Tracheostomy Tube
- Deflate the cuff. **Rationale:** *The client will have no airway if the cuff remains inflated. Double-check the balloon of the cuff inflation tube because it will be deflated if the cuff is deflated.*

7. Evaluate the client's ability to exhale around the tracheostomy tube.
   - Place your stethoscope over the client's neck and listen for air movement during respirations (i.e., an air leak).

Rationale: *The client needs to maintain an open airway by being able to breathe around the tracheostomy tube.*
- If no air leak is heard, notify the primary care provider. Do not place the speaking valve on the tracheostomy tube.

8. Place the speaking valve cap over the hub of the tracheostomy tube.
   - Monitor the client closely, comparing the data with baseline assessments.
   - Assess for ability to speak.
   - If assessments deteriorate from baseline, remove the speaking valve.

9. Remove and discard gloves.
   - Perform hand hygiene.

10. Apply clean gloves in preparation for removing the speaking valve.

11. Remove the speaking valve.
    - The amount of time that the client is able to tolerate the speaking valve will vary.

12. Reinflate the cuff, if needed.

13. Remove and discard gloves.
    - Perform hand hygiene.

14. Document all relevant information.
    - Document the amount, color, and consistency of the secretions; the amount of time the speaking valve was used; the client's ability to speak and swallow; and the client's tolerance of valve placement.

EVALUATION
- Conduct appropriate follow-up such as assessing respiratory status while the speaking valve is on (e.g., breath sounds, respiratory rate, and the use of accessory muscles for breathing) and ability to communicate with the speaking valve placement.
- Compare to baseline assessment data.
- Keep the primary care provider informed of the client's progress in using the speaking valve.

SKILL 27-2

Chapter **27** Review

FOCUSING ON CLINICAL THINKING

Consider This

1. The nurse informs you that the client frequently starts coughing when the inner cannula is removed. You are now performing tracheostomy care for this client. As you are cleaning the inner cannula, the client begins to cough and bring up secretions. What will you do?

2. You are assigned to provide nursing care for a client who had an emergency tracheostomy performed the previous day. What equipment will you ensure is available in the client's room?

See Focusing on Clinical Thinking answers on student resource website.

TEST YOUR KNOWLEDGE

1. The nurse is caring for a client with a tracheostomy who will begin to be weaned from the ventilator today. The goal is to remove the tracheostomy when the client is able to breathe independently. The client is anxious to be able to talk again. The nurse assesses the client to ensure that which type of tracheostomy tube is optimally in place?
   1. Cuffed tracheostomy tube
   2. Fenestrated tracheostomy tube
   3. Uncuffed tracheostomy tube
   4. Curved tracheostomy tube

2. The nurse is assisting with the insertion of a tracheostomy tube. After inserting the tube, the nurse ensures that which of the following is removed immediately?
   1. The inner cannula
   2. The outer cannula
   3. The obturator
   4. The flange

3. The nurse is caring for a client who has been in a chronic vegetative state. What type of tracheostomy tube would the nurse anticipate finding when assessing this client?
   1. Uncuffed tracheostomy tube
   2. Cuffed tracheostomy tube
   3. Fenestrated tracheostomy tube
   4. Plastic tracheostomy tube

4. The nurse is caring for a pediatric client with a tracheostomy. The nurse knows that this client will *not* require which of the following?
   1. Uncuffed tracheostomy tube
   2. Cuffed tracheostomy tube
   3. Fenestrated tracheostomy tube
   4. Inner cannula

5. The nurse is caring for a client who is 1 day postsurgery for radical neck resection secondary to cancer of the larynx. The client returned from surgery with a tracheostomy tube in place and is becoming increasingly frustrated with the inability to speak or be understood. Which would best meet the client's need?
   1. Paper and pencil so the client can write
   2. A fenestrated tracheostomy tube
   3. A speaking valve
   4. A communication board

6. The nurse is caring for a client with a new tracheostomy. The client is trying to tell the nurse something, but the nurse is unable to understand what the client is mouthing. The nurse offers paper and pencil, but the client is unable to write legibly enough for the nurse to understand. The client is becoming obviously frustrated. Which would be the nurse's best response?
   1. "Don't get upset. You'll be fitted with a speaking valve soon."
   2. "I know it's frustrating not being able to be understood. Let me go get a communication board to make this easier for you."
   3. "Don't try to talk. I will take good care of you and take care of everything you need."
   4. "I'm sorry I can't understand you. We'll try again later. Get some rest."

7. The nurse is preparing to perform tracheostomy care. Which action should the nurse complete prior to beginning the procedure?
   1. Tell the client to raise two fingers in the air to indicate pain or distress.
   2. Change the twill tape holding the tracheostomy in place.
   3. Clean the incision site.
   4. Check the tightness of the ties and knot.

8. The nurse is performing tracheostomy care. In what order will the nurse perform the following steps?
   1. Clean the incision site and tube flange.
   2. Clean the inner cannula.
   3. Suction the tracheostomy tube.
   4. Change the tracheostomy ties.
   5. Apply a sterile dressing.

9. The nurse is caring for a client who is beginning to use a speaking valve. Which is the best type of tracheostomy tube to use in conjunction with the speaking valve?
   1. Uncuffed tracheostomy tube
   2. Cuffed tracheostomy tube
   3. Fenestrated tracheostomy tube
   4. Curved tracheostomy tube

10. The nurse is caring for a client who has an order for a Shiley™ speaking valve. The nurse knows this valve is not appropriate for which client?
    1. A child
    2. One on a ventilator
    3. A geriatric client
    4. One who is sleepy

See Answers to Test Your Knowledge in Appendix A.

READINGS AND REFERENCES

References

Barnett, M. (2012). Back to basics: Caring for people with a tracheostomy. *Nursing & Residential Care, 14*, 390.

Frace, M. (2010). Tracheostomy care on the medical–surgical unit. *MEDSURG Nursing, 19*(1), 58–61.

Morris, L. L., Whitmer, A., & McIntosh, E. (2013). Tracheostomy care and complications in the intensive care unit. *Critical Care Nurse, 33*(5), 18–31. doi:10.4037/ccn2013518

Selected Bibliography

Berman, A., Snyder, S., & Frandsen, G. (2016). *Kozier & Erb's fundamentals of nursing: Concepts, practice, and process* (10th ed.). Upper Saddle River, NJ: Pearson.

Freeman, S. (2011). Care of adult patients with a temporary tracheostomy. *Nursing Standard, 26*(2), 49–56. doi:10.7748/ns2011.09.26.2.49.c8706

Grossbach, I., Stranberg, S., & Chlan, L. (2011). Promoting effective communication for patients receiving mechanical ventilation. *Critical Care Nurse, 31*(3), 46–60. doi:10.4037/ccn2010728

Hess, D. R., MacIntyre, N. R., Mishoe, S. C., Galvin, W. R., & Adams, A. B. (2012). *Respiratory care principles and practice* (2nd ed.). Sudbury, MA: Jones & Bartlett.

Nance-Floyd, B. (2011). Tracheostomy care: An evidence-based guide to suctioning and dressing changes. *American Nurse Today, 6*(7), 14–16.

Reed, C., Reineck, C., & Fonseca, I. (2011). Communicating with intubated patients: A new approach. *American Nurse Today, 6*(7), 34–35.

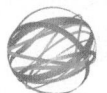 **28** Assisting with Mechanical Ventilation

When clients are unable to breathe effectively, they may require the assistance of a mechanical device called a **ventilator** that controls or assists with breathing. Their impaired breathing may be caused purposely by medications, such as anesthesia or neuromuscular blocking agents, or by a medical condition such as brain injury, neuromuscular degeneration, or respiratory failure. Respiratory failure can occur with congestive heart failure, chronic obstructive lung disease, or acute respiratory distress syndrome. Depending on the underlying cause of the impairment, mechanical ventilation may be temporary or long term, assistive or complete. The nurse assists respiratory therapy and medical staff team members in caring for the client on mechanical ventilation in acute, subacute, and community settings.

MECHANICAL VENTILATION

Historically, mechanical ventilators used negative pressure. The client's entire body was placed in a chamber up to the neck (an "iron lung"), or the chest was encircled in a shell. In this system, negative pressure (vacuum) expands the chest wall, drawing air into the lungs. When the vacuum is released, the client exhales passively. Negative pressure ventilator shells are still used in some parts of the United States, referred to as biphasic cuirass ventilation (BCV) because both inhalation and expiration can be controlled. With BCV, the client can eat, drink, and speak normally.

More commonly, machines used to deliver mechanical breathing use positive pressure, forcing the gas into the client's lungs. The gas is then expired passively due to the elastic recoil of the chest wall. These systems require a tube placed in the client's airway through which pressurized gas can be delivered. This tube can be an endotracheal tube (ETT) placed through the nose or the mouth, or a tracheostomy tube (see Chapters 26 ∞ and 27 ∞). *Note:* A client with an ETT will always have some method of mechanical ventilation, but many clients with tracheostomies breathe independently. A cuff around the portion of the tube in the client's trachea can be used to occlude that portion of the trachea so the ventilator's gas delivery does not leak out around the tube before inflating the lungs.

Characteristics of Positive Pressure Ventilators

Hand-controlled ventilators include bag-valve-mask devices used for emergency care or brief periods such as during transport of an intubated client when an electronic ventilator cannot be used. A bag-valve-mask is kept near every client who is intubated (see Chapter 30 ∞). Other noninvasive positive pressure respirators are those used for sleep apnea (see Chapter 25 ∞).

Mechanical ventilators can be used in acute, subacute, or home settings. Many parameters of breathing are controlled by the machine such as respiratory rate, duration of inspiration, inspiratory pressure, inspiratory volume, end-expiratory pressure, air/oxygen mix, and frequency and volume of mandatory sighs. The primary care provider may order these settings, or they may be managed by respiratory therapists and specially trained nurses according to guidelines based on client assessment of oxygen saturation and blood gases, lung assessment, and related data.

Complications of Mechanical Ventilation

Although a client is placed on a ventilator when that is the best mechanism for sustaining breathing and oxygenation, this invasive intervention also has its own risks and complications. In 2013, the Centers for Disease Control and Prevention issued guidelines for monitoring **ventilator-associated events (VAEs)**, situations in which the client's condition is worsening because of the use of a ventilator. VAEs include ventilator-associated condition (VAC), which is defined by worsening oxygenation plus a fever; infection-related ventilator-associated complication (IVAC), defined as a VAC with evidence of a respiratory infection such as purulent secretions; and ventilator-associated pneumonia (VAP). As many as 50% of clients on a ventilator in the hospital may have a VAE (Klompas, 2013). Clients who develop VAP may have up to 50% increased mortality (Chang, 2014). To maximize effectiveness and minimize the adverse impact of ventilators, nurses implement evidence-based care, strict compliance with infection control, and carefully designed routines for nutrition and hygiene. They also address the psychosocial concerns of clients and families.

Additional possible complications of mechanical ventilation include damage to the lungs from excessive pressure or volume, decreased cardiac output resulting from the increased thoracic pressure, hepatic dysfunction, nutritional deficiencies, and oxygen toxicity.

●○● NURSING PROCESS: CARING FOR THE CLIENT ON A MECHANICAL VENTILATOR

Check the client and the ventilator system when you first arrive on duty, after any changes in settings, and after any treatments or procedures. Depending on client condition and agency policy, reassess the client at regular intervals.

Caring for the Client on a Mechanical Ventilator

ASSESSMENT

Review the client record for the medical history and reason for mechanical ventilation.

Perform a head-to-toe assessment as with all clients. Also see Skill 3–11, Assessing the Thorax and Lungs, in Chapter 3 ∞.

Observe:

- *Airway:* Examine the ETT or tracheostomy tube to ensure it is in place and securely attached to the ventilator.
- *Breathing:* Check respiratory rate, use of accessory muscles, and oxygen saturation.
- *Skin and mucous membranes:* Note whether cyanosis or diaphoresis is present. **Rationale:** Cyanosis can indicate inadequate oxygenation. Clients who are approaching respiratory muscle fatigue may be diaphoretic.
- *Chest wall configuration* (e.g., kyphosis) and expansion.
- *Lung sounds:* Should be audible by auscultating the chest.

- *Presence of clinical signs of hypoxemia:* Check for tachycardia, tachypnea, restlessness, dyspnea, cyanosis, and confusion. Tachycardia and tachypnea are often early signs. Confusion is a later sign of severe oxygen deprivation. The nurse should always eliminate hypoxemia as a cause of any of these signs before treating them with other interventions.
- *Presence of clinical signs of elevated carbon dioxide level:* Check for hypertension, headache, lethargy, and tremor.

Determine:

- Vital signs, including oxygen saturation by pulse oximetry.
- Results of diagnostic studies such as chest x-ray, ventilation-perfusion scans, magnetic resonance imagery, and bronchoscopy.
- Hemoglobin, hematocrit, and complete blood count.
- Arterial blood gases (ABGs).
- Pulmonary function tests.

PLANNING

Review the orders for the ventilator settings—especially for oxygen percent, inspiratory/tidal volume, respiratory rate, and pressure limits or alarm settings. There are more than two dozen variations in control modes for ventilators, often used in combination (Table 28–1). Assist-control (AC) and synchronized intermittent mandatory ventilation (SIMV) are the most frequently used modes.

Positive end-expiratory pressure (PEEP) may be added to the ventilator settings to keep alveoli open and facilitate diffusion of oxygen into the blood. With PEEP, some amount of pressure above atmospheric pressure is kept in the airway at the end of the expiration so the alveoli cannot collapse. Common ventilator settings are shown in Table 28–2.

DELEGATION

Unlicensed assistive personnel (UAP) may provide basic care for clients on mechanical ventilation and collect routine data such as vital signs, but they do not adjust ventilator settings or perform sterile procedures such as suctioning. They report any ventilator alarms but do not assess the client or troubleshoot the system.

Caring for the Client on a Mechanical Ventilator—*continued*

INTERPROFESSIONAL PRACTICE

Caring for clients on a mechanical ventilator is always a team effort. Consult with a respiratory therapist for beginning and ongoing care of the client, especially if caring for a client on a respirator is not something you frequently do. In some agencies, the therapist establishes the initial settings and performs introductory client teaching. Often respiratory therapists perform all later setting changes. Determine agency policy. Although these therapists may verbally communicate their findings and plan to the health care team members, the nurse must also know where to locate their documentation in the client's medical record.

Equipment
- Prescribed type of ventilator
- Oxygen source
- Bag-valve-mask ventilator system
- Suctioning supplies (see Chapter 26 ∞)
- Ventilator setting flow sheet and medical record forms or access to the electronic record system
- Stethoscope
- Pulse oximeter and other vital signs monitors
- End-tidal carbon dioxide ($ETCO_2$) colorimetric measuring device ❶ or other system for measuring expired carbon dioxide level

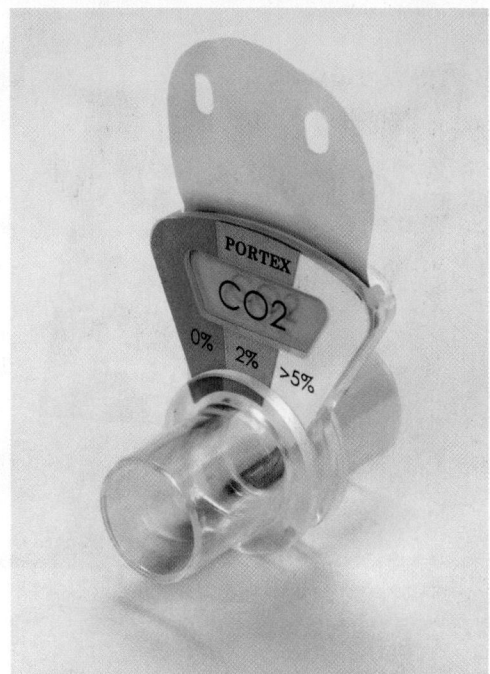

❶ $ETCO_2$ colorimetric measuring device.

IMPLEMENTATION
Preparation
- Review the manufacturer's manual for description of the ventilator controls and alarms if you are not adequately familiar with them (Table 28–3).
- Review the client record for data indicating the changes made in the client's ventilator settings over time and the client's tolerance of mechanical ventilation.

Performance
1. Prior to performing ventilator or client care, introduce self and verify the client's identity using agency protocol. Explain to the client what you are going to do, why it is necessary, and how he or she can participate. Discuss how the results will be used in planning further care or treatments.
2. Perform hand hygiene and observe other appropriate infection prevention procedures.
3. Provide for client privacy as needed.
4. Measure client temperature, pulse, blood pressure, and oxygen saturation using pulse oximetry. **Rationale:** *Changes in these vital signs may indicate either client improvement or inadequate ventilation requiring adjustments in ventilator settings.*
5. If indicated, obtain ABGs. In some cases, these are ordered routinely and in other cases only if the client's condition warrants. Blood for ABGs may be drawn by the nurse, respiratory therapist, or laboratory technologist, depending on agency policy. Repeat ABGs 30 minutes after changing the ventilator settings.
6. Confirm artificial airway tube placement by:
   - Auscultating lungs.
   - Measuring $ETCO_2$. Readings of 2% to 5% at end-expiration indicate the tube is in the trachea as opposed to the esophagus.
   - Check ETT placement by examining the length markings along the tube. Normally, the lips will be at the marks between 20 and 22 cm (7.9 and 8.7 in.). In some agencies the tube is marked with a pen at the confirmed length.
   - Check to see when the most recent chest x-ray was done and what position was documented for the tube.

7. Check the tube cuff inflation by listening over the trachea at the end of inspiration. No airflow should be heard. Usually, the respiratory therapist checks cuff inflation. It can be measured using a manometer and is generally 20 to 30 cm H_2O. Continuous monitoring and control of pressure has been shown to reduce VAP (Rouzé & Nseir, 2013). **Rationale:** *Proper cuff inflation helps prevent VAE by ensuring that secretions that collect above the cuff cannot leak down into the lungs.*
8. Suction the client if indicated. See Skill 26–1 (pages 598–600) and Skill 26–2 (pages 602–604). Use the bag valve mask to hyperventilate the client as indicated.
9. Once you have confirmed that the client's status does not require immediate intervention, examine the ventilator equipment and settings.
   - Tubing from the airway to the ventilator should be secured so it does not pull on the client's airway. This includes validating that there is adequate slack to allow the client to turn without pulling on the tubing.
   - Verify that ventilator settings are as ordered. ❷
   - Verify that ventilator alarms are set correctly and are active.
   - Check for condensation in the tubing. Newer systems warm the tubing so condensation is not a significant concern. If there is condensation in the tubing, empty it appropriately and discard. However, the closed system should not be opened unless absolutely necessary. Never empty fluid back into the humidifier, and use care that the fluid cannot run into the client's airway. **Rationale:** *Liquid in the tubing may be contaminated. Refill the humidifier if needed.*
10. Provide thorough oral care every 2 hours. Brush the teeth using a toothbrush and chlorhexidine gluconate or other antiseptic twice per day. Between brushings use tooth swabs and antiseptic to swab the client's mouth in all reachable areas (Sedwick, Lance-Smith, Reeder, & Nardi, 2012; Shi et al., 2013). Be certain to have suction ready in case it is needed. See the accompanying Practice Guidelines for preventing VAP.

Continued on page 620

SKILL 28–1

Caring for the Client on a Mechanical Ventilator—*continued*

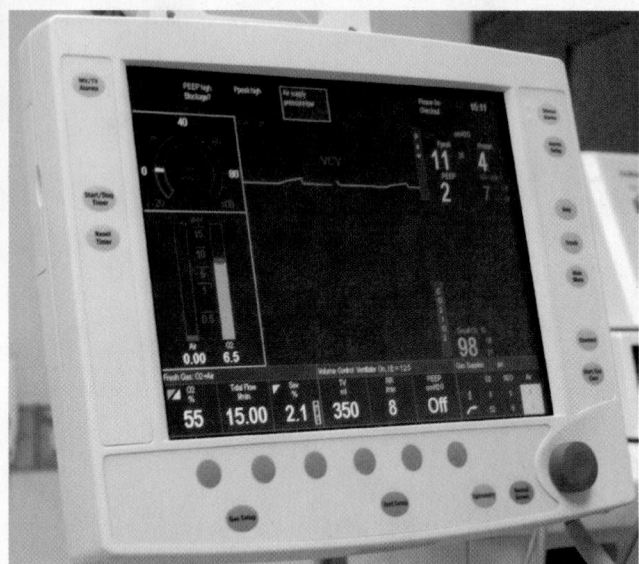

❷ Verify the ventilator settings and client data frequently.

Courtesy of Samuel Merritt University.

- Use a Yankauer suction tip to suction the mouth.
- Some ETTs have a lumen above the cuff to allow for continuous suction of secretions that could collect there. If this is not the case, use a small suction catheter to reach deeply alongside the ETT and suction secretions that pool above the cuff.
- If the client has an oral endotracheal airway, release the tape or holder, and move and resecure the tube to the opposite side of the mouth every 24 hours. **Rationale:** *This minimizes pressure on lips and oral mucosa. Recheck that the tube is correctly positioned after such a move.*

11. Administer medications as ordered to prevent complications of mechanical ventilation such as histamine receptor inhibitors to prevent gastric ulcers.
12. Administer pain or sedation medications as needed for comfort.
13. Institute actions to decrease complications such as deep venous thrombosis that may result from immobility related to the ventilator.
    - Perform range-of-motion exercises (see Chapter 13 ∞).

- Assist the client to change positions at least every 2 hours, keeping the head of the bed elevated to 30° to 45°.
- Assist the client to stand, walk, or sit in a chair as tolerated. Often only clients with a stable tracheostomy can accomplish this.
- Apply sequential compression devices to the lower limbs according to agency policy (see Skill 23–2 on page 570).
- If the client has a tracheostomy and can eat, encourage adequate intake of fluids and dietary fiber to promote gastrointestinal motility. For clients with an ETT, enteral feedings through a gastric tube are preferred over parenteral nutrition.
- Administer prophylactic anticoagulant medications according to agency policy.

14. Establish an effective method of communicating with the client who is intubated and cannot speak.
    - Explain everything you are doing even if it appears the client cannot hear or understand.
    - If the client requires eyeglasses, provide them.
    - If the client does not speak your language, provide a translator.
    - Ask yes/no questions when possible. Ask the client to nod the head if the answer is yes. Hand signals can also be used. Allow adequate time for the client to respond.
    - If the client can write, provide a writing pad or slate.
    - Be sure that the call light or bell is within reach at all times.
    - Acknowledge signs of frustration and attempt to determine and resolve the cause.
15. Document the ventilator settings and client parameters using checklists, flowcharts, and narrative notes as appropriate. Include results of settings changes, suctioning, activity, physical assessments, and laboratory data.

SAMPLE DOCUMENTATION

(Note that vital signs and ventilator settings would be recorded on flow sheets.)
10/1/2015 1530 ETT remains in place and secured, ETCO$_2$ 3%. Lungs clear to auscultation. Oral care provided. No signs of oral trauma or infection. Skin warm, no cyanosis. Active ROM all extremities. Turned to left side, head of bed @30 degrees. Skin dry & intact. No bowel sounds. Compression devices in place both calves. Indicates pain is 5 on scale of 0 to 10 by holding up fingers. Medicated IV with immediate reduction to pain level of 3. Family in to visit.
— T. Kourza, RN

EVALUATION

- Perform detailed follow-up based on findings that deviated from expected or normal for the client. Relate findings to previous assessment data if available.
- Report significant deviations from normal to the primary care provider.

- Determine if the client is making expected progress toward breathing independently.

TABLE 28–1	Selected Ventilator Control Modes

Mode	Features
Adaptive support ventilation (ASV)	Inspiratory pressure, inspiratory/expiratory ratio, and mandatory respiratory rate adjusted to maintain target volume and rate
Assist-control (AC)	Set volume with each client-triggered breath and set rate
Pressure control (PC)	Pressure-limited breath delivered at a set rate
Pressure-regulated volume control (PRVC); adaptive pressure ventilation (APV)	Pressure adjusted to deliver a set tidal volume
Pressure support ventilation (PSV)	Set pressure held during the entire inspiration
Synchronized intermittent mandatory ventilation (SIMV)	Set number of breaths and tidal volume while also allowing the client to take spontaneous breaths with a client-determined tidal volume and rate

TABLE 28–2   Common Initial Positive Pressure Ventilator Settings or Readings

Settings	Usual Range
Oxygen concentration (FiO$_2$*)	21% (room air, FiO$_2$ 0.21)—100% (FiO$_2$ of 1) to keep PaO$_2$ at greater than 60%
Flow rate	40–100 L/min
Tidal volume	10–12 mL/kg ideal body weight
Respiratory rate	10–12/min
Peak airway (inspiratory) pressure	Less than 0 cm H$_2$O
Plateau (end-inspiratory) pressure	Less than 30 cm H$_2$O
Sigh	1.5–2 times tidal volume; 6–8 times/hour if tidal volume less than 10–12 mL/kg and no PEEP
Inspiratory to expiratory ratio	Usually 1:2
Positive end-expiratory pressure (PEEP)	5 cm H$_2$O; used if PaO$_2$ less than 60 mmHg on FiO$_2$ of 0.6

*FiO$_2$ is the fraction of inspired oxygen and is expressed as a decimal, whereas oxygen concentration is expressed as a percentage.

TABLE 28–3   Ventilator Alarms

Type of Alarm	Possible Causes	Typical Settings (Chang & Hiers, 2014)
High pressure	A kink in the tubing Secretions in the ETT/airway Condensation in the tubing Client biting on the ETT Client coughing, gagging, or trying to talk Increased pressure in the airway due to bronchospasm or pneumothorax	10–15 cm H$_2$O greater than peak airway pressure
Low pressure	Ventilator tubing disconnected Dislodged ETT/tracheostomy	10–15 cm H$_2$O less than peak airway pressure
Low exhaled volume	Ventilator tubing disconnected Leak in cuff or inadequate cuff seal Anything that prevents the delivery of a full breath	100 mL less than tidal volume
High respiratory rate	Client anxiety or pain Hypoxia Hypercapnia Secretions in ETT/airway	10/min greater than observed frequency
Apnea	Disconnected equipment or client apnea	15- to 20-sec delay
High FiO$_2$	Inadvertent increase in delivery setting	5%–10% greater than setting
Low FiO$_2$	Disconnected O$_2$ source	5%–10% less than setting

LIFESPAN CONSIDERATIONS   Mechanical Ventilation

INFANTS AND CHILDREN
- Mechanical ventilation is used for children both in hospitals and in the home. Include the parents and other lay caregivers in all teaching and care instructions.
- When the child's condition is stable, provide age-appropriate activities such as play, art, and educational opportunities.

OLDER ADULTS
- Older clients may be at greater risk for oxygen toxicity, especially if they have chronic lung conditions. As with all clients, the lowest effective oxygen concentration should be used.
- Provide reassurance and emotional support, recognizing that the need for ongoing mechanical ventilation may be viewed by the client or family as a sign of deteriorating health and movement toward death.

Ambulatory and Community Settings   Mechanical Ventilation   **PATIENT-CENTERED CARE**

Long-term mechanical ventilation in the home is commonplace in many communities.
- Teach caregivers all of the interventions, emergency, and safety measures needed to provide effective client assistance.
- Assist caregivers in contacting local emergency agencies to inform them that a person in the home depends on a ventilator.

- Assist the client to determine if a backup power source is needed to run the ventilator should standard power be interrupted.
- Assist the client and family with community resources for obtaining needed equipment and disposal of biohazard waste. Ensure that they have extra supplies that might be needed in an emergency such as a bag-valve-mask system.

PRACTICE GUIDELINES

Preventing Ventilator-Associated Events

Preventing VAEs is an important nursing goal. Clients who develop VAEs have significantly greater mortality rates than clients who do not develop this infection. The Institute for Healthcare Improvement (2011) **ventilator bundle** identifies interventions that, when all are implemented simultaneously, can significantly reduce VAEs. The bundle components include (a) elevating the head of the bed, (b) reducing sedation daily while assessing readiness to extubate, (c) prophylaxis for peptic ulcer disease, (d) prophylaxis for deep venous thrombosis, and (e) daily oral care with chlorhexidine. Interventions to prevent or decrease VAE include the following:

- Maintain rigorous hand hygiene.
- Maintain the head of the bed at 30° to 45° unless contraindicated.
- Use oral (rather than nasal) endotracheal tubes if possible to reduce nasal or sinus colonization. Convert to a tracheostomy if long-term mechanical ventilation will be required.

- Provide oral care every 2 hours with toothbrushing twice a day and chlorhexidine gluconate rinses.
- Have the client be as physically active as possible: out of bed, performing weight-bearing and range-of-motion exercises.
- Do not change ventilator tubing or in-line suction catheter systems unless visibly soiled.
- Medicate for pain and anxiety.
- Maintain or enhance nutritional status. Gastric feedings should begin as soon as possible and be delivered through oral (rather than nasal) gastric tubes to reduce nasal or sinus colonization.
- Treat with appropriate antibiotics if VAP develops. The causative organisms could be *Streptococcus pneumoniae*, *Haemophilus influenzae*, *Pseudomonas*, *Klebsiella*, *Staphylococcus*, or *Enterobacter* species.

REMOVING THE CLIENT FROM A VENTILATOR

Clients should always be removed from a mechanical ventilator as soon as their conditions allow. Although the ventilator saves lives and permits procedures that would not otherwise be possible, the risk of adverse consequences occurring increases as the client is on the ventilator for extended periods of time. These consequences include those mentioned earlier, trauma to the airways, psychological distress related to dependence and limitations in mobility and interpersonal interactions, and cost.

One prospective, nonrandomized study of over 200 mechanically ventilated patients in an intensive care unit (ICU) demonstrated that nurse-driven, protocol-directed weaning shortened the time on ventilation and spent in the ICU and resulted in earlier initiation of weaning compared with usual physician-driven weaning. There was no difference in rates of reintubation, VAP, or hospital mortality between the groups. In addition, the ICU physicians had a positive attitude toward the implementation of the nurse-driven weaning protocol (Danckers et al., 2013).

Readiness for removal from the ventilator, which usually includes removal of the endotracheal tube and possibly the

tracheostomy, is projected based on several parameters (Box 28–1). Once the client meets the criteria, a series of trials may be needed to determine if the client can succeed breathing off the ventilator. Because these trials may involve progressive reductions in the amount of ventilatory support provided, the term **weaning** is often used to describe the process of gradual discontinuation of mechanical support.

Successful weaning is described as a minimum of 1 week with no ventilator. There is no one set of criteria that predicts the client's readiness to be weaned or whether weaning will succeed.

Clients are likely to have mixed emotions regarding removal from the ventilator. They may find the ventilator uncomfortable and restricting, but there is also a level of reassurance that the machine will breathe for them if they are unable. Weaning can be both an anxiety-producing and exciting experience. The client must be an active participant in the planning and implementation of weaning efforts. Systematic implementation of the weaning plan plus ongoing client communication and emotional support are needed for success. Teach the client relaxation techniques to assist with the process.

BOX 28–1   Common Criteria for Readiness for Weaning

- Client triggers ventilator 12 to 20 times per minute.
- Rapid shallow breathing index (respiratory rate/tidal volume) is less than 105.
- Cough/gag reflex is present.
- Tidal volume is greater than 7 mL/kg body weight.
- Vital signs are stable.

- Blood gases are within acceptable range, PO_2 is greater than 60 mmHg.
- FiO_2 is less than 0.5.
- P/F ratio is greater than 150 (PaO_2/FiO_2).
- PEEP is less than 8 cm H_2O.

●○● NURSING PROCESS: WEANING THE CLIENT FROM A VENTILATOR

Weaning the Client from a Ventilator

ASSESSMENT
Perform a thorough client assessment, paying particular attention to the respiratory system and all agency criteria used for weaning protocols such as those in Box 28–1.

PLANNING
Schedule the weaning trials when the client is rested and the client agrees. This is often done in the morning when the client is well rested. Inform the family as appropriate so they can provide emotional support.

DELEGATION
Adjusting ventilator settings is not delegated to UAP. If the UAP is caring for the client's basic needs, ensure that the UAP knows what data to gather and report to the nurse.

INTERPROFESSIONAL PRACTICE
Weaning clients from a mechanical ventilator is always a team effort. Consult with a respiratory therapist for beginning and ongoing weaning. Although these therapists may verbally communicate their findings and plan to the health care team members, the nurse must also know where to locate their documentation in the client's medical record.

Equipment
In addition to the existing ventilator equipment:
• Pulse oximeter
• Suctioning supplies
• Oxygen delivery system such as nasal cannula or mask for use after the ETT is removed

IMPLEMENTATION
Preparation
• Review the weaning protocol. Sometimes, the primary care provider prescribes the incremental steps and settings to be used. In other cases, a standardized protocol may be used. The nurse must be knowledgeable about the decisions that must be made at each step of the weaning process.
• If the client's condition permits, arrange for the client to sit in a chair during initial trials.

Performance
1. Prior to initiating weaning, introduce self and verify the client's identity using agency protocol. If the client has been on sedation, adjust the dose downward so the client is alert and can cooperate with instructions. Explain to the client what you are going to do, why it is necessary, and how he or she can participate. Discuss how the results will be used in planning further care or treatments.
2. Perform hand hygiene and observe other appropriate infection prevention procedures.
3. Provide for client privacy as needed.
4. Position the client upright as much as possible. **Rationale:** *This position promotes chest expansion.*
5. Suction the endotracheal tube above the cuff so that when the cuff is deflated, secretions do not fall into the airway.
6. Perform a spontaneous breathing trial according to agency policy. Several types of trials may be used.
   • *Pressure support:* The client controls the rate of respirations while the ventilator delivers positive pressure. The pressure is decreased gradually (manually or by computer). Once the pressure is below 5 to 6 cm H_2O without adverse reaction,

the client is breathing independently and does not require ventilator support.
   • *SIMV:* The client breathes at his or her own rate, but the number of breaths delivered by the ventilator automatically is reduced gradually to zero.
   • *Continuous positive airway pressure:* As the client breathes, a specific amount of pressure is kept in the airways at all times while the client breathes independently.
   • *T-piece:* Less commonly used, the ventilator is removed and humidified oxygen is delivered into the ETT while the client breathes spontaneously.
7. Monitor the client's response to the breathing trial. Findings should include:
   • No change in mental status.
   • Oxygen saturation greater than 85% (or according to agency policy).
   • ABGs within normal ranges for this client.
   • Pulse and BP within 20% of baseline.
   • Normal, symmetric chest wall expansion; no use of accessory muscles.
   • Respirations rate, depth, and rhythm within normal range.
   • Minimal signs of anxiety.
8. If the client shows signs of distress, resume the previous ventilator settings.
   • Reassess vital signs.
   • Reassure the client that it may take several trials to achieve success.
9. Document the details of each trial. Include the ventilator settings, length of time of the trial, and all client data.

EVALUATION
• Perform detailed follow-up based on findings that deviated from expected or normal for the client. Relate findings to previous assessment data if available.

• Report significant deviations from normal to the primary care provider.

Removing the Endotracheal Tube

Once the client is successfully weaned from the ventilator attached to an ETT, the tube may be removed. The term used to describe the removal is **extubation**. Although the client may welcome removal from the ventilation and the tube, it can also be an anxiety-producing time. The nurse explains what will happen during extubation, how the client can participate, and methods that will be used to reduce discomfort.

If the cuff on the ETT is inflated, the nurse suctions the oropharynx and the tube (see Skills 26–1 and 26–2 in Chapter 26 ∞) before deflating the cuff. This minimizes the secretions that remain, which

can slide back into the airway when the ETT is removed. Then, the cuff is deflated according to the manufacturer's instructions and the ETT is pulled out in one smooth continuous motion. This removal lasts only 1 to 2 seconds. Often the client will gag and cough immediately after removal. Monitor for any signs of laryngospasm (contraction of the muscles around the vocal cords), which usually lasts only a minute but can cause hypoxia in some clients. If indicated, apply oxygen by nasal cannula or mask (see Chapter 25 ∞).

Once the client is calm, offer mouth care and water to drink, if permitted. Remain with the client until he or she is comfortable and safety measures are in place such as having the call light within reach.

WHAT IF **Managing Ventilator-Related Events**

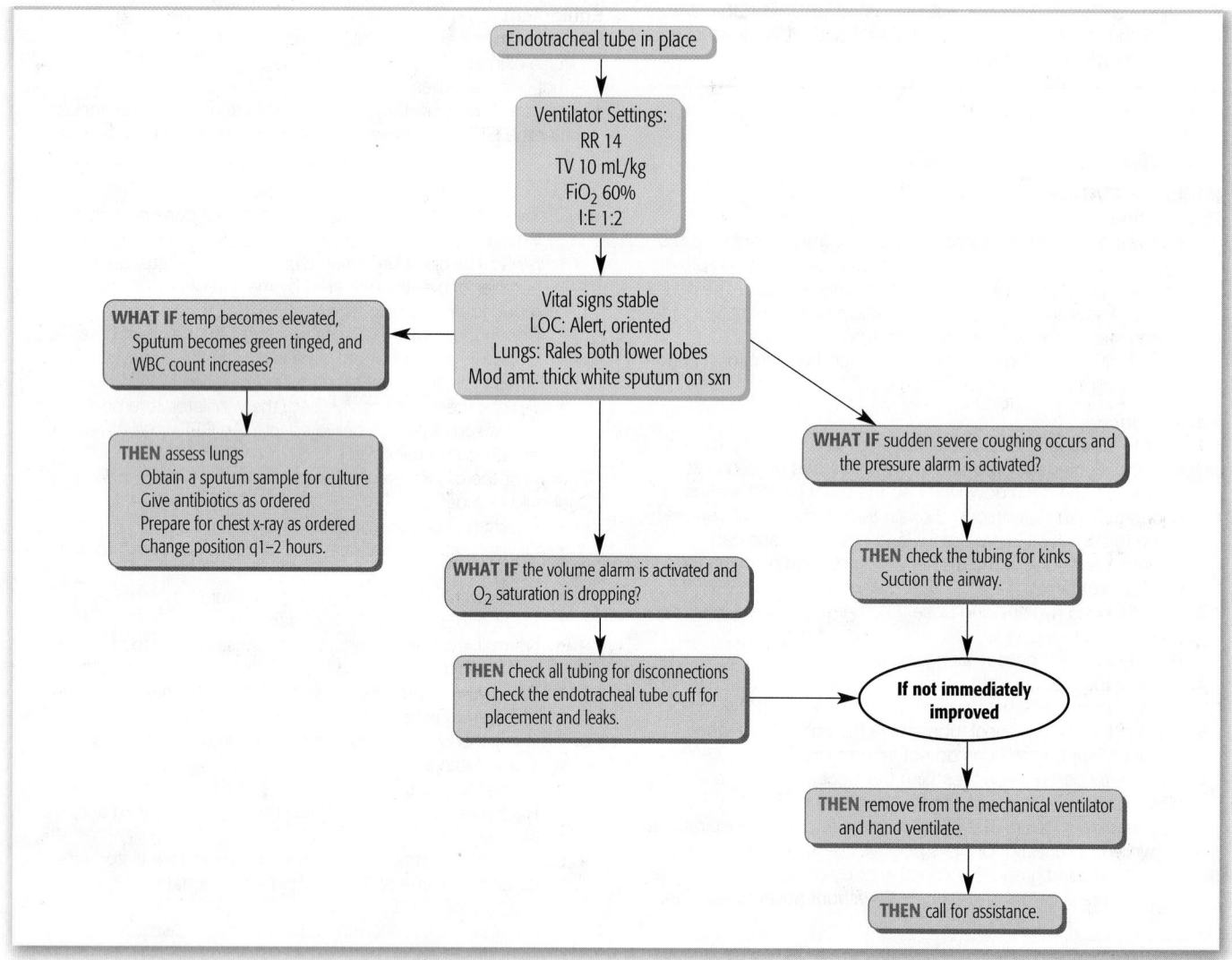

FOCUSING ON CLINICAL THINKING

Consider This

1. Your client's ventilator pressure alarms have been triggered about once per hour for the past few hours but every time you check, all settings appear correct and the client is resting comfortably. What steps might you need to take at this time?

2. You are working in a subacute hospital that specializes in care of clients who are dependent on mechanical ventilation. One of your assigned clients is believed to be an excellent candidate for permanent weaning off the ventilator, but refuses to allow the nurses to start the trial. What actions might you take? What data do you need and what would you say to the client?

See Focusing on Clinical Thinking answers on student resource website.

TEST YOUR KNOWLEDGE

1. The nurse is caring for a client on a ventilator set to allow the client to breathe at her own rate, but the ventilator delivers a specific number of breaths automatically. This setting is known as which of the following?
   1. Continuous positive airway pressure ventilation
   2. Synchronized intermittent mandatory ventilation
   3. Pressure support ventilation
   4. Assist-intermittent ventilation

2. Which action will the nurse do when beginning to wean the client from the ventilator?
   1. Progressively reduce ventilatory support provided.
   2. Increase the sedation required to prevent the client from fighting the ventilator.
   3. Alternate the ventilator's pressure settings from high to low.
   4. Allow the client to be off the ventilator at intervals such as to eat.

3. While caring for a client on mechanical ventilation, the nurse recognizes that the priority action to prevent atelectasis and pooling of secretions is which of the following?
   1. Reposition the client frequently.
   2. Suction the airway every 4 hours.
   3. Bathe the client daily.
   4. Monitor arterial blood gases.

4. The nurse is caring for a client who is intubated and unable to breathe independently. What is the nurse's priority action?
   1. Notify respiratory therapy of the need for a ventilator.
   2. Determine ventilator settings.
   3. Provide ventilation with a bag-valve-mask ventilation system.
   4. Assess the client's lung sounds.

5. The high-pressure alarm on the client's ventilator has been triggered almost hourly. When the alarm sounds, the nurse assesses the client and finds him resting comfortably, breathing easily, and with an oxygen saturation of 95%. The ventilator settings are set correctly. To what will the nurse attribute the alarm?
   1. Secretions in the airway
   2. Water in the ventilator tubing
   3. Kinked tubing
   4. The client coughing

6. The nurse is caring for a client requiring mechanical ventilation. The family asks the nurse why the ventilator tubing is secured to the bed linens. What would be the nurse's best response?
   1. "In order to prevent infection we don't want the tubing to lie on the floor."
   2. "If the ventilator becomes disconnected it keeps the tubing from falling on the floor."
   3. "Securing the tubing to the bed is our policy."
   4. "Securing the tubing to the bed keeps the weight of the tubing from causing pressure on the airway."

7. The unlicensed assistive personnel (UAP) offers to help provide care to a client on mechanical ventilation. What would be the nurse's best response?
   1. "Would you please decrease the oxygen percentage to 40%?"
   2. "Please suction the client's airway."
   3. "Please measure vital signs and oxygen saturation every 2 hours."
   4. "Please perform tracheostomy care."

8. The nurse is caring for a client requiring mechanical ventilation. The client has decreasing oxygen saturation, increasing respiratory acidosis, and restlessness. What is the nurse's priority action?
   1. Assess the placement of the endotracheal tube and breath sounds.
   2. Suction the airway.
   3. Call the primary care provider.
   4. Remove the endotracheal tube and begin hand bagging the client.

9. When caring for a client on mechanical ventilation, the nurse should report which assessment data to the primary care provider immediately?
   1. Oxygen saturation of 90% and respiratory rate of 28 breaths per minute
   2. Displacement of the endotracheal tube
   3. Flecks of blood in the endotracheal secretions
   4. Increased quantity of secretions

10. When documenting in the client's medical record, the nurse records which of the following related to the ventilator? Select all that apply.
    1. Color, quantity, and appearance of secretions when suctioning
    2. When the respiratory therapist changes the ventilator tubing
    3. Ventilator settings
    4. Vital signs, oxygen saturation, and assessment findings
    5. Length of tubing from the ventilator to the endotracheal tube

See Answers to Test Your Knowledge in Appendix A.

READINGS AND REFERENCES

References

Chang, D. W. (2014). Critical care issues in mechanical ventilation. In D. W. Chang (Ed.), *Clinical application of mechanical ventilation* (4th ed., pp. 489–515). Clifton Park, NY: Delmar.

Chang, D. W., & Hiers, J. H. (2014). Initiation of mechanical ventilation. In D. W. Chang (Ed.), *Clinical application of mechanical ventilation* (4th ed., pp. 212–240). Clifton Park, NY: Delmar.

Danckers, M., Grosu, H., Jean, R., Cruz, R. B., Fidellaga, A., Han, Q., . . . Khouli, H. (2013). Nurse-driven, protocol-directed weaning from mechanical ventilation improves clinical outcomes and is well accepted by intensive care unit physicians. *Journal of Critical Care, 28,* 433–441. doi:10.1016/j.jcrc.2012.10.012

Institute for Healthcare Improvement. (2011). *Implement the IHI ventilator bundle.* Retrieved from http://www.ihi.org/knowledge/Pages/Changes/ImplementtheVentilatorBundle.aspx

Klompas, M. (2013). Ventilator-associated events surveillance: A patient safety opportunity. *Current Opinion in Critical Care, 19,* 424–431. doi:10.1097/MCC.0b013e3283636bc9

Rouzé, A., & Nseir, S. (2013). Continuous control of tracheal cuff pressure for the prevention of ventilator-associated pneumonia in critically ill patients: Where is the evidence? *Current Opinion in Critical Care, 19,* 440–447. doi:10.1097/MCC.0b013e3283636b71

Sedwick, M. B., Lance-Smith, M., Reeder, S. J., & Nardi, J. (2012). Using evidence-based practice to prevent ventilator-associated pneumonia. *Critical Care Nurse, 32*(4), 41–51. doi:10.4037/ccn2012964

Shi, Z., Xie, H., Wang, P., Zhang, Q., Wu, Y., Chen, E., . . . Furness, S. (2013). Oral hygiene care for critically ill patients to prevent ventilator-associated pneumonia. *Cochrane Database of Systematic Reviews,* Issue 8, Art. No.: CD008367. doi:10.1002/14651858.CD008367.pub2

Selected Bibliography

Berry, A. M. (2013). A comparison of Listerine® and sodium bicarbonate oral cleansing solutions on dental plaque colonisation and incidence of ventilator associated pneumonia in mechanically ventilated patients: A randomised control trial. *Intensive and Critical Care Nursing, 29,* 275–281. doi:10.1016/j.iccn.2013.01.002

Branch-Elliman, W., Wright, S. B., Gillis, J. M., & Howell, M. D. (2013). Estimated nursing workload for the implementation of ventilator bundles. *BMJ Quality & Safety, 22,* 357–361. doi:10.1136/bmjqs-2012-001372

Burns, K. E. A., Meade, M., Lessard, M., Hand, L., Zhou, Q., Keenan, S., & Lellouche, F. (2013). Wean earlier and automatically with new technology (the WEAN Study). *American Journal of Respiratory and Critical Care Medicine, 187,* 1203–1211. doi:10.1164/rccm.201206-1026OC

Dale, C., Angus, J. E., Sinuff, T., & Mykhalovskiy, E. (2013). Mouth care for orally intubated patients: A critical ethnographic review of the nursing literature. *Intensive and Critical Care Nursing, 29,* 266–274. doi:10.1016/j.iccn.2012.09.003

Huang, C.-T., & Yu, C.-J. (2013). Conventional weaning parameters do not predict extubation outcome in intubated subjects requiring prolonged mechanical ventilation. *Respiratory Care, 58,* 1307–1314. doi:10.4187/respcare.01773

Jones, C. U., Kluayhomthong, S., Chaisuksant, S., & Khrisanapant, W. (2013). Breathing exercise using a new breathing device increases airway secretion clearance in mechanically ventilated patients. *Heart & Lung, 42,* 177–182. doi:10.1016/j.hrtlng.2012.12.009

MacIntyre, N. R. (2013). The ventilator discontinuation process: An expanding evidence base. *Respiratory Care, 58,* 1074–1082. doi:10.4187/respcare.02284

Micik, S., Besic, N., Johnson, N., Han, M., Hamlyn, S., & Ball, H. (2013). Reducing risk for ventilator associated pneumonia through nursing sensitive interventions. *Intensive and Critical Care Nursing, 29,* 261–265. doi:10.1016/j.iccn.2013.04.005

Nava, S. (2013). Behind a mask: Tricks, pitfalls, and prejudices for noninvasive ventilation. *Respiratory Care, 58,* 1367–1376. doi:10.4187/respcare.02457

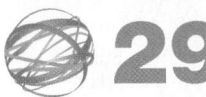 **29** **Caring for the Client with Chest Tube Drainage**

LEARNING OUTCOMES

At the completion of this chapter, the student will be able to:

1. Define the key terms used in the care of the client with a chest tube.
2. Recognize when it is appropriate to delegate aspects of the care of clients with chest tubes to unlicensed assistive personnel.
3. Verbalize the steps used in:
   a. Assisting with chest tube insertion.
   b. Maintaining chest tube drainage.
   c. Assisting with chest tube removal.
4. Demonstrate appropriate documentation and reporting of chest tube care.

SKILLS

Skill 29–1 Assisting with Chest Tube Insertion
Skill 29–2 Maintaining Chest Tube Drainage

Skill 29–3 Assisting with Chest Tube Removal

KEY TERMS

empyema, *627*
Heimlich chest drain valve, *629*

hemothorax, *627*
pleural effusion, *627*

pneumothorax, *627*
thoracostomy, *627*

tidaling, *628*
water-seal, *628*

Occasionally, excess fluid or air builds up in the narrow space between the parietal pleura, the membrane that lines the inside of the chest cavity, and the visceral pleura, which covers the entire surface of the lungs. The intrapleural pressure (between the membranes) is always lower than atmospheric pressure. Any buildup in the pleural space can destroy the negative pressure and impair the ability of the lungs to fully expand. This can cause a partial or full lung collapse. When the pleural space is filled with air, it is referred to as a **pneumothorax**. A **hemothorax** is the accumulation of blood in the pleural cavity, and a **pleural effusion** exists when excessive fluid accumulates in the pleural space. An **empyema** is a collection of pus in the pleural space, usually associated with a lung infection.

To remove the air, blood, fluid, or pus, a qualified health care provider (e.g., physician or advanced practice nurse) may perform a thoracentesis. Thoracentesis involves puncturing the pleural cavity with a large needle and syringe and aspirating the fluid or air. This can be done when the client is in the hospital or as an outpatient procedure. At the end of the thoracentesis, if the client has had recurrent pleural effusions or pneumothoraces, the provider may instill a chemical irritant such as talc to cause the pleura to seal together and prevent further accumulation or collapse. This procedure is known as pleurodesis.

If a thoracentesis is not effective at removing the air or fluid accumulation, and to reestablish the negative pressure between the pleura,

a chest tube may be inserted into the pleural space. Figure 29–1 ■ shows the proximity of the two pleural linings, their location within the chest cavity, and the placement of high and low chest tubes.

CHEST TUBES

Chest tubes are most commonly inserted through an intercostal space into the pleural cavity. Chest tubes used to remove air are usually inserted in the upper anterior chest (i.e., through the second intercostal space) because air rises within the pleural cavity. Tubes used to drain fluid collections from the pleural cavity are inserted more inferiorly, often in the fourth to sixth intercostal space (at the level of the nipple), and more posteriorly (see Figure 29–1).

Chest tube drainage is also required following open heart surgery and chest trauma to remove any blood pooling in the mediastinal cavity. Mediastinal chest tubes may differ from pleural chest tubes in that there are usually two placed in the anterior chest and they may be right-angled rather than straight.

The tube itself is a sterile, flexible catheter made of vinyl or silicone, about 50 cm (20 in.) long. A small-bore tube (size 12 to 20 French) can be used for small amounts of air, but larger tubes (size 24 to 40 French) may be needed for a hemothorax. When the chest tube is in place, the client is said to have had a **thoracostomy** performed. The chest tube is a temporary measure; once the lung is reinflated, the chest tube can be removed.

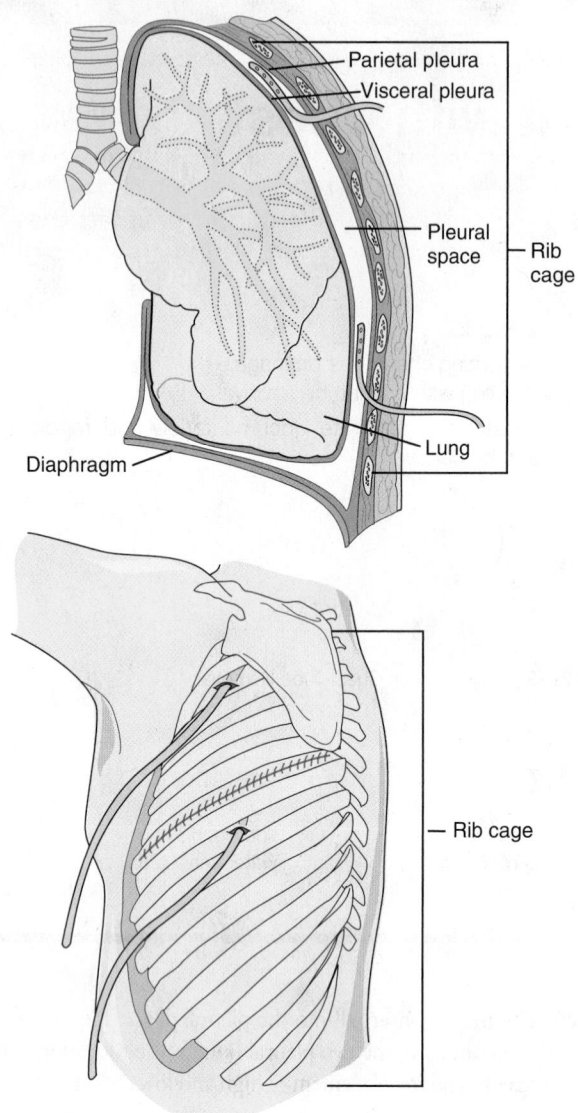

Placement of chest tubes.

Figure 29–1 ■ Chest tubes in the pleural spaces.

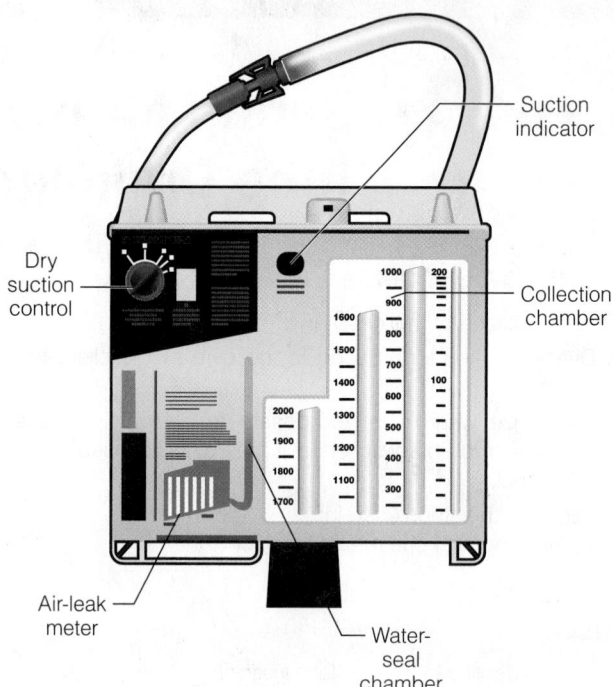

Figure 29–2 ■ A disposable chest drainage system. Fluid and blood collect in the white calibrated chambers. The red dial controls the suction, and the blue chamber indicates air leaks.

DRAINAGE SYSTEMS

Because the pleural cavity normally has negative pressure that allows lung expansion, any tube connected to it must be sealed so air or liquid cannot enter the space. The chest tube is connected either to a one-way valve, or to **water-seal** (underwater) or dry-seal drainage. In water-seal drainage, water in the bottom of the container prevents air from being sucked back into the chest tube and pleural cavity during inspiration.

Drainage systems use three mechanisms to drain fluid and air from the pleural cavity: positive expiratory pressure, gravity, and suction. When the pleural cavity contains air or fluid, a positive pressure develops during expiration. This positive pressure helps expel the air and some fluid from the space. Placing the drainage tubing so it descends from the insertion site on the chest wall to the collection chamber allows gravity to act as an evacuation force. Suction is used with the other two forces to enhance the removal of air or fluid in some drainage systems.

The collection chamber is calibrated and generally can hold at least 2 L of drainage (Figure 29–2 ■). It has a write-on surface that allows the nurse to mark the time, date, and amount of drainage. The collection tubing coming directly from the client's chest tube is connected to the collection chamber. If appropriate, an additional component may be connected to the system that allows for filtering of drained blood, which can then be reinfused into the client. See Chapters 18 ∞ and 33 ∞ for more information about transfusions and autotransfusions.

Several kinds of water-seal drainage systems are available. In the years before plastics and disposable supplies, glass bottles were used in tandem to provide the water seal, collection of drainage, and suction. Currently, disposable systems achieve the same effects by encompassing three chambers: the collection chamber with subchambers, the water-seal chamber, and the suction chamber. The exact combination of these features and the configuration of these chambers vary by manufacturer.

If a "wet" water seal is used, the chamber is filled with sterile fluid to the 2-cm line. The unit must be kept upright and the fluid level maintained in order for the seal to function correctly. The nurse should add or remove fluid as needed to keep the level at 2 cm. The level of the water should fluctuate with the client's respirations (**tidaling**). Bubbling signifies that air is being removed from the pleural space. It is a normal occurrence in clients with a pneumothorax or if the chest tube has just been inserted. Continuous or intermittent bubbling in the water-seal chamber, however, indicates an air leak within the system or a break in the tubing connection. In systems with an air leak meter, the degree of air leak can be monitored by noting the numbered column through which bubbling is noted. Some systems do not require a water seal. Instead, a one-way valve is used that can maintain a seal even if the unit is tipped over (dry seal).

Either wet or dry suction can be used with chest drainage systems. With wet suction, the suction control chamber is filled with sterile water to the desired level—often 20 cm H_2O. The tubing is then connected from the suction chamber to the suction device, which is turned on until gentle bubbling is seen in the chamber (usually 10 to 20 cm H_2O). Either a wall suction machine or a portable suction machine can be used. Turning the suction device higher will increase the amount of bubbling, but not the amount of suction applied to the chest tube. The amount of suction is controlled by the level of the water in the chamber. In dry systems, the amount of suction is set by the regulator dial instead of a water chamber. An indicator window in the system may display the word "Yes" or show a colored float to confirm that suction is active.

In recent years, mobile chest drains have allowed the client to move about with fewer restrictions and, in turn, have reduced the risks of immobility (i.e., deep venous thrombosis, pulmonary embolism). Mobile devices typically rely on gravity, not suction, for drainage. They are intended for use with the mobile client who is breathing spontaneously; they are not for clients who are ventilator dependent. A **Heimlich chest drain valve** may be used instead of a full collection system for clients who are ambulatory (Figure 29–3 ■). The Heimlich valve is a one-way flutter valve that allows air to escape from the chest cavity but prevents air from reentering. It consists of a piece of latex tubing inside a round plastic housing with connectors on both ends—a blue end that attaches to the chest tube and a clear end that allows the air to escape. The arrows or wording on the housing should always point away from the client. At each assessment, observe the inner valve carefully for movement during exhalation, indicating airflow through the device. The Heimlich valve has no reservoir and is not designed to collect fluid. The clear end may be attached to a collection bag, but the bag must be vented to allow the air to escape. Use of a mini-chest tube with Heimlich valve has been demonstrated to be an effective ambulatory treatment for spontaneous pneumothorax without hospitalization (Ho, Ong, Koh, Wong, & Raghuram, 2011).

Another device that can attach to the chest tube, called the Pneumostat, also has a one-way valve and, unlike the Heimlich valve, a small built-in collection chamber that typically holds only 30 mL of fluid. It is used exclusively for clients with a pneumothorax who usually have small amounts of fluid. Its design eliminates the risk

of incorrect attachment, as only one end of the valve can fit into the chest tube. The device comes with a clip that can be used to attach the device to the client's clothing (Figure 29–4 ■).

The Express Mini 500 (Figure 29–5 ■) has a relatively large (500 mL) collection chamber and a dry suction mechanism preset at 20 cm H_2O. The drain can be attached to a wall vacuum if needed. Its light weight reduces the pull on the chest tube, which results in less pain. Cloth straps allow the Mini to be worn over the shoulder

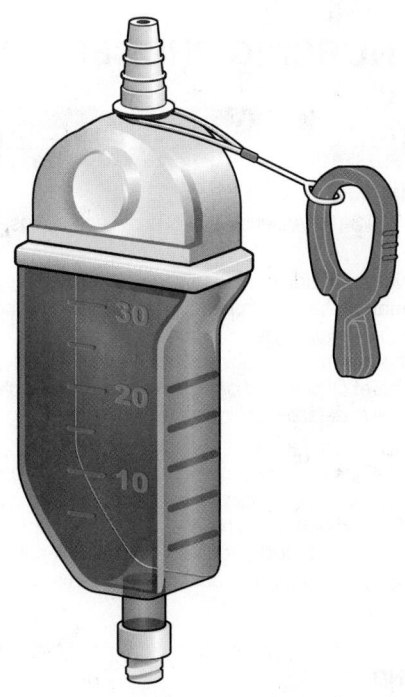

Figure 29–4 ■ The Pneumostat is an example of a device often used for clients with a pneumothorax. It uses a one-way valve and has a small collection chamber.

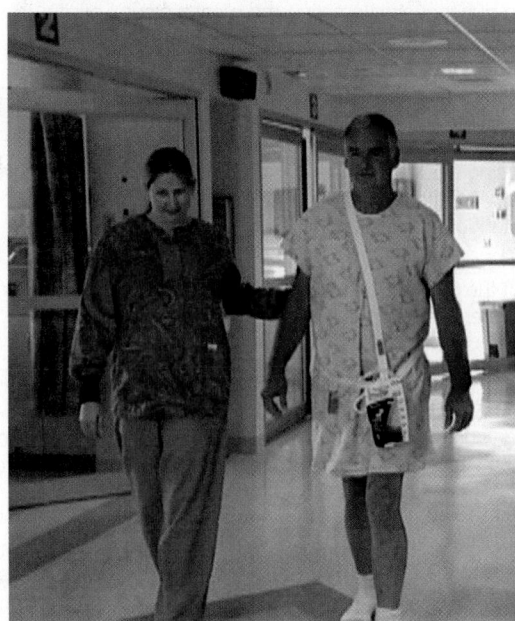

Figure 29–5 ■ A mobile chest drain system allows the client freedom of movement.

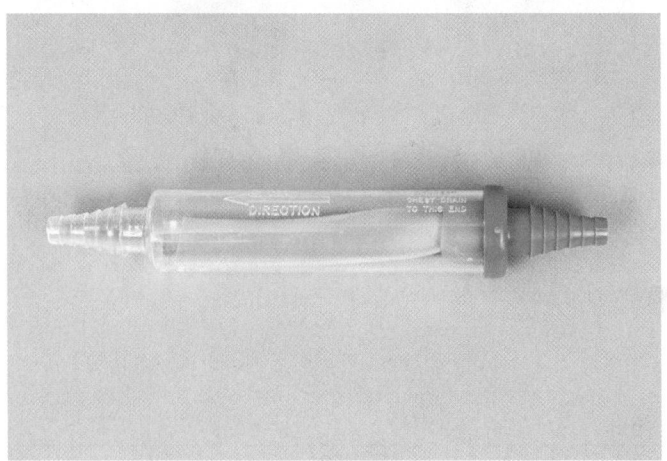

Figure 29–3 ■ Heimlich chest drain valve.

or at the waist when mobile, or hung from a bed rail or chair when at home.

Besides the various collection systems, there are also special long-term use chest tube catheters with valves that allow clients to drain pleural fluid as needed when they are at home. One example is the Pleurx˙ system, which can be used for those clients with chronic pleural effusions. When needed, the client attaches a disposable vacuum bottle to the end of the implanted catheter to drain the desired amount of fluid.

ASSISTING WITH CHEST TUBES

Chest tubes may be inserted and removed by the primary care provider or an advanced practice provider who may be an advanced practice nurse or a physician assistant (Morton & Fontaine, 2013). Both procedures require sterile technique and must be done without introducing air or microorganisms into the pleural cavity. After the insertion, an x-ray film is taken to confirm the position of the tube. The major objective of nursing care of clients with chest tubes is to facilitate drainage of fluid and air promoting lung reexpansion.

●○● NURSING PROCESS: ASSISTING WITH CHEST TUBE INSERTION

Assisting with Chest Tube Insertion

ASSESSMENT

See also Skill 3–11, Assessing the Thorax and Lungs, in Chapter 3 ∞. Obtain:

- Vital signs, including oxygen saturation, for baseline data. **Rationale:** *Changes in these parameters may indicate worsening of the initial problem or condition.*
- Breath sounds. Auscultate bilaterally for baseline data. **Rationale:** *Diminished or absent breath sounds after chest drainage is established indicate inadequate lung expansion.*

Examine the client for:

- Clinical signs of a pneumothorax before chest tube insertion. Signs include sharp pain on the affected side; weak, rapid pulse; pallor; vertigo; faintness; dyspnea; diaphoresis; excessive coughing; and blood-tinged sputum. Reexamine for these signs of a pneumothorax after chest tube insertion.

- Chest expansion (respiratory excursion). See Chapter 3 ∞, pages 93 and 95, and Figures ❶ and ❺ in Skill 3–11.
- Chest movements, such as retractions, flail chest, or paradoxical breathing.

Confirm:

- That informed consent for the procedure has been obtained from the client and/or family member by the primary care provider.
- Any known allergies to iodine, lidocaine, and tape. **Rationale:** *Povidone-iodine is used to cleanse the skin. Lidocaine is used to numb the skin area prior to chest tube insertion. The chest tube will be secured in place with tape.*

Review:

- The client's medication record for anticoagulant therapy. **Rationale:** *Anticoagulants (aspirin, Coumadin, or heparin) can increase incidence of blood loss.*

PLANNING

If the client is critically ill or a large volume of fluid is expected to drain immediately from the chest tube, ensure that oxygen, emergency airway supplies, and intravenous access are available.

Nurses must follow strict surgical aseptic technique when setting up chest drainage to prevent microorganisms from entering the system and subsequently entering the client's pleural cavity. To set up the drainage system (wet system):

- Open the packaged unit.
- Fill the water-seal chamber. The procedure will vary depending on the specifics of the actual device.
  - Remove the cap on the water-seal chamber. ❶
  - Using a 50-mL irrigating syringe with the plunger removed, fill the water-seal chamber with sterile water up to the 2-cm mark or as specified. ❷ Then reattach the cap.

  or

- Inject the required amount of water into the self-sealing port of the water-seal chamber using a syringe and needle. ❸

  or

- Use the prefilled bottle to instill the water into the chamber.
- If the primary care provider has ordered suction, remove the cap on the suction control chamber and fill the suction control chamber with sterile water or saline to the ordered level or according to agency policy, and replace the cap.

  or

- Set the suction control dial to the ordered amount.
- If no suction is ordered, leave the suction port open to allow air to escape (Frazer, 2012).
- Place the system in the rack supplied, or attach it to the bed frame.

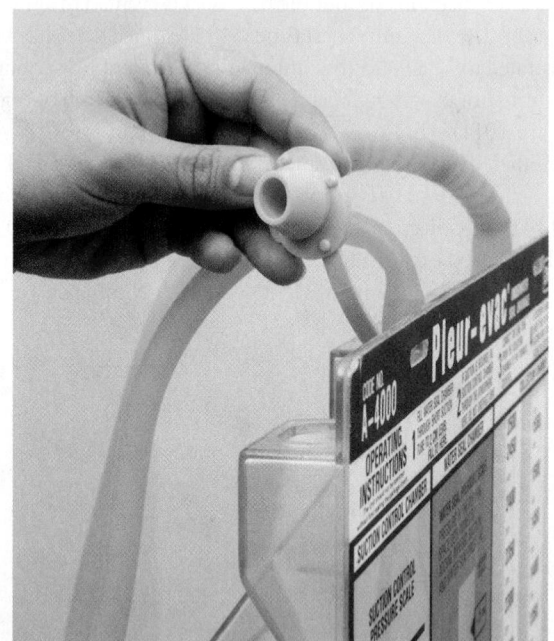

❶ Opening the water-seal filling port.

Assisting with Chest Tube Insertion—*continued*

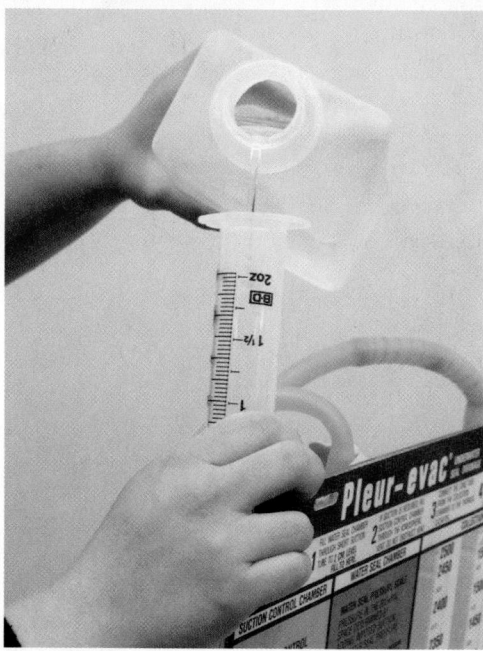

❷ Filling the water-seal chamber with sterile water.

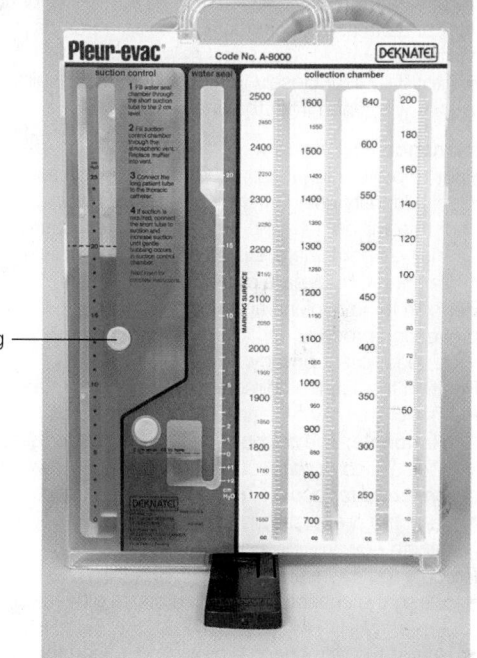

Self-sealing water-seal chamber port

❸ A three-chamber wet-suction/wet-seal disposable chest drainage system.

DELEGATION

Assisting the primary care provider with insertion of a chest tube is the role of the registered nurse and is not delegated to unlicensed assistive personnel (UAP).

INTERPROFESSIONAL PRACTICE

Assisting the primary care provider with insertion of a chest tube is within the scope of practice for those health care providers qualified to perform the insertion. Sometimes, technicians such as those who work in surgery or emergency settings may also be qualified to assist.

Equipment
- Sterile chest tube tray that includes:
  - Drapes
  - 10-mL syringe
  - Gauze sponges

- #22-gauge needle
- #25-gauge needle
- #11 blade scalpel
- Forceps
- Two padded or nontoothed tube clamps
- Extra 4×4 gauze sponges or other occlusive bandage material
- Split drain sponges
- Chest tubes of the appropriate size
- Trocar or hemostat
- Suture materials
- Drainage system (water or dry seal)
- Suction source, if ordered
- Sterile gloves (for primary care provider and nurse)
- Local anesthetic
- Skin cleansing solution (e.g., povidone-iodine)
- Adhesive or foam tape
- Petrolatum gauze (optional)

IMPLEMENTATION
Preparation
- Although the primary care provider will have already done initial client and family teaching, the nurse reinforces key elements. Review the technique of chest tube insertion and its purpose with the client and family. **Rationale:** *This reduces client anxiety and assists in efficiency of the procedure.*

- Confirm with the primary care provider the desired types and numbers of equipment needed. Primary care providers have personal preferences for styles and sizes of chest tubes, and needs vary with the purpose of the tube.

Continued on page 632

Assisting with Chest Tube Insertion—*continued*

- Premedicate the client for pain. Incorporate nonpharmacologic pain- and stress-reducing strategies as much as possible (see Chapter 9 ∞).
- Monitor the client closely to ensure that the respiratory status has not worsened from the analgesics.

Performance

1. Prior to performing the procedure, introduce self and verify the client's identity using agency protocol. Explain to the client what your role will be, why the procedure is necessary, and how he or she can participate. Discuss how the procedure will be used in planning further care or treatments.
2. Perform hand hygiene and observe other appropriate infection prevention procedures.
3. Provide for client privacy.
4. Position the client as directed by the primary care provider.
   - The client may be placed flat or in Fowler's position. **Rationale:** *The flat position is preferred for best access to the second or third intercostal space; a Fowler's position is preferred for access to the fourth to sixth intercostal space.*
   - Turn the client laterally so that the area receiving the tube is facing upward.
5. Prepare for the insertion.
   - Open the chest tube tray and sterile gloves on the overbed table.
   - Assist the primary care provider to clean the insertion site.
   - Assist the primary care provider with the local anesthetic as needed.
   - Participate in The Joint Commission's (2013) National Patient Safety Goal—Universal Protocol for Preventing Wrong Site, Wrong Procedure, Wrong Person Surgery, which requires preprocedure verification and a "time-out" to ensure that all members of the team agree about what is to be done and to whom.
6. Provide emotional support to the client as the primary care provider makes a small incision through the skin and muscle. Often, the practitioner will probe through the incision with a finger to ensure there are no underlying structures that may be damaged during insertion of the tube. The practitioner will use a trochar or hemostat to broaden and deepen the insertion site and then pass the tube into the chest. Monitor the client's condition and reaction to the procedure.
7. Dress the site. The primary care provider will usually place a purse-string suture to anchor the tube.
   - Apply sterile gloves and wrap the petrolatum gauze (if desired) around the chest tube at the insertion site.
   - Place split drain gauze around the chest tube, one from the top and one from the bottom.
   - Place several additional gauze squares and tape or occlusive bandage materials over the drain gauze. These form an airtight seal at the insertion site.
8. Secure the tube.
   - Assist with connecting the chest tube to the valve or drainage system.
   - Attach the longer tube from the collection chamber to the client's chest tube.
   - Remove and discard gloves.
   - Perform hand hygiene.
   - Tape the chest tube to the client's skin so that any pull on the tubing creates traction on the skin and not on the insertion site.
   - Tape all connections using spiral turns, but do not completely cover the collection tubing with tape. ❹ **Rationale:**

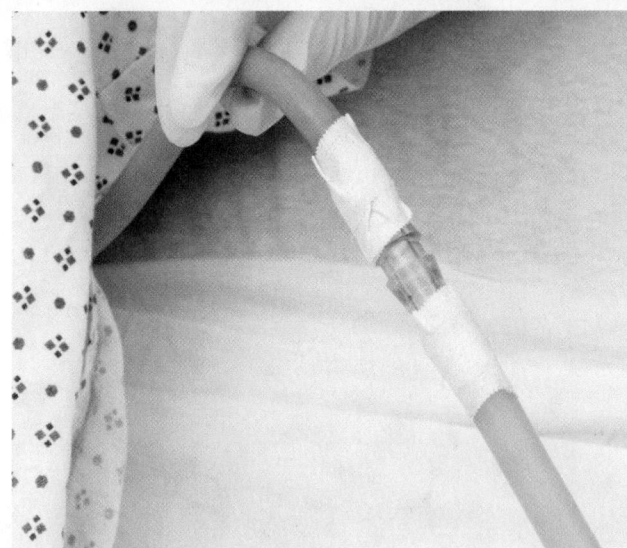

❹ Taped tubing connection with the connector exposed for observation of drainage.

Taping prevents inadvertent separation. Not covering all the collection tubing allows drainage to be seen.
   - Coil the excess drainage tubing next to the client, ensuring slack for the client to turn and move. **Rationale:** *This prevents kinking of the tubing and impairment of drainage.*
   - If suction is ordered, attach the remaining shorter tube from the suction chamber to the suction source, and turn it on. If wet suction is used, inspect the suction chamber for bubbling. Gentle bubbling indicates an appropriate suction level.
   - If suction has not been ordered, keep the shorter rubber tube unclamped. This maintains negative or equal pressure in the system.
9. When all drainage connections are complete, ask the client to take a deep breath and hold it for a few seconds, then slowly exhale. These actions facilitate drainage from the pleural space and lung reexpansion.
10. Prepare the client for a chest x-ray to check for placement of the tube and lung expansion.
11. Ensure client safety.
    - Keep chest tube clamps and petrolatum gauze at the bedside. See Skill 29–2 for actions to take if the tube becomes disconnected from the drainage system or the system breaks or cracks.
    - Assess the client for signs of a new or worsening pneumothorax.
    - Assess the client for signs of subcutaneous emphysema (collection of gas under the skin). Palpate around the dressing site for crackling indicative of subcutaneous emphysema. **Rationale:** *Subcutaneous emphysema can result from a poor seal at the chest tube insertion site.* This is not an emergency but should be reported, documented, and monitored. It should reabsorb in a few days.
    - Assess drainage, vital signs, and oxygen saturation every 15 minutes for the first hour and then as ordered. Mark the

Assisting with Chest Tube Insertion—*continued*

collection chamber with a line and the date and time. Report bleeding or drainage greater than 100 mL/h. The color or appearance of the chest tube drainage is discussed in Table 29–1.

12. Document the insertion in the client record using forms or checklists supplemented by narrative notes when appropriate. Include the name of the primary care provider, site of placement, type of tube, type of drainage system, characteristics of the immediate drainage, and other assessment findings.

SAMPLE DOCUMENTATION

5/12/2015 0130 32-Fr chest tube inserted into left chest by Dr. Novarty & connected to water-seal drainage unit. Suction at $-20\,cm\,H_2O$. Immediately drained 120 mL straw-colored fluid. Moderate coughing after insertion, eased in 10 minutes. All connections taped and tubing taped to chest wall. Tidaling with respirations noted. Client instructed re: positioning & care of tube & collection device. Client states understanding. VS 101°F, 100, 26, 170/94, SaO_2 97%. ————
—————————————————— J. Lygas, RN

EVALUATION

• Perform a detailed follow-up based on findings that deviated from expected or normal for the client. Relate findings to previous assessment data if available.

• Report significant deviations from normal to the primary care provider.

TABLE 29–1	Characteristics of Chest Tube Drainage

Description of Fluid	Indication
Blood tinged or bloody	Anticoagulant use Pulmonary infarct Trauma Malignancy Inflammation
Serous	Pleural fluid Plasma portion of blood indicating cessation of active bleeding
Cloudy	Infection or inflammation
Purulent (pus)	Empyema
Food particles	Esophageal rupture
Black	*Aspergillus* (fungal) infection
Low pH	Tuberculosis, malignancy

MANAGING A CLIENT WITH CHEST DRAINAGE

Once a client has had a chest tube inserted, the nurse maintains patency of the chest drainage system, facilitating lung reexpansion, and preventing complications associated with chest drainage (e.g., infection and bleeding).

●○● NURSING PROCESS: MAINTAINING CHEST TUBE DRAINAGE

Maintaining Chest Tube Drainage

ASSESSMENT

See Skill 3–11, Assessing the Thorax and Lungs, in Chapter 3 ∞, and see the assessments listed with Skill 29–1.

PLANNING

Review the client record for previous data regarding the condition, output, and client tolerance of the chest tube.

DELEGATION

Care of chest tubes is not delegated to UAP. However, the UAP may care for a client with a chest tube and aspects of the client's condition are observed during usual care and may be recorded by individuals other than the nurse. Abnormal findings must be validated and interpreted by the nurse.

INTERPROFESSIONAL PRACTICE

Maintaining chest tube drainage may be within the scope of practice for several health care providers, for example, respiratory therapists. Although these therapists may verbally communicate their findings and plan to the health care team members, the nurse must also know where to locate their documentation in the client's medical record.

Continued on page 634

SKILL 29-2

Maintaining Chest Tube Drainage—*continued*

Equipment
- Sterile gloves
- Two padded or nontoothed tube clamps if clamps are not integrated into the tubing system
- Petrolatum gauze (optional)
- 4×4 gauze sponges
- Split drain sponges
- Drainage system
- Skin cleansing solution (e.g., povidone-iodine)
- Adhesive or foam tape

IMPLEMENTATION
Preparation
- Determine when the last dressing change was performed.

Performance
1. Prior to performing the procedure, introduce self and verify the client's identity using agency protocol. Explain to the client what you are going to do, why it is necessary, and how he or she can participate. Discuss how the results will be used in planning further care or treatments.
2. Perform hand hygiene and observe other appropriate infection prevention procedures.
3. Provide for client privacy.
4. Assess the client.
   - Determine ease of respirations, breath sounds, respiratory rate and depth, oxygen saturation, and chest movements every 2 hours.
   - Observe the dressing site. Inspect the dressing for excessive and abnormal drainage, such as bleeding or foul-smelling discharge. Palpate around the dressing site for crackling indicative of subcutaneous emphysema. **Rationale:** *Subcutaneous emphysema can result from inadequate seal (air leak) at the chest tube insertion site.*
   - Determine level of discomfort with and without activity. **Rationale:** *Analgesics may need to be administered before the client moves or does deep-breathing and coughing exercises.*
   - Evaluate the impact of possible changes to the client's body image that occur when a person has tubes extending out from the body. It can be a frightening or disorienting experience for the client and family. There may be a fear of pulling the tubes out, pulling on them and causing pain, or having someone else accidentally pull on them. A nurse who is sensitive to this can offer a more comforting presence to the client.
5. Implement all necessary safety precautions.
   - Keep two 15- to 18-cm (6- to 7-in.) chest tube clamps within reach at the bedside or at the top of the client's bed to clamp the chest tube in an emergency.
   - Keep an extra drainage system unit available in the client's room. To change the drainage system, prepare the new system as described in Skill 29–1. If suction is being used, turn it off. Then:
     a. If the tubing system has no integrated clamp (❶A), clamp the chest tube close to the insertion site with two chest tube clamps placed in opposite directions (❶B).
     b. Apply sterile gloves. Disconnect the original collection tubing and connect the new system immediately.
     c. Reestablish the seals, remove the clamps, and reestablish suction as ordered.
   - Remove and discard gloves. Perform hand hygiene.
   - Keep the drainage system below chest level and upright at all times. **Rationale:** *Keeping the unit below chest level prevents backflow of fluid from the drainage chamber into the pleural space. Keeping the unit upright maintains the water seal.*
6. Maintain the patency of the drainage system.
   - Check that all connections are secured with tape. **Rationale:** *This ensures that the system is airtight.*

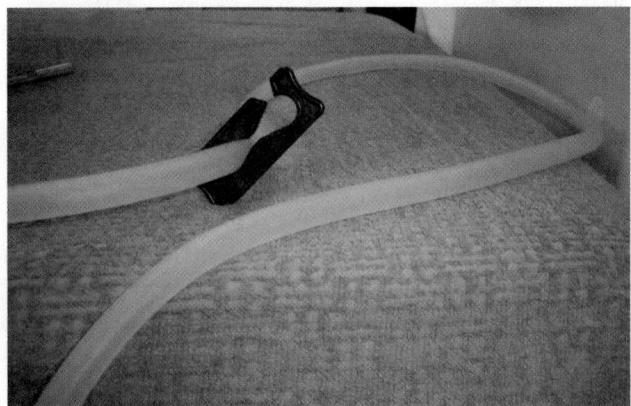

A

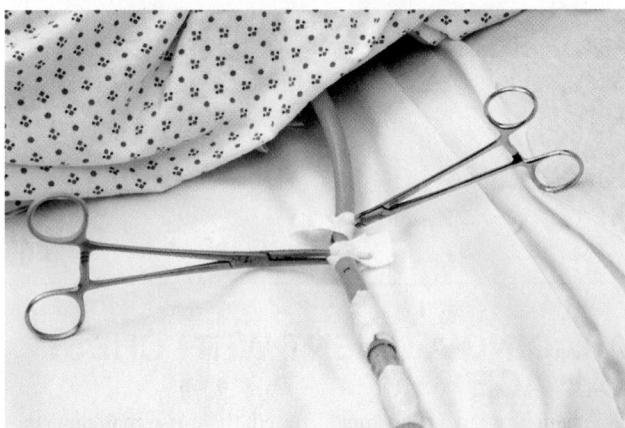

B

❶ Clamping a chest tube using *A,* an integrated clamp, or *B,* crossed clamps.

- Inspect the drainage tubing for kinks or loops dangling below the entry level of the drainage system.
- Coil the drainage tubing next to the client, ensuring enough slack for the client to turn and move. **Rationale:** *This prevents kinking of the tubing and impairment of the drainage system.* Be sure that there are no dependent loops of tubing between the bed surface and the collection device. **Rationale:** *This decreases the chances of clots forming in the tubing that can obstruct drainage.*
- Inspect the air vent in the system periodically to make sure it is not occluded. **Rationale:** *A vent must be present to allow air to escape. Obstruction of the air vent causes increased pressure in the system, which could result in pneumothorax.*
- Avoid any forceful manipulation of the tube. In some agencies, this includes stripping or milking the chest tubing. Stripping refers to compressing the chest tube between fingers and thumb, using a pulling motion down the rest of the tubing away from the chest wall. Milking involves squeezing, kneading, or twisting the tubing to create bursts

Maintaining Chest Tube Drainage—*continued*

of suction to move any clots. Stripping chest tubes may significantly increase negative pressure that could damage the pleural membranes and/or surrounding tissues, causing pain and impairing the client's recovery. If clots are present in the tubing, expert opinion recommends gently squeezing and releasing of small segments of the tubing between the fingers instead of stripping (Bauman & Handley, 2011; Kane, York, & Minton, 2013).

7. Assess fluid level fluctuations and bubbling in the drainage system.
   - Check for tidaling of the fluid level in the water-seal chamber as the client breathes. Normally, fluctuations of 5 to 10 cm (2 to 4 in.) occur until the lung has reexpanded. **Rationale:** *Tidaling reflects the pressure changes in the pleural space during inhalation and exhalation. The fluid level rises when the client inhales and falls when the client exhales. The absence of tidaling may indicate tubing obstruction from a kink, dependent loop, blood clot, or outside pressure (e.g., because the client is lying on the tubing), or it may indicate that full lung reexpansion has occurred.*
   - In suction drainage systems, the fluid line remains constant. To check for tidaling in suction systems, temporarily turn off the suction. Then observe the fluctuation.
   - Check for intermittent bubbling in the water of the water-seal chamber. **Rationale:** *Intermittent bubbling normally occurs when the system removes air from the pleural space, especially when the client takes a deep breath or coughs. Absence of bubbling may indicate that the drainage system is blocked or that the pleural space has healed and is sealed; this must be verified by x-ray. Continuous bubbling or a sudden change from an established pattern can indicate a break in the system (i.e., an air leak) and should be reported immediately.*
   - Check for gentle bubbling in the suction control chamber in wet systems. **Rationale:** *Gentle bubbling indicates proper suction pressure.*

8. Assess the drainage.
   - Inspect the drainage in the collection container at least every 15 minutes during the first 2 hours after chest tube insertion and every 2 hours thereafter.
   - Every 4 to 8 hours, mark the time, date, and drainage level on the collection chamber. ❷
   - Note any sudden change in the amount or color of the drainage.
   - If drainage exceeds 100 mL/h or if a color change indicates hemorrhage, notify the primary care provider immediately.

9. Watch for dislodgment of the tubes, and remedy the problem promptly.
   - If the chest tube becomes disconnected from the drainage system:
     a. Submerge the end of the chest tube 2 to 4 cm (about 1 to 2 in.) below the surface of a 250-mL bottle of sterile water or saline solution to form a fluid seal.
        or
        Have the client exhale fully. Clamp the chest tube close to the insertion site. **Rationale:** *The fluid seal or clamping prevents external air from entering the pleural space.*
        1. Apply sterile gloves. Quickly, clean the ends of the tubing with an antiseptic, reconnect them, and tape them securely.
        2. If clamped, unclamp the tube as soon as possible.
        3. Remove and discard gloves.
        4. Perform hand hygiene.

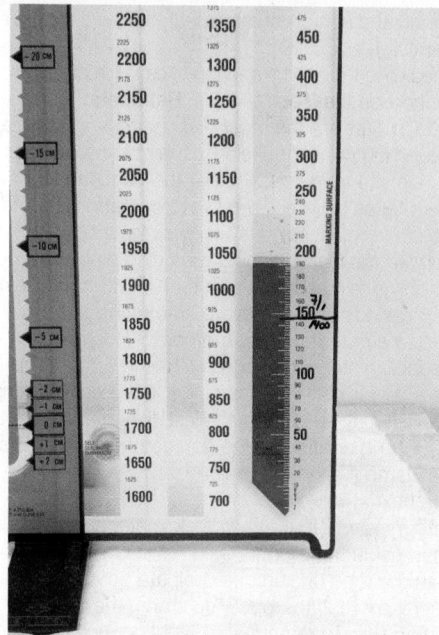

❷ Marking the date, time, and drainage level.

   b. Assess the client closely for respiratory distress (dyspnea, pallor, diaphoresis, blood-tinged sputum, or chest pain).
   c. Check vital signs every 10 minutes until stable.
   d. Document the incident in the client's medical record or other appropriate records according to the agency protocol.
   - If the chest tube becomes dislodged from the insertion site:
     a. Remove the dressing. If there is an air leak, tape sterile, dry gauze on only three sides to allow air to escape on exhalation (Frazer, 2012). **Rationale:** *Without an occlusive dressing, pleural air can escape and prevent a tension pneumothorax.*
     b. Have a coworker notify the primary care provider immediately.
     c. Remain with the client and assess for respiratory distress every 10 to 15 minutes or as the client's condition indicates.
     d. Prepare for replacement of the chest tube.
     e. Document the incident in the client's medical record or other appropriate records according to the facility's protocol.
   - If the wet drainage system is accidentally tipped over:
     a. Immediately return it to the upright position. Check the water level in the water-seal and suction control chambers and add water if indicated.
     b. Ask the client to take several deep breaths. **Rationale:** *Deep breaths help force air out of the pleural cavity that might have entered when the water seal was not intact.*
     c. Assess the client for respiratory distress.
     d. The system may need to be replaced. Notify the primary care provider if indicated.

10. If bubbling persists in the water-seal collection chamber or air leak chamber, determine its source. Continuous bubbling in the water-seal collection chamber normally occurs for only a few minutes after a chest tube is attached to drainage, because fluid and air initially rush out from the intrapleural space under high pressure.

Continued on page 636

Maintaining Chest Tube Drainage—*continued*

- To identify the source of an air leak, follow the next steps sequentially:
  a. Check the tubing connection sites. Tighten and retape any connection that seems loose. **Rationale:** *The tubing connection sites are the most likely places for leaks to occur.*
  b. If bubbling continues, clamp the chest tube near the insertion site, and see whether the bubbling stops while the client takes several deep breaths. **Rationale:** *Clamping the chest will determine whether the leak is proximal or distal to the clamp.* Chest tube clamping must be done for only a few seconds at a time. **Rationale:** *Clamping for long periods can aggravate an existing pneumothorax or lead to a recurrent pneumothorax.*
  c. If bubbling stops, proceed with the next step. The source of the air leak is above the clamp (i.e., between the clamp and the client). It may be either at the insertion site or inside the client.
  d. If bubbling continues, the source of the air leak is below the clamp (i.e., in the drainage system below the clamp). See next step.
- To determine whether the air leak is at the insertion site or internal (inside the client):
  a. With the tube unclamped, palpate gently around the insertion site. If the bubbling stops, the leak is at the insertion site. To remedy this situation, apply a petrolatum gauze and a 4×4 gauze around the insertion site, and secure these dressings with adhesive or foam tape.
  b. If the leak is not at the insertion site, it is internal and may indicate a dislodged tube or a new pneumothorax. In this instance, leave the tube unclamped, notify the primary care provider, and monitor the client for signs of respiratory distress.
- To locate an air leak below the chest tube clamp:
  a. Move the clamp a few inches farther down and keep moving it downward a few inches at a time. Each time the clamp is moved, check the water-seal collection chamber for bubbling. **Rationale:** *The bubbling will stop as soon as the clamp is placed between the air leak and the water-seal drainage.*
  b. Seal the leak when you locate it by applying tape to that portion of the drainage tube. Report and record the leak and what was done to correct it.
  c. If bubbling continues after the entire length of the tube is clamped, the air leak is in the drainage device. To remedy this situation, replace the drainage system according to agency protocol.

11. Take a specimen of the chest drainage as required.
    - Specimens of chest drainage may be taken from a disposable chest drainage system through the resealable connecting tubing or from a port in the collecting system.
12. Ensure essential client care.
    - Encourage deep-breathing and coughing exercises every 2 hours, if indicated (this may be contraindicated in clients with a lobectomy). Premedicate the client for pain as needed. Have the client sit upright to perform the exercises, and splint the tube insertion site with a pillow or with a hand to minimize discomfort. **Rationale:** *Deep breathing and coughing help remove accumulations from the pleural space, facilitate drainage, and help the lung to reexpand.*
    - Auscultate the client's chest at least every 4 hours. Breath sounds should be symmetric. **Rationale:** *Decreased breath sounds on the side of the chest tube could indicate that air or fluid is accumulating in the pleural space. If breath sounds are louder on the affected side, it could indicate that fluid is accumulated on the other side of the chest.*
    - Percuss the client's chest. A normal lung should have a resonant (hollow) sound. **Rationale:** *A dull or flat sound indicates fluid or solid tissue. Report any abnormal findings to the primary care provider.*
    - Check that the chest tube site dressing is dry and occlusive. The dressing does not need to be changed unless it is loose or wet. In some agencies, chest tube dressings are changed daily. **Rationale:** *A wet dressing could indicate a fluid leak around the tube.*
    - Examine the chest tube insertion site for signs of healing, skin irritation, or infection.
    - Reposition the client every 2 hours. When the client is lying on the affected side, place rolled towels on either side of the tubing. **Rationale:** *Position changes promote drainage, prevent complications, and provide comfort. Rolled towels prevent occlusion of the chest tube by the client's weight.*
    - Assist the client with range-of-motion exercises of the affected shoulder three times per day to maintain joint mobility.
    - Conduct regular pain assessments using a simple scoring system. If necessary, ask the primary care provider for more aggressive pain management (possibly patient-controlled analgesia). **Rationale:** *Pain will limit the client's mobility and will result in shallow breaths and incomplete lung expansion.*
    - When transporting and ambulating the client:
      a. Attach chest tube clamps to the client's gown for emergency use.
      b. Keep the water-seal unit below chest level and upright.
      c. Disconnect the drainage system from the suction apparatus before moving the client, and make sure the air vent is open. Or, if ordered, obtain a portable suction device.
13. Document findings in the client record using forms or checklists supplemented by narrative notes when appropriate. Record patency of chest tubes; type, amount, and color of drainage; presence of fluctuations; appearance of insertion site; laboratory specimens, if any were taken; respiratory assessments; client's vital signs and level of comfort; and all other nursing care provided to the client.

EVALUATION

- Perform detailed follow-up based on findings that deviated from expected or normal for the client. Relate findings to previous assessment data if available.
- Report significant deviations from normal to the primary care provider.

LIFESPAN CONSIDERATIONS **Maintaining Chest Tube Drainage**

OLDER ADULTS
- Coughing and deep-breathing exercises are particularly important because shallow breathing and decreased ability to cough may occur with aging.
- Encourage the client to take pain medication when needed. Older adults may be reluctant to take pain medication.
- Take special care of the client's skin due to the possibility of skin tears from tape and increased risk of skin breakdown over bony prominences as skin becomes thinner and less elastic.
- The older client is at increased risk for respiratory distress due to increased lung stiffness.

CLIENT TEACHING CONSIDERATIONS

Going Home with a Heimlich Valve

CARE OF THE CHEST TUBE AND VALVE
- Honking or "duck-like" sounds from the valve are normal.
- Movement of air or fluids should be visible through the valve.
- Check for signs and symptoms of infection daily. Check the chest tube insertion site for increased warmth or redness, pus-like drainage, swelling, or bleeding; or an oral temperature greater than 38°C (100.4°F).

GENERAL HYGIENE
- Instruct the client to shower with a waterproof dressing (plastic wrap) covering the chest tube insertion site and the valve.
- Tape all edges to keep the water out.
- Do not place the Heimlich valve directly in water.
- Do not block the tip of the valve that is open to air.

DRESSING CHANGE
- Wash around the tube insertion site with mild soap and water every other day (daily if drainage is noted at the site). Do not use soaps that contain lotion or heavy fragrances.
- Do not put lotions, powders, or ointment directly on the insertion site.
- Wear a split-drain gauze dressing around the insertion site.
- Prepare the skin with a skin barrier solution to protect it from tape.

- Tape the tube or valve to the skin so there is no pulling or kinking of the tube.
- The valve should never be closed with tape or an airtight dressing.

ACTIVITY
- There is no lifting restriction if only the chest tube is present. Instruct the client not to lift more than 5 to 10 lb for the next 4 weeks if a surgical incision is also present.
- Swimming or soaking in a bathtub or hot tub is prohibited while the chest tube is in place.

EMERGENCY SITUATIONS
- Call the primary care provider immediately if the valve breaks or becomes detached. The provider will give directions about how the valve is to be replaced or reattached.
- Call the primary care provider if experiencing an increase in pain that is unrelieved with medication.
- Call 911 immediately if experiencing sudden sharp chest pain or sudden onset of shortness of breath.
- Instruct the client and family to recognize the signs of infection, such as increased warmth or redness at the insertion site. The primary care provider should be notified if symptoms are present.

WHAT IF   Assessing Chest Tube Functioning

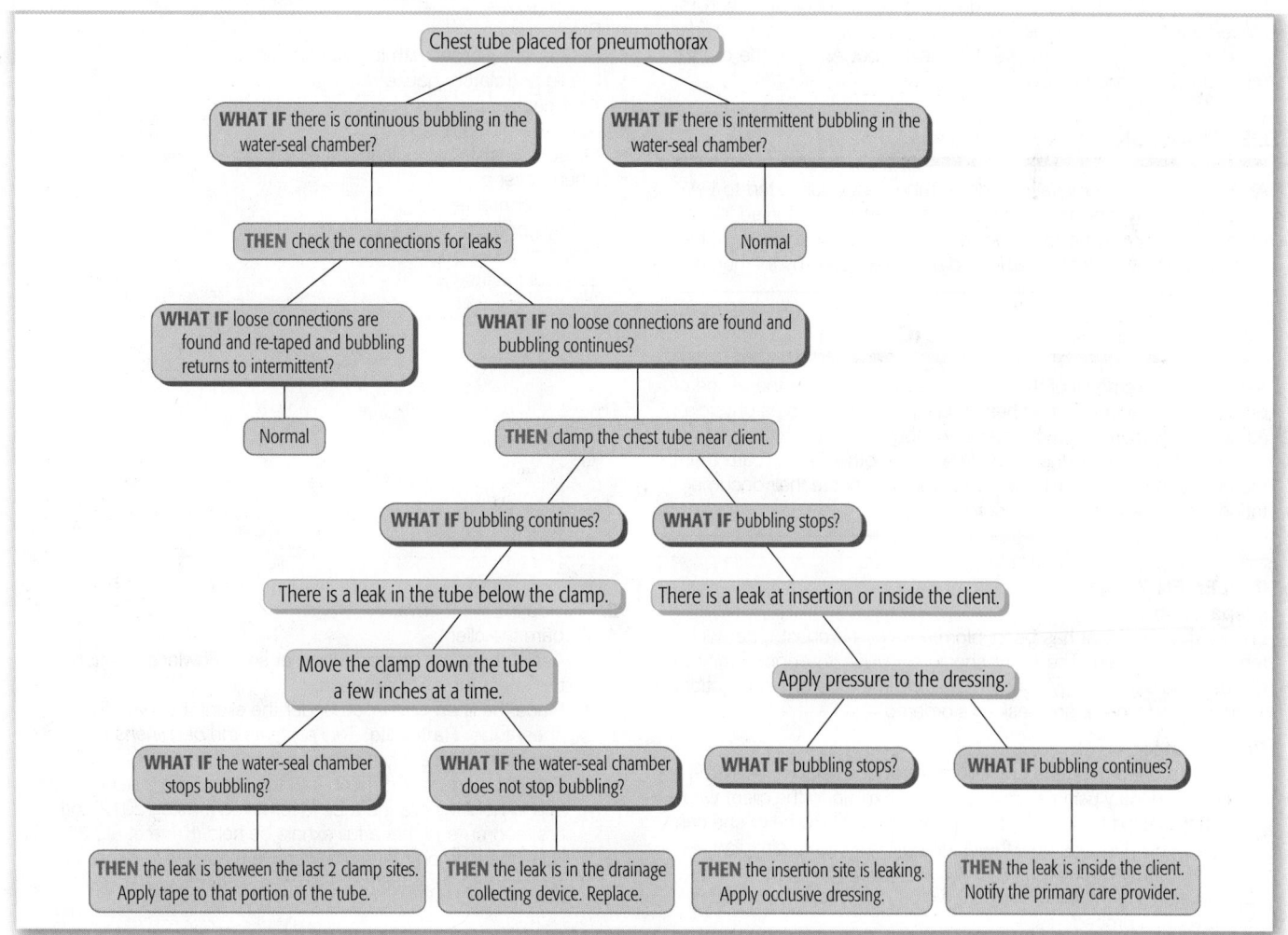

CHEST TUBE REMOVAL

Chest tube removal is the function of a physician or advanced practice provider. The chest tube may be removed when the underlying reason for its insertion has been corrected. Signs of this include:

- Minimal tube drainage (less than 50 mL in a 24-hour period).
- Lack of air leak for 24 to 48 hours.
- Chest x-ray shows reexpanded lung.
- Water seal not fluctuating.
- Respirations and lung sounds return to normal.
- Percussion of the chest reveals a resonant note.

The primary care provider may order that the tube be clamped and suction discontinued to determine if the client can tolerate being without it. If this is the case, assess the client every few minutes for signs of pneumothorax. Should signs appear, unclamp the tube or reestablish suction, and notify the primary care provider.

The procedure for removing the chest tube must be carried out in a way that minimizes the risk of allowing air to enter the chest cavity as the tube is pulled out.

●○● NURSING PROCESS: CHEST TUBE REMOVAL

SKILL 29–3

Assisting with Chest Tube Removal

ASSESSMENT

See Skill 3–11, Assessing the Thorax and Lungs, in Chapter 3 ∞ and see the assessments listed in Skill 29–1.

Prior to chest tube removal, review the client's laboratory results, because low platelets could cause excessive bleeding postprocedure.

Chest tube removal can be a very painful procedure. Determine when the client was last medicated for pain. Analgesia should be administered at least 30 minutes before the procedure to allow adequate time for it to take effect. In addition, using nonsteroidal anti-inflammatory drugs and deep-breathing relaxation exercises in conjunction with opioids can be more effective than opioids alone. At least one study has indicated that local application of ice to the skin surrounding the chest tube prior to removal results in less pain (Ertuğ & Ülker, 2012).

PLANNING

Often, a chest x-ray is done to determine if the original reason for placement of the chest tube has resolved. The primary care provider will determine when to remove the chest tube. Arrange the client's other activities around this.

DELEGATION

Assisting with the removal of a chest tube is not delegated to UAP. However, many effects of the removal may be observed during usual care and may be recorded by individuals other than the nurse. Abnormal findings must be validated and interpreted by the nurse.

INTERPROFESSIONAL PRACTICE

Assisting with removal of the chest tube may be within the scope of practice for specially trained health care providers such as physician assistants or surgical technicians. Although these providers may verbally communicate the procedure to the other health care team members, the nurse must also know where to locate their documentation in the client's medical record.

Equipment

- Clean gloves
- Sterile gloves
- Suture removal set with forceps and scissors
- Sterile petrolatum gauze
- 4×4 gauze sponges
- Adhesive or foam tape
- Moisture-resistant medical waste bag
- Linen-saver pad
- Sharps container
- Safety goggles
- Moisture-proof gowns
- Surgical masks

IMPLEMENTATION

Preparation

Ensure that the client has been informed that the chest tube will be removed and when. The client should be given the opportunity to discuss and express any concerns. Clamp the tube or stop suction, if ordered. Administer analgesics as ordered.

Performance

1. Prior to performing the procedure, introduce self and verify the client's identity using agency protocol. Explain to the client what you are going to do, why it is necessary, and how he or she can participate. Discuss how the results will be used in planning further care or treatments.
2. Perform hand hygiene and observe other appropriate infection prevention procedures.

3. Provide for client privacy.
4. Prepare the client:
   - Assist the client to a side-lying or semi-Fowler's position with the chest tube site exposed.
   - Place the linen-saver pad under the client, beneath the chest tube. **Rationale:** *This protects the bed linens and provides a place for the chest tube after removal.*
   - Some experts recommend that the client take a deep breath in and hold it while the tube is removed (Frazer, 2012); others recommend that a full exhale be held (Kane et al., 2013). Still others recommend the Valsalva maneuver—exhaling against the closed glottis (Bauman & Handley, 2011).

Assisting with Chest Tube Removal—*continued*

Rationale: *These techniques increase the intrathoracic pressure and prevent air from entering the pleural space.* Verify the preferred method with the provider who will be removing the chest tube and then instruct the client on how to hold the breath during removal.

5. Prepare the sterile field and supplies. Have the petrolatum gauze opened and ready for quick application.
6. Remove the dressing around the chest tube.
   - Apply clean gloves and dispose of the dressing in the moisture-proof medical waste bag.
   - Remove and discard gloves. Perform hand hygiene.
7. Assist with removal of the tube.
   - Apply sterile gloves.
   - Assist the client with the breathing technique and provide emotional support during the removal of the sutures and tube.
   - As the primary care provider removes the chest tube, either the provider or the nurse immediately applies the petrolatum gauze and covers it with dry gauze and adhesive or foam tape. **Rationale:** *This forms an airtight bandage.*
   - Remove all used equipment and place in appropriate medical waste containers.

   - Remove and discard gloves.
   - Perform hand hygiene.
8. Assess and monitor the client's response to tube removal.
   - Obtain vital signs every 15 minutes for the first hour and, if stable, then as indicated.
   - Auscultate lung sounds every hour for the first 4 hours to determine that the lung is remaining inflated.
   - Observe for signs of pneumothorax.
9. Document the date and time of removal, any drainage noted, and the client's response to the procedure in the client record using forms or checklists supplemented by narrative notes when appropriate.
10. Prepare the client for a chest x-ray 1 to 2 hours after chest tube removal and possibly again in 12 to 24 hours.

CLINICAL ALERT!

In some agencies, hydrocolloid dressings are applied to the tube removal site. In this case, the dressing should remain in place for 72 hours.

EVALUATION

- Perform detailed follow-up based on findings that deviated from expected or normal for the client. Relate findings to previous assessment data if available.
- Report significant deviations from normal to the primary care provider.

- The dressing should remain in place for 48 to 72 hours if there is only minimal drainage.

Chapter 29 Review

FOCUSING ON CLINICAL THINKING

Consider This

1. A client with a pneumothorax has had a chest tube inserted into the second intercostal space. After 1 hour, there is no drainage in the system. How do you explain this finding?
2. A client who had open heart surgery 48 hours ago has a chest tube in place that exits from the sixth intercostal space. Why is the chest tube in this place? Why might the chest tube stop draining?

3. The nurse on the off-going shift reports that there may be an air leak in the client's chest tube system, but the nurse did not have time to completely assess the problem. How would you proceed?

See Focusing on Clinical Thinking answers on student resource website.

TEST YOUR KNOWLEDGE

1. The nurse observes a gentle continuous bubbling in the water-seal column of the water-seal chest drainage system. This observation should prompt the nurse to do which action?
   1. Continue to monitor the client as usual; this is an expected outcome.
   2. Check the connections between the chest site and drainage tube, and where the drainage tube connects to the collection chamber.
   3. Decrease the suction to 15 cm of water and continue observing the system for any changes in bubbling during the next several hours.
   4. Remove half of the water from the water-seal chamber.

2. The client's chest tube is attached to a one-way flutter valve that allows air to escape the chest cavity and prevents air from reentering. The nurse would document this as:
   1. A Heimlich chest drain valve.
   2. A Pneumovax.
   3. A Pleurovac.
   4. A water seal.

3. When documenting that the client's water seal is fluctuating up and down with each inspiration and expiration, the nurse uses the proper term, which is:
   1. Bubbling.
   2. Tidaling.
   3. Fluttering.
   4. Alternating.

4. The nurse is caring for a client with a chest tube connected to water-seal drainage. The nurse may delegate which of the following tasks to unlicensed assistive personnel (UAP)?
   1. Milking the chest tube
   2. Measuring chest tube output
   3. Changing the chest tube drainage system
   4. Turning and positioning the client

5. A client with a chest tube and water-seal drainage system is breathing with more effort and at a faster rate than last observed 1 hour ago. The client's pulse rate has also increased. Which action should the nurse implement first?
   1. Check the drainage tubing to ensure that the client is not lying on it or kinking it.
   2. Increase the amount of suction in the system.
   3. Raise the drainage chamber to the level of the client's chest.
   4. Place two clamps on the chest tube to prevent any air leaks.

6. The nurse has just completed assisting with the insertion of a chest tube for a client with a hemothorax. During care after the primary care provider has left, which finding should be reported immediately?
   1. Drainage is bloody.
   2. Bubbling in the water seal stops.
   3. Preexisting subcutaneous emphysema is still present.
   4. There has been 300 mL of drainage in the collection system in the past hour.

7. The nurse is performing an initial assessment of a client with a chest tube in the fifth intercostal space. Which of the following findings would the nurse need to assess further? Select all that apply.
   1. Continuous bubbling in the water-seal chamber
   2. Respiratory rate of 18 breaths per minute
   3. The presence of subcutaneous emphysema
   4. Complaints of pain at the insertion site
   5. Serous drainage on the chest tube dressing the size of a bean

8. The nurse is caring for a client who has had a chest tube in place for 2 days. At the beginning of the shift, the nurse ensures that what equipment is at the bedside? Select all that apply.
   1. Chest tube clamps
   2. Plain 4×4 gauze
   3. Sterile petrolatum gauze
   4. Extra drainage system
   5. A sterile chest tube in the same size as the one inserted in the client

9. The client has a chest tube for a pneumothorax, which is noted to have continuous bubbling in the water-seal chamber. The nurse finds no loose connections. After clamping the chest tube near the client, the bubbling stops. The nurse's next action should be to:
   1. Apply pressure to the dressing around the chest tube insertion site.
   2. Move the clamp farther down the tube and note whether bubbling resumes.
   3. Replace the entire collection tubing and system.
   4. Increase the suction control until bubbling does not resume when the clamp is removed.

10. A nurse caring for a client with a chest tube accidentally disconnects the chest tube from the drainage tubing while turning the client from side to side. The initial nursing action is to:
    1. Call the primary care provider.
    2. Place the distal end of the tube in sterile water.
    3. Replace the drainage system.
    4. Place a sterile dressing over the chest tube insertion site.

See Answers to Test Your Knowledge in Appendix A.

READINGS AND REFERENCES

References

Bauman, M., & Handley, C. (2011). Chest-tube care: The more you know, the easier it gets. *American Nurse Today, 6*(9), 27–32.

Ertuğ, N., & Ülker, S. (2012). The effect of cold application on pain due to chest tube removal. *Journal of Clinical Nursing, 21*, 784–790. doi:10.1111/j.1365-2702.2011.03955.x

Frazer, C. (2012). Managing chest tubes. *Med-Surg Matters, 21*(1), 1, 10–12.

Ho, K. K., Ong, M. E. H., Koh, M. S., Wong, E., & Raghuram, J. (2011). A randomized controlled trial comparing minichest tube and needle aspiration in outpatient management of primary spontaneous pneumothorax. *American Journal of Emergency Medicine, 29*, 1152–1157. doi:10.1016/j.ajem.2010.05.017

The Joint Commission. (2013). *2014 National Patient Safety Goals*. Retrieved from http://www.jointcommission.org/standards_information/npsgs.aspx

Kane, C. J., York, N. L., & Minton, L. A. (2013). Chest tubes in the critically ill patient. *Dimensions of Critical Care Nursing, 32*(3), 111–117. doi:10.1097/DCC.0b013e3182864721

Morton, P. G., & Fontaine, D. K. (2013). *Essentials of critical care nursing: A holistic approach*. Philadelphia, PA: Wolters Kluwer Health/Lippincott Williams & Wilkins.

Selected Bibliography

Anand, R., Whelan, J., Ferrada, P., Duane, T., Malhotra, A., Aboutanos, M., & Ivatury, R. (2012). Thin chest wall is an independent risk factor for the development of pneumothorax after chest tube removal. *American Surgeon, 78*, 478–480.

Berman, A., Snyder, S., & Frandsen, G. (2016). *Kozier & Erb's fundamentals of nursing: Concepts, practice, and process* (10th ed.). Upper Saddle River, NJ: Pearson.

Coughlin, S., Emmerton-Coughlin, H., & Malthaner, R. (2012). Management of chest tubes after pulmonary resection: A systematic review and meta-analysis. *Canadian Journal of Surgery, 55*, 264–270. doi:10.1503/cjs.001411

Eisenberg, R., & Khabbaz, K. (2011). Are chest radiographs routinely indicated after chest tube removal following cardiac surgery? *American Journal of Roentgenology, 197*(1), 122–124. doi:10.2214/AJR.10.5856

Mann, A. (2012). Troubleshooting chest tubes: Learn how to assess, address and prevent potential problems. *Advance for Nurses*. Retrieved from http://nursing.advanceweb.com/continuing-education/ce-articles/troubleshooting-chest-tubes.aspx?CP=2

Shaw, D., & Frizelle, F. (2012). Avoidable complications following chest tube insertion. *New Zealand Medical Journal, 125*(1354), 12–14.

Woodward, C. S., Dowling, D., Taylor, R. P., & Savin, C. (2013). The routine use of chest radiographs after chest tube removal in children who have had cardiac surgery. *Journal of Pediatric Healthcare, 27*, 189–194. doi:10.1016/j.pedhc.2011.09.003

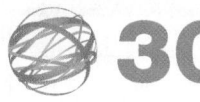 **30** Administering Emergency Measures to the Hospitalized Client

LEARNING OUTCOMES

At the completion of this chapter, the student will be able to:

1. Define key terms used in the skills of hospital emergency measures and cardiopulmonary resuscitation.
2. Identify indications for requesting a rapid response team or a cardiac/respiratory arrest team.
3. Describe the role of the nurse in initiating and participating in a cardiopulmonary arrest situation in a hospital.
4. Recognize when it is appropriate to delegate aspects of CPR to unlicensed assistive personnel.

5. Verbalize the steps used in:
   a. Clearing an obstructed airway.
   b. Performing rescue breathing.
   c. Administering external cardiac compressions.
   d. Administering automated external defibrillation.
6. Demonstrate appropriate documentation and reporting of emergency measures.

SKILLS

Skill 30–1 Clearing an Obstructed Airway
Skill 30–2 Performing Rescue Breathing

Skill 30–3 Administering External Cardiac Compressions
Skill 30–4 Administering Automated External Defibrillation

KEY TERMS

advanced cardiac life support (ACLS), *643*
asystole, *656*
automated external defibrillator (AED), *656*

basic life support (BLS), *643*
cardiopulmonary resuscitation (CPR), *642*
Code Blue, *642*
do not resuscitate (DNR), *643*

foreign body airway obstruction (FBAO), *643*
Heimlich maneuver, *644*
No Code Blue, *643*

pediatric advanced life support (PALS), *643*
rapid response teams (RRTs), *641*
respiratory arrest, *647*
ventricular fibrillation (VF), *656*

Medical emergencies of different types occur regularly in hospital, long-term care, outpatient, and community settings. Clients who are hospitalized may exhibit signs and symptoms indicating that their condition is deteriorating and immediate intervention beyond what the existing nursing staff can provide is required. Since the Institute for Healthcare Improvement (IHI) recommendation in 2004, hospitals have instituted **rapid response teams (RRTs)** to provide support when requested for clients experiencing potential life-threatening changes in their condition. The implementation of RRTs using an evidence-based practice framework can lead to decreased resuscitations, critical care transfers, overall mortality, and cost (Al-Qahtani et al., 2013; Leach & Mayo, 2013). If an arrest occurs, whether or not the RRT has been consulted, the nurse will need to institute cardiopulmonary resuscitation and request assistance from those health care providers in the agency designated to assist specifically with arrests.

RAPID RESPONSE TEAMS

Although the specific structure, duties, and name of the RRT vary by agency, the underlying concepts and purposes are the same. If nurses and other health care providers with advanced skills (especially critical care skills) can assist the client's nurse with assessment, diagnosis, and intervention of potentially life-threatening conditions, lives, time, and cost can be saved. Typically, two or more RRT members are available to respond within 5 minutes 24 hours per day, 7 days per week.

Team members always include experienced critical care nurses, but may or may not include medical doctors, advanced practice nurses, medical interns, respiratory therapists, physician assistants, and administrative personnel. In some cases, these nurses are assigned a lighter load of clients in their usual work setting so that, if called away, it is easier to cover their care. In other settings, those nurses do not have any assigned clients and make rounds on the nursing units routinely.

Client conditions most commonly triggering an RRT call are respiratory distress, low oxygen saturation, and hypotension. Table 30–1 lists guidelines for conditions warranting an RRT call. The nurse should be prepared to communicate client status to the RRT. The IHI recommends that the standardized method of doing this is to use the SBAR process: Situation, Background, Assessment, Recommendation (Table 30–2). See Chapter 1 ∞ for more information regarding the SBAR process and effective communication among health care team members.

TABLE 30–1	Triggers for Requesting a Rapid Response Team	

Condition	Parameter
Respiratory	Distress (e.g., accessory muscle use)
Oxygen saturation	SpO$_2$ less than 90% while on supplemental oxygen
Rate	Less than 8 or greater than 30
Skin color	Cyanosis or pallor
Cardiovascular	
Blood pressure	Systolic less than 80 or greater than 200 mmHg
Heart rate	Less than 40 and symptomatic or greater than 130 beats/min
Chest pain	
Urine output	Less than 100 mL in 4 hours
Laboratory values: sodium, potassium, glucose	Significantly outside normal range
Neuromuscular	
Seizure	
Sudden mental status change	Decreased level of consciousness (e.g., 2-point change on Glasgow Coma Scale)
Sudden loss of movement or weakness in an arm, leg, or the face	

TABLE 30–2	An SBAR Report from the RN to the Rapid Response Team

	SITUATION
	Name and location of client
	Brief subject of the call
S	Personal knowledge of status (e.g., vital signs, blood sugar, or other trigger)
	Why these are significant (how they have changed over what period of time)
	BACKGROUND
	Mental status
B	Medical diagnoses, reason for admission, procedures since admission
	Current active therapies (IVs/blood transfusions, medications, oxygen, ECG, wounds, gastrointestinal and urinary tubes)
	ASSESSMENT
A	Nurse's belief of what the problem is and how quickly the status is changing
	RECOMMENDATION
	Request to come see client or transfer client to another unit
R	Perform specific assessments or tests (x-ray, blood gases, cultures, ECG)
	Take other specific action (position client, give medications, call a code)

EMERGENCY MEASURES

The mission of the American Heart Association's (AHA) Emergency Cardiovascular Care (ECC) program is to "reduce disability and death from acute circulatory and respiratory emergencies, including stroke, by improving the chain of survival in every community and in every health care system" (2013). Outside of the hospital, AHA recommends Hands-Only CPR (call 911 and perform chest compressions only). The AHA still recommends compressions and breaths for infants and children and victims of drowning or drug overdose, or people who collapse due to breathing problems.

All health care workers are trained in **cardiopulmonary resuscitation (CPR)**, the techniques of providing effective chest compressions and rescue breathing in an attempt to restore oxygenation and circulation. The AHA issues revised standards for CPR every 5 years (e.g., 2010, 2015). CPR can be used in any setting. Aspects of CPR are indicated in cases of respiratory arrest (cessation of breathing only) or cardiac arrest, also referred to as cardiopulmonary, cardiorespiratory, or circulatory arrest. However, the events surrounding a cardiac or respiratory arrest in the hospital are somewhat different due to the presence of highly skilled health care workers and the availability of diagnostic and therapeutic services. Whether the nurse is a member of a specially trained arrest team or happens to discover a client who has arrested, it is a time of high anxiety and requires the nurse to recall the appropriate steps to take from memory.

Each health care facility has policies and procedures for announcing an arrest and initiating interventions. In many locations, a cardiac or respiratory arrest is called a **Code Blue**, and announcing the arrest may be referred to as "calling a code." The nurse is required to know how this is handled in each facility and each area within the facility. For example, there may be a special code button in the client's room, a special red or orange telephone at the nurse's station used only for such emergencies, or a specific phone number to call from any phone that links the caller directly to the facility phone operator. If a phone operator is called, the operator knows to answer immediately so that the code can be announced over the public address system to summon the arrest or rapid response team. Outside the hospital, the only resource may be the public emergency medical system (EMS) phone number, such as 911.

In most hospitals and some extended care facilities, specific personnel are designated as members of the Code Blue team. Individuals are needed to deliver chest compressions, perform rescue breathing, administer medications, and record the code activities. If possible, additional individuals should handle the emergency cart and equipment, support the family and clients who may be in the room, and care for the other clients of nurses participating in the code. One person must be designated as the code leader—the person who directs the activities of the other team members. An ideal code team would include a physician familiar with code procedures (e.g., an emergency department MD or intensivist—a physician who specializes in the care of critically ill clients, usually in an intensive care unit), a respiratory therapist, critical care nurses, an electrocardiography technician, a laboratory technician (to draw blood specimens), a pharmacist, a chaplain, and the client's nurse.

In addition to **basic life support (BLS)**, the term often used to refer to the CPR skill level required of all health care providers, those working in critical care areas may also be required to have certification in **advanced cardiac life support (ACLS)**. ACLS is a multiple-day training session appropriate for emergency medical technicians, paramedics, respiratory therapists, nurses, and other professionals who may need to respond to a cardiopulmonary emergency. The course includes content and practice in delivering medications, defibrillation, ventilation, and other skills often needed in such situations. The comparable course that focuses on children is **pediatric advanced life support (PALS)**.

Some clients have requested that they not be resuscitated in the event of an arrest. After discussion with the primary care provider, and following agency policies, the client record can be marked with the designation "**No Code Blue**," "no CPR," or "**do not resuscitate (DNR)**." Under most circumstances, if there is no DNR order in the record, all clients who arrest will have resuscitation efforts begun. A "slow code" and a "mini-code" are both illegal and unethical. Also see Chapter 34 ∞.

Throughout any emergency situation, the nurse must remember the person behind all of the technology and paraphernalia and maintain a personal connection by considering the client's spiritual and emotional needs. Seemingly small gestures such as holding a hand, making eye contact, or talking directly to them make a huge difference to clients. If their anxiety is relieved in any way, they are likely to do better—no matter what the outcome. To humanize health care is always a goal. Nursing *therapeutic presence* is the key. This should be extended to family members as well.

Obstructed Airway

There are several possible causes of airway obstruction and, as a result, several different methods for clearing an obstructed airway. Causes include:

- Aspirated food, a mucous plug, or foreign bodies, such as partial dentures. Food is the most common cause of **foreign body airway obstruction (FBAO)** or choking, particularly meat that has been ineffectively chewed.
- Unconsciousness or seizures, which cause the tongue to obstruct the airway.
- Severe trauma to the nose, mouth, or neck that produces blood clots that obstruct the airway, especially in an unconscious person.
- Acute edema of the trachea, from smoke inhalation, facial and neck burns, or anaphylaxis. In these instances, a tracheostomy is often indicated.

●○● NURSING PROCESS: OBSTRUCTED AIRWAY

Clearing an Obstructed Airway

ASSESSMENT

Foreign bodies may cause either partial (mild) or complete (severe) airway obstruction. When an airway is partially obstructed, the person may have either good air exchange or poor air exchange. If sufficient air is obtained, even though there is frequent wheezing between coughs, do not interfere with the person's attempts to breathe or expel the foreign object. Partial obstructions with inadequate air exchange are handled in the same manner as complete obstructions. The person with complete airway obstruction is unable to speak, breathe, or cough and may clutch at the neck.

PLANNING

A person can develop an obstructed airway at any time and the nurse must be prepared to help. In the hospital, all nurses and other available health care workers automatically work as a team to provide care to the client and to the nurse's other clients while the nurse is unavailable.

DELEGATION

Although unlicensed assistive personnel (UAP) cannot perform all aspects of a hospital code situation, they are trained in CPR and can perform FBAO techniques. If they are the first responders, UAP should call for help and initiate the intervention without waiting for a nurse.

INTERPROFESSIONAL PRACTICE

Clearing an obstructed airway is within the scope of practice for all health care providers. Each member of the health care team should know how to call for help and initiate the intervention.

Equipment
- Standard precautions (SP) supplies, including gloves, gowns, mask, and protective eyewear, should always be easily accessible.
- CPR mask or manual resuscitator (bag-valve-mask [BVM] device)

SKILL 30-1

Continued on page 644

Clearing an Obstructed Airway—*continued*

IMPLEMENTATION
Performance
Conscious Person

1. State your name and explain to the client that you are trained to help, what you are going to do, and how he or she can cooperate. Speak slowly, clearly, and with confidence.
2. Observe appropriate infection prevention procedures as much as possible.
3. Provide for as much privacy as is possible without interfering with the necessary individuals and activities. If another person is present and can participate, have that person get help. If family members are present, the nurse may request they leave for the moment. However, research also supports allowing family members to remain during emergencies (Jabre et al., 2013; Leske, McAndrew, & Brasel, 2013).
4. Give abdominal thrusts (**Heimlich maneuver**).
   - Stand or kneel behind the person, and wrap your arms around the person's waist.
   - Make a fist with one hand, ensuring the thumb lays across the folded fingers creating a flat surface on the thumb side of the fist. Place the thumb side of the fist just above the person's navel and below the xiphoid process. The thumb should not be tucked inside the fist. **Rationale:** *A protruding thumb could inflict injury.*
   - With the other hand, grasp the fist ❶ and press it into the person's abdomen with a firm, quick upward thrust. ❷ Avoid tightening the arms around the rib cage.
   - Deliver successive thrusts as separate and complete movements until the person's airway clears or the person becomes unconscious.
   - If the person becomes unconscious, lower the person carefully to the floor, supporting the head and neck to prevent injury.

Unconscious Person

5. Activate the emergency response system using "911" or the agency arrest code.
6. Apply clean gloves and other personal protective equipment as soon as possible.
7. Open the airway.
   - Tilt the person's head back, and lift the chin. **Rationale:** *This pulls the tongue away from the back of the throat.*
   - Remove an object only if you see it:
     a. If foreign material is visible in the mouth, it must be expediently removed. The finger sweep maneuver should be used only on unconscious individuals and with extreme caution. **Rationale:** *Foreign material can accidentally be pushed back into the airway, causing increased obstruction. In addition, the person may suddenly become responsive and bite the provider's fingers.*
     b. To remove solid material, insert the index finger of your free hand along the inside of the person's cheek and deep into the throat. With your finger hooked, use a sweeping motion to try to dislodge and lift out the foreign object. ❸
     c. After removing the foreign object, clear out liquid material, such as mucus, blood, or emesis, with suction.

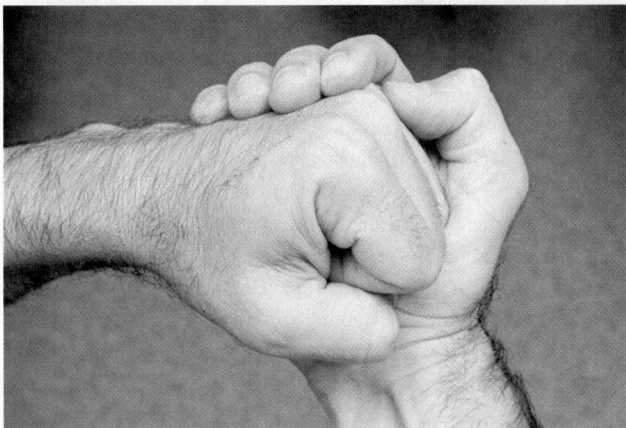

❶ The hand and fist position used for abdominal thrusts in a conscious person.

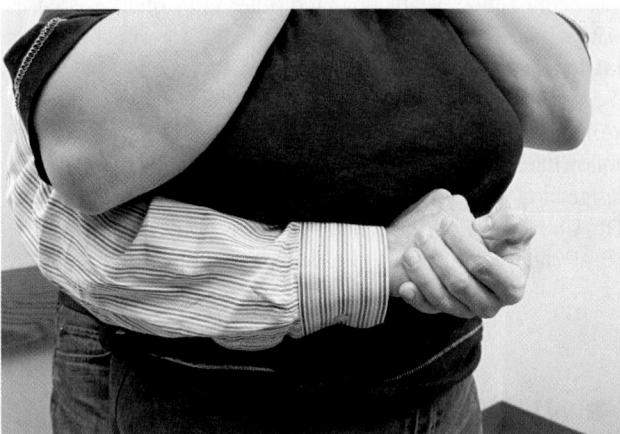

❷ The position to provide abdominal thrusts to a conscious person.

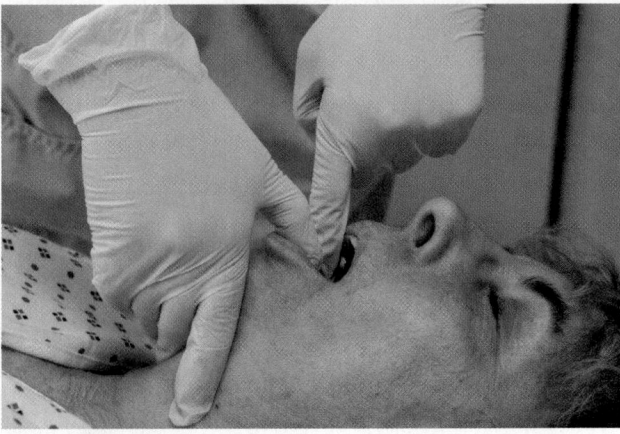

❸ The finger sweep maneuver.

Clearing an Obstructed Airway—*continued*

8. Provide ventilations.
- Apply a CPR resuscitation mask to the person's face (**❹**, *A* and *B*). If a mask is not available, insert the airway portion of a face shield into the person's mouth. **❹**, *C*
- Give one 1-second breath and observe for a visible chest rise.
- If unable to ventilate, retilt the head and repeat the breath.
- If successful, give a second 1-second breath.

9. If unsuccessful, proceed with full CPR (see Skills 30–2 through 30–4), chest compressions, repeating ventilation attempts, and foreign object checks until the airway clears or the person breathes.
- In the hospital setting, a person trained in airway interventions will take over responsibility for clearing the airway.
- When the emergency care is completed, remove and discard gloves and other personal protective equipment.
- Perform hand hygiene.

Variation: Chest Thrusts

Only chest thrusts are to be administered only to women in advanced stages of pregnancy and to markedly obese persons who cannot receive abdominal thrusts. Follow all steps above except substitute chest thrusts for the abdominal thrusts.

To administer chest thrusts:
- Place the thumb side of the fist on the middle of the breastbone (sternum), not on the xiphoid process.
- Grab the fist with the other hand and deliver a quick backward thrust.
- Repeat thrusts until the obstruction is relieved or the person becomes unconscious.

To administer chest thrusts to unconscious individuals lying on the floor:
- Position the person supine and kneel close to the side of the person's trunk.
- Position the hands as for cardiac compression with the heel of the hand on the lower half of the sternum (see Skill 30–3, step 7).
- Deliver five thrusts.

10. Document the date and time of the procedure, including the precipitating events and the person's response to the intervention.
- Describe the type of procedure, the duration of breathlessness, and the type and size of any foreign object.
- Note vital signs, any complications, medications administered, and type of follow-up care.

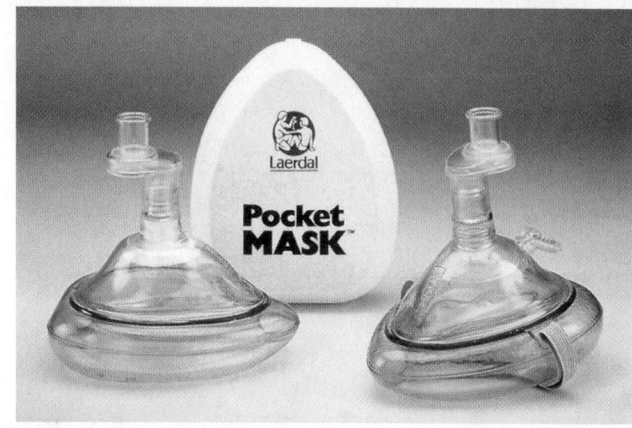

A

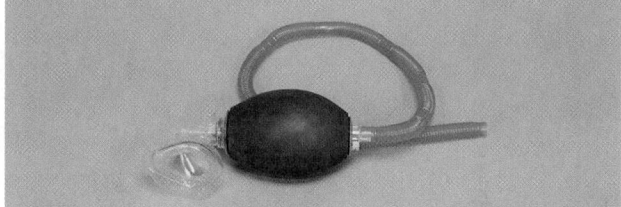

B

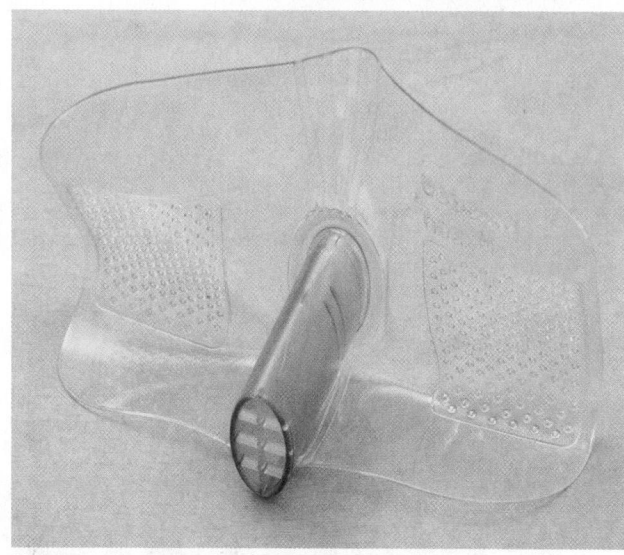

C

❹ Face masks: *A*, pocket mask with one-way valve; *B*, bag-valve-mask device; *C*, face shield.

EVALUATION
- Report the relevant events to the primary care provider.
- Conduct appropriate follow-up such as teaching or other interventions that could prevent an airway obstruction in the future.

LIFESPAN CONSIDERATIONS   Obstructed Airway

INFANTS

To administer a combination of back slaps and chest thrusts to infants:

1. Deliver back slaps.
   - Straddle the infant over your forearm with his or her head lower than the trunk.
   - Support the infant's head by firmly holding the jaw in your hand.
   - Rest your forearm on your thigh.
   - With the heel of the free hand, deliver five sharp slaps to the infant's back over the spine between the shoulder blades.

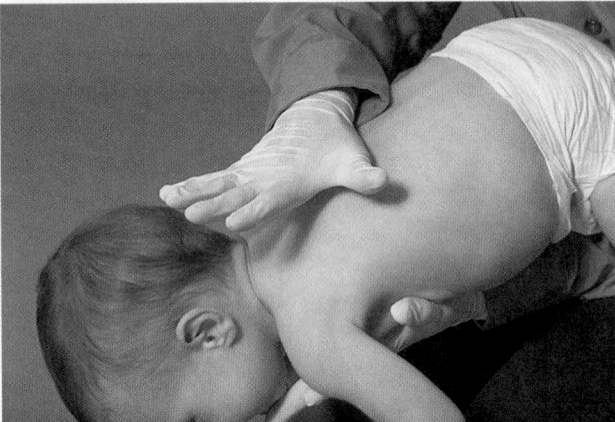

Infant back slaps.

2. Deliver chest thrusts.
   - Turn the infant as a unit to the supine position:
     a. Place the free hand on the infant's back.
     b. While continuing to support the jaw, neck, and chest with the other hand, turn and place the infant on the thigh with the baby's head lower than the trunk.
   - Using two fingers, administer five chest thrusts over the sternum in the same location as external chest compression for cardiac massage, one fingerwidth below the nipple line, 1 second each.

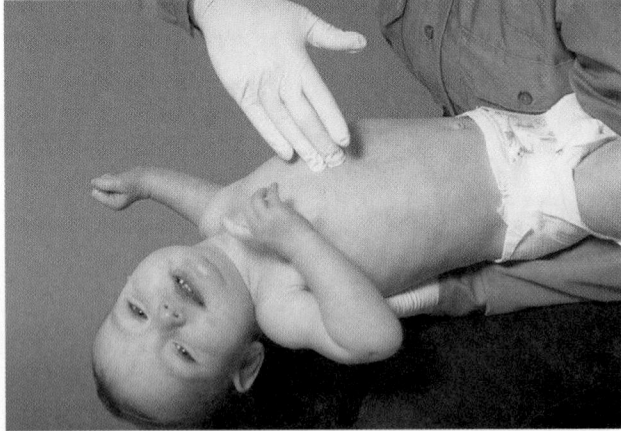

Infant chest thrusts.

- For a conscious infant, continue chest thrusts and back slaps until the airway is cleared or the infant becomes unconscious.
- If the infant is unconscious, begin CPR (see Skill 30–3).
  a. Begin chest compressions.
  b. Lift the jaw and tongue and check for foreign objects. If an object is noted, sweep it out with a finger.
  c. Assess the airway and give two breaths. As with adults, a mask or barrier should be used whenever possible. If unable to ventilate, retilt the infant's head and try to give two breaths.
  d. Repeat this sequence of chest compressions, foreign object checks, and breaths until the airway clears or the infant begins to breathe.

CHILDREN

- For conscious children over age 1 who are choking, perform the Heimlich maneuver as for adults (see Skill 30–1).

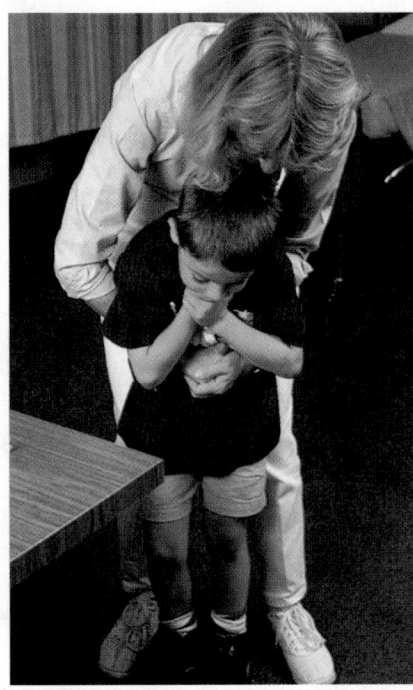

Conscious child abdominal thrusts.

OLDER ADULTS

- Older clients have a decreased gag reflex and therefore may be more prone to choking. Preventive measures, such as adjusting the consistency of food, proper fitting of dentures, and close surveillance of clients with a history of choking, may prevent an obstructed airway.
- Older clients can be injured by incorrect placement of the rescuer's hands. The sternum becomes more brittle with aging, and fracture of the sternum or ribs is more common.

- Stay with the individual.
- Any individual who receives intervention to treat an obstructed airway should seek immediate follow-up medical evaluation, even if the person remains conscious and the airway is cleared with abdominal thrusts.
- After removal of an airway obstruction at home, the person should receive a medical evaluation. The person may have aspirated foreign material, which can cause airway edema and infection.
- If the person becomes unconscious, activate the EMS.

FAMILY ROLE
- If a person has difficulty swallowing, teach the caregiver how to clear an obstructed airway.
- Young children are most likely to choke on objects such as small toys. Children do not understand the danger of placing objects in the mouth. Teach parents how to clear an obstructed airway, and emphasize the importance of keeping small objects away from young children.

Respiratory Arrest

A **respiratory arrest** is defined as the absence of breathing. It can be caused by an obstructed airway, suppression of the respiratory center of the brain due to medication overdose, poisoning, asphyxiation (suffocation), acid–base or electrolyte imbalance, seizure, drowning, trauma, or electric shock. The heart can continue to beat for only a few minutes after breathing stops.

In most situations involving adults, an arrest is primarily cardiac rather than respiratory. Thus, if the person is unresponsive and not breathing, the nurse will next check for a pulse. Unless the nurse is *absolutely certain* that only breathing has ceased, complete CPR should be initiated beginning with chest compressions (see Skill 30–3). Skill 30–2 describes the technique of rescue breathing, which can be used in the case of a respiratory arrest and concurrent with chest compressions in the case of a full arrest if trained and competent providers are present.

●○● NURSING PROCESS: RESPIRATORY ARREST

Performing Rescue Breathing

SKILL 30-2

PLANNING
The nurse should be prepared to deliver rescue breathing at any time. In the hospital, all nurses and other available health care workers automatically come to the nurse's assistance and work as a team to provide care to the person and to the other individuals while the nurse is unavailable.

DELEGATION

Although UAP cannot perform all aspects of a hospital code situation, they are trained in CPR and can perform rescue breathing techniques. If they are the first responders, UAP should call for help and initiate the intervention without waiting for a nurse.

INTERPROFESSIONAL PRACTICE

Performing rescue breathing is within the scope of practice for all health care providers. Each member of the health care team should know how to call for help and initiate the intervention.

Equipment
- SP supplies, including gloves, masks, gowns, and protective eyewear, should always be easily accessible.
- Emergency equipment such as intubation supplies should be centrally located.
- Pocket face mask with one-way valve or mouth shields, or BVM (commonly referred to as an Ambu bag) (see Figure ❹ in Skill 30–1).

IMPLEMENTATION
Performance
1. Recognize the presence of an emergency.
   - Determine that the person is unresponsive. ❶
   - Determine absence of normal breathing (i.e., no breathing or only gasping).
2. Call a "code" or follow agency protocol to call for assistance. If another person is present and can participate, have that person go get help. Tell the person to return and report that help has been called.
3. Take no more than 10 seconds to check for a pulse. To palpate the carotid artery, first locate the larynx, and then slide your fingers alongside it into the groove between the larynx and the neck muscles on the same side you are. ❷ Use gentle pressure. **Rationale:** *This avoids compressing the artery. The carotid pulse site is used because it is easy to reach and can often be palpated when more peripheral pulses, such as the radial, are imperceptible.*
   - If there is no pulse, begin CPR with compressions (see Skill 30–3).

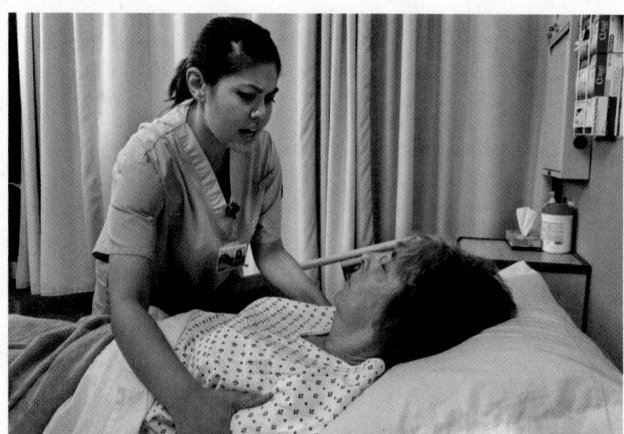

❶ Touch and gently shake the person while observing closely to determine that the person is not just sleeping. Rescue breathing should only be performed if the person is unresponsive and not breathing.

Continued on page 648

Performing Rescue Breathing—*continued*

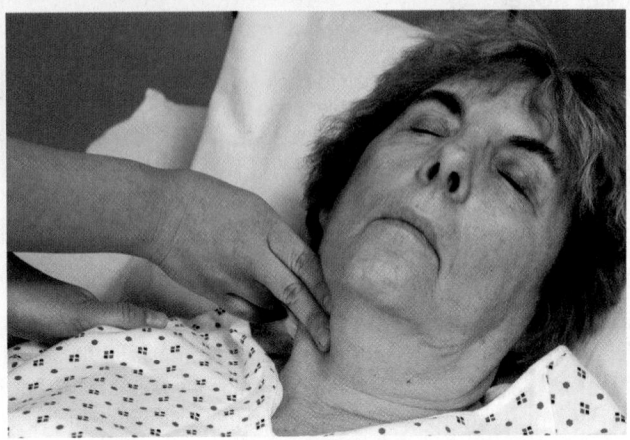

2 Checking the carotid pulse.

- If only a respiratory arrest exists, proceed with the steps below.
4. Observe appropriate infection prevention procedures, including applying clean gloves, as much as possible.
5. Provide for privacy. If family members are present, the nurse may request whether they prefer to remain or leave for the moment. Policies and procedures should be in place for a facilitator who can:
   - Explain the options to the family.
   - Support the family before, during, and after the event.
   - Support any family members' decisions not to be present.
   - Enforce contraindications for family presence such as extreme emotional behavior or interference with medical procedures.
6. Position the person appropriately.
   - If the person is lying on one side or face down, turn the person onto the back as a unit, while supporting the head and neck. If necessary to reach the person adequately, kneel beside the head.
7. Open the airway.
   - Use the head tilt–chin lift maneuver, or the jaw-thrust maneuver. A modified jaw thrust is used for individuals with suspected neck injury. In unconscious individuals, the tongue lacks sufficient muscle tone, falls to the back of the throat, and obstructs the pharynx. **3** Rationale: *Because the tongue is attached to the lower jaw, moving the lower jaw forward and tilting the head backward lifts the tongue away from the pharynx and opens the airway.*
   - If possible, insert an oropharyngeal (oral) airway (see Figure 26–1 in Chapter 26 ∞). **Rationale:** *This prevents the tongue from occluding the oropharynx.* Hold the airway with the curved end upward and insert as far as possible into the mouth to the end of the soft palate. Rotate the airway 180 degrees so the end is directed down the pharynx, gliding it over the tongue. The outer flange remains just outside the person's lips.

Head Tilt–Chin Lift Maneuver

- Place one hand palm downward on the forehead.
- Place the fingers of the other hand under the bony part of the lower jaw near the chin. The teeth should then be almost closed. The mouth should not be closed completely.
- Simultaneously press down on the forehead with one hand, and lift the person's chin upward with the other. **4** Avoid pressing

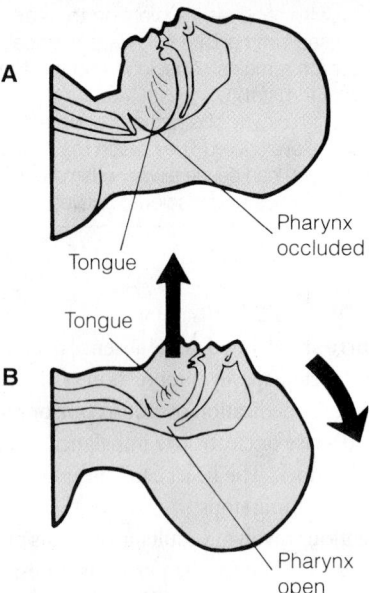

3 The position of an unconscious person's tongue: *A,* airway occluded; *B,* airway open.

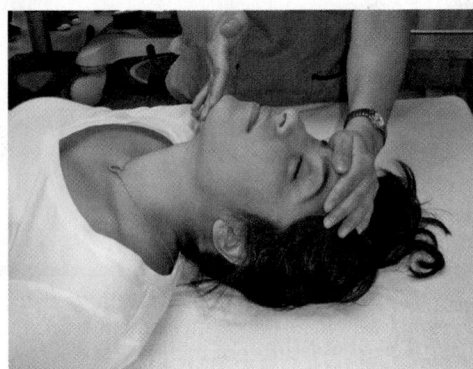

4 Head tilt–chin lift maneuver.

the fingers deeply into the soft tissues under the chin, or hyperextending the neck because too much pressure can obstruct the airway.
- Open the person's mouth by pressing the jaw downward with the thumb after tilting the head.
- Remove dentures if they cannot be kept in place. However, dentures that can be maintained in place make a mouth-to-mouth seal tighter should rescue breathing be required.

Jaw-Thrust Maneuver

- Kneel at the top of the person's head.
- Grasp the angle of the mandible directly below the earlobe between your thumb and forefinger on each side of the person's head.
- While tilting the head backward, lift the lower jaw until it juts forward and is higher than the upper jaw. **5**

Performing Rescue Breathing—*continued*

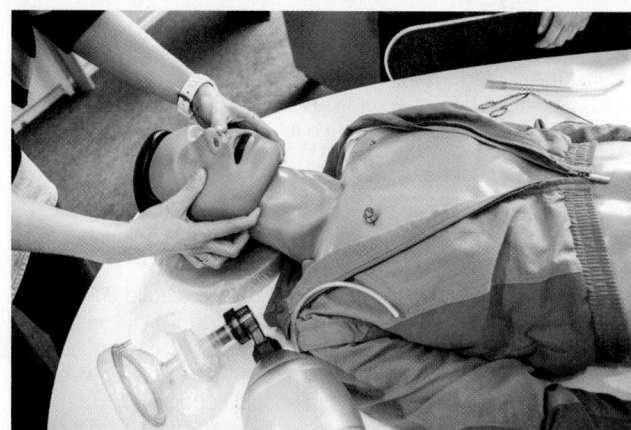

5 Jaw-thrust maneuver.
Arno Massee/Photo Researchers, Inc./Science Source.

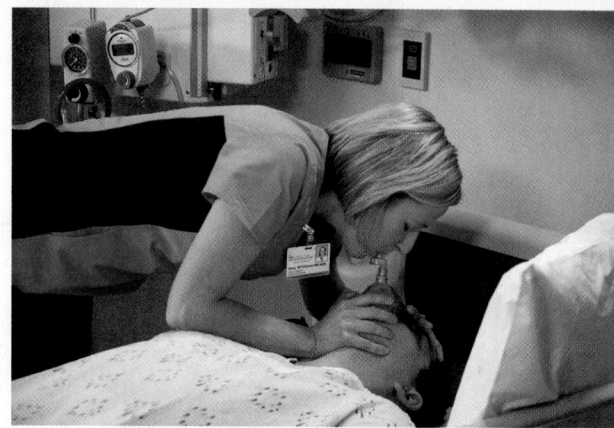

6 Mouth-to-mask rescue breathing.

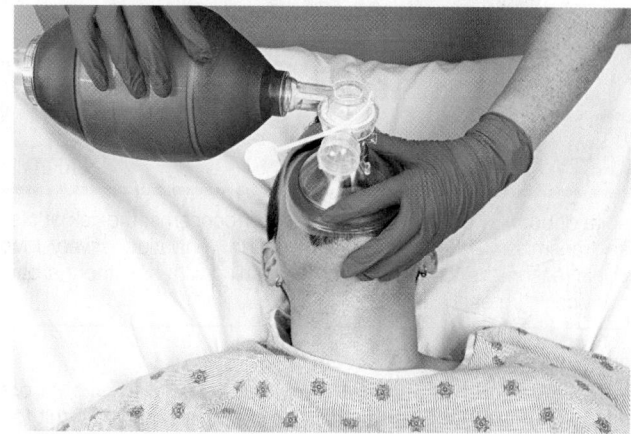

7 Bag-to-mask breathing.

- Rest your elbows on the surface on which the person is lying.
- Retract the lower lip with the thumbs prior to giving artificial respiration.
- If the person is suspected of having a spinal neck injury, do not hyperextend the neck.

8. Determine if the person has resumed breathing as a result of the opened airway. This takes 5 to 10 seconds.
   - Place your ear and cheek close to the person's mouth and nose.
   - Look at the chest and abdomen for rising and falling movement.
   - Listen for air escaping during exhalation.
   - Feel for air escaping against your cheek.
9. If no breathing is evident, provide rescue breathing.
   - Give two full breaths (1 second per breath). **Rationale:** *The 1-second time span allows adequate time to provide good chest expansion, and decreases the possibility of gastric distention. Excessive air volumes and rapid inspiratory flow rates can cause pharyngeal pressures that are great enough to open the esophagus, thus allowing air to enter the stomach.*
   - Ensure adequate ventilation by observing the person's chest rise and fall and by assessing the person's breathing as outlined in step 8.
   - If the initial ventilation attempt is unsuccessful, reposition the person's head and repeat the rescue breathing as above.
   - If the person still cannot be ventilated, proceed to clear the airway of any foreign bodies using the finger sweep if the foreign object is visible, abdominal thrusts, or chest thrusts described earlier in Skill 30–1.

Mouth-to-Mask Method
- If not already at hand, remove the mask from its case and push out the dome.
- Connect the one-way valve to the mask port.
- Position yourself at the top of the person's head, and open the airway using the head tilt–chin lift maneuver.
- Place the wider rim of the mask between the person's lower lip and chin. Place the rest of the mask over the face using your thumbs on each side of the mask to hold it in place. **6** **Rationale:** This keeps the mouth open under the mask.

Bag-Valve-Mask Method
- Use one hand to secure the mask at the top and bottom and to hold the person's jaw forward. Use the other hand to squeeze

and release the bag every 6 to 8 seconds (8 to 10 breaths per minute). **7** If two rescuers are available, one holds the head and mask in place while the second compresses the bag.

Mouth-to-Mouth Method
- *Only if a mask is not available,* perform mouth-to-mouth breathing using a face shield. Insert the airway portion of the shield into the person's mouth (see Figure **4** in Skill 30–1).
- Maintain the open airway by using the head tilt–chin lift maneuver.
- Pinch the person's nostrils with the index finger and thumb of the hand on the person's forehead. **Rationale:** *Pinching closes the nostrils and prevents resuscitation air from escaping through them.*
- Take a normal (not a deep) breath.
- Give each ventilation using 1 second per breath. **8** **Rationale:** *The 1-second time span allows adequate time to provide good chest expansion, and decreases the possibility of gastric distention. Excessive air volumes and rapid inspiratory flow rates can cause pharyngeal pressures that are great enough to open the esophagus, thus allowing air to enter the stomach.*
- Remove your mouth and allow the person to exhale passively.

Continued on page 650

Performing Rescue Breathing—*continued*

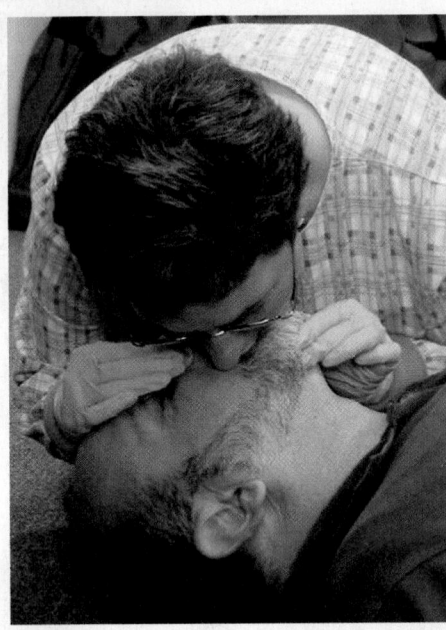

8 Mouth-to-mouth rescue breathing.
Courtesy Neal Shabashov.

SAFETY ALERT! | SAFETY

In spite of both lay and professional rescuer concerns, the risk of disease transmission through mouth-to-mouth ventilation is very low, and it is reasonable to initiate rescue breathing with or without a barrier device (Berg et al., 2010).

Mouth-to-Nose Method

This method can be used when there is an injury to the mouth or jaw or when the client is edentulous (toothless), making it difficult to achieve a tight seal over the mouth.

- Use a barrier device if a resuscitation mask is not available. Some face shields used for mouth-to-mouth breathing also are effective for mouth-to-nose breathing.

- Maintain the head tilt–chin lift position.
- Close the person's mouth by pressing the palm of your hand against the person's chin. The thumb of the same hand may be used to hold the bottom lip closed.
- Taking a normal breath, deliver two full breaths of 1 second each.
- Remove your mouth and allow the person to exhale passively. It may be necessary to separate the person's lips or to open the mouth for exhaling, since the nasal passages may be obstructed during exhalation.

10. After 2 minutes, recheck for the presence of a carotid pulse (Berg et al., 2010).
    - Take less than 10 seconds for this pulse check. Adequate time is needed since the person's pulse may be very weak and rapid, irregular, or slow but should not delay CPR. Compressions should never be delayed or interrupted for longer than 10 seconds.
11. If the carotid pulse is palpable, but breathing is not restored, repeat rescue breathing.
    - Inflate at the rate of 8 to 10 breaths per minute (1 breath every 6 to 8 seconds).
    - Deliver rescue breaths slowly but enough to make the person's chest rise.
    - If chest expansion fails to occur, ensure that the neck is not hyperextended and the jaw is lifted upward, or check again for the presence of obstructive material, fluid, or vomitus.
    - Reassess the carotid pulse every 2 minutes thereafter.
12. When the emergency care is completed, remove and discard gloves and other SP equipment.
    - Perform hand hygiene.
13. Document the date and time of the arrest, including the precipitating events, the duration of breathlessness, and the person's response to the breathing.
    - Notify the primary care provider of the relevant events if not already notified.

EVALUATION

In a health care setting, a review of the emergency event and the staff's response is commonly performed to see if there are indications for improvement in procedures. Mock arrests may be planned to assist the staff in practicing their skills.

LIFESPAN CONSIDERATIONS | Rescue Breathing

INFANTS AND CHILDREN
- Airway obstruction by a foreign body is the most common cause of respiratory arrest in children. Other common causes include suffocation, poisoning, or trauma.
- Acute epiglottitis can lead to upper airway obstruction in children. Symptoms usually occur suddenly and include drooling, difficulty swallowing, and a croaking sound with inspiration.

RESCUE BREATHING FOR INFANTS
- If the child is not breathing or only gasping, check for a brachial pulse. If the child is unresponsive and not breathing normally, and there are no signs of life, the nurse should begin CPR unless a pulse can definitely be felt within 10 seconds (Kleinman et al., 2010). See Skill 30–3.

- If there is a pulse but no breathing, begin ventilations. For infants, place one hand on the forehead and tilt the head back gently. Do not hyperextend the neck because this can cause the soft trachea to collapse.
- The jaw-thrust maneuver can also be used if a neck injury is suspected.
- When performing mouth-to-mouth breathing, cover both the mouth and nose of an infant.
- If an appropriate size mask and bag are available, they should always be used. The mask should reach from the bridge of the nose to the chin but not cover the eyes.
- Deliver 8 to 10 breaths per minute (1 breath every 6 to 8 seconds).

LIFESPAN CONSIDERATIONS **Rescue Breathing—***continued*

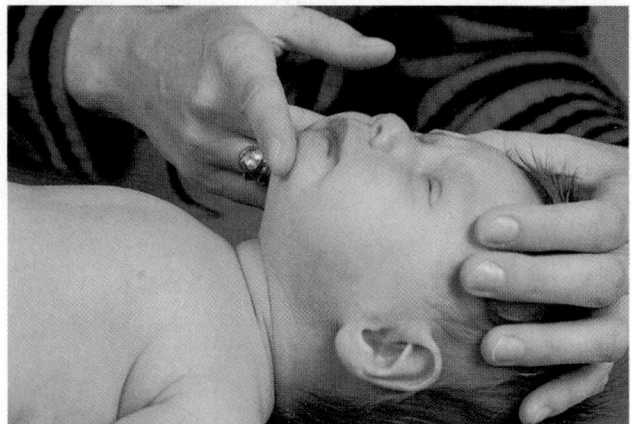

Infant head tilt–chin lift maneuver.

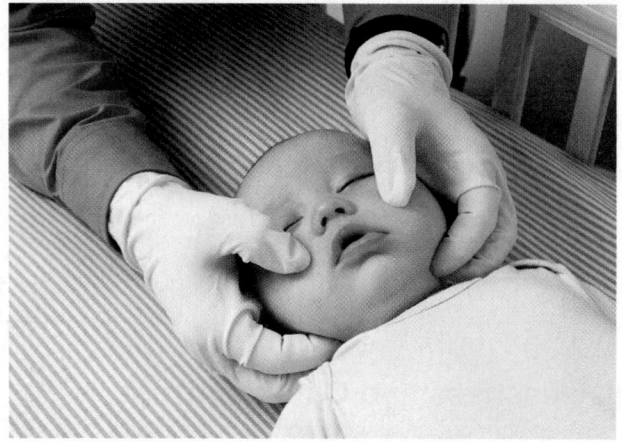

Infant jaw-thrust maneuver.

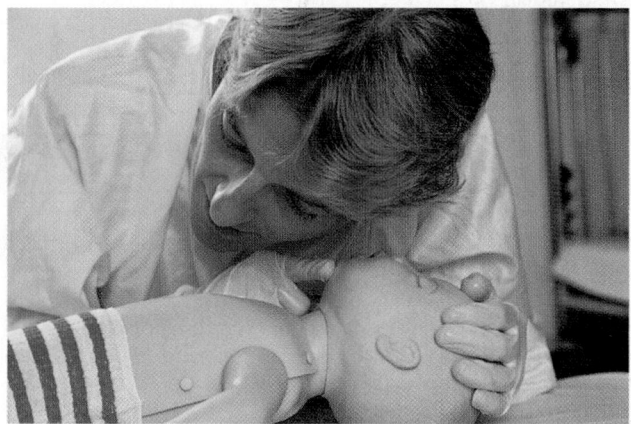

Infant assessment of breathing.

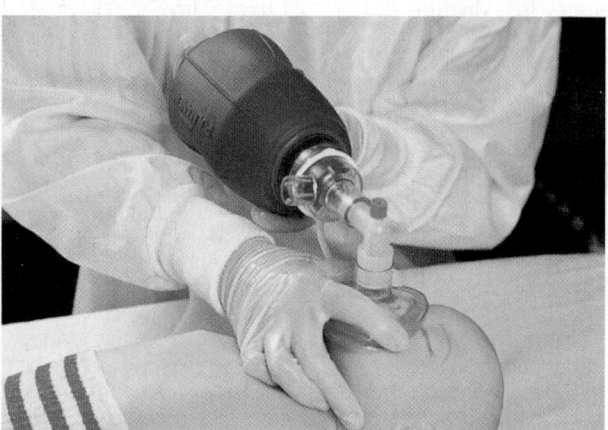

Infant bag-to-mask breathing.

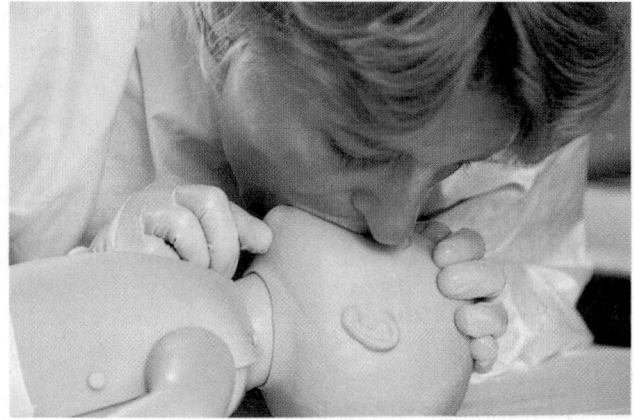

Infant mouth-to-mouth rescue breathing.

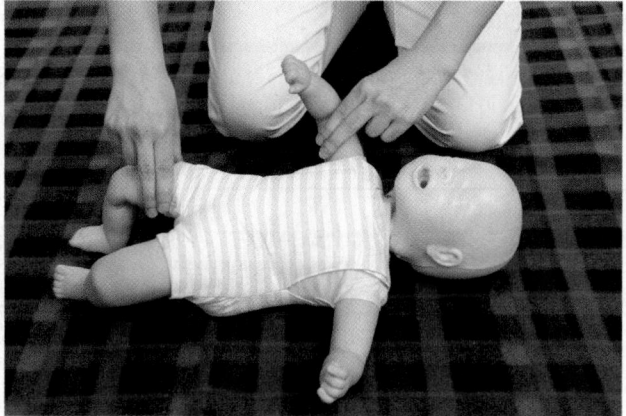

Checking the brachial pulse on an infant.
Roman Milert/Fotolia.

- If a person has cardiac or breathing problems, encourage the caregiver to learn CPR.
- Carry a pocket mask in the home care nursing bag at all times.
- Know how to activate the EMS. In most cases of respiratory arrest, the person will need oxygen, respiratory support, and ambulance transport to the emergency department.
- Assist the ambulance crew as needed and provide information about the person's history.

- Once the person is en route to the hospital, call the emergency department and give the report to the nurse in charge, including:
  - A brief health history.
  - Medications the person takes at home.
  - Findings prior to the respiratory arrest.
  - Duration of respiratory arrest and the person's response to resuscitation.
  - Vital signs.
- Provide emotional support to family members. If the person lives alone, contact family members, as needed.
- Notify the primary care provider.

Pulselessness and Cardiac Arrest

Several conditions can cause the heart to develop a lethal dysrhythmia or to stop beating. When blood supply to the heart muscle is interrupted, such as occurs during a myocardial infarction (heart attack), the heart may develop ventricular tachycardia or ventricular fibrillation. These rhythms are too rapid, uncoordinated, or inefficient to result in adequate perfusion or cardiac output to support life. Other causes of inadequate cardiac contraction that result in insufficient flow of blood throughout the body (pulselessness) include respiratory arrest, electric shock, electrolyte imbalances, and other cardiac diseases.

●○○● NURSING PROCESS: PULSELESSNESS AND CARDIAC ARREST

Administering External Cardiac Compressions

SKILL 30–3

ASSESSMENT

Pulselessness is generally detected as a result of assessment of an unconscious person. An unresponsive person is first examined for breathing (see Skill 30–2). If rescue breathing is indicated, the nurse's next step is to assess for a pulse. This is one of the areas in which BLS technique varies for lay rescuers when compared with health care providers. Although both health care providers and lay rescuers have been shown to be inaccurate in their assessment of the presence or absence of a carotid pulse (Kleinman et al., 2010), lay rescuers are no longer taught to do this assessment. In addition, even if breathing is absent, lay rescuers begin CPR with chest compressions. This recent change to the order of the steps of CPR minimizes the delay in reestablishing circulation that could occur due to the hesitancy and lack of expertise of lay rescuers performing mouth-to-mouth ventilations (Hazinski, 2010).

PLANNING

The nurse should be prepared to provide external cardiac compressions at any time.

DELEGATION

Although UAP cannot perform all aspects of a hospital code situation, they are trained in CPR and can perform external cardiac compression techniques. If they are the first responders, UAP should call for help and initiate the intervention without waiting for a nurse.

INTERPROFESSIONAL PRACTICE

Administering external cardiac compressions is within the scope of practice for all health care providers. Each member of the health care team should know how to call for help and initiate the intervention.

Equipment

- SP supplies, including gloves, masks, gowns, and protective eyewear, should always be easily accessible.
- Emergency equipment such as a defibrillator and intubation equipment should be centrally located.
- Face mask with one-way valve or mouth shields, or BVM (see Figure ❹ in Skill 30–1).
- A hard surface, such as a cardiac board, on which to place the person.

IMPLEMENTATION
Performance

1. Determine that the person is unresponsive.
2. If the person does not respond, call a "code" or follow agency protocol to call for assistance. If another person is present and can participate, have that person go get help. Tell the person to return and let you know that help has been called.

3. Observe appropriate infection prevention procedures, including applying clean gloves, as much as possible.
4. Provide for privacy. If family members are present, the nurse may request they leave for the moment. Family members should be allowed the option of remaining in the room

Administering External Cardiac Compressions—*continued*

(Jabre et al., 2013; Leske et al., 2013). Policies and procedures should be in place for a facilitator who can:

- Explain the options to the family.
- Support the family before, during, and after the event.
- Support any family members' decisions not to be present.
- Enforce contraindications for family presence such as extreme emotional behavior or interference with medical procedures.

5. Position the person appropriately if not already done.

- Place the person supine on a firm surface. **Rationale:** *Blood flow to the brain will be inadequate during CPR if the person's head is positioned higher than the thorax. A hard surface facilitates compression of the heart between the sternum and the hard surface.*
- If the person is in bed, place a cardiac board—preferably the full width of the bed—under the back. Some hospital beds that have pressure-distributing mattresses have a rapid-deflate mechanism for use during CPR. However, do not delay compressions to place the backboard or activate the rapid-deflate mechanism since neither has been shown to improve effectiveness of compressions (McEvoy, 2014). ❶ If necessary, place the person on the floor.
- If the person must be turned, turn the body as a unit while firmly supporting the head and neck so that the head does not roll, twist, or tilt backward or forward. **Rationale:** *Turning the person as a unit prevents further injury (if present) to the neck or spine.*

6. Position the hands on the sternum. Proper hand placement is essential for effective cardiac compression. Position the hands as follows:

- With the hand nearest the person's legs, use your middle and index fingers to locate the lower margin of the rib cage.
- Move the fingers up the rib cage to the notch where the lower ribs meet the sternum. ❷
- Place the heel of the other hand (nearest the person's head) along the lower half of the person's sternum, close to the index finger that is next to the middle finger in the costal-sternal notch. ❸ **Rationale:** *Proper positioning of the hands during cardiac compression helps prevent injury to underlying organs and the ribs. Compression directly over the xiphoid process can lacerate the person's liver.*
- Then place the first hand directly on top of the second hand. The fingers may be extended or interlaced (preferred). Compression occurs only on the sternum and through the heels of the hands.

7. Administer cardiac compression.

- Lock your elbows into position, straighten your arms, and position your shoulders directly over your hands. ❹
- For each compression, using the weight of your upper body, forcefully push straight down on the sternum. For an adult of normal size, depress the sternum at least 5 cm (2 in.). **Rationale:** *The muscle force of both arms is needed for adequate cardiac compression of an adult. The weight of your shoulders and trunk supplies power for compression. Extension of the elbows ensures an adequate and even force throughout compression.*
- Between compressions, completely release the compression pressure. However, do not lift your hands from the chest or change their position. **Rationale:** *Releasing the pressure allows the sternum to return to its normal position and allows the heart chambers to completely refill with blood. Leaving the hands on the chest prevents taking a malposition between compressions reducing effectiveness and possibly injuring the person.*
- Provide external cardiac compressions at the rate of at least 100 per minute. Push fast and maintain the rhythm

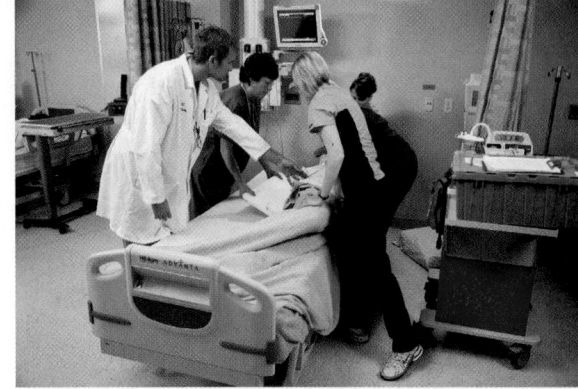

❶ Roll the person to one side and place the cardiac board beneath the thorax.

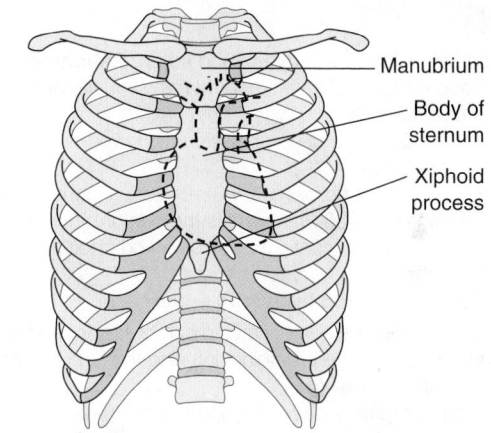

Manubrium

Body of sternum

Xiphoid process

❷ The sternum and ribs.

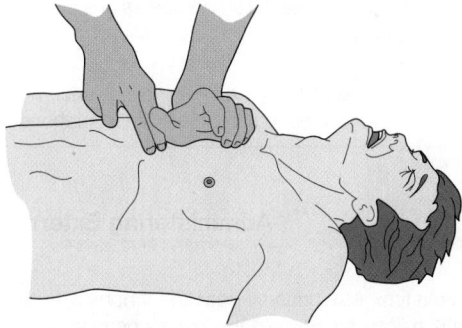

❸ Proper positioning of the hands during external cardiac compression.

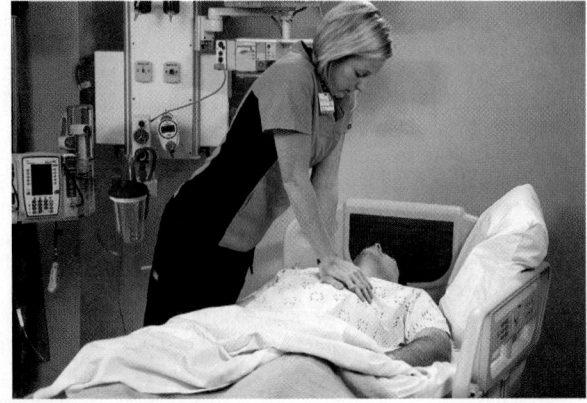

❹ Arm and hand position for external cardiac compression.

Continued on page 654

SKILL 30-3

Administering External Cardiac Compressions—*continued*

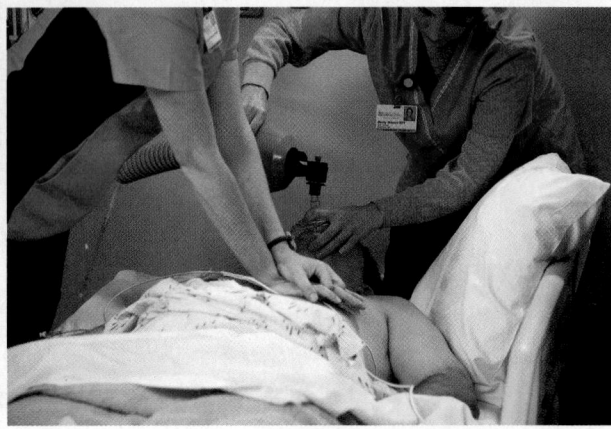

⑤ The rescuer performing compressions will pause for two breaths if there is no advanced airway in place.

by counting "one, two, three," and so on. **Rationale:** *The specified compression rate and rhythm simulate normal heart contractions.*

- Administer 30 external compressions followed by two rescue breaths.
- After five cycles (approximately 2 minutes) of compressions and breaths (ratio 30:2), reassess the person's carotid pulse. If there is no pulse, continue with CPR and check for the return of the pulse every few minutes.

Variation: CPR Performed by Two Rescuers

- One rescuer provides external cardiac compression, and the other can provide rescue breathing, inflating the lungs twice after every 30 compressions. ⑤
- Pause chest compressions for no longer than 10 seconds for the two breaths unless an advanced airway (e.g., endotracheal tube) is in place. If an advanced airway is in place, the compressing rescuer should deliver at least 100 compressions per

minute continuously, without pauses for ventilation. The rescuer delivering the rescue breaths should give 8 to 10 breaths per minute.
- Rescuers should switch positions after every five cycles, about 2 minutes. **Rationale:** *Changing positions should help prevent rescuers from becoming fatigued.*

8. When relieved from CPR:
   - Stand by to inform the team what has occurred and to assist as needed.
   - Provide emotional support to the person's family members and any others who may have witnessed the cardiac arrest. This is a frightening experience for others because it is often sudden and life threatening.
9. When the emergency care is completed, remove and discard gloves and other SP equipment.
   - Perform hand hygiene.
10. CPR is terminated only when one of the following events occurs:
    - Another trained individual takes over.
    - The person's heartbeat and breathing are reestablished.
    - Adjunctive life support measures are initiated.
    - A physician states that the person has died and that CPR is to be discontinued.
    - The rescuer becomes exhausted and there is no one to take over (this may occur when an arrest occurs outside the health care setting).
    Hospital resuscitation can take as long as 25 minutes to successfully achieve the return of the client's heartbeat (Nolan & Soar, 2012).
11. Document the date and time of the arrest, including the precipitating events, the duration of respiratory and cardiac arrest and resuscitation efforts, and the person's response.
    - Record any advanced cardiac life support interventions such as defibrillation or initiation of intravenous therapy.
    - Document vital signs, cardiac rhythm recordings, any complications, and type of follow-up care. Notify the primary care provider of the relevant events.

EVALUATION

In a health care setting, a review of the emergency event and the staff's response is commonly performed to see if there are indications for improvement in procedures. Mock cardiac arrests may be planned to assist the staff in practicing their skills.

LIFESPAN CONSIDERATIONS | Administering External Cardiac Compressions

INFANTS
- Place the infant on a firm, flat surface if possible. If none is available or the infant is being carried, hold the infant's head in your nondominant hand and rest the thorax along your forearm.
- Check carefully for airway obstruction in children with cardiac arrest. Cardiac arrest in children most often occurs after an initial respiratory arrest.
- To find the position for compressions, place your index finger on the sternum at the nipple line. Place your middle and ring fingers on the lower half of the sternum next to your index finger, then lift your index finger.
- Compress the chest at least one third the anterior-posterior diameter of the chest (about 4 cm [1.5 in.]) straight down using the pads of two fingers. Release the compression completely, keeping your fingers in the compression position while the other hand remains on the forehead, maintaining the open airway.
- Give compressions at a rate of at least 100 compressions/min with cycles of 30 compressions and two breaths if you are alone.

- If two rescuers are present, instead of the two-finger technique described above, one rescuer can encircle the infant's chest with both hands, fingers behind the thorax and the thumbs over the lower half of the sternum for compression. In this fashion, the heart is compressed from both front and back, resulting in more effective CPR. With two health care provider rescuers, the compression-ventilation ratio for infants becomes 15 compressions to 2 ventilations.

CHILDREN (AGES 1 YEAR TO PUBERTY)
- Check carefully for airway obstruction in children with cardiac arrest. Cardiac arrest in children most often occurs after an initial respiratory arrest.
- In children, to find the hand position for compressions, run your index and middle fingers up the ribs until you locate the sternal notch. With those two fingers on the lower end of the sternum, put the heel of the other hand on the sternum just above the location of the index finger.
- Use one or two hands for compressions, keeping the fingers off the chest. Compression depth is at least one third the

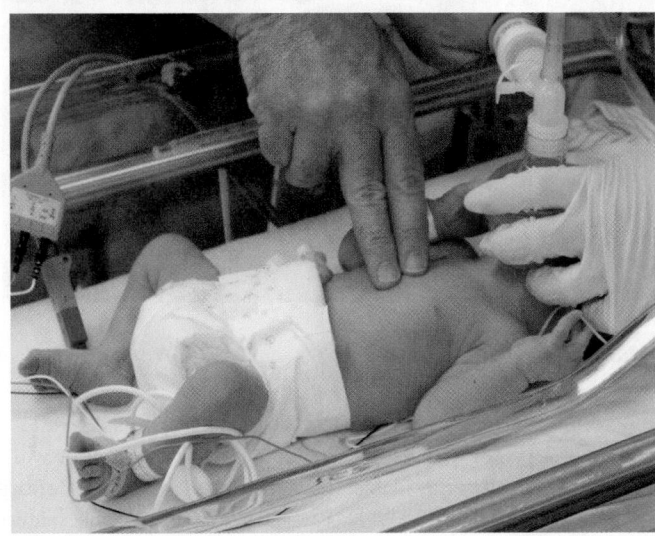

A

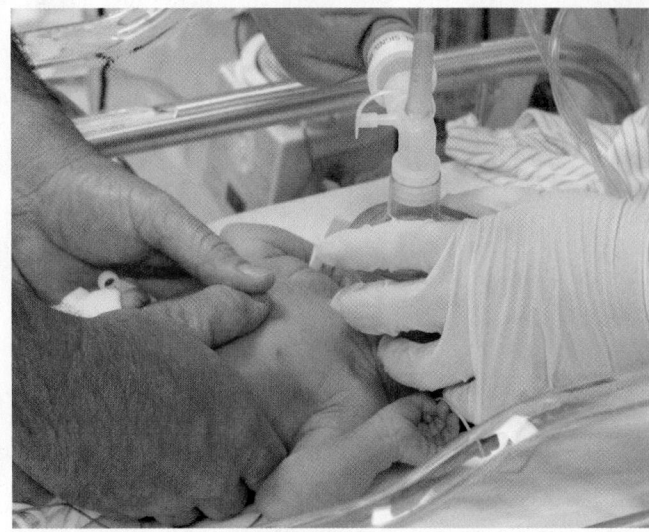

B

CPR on an infant.

anterior-posterior diameter of the chest (5 cm [2 in.]). Never lift the hand(s) off the chest.
- CPR for a child is given at the following rate: at least 100 compressions/min with cycles of 30 compressions and 2 breaths for single rescuers and 15 compressions to 2 breaths for two-rescuer CPR (Hazinski, 2010).

OLDER ADULTS
- Older clients are most likely to be injured by incorrect placement of the rescuer's hands. The sternum becomes more brittle with aging, and fracture of the sternum or ribs is more common.
- The older client may have an advance directive, or living will, expressing his or her wishes about life support.

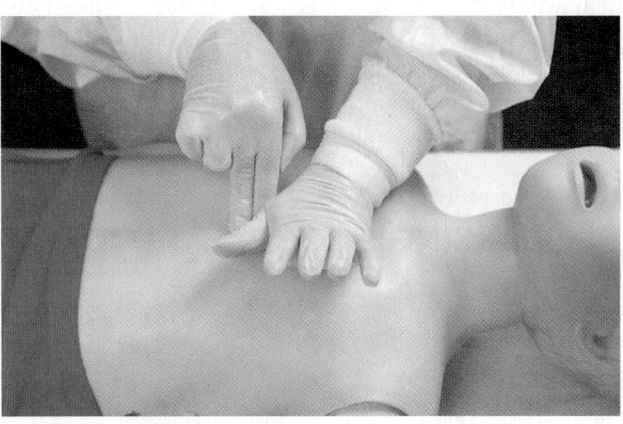

Locating the site for chest compressions on a child.

Ambulatory and Community Settings   **Administering External Cardiac Compressions**   EVIDENCE-BASED PRACTICE

- Always carry a pocket mask in the home care nursing bag.
- Survey the scene for safety hazards, presence of bystanders, and other individuals needing assistance.
- Call for help or have another person call for EMS or 911.
- The person who calls the local EMS must be able to impart all of the following information:
  - Location of the emergency
  - Telephone number from which the call is being made
  - What happened
  - Number of people needing assistance
  - Condition of the people needing assistance
  - What aid is being given
  - The EMS dispatcher may ask for additional information. Dispatchers will also give rescue skills instructions to the caller.
- If the rescuer is alone, summon help and then perform CPR.
- Have a bystander elevate the lower extremities (optional). This may promote venous return and augment circulation during external cardiac compressions.

- If a second person identifies himself or herself as a trained rescuer, have that person verify that EMS has been notified. If EMS has been notified, the second rescuer can help with CPR.
- After activating the emergency response system, continue resuscitation until the first responders arrive. If available, obtain and use an AED (see Skill 30–4). Be prepared to give a report to the crew and assist them as needed.
- While the person is en route to the hospital, contact the emergency department and report the following:
  - A brief health history
  - Medications the person takes at home
  - Findings prior to the cardiopulmonary arrest
  - Duration of the cardiopulmonary arrest and the person's response to resuscitation.
- Provide emotional support to family members. If the person is alone, contact family members or neighbors, as needed.
- Advise adults about preparing an advance directive for life support measures.
- Encourage caregivers or family members to learn CPR.

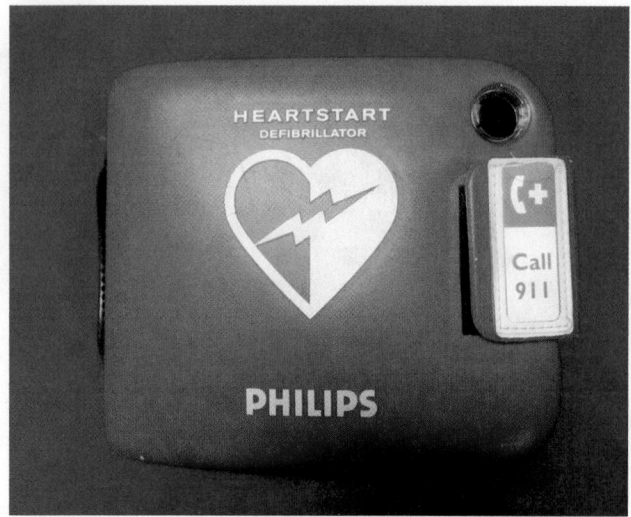

Figure 30–1 ■ An automated external defibrillator (AED).
Courtesy Neal Shabashov.

Automated External Defibrillation

The most common arrhythmia in sudden cardiac arrest is **ventricular fibrillation (VF)**, a quivering, nonperfusing, nonfunctional rhythm, which, if untreated, converts to **asystole** (no heartbeat). The best treatment for VF is electric shock defibrillation. Since the early 1990s it has become clear that, in both the hospital and community settings, early defibrillation provides the greatest chance for survival and can be implemented easily.

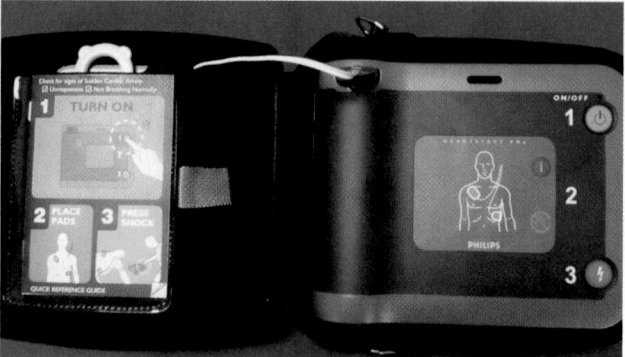

Figure 30–2 ■ AED instructions.
Courtesy Neal Shabashov.

For a person who is not already on a cardiac monitor with a manual defibrillator available, the **automated external defibrillator (AED)** is used. The AED is a relatively small, portable, battery-operated device that senses the cardiac rhythm through two adhesive pads (Figure 30–1 ■ and 30–2 ■). If the AED detects a rhythm that should be treated with electric shock, it indicates to the operator that a shock is advised. AEDs are commonly found in health clubs, restaurants, and many public locations where there is a relatively high likelihood of witnessed cardiac arrest (e.g., airports, casinos, sports facilities). Use of the AED is taught in most CPR classes—for both the lay rescuer and the professional rescuer.

●○○● NURSING PROCESS: AUTOMATED EXTERNAL DEFIBRILLATION

SKILL 30–4

Administering Automated External Defibrillation

ASSESSMENT
Determine that the person is unresponsive, has no breathing, and has no pulse.

PLANNING
An AED should be available on those nursing units where the full "crash cart" with defibrillator is not available.

DELEGATION
Any person who has been trained in its use can apply and activate the AED.

INTERPROFESSIONAL PRACTICE

Administering automated external defibrillation is within the scope of practice for all health care providers. Each member of the health care team should know how to call for help and initiate the intervention.

Equipment
- AED with all components including the automatic override key, event documentation module or tape, electrodes and cables, and charged battery pack. Brands and models differ in their features.

IMPLEMENTATION
Performance
1. Follow steps 1 through 9 of Skill 30–3. Traditional CPR must be performed until the AED can be attached.
2. Attach the AED.
   - Turn on the power of the AED (usually a green on/off button).
   - Apply the electrode pads to dry skin: one in the upper right chest near the clavicle, and the other in the lower left chest below the nipple. ❶ If the person has heavy chest hair, it may be necessary to quickly shave the hair. **Rationale:**

Heavy chest hair may prevent the pads from sticking to the chest and may also catch on fire during defibrillation.
   - Attach the cables to the box if necessary.
3. Initiate rhythm analysis. Be sure no one is touching the person. **Rationale:** *This ensures that the AED is reading only the person's cardiac electrical activity.* The analysis may take 5 to 15 seconds. In most models, this also charges the AED.
4. Defibrillate as indicated.
   - Before delivering the shock, state loudly "Clear" and visually check to ensure that no one is touching the person

Administering Automated External Defibrillation—*continued*

SKILL 30–4

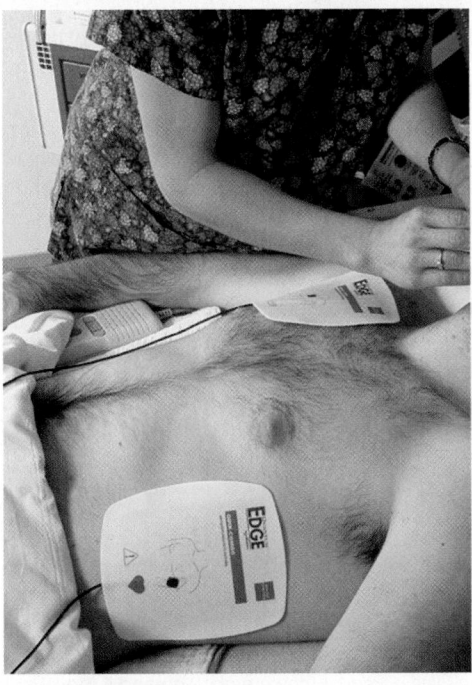

❶ Placement of AED electrode pads.

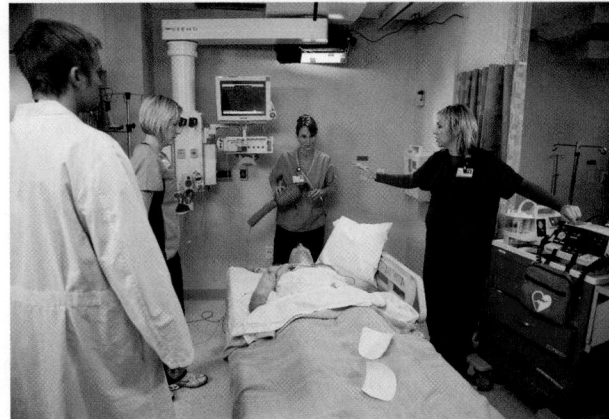

❷ The individual controlling the AED or defibrillator calls the "all clear" to be sure no one is touching the person or bed.

or anything that is touching the person (e.g., the bed). ❷
Rationale: *If a shock is delivered while someone is in contact with the person, that individual will also receive the shock.*

• Press the shock button and observe for the brief contraction of the person's muscles that indicates the shock has been delivered.

5. Resume CPR. The AED will automatically prompt to reanalyze the person in 2 to 3 minutes. Continue the sequence of CPR and defibrillation until the AED specifies that no shock is indicated, the person converts to a functional rhythm (pulse is felt or movement observed), or the code team takes over.
6. Document the events as in Skill 30–3 above including data provided by the AED. Attach electrocardiogram strips or other records made by the AED.

EVALUATION

In a health care setting, a review of the emergency event and the staff's response is commonly performed to see if there are indications for improvement in procedures. Review of the use of the AED may be indicated. Mock arrests may be planned to assist the staff in practicing their skills.

LIFESPAN CONSIDERATIONS | **Automated External Defibrillation**

INFANTS
• Use child-sized pads if available.
• A manual defibrillator is preferred. If a manual defibrillator is not available, an AED with pediatric dose attenuation is desirable. If neither is available, an AED without a dose attenuator may be used.

CHILDREN
• Use child-sized pads if available.
• Select a child shock dose (pediatric dose attenuator) on the AED if available. This may require turning a key or switch. If a child dose is not available, an AED without a dose attenuator may be used.

Ambulatory and Community Settings | **Automated External Defibrillation** | **EVIDENCE-BASED PRACTICE**

• Training in the use of an AED should be conducted in all health care facilities including clinics, long-term care facilities, and urgent care centers.
• AEDs can be used by trained lay rescuers.
• Use of the AED takes priority over CPR in *witnessed* arrest. The sequence of events is:
  • Confirm unresponsiveness and absence of breathing.
  • Activate the EMS notification system (e.g., call 911).
  • Start CPR until the AED can be attached.
  • Defibrillate if indicated.
  • Resume CPR for five cycles.

• For an *unwitnessed* arrest, the sequence of events is:
  • Confirm unresponsiveness, absence of breathing, and absence of pulse.
  • Activate the EMS notification system (e.g., call 911).
  • Perform CPR for five cycles.
  • Defibrillate with one shock.
  • Resume CPR without rechecking the rhythm.
• For a child with an unwitnessed arrest, perform five cycles (2 minutes) of CPR before using the AED.

FOCUSING ON CLINICAL THINKING

Consider This

1. You answer a client's call light and find the adult client coughing forcefully with the lunch tray thrown to the floor. On inspiration, there is an audible wheeze, the client's face is ruddy, and the eyes are wide. You ask: "Can you speak?" The client shakes the head "no" and continues to cough. When you approach the client and start to put your arms around the chest to attempt a Heimlich maneuver, the client waves the arms broadly, pushing you away. What should you do next?

2. You are administering medication to a person who suddenly has a generalized tonic-clonic seizure. At the end of the seizure, the person does not regain consciousness. Would you *first* (a) call the rapid response team, (b) call a code, (c) begin mouth-to-mouth resuscitation, (d) begin CPR, or (e) do something different?

3. You find a client slumped in the hospital bedside chair. The client is unresponsive to verbal stimuli and touch and is not breathing. After calling a code, establishing an open airway, and giving two breaths, you are unable to feel a carotid pulse. Describe your next steps.

4. After applying an AED and delivering a shock, a pulse check indicates that the heart has not resumed a normal rhythm. What steps should you take next?

See Focusing on Clinical Thinking answers on student resource website.

TEST YOUR KNOWLEDGE

1. If the agency has both a rapid response team and a Code Blue team, for which of the following clients would the nurse request the rapid response team's immediate intervention?
   1. A client complaining of severe postoperative incisional pain
   2. A client with no pulse who is not breathing
   3. A client complaining of chest pain, hypotension, and shortness of breath
   4. A client with a blood pressure of 164/96 mmHg

2. If the agency has both a rapid response team and a Code Blue team, for which of the following clients would the nurse call the arrest (Code Blue) team?
   1. A client with a blood pressure of 60/28 mmHg
   2. A client experiencing severe dyspnea secondary to asthma
   3. A client in atrial fibrillation
   4. An unconscious client in ventricular tachycardia

3. The nurse enters the client's hospital room and finds the client is not breathing and has no pulse. The client does not have a do-not-resuscitate order. What would the nurse's most immediate action be?
   1. Call the cardiac/respiratory arrest team.
   2. Begin CPR.
   3. Call a coworker for help.
   4. Get the crash cart.

4. A client has been found with no pulse or respirations. The cardiopulmonary arrest team has been called. What action is taken by the nurse while awaiting the team's arrival?
   1. Gather the client's medical record and medication administration record.
   2. Obtain the crash cart.
   3. Notify the client's primary care provider.
   4. Perform CPR.

5. The nurse sees on the cardiorespiratory monitor that the client's cardiac rhythm has changed from normal sinus rhythm to ventricular fibrillation. The nurse knows the most effective means of converting this rhythm is:
   1. CPR.
   2. Defibrillation.
   3. Oxygen.
   4. Precordial thump.

6. The nurse is dining in the hospital cafeteria when another patron stands and demonstrates the universal sign of choking. The nurse's first action should be to:
   1. Perform abdominal thrusts.
   2. Assign someone to call the emergency response system.
   3. Ask the person if they are choking and if they want help.
   4. Begin CPR.

7. The nurse observes a person collapse and stop breathing. The nurse would establish an airway by:
   1. Inserting an endotracheal tube.
   2. Inserting a finger to pull the tongue forward.
   3. Using the head tilt–chin lift maneuver.
   4. Using a modified jaw-thrust maneuver.

8. The nurse is performing cardiac compressions on a 4-year-old child with the assistance of another nurse. The nurses would deliver breaths and compressions at a ratio of:
   1. 30 compressions for 2 breaths.
   2. 15 compressions for 2 breaths.
   3. 5 compressions for 2 breaths.
   4. 5 compressions for 1 breath.

9. When applying an automated external defibrillator the nurse would:
   1. Connect the cable to the machine, apply the pads, and turn on the power.
   2. Turn on the power, apply the pads, and connect the cable.
   3. Turn on the power, connect the cable, and apply the pads.
   4. Connect the cable, turn on the power, and apply the pads.

10. When using an automated external defibrillator, it is important for the nurse to ensure that no one is touching the client:
    1. After connecting the cable to the machine.
    2. When the machine is plugged in.
    3. While applying the pads.
    4. While the machine analyzes the rhythm.

See Answers to Test Your Knowledge in Appendix A.

READINGS AND REFERENCES

References

Al-Qahtani, S., Al-Dorzi, H., Tamim, H., Hussain, S., Fong, L., Taher, S., . . . Arabi, Y. (2013). Impact of an intensivist-led multidisciplinary extended rapid response team on hospital-wide cardiopulmonary arrests and mortality. *Critical Care Medicine, 41*, 506–517. doi:10.1097/CCM.0b013e318271440b

American Heart Association (AHA). (2013). *CPR and first aid mission.* Retrieved from http://www.heart.org/HEARTORG/CPRAndECC/WhatisCPR/AboutUs/CPR-First-Aid-Mission_UCM_307510_Article.jsp

Berg, R. A., Hemphill, R., Abella, B. S., Aufderheide, T. P., Cave, D. M., Hazinski, M. F., . . . Swor, R. A. (2010). Part 5: Adult basic life support: 2010 American Heart Association Guidelines for Cardiopulmonary Resuscitation and Emergency Cardiovascular Care. *Circulation, 122*(Suppl. 3), S685–S705. doi:10.1161/CIRCULATIONAHA.110.970939

Hazinski, M. F. (Ed.). (2010). *Highlights of the 2010 American Heart Association Guidelines for CPR and ECC.* Dallas, TX: American Heart Association.

Jabre, P., Belpomme, V., Azoulay, E., Jacob, L., Bertrand, L., Lapostolle, F., . . . Adnet, F. (2013). Family presence during cardiopulmonary resuscitation. *New England Journal of Medicine, 368*, 1008–1018. doi:10.1056/NEJMoa1203366

Kleinman, M. E., de Caen, A. R., Chameides, L., Atkins, D. L., Berg, R. A., Berg, M. D., . . . Pediatric Basic and Advanced Life Support Chapter Collaborators. (2010). Part 10: Pediatric basic and advanced life support: 2010 international consensus on cardiopulmonary resuscitation and emergency cardiovascular care science with treatment recommendations. *Circulation, 122*, S466–S515. doi:10.1161/CIRCULATIONAHA.110.971093

Leach, L., & Mayo, A. M. (2013). Rapid response teams: Qualitative analysis of their effectiveness. *American Journal of Critical Care, 22*, 198–210. doi:10.4037/ajcc2013990

Leske, J. S., McAndrew, N. S., & Brasel, K. J. (2013). Experiences of families when present during resuscitation in the emergency department after trauma. *Journal of Trauma Nursing, 20*, 77–85. doi:10.1097/JTN.0b013e31829600a8

McEvoy, M. (2014). 6 surprising best resuscitation practices. *American Nurse Today, 9*(3), 20–25.

Nolan, J., & Soar, J. (2012). Duration of in-hospital resuscitation: When to call time? *Lancet, 380*(9852), 1451–1453. doi:10.1016/S0140-6736(12)61182-9

Selected Bibliography

Astroth, K. S., Woith, M. W., Stapleton, S. J., Degitz, R. J., & Jenkins, S. H. (2013). Qualitative exploration of nurses' decisions to activate rapid response teams. *Journal of Clinical Nursing, 22*, 2876–2882. doi:10.1111/jocn.12067

Bostock-Cox, B. (2012). Emergencies in general practice. *Practice Nurse, 42*(17), 22–25.

Chao, C., Lai, C., & Tan, C. (2012). Gastric perforation after Heimlich maneuver. *American Journal of Medicine, 125*(6), e7–e8.

Chapman, R., Watkins, R., Bushby, A., & Combs, S. (2013). Assessing health professionals' perceptions of family presence during resuscitation: A replication study. *International Emergency Nursing, 21*(1), 17–25. doi:10.1016/j.ienj.2011.10.003

Clark, A., Guzzetta, C., & O'Connell, K. (2013). Family presence during resuscitation attempts is associated with positive psychological effects for the observers. *Evidence Based Mental Health, 16*, 78. doi:10.1136/eb-2013-101354

Colbert, J., & Adler, J. (2013). Clinical decisions. Family presence during cardiopulmonary resuscitation—Polling results. *New England Journal of Medicine, 368*(26), e38. doi:10.1056/NEJMclde1307088

Craig, K., & Day, M. (2011). Are you up to date on the latest BLS and ACLS guidelines? *Nursing, 41*(5), 40–44. doi:10.1097/01.NURSE.0000395207.72990.df

Downar, J., & Kritek, P. (2013). Family presence during cardiac resuscitation. *New England Journal of Medicine, 368*, 1060–1062. doi:10.1056/NEJMclde1301020

Downar, J., Rodin, D., Barua, R., Lejnieks, B., Gudimella, R., McCredie, V., . . . Steel, A. (2013). Rapid response teams, do not resuscitate orders, and potential opportunities to improve end-of-life care: A multicentre retrospective study. *Journal of Critical Care, 28*, 498–503. doi:10.1016/j.jcrc.2012.10.002

Gulli, B., Piazza, G., & Rahm, S. J. (2012). *Health care provider CPR* (4th ed.). Burlington, MA: Jones & Bartlett.

Handley, A. (2013). At last, some research on choking. *Resuscitation, 84*, 413–414. doi:10.1016/j.resuscitation.2013.01.005

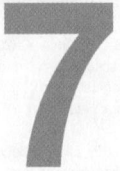
Applying the Nursing Process

This unit explores skills related to circulation and ventilation. Alterations in circulation and ventilation are often life threatening and require rapid and accurate intervention on the part of the nurse. All health care personnel should be competent in performing CPR and responding appropriately in an emergency situation. Nurses, who provide 24-hour care for the client, must be skilled in maintaining and promoting circulation and ventilation and know how to intervene promptly when problems arise.

CLIENT: Jamie   AGE: 20 Years   CURRENT MEDICAL DIAGNOSIS: Quadriplegia

Medical History: Jamie experienced a fracture of the third cervical vertebra after diving into the shallow end of a friend's swimming pool during a party to celebrate his high school graduation 2 years ago. He was initially admitted to the acute care facility and transferred to a rehabilitation facility once his neck fracture was stabilized. He has minimal shoulder function but is able to control his electric wheelchair by thrusting his shoulder forward or back. He has no other mobility in his extremities. He is largely dependent on a mechanical ventilator but can breathe independently for 5 to 10 minutes off the ventilator on good days if he is sitting upright. He has a tracheostomy in place

with a valve to allow him to talk. He was recently readmitted to the acute care facility secondary to left lower lobe pneumonia. He is on a positive pressure ventilator that is set for synchronized intermittent mandatory ventilation (SIMV).

Personal and Social History: Jamie lives with his parents in a two-story home that has been remodeled to allow him to go outside or around the first floor in his wheelchair. The dining room was converted into a bedroom for him. It has a hospital bed, oxygen, and a suctioning device.

Questions

Assessment

1. What does the nurse assess initially when caring for the client on a mechanical ventilator?
2. What assessment data indicate the client requires suctioning of the airway?

Analysis

3. List two possible nursing diagnoses that can be identified from the medical/personal history and assessment data above related to ventilation.

Planning

4. Based on the assessment data and the nursing diagnoses, identify one desired outcome related to the skills discussed in this unit.

Implementation

5. Describe nursing actions to be taken when suctioning the tracheostomy to prevent or reduce hypoxia during the procedure.

Evaluation

6. How will the nurse know if the expected outcome has been achieved?

See *Applying the Nursing Process* suggested answers on student resource website.

UNIT

8

Wounds and Injury Care

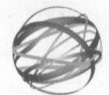

31 Performing Wound and Pressure Ulcer Care

LEARNING OUTCOMES

At the completion of this chapter, the student will be able to:

1. Define the key terms used in the skills of performing wound and pressure ulcer care.
2. Identify indications and contraindications for various types of wound care and dressings.
3. Identify assessment data pertinent to skin integrity and wounds.
4. Recognize when it is appropriate to delegate wound and pressure ulcer care to unlicensed assistive personnel.
5. Verbalize the steps used in:
   a. Assessing wounds and pressure ulcers.
   b. Performing a dry dressing change.
   c. Applying a transparent wound barrier.
   d. Applying a hydrocolloid dressing.
   e. Irrigating a wound.
   f. Assisting with a sitz bath.
   g. Performing a damp-to-damp dressing change.
   h. Using alginates on wounds.
   i. Applying bandages and binders.
6. Demonstrate appropriate documentation and reporting of wound and pressure ulcer care.

SKILLS

Skill 31–1 Assessing Wounds and Pressure Ulcers
Skill 31–2 Performing a Dry Dressing Change
Skill 31–3 Applying a Transparent Wound Barrier
Skill 31–4 Applying a Hydrocolloid Dressing
Skill 31–5 Irrigating a Wound
Skill 31–6 Assisting with a Sitz Bath
Skill 31–7 Performing a Damp-to-Damp Dressing Change
Skill 31–8 Using Alginates on Wounds
Skill 31–9 Applying Bandages and Binders

KEY TERMS

alginate, *682*
bandage, *685*
binder, *685*
debridement, *670*
dressings, *670*
eschar, *663*
friction, *663*
hydrocolloid, *676*
negative pressure wound therapy (NPWT), *684*
pressure ulcers, *663*
shearing force, *663*
sitz bath, *679*
sling, *685*
transparent wound barriers, *675*
wound, *662*

The skin serves a variety of functions, including protecting the individual from injury. Impaired skin integrity is not a frequent problem for most healthy people, but it is a threat to older adults and clients with restricted mobility, chronic illness, or trauma, and those undergoing invasive procedures. When the skin or underlying tissues are damaged, the inflammatory process of the individual's immune response acts to eliminate any foreign material, if possible, and prepare the injured area for healing. This injured body area is called a **wound**. The nurse plays an important role in assessing client risk for developing wounds, in preventing wounds, and in treating various types of wounds.

TYPES OF WOUNDS

Body wounds are either intentional or unintentional. *Intentional* traumas occur during therapy. Examples are operations or venipunctures. Although removing a tumor, for example, is therapeutic, the surgeon must cut into body tissues, thus traumatizing them. *Unintentional* wounds are accidental; for example, a person may fracture an arm in an automobile collision or have tissue breakdown from a metabolic condition such as diabetes or vascular disease. If the tissues are traumatized without a break in the skin, the wound is *closed*. The wound is *open* when the skin or mucous membrane surface is broken.

Wounds may be described according to how they are acquired (Table 31–1). They can also be described according to the likelihood and degree of wound contamination:

- *Clean wounds* are uninfected wounds in which there is minimal inflammation and the respiratory, alimentary, genital, and urinary tracts are not entered. Clean wounds are primarily closed wounds.

TABLE 31–1   Types of Wounds

Type	Cause	Description and Characteristics
Incision	Sharp instrument (e.g., knife or scalpel)	Open wound; deep or shallow. Once the edges have been sealed together as a part of treatment or healing, the incision becomes a closed wound.
Contusion	Blow from a blunt instrument	Closed wound, skin appears ecchymotic (bruised) because of damaged blood vessels
Abrasion	Surface scrape, either unintentional (e.g., scraped knee from a fall) or intentional (e.g., dermal abrasion to remove pockmarks)	Open wound involving the skin
Puncture	Penetration of the skin and often the underlying tissues by a sharp instrument, either intentional or unintentional	Open wound
Laceration	Tissues torn apart, often from accidents (e.g., with machinery)	Open wound; edges are often jagged
Penetrating wound	Penetration of the skin and the underlying tissues, usually unintentional (e.g., from a bullet or metal fragments)	Open wound

---

BOX 31–1   Classifying Wounds by Depth

- *Partial thickness:* confined to the skin, that is, the dermis and epidermis; heal by regeneration
- *Full thickness:* involving the dermis, epidermis, subcutaneous tissue, and possibly muscle and bone; require connective tissue repair.

- *Clean-contaminated wounds* are surgical wounds in which the respiratory, gastrointestinal, genital, or urinary tract has been entered. Such wounds show no evidence of infection.
- *Contaminated wounds* include open, fresh, accidental wounds and surgical wounds involving a major break in sterile technique or a large amount of spillage from the gastrointestinal tract. Contaminated wounds show evidence of inflammation.
- *Dirty* or *infected wounds* include wounds containing dead tissue and wounds with evidence of a clinical infection, such as purulent drainage.

Wounds, excluding pressure ulcers and burns, are classified by depth, that is, the tissue layers involved in the wound (Box 31–1).

Pressure Ulcers

Pressure ulcers (previously called decubitus ulcers, pressure sores, or bedsores) are reddened areas, sores, or ulcers of the skin over bony prominences. They are caused by interruption of the circulation to the tissue, resulting in localized ischemia. The tissue is caught between two hard surfaces, usually the surface of furniture such as the bed or chair and the bony skeleton. The ischemia deprives cells of oxygen and nutrients, and the waste products of metabolism accumulate. The tissue dies because of the resulting anoxia.

In addition to direct pressure as a cause of these ulcers, friction and shearing are major contributors. **Friction** is a force acting parallel to the skin surface. For example, sheets rubbing against skin create friction. Friction can abrade the skin, that is, remove the superficial layers, making it more prone to breakdown. **Shearing**

force is a combination of friction and pressure. It occurs commonly when a client sitting in bed tends to slide downward toward the foot of the bed. The skin and superficial tissues are relatively unmoving in relation to the bed surface, whereas the deeper tissues are firmly attached to the skeleton and move downward. This causes a shearing force in the area where the deeper tissues and the superficial tissues meet. The force damages the blood vessels and tissues in this area.

Much research has been conducted internationally regarding the prevention, diagnosis, and treatment of pressure ulcers. In 2009, a new classification system for pressure ulcers was published by the European Pressure Ulcer Advisory Panel and National Pressure Ulcer Advisory Panel. In this classification, the authors recommended that the term *category* be used to describe the different levels of ulcers although many organizations use the terms *stage* or *grade*. Category is preferred because it avoids the implication that ulcers change progressively from one level to another—which may not always be true. In this text, the term *category/stage* is used.

Both international and U.S. pressure ulcer panels agree to four categories/stages of pressure ulcers (Figure 31–1 ■). In the United States, two additional levels are used:

- *Unstageable/unclassified: full-thickness skin or tissue loss—depth unknown.* The actual depth of the ulcer is completely obscured by slough (yellow, tan, gray, green, or brown tissue) and/or **eschar** (tan, black, or brown necrotic tissue) but, once cleaned, it will be a category/stage III or IV ulcer. Stable (dry, adherent, intact without erythema or pus) eschar on the heels serves as "the body's natural (biological) cover" and should not be removed.
- *Suspected deep tissue injury—depth unknown.* Purple area of discolored intact skin or blood-filled blister. May be difficult to detect in individuals with dark skin tones. Evolution may include a thin blister over a dark wound bed. The wound may further evolve and become covered by thin eschar. Evolution may be rapid, exposing additional layers of tissue .even with optimal treatment.

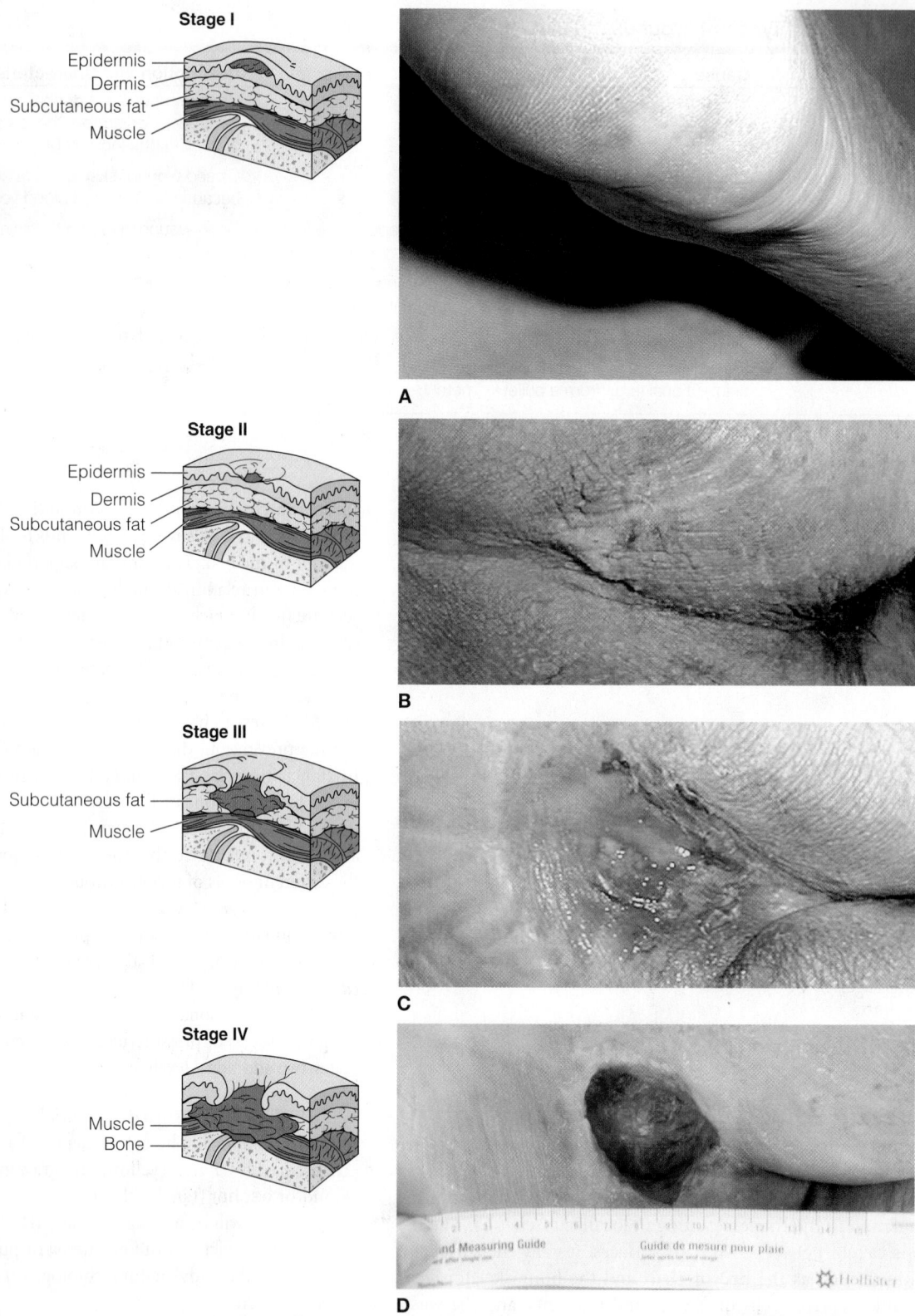

Figure 31–1 ■ Stages of pressure ulcers: *A,* Stage I: nonblanchable erythema signaling potential ulceration. *B,* Stage II: partial-thickness skin loss (abrasion, blister, or shallow crater) involving the epidermis and possibly the dermis. *C,* Stage III: full-thickness skin loss involving damage or necrosis of subcutaneous tissue that may extend down to, but not through, underlying fascia. The ulcer presents clinically as a deep crater with or without undermining of adjacent tissue. *D,* Stage IV: full-thickness skin loss with tissue necrosis or damage to muscle, bone, or supporting structures, such as a tendon or joint capsule. Undermining and sinus tracts may also be present. *E,* Unstageable/unclassified: full-thickness skin or tissue loss—depth unknown. Actual depth of the ulcer is completely obscured by slough (yellow, tan, gray, green, or brown) and/or eschar (tan, brown, or black) in the wound bed. *F,* Suspected deep tissue injury—depth unknown: purple or maroon localized area of discolored intact skin or blood-filled blister due to damage of underlying soft tissue from pressure and/or shear. Deep tissue injury may be difficult to detect in individuals with dark skin tones. Evolution may include a thin blister over a dark wound bed. The wound may further evolve and become covered by thin eschar.

Line art for *A–F* from "Clinical Practice Guideline, Pressure Ulcers in Adults: Prediction and Prevention," by U.S. Department of Health and Human Services (PPPPUA, Pub. No. 92-0047), 1992, Rockville, MD: Public Health Service. Reprinted with permission. Photos *A–F:* Courtesy of Cory Patrick Hartley, RN.

Unstageable/unclassified

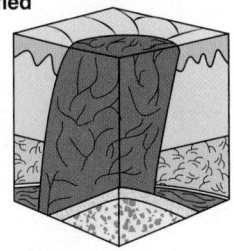

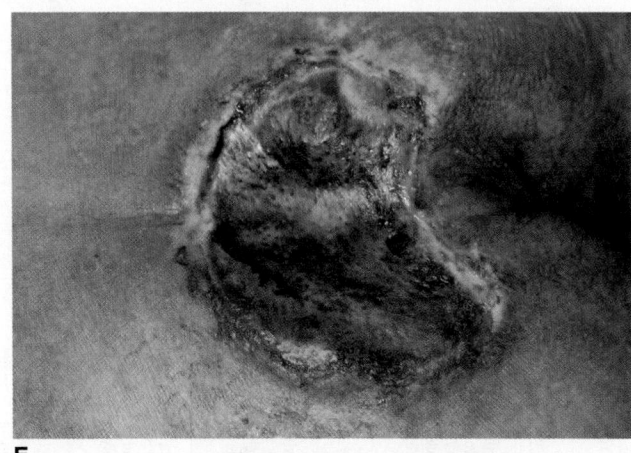

E

Suspected Deep Tissue Injury

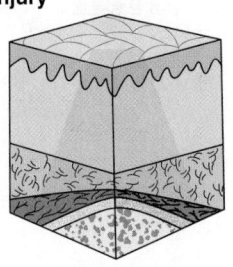

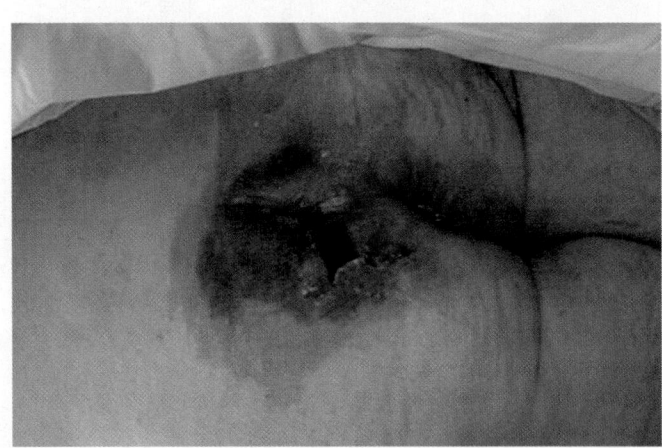

F

Figure 31–1 ■ *Continued.*

Preventing Pressure Ulcers

One of the National Patient Safety Goals for long-term care settings is prevention of pressure ulcers (The Joint Commission, 2013b). In addition, a *Healthy People 2020* objective is to reduce the rate of pressure ulcer–related hospitalizations among older adults (U.S. Department of Health and Human Services, 2013). Because most pressure ulcers are preventable, public health insurance—and increasing numbers of private health insurance companies—will no longer reimburse health care agencies for the cost of treating health care–associated pressure ulcers. In addition, development of a category/stage III or IV or unstageable pressure ulcer is considered a serious reportable event (National Quality Forum, 2013). Prevention requires early and regular assessment of clients' risk of developing a pressure ulcer. Assessment can be accomplished through use of a well-established risk assessment tool such as the Braden scale (see Figure 31–2 ■) or the Norton scale. In long-term care, assessment is performed on admission, weekly for the first month, and then every

3 months if the client's condition or risk factors are unchanged. Clients should be assessed in the acute care setting on admission and at least every 48 hours and more often, depending on how quickly their condition changes (Bates-Jensen, 2012).

Preventive measures to reduce the risks of developing pressure ulcers include manipulation of the environment, ongoing assessment, proper positioning and nutrition, meticulous hygiene, and instruction in preventing and protecting pressure areas. The nurse manipulates the environment when making the client's bed, providing a smooth, firm, wrinkle-free foundation on which the client can lie. Some clients may require a special mattress, such as an alternating pressure, egg-crate, or flotation mattress (available for beds and wheelchairs), to decrease pressure on body parts. See Table 10–2 in Chapter 10 ∞.

Sometimes, pressure ulcers occur in spite of preventive measures. See the accompanying Practice Guidelines for recommendations regarding treatment of pressure ulcers.

BRADEN SCALE FOR PREDICTING PRESSURE SORE RISK

Patient's Name _____ Evaluator's Name _____ Date of Assessment _____

SENSORY PERCEPTION Ability to respond meaningfully to pressure-related discomfort	1. Completely Limited: Unresponsive (does not moan, flinch, or grasp) to painful stimuli, due to diminished level of consciousness or sedation, OR limited ability to feel pain over most of body surface.	2. Very Limited: Responds only to painful stimuli. Cannot communicate discomfort except by moaning or restlessness, OR has a sensory impairment which limits the ability to feel pain or discomfort over 1/2 of body.	3. Slightly Limited: Responds to verbal commands but cannot always communicate discomfort or need to be turned, OR has some sensory impairment which limits ability to feel pain or discomfort in 1 or 2 extremities.	4. No Impairment: Responds to verbal commands. Has no sensory deficit which would limit ability to feel or voice pain or discomfort.
MOISTURE Degree to which skin is exposed to moisture	1. Constantly Moist: Skin is kept moist almost constantly by perspiration, urine, etc. Dampness is detected every time patient is moved or turned.	2. Moist: Skin is often but not always moist. Linen must be changed at least once a shift.	3. Occasionally Moist: Skin is occasionally moist, requiring an extra linen change approximately once a day.	4. Rarely Moist: Skin is usually dry; linen requires changing only at routine intervals.
ACTIVITY Degree of physical activity	1. Bedfast: Confined to bed.	2. Chairfast: Ability to walk severely limited or nonexistent. Cannot bear own weight and/or must be assisted into chair or wheelchair.	3. Walks Occasionally: Walks occasionally during day but for very short distances, with or without assistance. Spends majority of each shift in bed or chair.	4. Walks Frequently: Walks outside the room at least twice a day and inside room at least once every 2 hours during waking hours.
MOBILITY Ability to change and control body position	1. Completely Immobile: Does not make even slight changes in body or extremity position without assistance.	2. Very Limited: Makes occasional slight changes in body or extremity position but unable to make frequent or significant changes independently.	3. Slightly Limited: Makes frequent though slight changes in body or extremity position independently.	4. No Limitations: Makes major and frequent changes in position without assistance.
NUTRITION Usual food intake pattern	1. Very Poor: Never eats a complete meal. Rarely eats more than 1/3 of any food offered. Eats 2 servings or less of protein (meat or dairy products) per day. Takes fluids poorly. Does not take a liquid dietary supplement, OR is NPO and/or maintained on clear liquids or IV's for more than 5 days.	2. Probably Inadequate: Rarely eats a complete meal and generally eats only about 1/2 of any food offered. Protein intake includes only 3 servings of meat or dairy products per day. Occasionally will take a dietary supplement, OR receives less than optimum amount of liquid diet or tube feeding.	3. Adequate: Eats over half of most meals. Eats a total of 4 servings of protein (meat, dairy products) each day. Occasionally will refuse a meal, but will usually take a supplement if offered, OR is on a tube feeding or TPN regimen, which probably meets most of nutritional needs.	4. Excellent: Eats most of every meal. Never refuses a meal. Usually eats a total of 4 or more servings of meat and dairy products. Occasionally eats between meals. Does not require supplementation.
FRICTION AND SHEAR	1. Problem: Requires moderate to maximum assistance in moving. Complete lifting without sliding against sheets is impossible. Frequently slides down in bed or chair, requiring frequent repositioning with maximum assistance. Spasticity, contractures, or agitation leads to almost constant friction.	2. Potential Problem: Moves feebly or requires minimum assistance. During a move skin probably slides to some extent against sheets, chair, restraints, or other devices. Maintains relatively good position in chair or bed most of the time but occasionally slides down.	3. No Apparent Problem: Moves in bed and in chair independently and has sufficient muscle strength to lift up completely during move. Maintains good position in bed or chair at all times.	

Total Score _____

Figure 31–2 ■ Braden Scale for Predicting Pressure Sore Risk.

PRACTICE GUIDELINES

Treating Pressure Ulcers

- Minimize direct pressure on the ulcer. Reposition the client at least every 2 hours. Make a schedule, and record position changes on the client's chart. Provide devices to minimize or float pressure areas.
- Clean the pressure ulcer with every dressing change. The method of cleaning depends on the category/stage of the ulcer, products available, and agency protocol. Skill 31–5 details the steps involved in irrigating a wound.
- Clean and dress the ulcer using surgical asepsis. Use of povidone-iodine, acetic acid, sodium hypochlorite (Dakin solution), or hydrogen peroxide is controversial because they are

cytotoxic to tissue beds. Short-term use of these products may be indicated in extremely infected wounds (Bates-Jensen, Schultz, & Ovington, 2012).
- If the pressure ulcer is infected, obtain a sample of the drainage for culture and sensitivity to antibiotic agents (see Skill 4–9 in Chapter 4 ∞).
- Teach the client to move, even if only slightly, to relieve pressure.
- Provide range-of-motion (ROM) exercises and mobility out of bed as the client's condition permits.

●○● NURSING PROCESS: ASSESSING WOUNDS AND PRESSURE ULCERS

Assessing Wounds and Pressure Ulcers

SKILL 31–1

PLANNING

- Before assessing the wound, review the client record for information regarding the cause of the wound, the length of time the wound has been present, and previous treatment and response to treatment.
- Determine factors that may hinder wound healing:
  - *Malnutrition.* A poorly nourished person often has insufficient amounts of the protein, vitamins, and trace substances needed to synthesize wound-healing elements and to resist infection.
  - *Obesity.* Adipose tissue has a limited blood supply; thus, a client who is obese is more likely to acquire an infection and have poor wound healing.
  - *Medications.* Some medications may delay healing. Corticosteroids can suppress the inflammatory reaction. In addition, the prolonged use of antibiotics can increase the likelihood of infection from organisms that are resistant to that antibiotic.

- *Smoking.* Smoking reduces the amount of functional hemoglobin and causes peripheral vasoconstriction.
- *Compromised host.* A compromised host is a person at unusual risk for infection. For example, clients who have diabetes mellitus or cancer may be at increased risk for getting an infection.
- *Immobility.* Clients who cannot shift their own body position cannot relieve pressure areas independently. In addition, such clients may be incontinent of urine or stool. Ongoing moisture on skin can lead to skin breakdown; stagnant urine or stool can infect a wound.
- Determine results of laboratory tests pertinent to nutritional status and healing (e.g., wound culture, blood proteins, leukocyte count, and blood coagulation studies).
- Determine if the client requires premedication for pain or other pain management techniques prior to wound care (see Chapter 9 ∞).

DELEGATION

Assessment is not a skill delegated to unlicensed assistive personnel (UAP). However, UAP may observe the wound during usual care and must report abnormal findings to the nurse. Abnormal findings must be validated and interpreted by the nurse.

INTERPROFESSIONAL PRACTICE

Assessing wounds may be within the scope of practice for other health care providers. For example, in addition to nurses, both physical therapists and occupational therapists commonly assess wounds before, during, and after treatment. Although the therapists may verbally communicate their findings and plan to the health care team members, the nurse must also know where to locate their documentation in the client's medical record.

Equipment
- Clean gloves
- Sterile gloves (optional)
- Disposable millimeter ruler
- Paper or plastic for tracing the wound (optional)
- Sterile cotton tip applicator swabs
- Adequate lighting

IMPLEMENTATION
Preparation
If the wound is dressed or will be dressed after assessment, gather the appropriate additional supplies before beginning assessment.

Performance
1. Prior to performing the procedure, introduce self and verify the client's identity using agency protocol. Explain to the client what you are going to do, why it is necessary, and how he or she can participate. Discuss how the results will be used in planning further care or treatments.

Continued on page 668

Assessing Wounds and Pressure Ulcers—*continued*

2. Perform hand hygiene and observe other appropriate infection prevention procedures.
3. Provide for client privacy.
4. Position the client appropriately.
5. Apply clean gloves.
6. If necessary, remove the existing dressing (see Skill 31–2).
7. Assess the wound for:
   - *Appearance.* Inspect the wound itself for signs of healing and approximation (nearness) of the wound edges. Look for foreign bodies (soil, broken glass, shreds of cloth, or other foreign substances). If the wound is contaminated with foreign material, determine when the client last had a tetanus toxoid injection. A tetanus immunization or booster may be necessary.
   - *Drainage.* Observe the location, color, consistency, odor, and degree of saturation of dressings. Estimating the amount of wound drainage can be difficult. One recommendation is to describe the degree to which the dressing is saturated. Minimal drainage only stains the dressing, moderate drainage saturates the dressing without leakage prior to scheduled dressing changes, and heavy drainage overflows the dressing prior to scheduled changes. These terms, plus the description of the drainage and the amount and type of dressing material used, should be well understood by all care providers.
   - *Size.* To determine the length and width of the wound's surface area or its circumference, use a disposable measuring guide (❶, A). For irregularly shaped wounds, use paper or a transparent wound dressing, and trace and date the margins of the wounds. To measure an area located on a curved portion of the body, use a flexible measure (❶, B). Electronic devices allow tracings to be digitized for improved determination of total wound area (Hammond & Nixon, 2011).
   - *Depth/undermining.* To determine wound depth and extent of undermining, probe the deepest part of the wound with a sterile swab. If a calibrated swab is not available to measure the extent of undermining, place a second swab exactly parallel to the first and measure the distance from the edge of the wound to the tip of the exposed swab. ❷
   - *Swelling.* Palpate wound edges for tension and tautness of tissues; minimal to moderate swelling is normal in early stages of wound healing.
   - *Pain.* Expect severe to moderate pain for 3 to 5 days after surgery; persistent or increasing pain or sudden onset of severe pain may indicate internal hemorrhaging or infection.
   - *Drains or tubes.* Inspect drain security and placement, amount and character of drainage, and functioning of collecting apparatus, if present.
8. Determine the category/stage of a pressure ulcer.
   - Use the categories/stages described by the National Pressure Ulcer Advisory Panel. See Figure 31–1.
   - Request a consultation from a wound ostomy continence nurse if appropriate. **Rationale:** *Determining the initial level of pressure ulcer can be difficult. The surface evidence may not be truly indicative of underlying tissue damage. Eschar on the surface of the ulcer may require removal for complete assessment.*
9. Remove and discard gloves.
   - Perform hand hygiene.
10. Document the assessment and the client's response in the client record using forms or checklists supplemented by narrative notes when appropriate. Electronic health records will use a designated wound/skin documentation sheet. ❸

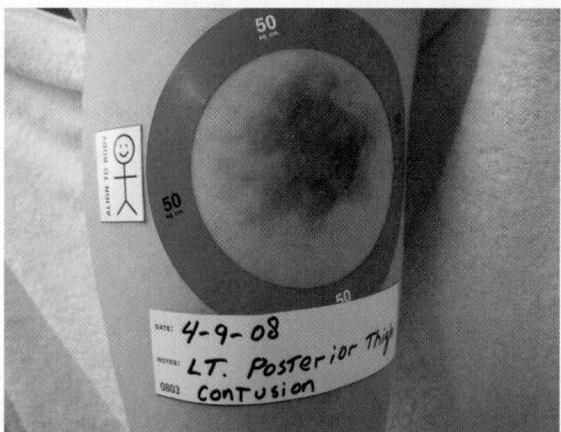

A

B

❶ Use of photo measuring guides provides documentation of scale and alignment with the body. *A,* This guide provides the diameter of the wound irrespective of camera distance. *B,* A flexible ruler (upper) is needed to prevent measurement error when assessing a wound on a curved part of the body. The red arrows indicate a difference of more than 0.5 cm between the two rulers.
Courtesy of KISS Healthcare, Inc.

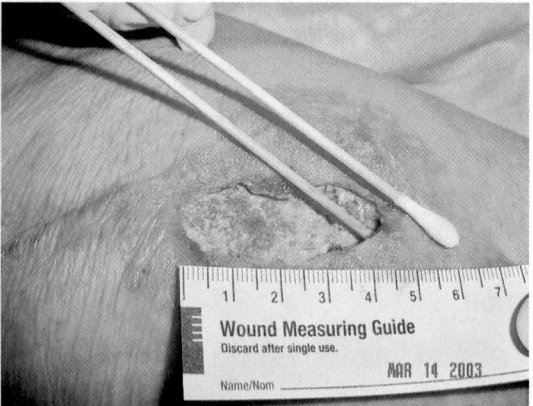

❷ Parallel swabs used to measure wound depth.
Courtesy of Cory Patrick Hartley, RN.

Assessing Wounds and Pressure Ulcers—*continued*

P Pressure Ulcer Risk and Staging - Sweda, Katherine

✓ 🖫 🚫 | 🖎 🗐 ⬆ ⬇ | 🔲 🔳 🖺

*Performed on: 08/17/2014   ▲▼ ▼   1758 ▲▼   CDT   By: Border, Cathy

Braden Assessme
Pressure Ulcer Sta
Push
Faculty Review

Pressure Ulcer Staging

Location

○ Hip, left   ○ Ankle, right
○ Hip, right   ○ Heel, left
○ Sacrum   ○ Heel, right
○ Ankle, left   ○ Other:

Appearance

☐ Black   ☐ White
☐ Pink   ☐ Other:
☐ Red
☐ Yellow

Size of Pressure Ulcer

Depth [_____ cm]   **Length** [_____ cm]   **Width** [_____ cm]

Description of Drainage in Ulcer

☐ Clear   ☐ Serous
☐ Bloody   ☐ Serosanguinous
☐ Green   ☐ Yellow
☐ Purulent   ☐ Other:

Drainage Amount

○ None   ○ Large
○ Scant   ○ Other:
○ Small
○ Moderate

Stage

○ I
○ II
○ III
○ IV
○ Unable to stage/necrotic
○ Other:

Staging Guide

Stage 1- Nonblanchable reddened area. Warmth, edema, induration, hardness, and/or pain may be present.

Stage 2- Partial thickness skin loss involving epidermis, dermis, or both. The ulcer is superficial and may present as an abrasion, blister, or shallow crater.

Stage 3- Full thickness skin loss involving damage to or necrosis of subcutaneous tissue, which may extend down to but not through underlying fascia.

Stage 4-Full thickness skin loss with extensive destruction, tissue necrosis, or damage to muscle, bone, or supporting structures.

In Progress

❸ Pressure ulcer documentation.

SAMPLE DOCUMENTATION

5/31/2015 1000 Wound on (R) hip 3×3 cm, 6 mm deep, draining minimal amt. thick yellow. No odor. Skin around wound erythematous but no undermining. Pain 0 on 0–10 scale ——— N. Jamaghani, RN

EVALUATION

- Perform follow-up assessments and interventions based on findings that deviate from expected or normal for the client. Relate findings to previous assessment data if available.

- Report significant deviations from normal to the primary care provider.

Reporting Wound Infections

The nurse must follow regulations regarding the reporting of wound infections to the agency infection prevention team. Many states have legislation requiring agencies to report health care–associated wound infections. These reports are sent to the National Healthcare Safety Network, a public health surveillance system maintained by the Centers for Disease Control and Prevention's Division of Healthcare Quality Promotion. Also see Chapter 7 ∞ regarding other aspects of infection prevention and control.

DRESSING WOUNDS

The purpose of the wound dressing must be determined before the proper type of dressing can be selected. **Dressings** are materials used to protect the wound, provide humidity to the wound surface, absorb drainage, prevent bleeding, immobilize, and hide the wound from view. The type of dressing is influenced by the location, size, and type of wound. In general, closed wounds (e.g., surgically secured) require dry dressings, whereas open wounds must be kept moist to allow for healing (Sussman, 2012).

Dressing Materials

Gauze, with or without absorbent padding, is commonly used to cover wounds (Figure 31–3 ■). Dressings with a nonadherent gauze surface on one or both sides minimize trauma to the wound during dressing changes. Examples are Adaptic, Cuticerin, Mepitel, petrolatum gauze, Urgotul, Tegapore, and Telfa. Exudate seeps through the surface and collects on the absorbent material on the other side or is sandwiched between the two nonadherent surfaces. Nonadherent dressings should not be used when wound **debridement** (removal of infected and necrotic tissue) is desired.

Larger and thicker gauze dressings, referred to as composite dressings, *surgipads*, or *abdominal (ABD) pads*, may be used to cover plain gauze and are, therefore, referred to as secondary dressings. They not only hold the other gauzes in place but also absorb and collect excess drainage. Surgipads are more absorbent on one side, and this side is placed toward the wound; the less absorbent, more protective side is placed outward to protect the wound from external contamination. The outer side is often indicated with a blue stripe.

More specialized types of wound dressings are described in Table 31–2. In addition to those listed, composite dressings, consisting of layers of two or more of the dressing types or ingredients, may be used. Commonly, the layer closest to the wound is a nonadherent substance, the middle layer is absorbent, and the outer layer controls moisture and gas exchange.

Dressing Changes

To guide dressing selection and changes, the nurse can use the RYB color code of wounds. This concept is based on the color of an open wound—red, yellow, or black (RYB)—rather than the depth or size of a wound. On this scheme, the goals of wound care are to protect (cover) red, cleanse yellow, and debride black.

Wounds that are red are usually in the late regeneration phase of tissue repair (i.e., developing granulation tissue). The nurse protects red wounds by (a) gentle cleansing (i.e., use of a noncytotoxic wound cleanser applied without pressure); (b) protecting periwound skin with alcohol-free barrier film; (c) filling dead space with hydrogel or alginate; (d) covering with an appropriate dressing such as transparent film, hydrocolloid dressing, or a clear absorbent acrylic dressing; and (e) changing the dressing as infrequently as possible.

Yellow wounds are characterized primarily by liquid to semiliquid "slough" that is often accompanied by purulent drainage or previous infection. The nurse cleanses yellow wounds to remove nonviable tissue. Methods used may include applying damp-to-damp normal saline dressings, irrigating the wound, using absorbent dressing materials such as impregnated hydrogel or alginate dressings, and consulting with the primary care provider about the need for a topical antimicrobial to minimize bacterial growth.

Debridement of nonviable tissue from a black wound must occur before the wound can be staged or heal. Debridement may be achieved in different ways: sharp, mechanical, chemical, and autolytic. In *sharp debridement*, a scalpel or scissors is used to separate and remove dead tissue (performed by a primary care provider or advanced practice nurse). *Mechanical debridement* is accomplished through scrubbing force or damp-to-damp dressings. *Chemical debridement* is more selective than sharp or mechanical techniques. Collagenase enzyme agents such as papain-urea are currently most recommended for this use. In *autolytic debridement*, dressings such as hydrocolloid and clear absorbent acrylic dressings trap the wound drainage against the eschar, and the body's own enzymes in the drainage break down the necrotic tissue. Fly larvae (maggots) can also be used to debride wounds, although many clients find them difficult to accept psychologically. Larval therapy can be extremely effective in cleansing chronic wounds because the maggots secrete enzymes that break down necrotic tissue (while leaving healthy tissue untouched), eat bacteria, and decrease bacterial growth through the rise in surface pH that results from their presence (Strohal, 2013).

When the eschar is removed, the wound is treated as yellow, then red. When more than one color is present, the nurse treats the most serious color first, that is, black, then yellow, then red.

Remember that even simple, clean wounds can be very distressing to the client. Some wounds are extremely large, with foul drainage and very unpleasant odors. Be sure that you are nonjudgmental and maintain a neutral facial expression when examining the wound. Nurses can help clients cope and heal by demonstrating acceptance and guiding clients to use correct imagery to promote innate healing abilities. Something as simple as having a client breathe deeply and slowly while picturing healthy, pink tissue growing from the inside out as the nurse is doing a dressing change can be a powerful healing tool.

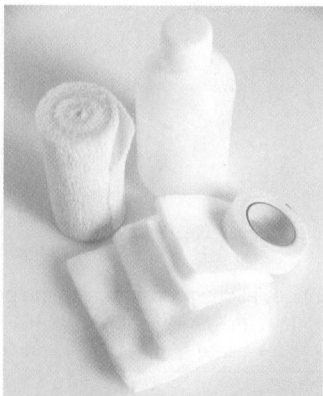

Figure 31–3 ■ Frequently used gauze dressing materials.
izo/Fotolia.

TABLE 31–2 Selected Types of Wound Dressings

Dressing	Description	Purpose	Indications	Examples
Transparent film	Adhesive plastic, semipermeable, nonabsorbent dressings allow exchange of oxygen between the atmosphere and wound surface. They are impermeable to bacteria and water.	To provide protection against contamination and friction; to maintain a clean moist surface that facilitates cellular migration; to provide insulation by preventing fluid evaporation; and to facilitate wound assessment	IV dressing Central line dressing Superficial wounds Pressure ulcers stage I	Bioclusive, Op-Site, Polyskin, Tegaderm
Impregnated nonadherent	Woven or nonwoven cotton or synthetic materials are impregnated with petroleum jelly, saline, zinc-saline, antimicrobials, or other agents. Require secondary dressings to secure them in place, retain moisture, and provide wound protection.	To cover, soothe, and protect partial- and full-thickness wounds without exudate	Postoperative dressing over staple/sutures Superficial burns	Adaptic, Aquaphor gauze, Carrasyn, Xeroform dressings
Hydrocolloids	Waterproof adhesive wafers, pastes, or powders. Wafers, designed to be worn for up to 7 days, consist of two layers. The inner adhesive layer has particles that absorb exudates and form a hydrated gel over the wound; the outer film provides an occlusive seal.	To absorb exudate; to produce a moist environment that facilitates healing but does not cause maceration of surrounding skin; to protect the wound from bacterial contamination, foreign debris, and urine or feces; and to prevent shearing	Pressure ulcers stages II–IV Autolytic debridement of eschar Partial-thickness wounds	Comfeel, DuoDERM, RepliCare, Restore, Tegasorb
Clear absorbent acrylic	Transparent absorbent wafer designed to be worn 5–7 days. The acrylic layer absorbs exudates and evaporates the excess off the transparent membrane.	To maintain a transparent membrane for easy wound bed assessment; to provide bacterial and shearing protection; to maintain moist wound healing; can be used with alginates to provide packing to deeper wound beds	Pressure ulcers Skin tears Venous stasis ulcers Surgical wounds Wounds undergoing chemical debridement	Tegaderm absorbent
Hydrogels	Glycerin or water-based nonadhesive jelly-like sheets, granules, or gels. Semipermeable to O_2 and CO_2 unless covered by a plastic film.	To liquefy necrotic tissue or slough, rehydrate the wound bed, and fill in dead space	Pressure ulcers Skin tears Partial-thickness wounds	Carrasyn, Elasto-Gel, NU-GEL, Purilon, Tegagel, Vigilon
Polyurethane foams	Nonadherent hydrocolloid dressings; these need to have their edges taped down or sealed. Require secondary dressings to obtain an occlusive environment. Surrounding skin must be protected to prevent maceration. Easy to cut and fit to the wound.	To absorb up to heavy amounts of exudate; to provide and maintain moist wound healing; to provide thermal insulation	Light to highly exudating wounds Pressure ulcers Skin tears Venous stasis ulcers Surgical wounds Wounds undergoing chemical debridement	Allevyn, Curafoam, Flexzan, Lyofoam, VigiFOAM
Alginates (exudate absorbers)	Nonadherent dressings of powder, beads or granules, ropes, sheets, or paste conform to the wound surface and absorb up to 20 times their weight in exudate; require a secondary dressing.	To provide a moist wound surface by interacting with exudate to form a gelatinous mass; to absorb exudate; to eliminate dead space or pack wounds; and to support debridement	Pressure ulcers Skin tears Venous stasis ulcers Surgical wounds Wounds undergoing chemical debridement agents	AlgiDerm, Curasorb, Debrisan, Kaltostat, Sorbsan
Collagen	Gels, pastes, powders, granules, sheets, and sponges are derived from animal sources—often cow or pig.	To assist with stopping bleeding; to help recruit cells into the wound and stimulate their proliferation to facilitate healing	Clean, moist wounds	Biostep, Cellerate RX, NU-GEL, Promogran

A general principle is that every effort should be made to keep sterile wounds sterile but that eventually, the surface of sterile wounds will become contaminated by the environment (which is, of course, not the same thing as being infected). Thus, in many agencies, both sterile and contaminated wounds can be dressed using clean rather than sterile technique. The main consideration for not using a sterile field and gloves is cost. The nurse should be skilled in both sterile and clean technique and choose the most appropriate method based on agency policy, available resources, and client need.

●○○● NURSING PROCESS: DRESSING WOUNDS

Performing a Dry Dressing Change

ASSESSMENT
- Before changing a dressing, review the client record for information regarding the cause of the wound, the length of time the wound has been present, and previous treatment and response to treatment.

- Determine allergies to wound cleaning agents, dressings, or tape; complaints of discomfort; the time of the last pain medication; and signs of systemic infection (e.g., elevated body temperature, diaphoresis, malaise, leukocytosis).

PLANNING
- If possible, schedule the dressing change at a time convenient for the client. Some dressing changes require only a few minutes, and others can take much longer. Dressing changes necessitated by a change in the wound or dressing condition may not be scheduled.
- Determine if the client requires premedication for pain or other pain management techniques prior to wound care (see Chapter 9 ∞).

SAFETY ALERT!   SAFETY

2014 The Joint Commission National Patient Safety Goals (2013a)

GOAL 3: IMPROVE THE SAFETY OF USING MEDICATIONS.
Label all medications, medication containers, and other solutions on and off the sterile field in perioperative and other procedural settings. Medications or other solutions in unlabeled containers are unidentifiable. Errors, sometimes tragic, have resulted from medications and other solutions removed from their original containers and placed into unlabeled containers.

DELEGATION

Due to the need for aseptic technique and assessment skills, most dressing changes are not delegated to UAP. In some states, UAP may apply dry dressings to clean, chronic wounds. UAP should observe an exposed wound or dressing during usual care and must report abnormal findings to the nurse. In some agencies, UAP may be permitted to reinforce the dressing (apply additional dry dressings over a saturated bandage), but this must be reported to the nurse as soon as possible. Assessment of the wound and abnormal findings must be validated and interpreted by the nurse.

Equipment
- Clean gloves
- Sterile gloves (optional)
- 4×4 gauze
- Hypoallergenic tape, tie tapes, or binder
- Bath blanket (if necessary)
- Moisture-proof bag
- Mask (optional)
- Acetone or another solution (if necessary to loosen adhesive)
- Sterile dressing set; if none is available, gather the following sterile items:
  - Drape or towel
  - Gauze squares
  - Container for the cleaning solution
  - Antimicrobial solution
  - Forceps
- Additional supplies required for the particular dressing (e.g., extra gauze dressings and ointment or powder, if ordered)

INTERPROFESSIONAL PRACTICE

Dressing wounds may be within the scope of practice for other health care providers. For example, in addition to nurses, both physical therapists and occupational therapists commonly dress wounds after treatment. Although the therapists may verbally communicate their findings and plan to the health care team members, the nurse must also know where to locate their documentation in the client's medical record.

IMPLEMENTATION
Preparation
- Acquire assistance for changing a dressing on a restless or confused adult. **Rationale:** *The person might move and contaminate the sterile field or the wound.*
- Make a cuff on the moisture-proof bag for disposal of the soiled dressings, and place the bag within reach. **Rationale:** *Making a cuff keeps the outside of the bag free from contamination by the soiled dressings and prevents subsequent contamination of the nurse's hands or of sterile instrument tips when discarding dressings or sponges. Placement of the bag within reach prevents the nurse from reaching across the sterile field and the wound and potentially contaminating these areas.*

Performance
1. Prior to performing the procedure, introduce self and verify the client's identity using agency protocol. Explain to the client what you are going to do, why it is necessary, and how he or she can

participate. Discuss how the results will be used in planning further care or treatments.
2. Perform hand hygiene and observe other appropriate infection prevention procedures.
3. Provide for client privacy. Assist the client to a comfortable position in which the wound can be readily exposed. Expose only the wound area and cover the rest of the client, if necessary. **Rationale:** *Undue exposure is physically and psychologically distressing to most people.*
4. Apply a face mask, as indicated. **Rationale:** *A mask may be worn for surgical dressing changes to prevent contamination of the wound by droplet spray from the nurse's respiratory tract.*
5. Remove outer dressings.
   - Apply clean gloves.
   - If adhesive tape was used, remove it by holding down the skin and pulling the tape gently but firmly toward the

Performing a Dry Dressing Change—*continued*

wound. **Rationale:** *Pressing down on the skin provides countertraction against the pulling motion. Tape is pulled toward the incision to prevent strain on the sutures or wound.*

- Use a solvent to loosen tape, if required. **Rationale:** *Moistening the tape with acetone or a similar solvent lessens the discomfort of removal, particularly from hairy surfaces.*
- Lift the dressing so that the underside is away from the client's face. **Rationale:** *The appearance and odor of the drainage may be upsetting to the client.*

6. Dispose of soiled dressings appropriately.
- Place the soiled dressing in the moisture-proof bag without touching the outside of the bag. **Rationale:** *Contamination of the outside of the bag is avoided to prevent the spread of microorganisms to the nurse and subsequently to others.*
- Remove gloves, dispose of them in the moisture-proof bag, and perform hand hygiene.

7. Remove inner dressings.
- Open the sterile dressing set, using aseptic technique (see Chapter 7 ∞).
- Place the sterile drape beside the wound or on the bedside table to form a sterile field. Open individual sterile equipment and place on the field. Apply sterile gloves (optional).
- Remove the underdressings with forceps or sterile gloves. **Rationale:** *Forceps or gloves are used to prevent contamination of the wound by the nurse's hands and contamination of the nurse's hands by wound drainage.*
- Assess the location, type (color, consistency), and odor of wound drainage, and the number of gauzes saturated or the diameter of drainage collected on the dressings.
- Discard the soiled dressings in the bag.
- After the dressings are removed, discard the forceps, or set them aside from the sterile field. **Rationale:** *These are now contaminated by the wound drainage.* Remove and discard sterile gloves if applied. Perform hand hygiene.

8. Assess the overall appearance of the wound and measure wound size (see Skill 31–1).

9. Clean the wound if indicated (also see Practice Guidelines).
- Clean the wound, using a new pair of forceps, clean gloves, and moistened swabs.
- Keep the forceps tips lower than the handles at all times. **Rationale:** *This prevents their contamination by fluid traveling up to the handle, coming in contact with nonsterile gloves, and then flowing back to the tips.*
- Clean with strokes from the top to the bottom, starting at the center and continuing to the outside. ❶

or

- Clean outward from the center of the wound. ❷ **Rationale:** *The wound is cleaned from the least to the most contaminated area.*
- Use a separate swab for each stroke, and discard each swab after use. **Rationale:** *This prevents the introduction of microorganisms to other wound areas.*
- Repeat the cleaning process until all drainage is removed.
- Remove and discard gloves.
- Perform hand hygiene.

10. Apply sterile dressings.
- Apply sterile dressings one at a time over the wound, using sterile forceps or sterile gloves. Start at the center of the wound and move progressively outward. The final surgipad

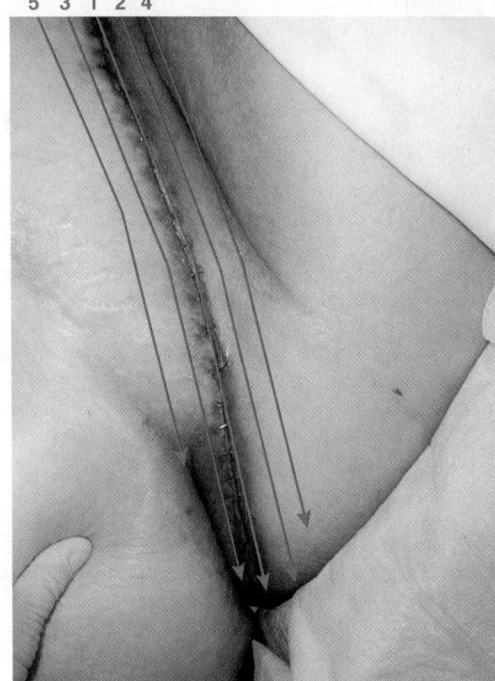

5 3 1 2 4

❶ Cleaning a wound from the midpoint outward and from top to bottom.
Courtesy of Cory Patrick Hartley, RN.

can be picked up by hand, touching only the outside, which is often marked by a blue line down the center.
- Remove and discard gloves if used.
- Perform hand hygiene.

11. Secure the dressing with tape, tie tapes, or a binder.
- Place the tape so that the dressing cannot be folded back to expose the wound. Place strips at the ends of the dressing, and space tapes evenly in the middle. ❸
- Ensure that the tape is long and wide enough to adhere to the skin but not so long or wide that it loosens with activity.
- Place the tape in the opposite direction from the body action, for example, across a body joint or crease, not lengthwise. ❹

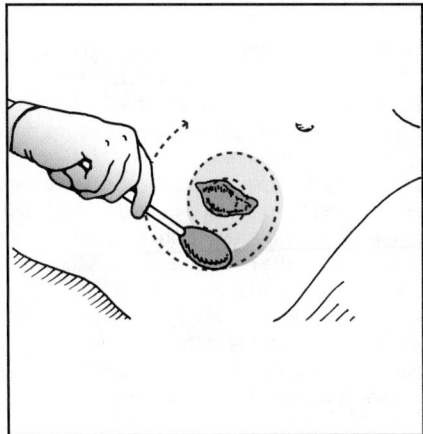

❷ Cleaning a wound from the center outward.

Continued on page 674

Performing a Dry Dressing Change—*continued*

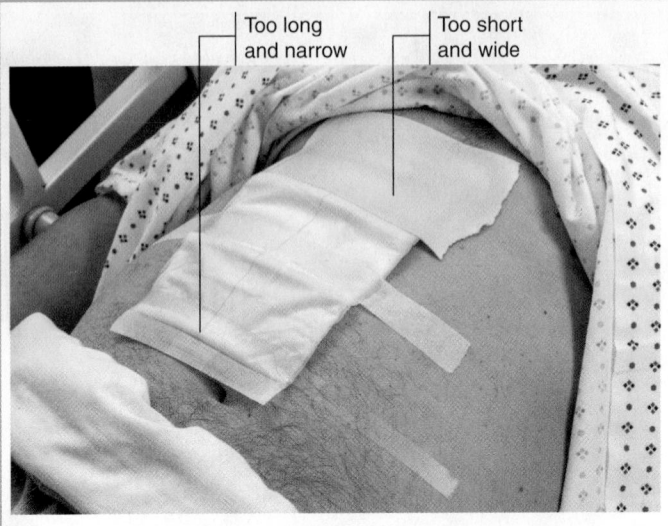

Too long and narrow | Too short and wide

❸ Taping the dressing.

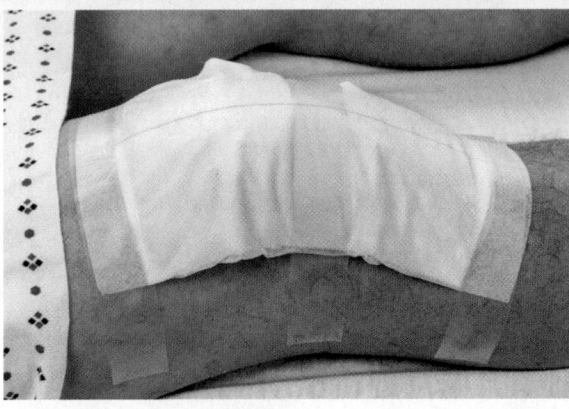

❹ Dressings over moving parts should be taped at a right angle to the joint movement.

- *Montgomery straps (tie tapes)* are commonly used for wounds requiring frequent dressing changes. ❺ **Rationale:** *These straps prevent the skin irritation and discomfort caused by removing the adhesive each time the dressing is changed.*
- For clients with tape allergies or other conditions in which tape should not be applied directly to the skin, wrap over the dressing and around the body part with rolled gauze, and tape only the gauze.

12. Document the dressing change and the client's response in the client record using forms or checklists supplemented by narrative notes when appropriate. Electronic health records will use a designated wound/skin documentation sheet (see Figure ❸ in Skill 31–1).

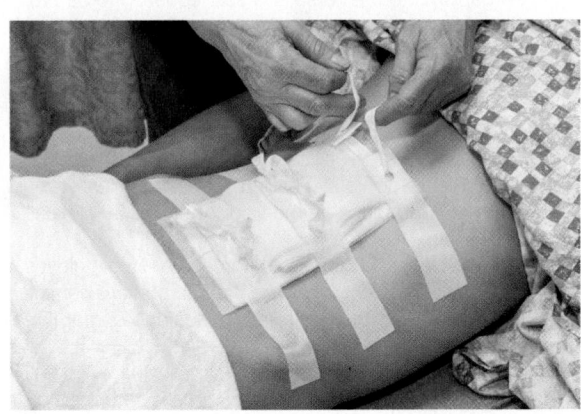

❺ Montgomery straps, or tie tapes, are used to secure large dressings that require frequent changing.

EVALUATION

- Perform follow-up based on findings that deviate from expected or normal for the client. Relate findings to previous assessment data if available.

- Report significant deviations from normal to the primary care provider.

Cleaning Wounds

- Follow standard precautions for personal protection. Wear gloves, gown, goggles, and mask as indicated.
- Use solutions such as isotonic saline or wound cleansers to clean or irrigate wounds. If antimicrobial solutions are used, make sure they are well diluted.
- Microwave heating of liquids for cleaning is not recommended. When possible, warm the solution to body temperature before use. **Rationale:** *Warming prevents lowering the wound temperature, which slows the healing process. Microwave heating could cause the solution to become too hot.*
- If a wound is grossly contaminated by foreign material, bacteria, slough, or necrotic tissue, clean the wound at every dressing change. **Rationale:** *Foreign bodies and devitalized tissue act as a focus for infection and can delay healing.*
- If a wound is clean, has little exudate, and reveals healthy granulation tissue, avoid repeated cleaning. **Rationale:** *Unnecessary cleaning can delay wound healing by traumatizing newly produced, delicate tissues; reducing the surface temperature of the wound; and removing exudate, which itself may have bactericidal properties.*

- Use gauze squares or nonwoven swabs that do not shed fibers. Avoid using cotton balls and other products that shed fibers onto the wound surface. **Rationale:** *The fibers become embedded in granulation tissue and can act as foci for infection. They may also stimulate "foreign body" reactions, prolonging the inflammatory phase of healing and delaying the healing process.*
- Clean superficial noninfected wounds by irrigating them with normal saline. **Rationale:** *The hydraulic pressure of an irrigating stream of fluid dislodges contaminating debris and reduces bacterial colonization.*
- Avoid drying a wound after cleaning it. **Rationale:** *This helps retain wound moisture.*
- Hold cleaning sponges with sterile forceps or with a sterile gloved hand.
- Clean from the wound in an outward direction to avoid transferring organisms from the surrounding skin into the wound.
- Consider not cleaning the wound at all if it appears to be clean.

SKILL 31-3

Transparent Wound Barriers

Transparent semipermeable membrane (TSM) dressings, called **transparent wound barriers** or transparent film, help retain wound moisture while allowing gases (oxygen, carbon dioxide) to pass into and away from the wound. They are occlusive in that they allow bathing without removing or changing the dressing, and microorganisms are repelled. An advantage of transparent wound barriers is that they do not adhere to wound surfaces and can be left in place for up to 1 week.

Applying a Transparent Wound Barrier

ASSESSMENT
See Skill 31–2.

PLANNING
See Skill 31–2.

DELEGATION

See Skill 31–2.

INTERPROFESSIONAL PRACTICE

See Skill 31–2.

Equipment
- Clean gloves
- Sterile gloves (optional)
- Hair scissors or clippers
- Alcohol or acetone
- Moisture-proof bag
- Sterile gauze and the wound-cleaning agents specified by the primary care provider or agency (e.g., sterile saline)
- Wound barrier dressing
- Scissors
- Paper tape

IMPLEMENTATION
Preparation
- Review the order regarding frequency and type of dressing change, and determine agency protocol about solutions used to clean the wound and whether clean or sterile technique is to be used. Many agencies recommend clean rather than sterile technique for chronic wounds such as a pressure ulcer.
- If possible, schedule the dressing change at a time convenient for the client. Some dressing changes require only a few minutes, and others can take much longer.

Performance
1. Prior to performing the procedure, introduce self and verify the client's identity using agency protocol. Explain to the client what you are going to do, why it is necessary, and how he or she can participate. Discuss how the results will be used in planning further care or treatments.
2. Perform hand hygiene and observe other appropriate infection prevention procedures.
3. Provide for client privacy. Assist the client to a comfortable position in which the wound can be readily exposed. Expose only the wound area and cover the rest of the client, if necessary. **Rationale:** Undue exposure is physically and psychologically distressing to most people.
4. Remove the existing dressing (see Skill 31–2, steps 5 through 7).
5. Assess the wound.
   - See Skill 31–1.
6. Thoroughly clean the skin area around the wound.
   - Apply clean gloves.
   - Clean the skin well with normal saline or a mild cleansing agent. Always rinse and dry the adjacent skin well before applying a dressing.
   - Clip the hair about 5 cm (2 in.) around the wound area if the amount of hair will prevent the dressing from sticking. Do not use a standard bladed razor because it can cause small nicks in the skin and create or spread infection.
   - Remove gloves and dispose of them in the moisture-proof bag.
   - Perform hand hygiene.
7. Clean the wound if indicated.
   - Apply clean or sterile gloves in accordance with agency protocol.

- Clean the wound with the prescribed solution.
- Dry the surrounding skin with dry gauze.
8. Apply the wound barrier.
   - Review the instructions on the barrier package. Remove part of the paper backing on the dressing. ❶
   - Apply the dressing at one edge of the wound site, allowing at least 2.5-cm (1-in.) coverage of the skin surrounding the wound.
   - Gently lay or press the barrier over the wound. Keep it free of wrinkles, but avoid stretching it too tightly. **Rationale:** *A stretched dressing restricts mobility and can pull loose easily.*
   - Remove and discard gloves.
   - Perform hand hygiene.
9. Reinforce the dressing only if absolutely needed. **Rationale:** *Additional dressing over the transparent barrier will constrict the flow of gases.*
   - Apply paper or other porous tape to "window frame" the edges of the dressing.
10. Assess the wound at least daily.
    - Determine the extent of serous fluid accumulation under the dressing, wound healing, and the need to repair the dressing.

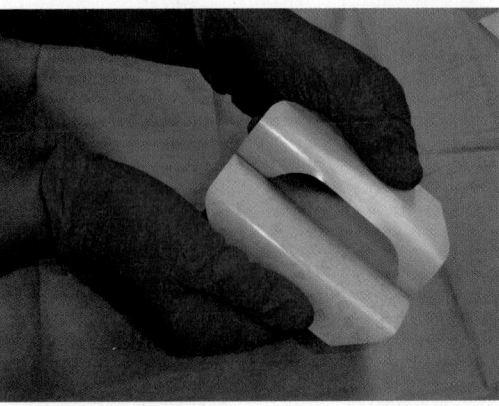

❶ Transparent wound dressing.

Continued on page 676

Applying a Transparent Wound Barrier—*continued*

- If excessive serum has accumulated, consider replacing the transparent wound barrier with a more absorbent type of dressing, such as hydrocolloid.
- If the dressing is leaking, remove it and apply another dressing.

11. Document the dressing change and the client's response in the client record using forms or checklists supplemented by narrative notes when appropriate. Electronic health records will use a designated wound/skin documentation sheet (see Figure ❸ in Skill 31–1).

CLINICAL ALERT!

To remove a TSM dressing, grasp one edge of the dressing and gently pull straight out to stretch it and release the adhesion. By stretching the dressing, the material expands and releases until the dressing is removed. To aid in lifting the dressing edge, press a small piece of tape onto a corner of the dressing and continue with the stretch release method of removal.

EVALUATION

- Perform follow-up based on findings that deviate from expected or normal for the client. Relate findings to previous assessment data if available.

- Report significant deviations from normal to the primary care provider.

Hydrocolloid Dressings

Hydrocolloid (a substance that forms a gel with water) dressings are frequently used for stasis and pressure ulcers. They are occlusive, allow bathing without removing or changing the dressing, and repel external microorganisms. They do not adhere to wound surfaces. They can remain in place for up to 1 week and are easily molded to fit the wound and body location. However, they are also opaque and do not allow easy examination of the wound. If microorganisms are present in the wound, the dressing can facilitate their growth. Therefore, they are not used on infected wounds.

Applying a Hydrocolloid Dressing

ASSESSMENT
See Skill 31–2.

PLANNING
See Skill 31–2.

DELEGATION
See Skill 31–2.

INTERPROFESSIONAL PRACTICE
See Skill 31–2.

Equipment
- Clean gloves
- Sterile gloves (optional)
- Hair scissors or clippers
- Alcohol or acetone
- Moisture-proof bag
- Sterile gauze and the wound-cleaning agents specified by the primary care provider or agency (e.g., sterile saline)
- Hydrocolloid dressing at least 3 to 4 cm (1.2 to 1.5 in.) larger than the wound on all four sides (Sussman, 2012) ❶
- Scissors
- Paper tape

❶ Hydrocolloid dressing.
SPL/Custom Medical Stock Photo.

IMPLEMENTATION
Preparation
- Review the order regarding frequency and type of dressing change, and determine agency protocol about solutions used to clean the wound and whether clean or sterile technique is to be used. Many agencies recommend clean rather than sterile technique for chronic wounds such as a pressure ulcer.
- Change the dressing if it leaks, is dislodged, or develops an odor. Otherwise, it may remain in place up to 1 week.

- If possible, schedule the dressing change at a time convenient for the client. Some dressing changes require only a few minutes and others can take much longer.

Performance
1. Prior to performing the procedure, introduce self and verify the client's identity using agency protocol. Explain to the client what you are going to do, why it is necessary, and how he or she can

Applying a Hydrocolloid Dressing—*continued*

participate. Discuss how the results will be used in planning further care or treatments.

2. Perform hand hygiene and observe other appropriate infection prevention procedures.

3. Provide for client privacy. Assist the client to a comfortable position in which the wound can be readily exposed. Expose only the wound area and cover the rest of the client, if necessary. **Rationale:** *Undue exposure is physically and psychologically distressing to most people.*

4. Remove the existing dressing (see Skill 31–2, steps 5 through 7).

5. Assess the wound.
   • See Skill 31–1.

6. Thoroughly clean the skin area around the wound.
   • Apply clean gloves.
   • Clean the skin well but gently with normal saline or a mild cleansing agent. Always rinse and dry the adjacent skin well before applying a dressing.
   • Clip the hair about 5 cm (2 in.) around the wound area if the amount of hair will prevent the dressing from sticking. Do not use a standard bladed razor because it can cause small nicks in the skin and create or spread infection.
   • Leave the residue that is difficult to remove on the skin. It will wear off in time. Attempts to remove residue can irritate the surrounding skin.

• Remove gloves and dispose of them in the moisture-proof bag.
• Perform hand hygiene.

7. Clean the wound if indicated.
   • Apply clean or sterile gloves in accordance with agency protocol.
   • Clean the wound with the prescribed solution.
   • Dry the surrounding skin with dry gauze.

8. Apply the dressing.
   • Follow the manufacturer's instructions for removing the adhesive backing and applying the dressing.
   • Remove and discard gloves.
   • Perform hand hygiene.
   • *Optional:* Apply tape to "window frame" the edges of the dressing or according to agency protocol. **Rationale:** *Taping prevents the dressing from sticking to bed linens and the edges from lifting.*

9. Assess and change the dressing as indicated.
   • Inspect the dressing at least daily for leakage, dislodgment, odor, and wrinkling.
   • Change the dressing if any of these signs are present.

10. Document the dressing change and the client's response in the client record using forms or checklists supplemented by narrative notes when appropriate. Electronic health records will use a designated wound/skin documentation sheet (see Figure ❸ in Skill 31–1).

EVALUATION

• Perform follow-up based on findings that deviate from expected or normal for the client. Relate findings to previous assessment data if available.

• Report significant deviations from normal to the primary care provider.

SKILL 31-4

TREATING WOUNDS

Sometimes, simply applying a dressing over a wound is not adequate to promote healing.

Newer biophysical agents may be used such as electrical stimulation, radio-frequency or electromagnetic fields, ultraviolet and laser light therapy, ultrasound, and hyperbaric oxygen. These agents have the ability to affect one or more of the barriers to healing (e.g., ischemia, infection, or moisture balance). These therapies may be selected and implemented by the wound specialist nurse in consultation with the primary care provider.

If the wound fails to heal due to infection or presence of debris in it, the wound may need more aggressive cleaning, such as can be done through irrigating or packing it with various materials. Also see Chapter 8 ∞ regarding the application of heat and cold to wounds.

Irrigating a Wound

Irrigation is the washing or flushing out of an area. Wound irrigation is performed using aseptic technique and normal saline or antiseptic solution.

●○● NURSING PROCESS: IRRIGATING A WOUND

Irrigating a Wound

ASSESSMENT

Review the client's record to determine:
• Previous appearance and size of the wound.
• Character of the exudate.

• Presence of pain and the time when pain medication was last administered.
• Clinical signs of systemic infection.
• Allergies to the wound irrigation agent or tape.

PLANNING

• Before irrigating a wound, determine (a) the type of irrigating solution, (b) the frequency of irrigations, and (c) the temperature of the solution.
• If possible, schedule the irrigation at a time convenient for the client. Some irrigations require only a few minutes, and others can take much longer.

• Determine if the client requires premedication for pain or other pain management techniques prior to wound care (see Chapter 9 ∞).

SKILL 31-5

Continued on page 678

Irrigating a Wound—*continued*

DELEGATION

Due to the need for aseptic technique and assessment skills, wound irrigations are not delegated to UAP. However, UAP may observe the wound and dressing during usual care and must report abnormal findings to the nurse. Abnormal findings must be validated and interpreted by the nurse.

INTERPROFESSIONAL PRACTICE

Irrigating wounds may be within the scope of practice for other health care providers. For example, in addition to nurses, physical therapists may irrigate wounds before treatment. Although the therapists may verbally communicate their findings and plan to the health care team members, the nurse must also know where to locate their documentation in the client's medical record.

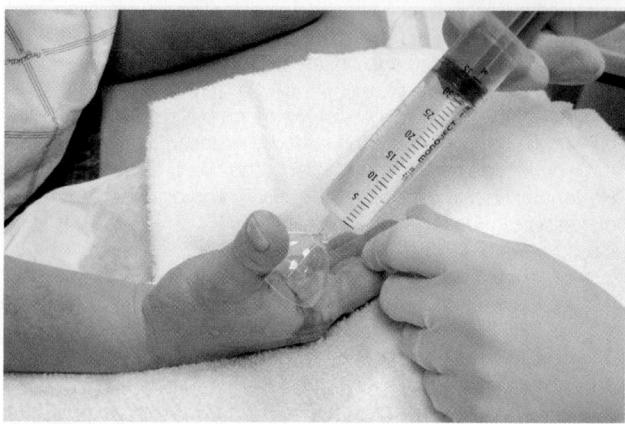

① A splash guard prevents contaminated fluid from spreading.
Courtesy of Cory Patrick Hartley, RN.

Equipment

Although a wound may already be contaminated, sterile equipment is usually used during irrigation to prevent the possibility of adding new nonresident microorganisms to the site. In settings outside of hospitals, some reusable supplies such as irrigating syringes or basins may be cleaned and used again for a specific wound.

- Sterile dressing equipment and dressing materials
- Sterile irrigation set or individual supplies, including:
  - Sterile syringe (e.g., a 30- to 60-mL syringe) with a catheter of an appropriate size (e.g., #18 or #19) or an irrigating tip syringe
  - Splash shield for syringe (optional) **①**

- Sterile graduated container for irrigating solution
- Basin for collecting the used irrigating solution
- Moisture-resistant sterile drape
- Moisture-resistant bag
- Irrigating solution, usually 200 mL (6.5 oz) of solution warmed to body temperature, according to the agency's or primary care provider's choice
- Goggles, gown, and mask
- Clean gloves
- Sterile gloves (optional)

IMPLEMENTATION

Preparation

Check that the irrigating fluid is at the proper temperature.

Performance

1. Prior to performing the procedure, introduce self and verify the client's identity using agency protocol. Explain to the client what you are going to do, why it is necessary, and how he or she can participate. Discuss how the results will be used in planning further care or treatments.
2. Perform hand hygiene and observe other appropriate infection prevention procedures.
3. Provide for client privacy.
4. Prepare the client.
   - Assist the client to a position in which the irrigating solution will flow by gravity from the upper end of the wound to the lower end and then into the basin.
   - Place the waterproof drape under the wound and over the bed.
   - Apply clean gloves and remove and discard the old dressing.
5. Measure and assess the wound and drainage (see Skill 31–1).
   - If indicated, clean the wound (see Skill 31–2, step 9).
   - Remove and discard gloves.
   - Perform hand hygiene.
6. Prepare the equipment.
   - Open the sterile dressing set and supplies.
   - Pour the ordered solution into the solution container.
   - Position the basin below the wound to receive the irrigating fluid.
7. Irrigate the wound.
   - Apply clean gloves.
   - Instill a steady stream of irrigating solution into the wound. Make sure all areas of the wound are irrigated.

- Use either a syringe with a catheter attached or an irrigating tip to flush the wound. **②**
- If you are using a catheter to reach tracts or crevices, insert the catheter into the wound until resistance is met. Do not force the catheter. **Rationale:** *Forcing the catheter can cause tissue damage.*
- Continue irrigating until the solution becomes clear (no blood or exudate is present).
- Dry the area around the wound. **Rationale:** *Moisture left on the skin promotes the growth of microorganisms and can cause skin irritation and breakdown.*
- Remove and discard gloves.
- Perform hand hygiene.

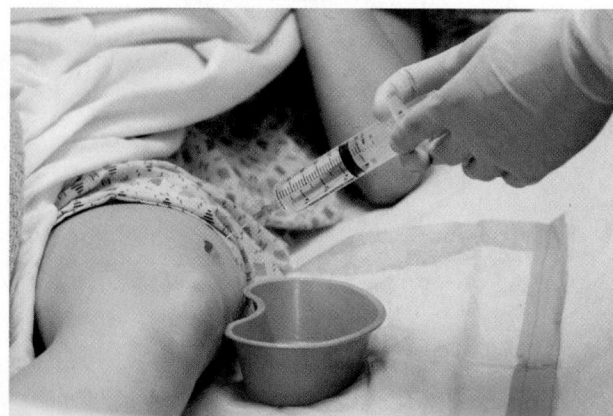

② Irrigating an open wound.

Irrigating a Wound—*continued*

8. Assess and dress the wound.
   - Assess the appearance of the wound again, noting in particular the type and amount of exudate still present and the presence and extent of granulation tissue.
   - Using sterile or clean technique, apply a sterile dressing to the wound based on the amount of drainage expected (see Table 31–2).
   - Remove and discard gloves.
   - Perform hand hygiene.
9. Document the irrigation and the client's response in the client record using forms or checklists supplemented by narrative notes when appropriate. Electronic health records will use a designated wound/skin documentation sheet (see Figure ❸ in Skill 31–1).

SAMPLE DOCUMENTATION

5/31/2015 1000 Wound on (R) hip 3×3 cm, 6 mm deep, draining minimal amt. thick yellow. No odor. Skin around wound erythematous. Pain 0 on 0–10 scale. Irrigated with NS until clear. Redressed using sterile technique. ———————————— N. Jamaghani, RN

EVALUATION

- Perform follow-up based on findings that deviate from expected or normal for the client. Relate findings to previous assessment data if available.
- Report significant deviations from normal to the primary care provider.

Sitz Baths

Another method of irrigating a wound is to immerse the body part in circulating warm water such as in a whirlpool bathtub. If the affected area is located in the perineal region, rather than immersing the entire body, the perineal area may be soaked in only a few inches of water by use of a **sitz bath**. The word *sitz* is German for *sit*. Sitz baths may be indicated for clients with hemorrhoids or anal fissures, for those who have had rectal surgery, following childbirth, or for many other perineal conditions involving pain, itching, or wounds.

●○● NURSING PROCESS: ASSISTING WITH A SITZ BATH

Assisting with a Sitz Bath

ASSESSMENT
Review the client's record to determine:
- Previous appearance and size of the wound.
- Character of any exudate.
- Presence of pain and the time when pain medication was last administered.

PLANNING
- Confirm the primary care provider's order for the length of time and frequency of the sitz baths. If possible, arrange the timing of the sitz baths to avoid interference with meals or visitors since the bath takes approximately 30 minutes.
- Because the nurse cannot remain with the client during the entire bath, ensure that the client is competent and safe to be left alone (with a call bell, of course).
- Determine if the client requires premedication for pain or other pain management techniques prior to wound care (see Chapter 9 ∞).

DELEGATION

Once the wound has been assessed and the safety of the client has been ensured, a sitz bath can be established and monitored by UAP. The nurse must confirm that the UAP knows which client reactions to the bath should be reported to the nurse. For example, the UAP should report any client complaints of dizziness, increased pain, or a burning sensation. The nurse will apply any dressings needed after the sitz bath is complete.

INTERPROFESSIONAL PRACTICE

Assisting the client with a sitz bath may be within the scope of practice for other health care providers such as physical therapists. Although the therapists may verbally communicate their findings and plan to the health care team members, the nurse must also know where to locate their documentation in the client's medical record.

Equipment
- Sitz bath (Some facilities have a built-in sitz bath similar to a bathtub. In most situations, a plastic, disposable, portable sitz bath is used. ❶ The system consists of the basin, solution bag, and tubing.)
- IV pole, door hook, or other means of hanging the solution bag above the level of the bath
- Clean client gown
- Bath towels
- Bath blanket
- Bath mat
- Solution or water source
- Clean gloves
- Moisture-resistant bag to hold used dressings, if needed

Continued on page 680

Assisting with a Sitz Bath—*continued*

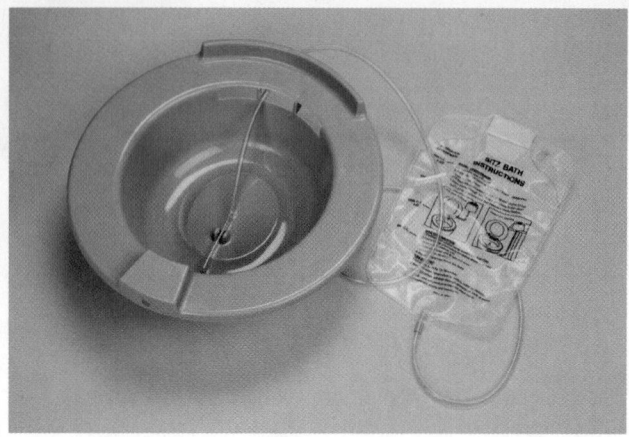

❶ A plastic, single-client sitz bath.

IMPLEMENTATION

Preparation

If the client has had sitz baths previously, determine if there were any difficulties and plan accordingly. Establish whether the client can walk to the bath or requires assistance with mobility.

Performance

1. Introduce self and verify the client's identity using agency protocol. Explain to the client what the sitz bath is, why it is necessary, and how he or she can participate. Discuss how the results will be used in planning further care or treatments.
2. Perform hand hygiene and observe other appropriate infection prevention procedures.
3. Provide for client privacy. If indicated, obtain a "Do Not Disturb" sign for the bathroom door.
4. Set up the sitz bath.
   - Place the disposable basin in the toilet. Generally, the tubing enters the front of the basin and drains at the rear.
   - Close the clamp on the tubing. Fill the solution bag with the desired amount of the ordered fluid at the required temperature—usually tap water warmed to 40°C to 43°C (105°F to 110°F) and hang above basin level.
   - Place the end of the tubing securely in the sitz bath channel designed to hold it in place.
   - If the ordered solution is plain warm tap water, fill the basin half full.
5. Position the client appropriately.
   - Assist the client to remove underclothing. If a dressing is present, apply clean gloves and remove and discard the dressing in the moisture-proof bag.

   - Assess the wound, if visible (see Skill 31–1).
   - Assist the client to sit securely on the sitz bath.
   - Cover the client with a gown and blankets as indicated so he or she does not chill.
6. Begin continuous slow flow of solution from the bag or show the client how to open the clamp as the solution in the basin cools. The solution will fill the basin and overflow into the toilet, bathing the treatment area. If necessary, return and refill the bag with additional solution.
7. Provide the client with a call bell or other means of requesting assistance. Be certain to tell the client when someone will return to assist with completion of the sitz bath. Generally, the fluid flow or soaking lasts 20 minutes.
8. When the sitz bath is finished, assist the client to rise. Apply clean gloves. Dry and dress the wound area as ordered.
9. Empty the sitz bath basin. Rinse, clean, and store it according to agency guidelines.
   - Remove and discard gloves.
   - Perform hand hygiene.
10. Document the bath, the wound condition, and the client's response in the client record using forms or checklists supplemented by narrative notes when appropriate. Electronic health records will use a designated wound/skin documentation sheet (see Figure ❸ in Skill 31–1).

EVALUATION

- Perform follow-up based on findings that deviate from expected or normal for the client. Relate findings to previous assessment data if available.

- Report significant deviations from normal to the primary care provider.

Packing a Wound

Various materials may be placed in a wound to facilitate formation of granulation tissue, removal of necrotic material, and healing by secondary intention. Continuous-thread 4×4 gauze without filling, medicated gauze, and narrow packing gauze may be ordered. Although gauze is much less expensive than advanced dressings (e.g., polymers, alginates, collagens), the cost per week can be higher due to the number of dressing changes required ("Wet-to-dry," 2011). Including the price of the dressing, gloves, saline, and tape,

the materials cost for a gauze dressing change twice per day versus an advanced dressing change three times per week is very similar. However, for clients at home, the cost per nurse home visit makes the gauze dressing almost five times as expensive. In addition, wounds have been shown to heal twice as quickly with advanced dressings compared to gauze. Practitioners should become familiar with the range and uses of advanced dressing materials. The selection of dressing materials must consider time, material cost, client comfort, and speed of wound healing.

●○●● NURSING PROCESS: PACKING A WOUND

Performing a Damp-to-Damp Dressing Change

ASSESSMENT

Review the client's record to determine:

- Previous appearance, size, and treatment of the wound.
- Character of any exudate.
- Presence of pain and the time when pain medication was last administered.
- Clinical signs of systemic infection.
- Allergies to medications or tape.

PLANNING

- Before packing a wound, determine the type of packing to be used and the frequency of dressing changes.
- If possible, schedule the dressing change at a time convenient for the client. Some packings require only a few minutes, and others can take much longer.
- Determine if the client requires premedication for pain or other pain management techniques prior to wound care (see Chapter 9 ∞).

DELEGATION

Due to the need for aseptic technique and assessment skills, wound packing is not delegated to UAP. However, UAP may observe the wound and dressing during usual care and must report abnormal findings to the nurse. Abnormal findings must be validated and interpreted by the nurse.

INTERPROFESSIONAL PRACTICE

Packing wounds may be within the scope of practice for other health care providers such as physical therapists. Although the therapists may verbally communicate their findings and plan to the health care team members, the nurse must also know where to locate their documentation in the client's medical record.

Equipment

- Sterile packing material
- Sterile dressing equipment and dressing materials
- Solution for wetting the packing (e.g., sterile saline)
- Sterile bowl
- Forceps or cotton-tipped applicators
- Moisture-proof bag
- Clean gloves
- Sterile gloves (optional)

IMPLEMENTATION

Performance

1. Prior to performing the procedure, introduce self and verify the client's identity using agency protocol. Explain to the client what you are going to do, why it is necessary, and how he or she can participate. Discuss how the results will be used in planning further care or treatments.
2. Perform hand hygiene and observe other appropriate infection prevention procedures.
3. Provide for client privacy and prepare the client. Assist the client to a comfortable position in which the wound can be readily exposed. Expose only the wound area and cover the rest of the client, if necessary. **Rationale:** *Undue exposure is physically and psychologically distressing to most people.*
4. Remove the existing dressing (see Skill 31–2, steps 5 through 7).
   - If the previous dressing adheres to any tissue during removal, soak it with sterile normal saline. **Rationale:** *This facilitates removal and prevents disruption of new granulation tissue.*
5. Assess the wound.
   - See Skill 31–1. For wounds that are being packed, it is particularly important to measure the depth of the wounds, including all crevices and tunnels (see Figure ❷ in Skill 31–1).
6. Clean the wound if indicated (see Skill 31–2, step 9).
7. Prepare the supplies.
   - Open the packages of the sterile dressing set, packing, and bowl.
   - Pour the ordered solution into the bowl.
   - Apply sterile or clean gloves according to agency policy.
   - Place the packing into the bowl and thoroughly saturate with solution unless contraindicated by manufacturer specification.
   - Wring out the packing until it is slightly moist. Avoid packing that is too wet. **Rationale:** *Excessively wet packing increases the risk for bacterial growth and may macerate the surrounding skin.*
8. Pack the wound with the damp packing.
   - Using sterile gloved fingers, forceps, or an applicator, pack into all depressions and grooves of the wound. Cover all exposed surfaces. **Rationale:** *Necrotic material is usually more prevalent in depressed wound areas and needs to be covered.*
   - Do not pack too tightly. **Rationale:** *Too tight application inhibits wound edges from contracting and compresses capillaries.*
   - Pack only to the edge of the wound. **Rationale:** *Overlapping the skin with moist packing can cause maceration of healthy tissue.*
   - Remove and discard gloves.
   - Perform hand hygiene.
9. Dress the wound.
   - If indicated, protect the surrounding skin with skin sealant or hydrocolloid dressing.
   - Apply 4×4 gauze or other absorbent dressings to protect the wound and take up excess drainage.
10. Document the dressing change and the client's response in the client record using forms or checklists supplemented by narrative notes when appropriate. Electronic health records will use a designated wound/skin documentation sheet (see Figure ❸ in Skill 31–1).

EVALUATION

- Perform follow-up based on findings that deviate from expected or normal for the client. Relate findings to previous assessment data if available.
- Report significant deviations from normal to the primary care provider.

USING ALGINATES

Alginate dressings are made from a type of seaweed and are capable of absorbing up to 20 times their weight in fluid. They come in both rope and sheet forms that conform to the wound shape and swell or become gel-like when activated. They can be used in both clean and infected draining wounds. To change a dressing on a wound using alginates, the existing alginate must be removed from the wound by lifting or irrigating and then the new alginate can be applied. A cover dressing is always needed over the alginate.

●○● NURSING PROCESS: USING ALGINATES

Using Alginates on Wounds

SKILL 31–8

ASSESSMENT
Review the client's record to determine:
- Previous appearance, size, and treatment of the wound.
- Character of exudate.
- Presence of pain and the time when pain medication was last administered.
- Clinical signs of systemic infection.
- Allergies to the alginate or tape.

PLANNING
- If possible, schedule the dressing change at a time convenient for the client. Packing some wounds with alginate requires only a few minutes, and others can take much longer.
- Determine if the client requires premedication for pain or other pain management techniques prior to wound care (see Chapter 9 ∞).

Equipment
- Alginate dressing
- Sterile dressing equipment and secondary dressing materials
- Solution for irrigation (e.g., sterile saline or water)
- Irrigating syringe
- Bowl
- Basin to collect irrigation
- Forceps or cotton-tipped applicators (optional)
- Moisture-proof bag
- Clean gloves
- Sterile gloves (optional)

DELEGATION

Due to the need for aseptic technique and assessment skills, alginate dressing changes are not delegated to UAP. However, UAP may observe the dressing during usual care and must report abnormal findings to the nurse. Abnormal findings must be validated and interpreted by the nurse.

INTERPROFESSIONAL PRACTICE

Using alginates with wounds may be within the scope of practice for other health care providers who perform wound care such as physical therapists. Although the therapists may verbally communicate their findings and plan to the health care team members, the nurse must also know where to locate their documentation in the client's medical record.

IMPLEMENTATION
Performance
1. Prior to performing the procedure, introduce self and verify the client's identity using agency protocol. Explain to the client what you are going to do, why it is necessary, and how he or she can participate. Discuss how the results will be used in planning further care or treatments.
2. Perform hand hygiene and observe other appropriate infection prevention procedures.
3. Prepare the client. Assist the client to a comfortable position in which the wound can be readily exposed.
4. Provide for client privacy. Expose only the wound area and cover the rest of the client, if necessary. **Rationale:** *Undue exposure is physically and psychologically distressing to most people.*
5. Prepare the supplies.
   - Open the sterile dressing set and supplies.
   - Pour the ordered solution into the solution container.
   - Position the basin below the wound to receive the irrigating fluid.

6. Remove the existing dressing and alginate.
   - Apply clean gloves. Remove and discard the outer secondary dressing in the moisture-proof bag.
   - Irrigate the wound with the prescribed solution until all of the alginate dressing has been removed.
   - If the alginate dressing does not remove easily with irrigation, either the secondary dressing is not maintaining a moist environment or the wound is no longer producing enough exudate to warrant alginate dressing.
7. Assess the wound.
   - See Skill 31–1.
8. Clean the wound if indicated (see Skill 31–2, step 9).
   - Remove and discard gloves.
   - Perform hand hygiene.
9. Pack the wound with the alginate.
   - Apply sterile gloves if alginate will be handled without instruments.
   - Pack the alginate into all depressions and grooves of the wound. Cover all exposed surfaces. ❶

Using Alginates on Wounds—*continued*

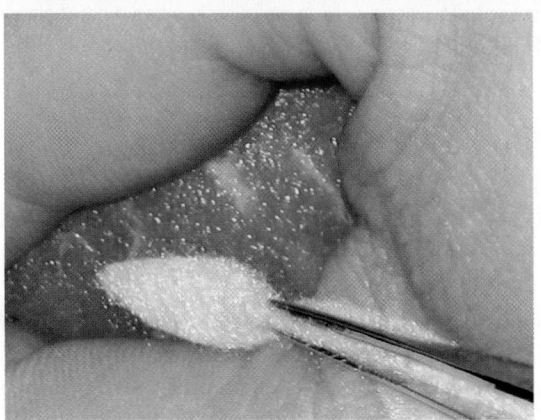

❶ Packing a wound with alginate.
Courtesy of Cory Patrick Hartley, RN.

10. Dress the wound.
    • Cover the alginate with petrolatum gauze, foam, or other secondary dressing that will keep the alginate in place and provide a moist wound environment.
    • Remove and discard gloves.
    • Perform hand hygiene.
11. Document the dressing change and the client's response in the client record using forms or checklists supplemented by narrative notes when appropriate. Electronic health records will use a designated wound/skin documentation sheet (see Figure ❸ in Skill 31–1).

EVALUATION

• Perform follow-up based on findings that deviate from expected or normal for the client. Relate findings to previous assessment data if available.

• Report significant deviations from normal to the primary care provider.

LIFESPAN CONSIDERATIONS | Wound Care

INFANTS
• The skin of infants is more fragile than that of older children and adults, and more susceptible to infection, shearing from friction, and burns. Keep skin hydrated by applying lotion daily.

CHILDREN
• Staphylococcus and fungus are two major infectious agents affecting the skin of children. Abrasions or small lacerations, commonly experienced by children, provide an entry in the skin for these organisms. Minor wounds should be cleansed with warm, soapy water, and covered with a sterile bandage.
• With more serious skin lesions, remind the child not to touch the wound, drains, or dressing. Cover with an appropriate bandage that will remain intact during the child's usual activities. Cover a transparent dressing with opaque material if viewing the site is distressing to the child. Restrain only when all alternatives have been tried and when absolutely necessary.
• For younger children, demonstrate wound care on a doll. Reassure the child that the wound will not be permanent and that nothing will fall out of the body.

OLDER ADULTS
• Hold wrinkled skin taut during application of a transparent dressing. Obtain assistance if needed.
• Skin of older adults is more fragile and can easily tear with removal of tape (especially adhesive tape). Use paper tape and tape remover as indicated, keeping tape use to the minimum required. Use extreme caution during tape removal. If possible, use conforming gauze bandage (e.g., Elastomull, Flexicon, Kerlix Lite, or Kling) to hold a dressing in place.
• Older adults who are in long-term care facilities often have immobility, malnutrition, and incontinence, all of which increase the risk for development of skin breakdown.
• Skin breakdown can occur as quickly as within 2 hours, so assessments should be done with each repositioning of the client.
• A thorough assessment of a client's heels should be done every shift. The skin can break down quickly from friction of movement in bed. Whenever possible, heels should be suspended off the mattress using pillows or other mechanisms.

CLIENT TEACHING CONSIDERATIONS

Wound and Skin Care

Perform appropriate client teaching for promoting wound healing and maintenance of healthy skin.

WOUND CARE
• Instruct the family about hygiene and medical asepsis, hand cleansing before and after dressing changes, and using a clean area for storage of dressing supplies.
• Instruct the client and family on where to obtain needed supplies. Be sensitive to the cost of dressings (e.g., transparent barriers are costly) and suggest less expensive alternatives if necessary. Be creative in the use of household items for padding pressure areas.

• Instruct the client and family in proper disposal of contaminated dressings. All contaminated items should be double-bagged in moisture-proof bags.

MAINTAINING INTACT SKIN
• Discuss the relationship between adequate nutrition (especially fluids, protein, vitamins B and C, iron, and calories) and healthy skin.
• Demonstrate appropriate positions for pressure relief.
• Establish a turning or repositioning schedule.
• Demonstrate application of appropriate skin protection agents and devices.
• Instruct to report persistent reddened areas.
• Identify potential sources of skin trauma and means of avoidance.

- Discuss the importance of adequate nutrition (especially fluids, protein, vitamins B and C, iron, and calories).
- Instruct in wound assessment and provide a mechanism for documenting.
- Emphasize the principles of asepsis, especially hand hygiene and proper methods of handling used dressings.
- Provide information about signs of wound infection and other complications to report.
- Reinforce appropriate aspects of pressure ulcer prevention.

- Demonstrate wound care techniques such as wound cleansing and dressing changes.
- Discuss pain control measures, if needed.
- Verify how the client may bathe with the wound (i.e., does the wound need to be covered with a waterproof barrier or should it be cleansed in the shower?).
- Drinking-quality tap water may be used to cleanse wounds instead of normal saline (Fernandez & Griffiths, 2012).

Negative Pressure Wound Therapy

Negative pressure wound therapy (NPWT), also termed vacuum-assisted closure (VAC), wound V.A.C., vacuum sealing, and topical negative pressure, refers to the use of suction equipment to apply negative pressure to a variety of wound types. This therapy has been shown to speed tissue generation, reduce swelling around the wound, and enhance wound healing by providing a moist and protected environment (Gabriel & Gupta, 2012). Sterile foam sponges are placed into a clean wound and covered with a transparent adhesive drape, and then a hole is cut in the drape to allow insertion of the vacuum tubing (Figure 31–4 ■). For maximum effectiveness the

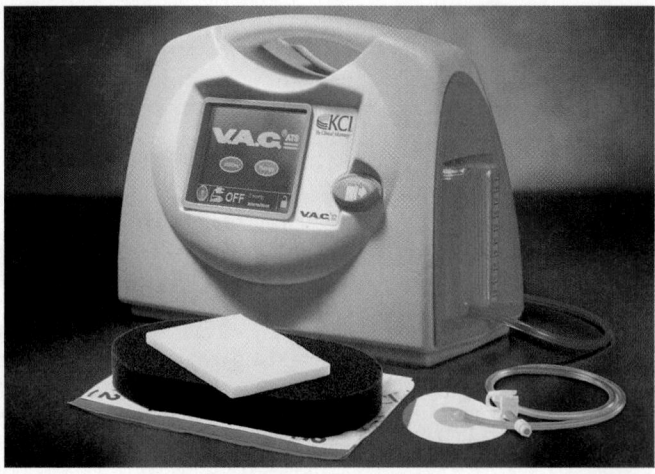

A

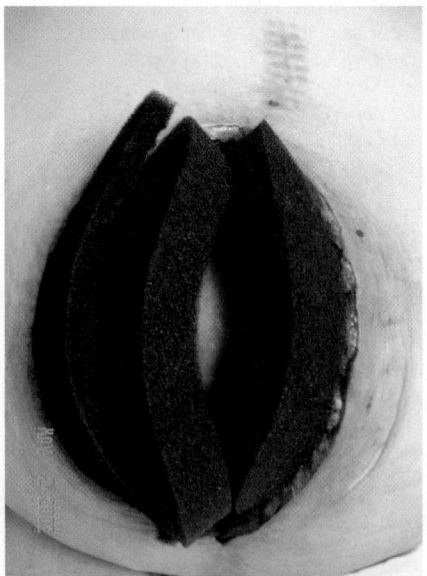

B

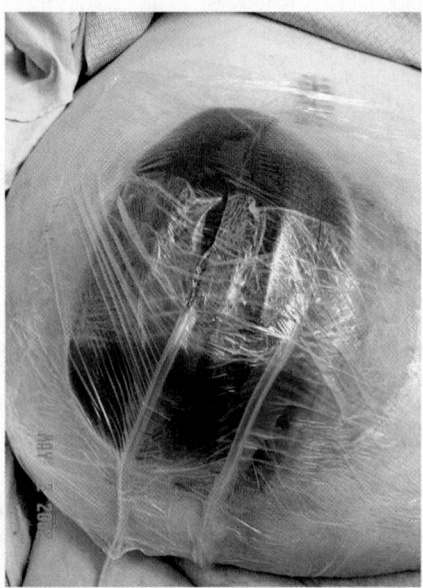

C

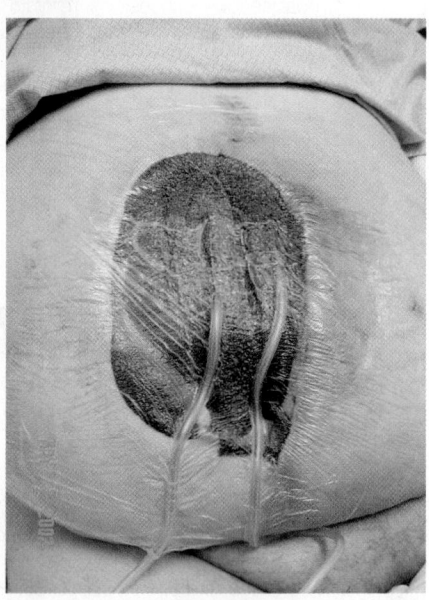

D

Figure 31–4 ■ Vacuum-assisted closure (VAC) system for wounds: *A,* therapy unit; *B,* foam strips laid into the wound; *C,* occlusive draping applied and suction tubing in place; *D,* finished dressing with negative pressure (suction) applied.
Photos *A,* V.A.C. ATS Therapy System Courtesy of KCI Licensing, Inc., San Antonio, TX; photos *B, C,* and *D;* Courtesy of Cory Patrick Hartley, RN.

vacuum is applied for almost 24 hours each day, and portable systems are available for ambulatory clients.

BANDAGES AND BINDERS

A **bandage** is a strip of cloth used to wrap some part of the body. Bandages are available in various widths, most commonly 1.5 to 7.5 cm (0.5 to 3 in.). Before applying a bandage, the nurse needs to know its purpose and to assess the area requiring support. General principles for bandaging are given in the accompanying Practice Guidelines.

Many types of materials are used for bandages. Gauze is one of the most commonly used; it is light and porous and readily molds to the body. It is also relatively inexpensive, so it is generally discarded when soiled. Gauze is frequently used to retain dressings on wounds and to bandage the fingers, hands, toes, and feet. It supports dressings and at the same time permits air to circulate; it can also be impregnated with petroleum jelly or other medications for application to wounds.

Elasticized bandages are applied to provide pressure to an area. They are commonly used to provide support and improve the venous circulation in the legs.

Applying bandages to various parts of the body involves one or more of five basic bandaging turns: circular, spiral, spiral reverse, recurrent, and figure eight. *Circular* turns are used to anchor bandages and to terminate them. Circular turns usually are not applied directly over a wound because of the discomfort the bandage would cause.

Spiral turns are used to bandage parts of the body that are fairly uniform in circumference (e.g., the upper arm or upper leg). *Spiral reverse* turns are used to bandage cylindrical parts of the body that are not uniform in circumference (e.g., the lower leg or forearm). *Recurrent* turns are used to cover distal parts of the body (e.g., the end of a finger, the skull, or the stump of an amputation). *Figure-eight* turns are

used to bandage an elbow, knee, or ankle, because they permit some movement after application.

A **binder** bandage is designed for a specific body part; for example, a **sling** is a binder shaped to support the elbow, lower arm, and hand. Binders are used to support large areas of the body, such as the abdomen or chest. Binders are made of muslin (plain-woven cotton fabric), flannel, or synthetic material that may or may not be elasticized. Some abdominal binders are made of an elasticized net-like material that fits the body contours and allows air to circulate around the body part.

PRACTICE GUIDELINES

Bandaging

- Whenever possible, bandage the part in its normal position, with the joint slightly flexed. **Rationale:** *This avoids putting strain on the ligaments and the muscles of the joint.*
- Pad between bandages and opposite skin surfaces or bony prominences. **Rationale:** *This prevents friction from the bandage against skin and consequent abrasion of the skin.*
- Always bandage body parts by working from the distal to the proximal end. **Rationale:** *This aids the return flow of venous blood.*
- Bandage with even pressure. **Rationale:** *This prevents interference with blood circulation.*
- Whenever possible, leave the end of the body part (e.g., the toe) exposed. **Rationale:** *This permits assessment of the adequacy of the blood circulation to the extremity.*
- Cover dressings with bandages at least 5 cm (2 in.) beyond the edges of the dressing. **Rationale:** *This prevents the dressing and wound from becoming contaminated.*

●○● NURSING PROCESS: BANDAGES AND BINDERS

Applying Bandages and Binders

ASSESSMENT

Assess the area to be bandaged or to which a binder is to be applied for:

- Swelling.
- Presence of and status of wounds (open wounds will require a dressing before a bandage or binder is applied).
- Presence of drainage (amount, color, odor, and viscosity).
- Adequacy of circulation (skin temperature, color, and sensation). Pale or cyanotic skin, cool temperature, tingling, and numbness can indicate impaired circulation.

- Presence of pain (location, intensity, onset, and quality). Determine:
- The client's ability to reapply the bandage or binder when needed.
- The client's ability to carry out activities of daily living (e.g., eat, dress, write, comb hair, bathe, or drive).

PLANNING

- If possible, schedule the bandaging at a time convenient for the client. Some bandages or bindings require only a few minutes to apply, and others can take much longer.
- Determine if the client requires premedication for pain or other pain management techniques (see Chapter 9 ∞).

DELEGATION

Application of binders can be delegated to UAP or family members/caregivers after the nurse has performed an initial assessment that these individuals can perform this skill safely. Application of bandages over wounds may be taught to clients or family members/caregivers for home care purposes.

SKILL 31-9

Continued on page 686

Applying Bandages and Binders—*continued*

INTERPROFESSIONAL PRACTICE

Applying bandages and binders may be within the scope of practice for other health care providers. For example, in addition to nurses, both physical therapists and occupational therapists commonly use these modalities. Although the therapists may verbally communicate their findings and plan to the health care team members, the nurse must also know where to locate their documentation in the client's medical record.

Equipment
- Clean bandage or binder of the appropriate material and size
- Padding, such as abdominal pads or gauze squares
- Tape, clips, or Velcro

IMPLEMENTATION
Performance

1. Prior to performing the procedure, introduce self and verify the client's identity using agency protocol. Explain to the client what you are going to do, why it is necessary, and how he or she can participate. Discuss how the results will be used in planning further care or treatments.
2. Perform hand hygiene and observe other appropriate infection prevention procedures.
3. Provide for client privacy.
4. Position and prepare the client appropriately.
   - Provide the client with support for the area to be bandaged. For example, if a hand needs to be bandaged, ask the client to place the elbow on a table, so that the hand does not have to be held up unsupported. **Rationale:** *Because bandaging takes time, holding up a body part without support can fatigue the client.*
   - Make sure that the area to be bandaged is clean and dry. Wash and dry the area if necessary. Perform wound care as indicated. **Rationale:** *Washing and drying remove microorganisms, which flourish in dark, warm, moist areas.*
   - Align the part to be bandaged with slight flexion of the joints, unless this is contraindicated. **Rationale:** *Slight flexion places less strain on the ligaments and muscles of the joint.*
5. Apply the bandage. Apply the beginning of the bandage to the most distal part of the body to be bandaged first. **Rationale:** *Wrapping from distal to proximal facilitates venous return and diminishes swelling.*

Circular Turns
- Hold the bandage in your dominant hand, keeping the roll uppermost, and unroll the bandage about 8 cm (3 in.). **Rationale:** *This length of unrolled bandage allows good control for placement and tension.*
- Hold the end down with the thumb of the other hand. ❶
- Encircle the body part a few times or as often as needed, making sure that each layer overlaps one half to two thirds of the previous layer. This provides even support to the area.
- The bandage should be firm, but not too tight. Ask the client if the bandage feels comfortable. A tight bandage can interfere with blood circulation, whereas a loose bandage does not provide adequate protection.
- Secure the end of the bandage with tape or clips if there is no Velcro fastener.

Spiral Turns
- Make two circular turns. **Rationale:** *Two circular turns anchor the bandage.*
- Continue spiral turns at about a 30° angle, each turn overlapping the preceding one by two thirds the width of the bandage. ❷
- Terminate the bandage with two circular turns, and secure the end as described for circular turns.

Spiral Reverse Turns
- Anchor the bandage with two circular turns, and bring the bandage upward at about a 30° angle.

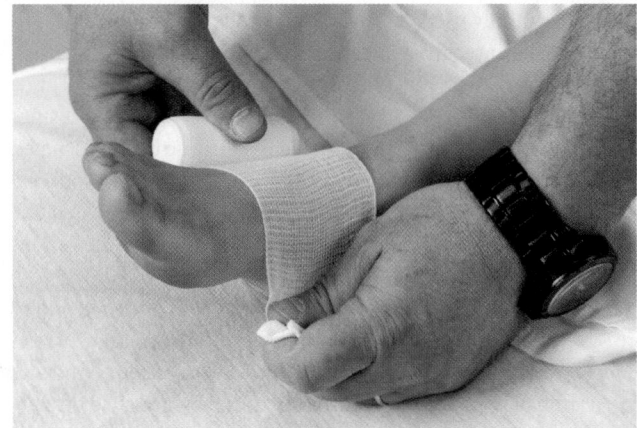

❶ Starting a bandage with circular turns.

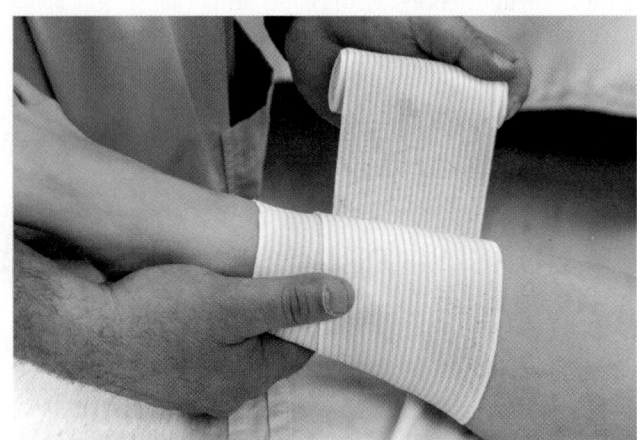

❷ Applying spiral turns.

- Place the thumb of your free hand on the upper edge of the bandage. ❸, A **Rationale:** *The thumb will hold the bandage while it is folded on itself.*
- Unroll the bandage about 15 cm (6 in.), and then turn your hand so that the bandage falls over itself. ❸, B
- Continue the bandage around the limb, overlapping each previous turn by two thirds the width of the bandage. Make each bandage turn at the same position on the limb so that the turns of the bandage will be aligned. ❸, C
- Terminate the bandage with two circular turns, and secure the end as described for circular turns.

Recurrent Turns
- Anchor the bandage with two circular turns.
- Fold the bandage back on itself, hold it with the thumb of the other hand, and bring it centrally over the distal end to be bandaged. ❹

Applying Bandages and Binders—*continued*

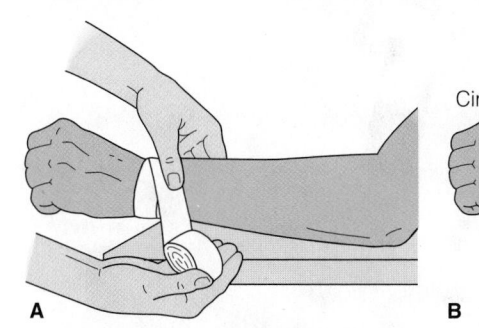
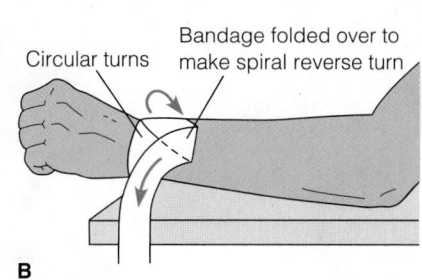

Circular turns

Bandage folded over to make spiral reverse turn

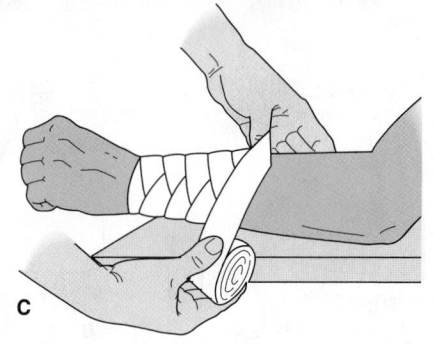

A   **B**   **C**

③ Applying spiral reverse turns.

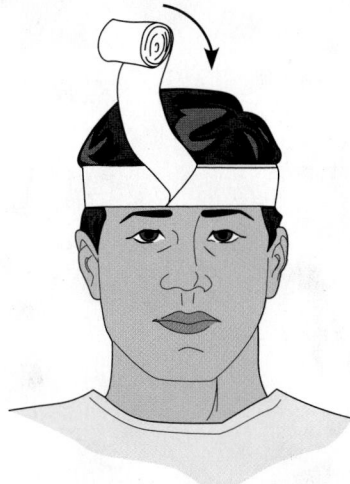

④ Starting a recurrent bandage.

- Bring the bandage back over the end to the right of the center bandage but overlapping it by two thirds the width of the bandage.
- Bring the bandage back on the left side, also overlapping the first turn by two thirds the width of the bandage.
- Continue this pattern of alternating right and left until the area is covered. Overlap the preceding turn by two thirds the bandage width each time.
- Terminate the bandage with two circular turns. **⑤** Secure the end appropriately.

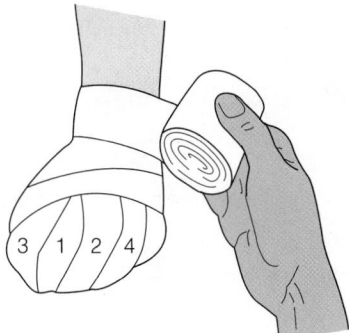

⑤ Completing a recurrent bandage.

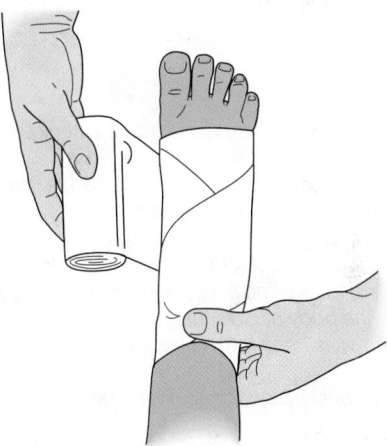

⑥ Applying a figure-eight bandage.

Figure-Eight Turns
- Anchor the bandage with two circular turns.
- Carry the bandage above the joint, around it, and then below it, making a figure eight. **⑥**
- Continue above and below the joint, overlapping the previous turn by two thirds the width of the bandage.
- Terminate the bandage above the joint with two circular turns, and then secure the end appropriately.

Arm Sling
- Ask the client to flex the elbow to an 80° angle or less, depending on the purpose. The thumb should be facing upward or inward toward the body. **Rationale:** *An 80° angle is sufficient to support the forearm, to prevent swelling of the hand, and to relieve pressure on the shoulder joint (e.g., to support the paralyzed arm of a client who has had a stroke whose shoulder might otherwise become dislocated). A more acute angle is preferred if there is swelling of the hand.*
- If a triangle is used, place one end of the unfolded binder over the shoulder of the uninjured side so that the binder falls down the front of the chest of the client with the point of the triangle (apex) under the elbow of the injured side. **⑦**
  - Take the upper corner, and carry it around the neck until it hangs over the shoulder on the injured side.
  - Bring the lower corner of the binder up over the arm to the shoulder of the injured side. Using a square knot, secure this corner to the upper corner at the side of the neck on the injured side. **Rationale:** *A square knot will not slip. Tying the knot at the*

Continued on page 688

SKILL 31-9

Applying Bandages and Binders—*continued*

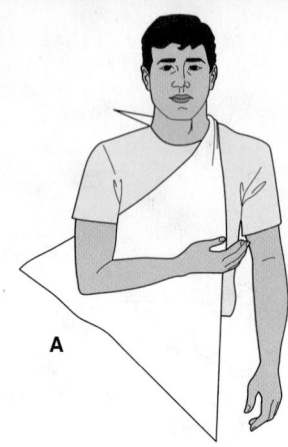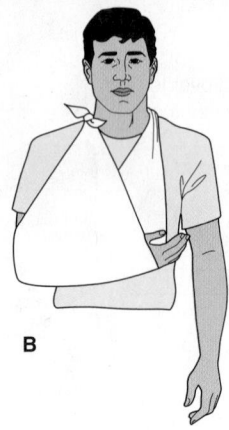

❼ A triangle arm sling.

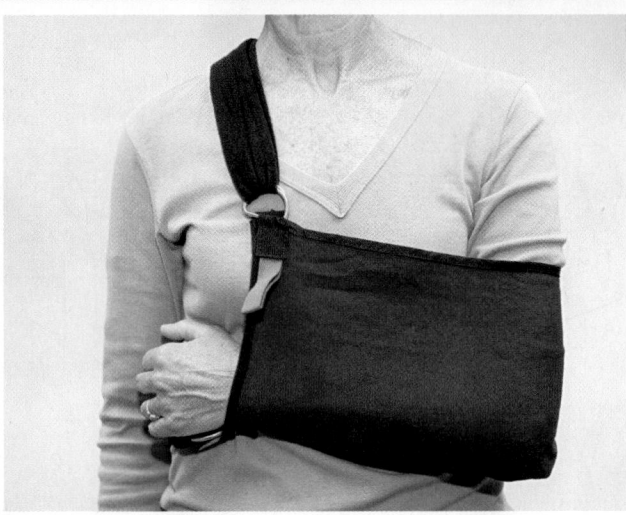

❽ A commercial arm sling.

side of the neck prevents pressure on the bony prominences of the vertebral column at the back of the neck.
• Fold the sling neatly at the elbow, and secure it with safety pins or tape. It may be folded and fastened at the front. ❼, B.
• If a commercial sling is used, it may also include a second strap that goes around the back of the client's chest from the finger end of the sling to the elbow. ❽ **Rationale:** *This strap holds the arm close to the body at all times, providing shoulder immobilization such as is used following a shoulder dislocation or surgery.*
• Make sure the wrist is supported. **Rationale:** *This maintains alignment.*
• Remove the sling periodically to inspect the skin for indications of irritation, especially around the site of the knot.

Straight Abdominal Binder
• Place the binder smoothly around the body. **Rationale:** *A binder placed too high interferes with respiration; one placed too low interferes with elimination and walking.*
• Apply padding over the iliac crests if the client is thin.
• Bring the ends around the client, overlap them, and secure them with clips or Velcro. ❾

6. Document the application of the bandage or binder and the client's response in the client record using forms or checklists supplemented by narrative notes when appropriate.

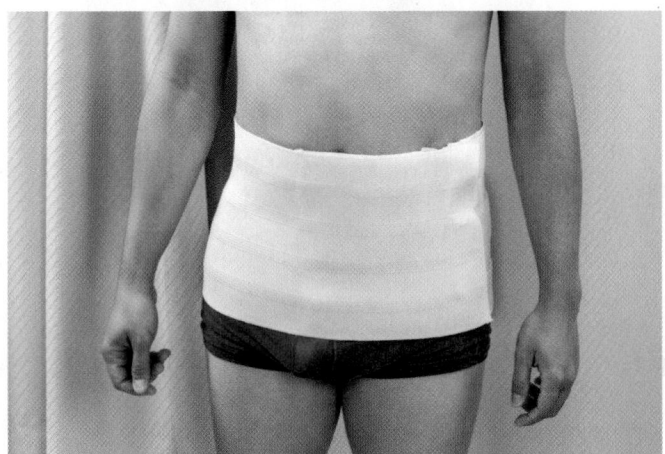

❾ A straight abdominal binder.

SAMPLE DOCUMENTATION

6/3/2015 1900 c/o severe sharp and cramping pain in shoulder when moving it. Commercial sling with shoulder immobilizer applied to l arm c̄ elbow flexed 60°. Upper extremity warm, no wounds or lesions, peripheral pulses strong, brisk capillary refill. Able to move fingers and wrist without pain. Client verbalizes understanding of need to request assistance with ADLs. ———————————— L. Morris, RN

EVALUATION
• Perform follow-up based on findings that deviate from expected or normal for the client. Relate findings to previous assessment data if available.

• Report significant deviations from normal to the primary care provider.

LIFESPAN CONSIDERATIONS   Applying Bandages and Binders

CHILDREN
- Allow the child to help with the procedure by holding supplies, opening boxes, counting turns, and so on.
- If a young client is apprehensive, demonstrate the procedure on a doll or stuffed animal.
- Encourage the child to decorate the bandage.
- Teach the caregivers to apply bandages and binders safely.

OLDER ADULTS
- Older clients may need extra support during the procedure, especially if arthritis, contractures, or tremors are present.
- Avoid constricting the client's circulation with a tight bandage or binder. Observe skin and bony prominences frequently for signs of impaired circulation. The risk for skin breakdown increases with age.

Ambulatory and Community Settings   Applying Bandages and Binders | PATIENT-CENTERED CARE |

- Assess the client's or caregiver's ability and willingness to perform the bandaging procedure.
- Ensure that the client has the proper supplies and knows how to obtain replacement supplies.
- The client should have two binders so that there is one to wear while the other is being washed. Bandages and binders should be washed inside a mesh laundry bag to keep them from becoming twisted and to prevent Velcro or hooks from catching on other laundry.

- Instruct the client's caregiver to:
  a. Cleanse hands thoroughly before handling dressing supplies and applying the bandage.
  b. Report skin breakdown, redness, pain, or pallor of the affected area.
  c. Check for adequate peripheral circulation after applying the bandage.

Chapter 31 Review

FOCUSING ON CLINICAL THINKING

Consider This

1. Your client has several different wounds of varying shapes and sizes. How would you document these in the client record?
2. You are in the client's home to change a dressing over a healing surgical wound that has significant drainage. How would you dispose of the soiled dressings?
3. What would be one appropriate use of a transparent semipermeable membrane dressing? Why?
4. Many practitioners apply paper tape around the four edges of a hydrocolloid dressing. Why would they do this?
5. You observe a colleague irrigating a wound using a 30-mL syringe with an #18-gauge needle attached. Why would this be correct or incorrect technique?

6. In preparing to perform a damp-to-damp dressing, the client record reveals that the dressings have been changed every 12 hours and that the client experiences significant pain during removal of the previous dressing. How would you proceed?
7. The client has a category/stage III pressure ulcer over the right trochanter. A recent journal article suggests you dress this with alginate. Assuming the primary care provider agrees, do you believe this would make an appropriate dressing? Why or why not?
8. What are four assessments that should be made for a client with a bandage or binder?

See Focusing on Clinical Thinking answers on student resource website.

TEST YOUR KNOWLEDGE

1. The nurse is aware that debridement of wounds is necessary to remove necrotic tissue called:
   1. Alginate.
   2. Eschar.
   3. Granulation.
   4. Drainage.

2. The nurse caring for a client with a fresh closed surgical wound knows that which is the best type of dressing for this wound?
   1. A dry sterile dressing
   2. A dry clean dressing
   3. A wet sterile dressing
   4. A wet clean dressing

3. The client has an ulcer with a large quantity of exudate. The nurse could apply what type of dressing to this wound? Select all that apply.
   1. Transparent film
   2. Impregnated nonadherent
   3. Polyurethane foam
   4. Alginate
   5. Hydrogel

4. While assessing the client's wound, the nurse finds that the wound appears yellow and recognizes that this indicates:
   1. Liquid to semiliquid slough resulting from infection requiring absorbent dressing.
   2. Late regeneration phase of tissue repair requiring no intervention.
   3. Necrotic tissue requiring debridement.
   4. Early regeneration phase of tissue repair requiring no intervention.

5. When assessing the client's pressure ulcer, the nurse sees a full-thickness ulcer with damage to the underlying muscle. The nurse will choose dressings appropriate for which type of pressure ulcer?
   1. Category/stage I
   2. Category/stage II
   3. Category/stage III
   4. Category/stage IV

6. Which of the following might the nurse delegate to unlicensed assistive personnel?
   1. Sterile postoperative dressing
   2. Dry dressings for a clean chronic wound
   3. Wound irrigation
   4. Wound packing

7. The nurse is caring for an older client in a long-term care facility. Which of the following assessment findings can the nurse document and report to the primary care provider on the next routine visit?
   1. Appearance of reddened area on sacrum
   2. Postoperative wound that has begun draining purulent material
   3. Appearance of a new venous stasis ulcer
   4. Persistent red area on left buttock

8. The nurse needs to irrigate a wound of a client in the hospital. The best time to perform this task would be:
   1. Before breakfast.
   2. After physician's rounds.
   3. After changing the wound dressing.
   4. After medicating the client for pain.

9. The nurse is applying an elastic bandage to the ankle of a client diagnosed with a sprain. When applying the dressing, where would the nurse *start* the bandage?
   1. Above the knee
   2. Above the ankle
   3. At the toes
   4. At the heel

10. The client had surgery on the shoulder and is not to move the arm for 1 week. The nurse applies a sling and recognizes it is the wrong size because:
    1. The strap around the waist needs to be tightened.
    2. The bottom of the sling stops in the center of the palm.
    3. The bottom of the sling stops at the wrist.
    4. The strap around the neck needs to be loosened.

See Answers to Test Your Knowledge in Appendix A.

READINGS AND REFERENCES

References

Bates-Jensen, B. M. (2012). Pressure ulcers: Pathophysiology, detection, and prevention. In C. Sussman & B. M. Bates-Jensen (Eds.), *Wound care: A collaborative practice manual for health professionals* (4th ed., pp. 230–277). Philadelphia, PA: Lippincott Williams & Wilkins.

Bates-Jensen, B. M., Schultz, G., & Ovington, L. G. (2012). Management of exudate, biofilms, and infection. In C. Sussman & B. M. Bates-Jensen (Eds.), *Wound care: A collaborative practice manual for health professionals* (4th ed., pp. 457–476). Philadelphia, PA: Lippincott Williams & Wilkins.

European Pressure Ulcer Advisory Panel and National Pressure Ulcer Advisory Panel. (2009). *Prevention and treatment of pressure ulcers: Quick reference guide*. Washington, DC: National Pressure Ulcer Advisory Panel.

Fernandez, R., & Griffiths, R. (2012). Water for wound cleansing. *Cochrane Database of Systematic Reviews*, Issue 2, Art. No.: CD003861. doi:10.1002/14651858 .CD003861.pub3

Gabriel, A., & Gupta, S. (2012). Management of the wound environment with negative pressure wound therapy. In C. Sussman & B. M. Bates-Jensen (Eds.), *Wound care: A collaborative practice manual for health professionals* (4th ed., pp. 765–780). Philadelphia, PA: Lippincott Williams & Wilkins.

Hammond, C., & Nixon, M. (2011). The reliability of a handheld wound measurement and documentation device in clinical practice. *Journal of Wound, Ostomy & Continence Nursing*, 38, 260–264. doi:10.1097/WON.0b013e318215fc60

The Joint Commission. (2013a). *National Patient Safety Goals effective January 1, 2014. Hospital accreditation program*. Retrieved from http://www.jointcommission.org/assets/1/6/HAP_NPSG_Chapter_2014.pdf

The Joint Commission. (2013b). *National Patient Safety Goals effective January 1, 2014: Long term care accreditation program*. Retrieved from http://www.jointcommission.org/assets/1/6/LT2_NPSG_Chapter_2014.pdf

National Quality Forum. (2013). *List of serious reportable events*. Retrieved from http://www.qualityforum.org/Topics/SREs/List_of_SREs.aspx

Strohal, R. (2013). Debridement. *EWMA Journal*, 13(1), 55–60.

Sussman, G. (2012). Management of the wound environment with dressings and topical agents. In C. Sussman & B. M. Bates-Jensen (Eds.), *Wound care: A collaborative practice manual for health professionals* (4th ed., pp. 502–521). Philadelphia, PA: Lippincott Williams & Wilkins.

U.S. Department of Health and Human Services. (2013). *Healthy people 2020: Topics and objectives*. Retrieved from http://healthypeople.gov/2020/topicsobjectives2020/objectiveslist.aspx?topicid=31

Wet-to-dry saline moistened gauze for wound dressing. (2011). *Wound Practice & Research*, 19(1), 48–49.

Selected Bibliography

Armour-Burton, T., Fields, W., Outlaw, L., & Deleon, E. (2013). The healthy skin project: Changing nursing practice to prevent and treat hospital-acquired pressure ulcers. *Critical Care Nurse*, 33(3), 32–40. doi:10.4037/ccn2013290

Barker, A., Kamar, J., Tyndall, T., White, L., Hutchinson, A., Klopfer, N., & Weller, C. (2013). Implementation of pressure ulcer prevention best practice recommendations in acute care: An observational study. *International Wound Journal*, 10(3), 313–320. doi:10.1111/j.1742-481X.2012.00979.x

Berman, A., Snyder, S., & Frandsen, G. (2016). *Kozier & Erb's fundamentals of nursing: Concepts, process, and practice* (10th ed.). Upper Saddle River, NJ: Pearson.

Blueman, D., & Blousfield, C. (2012). The use of larval therapy to reduce the bacterial load in chronic wounds. *Journal of Wound Care,*21, 244–253.

Coleman, S., Gorecki, C., Nelson, E., Closs, S., Defloor, T., Halfens, R., . . . Nixon, J. (2013). Patient risk factors for pressure ulcer development: Systematic review. *International Journal of Nursing Studies*, 50, 974–1003. doi:10.1016/j.ijnurstu.2012.11.019

Dowsett, C. (2012). Recommendations for the use of negative pressure wound therapy. *Wounds UK*, 8(2), 48–59.

Fagerdahl, A., Bostrom, L., Ulfvarson, J., & Ottoson, C. (2012). Risk factors for unsuccessful treatment and complications with negative pressure wound therapy. *Wounds: A Compendium of Clinical Research & Practice*, 24, 168–177.

Goosen, J., Mashiane, P., Mokopanele, T., Snyders, M., Biko, S., Ndjo, Y. M., and Lambrecht, N. (2013). Pearls for practice: Objective quantitative analysis of wound bed preparation for pressure ulcers and venous leg ulcers utilizing a hydroconductive wound dressing. *Ostomy Wound Management*, 59(4), 12.

Lang, D. P., Tho, P., & Ang, E. K. (2011). Effectiveness of the sitz bath in managing adult patients with anorectal disorders. *Japan Journal of Nursing Science*, 8, 115–128. doi:10.1111/j.1742-7924.2011.00175.x

Li, D., & Korniewicz, D. M. (2013). Determination of the effectiveness of electronic health records to document pressure ulcers. *MEDSURG Nursing*, 22(1), 17–25.

National Pressure Ulcer Advisory Panel. (2003). *Pressure ulcer scale for healing (PUSH): PUSH Tool 3.0*. Retrieved from http://www.npuap.org/PDF/push3.pdf

Ottosen, B. B., & Pedersen, B. D. (2013). Patients' experiences of NPWT in an outpatient setting in Denmark. *Journal of Wound Care*, 22, 197–206.

Ove, D., & Frandsen, D. (2013). Do certain support surfaces reduce the risk of pressure ulcers more than others? *Evidence-Based Practice*, 16(6), E15–E16.

Pieper, B., & National Pressure Ulcer Advisory Panel (NPUAP). (2012). *Pressure ulcers: Prevalence, incidence and implications for the future*. Washington, DC: NPUAP.

Rippon, M. M., Davies, P. P., & White, R. R. (2012). Taking the trauma out of wound care: The importance of undisturbed healing. *Journal of Wound Care, 21*, 359–368.

Sardina, D. (2013). Is your wound-cleansing practice up to date? *American Nurse Today, 8*(7), 37–38.

Scientific and Clinical Abstracts from the WOCN Society's 45th Annual Conference: Seattle, Washington, June 22–26, 2013. (2013). *Journal of Wound, Ostomy and Continence Nursing, 40*(Suppl. 3S), S1–S112.

Sussman, C., & Bates-Jensen, B. M. (2012). Skin and soft tissue anatomy and wound healing physiology. In C. Sussman & B. M. Bates-Jensen (Eds.), *Wound care: A collaborative practice manual for health professionals* (4th ed., pp. 17–52). Philadelphia, PA: Lippincott Williams & Wilkins.

Sweeney, I., Miraftab, M., & Collyer, G. (2012). A critical review of modern and emerging absorbent dressings used to treat exuding wounds. *International Wound Journal, 9*, 601–612. doi:10.1111/j.1742-481X.2011.00923.x

Upton, D. D., Stephens, D. D., & Andrews, A. A. (2013). Patients' experiences of negative pressure wound therapy for the treatment of wounds: A review. *Journal of Wound Care, 22*, 34–39.

Vig, S. S., Dowsett, C. C., Berg, L. L., Caravaggi, C. C., Rome, P. P., Birke-Sorensen, H. H., . . . Smith, J. J. (2011). Evidence-based recommendations for the use of negative pressure wound therapy in chronic wounds: Steps towards an international consensus. *Journal of Tissue Viability, 20*, S1–S18. doi:10.1016/j.jtv.2011.07.002

Wolvos, T. (2013). The use of negative pressure wound therapy with an automated volumetric fluid administration: An advancement in wound care. *Wounds: A Compendium of Clinical Research & Practice, 25*(3), 75–83.

Wood, L., & Hughes, M. (2013). Reviewing the effectiveness of larval therapy. *Journal of Community Nursing, 27*(2), 11–14.

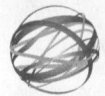

32 Orthopedic Care

LEARNING OUTCOMES

At the completion of this chapter, the student will be able to:

1. Define the key terms used in the skills of cast care and traction.
2. Identify indications for using plaster or synthetic splints and casts.
3. List nursing measures to care for and prevent problems for clients with casts.
4. List nursing measures to care for and prevent problems for clients in traction.
5. Recognize when it is appropriate to delegate care of clients with casts or traction to unlicensed assistive personnel.
6. List actions required for detecting and preventing neurovascular impairments and skin irritation due to casts.
7. Verbalize the steps used in:
   a. Providing initial cast care.
   b. Providing ongoing cast care.
   c. Caring for clients in skeletal traction.
8. Describe factors that affect nursing care of clients using orthotic devices (orthoses).
9. Demonstrate appropriate documentation and reporting of orthopedic nursing care.

SKILLS

Skill 32–1 Providing Initial Cast Care
Skill 32–2 Providing Ongoing Cast Care

Skill 32–2 Caring for Clients in Skeletal Traction

KEY TERMS

Various strategies can be used to immobilize and support parts of the musculoskeletal system to allow healing and encourage proper alignment. Nursing care of clients who are casted, splinted, or placed in traction, or who require orthotics will be addressed in this chapter.

CASTS

Casts are generally applied to immobilize a body part so that healing can take place without further injury. The degree of immobilization of the person varies with the type of cast. Some people are confined to bed, whereas others are able to resume most daily activities with only slight inconvenience from the cast. Although casts are applied for reasons other than fractures, this chapter focuses on clients who have fractures.

A **splint** is a partial cast that does not extend all the way around the limb and is commonly used for injuries of the finger, wrist, foot, and ankle. They can also be used on more proximal areas of the limbs. Splints (also called cast slabs in some countries) are frequently used at the onset of an injury to immobilize and protect the area and allow for swelling during the acute phase of the injury. Splints are faster and easier to apply than casts and are available preformed. Splints may also be used for chronic conditions to reduce pain and increase limb function. Generally, there are fewer complications with splints than with casts (Williams et al., 2013).

Cast Materials

Several synthetic materials are used to make casts: polyester and cotton, knitted fiberglass, fiberglass-free/latex-free materials, and thermoplastics. Synthetic casts dry quickly and are lightweight. Traditional gypsum plaster cast material is still used in situations where exact molding around a joint is desired (such as with serial

TABLE 32–1	Cast Materials		
Type of Material	**Description**	**Application**	**Setting Time and Weight-Bearing Restrictions**
Plaster (e.g., Gypsona, Specialist)	Open-weave cotton rolls or strips saturated with powdered calcium sulfate crystals (gypsum)	Applied after being soaked in tepid water for a few seconds until bubbling stops	Dries in 48 h; no weight bearing allowed until dry
Synthetics; polyester and cotton (e.g., Hygia Cast, Nemoa)	Open-weave polyester and cotton tape permeated with water-activated polyurethane resin	Applied after being soaked in cool water, 26°C (80°F); used within 2–3 min of soaking	Sets in 7 min; weight bearing allowed in 15 min
Fiberglass; water-activated (e.g., Scotchcast, Delta-Lite) or light-cured (e.g., Lightcast II); fiberglass-free/latex-free (e.g., Delta-Cast Elite, FlashCast Elite)	Open-weave fiberglass tape impregnated with water-activated polyurethane resin or photosensitive polyurethane resin	Applied after being immersed in tepid water for 10–15 sec or applied with gloves or silicone-type hand cream to keep it from sticking	Sets in 7–15 min; weight bearing allowed in 20–30 min; light-cured sets after being exposed for 3 min to a special ultraviolet lamp (curing), after which weight bearing is allowed immediately
Thermoplastic (e.g., Hexcelite, Orficast)	Knitted thermoplastic polyester fabric in rigid rolls	Applied after being heated in water at 76°C–82°C (170°F–180°F) for 3–4 min to make the rolls soft and pliable	Sets in 5 min; weight bearing allowed in 20 min
		Remove excess water by squeezing between towels before applying	

casting of a clubfoot) or when cutting a window in the cast is necessary to monitor a healing wound. Cast materials come in rolls that are soaked in water to begin activation and softening so they can be molded around the affected body part. As most cast materials dry (or cure), an exothermic reaction occurs. The heat that is produced is usually not harmful, but it is important to let clients know to expect this. The faster cast material hardens, the more heat is produced and the greater the chances of excessive heat or burning (Shuler & Bates, 2013). See Table 32–1 for descriptions and applications of various types of cast materials.

Padding Materials

Before the cast is applied, the affected area must be padded. **Stockinette**, a soft, flexible, tubular, cloth material, is placed over the body part before the cast material is applied. After the cast is applied, the distal end of the stockinette is folded back over the edge of the cast material to provide a smooth border (Figure 32–1 ■). *Cotton sheet wadding* or padding is often applied directly over the stockinette to pad bony prominences or between skin surfaces. Sheet wadding clings and molds to the contours of the limb. *Felt padding* may be needed over bony prominences or joints that are vulnerable to skin breakdown. If the synthetic cast will be placed in water for bathing, polypropylene stockinette and polyester padding must be used because they dry easily. Waterproof linings (such as Gore-Tex) have been used in some cases in which contact with urine may occur. Padding materials that resist growth of microorganisms are also available.

Types of Casts

The *long arm cast* or hanging arm cast (Figure 32–2A ■) extends from the axilla to the fingers of the hand, maintaining elbow flexion. It immobilizes the wrist, the radius, the ulna, and the humerus. The

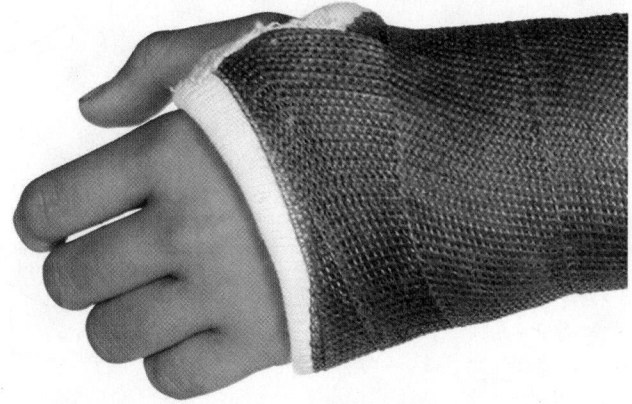

Figure 32–1 ■ White stockinette folded back over the cast to form a smooth edge.
Stacy Barnett/Shutterstock

short arm cast (Figure 32–2B) extends from below the elbow to the fingers. It immobilizes the wrist, the radius, and the ulna. The *shoulder spica cast* (Figure 32–2C) extends around the chest and along the entire arm to the fingers. The arm is usually abducted to immobilize the shoulder bones (e.g., the clavicle). **Spica** refers to any bandage that is applied in successive V-shaped crossings and is used to immobilize a limb, especially at a joint.

The *long*, or *full, leg cast* (Figure 32–2D) extends from above the knee to the toes. The *short leg cast* (Figure 32–2E) begins just below the knee and extends to the toes. The *hip spica cast* (Figure 32–2F) begins at waist level or above. It immobilizes the hip joint and the femur, extends down one entire leg, and may cover all or part of the second leg. A single spica covers one leg only. A double hip spica covers both legs to the toes. The *body cast* extends from the axillae to encompass the entire trunk. It is often used to immobilize the spine.

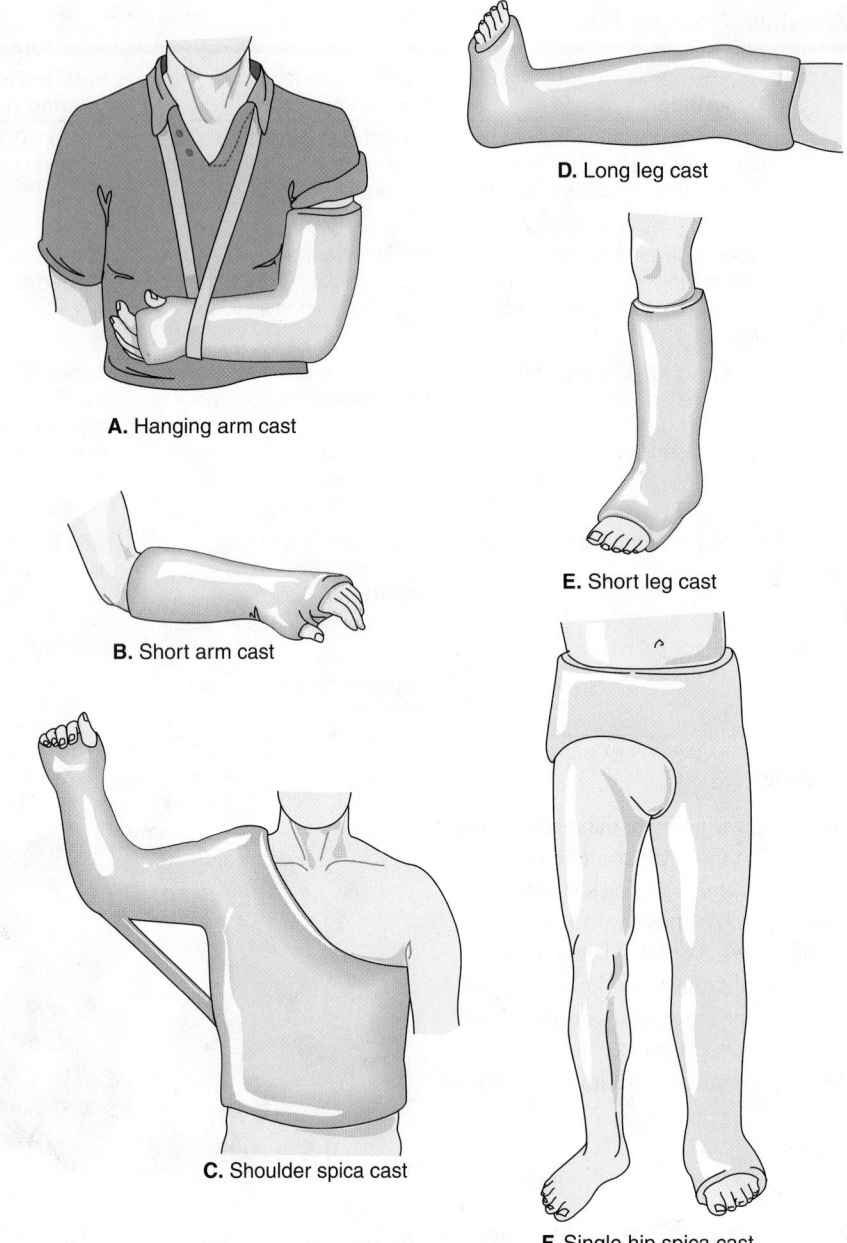

Figure 32–2 ■ Types of casts: *A*, long arm (hanging arm) cast; *B,* short arm cast; *C,* shoulder spica cast; *D,* long, or full, leg cast; *E,* short leg cast; *F,* single hip spica cast.

CARE FOR CLIENTS WITH CASTS

Essential nursing care for clients who have casts includes continual assessment and intervention to prevent pressure on underlying blood vessels, nerves, and the skin; to maintain the integrity of the cast itself; and to prevent problems associated with immobility. Common cast pressure areas are listed in Table 32–2. A fingerwidth should fit between the cast edge and the client's skin.

SAFETY ALERT!   SAFETY

Instruct clients to never stick anything inside their cast. Injury and infection can result.

Because a plaster cast and cast padding are porous and will absorb water or urine, every effort is made to keep the cast dry. Wet casts soften, which impairs their function; thus, tub baths and showers are contraindicated. Casts that become soiled with feces develop an irremovable odor. Elimination presents a particular problem for people with long leg, body, and hip spica casts. There is no effective way to clean a cast other than wiping it with a damp cloth. The best approach is to prevent soils and stains, especially those from food spills, urine, and feces.

Synthetic casts may, with the primary care provider's agreement, be immersed in water if polypropylene stockinette and padding were applied. The cast will dry in a few hours, which may be speeded through use of a handheld hair dryer on the cool temperature setting. In general, however, it is best to keep casts dry.

TABLE 32–2	Common Cast Pressure Areas		
Type of Cast	**Common Pressure Areas**	**Type of Cast**	**Common Pressure Areas**
Short arm cast	Radial styloid process Ulnar styloid process Joint at base of thumb	Long leg cast	Heel Achilles tendon Malleolus Popliteal artery behind knee Peroneal nerve at side of knee
Hanging arm cast	Radial styloid process Ulnar styloid process Olecranon Lateral epicondyle	Hip spica	As above for long leg cast Sacrum Iliac crests
Short leg cast	Heel Achilles tendon Malleolus		

●○● NURSING PROCESS: CARE FOR CLIENTS WITH CASTS

Providing Initial Cast Care

SKILL 32–1

ASSESSMENT

- Assess vital signs to establish the client's status both before and after cast application.
- Examine all extremities for edema, peripheral pulses, color, pain, and other signs of injury.
- Determine if the client has underlying diseases or conditions that would predispose to poor wound healing or create additional risks for complications from casts (e.g., diabetes, immune disorders, impaired mental status, or peripheral vascular disease).

PLANNING
DELEGATION

The nurse should perform baseline assessment of all new casts. Care of clients with stable casts may be delegated to unlicensed assistive personnel (UAP). The status of the cast is observed during usual care and may be recorded by individuals other than the nurse. However, assessment of complications from the cast requires the expertise of a nurse. Abnormal findings detected by UAP must be validated and interpreted by the nurse.

INTERPROFESSIONAL PRACTICE

Caring for casts may be within the scope of practice for other health care providers. For example, in addition to nurses, both physical therapists and occupational therapists commonly work with clients with casts. Although the therapists may verbally communicate their findings and plan to the health care team members, the nurse must also know where to locate their documentation in the client's medical record.

Equipment

- Pillows to support the casted areas
- Ice packs
- Pen

IMPLEMENTATION
Preparation
Review the client record to determine the reason for the cast and the initial status of the client's extremity. Examine the record regarding pain assessment findings and interventions.

Performance

1. Prior to performing the procedure, introduce self and verify the client's identity using agency protocol. Explain to the client what you are going to do, why it is necessary, and how he or she can participate. Discuss how the results will be used in planning further care or treatments.
2. Perform hand hygiene and observe other appropriate infection prevention procedures.
3. Provide for client privacy as indicated.
4. Assess the neurovascular status of the affected limbs.
   - Assess the toes or fingers for nerve and circulatory impairments every 30 minutes for 4 hours following cast application, and then every 3 hours for the first 24 to 48 hours or until all signs and symptoms of impairment are negative. Increase the frequency of neurovascular assessments in accordance with the client's condition (e.g., presence of

circulatory impairment). **Rationale:** *Rapid swelling under a cast can cause neurovascular problems, necessitating frequent neurovascular assessments by the nurse.*
5. Support and handle the cast appropriately.
   - Immediately after the cast is applied, place it on pillows. Avoid using plastic or rubber pillows. **Rationale:** *The pillows provide even pressure and support the curves of the cast and promote venous blood return, thereby decreasing the possibility of swelling. Plastic or rubber pillows do not allow the heat of a drying cast to dissipate and so cause discomfort.*
   - Until a cast has set or hardened (10 to 20 minutes), support the cast in the palms of your hands rather than with the fingertips, and extend your fingers so that your fingertips do not touch the plaster. **Rationale:** *Fingertip pressure can cause dents in unset plaster and subsequent skin pressure areas (Satryb, Wilson, & Patterson, 2011).*
   - When the cast is set, continue to handle the cast in your palms, but you may then wrap your fingers around the contour of the cast.

Continued on page 696

SKILL 32–1

Providing Initial Cast Care—*continued*

6. Implement measures to reduce swelling.
   - Control swelling by elevating arms or legs on pillows or, for a leg fracture, by elevating the foot of the bed. Immediately after injury and surgery, elevate the limb to 45° but not above heart level. Generally, three pillows are needed to achieve high elevation of a leg. As circulation improves and healing progresses, the elevation can be gradually reduced to two pillows (moderate elevation) and then to one pillow (low elevation). **Rationale:** *Swelling can cause neurovascular impairment.*
   - Apply ice packs to control perineal edema associated with a hip spica cast. Although ice packs are a less effective method of control than elevation, elevation of the area is obviously difficult.
   - Report excessive swelling and indications of neurovascular impairment to the primary care provider or nurse in charge. The primary care provider may **bivalve** a cast if it appears to be too tight. Bivalving a cast is cutting the cast partially or completely ❶ and wrapping with bandage material to hold it together. **Rationale:** *This relieves the pressure of the cast but still provides support.*

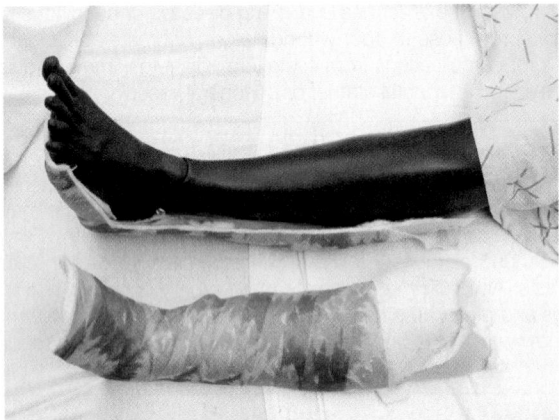

❶ Bivalved cast.

7. Use appropriate means to dry the plaster cast thoroughly.
   - Extremity plaster casts usually take 24 to 48 hours to dry completely; spica or body casts require 48 to 72 hours. Drying time depends on the temperature, humidity, size of the cast, and method used for drying. The cast is dry when it no longer feels damp. A dry cast feels dry, looks white and shiny, and is odorless, hard, and resonant when tapped. Synthetic casts take only 10 to 15 minutes to harden completely.
   - Expose the cast to the circulating air. Place sheets and blankets only over areas that do not have the cast.
   - Check agency policy about the recommended turning frequency for clients with different kinds of casts. **Rationale:** *Frequent turning promotes even drying of the cast.*
   - Turn the client with an extremity cast or body spica every 2 to 4 hours.
   - Use regular pillows. **Rationale:** *Plastic or rubber pillows hinder drying and do not allow the heat of a drying cast to dissipate.*

   - Avoid the use of artificial means to facilitate drying. These means include fans, hair dryers, infrared lamps, and electric heaters. **Rationale:** *Artificial methods dry the outer surface of the plaster cast while the inner portion remains soft and spongy. Such a cast cracks readily at points of strain. Natural methods dry the cast evenly.*

8. Monitor bleeding if an open reduction was done or if the injury was a compound fracture.
   - Monitor bloodstains or other drainage on the cast for 24 to 72 hours after surgery or injury or longer if necessary.
   - Outline the stained area with a pen at least every 8 hours if it is changing, and note the time and date so that any further bleeding can be determined.

9. Assess pain and pressure areas.
   - Never ignore any complaints of pain, burning, swelling, or pressure. If a client is unable to communicate, be alert to changes in temperament, restlessness, or fussiness that may indicate a problem. **Rationale: Compartment syndrome** *is a serious complication that can result when swelling and pressure within the closed fascial compartment build to dangerous levels, preventing nourishment from reaching nerve and muscle cells. If visible, the skin overlying the area may be red and hard. Apply ice, elevate, and notify the primary care provider immediately. An absent or diminished distal pulse necessitates immediate surgical action to allow expansion and blood flow and prevent nerve damage.*
   - Determine particularly whether the pain is persistent and if it occurs over a bony prominence or joint. See Table 32–2 for common pressure points associated with various casts.
   - Do not disregard a cessation of persistent pain or discomfort complaints from the client. **Rationale:** *Cessation of complaints can indicate nerve compression or a skin slough. When a skin slough occurs, superficial skin sensation is lost and the client no longer feels pain.*
   - When a pressure area under the cast is suspected, the primary care provider may either bivalve the cast so that all of the skin beneath the cast can be inspected or cut a window in the cast over only the area of concern. When a cast is windowed:
     a. Retain the piece (cast and padding) that was cut out. Some primary care providers order that it be taped back if there is no skin problem present, but that it be left out if a pressure area is present. **Rationale:** *Putting back the piece prevents window edema, which occurs when skin pressure at the window is not equal to that from the remainder of the cast.*
     b. Inspect the skin under the window at scheduled time intervals.

10. Document findings in the client record using forms or checklists supplemented by narrative notes when appropriate. Record each assessment (whether or not there are problems).

SAMPLE DOCUMENTATION

9/18/2015 1100 Cast still damp, elevated on one pillow. Fingers warm to touch, color pink, full ROM of fingers, no numbness or tingling. Arm pain at 2/10. Declined pain med. Will reassess in 30 minutes. ———————————————— E. Mitchell, RN

EVALUATION
- Perform detailed follow-up based on findings that deviated from expected or normal for the client. Relate findings to previous assessment data if available.

- Report significant deviations from normal to the primary care provider.

SKILL 32-2

●○● NURSING PROCESS: ONGOING CAST CARE

Providing Ongoing Cast Care

ASSESSMENT

- Perform a general head-to-toe assessment of the client.
- Determine if the client has underlying diseases or conditions that would predispose to poor wound healing or create additional risks for complications from casts (e.g., diabetes, immune disorders, impaired mental status, or peripheral vascular disease).

PLANNING
DELEGATION

Care of clients with stable casts may be delegated to UAP. The status of the cast is observed during usual care and may be recorded by individuals other than the nurse. However, assessment of complications from the cast requires the expertise of a nurse. Abnormal findings detected by UAP must be validated and interpreted by the nurse.

INTERPROFESSIONAL PRACTICE

Caring for casts may be within the scope of practice for other health care providers. For example, in addition to nurses, both physical therapists and occupational therapists commonly work with clients with casts. Although the therapists may verbally communicate their findings and plan to the health care team members, the nurse must also know where to locate their documentation in the client's medical record.

Equipment

Assemble any of the following equipment items necessary to complete client care:

- Pillows to support the casted areas
- Damp cloth
- Swab
- Alcohol, acetone, or nail polish remover
- Waterproof tape, adhesive strips, or moleskin
- Bib or towels
- Slipper (fracture) bedpan
- Plastic covering
- Soap and water
- Handheld blow dryer
- Mineral, olive, or baby oil
- Client lifting devices (e.g., Hoyer lift)

IMPLEMENTATION
Preparation

Review the client record to determine previous status of the cast and the client's extremities. Examine the record regarding pain assessment findings and interventions.

Performance

1. Prior to performing the procedure, introduce self and verify the client's identity using agency protocol. Explain to the client what you are going to do, why it is necessary, and how he or she can participate. Discuss how the results will be used in planning further care or treatments.
2. Perform hand hygiene and observe other appropriate infection prevention procedures.
3. Provide for client privacy as indicated.
4. Continue to assess the client for problems.
   - Assess the neurovascular status of the affected limb at regular intervals in accordance with agency protocol.
   - Inspect the skin near and under the cast edges whenever neurovascular assessments are made and/or whenever the client is turned.
   - Check the cast daily for a foul odor. **Rationale:** *This kind of odor may indicate skin excoriation from pressure or an infected area beneath the cast.*
5. Implement measures to prevent skin irritation at the edges of the cast.
   - Wash crumbs of plaster from the skin with a damp cloth and feel along the cast edges to check for rough edges or areas that press into the client's skin. **Rationale:** *As a plaster cast dries, small bits of plaster frequently break off from its rough edges. If they fall inside the cast, they can cause discomfort and irritation.*
   - Remove the resin of synthetic casting materials with a swab moistened with alcohol, acetone, or nail polish remover. Check the manufacturer's directions.

- When it is dry, cover any rough edges, and protect areas of the cast that may come in contact with urine. **Petal** the edges with small strips of waterproof tape or moleskin as follows:
   a. Cut several strips of 2.5-cm (1-in.) adhesive, 5 to 7.5 cm (2 to 3 in.) long. Then curve all corners of each strip. **Rationale:** *Square or pointed ends tend to curl.* ❶
   b. Insert one end of each strip as far as possible inside the cast, and bring the other end out over the cast edge. ❷
   c. Press the petals firmly against the plaster.
   d. Overlap successive petals slightly. ❸
6. Provide skin care to all areas vulnerable to pressure.
   - Examine all areas vulnerable to pressure and breakdown at least every 4 hours. For clients with sensitive skin or

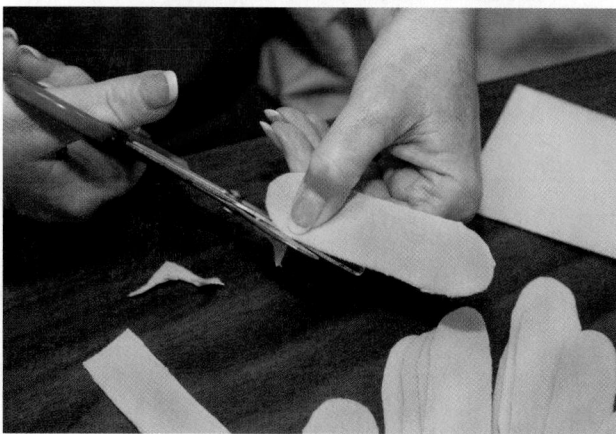

❶ Trim the corners of the strip to form oval ends.

Continued on page 698

SKILL 32-2

Providing Ongoing Cast Care—*continued*

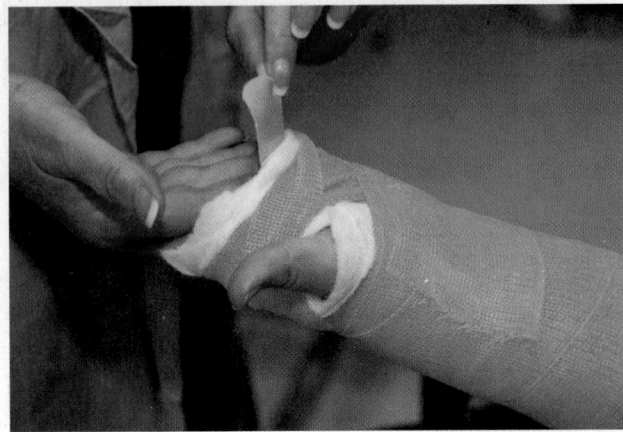

❷ Gently insert the strip under the cast and fold over the exposed edge.

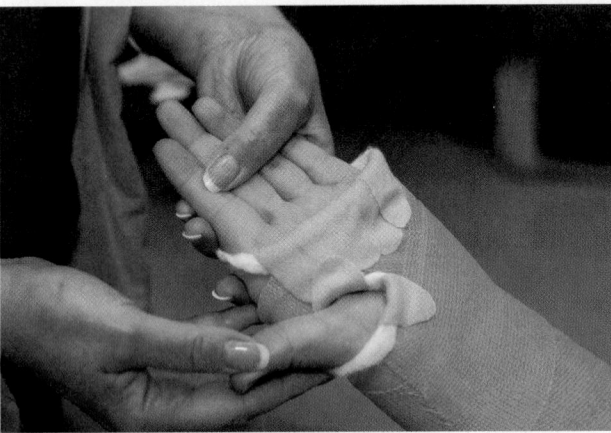

❸ Overlapping the strips ensures that there are no remaining exposed cast edges.

potential skin problems, provide care every 2 hours during the day and every 3 hours at night.
  a. Reach under the cast edges as far as possible and massage the area.
  b. Also provide skin care over all bony prominences not under the cast (e.g., the sacrum, heels, ankles, wrists, elbows, and feet). **Rationale:** *These are potential pressure areas if the client is confined to bed.*

7. Keep the cast clean and dry.
  • Place a bib or towel over a body cast to catch spills.

Plaster Cast
For elimination:
• Use a slipper (fracture) bedpan for people with long leg, hip spica, or body casts. **Rationale:** *The flat end placed correctly under the client's buttocks lessens the chance of spillage and minimizes the amount of lifting required by the client and/or nurse.*
• Before placing the client on the bedpan, tuck plastic or other waterproof material around the top of a long leg cast or around the perineal cutout. For a perineal cutout, funnel one end of the plastic into the bedpan.
• Remove the plastic when elimination is completed. **Rationale:** *If left in place, waterproof material makes the cast edge airtight and prevents evaporation of perspiration, which is irritating to the skin.*
• For people with long leg casts, keep the cast supported on pillows while the client is on the bedpan. **Rationale:** *If the cast dangles, urine may run down the cast.*

• For clients with hip spica casts, support both extremities and the back on pillows so that they are as high as the buttocks. **Rationale:** *This prevents urine from running back into the cast.*
• When removing the bedpan, hold it securely while the client is turning or lifting the buttocks. **Rationale:** *This prevents dripping and spilling.*
• After removing the bedpan, thoroughly clean and dry the perineal area.

Synthetic Cast
• Wash the soiled area with warm water and a mild soap.
• Thoroughly rinse the soap from the cast.
• Dry thoroughly to prevent skin maceration and ulceration under the cast.
• If the cast is immersed in water, dry the cast and underlying padding and stockinette thoroughly. First, blot excess water from the cast with a towel. Then, use a handheld blow dryer on the cool or warm setting, directing the air stream in a sweeping motion over the exterior of the cast for about 1 hour or until the client no longer feels a cold clammy sensation like that produced by a wet bathing suit. Specific actions depend on the type of liners used under the cast. **Rationale:** *This drying procedure is essential to prevent skin maceration and ulceration.*

8. Turn and position the client in correct alignment to prevent the formation of pressure areas.
  • Place pillows in such a way that:
    a. Body parts press against the edges of the cast as little as possible.
    b. Toes, heels, elbows, and so on are protected from pressure against the bed surface.
    c. Body alignment is maintained.
  • Plan and implement a turning schedule that will incorporate all of the possible positions. Generally, clients can be placed in lateral, prone, and supine positions unless surgical procedures or any other factors contraindicate them. Attach a trapeze to the overhead frame to enable the client to assist with moving (see Figure 32–3A ■ on page 702). **Rationale:** *Repositioning prevents pressure areas.*
  • Turn people with large casts or those unable to turn themselves at least once every 4 hours. If the person is at risk for skin breakdown, turn every 1 to 3 hours as needed.
  • When turning the client in a long leg cast to the unaffected side, place a pillow between the legs to support the cast.
  • In accordance with current safe client handling policies, request assistance from team members while the client is in the hospital or extended care facility. Use sufficient personnel to turn a person in a *damp* hip spica cast. When the cast is dry, the individual can usually turn with the assistance of the lifting device and one nurse.

9. Encourage range-of-motion (ROM) and isometric exercises.
  • Unless contraindicated, encourage active ROM exercises for all joints on the unaffected extremities, as well as the joints proximal and distal to the cast. If active exercises are contraindicated, implement active-assistive or passive exercises, depending on the client's abilities and disabilities (see Skill 13–1 in Chapter 13 ∞). **Rationale:** *Exercise helps prevent joint stiffness, muscle atrophy, and venous stasis.*
  • Encourage the client to move toes and/or fingers of the casted extremity as frequently as possible. **Rationale:** *Moving these extremities enhances peripheral circulation and decreases swelling and pain.*
  • Teach isometric (muscle-setting) exercises for extremities in a cast. **Rationale:** *Isometric exercises minimize muscle atrophy in the affected limb.*

Providing Ongoing Cast Care—*continued*

a. Teach the isometric exercises on the client's unaffected limb before the person applies it to the affected limb.

b. Demonstrate muscle palpation while the client is carrying out the exercise. **Rationale:** *Palpation enables the person to feel the changes that occur with muscle contraction and relaxation.*

• Determine if the client can be safely assisted out of bed. To protect both the nurse and the client, ensure that sufficient caregivers and equipment are available and properly used. Hospitals should have a designated process for the use of "lift teams" and devices (Gallagher, 2013). Zero-lift legislation has been passed in many states that mandates hospitals provide both lift equipment and trained lift teams.

10. Provide client teaching to promote self-care, comfort, and safety. (See the accompanying Client Teaching Considerations).

• Teach people immobilized in bed with large body casts ways to turn and to move safely by using a trapeze, the side rails, and other such devices.

• Instruct clients with leg casts about ways to walk effectively with crutches (see Skill 11–4 in Chapter 11 ∞).

• Instruct people with arm casts how to apply slings (see Skill 31–9 in Chapter 31 ∞).

• Teach clients how to resolve itching under the cast safely (see Client Teaching Considerations). Discourage the person from using objects to scratch under the cast. **Rationale:** *These objects can break the skin and cause an infection*

because bacteria flourish in the warm, dark, moist environment under the cast. Sticking objects under a cast can also cause folding or bunching of padding material and subsequent pressure and discomfort.

• When healing is complete and the cast is removed, the underlying skin is usually macerated, pale, flaky, and encrusted, since layers of dead skin have accumulated. Instruct clients to remove this debris gently and gradually.

a. Apply oil (e.g., mineral, olive, or baby oil).

b. Soak the skin in warm water and dry it.

c. Caution the client not to rub the area too vigorously. **Rationale:** Vigorous rubbing can cause bleeding or excoriation of fragile skin.

d. Repeat steps a and b for several days. **Rationale:** *Gradual removal of skin exudates reduces skin irritation.*

11. Document findings in the client record using forms or checklists supplemented by narrative notes when appropriate. Record each assessment (whether or not there are problems).

SAMPLE DOCUMENTATION

9/15/2015 1000 Cast intact, leg elevated on 2 pillows. Toes warm to touch, pink, capillary refill 2 seconds. Moves toes readily and fully; states no numbness or tingling. Pain 0/10. ————— B. Snyder, RN

EVALUATION

• Perform detailed follow-up based on findings that deviated from expected or normal for the client. Relate findings to previous assessment data if available.

• Report significant deviations from normal to the primary care provider.

LIFESPAN CONSIDERATIONS Cast Care

Children

• Teach parents of young children ways to prevent the child from placing small items inside the cast. Serious infections and damage to tissues can occur as a result of sticking anything inside the cast. Parents also need to ensure that the top of a body cast is covered during meals so that food does not fall inside the cast.

• If possible, allow the child to choose the color/pattern of the synthetic cast. Wearing a cast can cause disturbances in body image and self-concept. Education regarding cast care, how to adapt activities of daily living (ADLs), efficient ambulation, and what to expect as far as cast removal will help the child cope effectively.

• Reassure the child that the saw used for windowing, bivalving, and removing the cast is not painful. It rapidly vibrates back and forth rather than rotates, so injury from the blade is unlikely. The saw is rather loud and can scare children.
Consider whether another adult should be present to support the child during these procedures. Let the child keep the cast pieces when removed if desired and they are not needed.

OLDER ADULTS

• Older adults who are immobilized are at increased risk for skin breakdown and pressure ulcers.

• Wound healing may be slower in older than in younger clients.

• Older adults may be less able to manage the additional weight and imbalance caused by the cast.

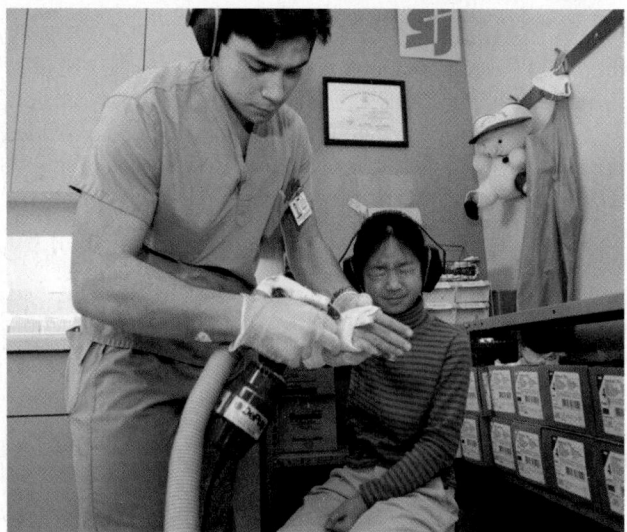

Both nurse and client can wear headsets to minimize the noise of the cast saw.
Jim Rankin/Getty Images

• Take appropriate steps in planning for use of crutches or other mobility aids to keep older adults moving safely.

Cast Care

- For itching, suggest that the client use a hair dryer on cool or an ice bag over the outside of the itching area. Emphasize the importance of *not* putting anything inside the cast, because serious infections and tissue damage can occur.
- Before discharge from the hospital, instruct the client to:
  a. Observe for indications of nerve or circulatory impairment, such as extreme coldness or blueness of toes or fingers; extreme continuous swelling of casted toes or fingers; numbness or tingling ("pins and needles" sensation) in casted toes or fingers; continuous complaints of pain; or inability to move the toes or fingers.
  b. Keep the plaster cast dry.
  c. Avoid strenuous activity and follow medical advice about exercise.
  d. Elevate the arm or leg frequently to prevent dependent edema.
  e. Move the toes or fingers frequently.
  f. Observe the skin around the cast edges frequently, and keep it clean and dry.
  g. Report any increase in pain; unexplained fever; foul odor from within the cast; decreased circulation; numbness; inability to move the fingers or toes; or a weakened, cracked, loose, or tight cast.
- Review modifications that may be necessary in clothing, toileting, sleeping, and other ADLs.
- When it is time for cast removal, reassure clients that the saw, though loud, oscillates rather than rotates, and is not dangerous. Skin under the cast will look macerated and pale, and hair growth can be increased. Depending on the length of time the cast has been worn, muscle atrophy can occur, leading to asymmetry of limbs. Muscles may regain strength through substantial physical effort although this is more likely in younger clients than in older adults.

TRACTION

Traction is a means of immobilization using a pulling force applied to a part of the body while a second force, called **countertraction**, pulls in the opposite direction. The pulling force is provided through a system of pulleys, ropes, and weights attached to the client. The countertraction is often achieved by elevating the foot or head of the bed and therefore is supplied by the client's body. People who are in traction are sometimes confined to bed for weeks or even months, though long-term traction is no longer widely used. Nursing care therefore involves ADLs, maintenance of the traction, and the prevention of problems related to immobility such as pressure ulcers.

Purposes of Traction

Traction is applied for several purposes:

- To reduce and/or immobilize a bone fracture for healing.
- To maintain proper bone alignment when operative fixation is not available for a period of time.
- To prevent soft tissue injury.
- To correct, reduce, or prevent deformities.
- To decrease muscle spasm and pain.
- To treat inflammatory conditions by immobilizing a joint (e.g., for arthritis or tuberculosis of a joint).

Types of Traction

The two major types of traction are skin and skeletal traction:

1. *Skin traction* is a pulling force applied to the skin and soft tissues through the use of tape or traction straps and a system of ropes, pulleys, and weights. The traction tape or strap is often made of vented foam rubber or cloth, and it may have either an adhesive or a nonadhesive backing. Adhesive skin traction is used for continuous traction. Nonadhesive skin traction is used intermittently; it can easily be removed and reapplied. The most common forms of skin traction are **Buck's extension** for presurgical stabilization of fractured hips (Figure 32–3A), and occasionally cervical for rotary subluxation of the first and second vertebrae. See the Practice Guidelines for care of the client in skin traction.

2. Skeletal traction is applied by inserting metal pins, wires, or tongs directly into or through a bone. The metal device is then attached to a system of ropes, pulleys, and weights by means of a metal frame attached to the bed. Skeletal traction can be applied to the skull, the proximal end of the ulna, the distal end of the femur, the proximal and distal ends of the tibia, and the calcaneus (heel bone). **Rationale:** *Because bone withstands greater stress than skin, weights heavier than those used for skin traction can be used (e.g., up to 16 kg [35 lb]).*

Traction setups are often named after their inventors. Figure 32–3 shows common varieties.

- The distal end of a **Thomas leg splint** and a **Pearson attachment** are attached to a weighted rope for suspension. The Pearson attachment supports the lower leg off the bed and permits the knee to be flexed (Figure 32–3B). The pin or wire drilled through the bone is attached to a spreader, which in turn is attached to ropes, pulleys, and weights. Countertraction is supplied mostly by the body's weight. A weighted rope attached to the proximal end of the Thomas splint, however, counterbalances the suspension weight. To prevent foot drop, a footplate is attached to the Pearson apparatus. To prevent skin breakdown, the ischial ring of the Thomas splint is padded. Sheepskin slings may be positioned along the Pearson attachment.
- **Skull tongs** (e.g., **Crutchfield**, Burton, Gardner–Wells, or Vinke) are secured to each side of the skull. The center metal bar is attached to ropes, pulleys, and weights and creates a traction pull along the long axis of the spine (Figure 32–3C).

Traction can be either continuous or intermittent. Continuous traction (skeletal or skin) is applied and released by a specially trained practitioner who is responsible for handling the affected part when it is not in traction. Intermittent traction (nonadhesive skin traction) can be applied and released by nursing personnel with the appropriate order. However, the primary care provider prescribes the amount of weight to be applied.

Traction Equipment

The following equipment is used for most skin and skeletal tractions:

- *Overhead frame:* This frame is attached to the hospital bed and provides a means for attachment of the traction apparatus. Each frame has at least two upright bars (one at each end of the bed) and one overhead bar.

PRACTICE GUIDELINES

Caring for the Client in Skin Traction

1. Determine the following: bruises and abrasions in the area where the traction is to be applied, any history of circulatory problems and skin allergies, mental and emotional status, and ability to understand activity restrictions.
2. Note the type of traction, and inspect the traction apparatus regularly, that is, whenever you are at the bedside or at prescribed intervals, such as every 2 hours (see Skill 32–2).
3. Maintain the client in the appropriate traction position.
   - Maintain the client in the supine position unless there are other orders. **Rationale:** *Changing position can change the body alignment and the amount of force supplied by the traction.*
   - Maintain body alignment when turning the client. In some cases, the person can turn to a lateral position if a pillow placed between the legs maintains body alignment. Refer to the client's record for information about permitted movement.
   - Provide a trapeze to assist the client to move and lift the body for back care if he or she is unable to turn.
   - Provide a fracture or slipper bedpan as required to minimize the client's movement during elimination.
4. Assess the neurovascular status of the affected extremity.
   - Conduct a neurovascular assessment 30 minutes following reapplication of the bandage, then every 2 hours for the first 24 hours. If the client's status is stable, then assess every 4 hours during the traction. If the client's status is unstable, continue assessments hourly.
5. Provide protective devices and measures to safeguard the skin.
   - Place heel protectors or sheepskins under the heels, sacrum, shoulders, and other pressure areas. See Table 32–2.
   - Change or clean the sheepskin lining at least weekly.
   - Massage the skin with rubbing alcohol or lotion every 4 hours, or if redness and signs of pressure appear, every 2 hours. **Rationale:** *Alcohol tends to toughen the skin and leave it less vulnerable to breakdown. Because alcohol is drying to the skin, however, lotion may be preferred for those who have dry skin (e.g., older adults).*
   - Make sure the spreader bar is wide enough to prevent the traction tape from rubbing on the client's bony prominences.
6. Remove only intermittent nonadhesive skin traction in accordance with agency protocol or orders.
   - To remove a nonadhesive skin traction:
     a. Remove the weights first.
     b. Unwrap the bandage and provide skin care.
     c. Rewrap the limb and slowly reattach the weights.
7. Teach the client ways to prevent problems associated with immobility.
   - Teach the client deep-breathing and coughing exercises to prevent hypostatic pneumonia (see Chapter 24 ∞).
   - Teach the client appropriate exercises to maintain and develop muscle tone, prevent muscle contracture and atrophy, and promote blood circulation:
     a. Range-of-motion exercises (discussed in Chapter 13 ∞) should be taught.
     b. Teach isometric exercises to strengthen the quadriceps that include tightening the knees. By pushing the knees down without moving them, the hamstring muscles are also strengthened. Tensing the buttocks and the inner thighs promotes stabilization of the hips. Tensing the inner thighs also helps stabilize the knees.
     c. Circulation to the extremities can be promoted by encouraging the client to flex and extend the feet as well as to perform the isometric exercises.
     d. Specific exercises to strengthen the biceps and triceps in preparation for using crutches can be taught as indicated. For example, raising the buttocks off the bed by pushing down with the arms develops the triceps, and pulling the body up with a trapeze develops the biceps.
8. Document findings in the client record using forms or checklists supplemented by narrative notes when appropriate.
9. Perform a detailed follow-up examination based on findings that deviated from expected or normal for the client. The client should be able to demonstrate usual ROM in all unaffected body joints, move all fingers or toes of the affected extremity, feel normal sensation and have normal skin color and temperature in all fingers or toes of the affected extremity, and be free of pressure signs (pallor, redness, increased warmth or tenderness) over pressure areas. Relate findings to previous assessment data if available. Report significant findings to the primary care provider.

TABLE 32–2   Traction Pressure Areas

Traction	Pressure Areas
Buck's extension	Skin over the tibia, if bandage slips; malleoli, hamstring tendon; heels; back
Russell traction	As above for Buck's extension; popliteal space due to sling; sole of foot due to footplate
Cervical head halter	Chin; occiput; ears; mandible
Thomas leg splint and Pearson attachment	Groin, popliteal space; Achilles tendon; heel; perineal nerve if splint misplaced
Halo-thoracic vest	Areas where jacket edges touch the skin; skin under vest

- *Trapeze:* Attached to the overhead frame, the trapeze can be used by the client for moving in bed, unless contraindicated by the client's health.
- *Firm mattress:* To maintain body alignment and the efficiency of the traction, a firm mattress is essential. Some beds are manufactured with a solid bottom instead of springs, to provide firm support. If a firm bed is not available, a bedboard can be used to provide the needed support.
- *Ropes, pulleys, weight hangers, and weights.*

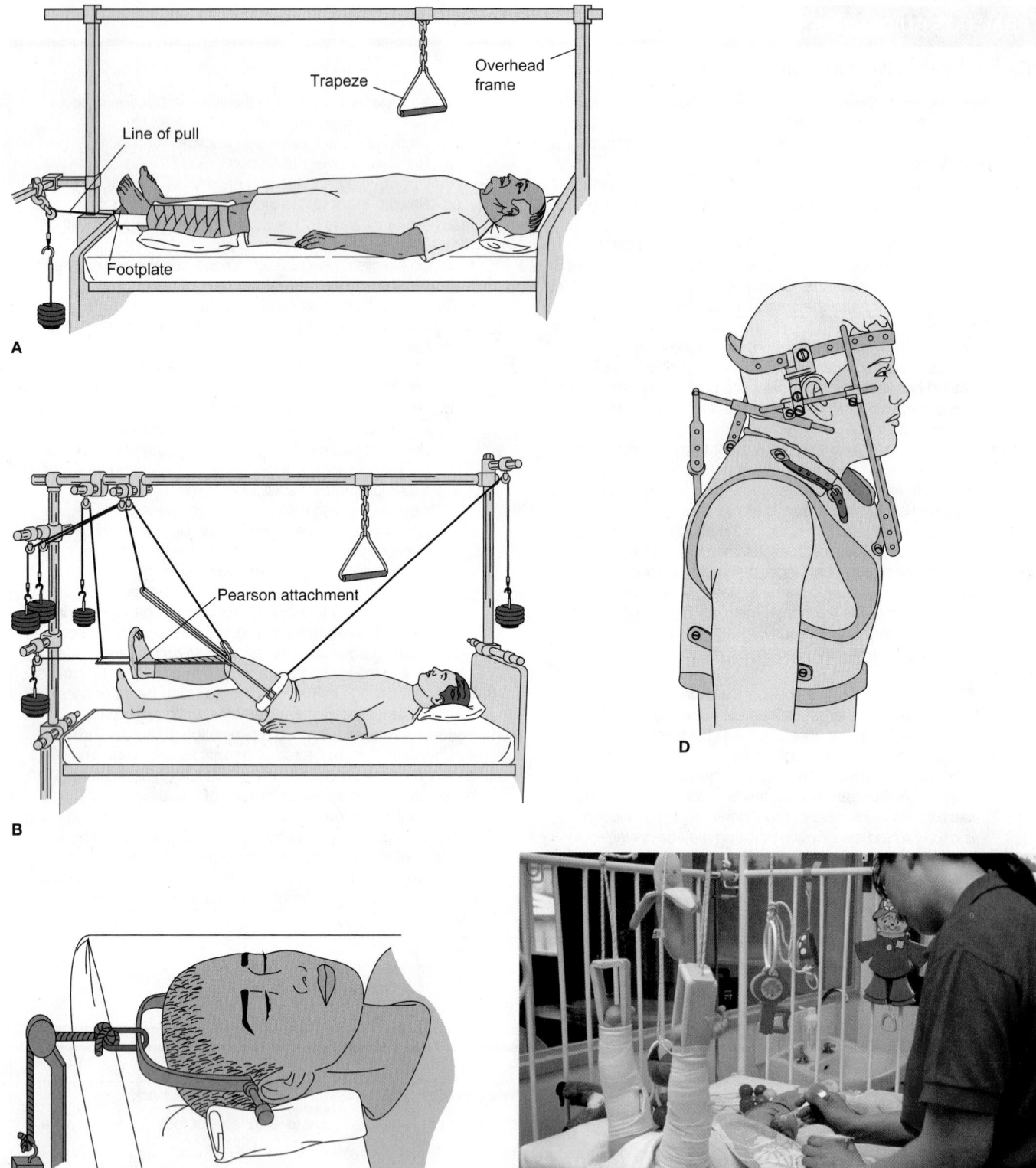

Figure 32–3 ■ *A,* Buck's extension for skin traction immobilizes hip fractures. It may be necessary to elevate the foot of the bed to prevent the client from sliding down. The standard foam boot cannot be used with a calf compression device for prevention of vascular problems. If the device must be used with Buck's traction, adhesive traction straps must be used instead. *B,* Thomas splint with Pearson attachment for fracture of the femur for balanced suspension skeletal traction. *C,* Gardner–Wells skull tongs for skeletal traction immobilizes fractures of cervical and upper thoracic vertebrae. *D,* halo-thoracic vest (external fixation) traction has a circular metal band secured by pins that penetrate the skull a fraction of an inch. The halo is attached to the vest by metal rods. The vest supports and suspends the weight of the entire apparatus around the chest. The advantage over other types of head and neck traction is that the client can sit, stand, and walk, thus decreasing problems associated with prolonged immobility. Keep a wrench of the appropriate type/size near the client at all times in case of emergency. *E,* Bryant's traction. Ensure that the sacrum is elevated sufficiently to allow the nurse to slip a hand between the child's buttocks and the bed.

●○● NURSING PROCESS: CARE OF THE CLIENT IN TRACTION

Caring for Clients in Skeletal Traction

ASSESSMENT

Assess:

- The neurovascular status of the affected extremity, that is, the status of peripheral pulses, color, amount of movement, temperature, capillary filling, edema, numbness, and sensation.
- The presence of pain in the area: exact location, degree, duration, and description of the pain (e.g., sharp, needle-like) and identification of any movement or activity that would initiate the pain.
- Clinical signs of thrombi and emboli (clot or other blockage of a blood vessel). Regularly assess the client's pulse, blood pressure, respirations, mental status, and breath sounds for evidence of emboli. Inspect the client's involved extremity for redness, swelling, and pain.
- Pressure areas for signs of skin irritation or breakdown. Note in particular (a) bony prominences (e.g., the heels, ankles, sacrum, elbows, chin, and shoulders) and (b) areas susceptible to pressure from the traction (e.g., the tibia for Buck's extension) as shown in Table 32–2 and Figure 32–3.
- Inflammation and drainage at the pin sites for skeletal traction.
- Presence of skin allergies.
- The skin for signs of infection or injury.

PLANNING

A physical therapist or orthopedic technician generally performs the initial setup of traction. Communicate with this person to establish the best time for the traction to be placed. The nurse is responsible for caring for the client in traction and ensuring that the traction is functioning properly.

DELEGATION

Care of clients in traction may be delegated to trained UAP. However, assessment and pin site care must be performed by the nurse.

INTERPROFESSIONAL PRACTICE

Establishing and maintaining traction may be within the scope of practice for other health care providers, especially physical therapists. Although the therapists may verbally communicate their findings and plan to the health care team members, the nurse must also know where to locate their documentation in the client's medical record.

Equipment

- Supplies for providing pin site care according to agency policy (e.g., normal saline, cotton-tipped swabs, gauze dressings, clean or sterile gloves)

IMPLEMENTATION

Preparation

Verify the primary care provider's orders. Determine the degree of movement permitted and any special precautions (e.g., bed positions permitted).

Performance

1. Prior to performing the procedure, introduce self and verify the client's identity using agency protocol. Explain to the client what you are going to do, why it is necessary, and how he or she can participate. Discuss how the results will be used in planning further care or treatments.
2. Perform hand hygiene and observe other appropriate infection prevention procedures.
3. Provide for client privacy.
4. Inspect the traction apparatus:
   - Is the appropriate countertraction provided? For example, is the foot of the bed elevated 2.5 cm (1 in.) for every 0.5 kg (1 lb) of traction or is the knee of the bed flexed 20° to 30°?
   - Are the correct weights applied? For example, Buck's traction should have no more than 2.3 kg (5 lb).
   - Is there free play of the ropes on the pulleys; that is, does the groove of the pulley support the rope? Are the knots positioned no closer than 30 cm (12 in.) to the nearest pulley?
   - Do all weights hang freely and not rest against or on the bed or floor when the bed is in the lowest position?
   - Are the ropes intact, that is, not frayed, knotted, or kinked between their points of attachment?
   - Are the ropes securely attached with slipknots and the short ends of ropes attached with tape?
   - Is the line of the traction straight and in the same plane as the long axis of the bone?
   - Are bedclothes and other objects free from the traction?
   - Is the spreader bar wide enough to prevent the traction tape from rubbing on bony prominences?
5. Maintain the client in the appropriate traction position. Check that the head, knee, and foot of the bed are properly elevated.
   - For clients with skull tongs or a halo ring (see Figure 32–3C and D), turn the client as a unit. Do not allow the neck to twist. A special bed and assistance from the lift team may be required (see Chapter 10 ∞).
   - If skull tongs or pins become dislodged, support the head, remove the weights, place sandbags or liter fluid bags on either side of the head to maintain alignment, and notify the primary care provider immediately.
6. Assess the neurovascular status of the affected extremity.
   - Conduct a neurovascular assessment every hour for the first 24 hours. If the client's status is stable, then assess every 4 hours during the traction. If the client's status is changing, continue assessments hourly.
7. Provide pin site care daily if indicated by the primary care provider's orders and agency protocol. Research studies have provided insufficient evidence to determine the best management of pin sites (Camathias, Valderrabano, & Oberli, 2013). Thus, all agency protocols should emphasize reduction of the potential for infection.
   - Carefully inspect the site. Regular inspection of the pin site ensures early detection of minor infections, as manifested by signs of serosanguineous drainage, crusting, swelling, and erythema.
   - Use clean or sterile technique as agency protocol dictates. **Rationale:** *Sterile technique is most often used in the hospital setting, clean technique in the ambulatory setting.*

Continued on page 704

Caring for Clients in Skeletal Traction—*continued*

- If in keeping with agency policy, remove crusts using normal saline or other agent such as diluted alcohol, povidone-iodine, or hydrogen peroxide recommended by the agency. Use a cotton-tipped swab with a gentle, rolling technique to reduce irritation to the tissue. **Rationale:** *Removing crusted secretions permits the pin site to drain freely. Initial crusts around pins do not create a problem and can serve as a barrier to infection, but accumulated crusts around external fixator pins may cause secondary infection.*
- If purulent (containing pus) drainage is present, notify the primary care provider and obtain specimens for culture and sensitivity (see Skill 4–9 in Chapter 4 ∞).
- Apply sterile ointment if ordered. Determine agency practices regarding pin site care; ointment could interfere with proper drainage.
- Loosely apply the gauze dressing around the pin site.

- Adjust frequency of care according to the amount of drainage. If no drainage is present, daily site care is adequate. If drainage is present, perform site care every 8 hours.
- Dispose of soiled equipment according to agency protocol.
- Remove and discard gloves if used.
- Perform hand hygiene.
8. Teach the client ways to prevent problems associated with immobility.
9. Document findings in the client record using forms or checklists supplemented by narrative notes when appropriate.

SAMPLE DOCUMENTATION

9/17/2015 1230 Traction maintained at 20 pounds with FOB ↑ 50 cm. Skin intact and pink, sensation present, no pain. Pin sites clean and dry without sign of infection. ————————— G. Merritt, RN

EVALUATION

- Perform follow-up based on findings that deviated from expected or normal for the client.
- Relate findings to previous assessment data if available.

- Report significant deviations from normal to the primary care provider.

LIFESPAN CONSIDERATIONS   Traction

INFANTS/CHILDREN

- Bryant's traction (Figure 32–3*E*) is an adaptation of a bilateral Buck's extension. It is used to stabilize fractured femurs or correct congenital hip dislocations in young children. The skin traction is applied to both the affected and the unaffected leg to maintain the position of the affected leg. A spreader bar attached to the strips or positioning of the pulleys maintains leg alignment. Unless otherwise ordered, the hips are flexed at right angles (90°) to the body with the knees extended, and the

buttocks are raised about 2.5 cm (1 in.). Pressure areas include skin over the tibia, malleoli, hamstring tendon, soles of feet, and upper back.

OLDER ADULTS

- Adhesive skin traction should not be used due to the fragility of older adults' skin.
- Skin breakdown can occur more easily with any form of traction in older adults than in younger clients.

Ambulatory and Community Settings   Traction

TEAMWORK AND COLLABORATION

- Cervical traction may be done in the home setting using electrical systems or over-the-door mechanical systems. Clients may be instructed to use the system several times a day for up to 30 minutes at a time. A physical therapist should establish the system and conduct initial client and family teaching. The nurse should reinforce proper technique and assess effectiveness during home or clinic visits.

- Clients in halo-thoracic vest traction (see Figure 32–3*D*) are ambulatory and need not be hospitalized. Client and family teaching regarding hygiene, care of the device, and when to contact health care providers must be reinforced.

ORTHOSES

Orthoses are orthotic braces that provide musculoskeletal support, balance (e.g., after a stroke), stretch, and comfort (Cervasio, 2011). Store-bought arch supports and prescription products such as molded ankle-foot orthoses and spinal braces (e.g., Wilmington and Boston) are all examples of these devices.

Spinal orthoses take the form of braces and are used to resist progression of scoliotic and kyphotic curves as well as to protect after trauma and fracture. Orthoses are used on lower extremities (Figure 32–4 ■) to manage contractures and support ambulation in those with neuromotor deficits (e.g., with cerebral palsy); to support hip, knee, and ankle joints; and to relieve pain (e.g., with plantar fasciitis). Foot orthoses help correct unbalanced pronation and supination. This, in turn, helps to control the stabilization and mechanics of the whole body. Orthoses are also used to support and increase

comfort for those with tendinitis and chronic degeneration from overuse of the elbow, wrist, hand, and fingers.

Nursing responsibilities for clients with orthotic devices are mostly educative, and focused on application and maintenance of the device, duration/intervals of wearing, comfort, careful skin care and monitoring, and assisting with any other particular instructions from the manufacturer and/or prescriber. An accurate fit is essential, and professional orthotists offer adjustments to fine-tune orthoses as needed. Most orthoses can be washed with mild soap and warm water and then air-dried. They should be kept away from sources of high heat (prolonged sunlight, heaters) and should not be exposed to chemicals such as bleach or acetone. Ensuring client understanding of instructions is essential for proper use and efficacy of orthotic devices. A summary of important considerations and family teaching points appears in Client Teaching Considerations.

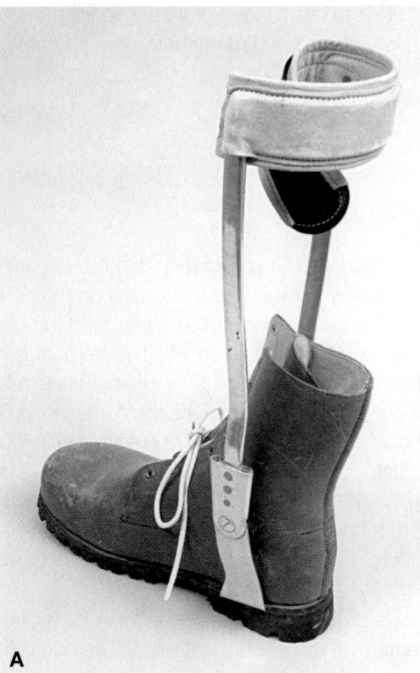

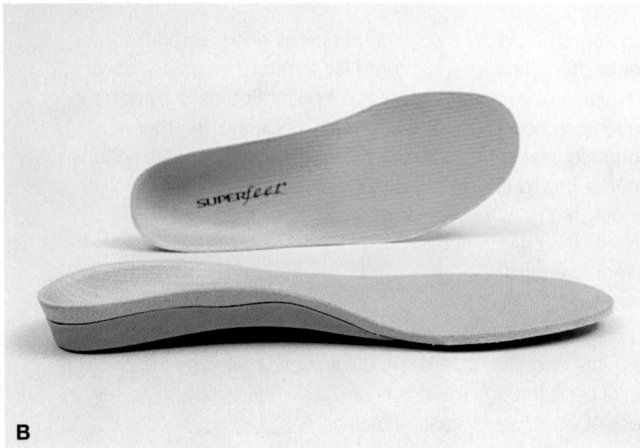

A

B

Figure 32–4 ■ Examples of orthoses: *A,* an ankle-foot orthotic that stops below the knee but supports the ankle; *B,* a foot orthotic that slips inside a shoe or sneaker to correct alignment.

CLIENT TEACHING CONSIDERATIONS

Caring for Clients with Orthoses

- In general, orthoses must fit snugly, and skin care and monitoring are essential. Any red or open areas must be covered with a thin sterile bandage and checked every 2 to 3 hours. If healing is slow (more than 3 days), the primary care provider and orthotist should be consulted. Open areas might need time and exposure to air in order to heal completely. Any burning sensation under or near an orthotic device is an important warning sign requiring follow-up with the primary care provider and orthotist.
- Applying lotion to skin under orthoses is contraindicated (unless skin is very dry) because soft skin may be more prone to breakdown (Cervasio, 2011).
- For orthoses that support the thoracolumbosacral area, a cotton undershirt should be worn underneath. It is important to make

sure the shirt is clean, dry, and free of wrinkles. Any tender, raw area or red mark that does not fade within 20 minutes should be reported to the orthotist.
- As children grow, they need periodic adjustments in (or replacement of) their orthoses. Ill-fitting orthoses (in any client) will cause problems with balance, support, and comfort.
- Orthotic devices must be carefully maintained to ensure efficacy and client safety. Support sections of braces should be cleaned with mild soap and water and then carefully dried. Joint hinges (found in ankle-foot, knee-ankle-foot, and hip-knee-ankle-foot orthoses) should be periodically oiled with a household lubricant such as 3-IN-ONE oil. Any joint screws should be checked periodically to make sure they are tight.

Chapter **32** Review

FOCUSING ON CLINICAL THINKING

Consider This

1. A teenager is to be casted for a severe fracture of the elbow with significant tissue swelling and a break in the skin. The primary care provider plans to cast the elbow in a 45° flexed position for several days and then recast in a 90° flexed position. When told that a plaster cast will be used, the client is upset, insisting that a colorful synthetic cast will be easier to care for and allow showering. What data will you use to explain the choice of plaster to the client?

2. You are visiting your older client in the home to check on a casted fracture of the wrist. The fingers appear swollen, somewhat dusky in color, and cool. What further assessments are indicated, and what actions would you take?

3. Your young client has been placed in Buck's traction. While assessing the response to treatment, the client complains of being "bored lying flat on my back all day" and wants you to remove the apparatus. What will you say? What will you do?

4. The hospitalized client in skeletal traction for a fractured femur has slid down to the end of the bed. Describe how you would reposition the client.

See Focusing on Clinical Thinking answers on student resource website.

TEST YOUR KNOWLEDGE

1. The nurse is caring for a 43-year-old client who has required 2 weeks of traction for a fractured left femur. The client is now complaining of sharp left-sided chest pain rated as 8/10 without radiation and accompanying shortness of breath. In order of importance, place a 1, 2, and a 3 beside the appropriate actions the nurse should take in this situation:
   1. Notify the primary care provider.
   2. Notify the charge nurse.
   3. Apply oxygen.
   4. Administer nitroglycerin.

2. The nurse is caring for a client who sustained a compound fracture of the ulna. After the bone is set, the wound created by the perforation of bone through the skin is dressed. The nurse anticipates the use of what type of casting material? _____

3. The nurse is admitting a client who just had a long leg cast applied. The nurse will assess this client for nerve and circulatory impairment every:
   1. 10 minutes for 4 hours.
   2. 1 hour for 8 hours.
   3. 30 minutes for 2 hours.
   4. 30 minutes for 4 hours.

4. The nurse is assessing a client with a new cast applied to the leg for neurosensory and circulatory impairment. Which of the following signs would indicate impairment and the need to notify the primary care provider?
   1. Toes on both feet are cold to touch.
   2. Capillary refill time in the casted toes is 3 seconds.
   3. The toes of the casted leg are pale.
   4. The toes of the casted leg are edematous.

5. The nurse is providing discharge teaching for a client who had a synthetic cast applied to a fractured left arm. The nurse recognizes that discharge teaching has been effective when the client states:
   1. "If my cast gets dirty I should come to the emergency department to have it changed."
   2. "When I shower I don't need to do anything special because it is okay for this casting material to get wet."
   3. "When I shower I should cover the cast with a plastic bag."
   4. "I should not clean my cast with a wet cloth if it gets dirty."

6. The nurse is admitting a client with a plaster cast newly applied to the right leg. Once the client is moved to the bed, the nurse positions the client by:
   1. Elevating the foot and head of the bed with the client lying supine.
   2. Placing the casted leg on pillows with the foot of the bed elevated with the client lying supine.
   3. Placing the casted leg in balanced suspension traction.
   4. Placing the casted leg on pillows with the client lying on the left side.

7. A nurse, working in the emergency department, is teaching the client with a newly placed synthetic cast on the right leg how to care for the cast at home. The nurse recognizes the client understood the teaching when which statement is made?
   1. "I should call my doctor if the pain increases a lot or if my toes get cold, pale, or feel like they are asleep."
   2. "I should go home and sit in my recliner with ice applied to the cast."
   3. "I can walk as much as I want as long as I use crutches and don't put weight on my injured foot."
   4. "I should use a hair dryer when I get home to help the cast dry faster."

8. The nurse is providing discharge teaching for a client with a newly casted left arm. The client says, "I've heard these things itch. Is it okay if I use the handle of a wooden spoon to scratch inside the cast since that wouldn't be pointy or scratch the skin?" The nurse's best response would be:
   1. "Yes, that would be okay since it wouldn't cause any skin damage."
   2. "No, don't use anything inside the cast. Instead use a hair dryer on cool or a vacuum cleaner on reverse, or put an ice bag over the area that itches."
   3. "No, you shouldn't put anything into the cast."
   4. "Don't worry; you won't experience any itching with a synthetic cast."

9. The nurse is working on the pediatric unit caring for a child with cerebral palsy who wears an orthotic device. When the orthotic device is removed, the nurse notices a red area under the device. The nurse's priority action will be to:
   1. Notify the orthotist.
   2. Apply lotion to the area.
   3. Teach the mother to rub the area to improve circulation.
   4. Reassess the area in 20 minutes.

10. The mother of a child wearing knee-ankle-foot braces informs the nurse that she applied 3-IN-ONE oil to the hinges of the child's braces. The nurse's best response would be:
    1. "That's a good idea. How often do you do that?"
    2. "I know you were trying to do what you thought was best for your child, but it would be better if you let the orthotist take care of things like that."
    3. "You really shouldn't do that. You could damage the brace."
    4. "Why did you do that?"

See Answers to Test Your Knowledge in Appendix A.

READINGS AND REFERENCES

References

Camathias, C., Valderrabano, V., & Oberli, H. (2013). Routine pin tract care in external fixation is unnecessary: A randomised, prospective, blinded controlled study. *Injury, 43*, 1969–1973. doi:10.1016/j.injury.2012.08.010

Cervasio, K. (2011). Lower extremity orthoses in children with spastic quadriplegic cerebral palsy: Implications for nurses, parents, and caregivers. *Orthopaedic Nursing, 30*, 155–161. doi:10.1097/NOR.0b013e31821b6c18

Gallagher, S. (2013). *Implementation guide to the safe patient handling and mobility interprofessional national standards*. Silver Spring, MD: American Nurses Association.

Satryb, S. A., Wilson, T. J., & Patterson, M. M. (2011). Casting: All wrapped up. *Orthopaedic Nursing, 30*, 37–41. doi:10.1097/NOR.0b013e31820574f9

Shuler, F. D., & Bates, C. M. (2013). Skin temperatures generated following plaster splint application. *Orthopedics, 36*, 364–367. doi:10.3928/01477447-20130426-06

Williams, K. G., Smith, G., Luhmann, S. J., Mao, J., Gunn, J. D., & Luhmann, J. D. (2013). A randomized controlled trial of cast versus splint for distal radial buckle fracture: An evaluation of satisfaction, convenience, and preference. *Pediatric Emergency Care, 29*, 555–559. doi:10.1097/PEC.0b013e31828e56fb

Selected Bibliography

American Nurses Association. (2013). *Safe patient handling and mobility: Interprofessional national standards*. Silver Spring, MD: Author.

Beaty, J. A., & Murphy, A. L. (2013). Effectiveness of a flex orthotic splint on hand range of motion for older adults: A pilot study. *Physical & Occupational Therapy in Geriatrics, 31*, 159–167. doi:10.3109/02703181.2013.769481

Even, J., Richards, J., Crosby, C., Kregor, P., Mitchell, E., Jahangir, A., . . . Obremskey, W. (2012). Preoperative skeletal versus cutaneous traction for femoral shaft fractures treated within 24 hours. *Journal of Orthopaedic Trauma, 26*(10), e177–e182.

Handoll, H., Queally, J., & Parker, M. (2011). Pre-operative traction for hip fractures in adults. *Cochrane Database of Systematic Reviews*, Issue 12, Art. No.: CD000168. doi:10.1002/14651858.CD000168.pub3

Reed, C., Carroll, L., Baccari, S., & Shermont, H. (2011). Spica cast care: A collaborative staff-led education initiative for improved patient care. *Orthopaedic Nursing, 30*, 353–360. doi:10.1097/NOR.0b013e318237105a

Seidl, K., Bunke, J., Gallagher, S., McGinley, L., Muir, M., Race, E., & Short, M. (2011). Safe patient handling and the lift team concept. *Bariatric Nursing and Surgical Patient Care, 6*, 57–64. doi:10.1089/bar.2011.9964

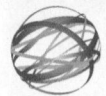

33 Performing Perioperative Care

LEARNING OUTCOMES

At the completion of this chapter, the student will be able to:

1. Define the key terms used in the skills for perioperative care.
2. Describe the phases of the perioperative period.
3. Describe essential aspects of preparing a client for surgery.
4. List the four dimensions of preoperative teaching that have been identified as important to clients.
5. Compare and contrast the traditional antiseptic surgical scrub and the antiseptic hand rub.
6. Describe essential aspects of preparing to receive the postoperative client from the postanesthesia room.
7. Describe ongoing postoperative nursing care.
8. Identify the clinical signs of potential postoperative complications and describe nursing interventions to prevent them.

9. Recognize when it is appropriate to delegate perioperative care skills to unlicensed assistive personnel.
10. Verbalize the steps used in:
    a. Conducting preoperative teaching.
    b. Performing a surgical hand antisepsis/scrub.
    c. Applying a sterile gown and sterile gloves (closed method).
    d. Managing gastrointestinal suction.
    e. Cleaning a sutured wound and changing a dressing on a wound with a drain.
    f. Maintaining closed wound drainage.
    g. Removing sutures.
11. Demonstrate appropriate documentation and reporting of perioperative skills.

SKILLS

Skill 33–1 Conducting Preoperative Teaching
Skill 33–2 Performing a Surgical Hand Antisepsis/Scrub
Skill 33–3 Applying a Sterile Gown and Sterile Gloves (Closed Method)
Skill 33–4 Managing Gastrointestinal Suction

Skill 33–5 Cleaning a Sutured Wound and Changing a Dressing on a Wound with a Drain
Skill 33–6 Maintaining Closed Wound Drainage
Skill 33–7 Removing Sutures

KEY TERMS

circulating nurse, *717*
closed wound drainage system, *734*
continuous suction, *724*
continuous sutures, *736*
drains, *734*
Hemovac, *734*
intermittent suction, *724*

interrupted sutures, *736*
intraoperative phase, *708*
Jackson–Pratt, *734*
penrose drain, *734*
perioperative period, *708*
postanesthesia care unit (PACU), *708*
postanesthesia room (PAR), *708*

postoperative phase, *708*
preoperative phase, *708*
recovery room (RR), *708*
registered nurse first assistant (RNFA), *717*
retention sutures, *736*
scrub person, *717*
staples, *736*

surgical hand antisepsis, *717*
suture, *736*
wound dehiscence, *727*
wound evisceration, *727*

Surgery is a unique experience of a planned physical alteration encompassing three phases: preoperative, intraoperative, and postoperative. These three phases are together referred to as the **perioperative period**. Perioperative nursing is practiced in hospital-based inpatient and outpatient surgical/laser/endoscopy suites, physician office–based surgical suites (outpatient), and freestanding outpatient/ambulatory surgical centers. Outpatient procedures do not require an overnight hospital stay. The client goes to the outpatient site the day of surgery, has the procedure, and leaves the same day.

The **preoperative phase** begins when the decision to have surgery is made and ends when the client is transferred to the operating table. The nursing activities associated with this phase include assessing the client, identifying potential or actual health problems, planning specific care based on the individual's needs to prepare the client for surgery, and providing preoperative teaching for the client, the family, and significant others.

The **intraoperative phase** begins when the client is transferred to the operating table and ends when the client is admitted to the **postanesthesia care unit (PACU)**, also called the **postanesthesia room (PAR)** or **recovery room (RR)**. The nursing activities related to this phase include a variety of specialized procedures designed to create and maintain a safe therapeutic environment for the client and the health care personnel. These activities include interventions that provide for the client's safety, maintaining an aseptic environment, ensuring proper functioning of equipment, and providing the surgical team with the instruments and supplies needed during the procedure.

The **postoperative phase** begins with the admission of the client to the PAR and ends when healing is complete. During the postoperative phase, nursing activities include assessing the client's response (physiological and psychological) to surgery, performing interventions to facilitate healing and prevent complications, teaching and providing support to the client and the client's support people, and planning for home care. The goal is to assist the client to achieve the most optimal health status possible.

PREPARING A CLIENT FOR SURGERY

The overall goal in the preoperative period is to ensure that the client is mentally and physically prepared for surgery. Planning should involve the client, the family, and significant others. Preoperative care planning and teaching interventions are usually done on an outpatient basis either in person or via a telephone interview by the perioperative nurse.

Preoperative Consent

Prior to any surgical procedure, informed consent is required from the client or legal guardian. Informed consent implies that the client has been informed and involved in decisions affecting his or her health. The surgeon is responsible for obtaining the informed consent by providing the following information to the client or legal guardian:

- The nature of and the reason for the surgery
- All available options and the risks associated with each option
- The risks of the surgical procedure and its potential outcomes or complications
- The name and qualifications of the surgeon performing the procedure
- The right to refuse consent or later withdraw consent

The surgeon documents the informed consent conversation with the client or legal guardian in the preoperative progress note.

The surgical consent form, provided by the agency, protects the client from incorrect or unwanted procedures and the surgeon and agency from litigation related to unauthorized surgeries or uninformed clients. This consent form becomes part of the client's medical record and goes to the operating room with the client. The RN ensures consent is in the client's chart prior to releasing the client to surgery.

Although the surgeon maintains legal responsibility for ensuring that the client is giving informed consent, the nurse may witness the client's signature on the agency consent form. In doing so, the nurse ensures that the consent form is signed and serves as a witness to the signature, not to the fact that the client is informed. If the nurse assesses that the client does not understand the procedure to be performed, the surgeon is contacted and requested to speak with the client before surgery can proceed.

Informed consent is only possible when the client understands the provided information, that is, speaks the language and is conscious, mentally competent, and not sedated. A minor may not give informed consent. Specific guidelines regarding consent for minors vary among the states. Nurses must be aware of their responsibilities regarding consent and of the particular facility's policies.

Preoperative Assessment

Preoperative assessment includes collecting and reviewing physical, psychological, and social client data to determine the client's needs throughout the three perioperative phases. The perioperative nurse collects the data by interviewing the client in the presurgical care unit or by telephone prior to the day of surgery. When data cannot be collected directly, the perioperative nurse uses other data sources such as the nursing admission assessment. Forms vary considerably among agencies. Box 33–1 summarizes essential preoperative information that should be included.

| **BOX 33–1** | **Preoperative Assessment Data** |

- *Current health status.* Essential information includes general health status and the presence of any chronic diseases, such as diabetes or asthma, that may affect the client's response to surgery or anesthesia. Note any physical limitations that may affect the client's mobility or ability to communicate after surgery, as well as any prostheses such as hearing aids or contact lenses.
- *Allergies.* Include allergies to prescription and nonprescription drugs, food allergies, and allergies to tape, latex, soaps, or antiseptic agents. Some food allergies may indicate a potential reaction to drugs or substances used during surgery or diagnostic procedures; for example, an allergy to seafood alerts the nurse to a potential allergy to iodine-based dyes or soaps commonly used in hospitals.
- *Medications.* List all current medications (prescribed and over the counter). It may be vital to maintain a blood level of some medications (e.g., anticonvulsants) throughout the surgical experience; others, such as anticoagulants or aspirin, increase the risks of surgery and anesthesia and need to be discontinued several days prior to surgery. It is important to include in the list any herbal remedies the client currently takes.
- *Previous surgeries.* Previous surgical experiences may influence the client's physical and psychological responses to surgery or may reveal unexpected responses to anesthesia.
- *Mental status.* The client's mental status and ability to understand and respond appropriately can affect the entire perioperative experience. Note any developmental disabilities, mental illness, history of dementia, or excessive anxiety related to the procedure.
- *Understanding of the surgical procedure and anesthesia.* The client should have a good understanding of the planned procedure and what to expect during and after surgery as well as the expected outcome of the procedure.
- *Smoking.* Smokers may have more difficulty clearing respiratory secretions after surgery, increasing the risk of postoperative complications such as pneumonia, atelectasis, and delayed wound healing.
- *Obstructive sleep apnea (OSA).* The majority of adults do not know if they have OSA, which puts them at risk for postoperative pulmonary complications. Furthermore, when asked if they have sleep apnea, clients often state that they do not have a sleeping problem. Lakdawala (2011) points out that, because many clients do not fully understand OSA, The Joint Commission recommends using a sleep apnea screening tool for the perioperative area (p.16).
- *Alcohol and other mind-altering substances.* Use of substances that affect the central nervous system, liver, or other body systems can affect the client's response to anesthesia and surgery, and postoperative recovery.
- *Coping.* Clients with a healthy self-concept who have successfully employed appropriate coping mechanisms in the past are better able to deal with the stressors associated with surgery.
- *Social resources.* Determine the availability of family or other caregivers as well as the client's social support network. These resources are important to the client's recovery, particularly for the client undergoing same-day or short-stay surgery.
- *Cultural and spiritual considerations.* Culture and spirituality influence the client's response to surgery; respecting cultural and spiritual beliefs and practices can reduce preoperative anxiety and improve recovery.

PHYSICAL ASSESSMENT

Preoperatively, the nurse performs a brief but complete physical assessment, paying particular attention to systems (e.g., cardiac, respiratory, or renal) that could affect the client's response to anesthesia or surgery. A brief or "mini" mental status examination provides valuable baseline data for evaluating the client's mental status and alertness after surgery. It is also important to evaluate the client's ability to understand what is happening. For example, assessments of hearing and vision help guide perioperative teaching. Respiratory and cardiovascular assessments not only provide baseline data for evaluating the client's postoperative status, but also may alert care providers to a problem (e.g., a respiratory infection or irregular pulse rate) that may affect the client's response to surgery and anesthesia. Other systems (gastrointestinal, genitourinary, and musculoskeletal) are examined to provide baseline data.

SCREENING TESTS

The surgeon and/or anesthesiologist orders preoperative diagnostic and laboratory tests. Abnormalities may warrant treatment prior to surgery or delay the surgery. The nurse's responsibility is to review the orders carefully, to see that they are implemented, and to ensure that the results are obtained and in the client's record prior to surgery. Table 33–1 lists routine preoperative screening tests. In addition to these routine tests, diagnostic tests directly related to the client's disease are usually appropriate (e.g., gastroscopy to clarify the pathologic condition before gastric surgery).

Planning for Home Care

For the perioperative client, discharge planning begins before admission for the planned procedure. Early planning to meet the discharge needs of the client is particularly important for outpatient procedures, because these clients are generally discharged within hours after the procedure is performed.

Discharge planning incorporates an assessment of the client's, family's, and significant others' abilities and resources for care, their financial resources, and the need for referrals and home health services. The extent of discharge planning and home care will vary significantly for clients having different types of surgery.

Physical Preparation

Preoperative preparation includes the following areas: nutrition and fluids, elimination, hygiene, medications, sleep, care of valuables and prostheses, special orders, surgical skin preparation, temperature, safety protocols, vital signs, and preventing venous thromboembolism. In many agencies a preoperative checklist is used on the day of surgery (Figure 33–1 ■). The nurse completes the agency's preoperative checklist following appropriate documenting procedures. All pertinent records (laboratory records, x-ray films, consents) must be available for perioperative personnel to refer to them and all physical preparation must be completed to ensure client safety.

NUTRITION AND FLUIDS

Adequate hydration and nutrition promote healing. Nurses need to identify and record any signs of malnutrition or fluid imbalance. If the client is on intravenous (IV) fluids or on measured fluid intake, nurses must ensure that the fluid intake and output are accurately measured and recorded.

The order "NPO after midnight" has been a long-standing tradition because it was believed that anesthetics depress gastrointestinal functioning and there was a danger the client would vomit and aspirate during the administration of a general anesthetic. Reevaluation and research, however, do not support this tradition. As a result, the American Society of Anesthesiologists (ASA) revised its practice guidelines for preoperative fasting in healthy clients undergoing elective procedures. According to the ASA (2011), the current guidelines allow for:

- The consumption of clear liquids up to 2 hours before elective surgery requiring general anesthesia, regional anesthesia, or sedation-analgesia.
- A light breakfast (e.g., tea and toast) 6 hours before the procedure.
- A heavier meal (fried or fatty foods) 8 hours before surgery.

TABLE 33–1 Routine Preoperative Screening Tests

Test	Rationale
Complete blood count (CBC)	Red blood cells (RBCs), hemoglobin (Hgb), and hematocrit (Hct) are important to the oxygen-carrying capacity of the blood White blood cells (WBCs) are an indicator of immune function
Blood grouping and crossmatching	Determined in case blood transfusion is required during or after surgery
Serum electrolytes (Na^+, K^+, Ca^{2+}, Mg^{2+}, Cl^-, HCO_3^-)	To evaluate fluid and electrolyte status
Fasting blood glucose	High levels may indicate undiagnosed diabetes mellitus
Blood urea nitrogen (BUN) and creatinine	To evaluate renal function
ALT, AST, LDH, and bilirubin	To evaluate liver function
Serum albumin and total protein	To evaluate nutritional status
Urinalysis	To determine urine composition and possible abnormal components (e.g., protein or glucose) or infection
Chest x-ray	To evaluate respiratory status and heart size
Electrocardiogram (ECG) (all clients over 40 years of age and/or clients with preexisting cardiac conditions)	To identify preexisting cardiac problems or disease
Pregnancy test (all female clients of childbearing age)	To identify if the client is pregnant

MEDICAL DOCUMENTATION	INITIALS
History and Physical completed and in chart	
Lab studies/reports in chart	
EKG report in chart	
Chest x-ray report in chart	
Operative Permit completed, signed, and witnessed in chart	
Surgical site verified	
Surgical side: _____ Left _____ Right _____ Bilateral _____ NA	
Anesthesia Permit completed, signed, and witnessed in chart	
Medication Reconciliation Form completed and signed	
PREOPERATIVE PREPARATION	
Identification bracelet accurate and affixed to wrist or ankle prior to transport	
Allergies checked, allergies bracelet on, and allergy sticker on chart	
Copy of Advanced Directive on chart	
Jewelry, hairpieces, hairpins, contact lenses, glasses, prosthesis, underwear, money removed	
Vital signs taken and recorded	
Time taken: _____ BP _____ Temp _____ HR _____ Resp _____ O2 Sat _____	

Dentures: ☐ *Full*: ☐ Upper ☐ Lower ☐ *Partial*: ☐ Upper ☐ Lower
       ☐ Other: _____
       ☐ Removed: ☐ Sent home ☐ Left at bedside
       ☐ Left in place as requested by: ☐ Anesthesiologist ☐ Client	

Client NPO ☐ yes since _____ ☐ No	
If no: O.R. notified (Time)_____ (Whom)_____	
Voided. Time _____	
Medication sheets on chart	
Most recent nursing assessment attached	

INITIALS	SIGNATURE AND TITLE

Figure 33–1 ■ Sample nursing preoperative checklist.

ELIMINATION

Enemas before surgery are no longer routine, but cleansing enemas may be ordered if bowel surgery is planned. The enemas help prevent postoperative constipation and contamination of the surgical area (during surgery) by feces. After surgery involving the intestines, peristalsis often does not return for 24 to 48 hours.

Prior to surgery an in-and-out/straight catheterization or an indwelling Foley catheter may be ordered to ensure that the bladder remains empty. This helps prevent inadvertent injury to the bladder, particularly during pelvic surgery. If the client does not have a catheter, it is important to empty the bladder prior to receiving preoperative medications.

HYGIENE

In some settings, clients are asked to bathe or shower the evening or morning of surgery (or both). The purpose of hygienic measures is to reduce the risk of wound infection by reducing the amount of bacteria on the client's skin. The bath includes a shampoo whenever possible.

The client's nails should be trimmed and free of polish, and all cosmetics should be removed so that the nail beds, skin, and lips are visible when circulation is assessed during the perioperative phases.

Intraoperatively the client will be required to wear a surgical cap. The surgical cap contains the client's hair and any microorganisms on the hair and scalp.

Before going into the operating room, and while in the holding area, the client should remove all hairpins and clips because they may cause pressure or accidental damage to the scalp when the client is unconscious. The client also removes personal clothing and puts on an operating room gown.

MEDICATIONS

The anesthetist or anesthesiologist may order routinely taken medications to be held the day of surgery. However, recent studies recommend continuing beta-blocker therapy for all clients taking a beta-blocker before admission for surgery (Elliott, 2013).

In some settings, preoperative medications are given to the client prior to going to the operating room. Commonly used preoperative medications include the following:

- *Sedatives* and *tranquilizers* such as lorazepam (Ativan) are administered by IV 15 to 20 minutes before surgery or by the intramuscular route 2 hours prior to the procedure (Adams & Urban, 2013) to reduce anxiety and ease anesthetic induction.
- *Opioid analgesics* such as morphine provide client sedation and reduce the required amount of anesthetic.
- *Anticholinergics* such as atropine, scopolamine, and glycopyrrolate (Robinul) reduce oral and pulmonary secretions and prevent laryngospasm.
- *Antiemetic agents* such as ondansetron (Zofran) are administered parenterally (IV) 30 minutes before the end of surgery to prevent nausea and vomiting (Adams & Urban, 2013).
- *Histamine-receptor antihistamines* such as cimetidine (Tagamet) and ranitidine (Zantac) reduce gastric fluid volume and gastric acidity.
- *Neurolept analgesic* agents such as Innovar induce general calmness and sleepiness.

Preoperative medications must be given at a scheduled time or "on call," that is, when the operating room notifies the nurse to give the medication.

SLEEP

Nurses should do everything to help the client sleep the night before surgery. Often a sedative is ordered. Adequate rest helps the client manage the stress of surgery and helps healing. Oral benzodiazepines may be given several days prior to surgery to relieve anxiety and enhance rest (Adams & Urban, 2013).

VALUABLES

Valuables such as jewelry and money should be sent home with the client's family or significant other. If valuables and money cannot be sent home, they need to be labeled and placed in a locked storage area per the agency's policy. Removing jewelry also means removing body-piercing jewelry because there is a risk of injury from burns if an electrosurgical unit is used. If a client wishes not to remove or is unable to remove a wedding band, the nurse can tape it in place. Wedding bands must be removed, however, if there is danger of the fingers swelling after surgery. Situations warranting removal include surgery on or cast application to an arm, or a mastectomy that involves removal of the lymph nodes. (Mastectomies may cause edema of the arm and hand.)

PROSTHESES

All prostheses (artificial body parts, such as partial or complete dentures, contact lenses, artificial eyes, and artificial limbs) and eyeglasses, wigs, and false eyelashes must be removed before surgery. Hearing aids are often left in place and the operating room personnel notified.

In some hospitals, dentures are placed in a locked storage area; in others they are placed in labeled containers and kept at the client's bedside. Partial dentures can become dislodged and obstruct an unconscious client's breathing. The nurse also checks for the presence of chewing gum or loose teeth. Loose teeth are a common problem with 5- or 6-year-olds undergoing tonsillectomy because they can become dislodged and aspirated during anesthesia.

Culturally Responsive Care | **PATIENT-CENTERED CARE**

Body Piercing and Dermal Implants

Diccini, Malheiro Da Costa Nogueira, and Sousa (2009) write that body piercing is an ancient practice documented throughout the ages. For example, the Mayan civilization in A.D. 700 used body piercing commonly in the practice of their religion. Egyptian royalty and Roman soldiers pierced the nipples and genitalia (p. 161). And, in recent years the practice of body piercing has increased worldwide.

The most common sites for piercing are the earlobes, ear cartilage, tragus, nasal septum, eyebrow, tongue, lips, navel, breast nipples, and genitalia. Nurses need to assess the client for piercing, because piercings can produce medical complications such as bleeding, skin tears, or infections. Body piercing can affect client safety in the preoperative, intraoperative, and postoperative phase.

Moving the client from the bed to the stretcher and operating room table may place the client at risk for skin tears when the piercings are left in place. Clapham and Crooke (2011) report of anesthetic complications with tongue piercings relating to airway management and endotracheal intubation. Body piercing can also place the client and operating room staff at risk for electrical burns if the piercings are not removed. Thus, the client or nurse must remove the piercings prior to being transported to surgery.

New forms of body decoration have recently emerged in the form of subdermal, transdermal, and microdermal implants, which cannot be removed. Wanzer and Hicks (2012) describe the implants: For the subdermal implants a pocket is created under the skin and a decorative shape made of silicone, Teflon, or metal is embedded to create a silhouette of the molded shape on the surface of the skin. The transdermal and microdermal implants have a footplate (or anchor) inserted into the epidermis with a thin piece of metal protruding from the skin. A piece of jewelry is then attached to this metal (p. C5).

One safety concern for the perioperative client with a subdermal implant is maintaining skin integrity because skin completely covers the implant. The transdermal and microdermal implants, however, create more safety concerns because of the protruding metal post. The safety risks relate to skin integrity as the client is transferred and positioned and potential burn risks if electrocautery is used during the surgery.

SPECIAL ORDERS

The nurse checks the surgeon's orders for special requirements (e.g., the insertion of a nasogastric tube prior to surgery; the administration of medications, such as insulin; or the application of antiemboli stockings). For the skill of inserting a nasogastric tube, see Skill 19–2 in Chapter 19 ∞.

SKIN PREPARATION

Sometimes the client may need to use antimicrobial disposable wipes to wash the surgical area the night before and the morning of surgery. In most agencies, skin preparation is carried out during the intraoperative phase. The surgical site is cleansed with an antimicrobial to remove soil and reduce the resident microbial count to subpathogenic levels. The purpose of a surgical skin preparation is to reduce the risk of surgical site infections (SSIs), the most common type of health care–associated infection in the surgical population (Zinn et al., 2013, p. 552). Removal of hair from the surgical site is performed only when necessary, for example, if it interferes with the surgical procedure. Personnel skilled in hair removal should use techniques that preserve skin integrity such as electric clippers to reduce the risk of traumatizing the skin during hair removal. Razors can disrupt skin integrity so hair removal with a razor is not recommended. Skin trauma and abrasions increase the risk of microorganisms colonizing the surgical site. If hair is to be removed, it is done as close to the time of surgery as possible and not in the vicinity of the sterile field to avoid dispersal of loose hair and potential contamination of the sterile field.

TEMPERATURE

Surgical clients are at risk of losing body heat; therefore, temperature management is an important aspect of perioperative client safety and comfort. Approximately 70% of surgical clients develop inadvertent or unplanned hypothermia during the perioperative period (Wu, 2013, p. 302). Hypothermia has many possible causes, including minimal clothing (i.e., only a hospital gown), inactivity while in the holding area, skin exposure during insertion of an IV and during surgery, and intentionally low temperatures in the OR. In addition, the administration of anesthesia impairs both thermoregulation and the ability of the body to generate and retain heat (Bernard, 2013; Wu, 2013). Clients with extremes in body weight or condition are at risk for hypothermia because of body surface area to weight ratios (Lynch, Dixon, Leary, & Holm, 2010, p. 557). Complications associated with perioperative hypothermia include increased blood loss, delayed wound healing, increased risk of SSI, and increased length of stay in the hospital. It is important for the client's temperature to be assessed during the entire perioperative experience to prevent unintended hypothermia. Researchers recommend prewarming or warming to reduce the complications of hypothermia. One method is to use a forced-air warming system, which consists of a power unit that generates warmed air and a fan that blows the warmed air through a hose into a disposable blanket that has direct contact with the client (Wu, 2013, p. 303). This method of warming can be started in the presurgical area and used throughout surgery and on into the PACU (Bernard, 2013). Studies have shown that warming improves postoperative recovery; however, it has not yet become a routine part of preoperative preparation (Wu, 2013).

SAFETY PROTOCOLS

The Joint Commission established the Universal Protocol for Preventing Wrong Site, Wrong Procedure, and Wrong Person Surgery in 2004. This protocol involves three steps. The first step requires preoperative verification. The frequency and scope of the verification process depends on the type and complexity of the procedure. Possibilities include when the procedure is scheduled, at the time of

---

SAFETY ALERT! | **SAFETY**

2014 The Joint Commission National Patient Safety Goals (2013)

UNIVERSAL PROTOCOL FOR PREVENTING WRONG SITE, WRONG PROCEDURE, AND WRONG PERSON SURGERY

- Conduct a preprocedure verification process. **Rationale:** *Hospitals should always make sure that any procedure is what the patient needs and is performed on the right person.*
- Mark the procedure site.
- A time-out is performed before the procedure. **Rationale:** *The purpose of the time-out is to conduct a final assessment to ensure that the correct patient, site, and procedure have been identified.*

---

preadmission testing and assessment, at the time of admission for the procedure, and before the client leaves the preprocedure area or enters the procedure room (The Joint Commission, 2013, p. 13).

The second step involves marking of the operative site. The protocol does not specify the type of mark; however, The Joint Commission does require that the surgical site marking method be consistent throughout the facility and encourages client involvement. The facility chooses its own surgical site method (e.g., the client's initials, surgeon's initials, or the word "YES"). The essential focus is that the mark is unambiguous and a clear communication to all involved. The mark must be permanent and visible after the client has been prepped and draped for surgery. There is no clear consensus on who should mark the site. Because the mark is a communication tool about the client for members of the team, The Joint Commission (2013) suggests that the individual who knows the most about the client should mark the site. In most cases, that will be the person performing the procedure (p. 15).

The third step is called "time-out." Before surgery begins, the surgical team takes a time-out to conduct a final verification of the correct client, procedure, and site. Any questions or concerns must be resolved before the procedure can begin.

VITAL SIGNS

Preoperatively assess and document vital signs for baseline data. Report any abnormal findings, such as elevated blood pressure or elevated temperature.

PREVENTING VENOUS THROMBOEMBOLISM

A goal of a coalition of health care organizations called the Surgical Care Improvement Project (SCIP) is to reduce the incidence of surgical complications. SCIP recommends preventive pharmacologic and mechanical therapies to prevent venous thromboembolism (VTE) (Larkin, Mitchell, & Petrie, 2012). The mechanical therapies include antiemboli (elastic) stockings and intermittent pneumatic compression devices (see Chapter 23 ∞).

PREOPERATIVE TEACHING

The major nursing activity to ensure that the client is prepared for surgery is preoperative teaching. Studies have shown that preoperative teaching reduces clients' anxiety, improves pain control, and increases client satisfaction with the surgical experience. Effective preoperative teaching also facilitates the client's successful and early return to work and other activities of daily living (ADLs). Four dimensions of preoperative teaching have been identified as important to clients:

1. *Information, including what will happen to the client, when and what the client will experience, such as expected sensations and discomfort.* The nurse needs to listen carefully and attentively to the client to identify specific concerns and fears. Pain assessment and management are important to explain to the client because there will be discomfort after the procedure.

    Explain that the surgeon will order pain medication. Describe the 0-to-10 pain scale and how this is used to assess the client's level of pain. Stress the importance of working together to manage the pain because clients are able to move around easier and ambulate sooner when their pain is controlled. It is important for surgical clients to know their rights and have elevated

BOX 33–2   Preoperative Instructions

PREOPERATIVE REGIMEN

- Explain the need for preoperative tests (e.g., laboratory, x-ray, ECG).
- Discuss bowel preparation, if required.
- Discuss skin preparation, including operative area and preoperative bath or shower.
- Discuss preoperative medications, if ordered.
- Explain individual therapies ordered by the primary care provider, such as IV therapy, the insertion of a urinary catheter or nasogastric tube, use of a spirometer, or antiemboli stockings.
- Discuss the visit by the anesthetist.
- Explain the need to restrict food and oral fluids before surgery.
- Provide a general timetable for perioperative events, including the time of surgery.
- Discuss the need to remove jewelry, makeup, and all prostheses (e.g., eyeglasses, hearing aids, complete or partial dentures, wig) immediately before surgery.
- Inform the client about the preoperative holding area, and give the location of the waiting room for support people.
- Teach deep-breathing and coughing exercises, leg exercises, ways to turn and move (see Skill 33–1), and splinting techniques.
- Complete the preoperative checklist.

POSTOPERATIVE REGIMEN

- Discuss the PAR routines and emergency equipment.
- Review type and frequency of assessment activities.
- Discuss pain management.

- Explain usual activity restrictions and precautions related to getting up for the first time postoperatively.
- Describe usual dietary alterations.
- Discuss postoperative dressings and drains.
- Provide an explanation and tour of the intensive care unit if the client is to be transferred there postoperatively.

OUTPATIENT SURGICAL CLIENTS

- Review all instructions in the preoperative and postoperative regimen.
- Confirm place and time of surgery, including when to arrive (e.g., 1 to 1.5 hours before scheduled surgery) and where to register (e.g., reception desk).
- Discuss what to wear (e.g., clients having hand surgery should wear a garment with large sleeve openings to fit over a bulky dressing; all clients need to leave valuables at home).
- Explain the need for a responsible adult to drive or accompany the client home.
- Discuss discharge criteria and how long the client should expect to stay postoperatively.
- Discuss medications, including specific preoperative medications and the client's current medication regimen.
- Communicate by telephone the evening before surgery to confirm time of surgery and arrival time.
- Communicate by telephone within 48 hours postoperatively to evaluate surgical outcomes and identify any problems or complications.

---

expectations as to what is possible for them in terms of pain relief after surgery. Minorities and poor people are at risk for inadequate pain control, and nurses must be vigilant to prevent undertreatment in these clients.

2. *Psychosocial support to reduce anxiety.* The nurse provides support by actively listening and providing accurate information. It is important to correct any misunderstandings the client may have.

3. *The roles of the client and support people in preoperative preparation, during the surgical procedure, and during the postoperative phase.* Understanding his or her role during the perioperative experience increases the client's sense of control and reduces anxiety. This includes what will be expected of the client, desired behaviors, self-care activities, and what the client can do to facilitate recovery.

4. *Skills training.* This includes moving, deep breathing, coughing, splinting incisions with the hands or a pillow, and using an incentive spirometer.

If the client is scheduled for outpatient surgery, preoperative teaching is often provided before the day of surgery using some combination of videos and verbal and written instructions. The client may have an appointment with the outpatient perioperative nurse (usually scheduled to coincide with preoperative diagnostic testing) to discuss preoperative concerns and implement the teaching plan. Written instructions are always provided to reinforce verbal teaching. Teaching is further reinforced when the client is admitted on the day of surgery and before discharge from the PAR. Preoperative instructions are summarized in Box 33–2.

When the client is a child, addressing the fears and anxieties of both the child and the family is vital. Both parents and the child need to know what to expect and to be able to express their concerns. Parents should be considered members of the perioperative team and allowed to participate in providing as much care as possible.

Skill 33–1 provides guidelines for teaching clients about moving, leg exercises, deep breathing, and coughing. See Box 33–3 for outcomes of successful preoperative teaching.

BOX 33–3   Outcomes of Effective Preoperative Teaching

MOVING

- To maintain blood circulation
- To stimulate respiratory function
- To decrease stasis of gas in the intestine
- To facilitate early ambulation

LEG EXERCISES

- To stimulate blood circulation, thereby preventing venous thromboembolism

DEEP BREATHING AND COUGHING

- To facilitate lung aeration, thereby preventing atelectasis and pneumonia

●○● NURSING PROCESS: CONDUCTING PREOPERATIVE TEACHING

Conducting Preoperative Teaching

ASSESSMENT
Assess:
- Vital signs.
- Discomfort.
- Temperature and color of feet and legs.
- Breath sounds.
- Presence of dyspnea or cough.

- Learning needs of the client.
- Anxiety level of the client.
- Client experience with previous surgeries and anesthesia.
- Incidence of postoperative nausea, vomiting, or other reaction to previous anesthesia.

PLANNING
Before beginning to teach moving, leg exercises, deep-breathing exercises, and coughing, determine (a) the type of surgery, (b) the time of the surgery, (c) the name of the surgeon, (d) the preoperative orders, and (e) the agency's practices for preoperative care. Also, verify that the primary care provider has completed the medical history and physical examination and that the client or the family has signed the consent form.

DELEGATION

Assessment of the learning needs of the client and his or her support people and determining the teaching content and appropriate strategies for teaching require application of professional knowledge and critical thinking. Preoperative teaching is conducted by the nurse and is not delegated to unlicensed assistive personnel (UAP). The UAP, however, can reinforce teaching, assist the client with the exercises, and report to the nurse if the client is unable to perform the exercises.

INTERPROFESSIONAL PRACTICE

Teaching moving, leg exercises, deep breathing, and coughing may be within the scope of practice for other health care providers. For example, in addition to nurses, both respiratory therapists and physical therapists may teach this information to the client. Although the therapists may verbally communicate their findings and plan to the health care team members, the nurse must also know where to locate their documentation in the client's medical record.

Equipment
- Pillow
- Teaching materials (e.g., audiovisual, written materials) if available at the agency

IMPLEMENTATION
Preparation
Ensure that potential distracters (e.g., pain, TV, visitors) to teaching are not present. Family and significant others should be included in the teaching plan, if appropriate.

Performance
1. Prior to performing the procedure, introduce self and verify the client's identity using agency protocol. Explain to the client what you are going to teach and the importance of the client's participation in the exercises he or she is going to be taught.
2. Perform hand hygiene and observe other appropriate infection prevention procedures.
3. Provide for client privacy.
4. Show the client ways to turn in bed and to get out of bed.
   - Instruct a client who will have a right abdominal incision or a right-sided chest incision to turn to the left side of the bed and sit up as follows:
     a. Flex the knees.
     b. Splint the wound by holding the left arm and hand or a small pillow against the incision.
     c. Turn to the left while pushing with the right foot and grasping a partial side rail on the left side of the bed with the right hand.
     d. Come to a sitting position on the side of the bed by using the right arm and hand to push down against the mattress and swinging the feet over the edge of the bed.
   - Teach a client with a left abdominal or left-sided chest incision to perform the same procedure but splint with the right arm and turn to the right.
   - For clients with orthopedic surgery (e.g., hip surgery), use special aids, such as a trapeze, to assist with movement.

5. Teach the client the following three leg exercises:
   - Alternate dorsiflexion and plantar flexion of the feet. **Rationale:** *This exercise is sometimes referred to as calf pumping, because it alternately contracts and relaxes the calf muscles, including the gastrocnemius muscles.* ❶
   - Flex and extend the knees, and press the backs of the knees into the bed while dorsiflexing the feet. ❷ Instruct clients who cannot raise their legs to do isometric exercises that contract and relax the muscles.
   - Raise and lower the legs alternately from the surface of the bed. Flex the knee of the stable leg and extend the knee of the moving leg. ❸ **Rationale:** *This exercise contracts and relaxes the quadriceps muscles.*
6. Demonstrate deep-breathing (diaphragmatic) exercises as follows:
   - Place your hands palms down on the border of your rib cage, and inhale slowly and evenly through the nose until the greatest chest expansion is achieved. ❹
   - Hold your breath for 2 to 3 seconds.
   - Then exhale slowly through the mouth.
   - Continue exhalation until maximum chest contraction has been achieved.
7. Help the client perform deep-breathing exercises.
   - Ask the client to assume a sitting position.
   - Place the palms of your hands on the border of the client's rib cage to assess respiratory depth.
   - Ask the client to perform deep breathing, as described in step 6.
8. Instruct the client to cough voluntarily after five deep inhalations.
   - Ask the client to inhale deeply, hold the breath for a few seconds, and then cough once or twice.

Continued on page 716

Conducting Preoperative Teaching—*continued*

Anterior View

Quadriceps muscles

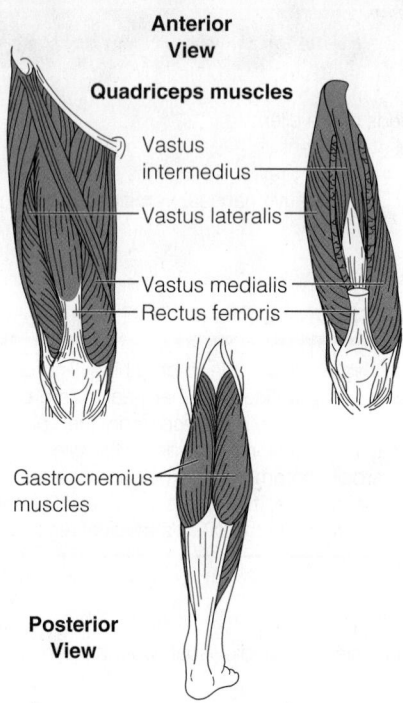

- Vastus intermedius
- Vastus lateralis
- Vastus medialis
- Rectus femoris

Gastrocnemius muscles

Posterior View

❶ Leg muscles: anterior and posterior views.

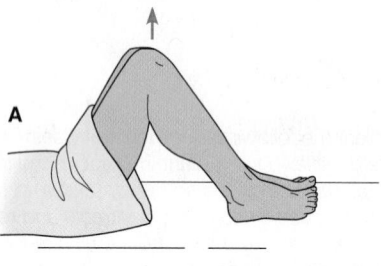

A

B

C

❷ Flexing and extending the knees.

- Ensure that the client coughs deeply and does not just clear the throat.
9. If the incision will be painful when the client coughs, demonstrate techniques to splint the abdomen.
   - Show the client how to support the incision by placing the palms of the hands on either side of the incision site or directly over the incision site, holding the palm of one hand over the other. **Rationale:** *Coughing uses the abdominal and other accessory respiratory muscles. Splinting the*

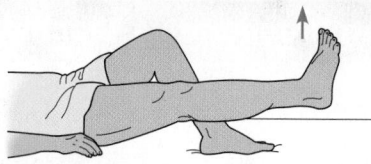

❸ Raising and lowering the legs.

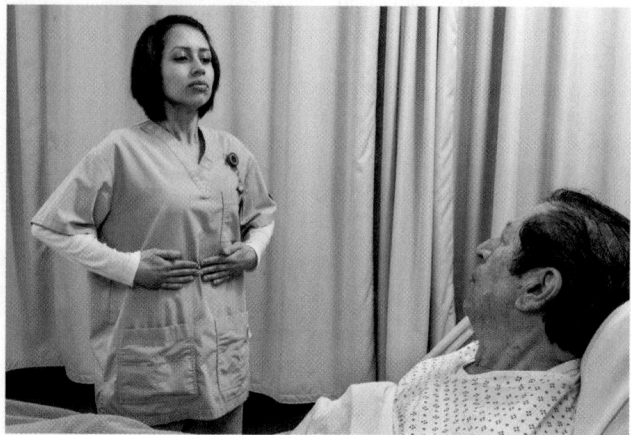

❹ Demonstrating deep breathing.

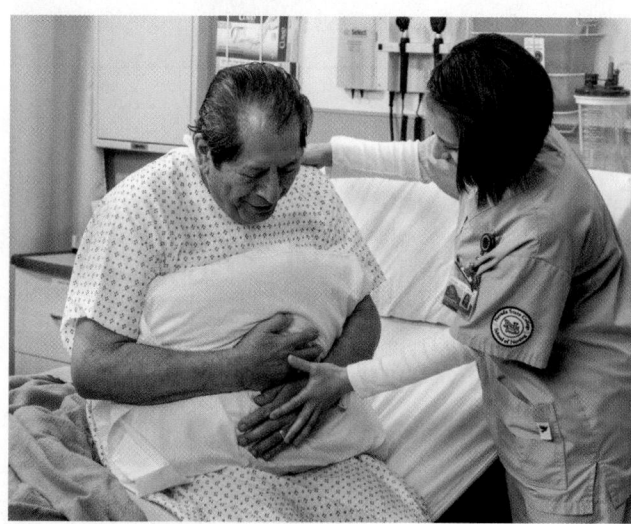

❺ Splinting an incision with a pillow while coughing.

incision may reduce pain while coughing if the incision is near any of these muscles.
   - Show the client how to splint the abdomen with clasped hands and a firmly rolled pillow held against the client's abdomen. ❺
10. Inform the client about the expected frequency of these exercises.
    - Instruct the client to start the exercises as soon after surgery as possible.
    - Encourage clients to carry out deep breathing and coughing at least every 2 hours, taking a minimum of five breaths at each session. Note, however, that the number of breaths and frequency of deep breathing vary with the client's condition. People who are susceptible to pulmonary problems may need deep-breathing exercises every hour. People

Conducting Preoperative Teaching—*continued*

with chronic respiratory disease may need special breathing exercises (e.g., pursed-lip breathing, abdominal breathing, or exercises using various kinds of incentive spirometers). See Chapter 24 ∞.

- Document the teaching and all assessments. Some agencies may have a preoperative teaching flow sheet. Check agency policy.

SAMPLE DOCUMENTATION

3/19/2015 0900 Instructed how to splint abdomen while deep breathing and coughing. Able to perform correctly. Stated that he will use this technique after surgery. —————————— A. Moore, RN

EVALUATION

Document the outcome of the teaching plan such as:

- Client's demonstrated ability to perform moving, leg exercises, deep-breathing, and coughing exercises.

- Client's verbalization of key information presented.

LIFESPAN CONSIDERATIONS | Preoperative Teaching

CHILDREN

- Parents need to know what to expect and to be able to express their concerns.
- Separation from parents often is the child's greatest fear; the time of separation should be minimized and parents allowed to interact with the child both immediately preceding and following the surgery.
- Teaching and communicating with children (both timing and content) should be geared to the child's developmental level and cognitive abilities (e.g., "You will have a sore tummy").
- Play is an effective teaching tool with children (e.g., the child can put a bandage on an incision on a doll).

OLDER ADULTS

- Assess hearing ability to ensure the older client hears the necessary information.
- Assess short-term memory. Presenting one focused idea at a time and repeating or reinforcing information may be necessary.
- Older adults are at greater risk for postoperative complications, such as pneumonia. Reinforce moving and deep-breathing and coughing exercises.

- Assess potential postoperative needs at this time. Arrangements can be made preoperatively to obtain necessary items. Examples are medical equipment, such as walkers, raised toilet seats, and bed trapezes; Meals-on-Wheels; and help with transportation.
- If the older adult client will need to be in extended care for a period of time after surgery, this is the time to initiate these plans.
- Assess the client for risk of pressure ulcer development postoperatively, and be extra attentive to use of proper padding and support devices to prevent injury during positioning and transfers in the operating room. Risks are:
  - Older age.
  - Poor nutritional status.
  - History of diabetes or cardiovascular problems.
  - History of taking steroids, which cause increased bruising and skin breakdown.

INTRAOPERATIVE PHASE

The intraoperative nurse uses the nursing process to design, coordinate, and deliver care to meet the identified needs of clients whose protective reflexes or self-care abilities are potentially compromised because they are having operative or other invasive procedures.

Intraoperative interventions are carried out by the circulating nurse, the scrub person, and the registered nurse first assistant. The **circulating nurse** coordinates activities and manages client care by continually assessing client safety (e.g., client positioning) and by monitoring aseptic practice and the environment (e.g., temperature, humidity, and lighting). The Association of Operating Room Nurses (AORN) recommends that the circulating nurse must always be a perioperative RN and that a minimum of one perioperative RN circulator should be dedicated to each client undergoing a surgical procedure (AORN, 2011, 2012b). The **scrub person** is usually a UAP but can be an RN, LPN, or certified surgical technologist (CST). They wear sterile gowns, gloves, caps, and eye protection. Their role is to assist the surgeons. Their responsibilities include draping the client with sterile drapes and handling sterile instruments and supplies. The **registered nurse first assistant (RNFA)** has additional

education and training and functions in an expanded perioperative nursing role. The RNFA assists the surgeon by controlling bleeding, using instruments, handling and cutting tissue, and suturing during the procedure (AORN, 2012a). The circulating nurse and the scrub person are responsible for accounting for all sponges, needles, and instruments at the close of surgery. This precaution prevents foreign bodies from being left inside the client.

Surgical Hand Antisepsis

The term **surgical hand antisepsis** refers to the antiseptic surgical scrub or antiseptic hand rub that is performed before applying (i.e., putting on) sterile gloves and gowns preoperatively. The purpose of the surgical hand scrub is to remove microorganisms from the nails, hands, and forearms to a minimum and prevent microbial regrowth.

The surgical hand scrub has been the traditional method used for surgical antisepsis. This includes scrubbing the hands for 5 to 10 minutes. The use of a brush, however, can have harmful effects on the skin. For instance, the brush can lead to skin abrasion and dermatitis and can increase skin shedding (Weight, Lee, & Palmer, 2010). In 2004, the

AORN recommended that an FDA-approved waterless, alcohol-based hand-rub product could also be used for surgical hand antisepsis. The use of a brush is not needed with the hand rub when alcohol-based products are used. In addition, they also contain ingredients such as conditioners and moisturizers that help protect the skin.

There are two types of traditional surgical scrubs: the stroke-count scrub and the timed scrub. They both take about 5 minutes to complete. The stroke-count scrub involves a specific number of cleaning strokes for each aspect of the hands and arms. With the timed scrub, each area is scrubbed for a specific length of time. The fingers and hands are scrubbed, then the arms to 5 cm (2 in.) above each elbow. Most agencies have specific recommended protocols regarding the surgical hand scrub. The protocol usually follows the scrub agent manufacturers' recommendations. The surgical hand antisepsis/scrub is performed in operating rooms, delivery rooms, burn units, and special diagnostic areas.

●○● NURSING PROCESS: PERFORMING SURGICAL HAND ANTISEPSIS/SCRUB

SKILL 33–2

Performing a Surgical Hand Antisepsis/Scrub

ASSESSMENT

Assess:
- Nails, which should be short, clean, and free of nail polish. No artificial nails. **Rationale:** *Short nails prevent glove punctures or tears. Chipped nail polish harbors bacteria. Fungal growth can occur under artificial nails.*
- Cuticles, hands, and forearms. **Rationale:** *Cuts, abrasions, hangnails, and so on (e.g., breaks in skin integrity) may contain pathogens and increase the risk of infection.*

PLANNING

Determine the type and length of time for the surgical hand antisepsis/scrub per agency protocol.

DELEGATION

Surgical hand antisepsis/scrub is performed by a perioperative nurse or RNFA. It can be, however, delegated to a LVN/LPN or CST in some agencies. The AORN (2011) believes that individuals who are not licensed to practice professional nursing and who perform in the role of scrub person are performing a delegated technical function under the supervision of a perioperative RN.

Equipment
- Deep sink with foot, knee, or elbow controls
- Antimicrobial solution
- Nail-cleaning tool, such as a file or orange stick
- Surgical scrub brush
- Sterile towels for drying the hands

IMPLEMENTATION

Preparation

Ensure that the entire surgical attire is in place (i.e., shoe covers; cap, which should completely cover all the hair; face mask; and protective eyewear).

Performance

1. Prepare for the surgical hand antisepsis/scrub.
   - Remove wristwatch, bracelets, and all rings. Ensure that fingernails are trimmed. **Rationale:** *Jewelry and long fingernails harbor microorganisms. Removal of jewelry permits full skin contact with the antimicrobial agent.*
   - Turn on the water, using the foot, knee, or elbow control, and adjust the temperature to lukewarm. **Rationale:** *Warm water removes less protective oil from the skin than hot water. Soap irritates the skin more when hot water is used.*
2. Wash hands.
   - Wet the hands and forearms under running water, holding the hands above the level of the elbows so that the water runs from the fingertips to the elbows. **Rationale:** *The hands will become cleaner than the elbows. The water should run from the least contaminated to the most contaminated area.*
   - Apply 2 to 4 mL (1 tsp) antimicrobial solution to the hands.
   - Use firm, rubbing, and circular movements to wash the palms and backs of the hands, the wrists, and the forearms. Interlace the fingers and thumbs, and move the hands back and forth. ❶ ❷ ❸ Continue washing for 20 to 25 seconds. **Rationale:** *Circular strokes clean most effectively, and rubbing ensures a thorough and mechanical cleaning action. (Other areas of the hands still need to be cleaned, however.)*
   - Hold the hands and arms under the running water to rinse thoroughly, keeping the hands higher than the elbows. **Rationale:** *The nurse rinses from the cleanest to the least clean area.*

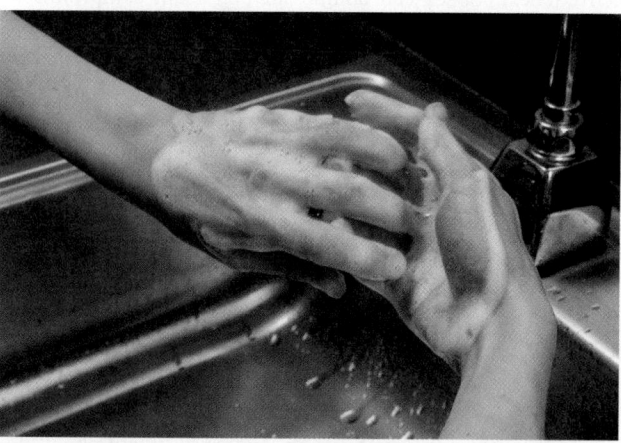

❶ Using circular movements to wash the palms.

Performing a Surgical Hand Antisepsis/Scrub—*continued*

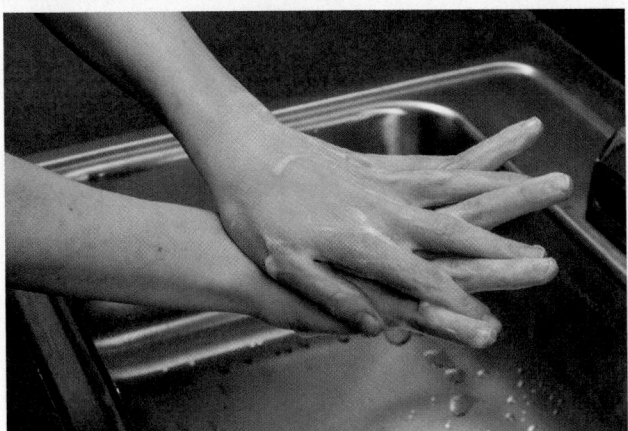

❷ Washing the backs of the hands.

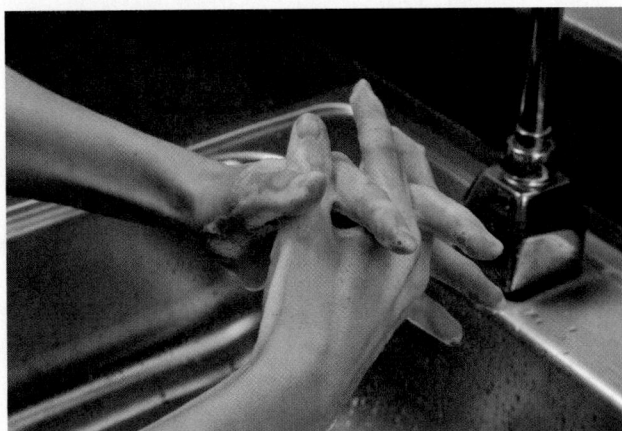

❸ Interlacing the fingers during hand washing.

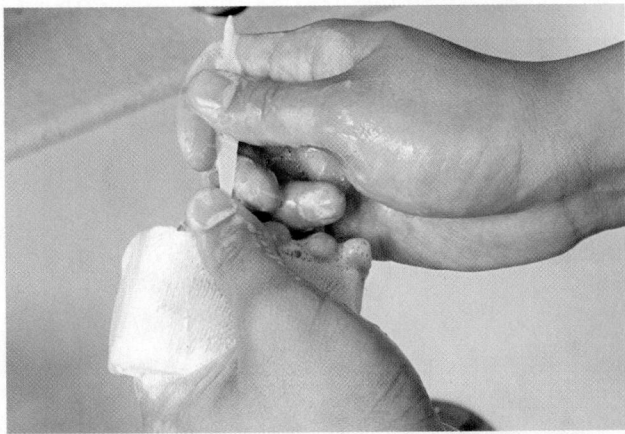

❹ Cleaning fingernails.

- Check the nails, and clean them with a file or orange stick if necessary. Rinse the nail tool after each nail is cleaned. ❹ **Rationale:** *Sediment under the nails is removed more readily when the hands are moist. Rinsing the nail tool after cleaning each nail prevents the transmission of sediment from one nail to another.*

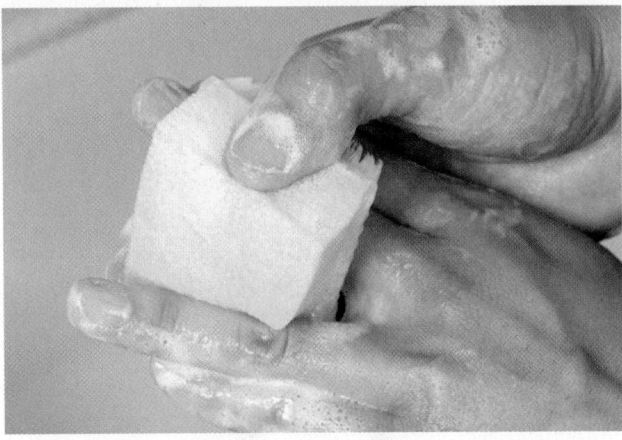

❺ Scrubbing the side of a finger.

3. Perform surgical hand antisepsis/scrub (with brush/sponge).
   - Apply the antimicrobial agent to wet hands and forearms and lather the hands again. Using a scrub brush or sponge, scrub each hand. Visualize each finger and hand as having four sides. Wash all four sides effectively. ❺ Repeat this process for the opposite fingers and hand. **Rationale:** *Scrubbing loosens bacteria, including those in the creases of the hands.*
   - Using the scrub brush or sponge, scrub from the wrists to 5 cm (2 in.) above each elbow. Visualize each arm as having four sides. Using agency protocol (e.g., scrubbing by number of strokes or length of time), wash all parts of the arms: lower forearm, upper forearm, and antecubital space to marginal area above elbows. Continue to hold the hands higher than the elbows. **Rationale:** *Scrubbing thus proceeds from the cleanest area (hands) to the least clean area (upper arm).*
   - Discard the scrub brush or sponge.
   - Rinse hands and arms thoroughly so that the water flows from the hands to the elbows. **Rationale:** *Rinsing removes resident and transient bacteria and sediment.*
   - Avoid splashing water onto surgical attire. **Rationale:** *A sterile gown put over wet or damp surgical attire would be considered contaminated.*
   - If a longer scrub is required, use a second brush and scrub each hand and arm with the antimicrobial agent for the recommended time.
   - Discard the second brush, and rinse hands and arms thoroughly.
   - Turn off the water with the foot or knee pedal.
   - Keeping hands elevated and away from the body, enter the operating room by backing into the room. **Rationale:** *This position of the hands maintains the cleanliness of the hands, and backing into the room prevents accidental contamination.*
4. Dry the hands and arms.
   - Use a sterile towel to dry one hand thoroughly from the fingers to the elbow. ❻ Use a rotating motion. Use a second sterile towel to dry the second hand in the same manner. In some agencies, towels are of a sufficient size that one half can be used to dry one hand and arm and the second half for the second hand and arm. **Rationale:** *The nurse dries the hands (the cleanest area) to the least clean area. Using a new towel or the opposite end of a towel prevents the transfer of microorganisms from one elbow (least clean area) to the other hand (cleanest area).*

Continued on page 720

Performing a Surgical Hand Antisepsis/Scrub—*continued*

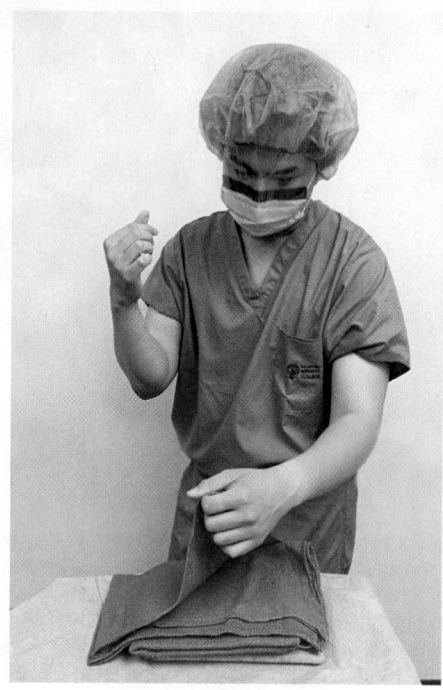

⑥ Picking up a sterile towel to dry hands and arms.

* Discard the towel(s).
* Keep the hands in front and above the waist. **Rationale:**
  *This position maintains the cleanliness of the hands and
  prevents accidental contamination.*

Variation: Surgical Hand Antisepsis/Hand Scrub Using Alcohol-Based Surgical Hand Rub

* Prepare for the surgical hand antisepsis/scrub and wash hands
  (see steps 1 and 2 above).
* Dry hands and forearms thoroughly with a paper towel.
* Follow the manufacturer's directions for use of the brushless surgical hand antisepsis product. Following is an example of how to
  use one brushless product. Note, however, that many products
  are available and it is imperative to use a product according to
  the manufacturer's guidelines. **Rationale:** *Following the manufacturer's guidelines helps ensure effective surgical hand antisepsis, which is needed to prevent surgical site infections.*
* Using a foot pump, dispense one pump (2 mL) of the surgical
  hand rub product into the palm of one hand. **⑦ Rationale:** *A
  foot pump avoids contamination of the hands.*
* Dip fingertips of the opposite hand into the hand rub product
  and work under the fingernails. **⑧** Spread the remaining hand
  rub product over the hand and up to just above the elbow.
* Dispense another pump (2 mL) of the surgical hand rub product
  into the palm of the opposite hand and repeat the procedure.
* Dispense a final pump (2 mL) of hand rub product into either
  hand and reapply to all aspects of both hands up to the
  wrists. **⑨**
* Rub thoroughly until dry. Do not use towels.

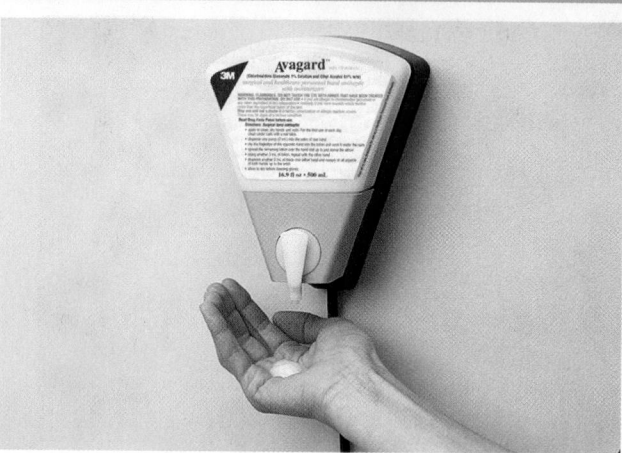

⑦ Dispensing hand rub.
Courtesy 3M.

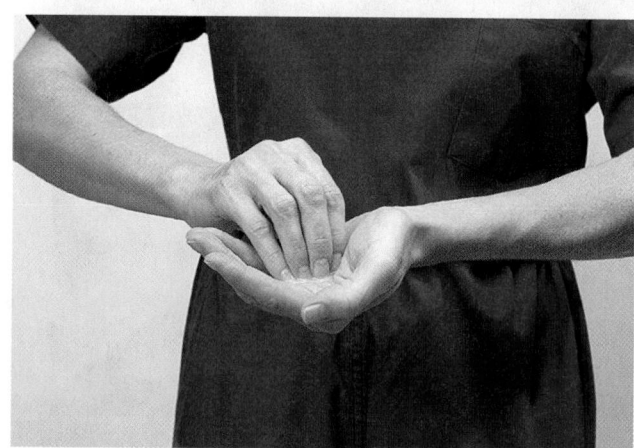

⑧ Dip fingertips into hand prep.
Courtesy 3M.

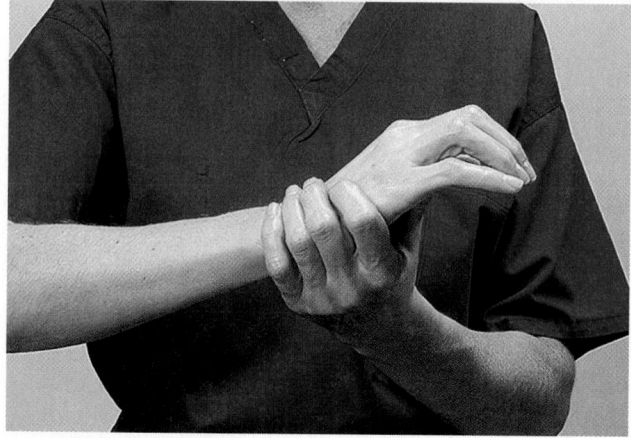

⑨ Reapply hand rub to both hands up to wrists.
Courtesy 3M.

EVALUATION

There is no traditional evaluation of the effectiveness of the individual
nurse's hand hygiene. Institutional quality control departments monitor the
occurrence of client infections and investigate those situations in which
health care providers are implicated in the transmission of infectious
organisms. Research has repeatedly shown the positive impact of careful
hand hygiene on client health associated with prevention of infection.

Applying a Sterile Gown and Sterile Gloves

Sterile gowning and closed gloving are chiefly carried out in operating or delivery rooms, where surgical asepsis is necessary. The closed method of gloving can be used only when a sterile gown is worn because the gloves are handled through the sleeves of the gown. Before these procedures, the nurse applies a hair cover and a mask, and performs a surgical hand antisepsis/scrub.

Skill 33–3 describes the steps in applying a sterile gown and sterile gloves by the closed method.

●○● NURSING PROCESS: APPLYING A STERILE GOWN AND STERILE GLOVES

Applying a Sterile Gown and Sterile Gloves (Closed Method)

SKILL 33-3

ASSESSMENT
Review the client's record and orders to determine exactly what procedure will be performed that requires sterile gloves. Check the client record and ask about latex allergies. Use nonlatex gloves whenever possible.

PLANNING
Think through the procedure, planning which steps need to be completed before the gloves and gown can be applied. Determine what additional supplies are needed to perform the procedure for this client. Always have an extra pair of sterile gloves available.

DELEGATION

Applying a sterile gown and sterile gloves is performed by a perioperative nurse or RNFA. It can be, however, delegated to an LVN/LPN or CST in some agencies.

Equipment
• Sterile pack containing a sterile gown and sterile gloves

IMPLEMENTATION
Preparation
• Ensure the sterility of the sterile pack.

Performance
1. Perform surgical hand antisepsis/scrub (see Skill 33–2).

Applying a Sterile Gown
1. Apply the sterile gown.
   • Grasp the sterile gown at the crease near the neck, hold it away from you, and permit it to unfold freely without touching anything, including the uniform. **Rationale:** *The gown will be unsterile if its outer surface touches any unsterile objects.*
   • Put the hands inside the shoulders of the gown without touching the outside of the gown.
   • Work the hands down the sleeves only to the beginning of the cuffs. ❶
   • Have a coworker wearing a hair cover and mask reach inside the arm seams and pull the gown over the shoulders.
   • The coworker grasps the neck ties without touching the outside of the gown and pulls the gown upward to cover the neckline of the scrub person's uniform in front and back. The coworker ties the neck ties. ❷ Completion of gowning continues on page 722.

Applying Sterile Gloves (Closed Method)
1. Open the sterile glove wrapper while the hands are still covered by the sleeves. ❸
2. Put the glove on the nondominant hand. Figures ❹, ❺, and ❻ show a right-handed person.
   • With the dominant hand, pick up the opposite glove with the thumb and index finger, handling it through the sleeve.
   • Position the dominant hand palm upward inside the sleeve. Lay the glove on the opposite gown cuff, thumb side down, with the glove opening pointed toward the fingers. ❹
   • Use the nondominant hand to grasp the cuff of the glove through the gown cuff, and firmly anchor it.
   • With the dominant hand working through its sleeve, grasp the upper side of the glove's cuff and stretch it over the cuff of the gown.

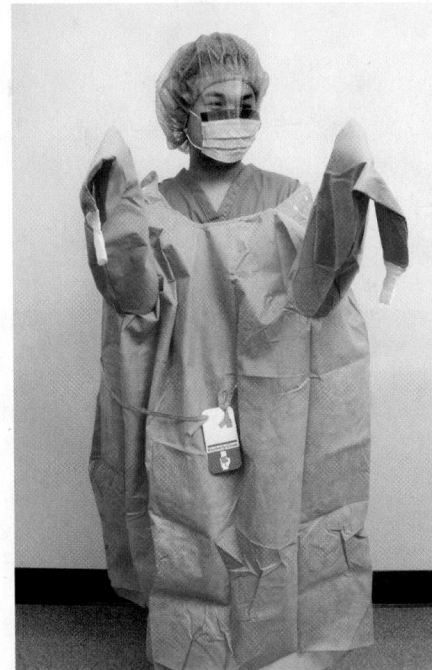

❶ Working the hands down the sleeves of a sterile gown.

   • Pull the sleeve up to draw the cuff over the wrist as you extend the fingers of the nondominant hand into the glove's fingers. ❺
3. Put the glove on the dominant hand.
   • Place the fingers of the gloved hand under the cuff of the remaining glove.
   • Place the glove over the cuff of the second sleeve.
   • Extend the fingers into the glove as you pull the glove up over the cuff. ❻

Continued on page 722

Applying a Sterile Gown and Sterile Gloves (Closed Method)—*continued*

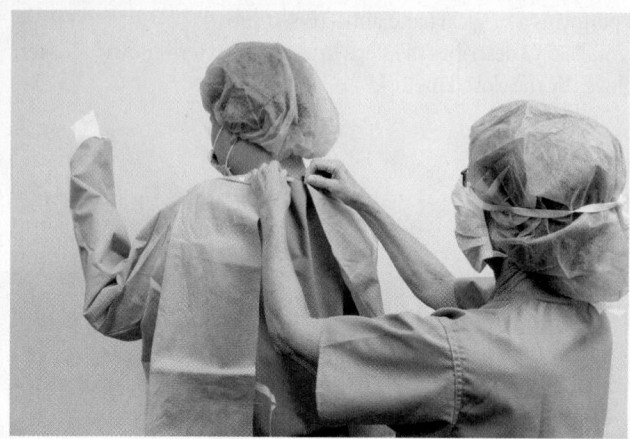

❷ Coworker ties the neck ties of the sterile gown.

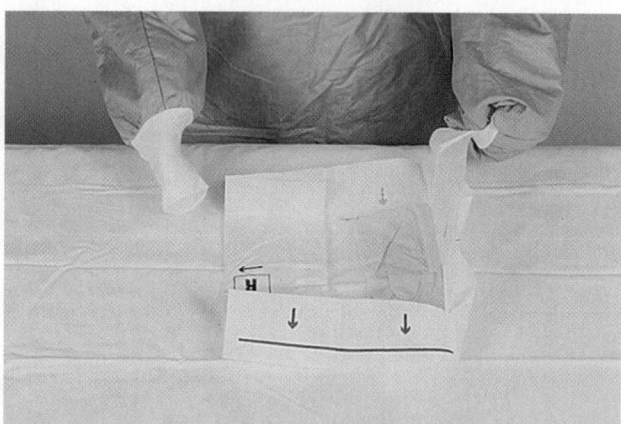

❸ Opening the sterile glove wrapper.

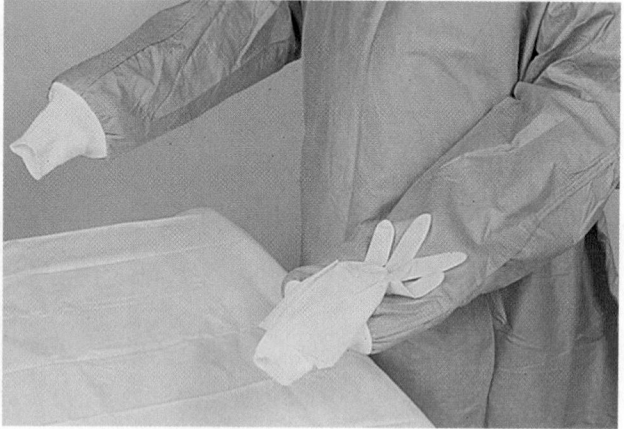

❹ Positioning the first sterile glove for the nondominant hand.

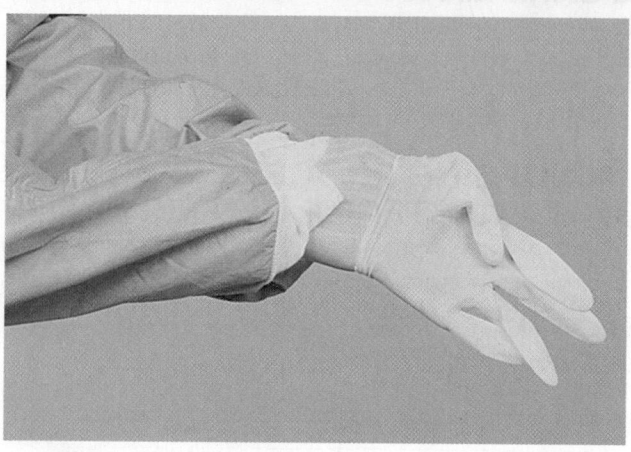

❺ Pulling on the first sterile glove.

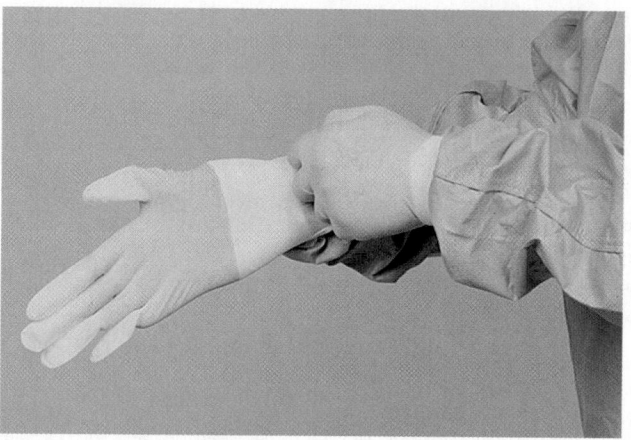

❻ Extending the fingers into the second glove of the dominant hand.

Completion of Gowning

1. Complete gowning as follows:

- Have a coworker hold the waist tie of your gown, using sterile gloves or a sterile forceps or drape. **Rationale:** *This approach keeps the ties sterile.*
- Make a three-quarter turn, then take the tie and secure it in front of the gown.

or

- Have a coworker take the two ties at each side of the gown and tie them at the back of the gown, making sure that the scrub person's uniform is completely covered.
- When worn, sterile gowns should be considered *sterile* in front from the waist to the shoulder. Once the nurse approaches a table, the gown is considered contaminated from the waist or table down, whichever is higher. The sleeves should be considered sterile from the cuff to 5 cm (2 in.) above the elbow, since the arms of a scrubbed person must move across a sterile field. Moisture collection and friction areas such as the neckline, shoulders, underarms, back, and sleeve cuffs should be considered unsterile.

EVALUATION

Conduct any follow-up indicated during care of the client.

PREPARING FOR THE POSTOPERATIVE CLIENT

While the client is in the operating room, the client's bed and room are prepared for the postoperative phase. In some agencies, the client is brought back to the unit on a stretcher and transferred to the bed in the room. (See Chapter 6 ∞ for information on making a surgical bed.) In other agencies, the client's bed is brought to the surgery suite, and the client is transferred there. In the latter situation, the bed needs to be made with clean linens as soon as the client goes to surgery so that it can be taken to the operating room when needed. In addition, the nurse must obtain and set up any special equipment, such as an IV pole, suction, oxygen equipment, and orthopedic appliances (e.g., traction). If these are not requested on the client's record, the nurse should consult with the perioperative nurse or surgeon.

POSTOPERATIVE PHASE

Nursing during the postoperative phase is especially important for the client's recovery because anesthesia impairs the ability of clients to respond to environmental stimuli and to help themselves, although the degree of consciousness of clients will vary. Moreover, surgery itself traumatizes the body by disrupting protective mechanisms and homeostasis.

Immediate Postanesthetic Care

Recovery of surgical clients who required anesthesia is performed in the PACU or RR. PACU nurses, often certified by the American Society of PeriAnesthesia Nurses (ASPAN), have specialized skills to care for clients recovering from anesthesia and surgery (Figure 33–2 ■).

During the immediate postanesthetic stage, an unconscious client is positioned on the side, with the face slightly down. A pillow is not placed under the head. In this position, gravity keeps the tongue forward, preventing occlusion of the pharynx and allowing drainage of mucus or vomitus out of the mouth rather than down the respiratory tree.

The nurse ensures maximum chest expansion by elevating the client's upper arm on a pillow. The upper arm is supported because the pressure of an arm against the chest reduces chest expansion potential. An artificial airway is maintained in place, and the client is suctioned as needed until cough and swallowing reflexes return. Generally the client spits out an oropharyngeal airway when coughing returns. Endotracheal tubes are not removed until clients are awake and able to maintain their own airway. The client is then helped to turn, cough, and take deep breaths, provided that vital signs are stable. When spinal anesthesia is used, the client may be required to remain flat for a specified period. Assessment of the client in the immediate postanesthetic period is summarized in Box 33–4.

The return of the client's reflexes, such as swallowing and gagging, indicates that anesthesia is ending. Time of recovery from anesthesia varies with the kind of anesthetic agent used, its dosage, and the individual's response to it. Nurses should arouse clients by calling them by name, and in a normal tone of voice repeatedly telling them that the surgery is over and that they are in the PACU.

The PACU nurse uses specific criteria, developed by the anesthesia department, to evaluate client readiness for discharge from the PACU. Aldrete and Kroulik (1970) were the first to introduce a postanesthetic recovery score (PARS), also called the Aldrete Score, to provide an objective scoring system to help in the discharge decision-making process. The original Aldrete scoring system included assessment of muscle activity, respiration, circulation, consciousness, and color. In 1995, this scoring system was revised to

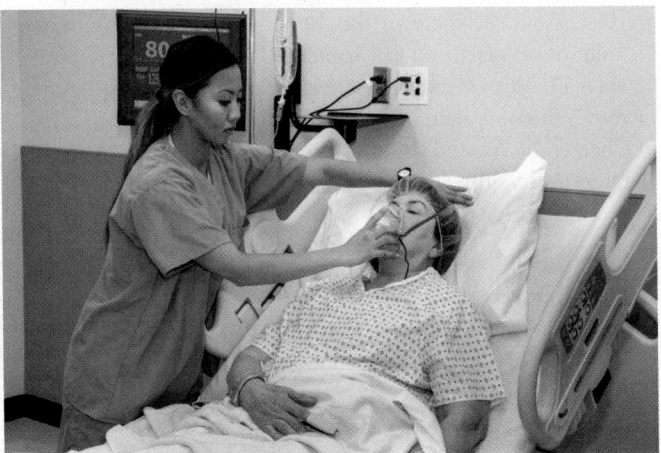

Figure 33–2 ■ The PACU nurse provides constant assessment and care for clients recovering from anesthesia and surgery.

BOX 33–4	**Immediate Postanesthetic Phase**

CLINICAL ASSESSMENT
- Adequacy of airway
- Oxygen saturation
- Adequacy of ventilation
  - Respiratory rate, rhythm, and depth
  - Use of accessory muscles
  - Breath sounds
- Cardiovascular status
  - Heart rate and rhythm
  - Peripheral pulse amplitude and equality
  - Blood pressure
  - Capillary filling
- Level of consciousness
  - Not responding
  - Arousable with verbal stimuli
  - Fully awake
  - Oriented to time, person, and place
- Presence of protective reflexes (e.g., gag, cough)
- Activity, ability to move extremities
- Skin color (pink, pale, dusky, blotchy, cyanotic, jaundiced)
- Fluid status
  - Intake and output
  - Status of IV infusions (type of fluid, rate, amount in container, patency of tubing)
  - Signs of dehydration or fluid overload
- Condition of operative site
  - Status of dressing
  - Drainage (amount, type, and color)
- Patency of and character and amount of drainage from catheters, tubes, and drains
- Discomfort (i.e., pain) and its type, location, and severity; nausea; vomiting
- Safety (i.e., necessity for side rails, call light within reach)

TABLE 33–2 Aldrete Postanesthetic Recovery Score

Activity	Respiration	Circulation	Consciousness	Oxygen Saturation
2: Moves all extremities voluntarily/on command	2: Breathes deeply and coughs freely	2: BP ± 20 mm Hg of preanesthetic level	2: Full awake	2: Maintains value >90% on room air
1: Some weakness in movement of extremities	1: Dyspneic, shallow or limited breathing (splinting)	1: BP ± 20–50 mm Hg of preanesthetic level	1: Arousable on calling	1: Requires oxygen to maintain value >90%
0: Unable to move extremities	0: Apneic	0: BP ± 50 mm Hg of preanesthetic level	0: Not responding	0: Value <90% with supplemental oxygen

Source: Adapted from "A Postanesthetic Recovery Score," by J. A. Aldrete and D. Kroulik, 1970, *Anesthesia and Analgesia, 49*(6), pp. 924–934; *Anesthesiology,* 2nd ed., by D. Longnecker, D. L. Brown, M. F. Newman, and W. Zapol, 2012, New York, NY: McGraw-Hill; and "New Criteria for Fast-Tracking After Outpatient Anesthesia: A Comparison with the Modified Aldrete's Scoring System," by P. F. White and D. Song, 1999, *Anesthesia and Analgesia, 88*, pp. 1069–1072.

replace the assessment of color with oxygen saturation and is called the Modified Aldrete. A rating of 0 to 2 is given to each assessment, depending on its absence or presence. The numbers given to each assessment are added up with a score of 10 indicating that the client is in the best possible condition. Many PACUs require a score of 9 for discharge. Table 33–2 is one example of an Aldrete PARS.

A number of scoring systems have been developed and there is no consensus regarding which specific assessments should be used to determine readiness for discharge (Phillips, Haesler, Street, & Kent, 2011). The ASPAN standards do not require use of a scoring system. However, each facility should develop assessment and discharge criteria and may include a postanesthesia scoring system as a component of the discharge criteria (ASPAN, 2012). It is important for the nurse to use critical thinking and nursing judgment along with the discharge criteria.

Clients are usually discharged from the PACU when:

- They are conscious and oriented.
- They are able to maintain a clear airway and deep breathe and cough freely.
- Vital signs have been stable or consistent with preoperative vital signs for at least 30 minutes.
- Protective reflexes (e.g., gag, swallowing) are active.
- They are able to move all extremities.
- Intake and urinary output are adequate.
- They are afebrile or a febrile condition has been attended to.
- Dressings are dry and intact; there is no overt drainage.

Once the health status has stabilized, the client is returned to the nursing unit or the outpatient surgery discharge area.

ONGOING POSTOPERATIVE NURSING CARE

As soon as the client returns to the nursing unit, the nurse conducts an initial assessment. The sequence of these activities varies with the situation. For example, the nurse may need to check the primary care provider's "stat" orders before conducting the initial assessment; in such a case, nursing interventions to implement the orders can be carried out at the same time as assessment.

The nurse consults the surgeon's postoperative orders to learn the following:

- Food and fluids permitted by mouth
- IV solutions and IV medications
- Position in bed

- Medications ordered (e.g., analgesics, antibiotics)
- Laboratory tests
- Intake and output, which in some agencies are monitored for all postoperative clients
- Activity permitted, including ambulation

The nurse also checks the PACU record for the following data:

- Operation performed
- Presence and location of any drains
- Anesthetic used
- Postoperative diagnosis
- Estimated blood loss
- Medications administered in the PACU

Many hospitals have postoperative protocols for regular assessment of clients. In some agencies, assessments are made every 15 minutes until vital signs stabilize, every hour for the next 4 hours, then every 4 hours for the next 48 hours. It is important that the assessments be made as often as the client's condition requires.

Assessment continues throughout the postoperative period. See Box 33–5 for postoperative assessment guidelines and Table 33–3 regarding potential postoperative problems. Nursing interventions designed to prevent these problems include early ambulation, deep-breathing and coughing exercises, adequate hydration, leg exercises, monitoring fluid intake and output, and early recognition of signs of complications.

Skills commonly implemented in the postoperative period are discussed elsewhere in this book. For example, IV therapy techniques are discussed in Chapter 18, parenteral medications in Chapter 17 ∞, pain management in Chapter 9 ∞, assisting clients to move and ambulate in Chapter 11 ∞, promoting circulation in Chapter 23 ∞, and breathing exercises in Chapter 24 ∞. This chapter includes the skills of managing gastrointestinal suction and surgical wound care.

Suction

Some clients return from surgery with a gastric or intestinal tube in place and orders to connect the tube to suction. The suction ordered can be continuous or intermittent. **Intermittent suction** is applied when a single-lumen gastric tube (Levin tube) is used to reduce the risk of damaging the mucous membrane near the distal port of the tube. **Continuous suction** may be applied if a double-lumen tube (Salem sump tube) is in place (Figure 33–3 ∎ on p. 728). Fluids and electrolytes must be replaced intravenously when gastric suction or continuous

BOX 33–5 Postoperative Assessment Guidelines

Assess:
- *Level of consciousness.* Assess orientation to time, place, and person. Most clients are fully conscious but drowsy when returned to their room or area. Assess reaction to verbal stimuli and ability to move extremities.
- *Vital signs.* Take the client's vital signs (pulse, respiration, blood pressure, and oxygen saturation level) every 15 minutes until stable or in accordance with agency protocol. Compare initial findings with PACU data. In addition, assess the client's lung sounds and assess for signs of common circulatory problems such as postoperative hypotension, hemorrhage, or shock. Hypovolemia due to fluid losses during surgery is a common cause of postoperative hypotension. Hemorrhage can result from insecure ligation of blood vessels or disruption of sutures. Massive hemorrhage or cardiac insufficiency can lead to shock postoperatively.
- *Skin color and temperature,* particularly that of the lips and nail beds. The color of the lips and nail beds is an indicator of tissue perfusion (passage of blood through the vessels). Pale, cyanotic, cool, and moist skin may be a sign of circulatory problems.

CLINICAL ALERT!

Older clients may not show the classic signs of infection (e.g., fever, tachycardia, increased WBC count); instead there may be an abrupt change in their mental status.

- *Comfort.* Assess pain with the client's vital signs and as needed between vital sign measurements. Assess the location and intensity of the pain. Do not assume that reported pain is incisional; other causes may include muscle strains, flatus, and angina. Evaluate the client for objective indicators of pain: pallor, perspiration, muscle tension, and reluctance to cough, move, or ambulate. Determine when and what analgesics were last administered and assess the client for any side effects of medication such as nausea and vomiting.
- *Fluid balance.* Assess the type and amount of IV fluids, flow rate, and infusion site. Monitor the client's fluid intake and output. In addition to watching for shock, assess the client for signs of circulatory overload and monitor serum electrolytes. Anesthetics and surgery affect the hormones regulating fluid and electrolyte balance (aldosterone and antidiuretic hormone in particular), placing the client at risk for decreased urine output and fluid and electrolyte imbalances.
- *Dressing and bedclothes.* Inspect the client's dressings and bedclothes underneath the client. Excessive bloody drainage on dressings or on bedclothes, often appearing underneath the client, can indicate hemorrhage. The amount of drainage on dressings is recorded by describing the diameter of the stains or by denoting the number and type of dressings saturated with drainage. Later, when dressings are changed, inspect the wound for signs of localized infection.
- *Drains and tubes.* Determine color, consistency, and amount of drainage from all tubes and drains. All tubes should be patent, and tubes and suction equipment should be functioning. Drainage bags must be hanging properly.
- *Any difficulties with voiding and/or bladder distention.*
- *Return of peristalsis.* Auscultate the client's abdomen to confirm the return of peristalsis. Note the passage of flatus and stool.
- *Tolerance of food and fluids ingested.*

TABLE 33–3 Potential Postoperative Problems

Problem	Description	Cause	Clinical Signs	Preventive Interventions
RESPIRATORY				
Pneumonia	Inflammation of the alveoli	Infection, toxins, or irritants causing inflammatory process Immobility and impaired ventilation, resulting in atelectasis and promote growth of pathogens	Elevated temperature, cough, expectoration of blood-tinged or purulent sputum, dyspnea, chest pain	Deep-breathing exercises and coughing, moving in bed, early ambulation
Atelectasis	A condition in which alveoli collapse and are not ventilated	Mucous plugs blocking bronchial passageways, inadequate lung expansion, analgesics, immobility	Dyspnea, tachypnea, tachycardia; diaphoresis, anxiety; pleural pain, decreased chest wall movement; dull or absent breath sounds; decreased oxygen saturation	Deep-breathing exercises and coughing, moving in bed, early ambulation
Pulmonary embolism	Blood clot that has moved to the lungs and blocks a pulmonary artery, thus obstructing blood flow to a portion of the lung	Stasis of venous blood from immobility, venous injury from fractures or during surgery, use of oral contraceptives high in estrogen, preexisting coagulation or circulatory disorder	Sudden chest pain, shortness of breath, cyanosis, shock (tachycardia, low blood pressure)	Turning, ambulation, anti-emboli stockings, sequential compression devices (SCDs)

Continued on page 726

TABLE 33–3 | Potential Postoperative Problems (*continued*)

Problem	Description	Cause	Clinical Signs	Preventive Interventions
CIRCULATORY				
Hypovolemia	Inadequate circulating blood volume	Fluid deficit, hemorrhage	Tachycardia, decreased urine output, decreased blood pressure	Early detection of signs; fluid and/or blood replacement
Hemorrhage	Internal or external bleeding	Disruption of sutures, insecure ligation of blood vessels	Overt bleeding (dressings saturated with bright blood; bright, free-flowing blood in drains or chest tubes), increased pain, increasing abdominal girth, swelling or bruising around incision	Early detection of signs
Hypovolemic shock	Inadequate tissue perfusion resulting from markedly reduced circulating blood volume	Severe hypovolemia from fluid deficit or hemorrhage	Rapid weak pulse, dyspnea, tachypnea; restlessness and anxiety; urine output less than 30 mL/h; decreased blood pressure; cool, clammy skin, thirst, pallor	Maintain blood volume through adequate fluid replacement; prevent hemorrhage; early detection of signs
Thrombophlebitis	Inflammation of the veins, usually of the legs and associated with a blood clot	Slowed venous blood flow due to immobility or prolonged sitting; trauma to vein, resulting in inflammation and increased blood coagulability	Aching, cramping pain; affected area is swollen, red, and hot to touch; vein feels hard; discomfort in calf when foot is dorsiflexed (Homans' sign) or when client walks	Early ambulation, leg exercises, antiemboli stockings, SCDs, adequate fluid intake
Thrombus	Blood clot attached to wall of vein or artery (most commonly the leg veins)	Thrombophlebitis for venous thrombi; disruption or inflammation of arterial wall for arterial thrombi	*Venous:* same as thrombophlebitis *Arterial:* pain and pallor of affected extremity; decreased or absent peripheral pulses	*Venous:* same as thrombophlebitis *Arterial:* maintain prescribed position; early detection of signs
Embolus	Foreign body or clot that has moved from its site of formation to another area of the body (e.g., the lungs, heart, or brain)	Venous or arterial thrombus; broken IV catheter, fat, or amniotic fluid	In venous system, usually becomes a pulmonary embolus (see pulmonary embolism); signs of arterial emboli may depend on the location	Turning, ambulation, leg exercises, SCDs; careful maintenance of IV catheters
URINARY				
Urinary retention	Inability to empty the bladder with excessive accumulation of urine in the bladder	Depressed bladder muscle tone from narcotics and anesthetics; handling of tissues during surgery on adjacent organs (rectum, vagina)	Fluid intake larger than output; inability to void or frequent voiding of small amounts, bladder distention, suprapubic discomfort, restlessness	Monitoring of fluid intake and output, interventions to facilitate voiding, urinary catheterization as needed
Urinary tract infection	Inflammation of the bladder, ureters, or urethra	Immobilization and limited fluid intake, instrumentation of the urinary tract	Burning sensation when voiding, urgency, cloudy urine, lower abdominal pain	Adequate fluid intake, early ambulation, aseptic straight catheterization only as necessary, good perineal hygiene
GASTROINTESTINAL				
Nausea and vomiting		Pain, abdominal distention, ingesting food or fluids before return of peristalsis, certain medications, anxiety	Complaints of feeling sick to the stomach, retching or gagging	IV fluids until peristalsis returns; then clear fluids, full fluids, and regular diet; antiemetic drugs if ordered; analgesics for pain

TABLE 33–3 Potential Postoperative Problems (*continued*)

Problem	Description	Cause	Clinical Signs	Preventive Interventions
Constipation	Infrequent or no stool passage for abnormal length of time (e.g., within 48 hours after solid diet started)	Lack of dietary roughage, analgesics (decreased intestinal motility), immobility	Absence of stool elimination, abdominal distention, and discomfort	Adequate fluid intake, high-fiber diet, early ambulation
Tympanites	Retention of gases within the intestines	Slowed motility of the intestines due to handling of the bowel during surgery and the effects of anesthesia	Obvious abdominal distention, abdominal discomfort (gas pains), absence of bowel sounds	Early ambulation; avoid using a straw, provide ice chips or water at room temperature
Postoperative ileus	Intestinal obstruction characterized by lack of peristaltic activity	Handling the bowel during surgery, anesthesia, electrolyte imbalance, wound infection	Abdominal pain and distention; constipation; absent bowel sounds; vomiting	Early ambulation; chewing gum; early oral intake and feeding
WOUND Wound infection	Inflammation and infection of incision or drain site	Poor aseptic technique; laboratory analysis of wound swab identifies causative microorganism	Purulent exudate, redness, tenderness, elevated body temperature, wound odor	Keep wound clean and dry, use surgical aseptic technique when changing dressings
Wound dehiscence	Separation of a suture line before the incision heals	Malnutrition (emaciation, obesity), poor circulation, excessive strain on suture line	Increased incision drainage, tissues underlying skin become visible along parts of the incision	Adequate nutrition, appropriate incisional support, and avoidance of strain
Wound evisceration	Extrusion of internal organs and tissues through the incision	Same as for wound dehiscence	Opening of incision and visible protrusion of organs	Same as for wound dehiscence
PSYCHOLOGICAL Postoperative depression	Mental disorder characterized by altered mood	Weakness, surprise nature of emergency surgery, news of malignancy, severely altered body image, other personal matter; may be a physiological response to some surgeries	Anorexia, tearfulness, loss of ambition, withdrawal, rejection of others, feelings of dejection, sleep disturbances (insomnia or excessive sleeping)	Adequate rest, physical activity, opportunity to express anger and other negative feelings

---

Ambulatory and Community Settings **Postoperative Instructions** | PATIENT-CENTERED CARE |

Adults want information about activities they normally perform while they are recovering at home. This is important information for all surgical clients and particularly clients having outpatient surgery. Discuss the following areas:

- *Food.* Eat small portions at first because anesthesia and pain medications slow gastric emptying.
- *Bowel movements.* Constipation occurs frequently as a result of decreased gastrointestinal motility due to many causes (e.g., anesthesia, decreased activity, pain medications). Discuss strategies to prevent constipation.
- *Sexual activity.* Intimacy such as gentle hugging and kissing is allowed for clients when they feel like it. Full sexual intercourse cannot be resumed until wound soreness and tenderness are resolved, approximately 2 to 4 weeks. Check with the surgeon for gynecologic procedures.

- *Wound care.* Discuss wound care, including the signs and symptoms of infection and when to notify the surgeon.
- *Lifting.* Be specific about weight limits, if appropriate. Relate the weight limit to everyday items (e.g., a gallon of milk weighs approximately 8 pounds).
- *Pain.* Provide information about the client's pain medications. Ask the client to describe his or her daily activities, and discuss ways to avoid or reduce painful activities.
- *Bathing.* Check with the surgeon because some prefer the wound to be kept dry. There is no evidence that water on a closed wound is harmful or interferes with wound healing. If allowed, instruct the client to shower, letting the warm water wash over the incision and gently patting the incision dry.
- *Activities.* Advise the client that he or she will tire easily and to plan short activities with frequent rest breaks.

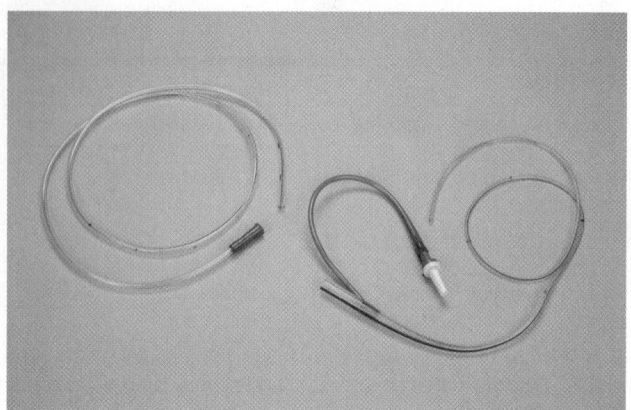

Figure 33–3 ■ Nasogastric tubes used for gastric decompression. *Left:* Levin (single-lumen) tube. *Right:* Salem sump (double-lumen) tube with antireflux valve.

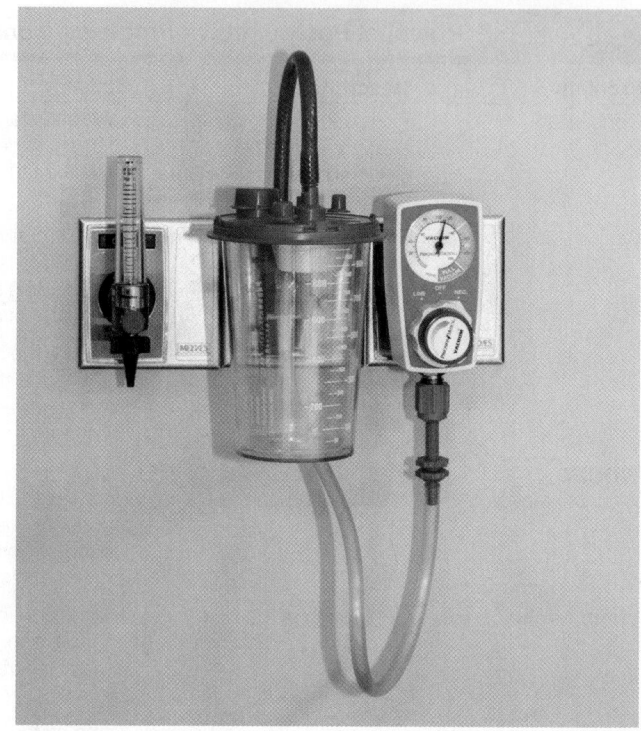

Figure 33–4 ■ Wall suction unit for generating negative pressure for nasogastric suction.

drainage is ordered. Nasogastric tubes may be irrigated if the lumen becomes clogged. They are generally irrigated before and after tube feedings or the instillation of medications. Nasogastric irrigation may require a surgeon's order, particularly following gastrointestinal surgery. Skill 33–4 describes the management of gastrointestinal suction.

Suction may also be applied to other drainage tubes such as chest tubes or a wound drain. The type and amount of suction is ordered by the surgeon. Most agencies have wall suction units available (Figure 33–4 ■). A suction regulator with a drainage receptacle connects to a wall outlet that provides negative pressure. Check the receptacle frequently to prevent excess drainage from interfering

with the suction apparatus; empty or change the receptacle according to agency policy. Portable electric suction units or pumps (e.g., the Gomco pump) may be used in the home or when wall suction is not available.

●○● NURSING PROCESS: SUCTION

SKILL 33–4

Managing Gastrointestinal Suction

ASSESSMENT
Assess:
- Presence of abdominal distention on palpation.
- Bowel sounds.
- Abdominal discomfort.
- Vital signs for baseline data.
- Amount and characteristics of drainage.

PLANNING
Before initiating gastric suction, determine (a) whether the suction is continuous or intermittent; (b) the ordered suction pressure (a low suction pressure is between 80 and 100 mmHg, and a high pressure is between 100 and 120 mmHg); and (c) whether there is an order to irrigate the gastrointestinal tube, and if so, the type of solution to use.

DELEGATION

Managing gastrointestinal suction requires application of knowledge and problem solving and is not delegated to UAP. The UAP, however, can assist with emptying the drainage receptacle and reporting changes in amount and/or color of the drainage to the nurse.

Equipment
Initiating Suction
- Gastrointestinal tube in place in the client
- Basin

- 50-mL syringe with an adapter
- Stethoscope
- Suction device for either continuous or intermittent suction
- Connector and connecting tubing
- Clean gloves

Maintaining Suction
- Graduated container as required to measure gastric drainage
- Basin of water
- Cotton-tipped applicators
- Ointment or lubricant
- Clean gloves

Irrigation
- Clean gloves
- Stethoscope
- Disposable irrigating set containing a sterile 50-mL syringe, moisture-resistant pad, basin, and graduated container
- Sterile normal saline (500 mL) or the ordered solution

Managing Gastrointestinal Suction—*continued*

IMPLEMENTATION
Performance

1. Prior to performing the procedure, introduce self and verify the client's identity using agency protocol. Explain to the client what you are going to do, why it is necessary, and how he or she can participate. Discuss the purpose(s) of the gastrointestinal suction.

2. Perform hand hygiene and observe other appropriate infection prevention procedures (e.g., clean gloves).

3. Provide for client privacy.

Initiating Suction

4. Position the client appropriately.
   • Assist the client to a semi-Fowler's position if it is not contraindicated. **Rationale:** *In the semi-Fowler's position, the tube is not as likely to lie against the wall of the stomach and will therefore suction most efficiently. The semi-Fowler's position also prevents reflux of gastric contents, which could lead to aspiration.*

5. Confirm that the tube is in the stomach.
   • Perform hand hygiene.
   • Apply clean gloves.
   • Check agency protocol for preferred methods to verify placement because clinical practice varies across health regions:

   a. The method of inserting air into the tube with the syringe and listening with a stethoscope over the stomach (just below the xiphoid process) for a swish of air is often used at the bedside; however, a similar gurgling sound can be heard when the tube is incorrectly placed in the lungs or esophagus (Lemyze, 2010) and recent evidence does not support this practice. For example, Tho, Mordiffi, Ang, and Chen (2011) found that there is "no evidence that supports the method of auscultation to confirm correct NG tube placement in the absence of aspirate" (p. 51). Furthermore, Boeykens, Steeman, and Duysburgh (2014) evaluated the auscultatory method and the pH measurement method and concluded that the auscultatory method was unreliable.

   b. Aspirate to obtain stomach contents. Secretions from the stomach are usually greenish but can be colorless with shreds of mucus. Distinguishing between respiratory and gastric secretions is subjective.

   c. Check the acidity of gastric aspirate using a pH test strip. Gastric secretions often have a pH of 5 or less. The pH of the aspirate will increase if the client is on acid-inhibiting medication.

   d. X-ray examination is considered the gold standard for determining placement, especially for high-risk clients (e.g., those who are critically ill, dysphagic, or unconscious).

   • Remove and discard gloves.
   • Perform hand hygiene.

6. Set and check the suction.
   • Connect the appropriate suction regulator to the wall suction outlet and the collection device to the regulator. Intermittent suction regulators generally are used with single-lumen tubes and apply suction for a set interval (15 to 60 seconds), followed by an interval of no suction. Intermittent suction is set at 80 to 100 mmHg or as ordered by the primary care provider. Check the suction level by occluding the drainage tube and observing the regulator dial during a suction cycle. Continuous suction regulators are used with double-lumen (e.g., Salem sump) nasogastric tubes. Set continuous suction as ordered by the primary care provider, or at 60 to 120 mmHg.
   • If using a portable suction machine, turn on the machine and regulate the suction as above. The Gomco pump has two settings: low intermittent for single-lumen tubes, and high for double-lumen tubes.
   • Test for proper suctioning by holding the open end of the suction tube to the ear and listening for a sucking noise or by occluding the end of the tube with a thumb.

7. Establish gastric suction.
   • Connect the gastrointestinal tube to the tubing from the suction by using the connector.
   • If a Salem sump tube is in place, connect the larger lumen to the suction equipment. This double-lumen tube has a smaller tube running inside the primary suction tube. **Rationale:** *The smaller tube provides a continuous flow of atmospheric air through the drainage tube at its distal end and prevents excessive suction force on the gastric mucosa at the drainage outlets. Damage to the gastric mucosa is thus avoided.*
   • Always keep the air vent tube of a Salem sump tube open and above the level of the stomach when suction is applied. **Rationale:** *Closing the vent would stop the sump action and cause mucosal damage. Keeping the end of the air vent tube higher than the stomach prevents reflux of gastric contents into the air lumen of the tube.*
   • After suction is applied, watch the tubing for a few minutes until the gastric contents appear to be running through the tubing into the receptacle. A Salem sump tube makes a soft, hissing sound when it is functioning correctly.
   • If the suction is not working properly, check that all connections are tight and that the tubing is not kinked.
   • Coil and pin the tubing to the client's gown so that it does not loop below the suction bottle. **Rationale:** *If the tubing falls below the suction bottle, the suction may be obstructed because of the pressure required to push the fluid against gravity.*

8. Assess the drainage.
   • Observe the amount, color, odor, and consistency of the drainage. Normal gastric drainage has a mucoid (resembling mucus) consistency and is either colorless or yellow-green because of the presence of bile. A coffee-ground color and consistency may indicate bleeding.
   • Test the gastric drainage for pH and blood when indicated. A client who has had gastrointestinal surgery can be expected to have some blood in the drainage.

Maintaining Suction

9. Assess the client and the suction system regularly.
   • Assess the client every 30 minutes until the system is running effectively and then every 2 hours, or as the client's health indicates, to ensure that the suction is functioning properly. If the client complains of fullness, nausea, or epigastric pain or if the flow of gastric secretions is absent in the tubing or in the collection bottle, ineffective suctioning or blockage of the nasogastric tube is likely.
   • Inspect the suction system for patency of the system (e.g., kinks or blockages in the tubing) and tightness of the connections. **Rationale:** *Loose connections can permit air to enter and thus decrease the effectiveness of the suction by decreasing the negative pressure.*

10. Relieve blockages if present.
    • Perform hand hygiene.
    • Apply clean gloves.
    • Check the suction equipment. To do this, disconnect the nasogastric tube from the suction over a collecting basin (to collect gastric drainage), and then, with the suction on, place the end of the suction tubing in a basin of water. If water is drawn into the drainage bottle, the suction equipment is functioning properly, but the nasogastric tube is either blocked or positioned incorrectly.

Continued on page 730

Managing Gastrointestinal Suction—*continued*

- Reposition the client (e.g., to the other side) if permitted. **Rationale:** *This may facilitate drainage.*
- Rotate the nasogastric tube and reposition it. This step is contraindicated for clients with gastric surgery. **Rationale:** *Moving the tube may interfere with gastric sutures.*
- Irrigate the nasogastric tube as agency protocol states or on the order of the primary care provider (see steps 14 to 16).
- Remove and discard gloves.
- Perform hand hygiene.

11. Prevent reflux into the vent lumen of a Salem sump tube. **Rationale:** *Reflux of gastric contents into the vent lumen may occur when stomach pressure exceeds atmospheric pressure. In this situation, gastric contents follow the path of least resistance and flow out the vent lumen rather than the drainage lumen.* To prevent reflux:
    - Place the vent tubing higher than the client's stomach to prevent gastric fluid backup into the blue lumen air vent.
    - Keep the drainage lumen free of particulate matter that may obstruct the lumen (see steps 14 to 16 for irrigating a nasogastric tube).

12. Ensure client comfort.
    - Clean the client's nares as needed, using the cotton-tipped applicators and water. Apply a water-soluble lubricant or ointment.
    - Provide mouth care every 2 to 4 hours and as needed. Some postoperative clients are permitted to suck ice chips or a moist cloth to maintain the moisture of the oral mucous membranes.

13. Change the drainage receptacle according to agency policy.
    - Clamp the nasogastric tube and turn off the suction.
    - Apply clean gloves.
    - If the receptacle is marked with lines to indicate the amount of drainage, determine the amount of drainage.
    - Disconnect the receptacle.
    - Inspect the drainage carefully for color, consistency, and presence of substances (e.g., blood clots).
    - Replace the full receptacle and attach a new receptacle to the suction. Check agency policy.
    - Turn on the suction and unclamp the nasogastric tube.
    - Observe the system for several minutes to make sure function is reestablished.
    - Remove and discard gloves.
    - Perform hand hygiene.
    - Go to step 17.

Irrigating a Gastrointestinal Tube

14. Prepare the client and the equipment.
    - Place the moisture-resistant pad under the end of the gastrointestinal tube.
    - Turn off the suction.
    - Apply clean gloves.
    - Disconnect the gastrointestinal tube from the connector.
    - Determine that the tube is in the stomach. See step 5. **Rationale:** *This ensures that the irrigating solution enters the client's stomach.*

15. Irrigate the tube.
    - Draw up the ordered volume of irrigating solution in the syringe; 30 mL of solution per instillation is usual, but up to 60 mL may be given per instillation if ordered.
    - Attach the syringe to the nasogastric tube and slowly inject the solution.
    - Gently aspirate the solution. **Rationale:** *Forceful withdrawal could damage the gastric mucosa.*
    - If you encounter difficulty in withdrawing the solution, inject 20 mL of air and aspirate again, and/or reposition the client or the nasogastric tube. **Rationale:** *Air and repositioning may move the end of the tube away from the stomach wall.* If aspirating difficulty continues, reattach the tube and set to intermittent low suction, and notify the nurse in charge.
    - Repeat the preceding steps until the ordered amount of solution is used.
    - *Note:* A Salem sump tube can also be irrigated through the vent lumen without interrupting suction. However, only small quantities of irrigant can be injected via this lumen compared to the drainage lumen.
    - After irrigating a Salem sump tube, inject 10 to 20 mL of air into the vent lumen while applying suction to the drainage lumen. **Rationale:** *This tests the patency of the vent and ensures sump functioning.*

16. Reestablish suction.
    - Reconnect the nasogastric tube to suction.
    - If a Salem sump tube is used, inject the air vent lumen with 10 mL of air after reconnecting the tube to suction.
    - Observe the system for several minutes to make sure it is functioning.
    - Remove and discard gloves.
    - Perform hand hygiene.

17. Document all relevant information.
    - Record the time suction was started. Also record the pressure established, the color and consistency of the drainage, and nursing assessments.
    - During maintenance, record assessments, supportive nursing measures, and data about the suction system.
    - When irrigating the tube, record verification of tube placement; the time of the irrigation; the amount and type of irrigating solution used; the amount, color, and consistency of the returns; the patency of the system following the irrigation; and nursing assessments.

SAMPLE DOCUMENTATION

3/20/2015 1300 Returned from PACU. Salem sump tube in place and connected to low continuous suction. Placement verified. Draining small to moderate amount of tannish fluid. ——— R. Martinez, RN

EVALUATION

- Conduct appropriate follow-up such as relief of abdominal distention or discomfort, bowel sounds, character and amount of gastric drainage, integrity of nares, hydration of oral mucous membranes, patency of tube, and system functioning.
- Compare to previous findings if available.
- Report significant deviations from normal to the primary care provider.

PATIENT-CENTERED CARE

Instruct the caregiver to:
- Maintain suction as ordered; do *not* increase or decrease the suction without instructions from the nurse or primary care provider.
- Offer mouth care every 2 hours.

- Avoid tension and pulling on the tube by securing it to the gown.
- Check the patency of the tube if nausea or vomiting occurs.
- Report an increasing amount of or bloody drainage.

Wound Care and Surgical Dressings

Most clients return from surgery with a sutured wound covered by a dressing, although in some cases the wound may be left unsutured. Dressings are inspected regularly to ensure that they are clean, dry, and intact. Excessive drainage may indicate hemorrhage, infection, or an open wound.

When dressings are changed, the nurse assesses the wound for appearance, size, drainage, swelling, pain, and the status of a drain or tubes. Details about these assessments are outlined in Practice Guidelines.

Not all surgical dressings require changing. Sometimes, surgeons in the operating room apply a dressing that remains in place until the sutures are removed and no further dressings are required. In many situations, however, surgical dressings are changed regularly to prevent the growth of microorganisms.

In some instances a client may have a **Penrose drain** (flat, thin rubber tube) inserted. The Penrose drain allows for fluid to flow from the wound. Because there is no collection device, be prepared to change the dressing more often. In this situation, the main surgical incision is considered cleaner than the surgical drain incision made for the Penrose drain insertion because there is usually considerable drainage. The main incision is therefore cleaned *first*, and under no

PRACTICE GUIDELINES

Assessing Surgical Wounds

- *Appearance.* Inspect the color of the wound and surrounding area and approximation of wound edges.
- *Size.* Note size and location of dehiscence, if present.
- *Drainage.* Observe location, color, consistency, odor, and degree of saturation of dressings. Note the number of gauzes saturated or the diameter of drainage on the gauze.
- *Swelling.* Observe the amount of swelling; minimal to moderate swelling is normal in early stages of wound healing.
- *Pain.* Expect severe to moderate postoperative pain for 3 to 5 days; persistent severe pain or sudden onset of severe pain may indicate internal hemorrhaging or infection.
- *Drains or tubes.* Inspect drain security and placement, amount and character of drainage, and functioning of collecting apparatus, if present.

circumstances are materials that were used to clean the drain incision used subsequently to clean the main incision. In this way, the main incision is kept free of the microorganisms around the drain incision. Cleaning a wound and applying a sterile dressing are detailed in Skill 33–5.

●○● NURSING PROCESS: WOUND CARE AND SURGICAL DRESSINGS

Cleaning a Sutured Wound and Changing a Dressing on a Wound with a Drain

SKILL 33-5

ASSESSMENT
Assess:
- Client allergies to wound cleaning agents.
- The appearance and size of the wound.
- The amount and character of exudates.

- Client complaints of discomfort.
- The time of the last pain medication.
- Signs of systemic infection (e.g., elevated body temperature, diaphoresis, malaise, leukocytosis).

PLANNING
Before changing a dressing, determine any specific orders about the wound or dressing.

DELEGATION

Cleaning a newly sutured wound, especially one with a drain, requires application of knowledge, problem solving, and aseptic technique. As a result, this procedure is not delegated to UAP. The nurse can ask the UAP to report soiled dressings that need to be changed or if a dressing has become loose and needs to be reinforced. The nurse is responsible for the assessment and evaluation of the wound.

Equipment
- Bath blanket (if necessary)
- Moisture-resistant biohazard bag

- Mask (optional)
- Clean gloves
- Sterile gloves
- Sterile dressing set; if not available, gather the following sterile items:
  - Drape or towel
  - Gauze squares
  - Container for the cleaning solution
  - Cleaning solution (e.g., normal saline)
  - Two pairs of forceps
  - Gauze dressings and surgipads
  - Applicators or tongue blades to apply ointments
- Additional supplies required for the particular dressing (e.g., extra gauze dressings and ointment, if ordered)
- Tape, tie tapes, or binder

Continued on page 732

Cleaning a Sutured Wound and Changing a Dressing on a Wound with a Drain—*continued*

IMPLEMENTATION

Preparation

Prepare the client and assemble the equipment.

- Obtain assistance for changing a dressing on a restless or confused adult. **Rationale:** *The person might move and contaminate the sterile field or the wound.*
- Assist the client to a comfortable position in which the wound can be readily exposed. Expose only the wound area, using a bath blanket to cover the client, if necessary. **Rationale:** *Undue exposure is physically and psychologically distressing to most people.*
- Make a cuff on the biohazard bag for disposal of the soiled dressings, and place the bag within reach. **Rationale:** *The cuff helps keep the outside of the bag free from contamination by the soiled dressings and prevents subsequent contamination of the nurse's hands or of sterile instrument tips when discarding dressing or sponges. Placement of the bag within reach prevents the nurse from reaching across the sterile field and the wound and potentially contaminating these areas.*
- Apply a face mask, if required. **Rationale:** *Some agencies require that a mask be worn for surgical dressing changes to prevent contamination of the wound by droplet spray from the nurse's respiratory tract.*

Performance

1. Prior to performing the procedure, introduce self and verify the client's identity using agency protocol. Explain to the client what you are going to do, why it is necessary, and how he or she can participate. Discuss how the results will be used in planning further care or treatments.
2. Perform hand hygiene and observe other appropriate infection prevention procedures.
3. Provide for client privacy.
4. Remove binders (see Chapter 31 ∞) and tape.
   - Remove binders, if used, and place them aside. Untie tie tapes, if used. Montgomery straps (tie tapes) are commonly used for wounds requiring frequent dressing changes. ❶ **Rationale:** *These straps prevent skin irritation and discomfort caused by removing the adhesive each time the dressing is changed.*
   - If adhesive tape was used, remove it by holding down the skin and pulling the tape gently but firmly toward the wound. **Rationale:** *Pressing down on the skin provides countertraction against the pulling motion. Tape is pulled toward the incision to prevent strain on the sutures or wound.*

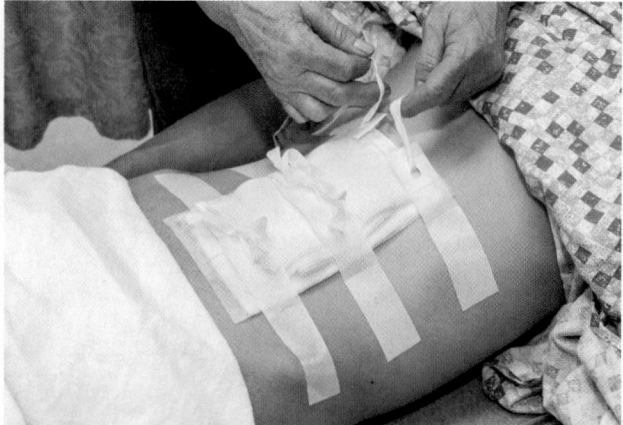

❶ Montgomery straps holding the dressing.

5. Remove and dispose of soiled dressings appropriately.
   - Apply clean gloves, and remove the outer abdominal dressing or surgipad.
   - Lift the outer dressing so that the underside is *away* from the client's face. **Rationale:** *The appearance and odor of the drainage may be upsetting to the client.*
   - Place the soiled dressing in the biohazard bag without touching the outside of the bag. **Rationale:** *Contamination of the outside of the bag is avoided to prevent the spread of microorganisms to the nurse and subsequently to others.*
   - Remove the underdressings, taking care not to dislodge any drains. If the gauze sticks to the drain, support the drain with one hand and remove the gauze with the other.
   - Assess the location, type (color, consistency), and odor of wound drainage, and the number of gauzes saturated or the diameter of drainage collected on the dressings.
   - Discard the soiled dressings in the bag as before.
   - Remove and discard gloves in the moisture-resistant bag.
   - Perform hand hygiene.
6. Set up the sterile supplies.
   - Open the sterile dressing set, using surgical aseptic technique.
   - Place the sterile drape beside the wound.
   - Open the sterile cleaning solution, and pour it over the gauze sponges in the plastic container.
   - Apply sterile gloves.
7. Clean the wound, if indicated.
   - Clean the wound, using your gloved hands or forceps and gauze swabs moistened with cleaning solution.
   - If using forceps, keep the forceps tips lower than the handles at all times. **Rationale:** *This prevents their contamination by fluid traveling up to the handle and nurse's wrist and back to the tips.*
   - Use the cleaning methods illustrated and described in ❷ or one recommended by agency protocol.
   - Use a separate swab for each stroke, and discard each swab after use. **Rationale:** *This prevents the introduction of microorganisms to other wound areas.*
   - If a drain is present, clean it next, taking care to avoid reaching across the cleaned incision. Clean the skin around the drain site by swabbing in half or full circles from around the drain site outward, using separate swabs for each wipe ❷, C.
   - Support and hold the drain erect while cleaning around it. Clean as many times as necessary to remove the drainage.
   - Dry the surrounding skin with dry gauze swabs as required. Do not dry the incision or wound itself. **Rationale:** *Moisture facilitates wound healing.*
8. Apply dressings to the drain site and the incision.
   - Place a precut 4×4 gauze snugly around the drain, ❸ or open a 4×4 gauze to 4×8, fold it lengthwise to 2×8, and place it around the drain so that the ends overlap. **Rationale:** *This dressing absorbs the drainage and helps prevent it from excoriating the skin. Using precut gauze or folding it as described, instead of cutting the gauze, prevents any threads from coming loose and getting into the wound, where they could cause inflammation and provide a site for infection.*
   - Apply the sterile dressings one at a time over the drain and the incision. Place the bulk of the dressings over the drain area and below the drain, depending on the client's usual position. **Rationale:** *Layers of dressings are placed for best absorption of drainage, which flows by gravity.*
   - Apply the final surgipad.

Cleaning a Sutured Wound and Changing a Dressing on a Wound with a Drain—*continued*

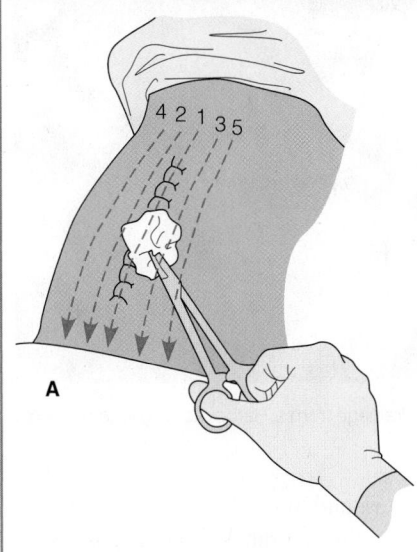

A

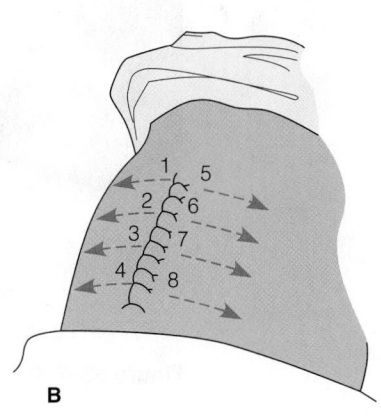

B

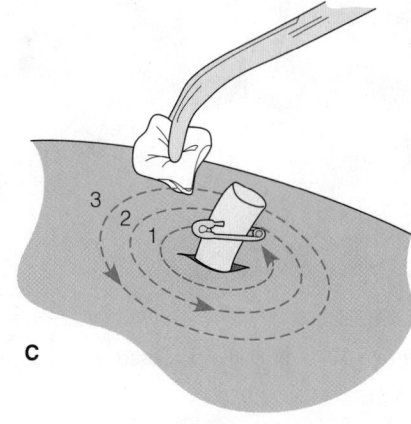

C

❷ Methods of cleaning surgical wounds: *A,* cleaning the wound from top to bottom, starting at the center; *B,* cleaning a wound outward from the incision; *C,* cleaning around a Penrose drain site. For all methods, a clean sterile swab is used for each stroke.

- Remove and discard gloves. Secure the dressing with tape or ties.
- Perform hand hygiene.

9. Document the procedure and all nursing assessments.

SAMPLE DOCUMENTATION

3/21/2015 1100 Abdominal dressing changed. Small amount of serosanguineous drainage—size of a half dollar—in middle of dressing. Incision approximated with slight redness at edges. Sutures intact. Tolerated well.————————————— S. Jones, RN

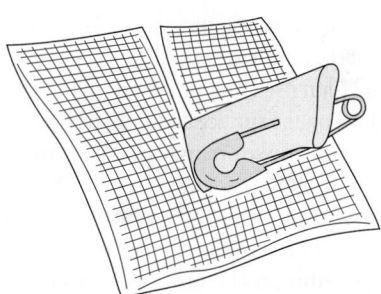

❸ Precut gauze in place around a Penrose drain.

EVALUATION

- Conduct appropriate follow-up, such as amount of granulation tissue or degree of healing; amount of drainage and its color, consistency, and odor; presence of inflammation; and degree of discomfort associated with the incision or drain site.
- Compare to previous findings, if available.
- Report significant deviations from normal to the primary care provider.

Ambulatory and Community Settings   **Cleaning a Sutured Wound** | PATIENT-CENTERED CARE |

Instruct caregivers to:

- Provide pain medication approximately 30 minutes before the procedure if the wound care causes pain or discomfort.
- Wash hands thoroughly and dry prior to handling wound care supplies and providing wound care.
- Clean and wipe dry a flat surface for the sterile field.
- Keep pets out of the area when setting up for and performing sterile procedures.
- Acquire all needed supplies before starting a sterile procedure.
- Maintain sterile or clean technique as instructed.

- Handle all sterile supplies from the outside of the wrapper or the edges.
- Not touch the parts of supplies or equipment that will touch the client.
- Avoid skin injury by using paper tape or Montgomery straps instead of adhesive tape.
- Report any increasing wound drainage, pain, redness, swelling, or opening or gaping of wound edges.
- Place any soiled dressing materials in a waterproof bag and dispose of it according to public health recommendations.

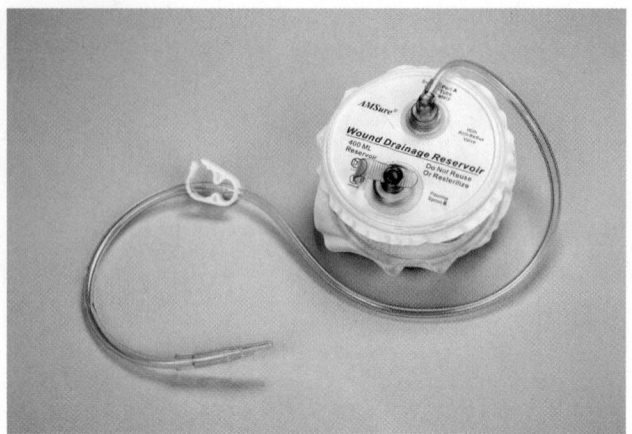

Figure 33–5 ■ Hemovac closed wound drainage system.

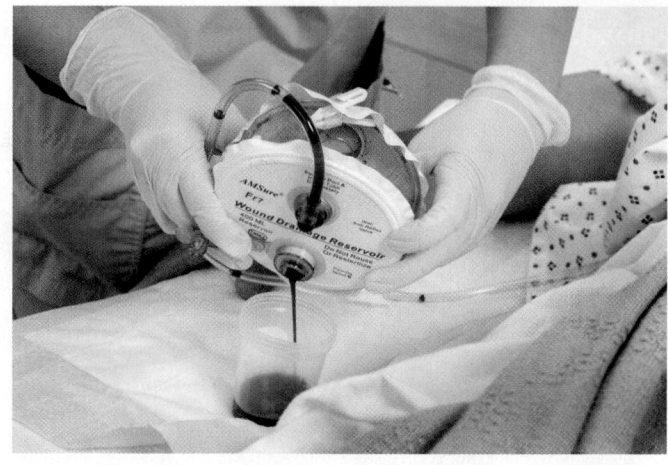

Figure 33–7 ■ Emptying drainage from a Hemovac drainage system.

Wound Drains and Suction

Surgical **drains** are inserted to permit the drainage of excessive serosanguineous fluid and purulent material and to promote healing of underlying tissues. These drains may be inserted and sutured through the incision line, but they are most commonly inserted through drain incisions a few centimeters away from the incision line so that the incision itself may be kept dry. Without a drain, some wounds would heal on the surface and trap the discharge inside, and an abscess might form. These drains (e.g., the Penrose drain) have an open end that drains onto a dressing.

A **closed wound drainage system** consists of a drain connected to either an electric suction or a portable drainage suction, such as a **Hemovac** (Figure 33–5 ■) or **Jackson–Pratt** (Figure 33–6 ■). The closed system reduces the potential entry of microorganisms into the wound through the drain. The drainage tubes are sutured in place and connected to a reservoir. For example, the Jackson–Pratt drainage tube is connected to a reservoir that maintains constant low suction. These portable wound suction devices also provide for accurate measurement of the drainage.

The surgeon inserts the wound drainage tube during surgery. Generally, the suction is discontinued from 3 to 5 days postoperatively or when the drainage is minimal. Nurses are responsible for maintaining the wound suction, which hastens the healing process by draining excess exudates that might otherwise interfere with the formation of granulation tissue.

Closed wound drainage systems have directions for use printed on the drainage container. When emptying the container, the nurse should wear gloves and avoid touching the drainage port (Figure 33–7 ■). To reestablish suction, the nurse places the container on a solid, flat surface with the port open. The palm of one hand presses the top and bottom together while the other hand cleanses the opening and plug with an alcohol swab (Figure 33–8 ■). Replace the drainage plug before releasing hand pressure to reestablish the vacuum necessary for the closed drainage system to work. Skill 33–6 describes how to maintain a closed wound drainage system.

Another type of closed wound drainage system is used postoperatively to collect, filter, and allow for reinfusion of autologous blood. Autologous blood transfusion is the collection of a client's own blood or blood components. Allogenic or homologous

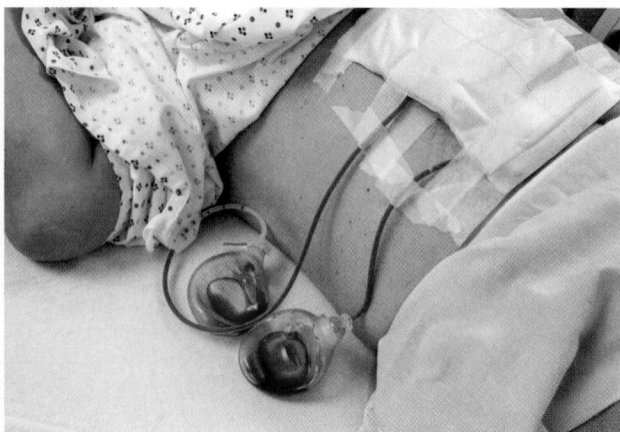

Figure 33–6 ■ Two Jackson–Pratt devices compressed to facilitate collection of exudates.

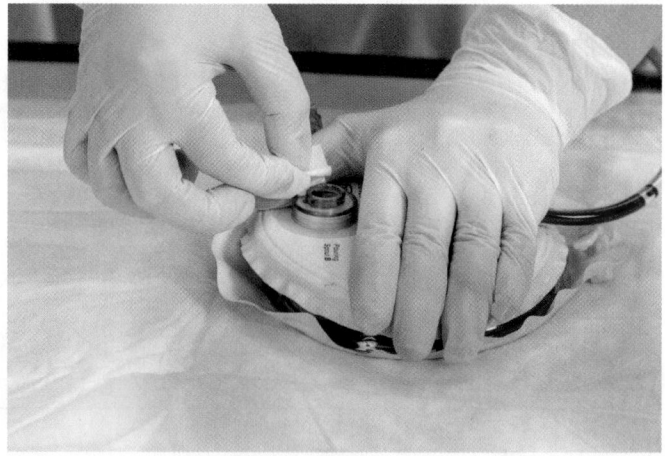

Figure 33–8 ■ With one hand, press the top and bottom together. With the other hand, clean the opening and plug with an alcohol swab. Replace the plug before releasing the hand.

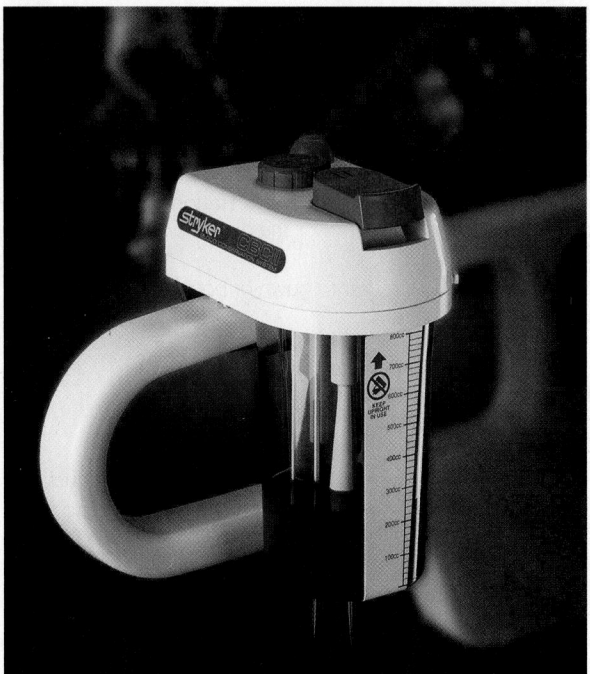

Figure 33–9 ■ A Stryker® closed wound drainage system often used for postoperative reinfusion in clients with knee or hip arthroplasty.
Courtesy of Stryker Instruments/Peterson.

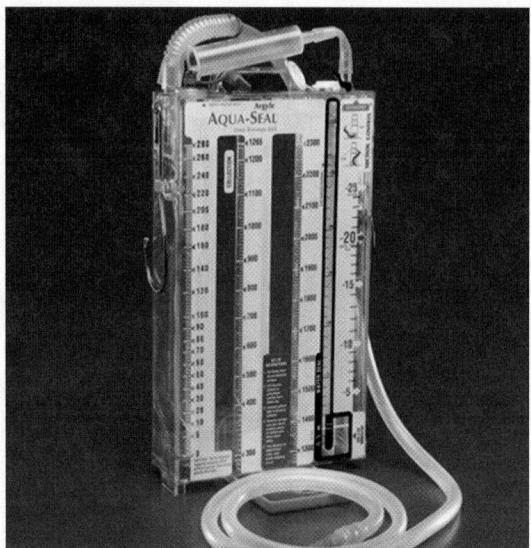

Figure 33–10 ■ An Aqua-Seal™ autotransfusion-ready chest drainage unit.
Dover, Kendall, Monoject, Shiley, Aqa-Seal, Kangaroo and Argyle are trademarks of a Covidien company. Image provided courtesy of Covidien. © 2014 Covidien.

transfusion is transfusion of blood collected from someone other than the client. This blood recovery system or autotransfusion may be used after knee or hip arthroplasty (Figure 33–9 ■) or as a chest drainage unit after cardiothoracic surgery or traumatic chest injury (Figure 33–10 ■).

Guidelines for the transfusion of the autologous (sometimes called shed or salvaged) blood are per institutional protocol. The blood should be administered no more than 6 hours from initial collection. Protocol may include number of hours or amount of drained blood (e.g., reinfuse at 4 hours or 400 mL). Studies have shown that reinfusion drains reduce the need for allogenic blood transfusion after hip and knee arthroplasty.

●○● NURSING PROCESS: WOUND DRAINS AND SUCTION

Maintaining Closed Wound Drainage

ASSESSMENT
Assess:
- Amount, color, consistency, clarity, and odor of the drainage.
- Discomfort around the area of the drain.
- Clinical signs of infection (e.g., elevated body temperature).
- Tube patency (e.g., movement of drainage through tube to collection device; connection sites intact).

PLANNING

DELEGATION

Assessment of the wound, wound drainage, and patency of the wound suction requires application of knowledge and problem solving and is the responsibility of the nurse and is not delegated to UAP. The UAP, however, can empty the drainage unit, measure the drainage, and record the amount on the intake and output record. The nurse must ensure that the UAP knows how to empty the unit without contaminating it.

Equipment
- Clean gloves
- Calibrated drainage receptacle
- Moisture-resistant pad
- Alcohol sponge
- Closed wound drainage system (e.g., Hemovac or Jackson–Pratt)

IMPLEMENTATION
Preparation
Determine the type and placement of the client's closed wound drainage.

Performance
1. Prior to performing the procedure, introduce self and verify the client's identity using agency protocol. Explain to the client what

SKILL 33-6

Continued on page 736

Maintaining Closed Wound Drainage—*continued*

you are going to do, why it is necessary, and how he or she can participate. Discuss how the results will be used in planning further care or treatments.

2. Perform hand hygiene and observe other appropriate infection prevention procedures.
3. Provide for client privacy.
4. Empty the drainage unit.
   • Apply clean gloves.
   • Place the Hemovac or Jackson–Pratt unit on the waterproof pad.
   • Open the plug of the drainage unit.
   • Invert the unit and empty it into the collecting receptacle (see Figure 33–7).
5. Reestablish suction.

Hemovac
• Place the unit on a solid, flat surface with the port open.
• Place the palm of a hand on the unit and press the top and the bottom together.
• While holding the top and bottom together, cleanse the opening and plug with an alcohol swab (see Figure 33–8).
• Replace the drainage plug before releasing hand pressure. **Rationale:** *This reestablishes the vacuum necessary for the closed drainage system to work.*

Jackson–Pratt
• Compress the bulb with the port open.
• While maintaining tight compression on the bulb, cleanse the ends of the emptying port.
• Insert the plug into the emptying port. **Rationale:** *This reestablishes the vacuum necessary for the closed drainage system to work.*

6. Secure the unit to the client's gown or position the suction unit on the bed.
   • Ensure that the unit is below the level of the wound. **Rationale:** *This facilitates drainage.*
7. Remove and discard gloves.
   • Perform hand hygiene.
8. Document all relevant information.
   • Record the emptying of the drainage unit and the nursing assessments.
   • Record the amount and type of drainage on the intake and output record.

EVALUATION
• Conduct appropriate follow-up, such as amount of drainage and its color, clarity, consistency, and odor; increased or decreased discomfort; and clinical signs of infection.

• Compare to previous findings if available.
• Report significant deviations from normal to the primary care provider.

Ambulatory and Community Settings   **Closed Wound Drainage System**   PATIENT-CENTERED CARE

• Schedule regular nursing visits to teach wound care and to observe the drainage site.
• Teach the client or a caregiver to empty, measure, and record the drainage at least once daily.
• Instruct the caregiver to observe the wound daily for signs of infection, such as redness, edema, tenderness, or purulent drainage. The client's temperature should be measured twice daily. **Rationale:** *Elevated temperature can indicate infection.*

• Ensure that the client has the proper supplies and knows how to obtain new items as needed.
• Notify the primary care provider of excess drainage, signs of infection, or occlusion of the tube.
• Determine when the surgeon plans to remove the drain, and help the client keep the appointment.

Sutures

A **suture** is a thread used to sew body tissues together. Sutures used to attach tissues beneath the skin are often made of an absorbable material that disappears in several days. Skin sutures, by contrast, are made of a variety of nonabsorbable materials, such as silk, cotton, linen, wire, nylon, and Dacron (polyester fiber). Wire clips or **staples** are also available. Usually, sutures and staples are removed 7 to 10 days after surgery.

There are various methods of suturing. Skin sutures can be broadly categorized as either **interrupted sutures** (each stitch is tied and knotted separately) or **continuous sutures** (one thread runs in a series of stitches and is tied only at the beginning and at the end of the run). Common methods of suturing are illustrated in Figure 33–11 ■.

Retention sutures are very large sutures used in addition to skin sutures for some incisions (Figure 33–12 ■). They attach underlying tissues of fat and muscle as well as skin and are used to support

incisions in individuals who are obese or when healing may be prolonged. They are frequently left in place longer than skin sutures (14 to 21 days) but in some instances are removed at the same time as the skin sutures. To prevent these large sutures from irritating the incision, the surgeon may place rubber tubing over them or a roll of gauze under them extending down the incision line.

The primary care provider orders the removal of sutures. Agency policies about removal of retention sutures vary. In some agencies, only primary care providers remove sutures; in others, RNs and nursing students with appropriate supervision may do so. The nurse should verify whether they are to be removed and who may remove them.

Sterile technique and special suture scissors are used to remove sutures. The scissors have a curved cutting tip that readily slides under the suture (Figure 33–13 ■). Wire clips or staples are removed with a special instrument that squeezes the center of the clip to remove it from the skin (Figures 33–14 ■ and 33–15 ■).

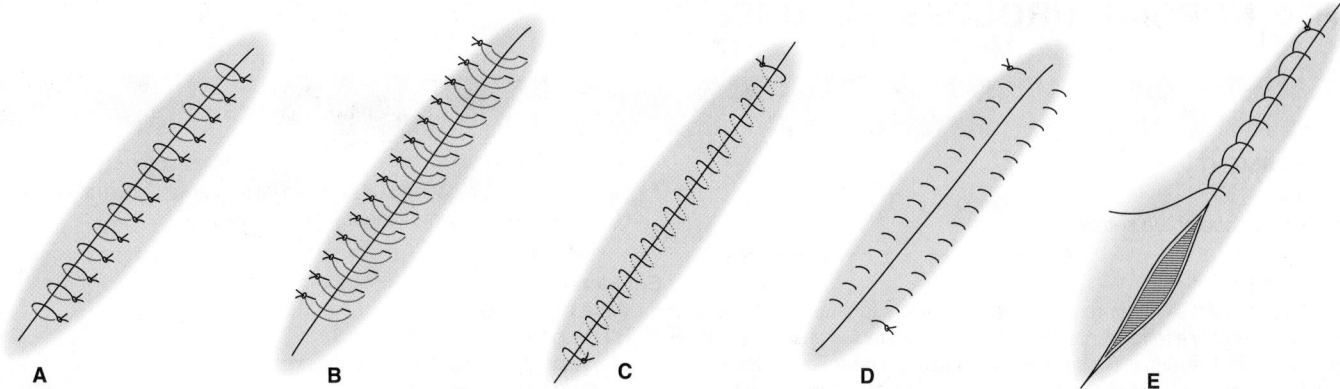

Figure 33–11 ■ Common sutures: *A,* plain interrupted; *B,* mattress interrupted; *C,* plain continuous; *D,* mattress continuous; *E,* blanket continuous.

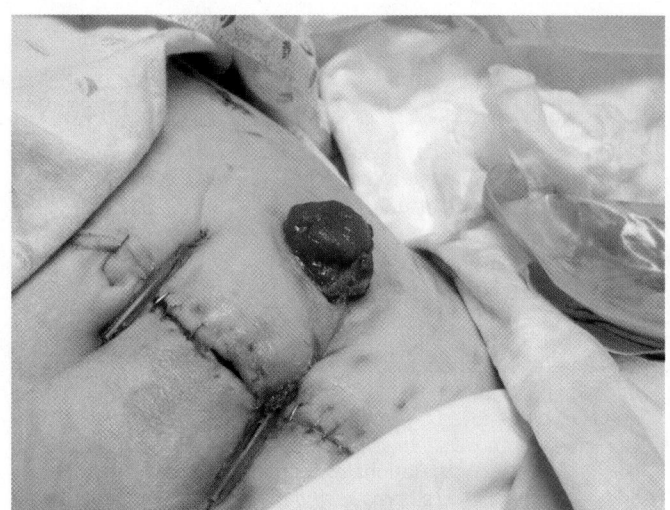

Figure 33–12 ■ A surgical incision with retention sutures.
B. Slavin/Custom Medical Stock Photo.

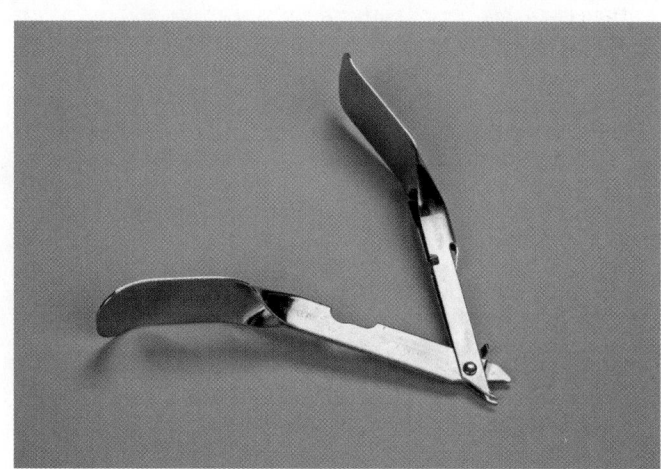

Figure 33–14 ■ Staple remover.

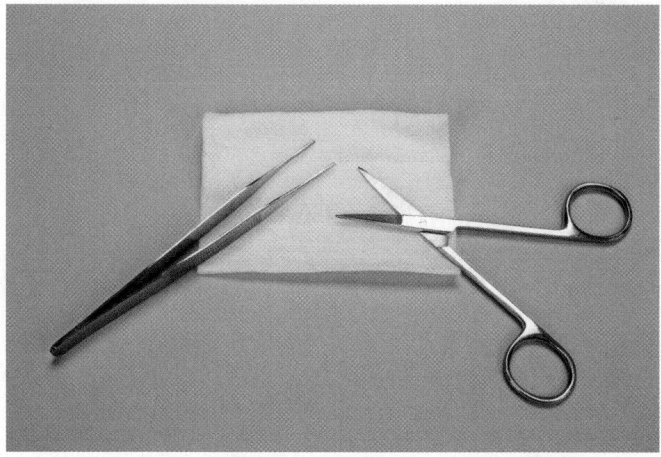

Figure 33–13 ■ Contents of a suture removal tray.

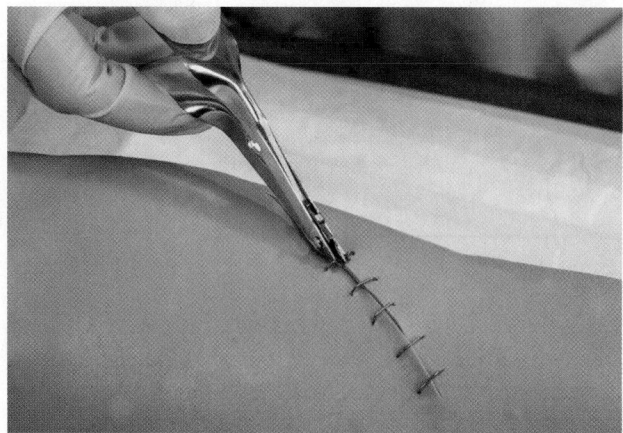

Figure 33–15 ■ Removing surgical clips or staples.

●○○● NURSING PROCESS: SUTURES

Removing Sutures

ASSESSMENT
Assess:
- Appearance of the suture line.
- Factors contraindicating suture removal (e.g., nonuniformity of closure, inflammation, presence of drainage).

PLANNING
Before removing skin sutures, verify (a) the orders for suture removal (many times only *alternate* interrupted sutures or staples are removed one day and the remaining sutures or staples are removed a day or two later); (b) whether a dressing is to be applied following the suture removal; and (c) when the client may bathe or shower. Some primary care providers prefer no dressing; others prefer a small, light gauze dressing to prevent friction by clothing.

Equipment
- Waterproof bag
- Sterile gloves
- Sterile dressing equipment including:
  - Sterile suture scissors
  - Sterile hemostat or forceps
  - Sterile butterfly tape or Steri-Strips (thin adhesive strips) (optional)
  - Tape (if a dressing is to be applied)

DELEGATION

Removal of sutures or staples requires application of knowledge and problem solving and is not delegated to UAP.

IMPLEMENTATION
Performance
1. Prior to performing the procedure, introduce self and verify the client's identity using agency protocol. Explain to the client what you are going to do, why it is necessary, and how he or she can participate. Inform the client that suture removal may produce slight discomfort, such as a pulling or stinging sensation, but should not be painful.
2. Perform hand hygiene and observe other appropriate infection prevention procedures.
3. Provide for client privacy.
4. Remove dressings and clean the incision.
   - Clean the suture line with an antimicrobial solution before and after suture removal. **Rationale:** *This is generally done as a prophylactic measure to prevent infection.*
   - Apply sterile gloves.
5. Remove the sutures.

Plain Interrupted Sutures
- Grasp the suture at the knot with a pair of forceps.
- Place the curved tip of the suture scissors under the suture as close to the skin as possible, either on the side opposite the knot ❶ or directly under the knot. Cut the suture. **Rationale:** *Sutures are cut as close to the skin as possible on one side of*

the visible part because the visible suture material is contaminated with skin bacteria and must not be pulled beneath the skin during removal. Suture material that is beneath the skin is considered free from bacteria.
- With the forceps or hemostat, pull the suture out in one piece. Inspect carefully to make sure that all suture material is removed. **Rationale:** *Suture material left beneath the skin acts as a foreign body and causes inflammation.*
- Discard the suture onto a piece of sterile gauze or into the moisture-resistant bag, being careful not to contaminate the forceps tips. Sometimes, the suture sticks to the forceps and needs to be removed by wiping the tips on a sterile gauze.
- Continue to remove *alternate* sutures, such as the third, fifth, seventh, and so forth. **Rationale:** *Alternate sutures are removed first so that remaining sutures keep the skin edges in close approximation and prevent any dehiscence from becoming large.*
- If no dehiscence occurs, remove the remaining sutures. If wound dehiscence (separation of an incision) does occur, do not remove the remaining sutures, and report the dehiscence to the nurse in charge.
- If Steri-Strips are ordered by the surgeon or a little wound dehiscence occurs, apply a sterile Steri-Strip over the wound or gap:
   a. Attach the Steri-Strip to one side of the incision.
   b. Press the wound edges together.
   c. Attach the Steri-Strip to the other side of the incision.
      Rationale: *The Steri-Strip (a thin strip of sterile, nonwoven, porous fabric tape) holds the wound edges as close together as possible and promotes healing. Some primary care providers order Steri-Strip application to provide additional support to the healing wound.*
- If a large dehiscence occurs, cover the wound with sterile gauze and report the problem immediately to the nurse in charge or primary care provider.

Mattress Interrupted Sutures
- When possible, cut the visible part of the suture close to the skin, at A and B in ❷, opposite the knot and remove this small visible piece. Discard it as described above. In some sutures, the visible part opposite the knot may be so small that it can be cut only once.
- Grasp the knot (C) with forceps. Remove the remainder of the suture beneath the skin by pulling out in the direction of the knot.

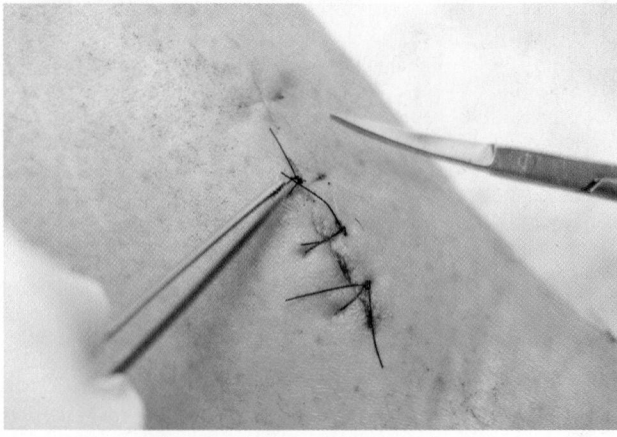

❶ Removing a skin suture.

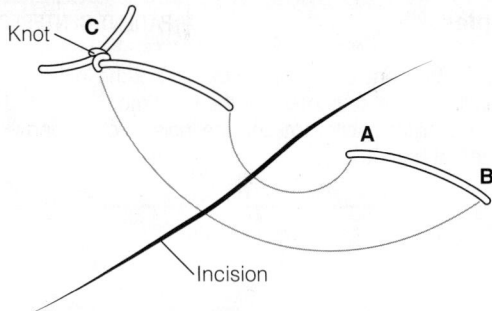

2 Mattress interrupted sutures.

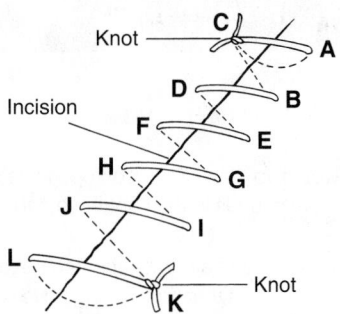

3 Plain continuous sutures.

Plain Continuous Sutures
- Cut the thread of the first suture opposite the knot at A in **3**. Then cut the thread of the second suture on the same side at B.
- Grasp the knot (C) with the forceps and pull. **Rationale:** *This removes the first stitch and the piece of thread beneath the skin, which is attached to the second stitch.*
- Discard the suture.
- Cut off the visible part of the second suture at D, and discard it.
- Grasp the suture at E and pull out the underlying loop between D and E.
- Cut the visible part at F and remove it.
- Repeat the above two steps at G through J, until the last knot is reached. Note that after the first stitch is removed, each thread is cut down the same side, below the original knot.
- Cut the last suture at L and pull out the last suture at K.

Blanket Continuous Sutures
- Cut the threads that are opposite the looped blanket edge; for example, cut at A through F in **4**.
- Pull each stitch out at the looped edge.

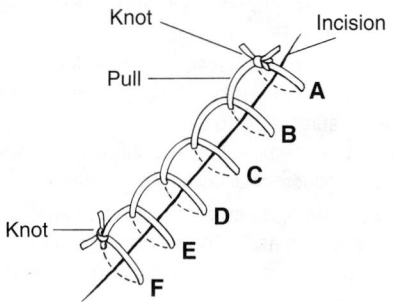

4 Blanket continuous sutures.

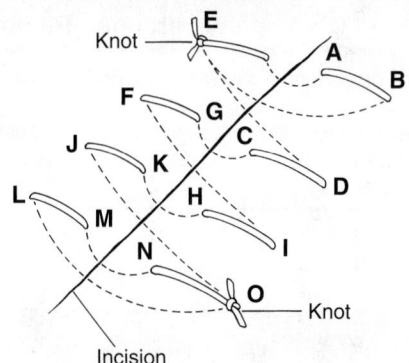

5 Mattress continuous sutures.

Mattress Continuous Sutures
- Cut the visible suture at both skin edges opposite the knot, at A and B in **5**, and the next suture opposite the knot (at C and D). Remove and discard the visible portions as described above.
- Pull the first suture out by the knot at E.
- Lift the second suture between F and G to pull out the underlying suture between G and C. Cut off the visible part at F as close to the skin edge as possible.
- Go to the opposite side between H and I. Lift out the suture between F and I and cut off all the visible part close to the skin at H.
- Lift the suture between J and K to pull out the suture between H and K and cut the suture close to the skin at J.
- Repeat the above two steps, working from side to side of the incision until the last suture is reached.
- Cut the visible suture opposite the knot at L and M. Pull out all remaining pieces of suture at O.
6. Clean and cover the incision.
   - Clean the incision again with antimicrobial solution.
   - Apply a small, light, sterile gauze dressing if any small dehiscence has occurred or if this is agency practice.
7. Remove and discard gloves.
   - Perform hand hygiene.
8. Instruct the client about follow-up wound care.
   - Generally, if a wound is dry and healing well, the person can take showers in a day or two.
   - Instruct the client to contact the primary care provider if increased redness, drainage, or open areas are observed.
9. Document the suture removal; number of sutures removed; appearance of the incision; application of a dressing, Steri-Strips, or butterfly tapes (if appropriate); client teaching; and client tolerance of the procedure.

Variation: Removing Staples
- Repeat steps 1 through 4.
- Place the lower tips of the sterile staple remover under the staple.
- Squeeze the handles together until they are completely closed (see Figures 33–14 and 33–15). **Rationale:** *Pressing the handles together causes the staple to bend in the middle and pulls the edges of the staple out of the skin.* Do not lift the staple remover when squeezing the handles.
- When both ends of the staple are visible, gently move the staple away from the incision site.
- Hold the staple remover over a disposable container, and release the staple remover handles which releases the staple.
- Repeat steps 6 through 8.

EVALUATION
- Conduct appropriate follow-up, such as status of suture line, any wound separation, or discharge.
- Compare to previous findings, if available.
- Report significant deviations from normal to the primary care provider.

- Perform the procedure in a well-lighted, private area of the home.
- Instruct the client to observe the incision daily and call the health care provider if increased redness, drainage, or open areas are observed.

- Provide instructions and supplies for care of the incision, and tell the client when to shower for the first time.
- Assess the client's ability to keep the incision clean and protected at home.

Chapter 33 Review

FOCUSING ON CLINICAL THINKING

Consider This

1. The client does not understand English, and preoperative teaching needs to be done. What would you do?
2. Your client returned from surgery with a Salem sump tube in place and connected to suction. You note that gastric contents are coming out of the blue air vent of the tube. What would you do?

3. What action would you take if the postoperative client has diminished breath sounds in the right base and a respiratory rate of 24/min?
4. The UAP informs you that a client, who had major abdominal surgery 4 days ago, said that "something gave way" and the client felt a "popping" sensation in his incision. What would you do?

See Focusing on Clinical Thinking answers on student resource website.

TEST YOUR KNOWLEDGE

1. During a dressing change of a postoperative client, the nurse observes separation of the incision. What term does the nurse use to record this observation?
   1. Infection
   2. Dehiscence
   3. Evisceration
   4. Approximation
2. The nurse is assisting the surgeon by using instruments, handling and cutting tissue, and suturing during which phase of the perioperative period?
   1. Preoperative
   2. Postoperative
   3. Intraoperative
   4. Perioperative
3. The nurse is providing preoperative teaching and includes which of the following? Select all that apply.
   1. Information
   2. Psychosocial support
   3. Skills training
   4. Physiological support
   5. Role of the client
4. The nurse is preparing to provide an in-service on hand hygiene for the nurses in the operating room. The nurse will explain that the use of a brush:
   1. Helps to reduce microbial counts.
   2. May increase shedding of skin.
   3. Is necessary when using alcohol-based products.
   4. Helps to reduce skin damage.

5. The nurse is encouraging a 1-day postoperative client to get out of bed. The client says, "It hurts when I move. Why can't I just lie here until it doesn't hurt so much?" What is the nurse's best response?
   1. "Getting up and moving as soon as possible reduces the risk of breathing problems, urinary tract infections, and blood clots."
   2. "Getting up and moving as soon as possible reduces the risk of respiratory and circulatory complications as well as the risk of UTI."
   3. "Early ambulation prevents complications of the respiratory, renal, and circulatory systems."
   4. "Moving prevents complications such as hemorrhage and wound infection."
6. The nurse is preparing to conduct preoperative teaching with the client and family. Prior to beginning the teaching session it is important for the nurse to assess all of the following except:
   1. The client's understanding of the surgery to be performed.
   2. The client's surgical history.
   3. The family's agreement that the surgery is needed.
   4. The client's educational level.
7. The nurse is preparing to enter the operating room during a surgical procedure to assist the surgeon. In dressing to enter the room, the nurse puts on the following apparel in which order?
   1. Sterile gown
   2. Sterile gloves
   3. Mask
   4. Shoe covers

8. The client enters the postanesthesia care unit (PACU) with a single-lumen gastric tube in place. The nurse expects the surgeon to write an order for gastric suction at what type of suction?
1. Continuous suction
2. Intermittent suction
3. Continuous suction for a while and then change to intermittent suction
4. Intermittent suction for a while and then change to continuous suction

9. The nurse is caring for a client with a Jackson–Pratt drainage unit in place. The nurse is preparing to empty the drainage. Put the following steps in the correct order in which the nurse should perform them.
1. Invert the unit.
2. Compress the bulb to reestablish suction.
3. Open the plug.
4. Place the drain on a waterproof pad.
5. Clean the end of the port with alcohol.

10. After receiving an order to remove the client's sutures, the nurse assesses the wound. Which of the following would contraindicate the order?
1. Drainage from the wound
2. Moisture at the wound site
3. A light red line marking the incision
4. Half of the sutures are gone

See Answers to Test Your Knowledge in Appendix A.

READINGS AND REFERENCES

References

Adams, M. P., & Urban, C. Q. (2013). *Pharmacology: Connections to nursing practice* (2nd ed.). Upper Saddle River, NJ: Pearson Education.

Aldrete, J. A., & Kroulik, D. (1970). A postanesthetic recovery score. *Anesthesia and Analgesia, 49*(6), 924–934.

American Society of Anesthesiologists. (2011). Practice guidelines for preoperative fasting and the use of pharmacologic agents to reduce the risk of pulmonary aspiration: Application to healthy patients undergoing elective procedures: An updated report by the American Society of Anesthesiologists Committee on Standards and Practice Parameters. *Anesthesiology 114*, 495–511. doi:10.1097/ALN.0b013e3181fcbfd9

American Society of PeriAnesthesia Nurses. (2012). *What discharge scoring system does ASPAN recommend?* Retrieved from http://www.aspan.org/ClinicalPractice/FAQs/tabid/14107/Default.aspx#30

Association of Operating Room Nurses. (2011). *Position statement: Allied health care providers and support personnel in the perioperative practice setting.* Retrieved from http://www.aorn.org/Clinical_Practice/Position_Statements/Position_Statements.aspx

Association of Operating Room Nurses. (2012a). *AORN position statement on RN first assistants.* Retrieved from http://www.aorn.org/Clinical_Practice/Position_Statements/Position_Statements.aspx

Association of Operating Room Nurses. (2012b). *Position statement: One perioperative registered nurse circulator dedicated to every patient undergoing a surgical or other invasive procedure.* Retrieved from http://www.aorn.org/Clinical_Practice/Position_Statements/Position_Statements.aspx

Bernard, H. (2013). Patient warming in surgery and the enhanced recovery. *British Journal of Nursing, 22*, 319–325.

Boeykens, K., Steeman, E., & Duysburgh, I. (2014). Reliability of pH measurement and the auscultatory method to confirm the position of a nasogastric tube. *International Journal of Nursing Studies, 51*(11), 1427–1433. doi:10.1016/j.ijnurstu.2014.03.004

Clapham, E., & Crooke, J. (2011). The patient with a pierced tongue. *Journal of Perioperative Practice, 21*, 156–157.

Diccini, S., Malheiro Da Costa Nogueira, A., & Sousa, V. D. (2009). Body piercing among Brazilian surgical patients. *AORN Journal, 89*, 161–165. doi:10.1016/j.aorn.2008.07.003

Elliott, W. T. (2013). Do perioperative beta-blockers reduce mortality? *Critical Care Alert*, pp. 1–2.

The Joint Commission. (2013). *National Patient Safety Goals effective January 1, 2014. Hospital accreditation program.* Retrieved from http://www.jointcommission.org/assets/1/6/HAP_NPSG_Chapter_2014.pdf

Lakdawala, L. (2011). Creating a safer perioperative environment with an obstructive sleep apnea screening tool. *Journal of PeriAnesthesia Nursing, 26*(1), 15–24. doi:10.1016/j.jopan.2010.10.004

Larkin, B., Mitchell, K., & Petrie, K. (2012). Translating evidence to practice for mechanical venous thromboembolism prophylaxis. *AORN Journal, 96*(5), 513–527. doi:10.1016/j.aorn.2012.07.011

Lemyze, M. (2010). The placement of nasogastric tubes. *Canadian Medical Association Journal, 182*, 802. doi:10.1503/cmaj.091099

Longnecker, D., Brown, D. L., Newman, M. F., & Zapol, W. (2012). *Anesthesiology* (2nd ed.). New York, NY: McGraw-Hill.

Lynch, S., Dixon, J., Leary, D., & Holm, R. (2010). Reducing the risk of unplanned perioperative hypothermia. *AORN Journal, 92*(5), 553–565. doi:10.1016/j.aorn.2010.06.015

Phillips, N. M., Haesler, E., Street, M., & Kent, B. (2011). Post-anaesthetic discharge scoring criteria: A systematic review. *JBI Library of Systematic Reviews 9*(41), 1679–1713. doi:10.11124/jbisrir-2011-110

Tho, P., Mordiffi, S., Ang, E., & Chen, H. (2011). Implementation of the evidence review on best practice for confirming the correct placement of nasogastric tube in patients in an acute care hospital. *International Journal of Evidence-Based Healthcare, 9*(1), 51–60. doi:10.1111/j.1744-1609.2010.00200.x

Wanzer, L., & Hicks, R. (2012). Identifying and minimizing risks for surgical patients with dermal implants. *AORN Journal, 96*(4), C5–C6. doi:10.1016/S0001-2092(12)00948-9

Weight, C. J., Lee, M. C., & Palmer, J. S. (2010). Avagard hand antisepsis vs. traditional scrub in 3600 pediatric urologic procedures. *Urology, 76*, 15–17.

White, P. F., & Song, D. (1999). New criteria for fast-tracking after outpatient anesthesia: A comparison with the modified Aldrete's scoring system. *Anesthesia and Analgesia, 88*, 1069–1072.

Wu, X. (2013). The safe and efficient use of forced-air warming systems. *AORN Journal, 97*, 302–308. doi:10.1016/j.aorn.2012.12.008

Zinn, J., Jenkins, J. B., Harrelson, B., Wrenn, C., Haynes, E., & Small, N. (2013). Differences in intraoperative prep solutions: A retrospective chart review. *AORN Journal, 97*, 552–558. doi:10.1016/j.aorn.2013.03.006

Selected Bibliography

Alexander-Magalee, M. A. (2010). Pre-op prep for the pros. *Nursing Made Incredibly Easy!, 8*(3), 14–17.

Allen, G. (2010). Evidence for Practice. *AORN Journal, 91*, 300–306. doi:10.1016/j.aorn.2009.11.060

Berman, A., Snyder, S., & Frandsen, G. (2016). *Kozier & Erb's fundamentals of nursing: Concepts, process, and practice* (10th ed.). Upper Saddle River, NJ: Pearson.

Cosh, J. (2012). Breaking the fast. *Nursing Standard, 26*(24), 22–23.

Graling, P. R., & Vasaly, F. W. (2013). Effectiveness of 2% CHG cloth bathing for reducing surgical site infections. *AORN Journal, 97*, 547–551. doi:10.1016/j.aorn.2013.02.009

Hewkin, K. (2011). The importance of disinfection prior to surgery. *British Journal of Nursing, 20*, 964.

Lobley, S. N. (2013). Factors affecting the risk of surgical site infection and methods of reducing it. *Journal of Perioperative Practice, 23*(4), 77–81.

Memtsoudis, S. G., Besculides, M. C., & Mazumdar, M. (2013). A rude awakening: The perioperative sleep apnea epidemic. *New England Journal of Medicine, 368*, 2352–2353. doi:10.1056/NEJMp1302941

Reimer-Kent, J. (2010). NPO after midnight is not best practice. *Canadian Journal of Cardiovascular Nursing, 20*(1), 22–23.

Taylor, S., Allan, K., McWilliam, H., Manara, A., Brown, J., Toher, D., & Rayner, W. (2014). Confirming nasogastric tube position with electromagnetic tracking versus pH or X-ray and tube radio-opacity. *British Journal of Nursing, 23*(7), 352–358.

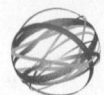

34 End-of-Life Care

LEARNING OUTCOMES

At the completion of this chapter, the student will be able to:

1. Define the key terms used in the skills of caring for clients at the end of life.
2. Describe the role of the nurse in working with families or caregivers of clients who are dying.
3. List clinical signs of impending and actual death.
4. Recognize when it is appropriate to delegate end-of-life care to unlicensed assistive personnel.

5. Verbalize the steps used in:
   a. Meeting the physiological needs of the client who is dying.
   b. Performing postmortem care.
6. Demonstrate appropriate documentation and reporting of end-of-life care.

SKILLS

Skill 34–1 Meeting the Physiological Needs of the Dying Client
Skill 34–2 Performing Postmortem Care

KEY TERMS

Nurses may interact with dying clients and their families or caregivers in a variety of settings, from a fetal demise (death of an unborn child), to the adolescent victim of an accident, to the older client who finally succumbs to a chronic illness. Death can be viewed as a person's final opportunity to experience life in ways that bring significance and fulfillment. It is the nurse's role to provide or facilitate physical, emotional, and spiritual care of the dying client and the client's family.

Caring for the dying and the **bereaved** (those individuals mourning the dead) is one of the nurse's most complex and challenging responsibilities, bringing into play all skills needed for holistic physiological and psychosocial care (Figure 34–1 ■). This chapter emphasizes physical care. It is beyond the scope of the chapter to address, in detail, theoretical concepts such as grief and grieving or legal aspects such as the process of organ donation and living wills. The reader is referred to a fundamentals or concepts book for additional material.

DEFINITIONS OF DEATH

The traditional clinical signs of death were cessation of the apical pulse, respirations, and blood pressure, also referred to as **heart-lung death**. However, since the advent of artificial means to maintain respirations and blood circulation, identifying death is more difficult. In 1968, the World Medical Assembly adopted the following guidelines for physicians as indications of death:

- Total lack of response to external stimuli
- No muscular movement, especially breathing
- No reflexes

- Flat encephalogram (brain waves).

The Uniform Determination of Death Act, passed in 1981 for all U.S. states, specifies that death has occurred when there is irreversible termination of cardiac and respiratory function or irreversible cessation of all brain (including brainstem) functioning. In instances in which artificial life support is used, absence of brain waves for at least 24 hours is an indication of death. Only then can a physician pronounce death, and only after this pronouncement can life-support systems be shut off.

Another definition of death is **cerebral death** or **higher brain death**, which occurs when the cerebral cortex is irreversibly destroyed. In this case, there is "a clinical syndrome characterized by the permanent loss of cerebral and brainstem function, manifested by absence of responsiveness to external stimuli, absence of cephalic reflexes, and apnea. An isoelectric electroencephalogram for at least 30 minutes in the absence of hypothermia and poisoning by central nervous system depressants supports the diagnosis" (*Stedman's Medical Dictionary for the Health Professions and Nursing*, 2012). People who support this definition of death believe the cerebral cortex, which holds the capacity for thought, voluntary action, and movement, is the individual.

These definitions of death are differentiated from a **persistent vegetative state (PVS)** in which the person has lost cognitive function and awareness but respiration and circulation remain. Individuals in a PVS may have a variety of facial, eye, and limb movements but do not interact purposefully with their environment.

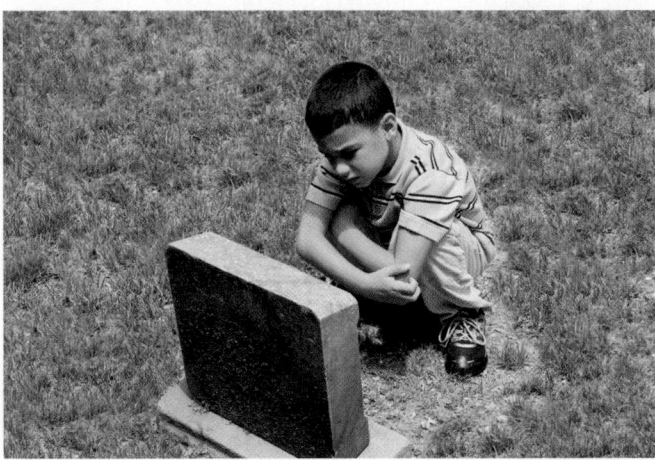

Figure 34–1 ■ Children experience the same emotions of grief as adults.
Juan Silva/Getty Images.

DEATH-RELATED RELIGIOUS AND CULTURAL PRACTICES

Cultural and religious traditions and practices associated with death, dying, and the grieving process help people cope with these experiences. Nurses are often present throughout the dying process and at the moment of death. Knowledge of the client's religious and cultural heritage helps nurses provide individualized care to clients and their families, even though they may not participate in the rituals associated with death.

Members of certain ethnic groups may request that health professionals not reveal the prognosis to dying clients. They believe the person's last days should be free of worry. Other cultures prefer that a family member (preferably a male in some cultures) be told the diagnosis so that the client can be tactfully informed by a family member in gradual stages or not be told at all. Nurses also need to determine whom to call, and when, as the impending death draws near.

Beliefs about autopsy, organ donation, cremation, prolonging life, and preparation of the body are closely allied to the person's religion. Autopsy, for example, may be prohibited, opposed, or discouraged by Islam, Jehovah's Witnesses, Orthodox Judaism, and Rastafarianism. These same religions prohibit the removal of body parts, or dictate that all body parts be given appropriate burial. Some groups, such as Hindus, may oppose autopsy based on not wanting non-Hindus to touch the body (Carpenter et al., 2011). Organ donation is prohibited by Jehovah's Witnesses and Muslims, whereas Buddhists in America consider it an act of mercy and encourage it. In general, the most significant factor in the decision to donate a family member's organs is how religious the consenter is (Ashkenazi & Klein, 2012). Cremation is discouraged, opposed, or prohibited by the Baha'i, Mormon, Eastern Orthodox, Islamic, and Roman Catholic faiths. Buddhists, Hindus, Shintos, and Sikhs, in contrast, prefer cremation. Prolongation of life is generally encouraged; however, some religions, such as Christian Science, are unlikely to recommend medical means to prolong life, and the Jewish faith generally opposes prolonging life after irreversible brain damage. In hopeless illness, Buddhists may permit euthanasia.

Nurses need to be knowledgeable about the client's death-related rituals, such as last rites, chanting at the bedside, and other

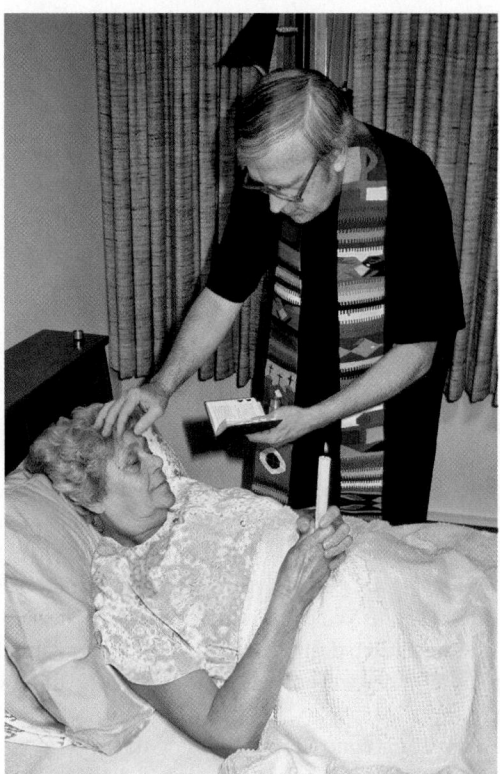

Figure 34–2 ■ Catholic clients may request last rites or the sacrament of the sick.
Dennis MacDonald/PhotoEdit.

practices, such as special procedures for washing, dressing, positioning, shrouding, and attending the dead (Figure 34–2 ■). For example, certain cultures retain their native customs in which family members of the same sex wash and prepare the body for burial and cremation. Muslims also customarily turn the body of the dying and the dead so that the face is toward Mecca. In several religions, the body cannot be left unattended until burial and individuals may be hired to sit with the body if family members do not perform this duty. Nurses need to ask family members about their preferences and verify who will carry out these activities. Burial clothes and other cultural or religious items are often important symbols for the funeral. For example, Mormons are often dressed in their "temple clothes." Some Native Americans may be dressed in elaborate apparel and jewelry and wrapped in new blankets with money. The nurse must ensure that any ritual items present in the health care agency be returned to the family or to the funeral home.

HELPING CLIENTS DIE WITH DIGNITY

Nurses need to ensure that the client is treated with dignity, that is, with honor and respect. Clients who are dying often feel they have lost control over their lives and over life itself. Helping clients die with dignity involves maintaining their humanity, consistent with their values, beliefs, and culture. By introducing options available to the client and significant others, nurses can restore and support feelings of control. Some choices that clients can make are the location of care (e.g., hospital, home, or hospice facility), times of appointments with health professionals, activity schedule, use of health resources, and times of visits from relatives and friends.

Clients may want to manage the events preceding death so they can die peacefully. Nurses can help clients to determine their own physical, psychological, and social priorities. Dying people often strive for self-fulfillment more than for self-preservation, and may need to find meaning in continuing to live while suffering. Part of the nurse's challenge, then, is to support the client's will and hope.

Verbalization about the impending death is an opportunity for the nurse to play a central and gratifying role in the client's and family's lives. Although it may be uncomfortable discussing death, steps can be taken to make such discussions easier for both the nurse and the client. Strategies include the following:

- Identify your personal feelings about death and how they may influence interactions with clients. Acknowledge personal fears about death, and discuss them with a friend or colleague.
- Focus on the client's needs. The client's or family's fears and beliefs may be different from the nurse's. It is important for the nurse to avoid imposing personal fears and beliefs on the client or family.
- Talk to the client or the family about how the client usually copes with stress. Clients will use their usual coping strategies for dealing with impending death. For example, if they are usually quiet and reflective, they will become more quiet and withdrawn when facing terminal illness.
- Establish a communication relationship that shows concern for and commitment to the client. Communication strategies that let the client know you are available to talk about death include the following:
  a. Describe what you see, for example, "You seem sad. Would you like to talk about what's happening to you?"
  b. Clarify your concern, for example, "I'd like to better understand how you feel and how I may help you."
  c. Acknowledge the client's struggle, for example, "It must be difficult to feel so uncomfortable. I would like to help you be more comfortable."
  d. Provide a caring touch. Holding the client's hand or offering a comforting massage can encourage the client to verbalize feelings.
- Determine what the client knows about the illness and prognosis. Use language the client can understand, not medical jargon.
- Respond with honesty and directness to the client's questions about death. Balance realistic expectations with the need for hope.
- Make time to be available to the client to provide support, listen, and respond.

HOSPICE AND PALLIATIVE CARE

Hospice care focuses on support and care of the dying person and family, with the goal of facilitating a peaceful and dignified death. Hospice care is based on holistic concepts, emphasizes care to improve quality of life rather than cure, supports the client and family through the dying process, and supports the family through bereavement. Assessing the needs of the client's family is just as important as caring for the client who is receiving hospice care (Figure 34–3 ■). As the condition of the client deteriorates, attention should be focused on the caregivers to ensure that they are receiving support and resources as these changes occur. If the hospice team meets regularly, these changes can be discussed and interventions initiated. Thorough assessment and ongoing evaluation can help indicate when modifications in the plan of care are needed. Hospice care can be delivered

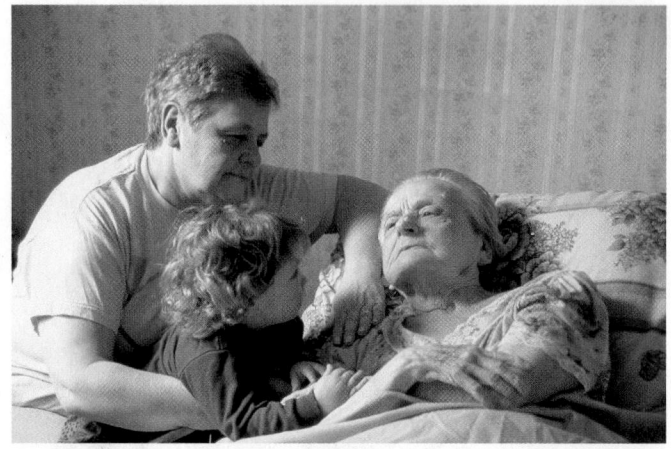

Figure 34–3 ■ Family members may be closely involved in both physical and psychological support of the dying.
Jeff Greenberg/PhotoEdit.

almost anywhere: in the home, a long-term care facility, a dedicated freestanding hospice center, or a section of an acute care hospital. Although 70% of Californians polled in 2011 stated that they would prefer to die at home, only 32% of the state's deaths occurred there. However, that is significantly higher than the 13% of Californians who died at home in 1989 (California Healthcare Foundation, 2012). The data differs for seniors nationally. Only 25% of Medicare clients died in the hospital and over 47% used hospice services (Goodman et al., 2013).

Palliative care, as described by the World Health Organization (WHO), "is an approach that improves the quality of life of clients and their families facing the problems associated with life-threatening illness, through the prevention and relief of suffering by means of early identification and impeccable assessment and treatment of pain and other problems, physical, psychosocial and spiritual. Palliative care:

- provides relief from pain and other distressing symptoms;
- affirms life and regards dying as a normal process;
- intends to neither hasten nor postpone death;
- integrates the psychological and spiritual aspects of client care;
- offers a support system to help clients live as actively as possible until death;
- offers a support system to help the family cope during the client's illness and in their own bereavement;
- uses a team approach to address the needs of clients and their families, including bereavement counseling, if indicated;
- will enhance quality of life, and may positively influence the course of illness;
- is applicable early in the course of illness, in conjunction with other therapies that are intended to prolong life, such as chemotherapy or radiation therapy, and includes those investigations needed to better understand and manage distressing clinical complications." (n.d.)

This care may differ from hospice in that the client is not necessarily believed to be imminently dying. Both hospice and palliative care can include **end-of-life care**, that is, the care provided in the final weeks before death. Client priorities at the end of life focus on ensuring that the family is not overburdened by financial or care decisions, being kept comfortable, and having others to support them (California Healthcare Foundation, 2012).

●○● NURSING PROCESS: CARING FOR CLIENTS AT THE END OF LIFE

The major nursing responsibility for clients who are dying is to assist the client to a peaceful death. Responsibilities that are more specific are to:

- Minimize loneliness, fear, and depression.
- Maintain the client's sense of security, self-confidence, dignity, and self-worth.

- Help the client accept losses.
- Provide physical comfort.

SKILL 34–1

Meeting the Physiological Needs of the Dying Client

ASSESSMENT

Determine if the client has a living will, durable power of attorney for health care, or other advance directive that describes preferences for end-of-life care and decision making. If there is a document, a copy must be kept with the medical record so that all staff are aware of the information. The nurse must be familiar with the specifics including who can legally make decisions for the client's care; what preferences have been expressed for pain relief, nutrition, and hydration; and details related to organ donation.

Nursing care and support for the dying client and family include making an accurate assessment of the physiological signs of approaching death. In addition to signs related to the client's specific disease, certain other physical signs are indicative of impending death. The four main characteristic changes are loss of muscle tone, slowing of the circulation, changes in respirations, and sensory impairment. Clinical Manifestations on page 747 lists indications of impending clinical death.

As death approaches, the nurse assists the family and other significant people to prepare. Depending in part on knowledge of the person's state of awareness, the nurse asks questions that help identify ways to provide support during the period before and after death. In particular, the nurse needs to know what the family expects to happen when the person dies so accurate information can be given at the appropriate depth. See Box 34–1 on page 747 for sample interview questions. When the family members know what to expect, they may be better able to support the dying person and others who are grieving. In addition, they may be able to make certain decisions about events surrounding the death such as whether they will want to view the body after death.

PLANNING

Major goals for clients who are dying are (a) maintaining physiological and psychological comfort and (b) achieving a dignified and peaceful death, which includes maintaining personal control and accepting declining health status. When planning care with these clients, the Dying Person's Bill of Rights (Box 34–2 on page 747) can be a useful guide.

DELEGATION

Comfort measures and supportive care strategies for care of clients at the end of life are often delegated to unlicensed assistive personnel (UAP). The nurse reviews with the UAP those measures and strategies needed for a specific client. The UAP must inform the nurse if the client appears in unanticipated or unrelieved distress.

INTERPROFESSIONAL PRACTICE

Caring for the dying is a nurse role. However, other health care providers may also provide aspects of the care. For example, the dietitian may consult regarding the client's diet, and physical and respiratory therapists may provide palliative treatments. Although these providers may verbally communicate their findings and plan to the health care team members, the nurse must also know where to locate their documentation in the client's medical record.

Equipment

- Needed equipment depends on the specific comfort measures being provided. Items may include medications, linens, and hygiene supplies.

IMPLEMENTATION

Preparation

The physiological needs of people who are dying are related to a slowing of body processes and to homeostatic imbalances. Interventions include providing personal hygiene measures; controlling pain; relieving respiratory difficulties; assisting with movement, nutrition, hydration, and elimination; and providing measures related to sensory changes.

Performance

1. Introduce self and verify the client's identity using agency protocol. Explain to the client what you are going to do, why it is necessary, and how he or she can participate. Discuss how the results will be used in planning further care or treatments.
2. Perform hand hygiene and observe other appropriate infection prevention procedures.
3. Provide for client privacy depending on the specific interventions.

4. Perform bathing/hygiene.
   - Provide frequent baths and linen changes if the client is diaphoretic or incontinent, or if there is a need for odor control. **Rationale:** The *dying may have wounds, fever, or loss of sphincter control that are both uncomfortable when substances are left on the skin and cause distressing smells.*
   - Give mouth care as needed for dry mouth, to remove secretions, and to provide comfort.
   - Apply moisturizing creams and lotions for dry skin, and moisture-barrier skin preparations for clients who are incontinent.
   - Cleanse skin areas around wounds or that collect wound drainage.
5. Provide pain control.
   - Pain control is essential to enable clients to maintain some quality in their life and their daily activities, including eating,

Continued on page 746

Meeting the Physiological Needs of the Dying Client—*continued*

moving, and sleeping. Many drugs have been used to control the pain associated with terminal illness such as morphine, heroin, methadone, and alcohol.

- Usually the primary care provider determines the dosage, but the client's opinion should be considered; the client is the one ultimately aware of personal pain tolerance. Because primary care providers usually prescribe a range for the dosage of pain medication, nurses use their own judgment as to the specific amount and frequency of pain medication needed to provide client relief.
- Because of decreased blood circulation, if analgesics cannot be administered orally, they are given topically, by intravenous infusion, sublingually, or rectally, rather than subcutaneously or intramuscularly. **Rationale:** *Subcutaneous or intramuscular injections given to clients with impaired circulation will not reach the desired receptors and, thus, will be ineffective.*
- Clients on narcotic pain medications also require implementation of a protocol to treat opioid-induced constipation. See Chapter 9 ∞ for more on pain management.
- Under periods of stress, the brain releases endorphins, morphine-like substances that modulate pain perception. Although studied primarily in animal models and in near-death experiences, some scientists believe that large amounts of endorphins may be released at the time of death. This could explain the seemingly peaceful sense of dissociation from the reality of pain, floating outside the body, seeing a tunnel, or moving toward the light that is expressed by some individuals.

6. Provide respiratory support.
   - For clients with difficulty clearing their own airway, place in Fowler's position if conscious, lateral position if unconscious. **Rationale:** *Fowler's position makes breathing easier. The lateral position allows secretions to drain out rather than entering the client's airway.*
   - Perform oral throat suctioning as needed, especially for conscious clients who express discomfort.
   - Apply nasal oxygen for clients who are hypoxic. **Rationale:** *Supplemental oxygen may relieve the signs and symptoms of oxygen deprivation such as confusion.*
   - Anticholinergic medications (e.g., atropine, hyoscine hydrobromide) may be indicated to help dry secretions. Note that noisy respirations, sometimes referred to as the *death rattle*, are believed to be more distressing to those who have to listen to the sounds than the condition is for the dying client (Lokker, van Zuylen, van der Rijt, & van der Heide, 2014).
   - For clients who have air hunger (the sensation of needing to breathe), open windows or use a fan to circulate air. Morphine may be indicated in an acute episode.

7. Assist with movement.
   - Assist the client out of bed periodically, if able.
   - Regularly change the client's position.
   - Support the client's position with pillows, blanket rolls, or towels as needed.
   - Elevate the client's legs when sitting up.
   - Implement a pressure ulcer prevention program and use pressure-relieving surfaces as indicated.

8. Provide nutrition and hydration as indicated.
   - Administer antiemetics to treat nausea.
   - Encourage favorite foods as tolerated.

- Support family members who may be very concerned that their loved one is not eating or drinking sufficiently or who believe that failure to push nutrition signifies giving up and failure.
- In some states, a feeding tube cannot be removed from a person in a PVS without a prior directive from the client. In other states, the removal is allowed at the family's request or with a physician's order.
- Teach family that clients with dehydration and alterations in electrolytes at the end of life may not experience discomfort. In addition, dehydration actually reduces secretions and the need for elimination.

9. Assist with elimination.
   - For constipation, provide dietary fiber as tolerated, stool softeners or laxatives as needed.
   - Perform meticulous skin care in response to incontinence of urine or feces.
   - Keep the bedpan, urinal, or commode chair nearby and the call light within reach for assistance with elimination.
   - Use absorbent pads under incontinent clients; change linen as often as needed.
   - Urinary catheterization may be performed, if necessary.
   - Keep the room as clean and odor-free as possible.

10. Be aware of sensory changes.
    - Check the client's preference for a light or dark room. Position the client to be able to view the television, favorite items or photos, or a window as desired.
    - Hearing is not diminished; speak clearly and do not whisper. Use music as desired.
    - Touch sensation is diminished, but the client will feel pressure.
    - Provide a gown, clothing, and bedding that feels and looks as the client prefers.
    - Facilitate client interaction with others as desired. This may require flexing agency rules regarding visiting hours or the presence of pets. Advocate for the client as much as possible about these.
    - Implement a pain management protocol if indicated; provide treatment or medication for other sensory alterations such as itching.

11. Family members should be encouraged to participate in the physical care of the dying person as much as they wish to and are able. The nurse can suggest they assist with bathing, speak or read to the client, and hold hands. The nurse must, however, have no specific expectations for family members' participation. Those who feel unable to care for or be with the dying person also require support from the nurse and from other family members. They should be shown an appropriate waiting area if they wish to remain nearby.

CLINICAL ALERT!

Sometimes, it seems as if the client is "holding on," possibly out of concern for the family not being ready. It may be therapeutic for both the client and the family for the family to verbally give permission to the client to "let go," to die when he or she is ready. This is a painful process, and the nurse must be prepared to encourage and support the family through saying their last good-byes.

Meeting the Physiological Needs of the Dying Client—*continued*

12. Consider how routine care should be modified based on the dying client. Often vital signs are measured less frequently, blood and other laboratory tests are no longer performed, and active, invasive, or expensive treatment measures (such as antibiotics for infection) are suspended. Caring for dying clients who have agreed to organ donation can also be complex in terms of determining which medications, treatments, or equipment must be continued until the time for harvesting the organs has arrived.

13. Document all client care, especially the effectiveness of symptom management activities.

SAMPLE DOCUMENTATION

2/20/2015 23:30

S "I am so tired. Please don't make me turn right now. Could you give me some ice chips?"

O Lotion and massage to reachable back and extremities. Repositioned slightly to shift weight off bony prominences. Ice chips given and placed within reach.

A Care modified to support dying client autonomy.

P Turn q3h instead of q2h if the client prefers. Reinforce need to assess and treat dependent skin areas. Assess need for analgesics before each turn. Request pressure-reducing mattress. ———————————— S. Amber, RN

EVALUATION

It can be difficult to evaluate accurately the effectiveness of care for the client during the dying process. Use symptom management rating scales whenever possible to track changes. Keep the primary care provider informed regularly of the client's status.

CLINICAL MANIFESTATIONS

Impending Clinical Death

LOSS OF MUSCLE TONE
- Relaxation of the facial muscles (e.g., the jaw may sag)
- Difficulty speaking
- Difficulty swallowing and gradual loss of the gag reflex
- Decreased activity of the gastrointestinal tract, with subsequent nausea, accumulation of flatus, abdominal distention, and retention of feces, especially if narcotics or tranquilizers are being administered
- Possible urinary and rectal incontinence due to decreased sphincter control
- Diminished body movement

SLOWING OF THE CIRCULATION
- Diminished sensation
- Mottling and cyanosis of the extremities
- Cold skin, first in the feet and later in the hands, ears, and nose (the client, however, may feel warm if there is a fever)

- Slower and weaker pulse
- Decreased blood pressure

CHANGES IN RESPIRATIONS
- Rapid, shallow, irregular, or abnormally slow respirations
- Noisy breathing, referred to as the death rattle, due to collecting of mucus in the throat
- Mouth breathing, dry oral mucous membranes

SENSORY IMPAIRMENT
- Blurred vision
- Impaired senses of taste and smell
- Various consciousness levels may exist just before death. Some clients are alert, whereas others are drowsy, stuporous, or comatose. Hearing is thought to be the last sense lost.

| BOX 34–1 | Assessment Interview |

Ask the spouse, partner, or significant others of the dying client:
- Have you ever been close to someone who was dying before?
- What have you been told about what may happen when death occurs?
- Do you have questions about what may happen at the time of death?

- How do you think you would like to say good-bye?
- How are you taking care of yourself during these times?
- Whom can you turn to for help and support at this time?
- Is there anyone you would like us to contact now or when the death occurs?

| BOX 34–2 | The Dying Person's Bill of Rights |

I have the right to be treated as a living human being until I die.
I have the right to maintain a sense of hopefulness however changing its focus may be.
I have the right to express my feelings and emotions about my approaching death in my own way.
I have the right to participate in decisions concerning my care.
I have the right to expect continuing medical and nursing attention even though cure goals must be changed to comfort goals.
I have the right not to die alone.
I have the right to be free from pain.
I have the right to have my questions answered honestly.
I have the right not to be deceived.

I have the right to have help from and for my family in accepting my death.
I have the right to die in peace and with dignity.
I have the right to retain my individuality and not be judged for my decisions which may be contrary to the beliefs of others.
I have the right to be cared for by caring, sensitive, knowledgeable people who will attempt to understand my needs and will be able to gain some satisfaction in helping me face my death.

From "The Dying Person's Bill of Rights," by A. J. Barbus, 1975, created at the Terminally Ill Patient and the Helping Person Workshop, Lansing, MI: South Western Michigan Inservice Education Council.

Caring for the Dying Client

Caregivers of a dying person need ongoing support and ongoing teaching as the client's condition changes. Some of these teaching needs include:

- Ways to feed the client when swallowing becomes difficult.
- Ways to transfer and reposition the client safely.
- Ways to communicate if verbalization becomes more difficult.

- Nonpharmacologic methods of pain control.
- Comfort measures, such as frequent oral care and frequent repositioning.
- Who to contact for different sources of support (e.g., respite care, pharmacies that deliver to the home, information about interpreting changes in the client's condition).

Ambulatory and Community Settings **Caring for the Dying**   PATIENT-CENTERED CARE

People facing death may need help accepting that they have to depend on others. Some dying clients require only minimal care; others need continuous attention and services. People need help, well in advance of death, in planning for the period of dependence. They need to consider what will happen and how and where they would like to die.

A major factor in determining whether a person will die in a health care facility or at home is the availability of willing and able caregivers. If the dying person wishes to be at home, and family or others can provide care to maintain symptom control, the nurse should facilitate a referral to outpatient hospice services. Hospice staff and nurses will then conduct a full assessment of the home and care providers' skills.

Although the original hospice was a freestanding facility, according to the National Hospice and Palliative Care Organization (2013), the largest segment of hospice care in the United States is delivered in the home (41.5% of hospice cases). The hospice concept is also implemented in hospice centers (27.4% of cases), palliative care areas in acute care hospitals (6.6% of cases), and designated locations within long-term care facilities (24.5% of cases). Most insurance policies, including Medicare, cover hospice services. In 2011, approximately 45% of all deaths in the United States occurred under hospice care.

CARE OF THE CLIENT AFTER DEATH

Sometimes, the organs of someone in a PVS, declared to have brain death, or who has been pronounced dead will be donated for research or transplantation. Because tissue donation may only be possible if certain activities are performed prior to cessation of circulation and breathing, it is extremely important that the possibility of donation be determined as soon as the client meets the donation criteria. In many states, if there is no valid donor document indicating that the person wished to donate some or all of the body tissues, health care workers are required to discuss the option of organ donation with the survivors. Survivors are obliged to grant or withhold donation in accordance with their knowledge of the donor's views on anatomic gifts. The details regarding this process of requesting donation from family members and other legal aspects of organ donation vary by state. The nurse needs to be familiar with the appropriate legislation and agency policy.

Nursing personnel may be responsible for care of a body after death (**postmortem care**). Postmortem care should be carried out according to the policy of the hospital or agency. Because care of the body may be influenced by religious law, the nurse should check the client's religion and make every attempt to comply. After the client dies, the family should be encouraged to view the body (with or without a nurse present), because this has been shown to facilitate the grieving process (Williams, Lewis, Burgio, & Goode, 2012). They may wish to clip a lock of hair as a remembrance. Children should be included in the events surrounding the death if they wish to.

In some situations, it may be desirable to perform a postmortem examination (autopsy), also referred to as a necropsy. If the cause of death is unknown or suspicious, the family or primary care provider may wish to have this examination performed in an effort to determine the cause. If the person died outside of a hospital, in an emergency department, or within 24 hours of admission to the hospital, the death may be considered a case for investigation or clearance by the medical examiner or **coroner**. A coroner is a physician who is authorized by the county or other government agency to determine causes of deaths under unusual circumstances. If an autopsy is requested by this authority, family consent may not be needed. If there are religious objections to the autopsy, the procedure can sometimes be modified (Carpenter et al., 2011).

●○● NURSING PROCESS: POSTMORTEM CARE

Postmortem care must be performed promptly. **Rigor mortis**, stiffening of the body, occurs about 2 to 4 hours after death. It results from a lack of adenosine triphosphate, which causes the muscles to contract, which in turn immobilizes the joints. Rigor mortis starts in the involuntary muscles (heart, bladder, and so on), then progresses to the head, neck, and trunk, and finally reaches the extremities.

Performing Postmortem Care

ASSESSMENT

If the death is expected, cessation of breathing and heartbeat generally signal the beginning of the postmortem phase of care. In the case of witnessed sudden death, such as in an emergency department, the physician will determine when lifesaving activities are to cease. In some states, specially trained nurses are permitted to pronounce a client as having died depending on the location and whether or not the death was expected (Weaver, 2011). Determine whether nurses can perform this requirement in your agency.

PLANNING

Before beginning postmortem care, determine any special circumstances that will influence the care. For example, if an autopsy will be performed, certain dressings or tubes may need to be left in place rather than removed for traditional body preparation.

DELEGATION

Postmortem care can be delegated to UAP after the activities described above have been completed so that the UAP knows what tubes or other medical devices can be removed or other special care provided.

INTERPROFESSIONAL PRACTICE

Postmortem care is a nursing role; however, other health care providers are not prohibited from participating.

Equipment
- Shroud ① or other linens used by the agency to wrap the body
- Washcloths, towels
- Absorbent pads

- Clean gloves and any other personal protective equipment as indicated by the client's condition
- Gown for the client (if the family will be viewing the body)
- Bags for personal belongings and the medical record document used to record transfer of the belongings and valuables

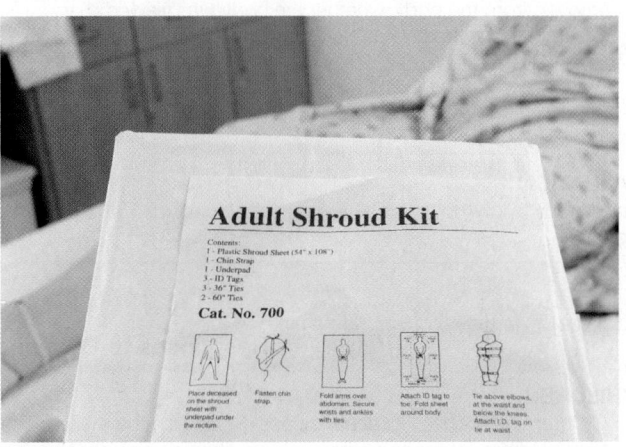

① Shroud contents.

IMPLEMENTATION
Preparation
- Consider whether more than one person or lifting devices are needed to perform the postmortem care since turning the body is involved. For caregivers who are performing postmortem care for the first time, it is especially advised that at least two caregivers work together to provide the care.
- Postmortem care can be time consuming. Arrange for someone to cover the caregiver's other clients during this time.

Performance
1. Observe appropriate infection prevention procedures. Apply clean gloves.
2. Because the deceased person's family often wants to view the body immediately after death, and because it is important that the deceased appear natural and comfortable, nurses need to position the body, place dentures in the mouth, and close the eyes and mouth before rigor mortis sets in.
   - Normally, the body is placed in a supine position with the arms either at the sides, palms down, or across the abdomen.
   - After blood circulation has ceased, the red blood cells break down, releasing hemoglobin, which discolors the surrounding tissues. This discoloration, referred to as **livor mortis**, appears in the lowermost or dependent areas of the body. One pillow is placed under the head and shoulders to prevent blood from settling in and discoloring the face.
   - Close the eyelids and hold in place for a few seconds so they remain closed.
   - Dentures are usually inserted to help give the face a natural appearance. The mouth is then closed.
     If the body will be viewed in the hospital:

- Place a clean gown on the client, and arrange the hair.
- Adjust the top bed linens neatly to cover the client to the shoulders.
- Provide tissues, soft lighting, and chairs for the family.
- All equipment, soiled linen, and supplies should be removed from the bedside.
3. Some agencies require that all tubes in the body remain in place; in other agencies, tubes may be cut to within 2.5 cm (1 in.) of the skin and taped in place; in others, all tubes may be removed. In some cases, if a central IV line is in place, it may be left to assist with the process of preserving the body (embalming). Use the same careful handling you would use with a living body. **Rationale:** *As the body cools, the skin loses its elasticity and can easily be broken when removing dressings and adhesive tape.*
4. Soiled areas of the body are washed; however, a complete bath is not necessary because the body will be washed by the mortician (also referred to as an undertaker), a person trained in care of the dead.
5. Absorbent pads are placed under the buttocks to take up any feces and urine released because of relaxation of the sphincter muscles.
6. Remove all jewelry, except a wedding band in some instances, which is taped to the finger.
7. The deceased's wrist identification tag is left on. After the body has been viewed by the family, additional identification tags are applied. **Rationale:** *Mislabeling can create legal problems if the body is inappropriately identified and prepared incorrectly for burial or a funeral.*

Continued on page 750

Performing Postmortem Care—*continued*

8. Wrap the body in a **shroud**, a large piece of plastic or cotton material used to enclose a body after death. ❷ Apply additional identification to the outside of the shroud.
   - If the dentures were placed in the mouth for the viewing, secure the jaw with a strap or remove them so they do not fall out as the mouth muscles relax.
   - Remove and discard gloves.
   - Perform hand hygiene.
9. Arrange for transport of the body to the morgue if a mortician will not pick it up from the client's room.
10. Document the postmortem care in the client record and on forms designed for this purpose. Include what items were removed from the body, whether the body was viewed by the family, and whether the body was taken to the morgue or picked up from the room.

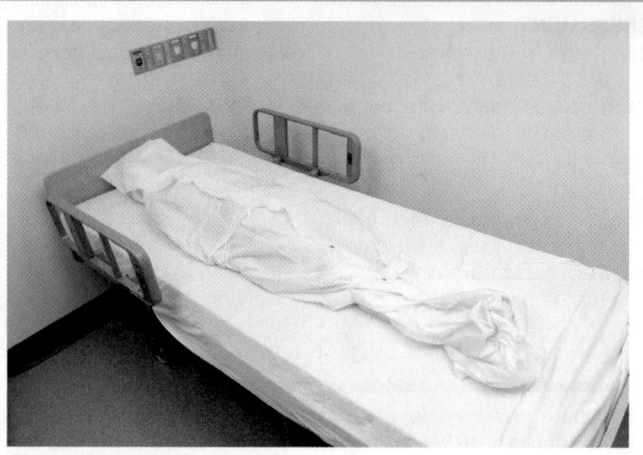

❷ A body wrapped in a shroud.

EVALUATION
Conduct any follow-up that is required related to handling the client's belongings.

LIFESPAN CONSIDERATIONS **Responses to Own and Others' Death**

CHILDREN
- Children's responses to death or loss depend on the messages they get from adults and others around them as well as their understanding of death. When adults are able to cope effectively with a death, they are more likely to be able to support children through the process.
- Comprehension of death evolves as the person develops:
  - *From infancy to 5 years:* Does not understand the concept of death. An infant's sense of separation forms a basis for later understanding of loss and death. Believes death is reversible, a temporary departure, or sleep.
  - *From 5 to 9 years:* Understands that death is final. Believes own death can be avoided. Associates death with aggression or violence. Believes wishes or unrelated actions can be responsible for death.
  - *From 9 to 12 years:* Understands death as the inevitable end of life. Begins to understand own mortality, expressed as interest in afterlife or as fear of death.
  - *From 12 to 18 years:* Fears a lingering death. May fantasize that death can be defied, acting out defiance through reckless behaviors (e.g., dangerous driving, substance abuse). Seldom thinks about death, but views it in religious and philosophic terms. May seem to reach "adult" perception of death, but be emotionally unable to accept it. May still hold concepts from previous developmental stages.

- One of the saddest situations is that of parents who experience the death of a child. They will likely feel shock, disbelief, and many other emotions. The nurse supports the parents by giving concrete and specific information about the child's condition, arranging for the parents to be close to the child for as much extended time as they desire, and facilitating parent participation in the child's care (Ball & Bindler, 2014). The challenges of providing "competent, compassionate, and consistent care that meets their physical, emotional, and spiritual needs" to dying children and their families has been well described in a report by the Institute of Medicine (Field & Behrman, 2003), available to read free online.

OLDER ADULTS
- Older adults who are dying often have a need to know that their lives had meaning. An excellent way to assure them of this is to make audiotapes or videotapes of them telling stories of their lives. This gives the client a sense of value and worth and lets him or her know that family members and friends will also benefit from it. Doing this with children and grandchildren often eases communication and support during this difficult time.
- Older adults fear prolonged illness and see death as having multiple meanings (e.g., freedom from pain, or reunion with already deceased family members).

CARING FOR THE CAREGIVER

Caregivers, both professionals and support persons, also respond to the impending and actual death. For example, performing postmortem care is always distressing to the caregiver—that is a normal response to the end of life. Professional caregivers, including nurses, may experience role strain due to repeated interactions with dying clients and their families. Although most nurses who work in oncology, hospice, intensive care, emergency, or other areas where client deaths are common have chosen such assignments, there can still be a sense of failure when clients die. Just as there must be support systems for grieving clients, there must also be support systems for grieving health care professionals. This is especially true because nurses may feel as though they should suppress demonstrating grief when, at the same time, they encourage clients to express similar feelings (Davenport & Hall, 2011).

Resources for caregivers include the clergy, social services, activities such as attending memorials, having planned staff counseling and remembrance sessions, and caregivers talking with each other about the deaths and their feelings. More research on grieving among caregivers is needed to demonstrate effective prevention of unhealthy grief and associated burnout.

FOCUSING ON CLINICAL THINKING

Consider This

1. If you have never touched a dead person before, it can be quite a frightening and emotional experience. How do you think it would be best to prepare? What do you think your reactions might be? Talk to others who have and see what they say. If you have had this experience already, try to remember what helped you get through that first time and imagine how you can support someone else through it.

2. Quite often, a dying person is in pain. How do you balance the need to give enough medication to relieve a client's suffering against the possibility that the dose will also shorten the person's life?

3. Think about the death-related practices in your own culture. How might you use these to find a way to support someone who is dying and has very different cultural beliefs or practices? For example, do you believe in heaven? What if your client feels differently from you and wants to discuss this? How would you respond if the client wants you to pray with him or her and you are of different religious beliefs?

See Focusing on Clinical Thinking answers on student resource website.

TEST YOUR KNOWLEDGE

1. While providing care for the client after death, which action by the nurse prevents livor mortis of the face?
   1. Turning the client in a lateral position
   2. Lowering the head of the bed below heart level
   3. Elevating the head on a pillow
   4. Applying ice packs to the face and shoulder area

2. The nurse knows that higher brain death has occurred when which of the following occurs?
   1. The cerebral cortex is irreversibly destroyed.
   2. The frontal lobe is irreversibly destroyed.
   3. The medulla is irreversibly destroyed.
   4. The brainstem is irreversibly destroyed.

3. While performing assessment of a terminal client, the nurse notes the client has lost muscle tone and has increased capillary refill time. The nurse knows these and what other sign indicate impending death?
   1. Slowing heart rate
   2. Increase in blood pressure
   3. Sensory impairment
   4. Increased desire to have the family at the bedside

4. The nurse enters a client's room to find the client has died. Because the nurse finds rigor mortis, the nurse knows the client most likely died at least how long ago?
   1. 30 minutes ago
   2. 1 hour ago
   3. 2 hours ago
   4. 8 hours ago

5. The dying client in a two-bed room (with a roommate) is requesting to see her 4-year-old child, but hospital policy does not allow anyone under the age of 12 in the client rooms due to risk of infection. Assuming that neither the client nor the roommate has a condition contagious to the child and that the child is healthy, the nurse, recognizing that death is impending for this client, takes which action?
   1. Allows the child and mother to visit in the room in spite of policy.
   2. Moves the client to a space where the child can visit with the mother.
   3. Informs the client that children are not allowed to visit.
   4. Takes the client to the window to view the child outside.

6. The nurse delegates postmortem care to the UAP but knows it is the nurse's responsibility to explain which priority information?
   1. How to bathe the body
   2. How to wrap the body
   3. Which medical devices must be left in place
   4. How to place proper identifiers on the body

7. A priority item for the nurse documenting postmortem care includes which of the following?
   1. Medical diagnosis
   2. Time of death
   3. Items remaining on the body
   4. Client's final words

8. When performing postmortem care for a client who died in the emergency department, the nurse should not remove which item?
   1. Blood from the client's face and hair
   2. Pieces of glass in the client's hair and clothing
   3. The client's clothing
   4. The urinary catheter

9. The nurse is caring for a terminal client whose wife is quietly sitting at the bedside. Which statement by the nurse involves the wife in caring for the client?
   1. "I'm going to change your husband's pajamas and give him a bath. Would you like to participate?"
   2. "Your husband might feel better if he was bathed. Do you want to do it?"
   3. "I'm going to change your husband's pajamas and give him a bath. You should help me."
   4. "Your husband would feel better if you bathed him."

10. A terminally ill client with a do-not-resuscitate order has become progressively unable to swallow and has stopped eating. The nurse is called to the room by the client's adult child, who has been feeding the client, because the client is choking. After suctioning and settling the client, what statement by the nurse made privately to the family member would be most supportive?
    1. "Your mother has a do-not-resuscitate order. You shouldn't feed her."
    2. "It can be difficult to watch someone you love not eating."
    3. "Don't feel badly. What's done is done."
    4. "Don't try to feed her again, it only makes things worse."

See Answers to Test Your Knowledge in Appendix A.

READINGS AND REFERENCES

References

Ashkenazi, T., & Klein, M. (2012). Predicting willingness to donate organs according to the demographic characteristics of the deceased's family. *Progress in Transplantation, 22,* 304–311. doi:10.7182/pit2012955

Ball, J., & Bindler, R. (2014). *Child health nursing: Partnering with children and families* (3rd ed.). Upper Saddle River, NJ: Pearson.

Barbus, A. J. (1975). *The dying person's bill of rights.* Created at the Terminally Ill Patient and the Helping Person Workshop. Lansing, MI: South Western Michigan Inservice Education Council.

California Healthcare Foundation. (2012). *Final chapter: Californians' attitudes and experiences with death and dying.* Retrieved from http://www.chcf.org/publications/2012/02/final-chapter-death-dying

Carpenter, B., Tait, G., Adkins, G., Barnes, M., Naylor, C., & Begum, N. (2011). Communicating with the coroner: How religion, culture, and family concerns may influence autopsy decision making. *Death Studies, 35,* 316–337. doi:10.1080/07481187.2010.520506

Davenport, L. A., & Hall, J. M. (2011). To cry or not to cry: Analyzing the dimensions of professional vulnerability. *Journal of Holistic Nursing, 29,* 180–189. doi:10.1177/0898010110393356

Field, M. J., & Behrman, R. E. (Eds.). (2003). *When children die: Improving palliative and end-of-life care for children and their families.* Washington, DC: National Academies Press. Retrieved from http://www.nap.edu/catalog/10390.html

Goodman, D. C., Fisher, E. S., Wennberg, J. E., Skinner, J. S., Chasan-Taber, S., & Bronner, K. K. (2013). *Tracking improvement in the care of chronically ill patients: A Dartmouth Atlas brief on Medicare beneficiaries near the end of life.* Retrieved from http://www.dartmouthatlas.org/downloads/reports/EOL_brief_061213.pdf

Lokker, M. E., van Zuylen, L., van der Rijt, C. C., & van der Heide, A. (2014). Prevalence, impact, and treatment of death rattle: A systematic review. *Journal of Pain and Symptom Management,47,* 105–122. doi:10.1016/j.jpainsymman.2013.03.011

National Hospice and Palliative Care Organization. (2013). *NHCPO facts and figures: Hospice care in America.* Alexandria, VA: Author. Retrieved from http://www.nhpco.org/hospice-statistics-research-press-room/facts-hospice-and-palliative-care

Stedman's medical dictionary for the health professions and nursing (7th ed.). (2012). Philadelphia, PA: Lippincott Williams & Wilkins.

Weaver, S. (2011). Your final assessment: Determination of death. *Nursing, 41*(2), 60–62. doi:10.1097/01.NURSE.0000392915.99282.b8

Williams, B. R., Lewis, D. R., Burgio, K. L., & Goode, P. S. (2012). "Wrapped in Their Arms:" Next-of-kin's perceptions of how hospital nursing staff support family presence before, during, and after the death of a loved one. *Journal of Hospice and Palliative Nursing,14,* 541–550. doi:10.1097/NJH.0b013e31825d2af1

World Health Organization. (n.d.). *WHO definition of palliative care.* Retrieved from http://www.who.int/cancer/palliative/definition/en

Selected Bibliography

Berman, A., Snyder, S., & Frandsen, G. (2016). *Kozier & Erb's fundamentals of nursing: Concepts, process, and practice* (10th ed.). Upper Saddle River, NJ: Pearson.

Bernat, J. L. (2013). Determining death in uncontrolled DCDD organ donors. *Hastings Center Report, 43*(1), 30–33. doi:10.1002/hast.129

Bülow, H., Sprung, C., Baras, M., Carmel, S., Svantesson, M., Benbenishty, J., . . . Nalos, D. (2012). Are religion and religiosity important to end-of-life decisions and patient autonomy in the ICU? The Ethicatt study. *Intensive Care Medicine, 38,* 1126–1133. doi:10.1007/s00134-012-2554-8

Cohen, J., Van Landeghem, P., Carpentier, N., & Deliens, L. (2013). Different trends in euthanasia acceptance across Europe. A study of 13 Western and 10 Central and Eastern European countries, 1981–2008. *European Journal of Public Health, 23,* 378–380. doi:10.1093/eurpub/cks186

Corr, C. A., & Corr, D. M. (2013). *Death and dying: Life and living* (7th ed.). Belmont, CA: Wadsworth Cengage.

Das, A. (2013). Spousal loss and health in late life: Moving beyond emotional trauma. *Journal of Aging & Health, 25,* 221–242. doi:10.1177/0898264312464498

Dhanani, S., Hornby, L., Ward, R., & Shemie, S. (2012). Variability in the determination of death after cardiac arrest: A review of guidelines and statements. *Journal of Intensive Care Medicine, 27,* 238–252. doi:10.1177/0885066610396993

Hart, J. L., Kohn, R., & Halpern, S. D. (2012). Perceptions of organ donation after circulatory determination of death among critical care physicians and nurses: A national survey. *Critical Care Medicine, 40,* 2595–2600. doi:10.1097/CCM.0b013e3182590098

Heuberger, R. (2012). Artificial feeding and hydration in persons nearing death. *Clinical Nutrition Insight, 38*(10), 1–3.

Kellehear, A. (2013). Vigils for the dying: Origin and functions of a persistent tradition. *Illness, Crisis & Loss, 21*(2), 109–124. doi:10.2190/IL.21.2.c

Kübler-Ross, E. (1978). *To live until we say good-bye.* Englewood Cliffs, NJ: Prentice Hall.

Munjal, K. G., Wall, S. P., Goldfrank, L. R., Gilbert, A., Kaufman, B. J., & Dubler, N. (2013). A rationale in support of uncontrolled donation after circulatory determination of death. *Hastings Center Report, 43*(1), 19–26. doi:10.1002/hast.113

Padela, A. I., Arozullah, A., & Moosa, E. (2013). Brain death in Islamic ethico-legal deliberation: Challenges for applied Islamic bioethics. *Bioethics, 27,* 132–139. doi:10.1111/j.1467-8519.2011.01935.x

Shah, S. K., Truog, R. D., & Miller, F. G. (2011). Death and legal fictions. *Journal of Medical Ethics, 37,* 719–722. doi:10.1136/jme.2011.045385

Smith-Stoner, M., & Hand, M. W. (2012). Expanding the concept of patient care: Analysis of postmortem policies in California hospitals. *MEDSURG Nursing,21,* 360–366.

Teitelbaum, J., & Shemi, S. (2011). Neurologic determination of death. *Neurologic Clinics, 29,* 787–799. doi:10.1016/j.ncl.2011.08.003

Tonti-Filippini, N. (2012). Religious and secular death: A parting of the ways. *Bioethics, 26,* 410–421. doi:10.1111/j.1467-8519.2011.01882.x

Whitman, H. H., & Lukes, S. J. (1975). Behavioral modification for terminally ill patients. *American Journal of Nursing,75*(1), 98–101.

Wiener, L., McConnell, D. G., Latella, L., & Ludi, E. (2013). Cultural and religious considerations in pediatric palliative care. *Palliative & Supportive Care, 11,* 47–67. doi:10.1017/S1478951511001027

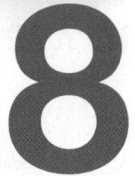

Applying the Nursing Process

This unit explores skills related to wound and injury care. Caring for clients following surgery or a traumatic injury, or with pressure ulcers, requires the nurse to have skills related to wound care. Also included in this unit is care of the client who is at the end of life. Health care providers recognize that death is not always a failure and clients in this stage of the life cycle require unique and thoughtful care planning to make their final days as comfortable as possible.

CLIENT: Will   AGE: 18 Years   CURRENT MEDICAL DIAGNOSIS: Fractured Left Radius and Ulna, Multiple Lacerations and Abrasions

Medical History: Will was skateboarding at a local skateboard park and was imitating a move he saw when he watched the Olympics. After making two successful flips in the air, he lost his balance and landed hard. He fractured both the radius and ulna of his left arm, requiring open reduction and placement of pins and plates. After surgery, his arm was placed in a plaster cast with a window to allow observation of the 10-cm (4-in.) incision on his forearm. He also has a 7.5-cm (3-in.) laceration with nine stitches on his left knee, a 10- × 5-cm (4- × 2-in.) hematoma on his right anterior thigh, an abrasion that covers his entire right knee, and multiple small abrasions and contusions on all of his extremities and left trunk. He is otherwise healthy and was heard comforting his mother by saying, "At least I was wearing a helmet, Mom!"

Personal and Social History: Will attends public school and will graduate this year. He lives with his parents, older brother, and younger sister. His friends and girlfriend visit often.

Questions

Assessment

1. Describe essential assessments made by the nurse when caring for Will after he returns from the operating room related to his casted left arm.
2. What wound assessments would the nurse make while caring for Will?

Analysis

3. List two possible nursing diagnoses that can be identified in the medical/personal history and assessment data above.

Planning

4. Based on the assessment data and nursing diagnoses, identify one desired outcome.
5. Identify the action verb, measurable criteria, and time line for the outcome.

Implementation

6. In preparing Will and his parents for discharge, what teaching will the nurse provide related to cast and wound care?
7. Describe nursing actions to be taken when changing Will's dressings on his left forearm incision and the laceration on his left knee.
8. When Will returns a week later for follow-up care, the doctor writes an order to remove his sutures. What assessment findings would cause the nurse to consult the physician to suggest the sutures remain in place longer?

Evaluation

9. Write a sample charting note describing the evaluation of the care plan.

See *Applying the Nursing Process* suggested answers on student resource website.

Appendix A Answers to Test Your Knowledge

Chapter 1: Foundational Skills

1. **Answer:** 1, 2, 3, 4, and 5 **Rationale:** Proper use of alcohol-based products includes following these steps: Apply a palmful of product into a cupped hand—enough to cover all surfaces of both hands (option 1); rub palms together (option 2); interlace fingers palm to palm (option 3); rub palms against back of hands (option 4); and rub all surfaces of each finger with opposite hand (option 5); continue until product is dry—about 20 to 30 seconds, not 10 to 15 seconds as stated incorrectly in option 6. **Cognitive Level:** Applying **Client Need:** Safe and Effective Care Environment **Nursing Process:** Implementation **Learning Outcome:** 1-5b

2. **Answer:** 1, 3, and 4 **Rationale:** Nails should be kept short (option 1). Most agencies do not permit health care workers in direct contact with clients to have any form of artificial nails, making option 2 incorrect. Squarely filed nails (option 3) and intact cuticles (option 4) are correct answers because they do not pose any risk of harm to either the client or nurse. **Cognitive Level:** Applying **Client Need:** Safe and Effective Care Environment **Nursing Process:** Planning **Learning Outcome:** 1-5a and b

3. **Answer:** 3 **Rationale:** Moist skin becomes chapped readily as does dry skin that is rubbed vigorously. Chapping produces lesions. Dry hands and arms thoroughly with a paper towel without scrubbing. Adjust the water flow so that the water is warm. Warm water removes less of the protective oil of the skin than hot water (option 1). Use firm, rubbing, and circular movements to wash the palm, back, and wrist of each hand. Be sure to include the heel of the hand. Interlace the fingers and thumbs, and move the hands back and forth (option 2). Use a new paper towel to grasp a hand-operated control. This prevents the nurse from picking up microorganisms from the faucet handles (option 4). **Cognitive Level:** Applying **Client Need:** Safe and Effective Care Environment **Nursing Process:** Implementation **Learning Outcome:** 1-5b

4. **Answer:** 3 **Rationale:** Caring for a diaphoretic client with chest pain does not require the implementation of standard precautions. SP apply to blood; all body fluids, including excretions and secretions except sweat; nonintact (broken) skin; and mucous membranes. Options 1, 2, and 4 deal with some or all of the above and are incorrect answers. **Cognitive Level:** Applying **Client Need:** Safe and Effective Care Environment **Nursing Process:** Implementation **Learning Outcome:** 1-3

5. **Answer:** 2 **Rationale:** If the nurse wears prescription glasses, goggles must still be worn over the glasses to provide shielding around the sides of the glasses. Disposable gloves are worn to protect the hands when the nurse is likely to handle any potentially infective material or objects (option 1). Sterile gowns may be indicated when the nurse changes the dressings of a client with extensive wounds, i.e., burns (option 3). Hands should be washed after removing gloves because gloves may have holes that can allow microorganisms in or the hands may become contaminated during removal (option 4). **Cognitive Level:** Applying **Client Need:** Safe and Effective Care Environment **Nursing Process:** Evaluation **Learning Outcome:** 1-4

6. **Answer:** 4 **Rationale:** Unlicensed assistive personnel (UAP) may be delegated the task of assisting the nurse or other health care provider with some skills. However, if these activities require the assistant to perform skills not generally expected of UAP, such as sterile technique, they may not be delegated to the UAP. Reviewing the primary care provider's order for the procedure, if available (option 1); measuring and recording vital signs and assessing for pertinent health factors before the procedure (option 2); and arranging for someone to care for other clients if necessary (option 3) are all correct actions. **Cognitive Level:** Applying **Client Need:** Safe and Effective Care Environment **Nursing Process:** Evaluation **Learning Outcome:** 1-5d

7. **Answer:** 1, 2, 3, and 5 **Rationale:** For each procedure include the exact procedure performed and the date and time it was performed (option 1); client's reaction to and tolerance of the procedure (option 2); any measurements taken (option 3); and all client teaching done prior to, during, and following the procedure (option 5). Details regarding disposal of used supplies need not be charted in the client record (option 4). **Cognitive Level:** Applying **Client Need:** Safe and Effective Care Environment **Nursing Process:** Evaluation **Learning Outcome:** 1-7

8. **Answer:** 1 **Rationale:** If wearing a gown, pull the gloves up to cover the cuffs of the gown. If not wearing a gown, pull the gloves up to cover the wrists. To be effective, a mask must cover both the nose and the mouth, because air moves in and out of both (option 2). When applying a gown, overlap the gown at the back as much as possible, and fasten the waist ties or belt; overlapping securely covers the uniform at the back (option 3). A clean mask should be applied, not one hanging from around the neck that may have been contaminated. **Cognitive Level:** Applying **Client Need:** Safe and Effective Care Environment **Nursing Process:** Evaluation **Learning Outcome:** 1-4

9. **Answer:** 2 **Rationale:** A health care–associated infection is an infection that may have originated in any health care setting including the home. This client's infection is likely to have been caused by the indwelling catheter. A nosocomial infection is an infection that was likely to have originated while in the hospital. This client developed an infection while at home, so this term does not apply (option 1). This infection is most likely bacterial in origin, which would rule out a viral infection (option 3) or a fungal infection (option 4). **Cognitive Level:** Applying **Client Need:** Safe and Effective Care Environment **Nursing Process:** Assessment **Learning Outcome:** 1-1

10. **Answer:** 4 **Rationale:** The nurse should wear a clean uniform, even if it is not a favorite because the uniform comes in contact with pathogens throughout the day and wearing a dirty uniform puts the clients the nurse cares for at risk of cross-infection (option 4). Although the uniform may look and smell clean, pathogens are invisible and can still reside in the material (option 1). Spraying the uniform with a disinfectant may kill some pathogens, but it will not be effective in killing most pathogens and puts the clients the nurse cares for while wearing this uniform at risk for infection (option 2). Wearing either the pants or the top of a soiled uniform still puts clients at risk for cross contamination and is not professional or appropriate (option 3). **Cognitive Level:** Analyzing **Client Need:** Safe and Effective Care Environment **Nursing Process:** Planning **Learning Outcome:** 1-3

Chapter 2: Vital Signs

1. **Answer:** 1, 3, and 4 **Rationale:** Unless the client is unstable, UAP can take initial vital signs on a newly admitted client or a client returning from dialysis (options 1 and 3). Measurement of a client's temperature can be delegated to UAP (option 4). UAP, however, may not assess, so the nurse needs to assess the apical pulse for rhythm and rate. Although UAP can count the rate, they cannot assess for regularity. However, remember that UAP can do this data collection, but an

assessment needs to be completed by a registered nurse (option 2). UAP cannot be delegated vital signs for unstable clients (option 5). **Cognitive Level:** Applying **Client Need:** Safe and Effective Care Environment **Nursing Process:** Planning **Learning Outcome:** 2-3

2. **Answer:** 1 **Rationale:** The arm should be at the level of the heart and not above the level of the heart. An arm at shoulder level gives an erroneously low reading. Option 2 describes the correct height for the arm while taking blood pressure. Waiting 1 to 2 minutes before repeating an assessment prevents an erroneously high systolic or low diastolic reading (option 3). Assessing immediately after a meal or while a client smokes can also cause an erroneously high blood pressure, so resting before measuring is the correct technique (option 4). **Cognitive Level:** Applying **Client Need:** Health Promotion and Maintenance **Nursing Process:** Evaluation **Learning Outcome:** 2-5d

3. **Answer:** 1 **Rationale:** An average pulse rate for a teenager is 75, not 100, beats per minute. An average heart rate of 100 beats per minute would describe a child between the ages of 5 and 8. An average range of respirations for a newborn is 30 to 80 breaths per minute (option 2). An average pulse range for a 1-year-old is 80 to 140 beats per minute (option 3). An average respiration rate for an older adult is 16 breaths per minute (option 4). **Cognitive Level:** Applying **Client Need:** Health Promotion and Maintenance **Nursing Process:** Evaluation **Learning Outcome:** 2-6

4. **Answer:** 3 **Rationale:** In hypertension stage 1, the systolic reading falls between 140 and 159 mmHg or the diastolic reading falls between 90 and 99. A normal blood pressure reading (option 1) is a systolic reading of less than 120 mmHg, and a diastolic reading of less than 80 mmHg. In prehypertension (option 2), the systolic is between 120 and 139 mmHg or the diastolic is between 80 and 89 mmHg. In hypertension stage 2 (option 4), the systolic reading is greater than 160 mmHg or the diastolic is greater than 100 mmHg. **Cognitive Level:** Remembering **Client Need:** Health Promotion and Maintenance **Nursing Process:** Diagnosis **Learning Outcome:** 2-7d

5. **Answer:** 2 **Rationale:** Rectal thermometers provide a reliable measurement, but the presence of stool may interfere with thermometer placement. Oral temperature readings are accessible and convenient, but can be inaccurate if the client has just ingested hot or cold food or fluid or been smoking (option 1). A temporal artery measurement is safe, noninvasive, and very fast (option 3). A tympanic membrane measurement is readily accessible, reflects the core temperature, and is very fast as well (option 4). **Cognitive Level:** Applying **Client Need:** Health Promotion and Maintenance **Nursing Process:** Evaluation **Learning Outcome:** 2-8

6. **Answer:** 4 **Rationale:** In this instance, the nurse needs an accurate assessment of the pulse rate and rhythm before administering a medication that affects heart rate, digoxin, so an apical pulse needs to be auscultated for a full minute prior to administration because it is the most accurate means of assessing the pulse. Options 1, 2, and 3 are incorrect because peripheral pulse assessment is less accurate than apical pulse assessment. **Cognitive Level:** Applying **Client Need:** Health Promotion and Maintenance **Nursing Process:** Assessment **Learning Outcome:** 2-2b

7. **Answer:** 3 **Rationale:** The symptoms provided describe tachypnea or quick shallow breaths; intercostal retractions, or indrawing between the ribs; hemoptysis, or the presence of blood in the sputum; and stridor, or a shrill, harsh sound heard during inspiration with laryngeal obstruction. Bradypnea is abnormally slow respirations (options 1 and 2). Substernal retractions are indrawing below the xiphoid process (options 2 and 4), and wheezing is a high-pitched whistling sound (option 4). **Cognitive Level:** Applying **Client Need:** Health Promotion and Maintenance **Nursing Process:** Assessment **Learning Outcome:** 2-11

8. **Answer:** 4 **Rationale:** Release the valve on the cuff carefully so that the pressure decreases at the rate of 2 to 3 mmHg per second. If the rate is faster or slower, an error in measurement may occur. The client should be positioned appropriately. The adult client should be sitting unless otherwise specified. Both feet should be flat on the floor. Sitting with legs crossed at the knee results in elevated systolic and diastolic blood pressures (option 1). Wrap the deflated cuff evenly around the upper arm. Locate the brachial artery and apply the center of the bladder directly over the artery (option 2). Pump the cuff until the sphygmomanometer reads 30 mmHg above the point where the brachial pulse disappeared (option 3). **Cognitive Level:** Applying **Client Need:** Health Promotion and Maintenance **Nursing Process:** Evaluation **Learning Outcome:** 2-4d

9. **Answer:** 1 **Rationale:** Apply the sensor and connect it to the pulse oximeter. Make sure the LED and photodetector are accurately aligned, that is, opposite each other on either side of the finger, toe, nose, or earlobe. It may be necessary to remove dark nail polish because it can interfere with accurate measurements (option 2). Inspect and move or change the location of an adhesive toe or finger sensor every 4 hours and a spring-tension sensor every 2 hours (option 3). Compare the pulse rate indicated by the oximeter to the radial pulse periodically. A large discrepancy between the two values may indicate oximeter malfunction or poor perfusion to the area measured by the oximeter (option 4). **Cognitive Level:** Applying **Client Need:** Health Promotion and Maintenance **Nursing Process:** Implementation **Learning Outcome:** 2-4b

10. **Answer:** 2 **Rationale:** Document the respiratory rate, depth, rhythm, and character on the appropriate record. Arterial blood gases are not generally documented as part of the postprocedure assessment of respirations (option 4). **Cognitive Level:** Applying **Client Need:** Health Promotion and Maintenance **Nursing Process:** Assessment **Learning Outcome:** 2-12

Chapter 3: Health Assessment

1. **Answer:** 3 **Rationale:** Percussion can indicate whether tissue is fluid filled, air filled, or solid. Dullness is a thudlike sound produced by dense tissue such as the liver, spleen, or heart (option 3). Tympany is a musical or drumlike sound produced from an air-filled stomach (option 1). Flatness is an extremely dull sound produced by very dense tissue, such as muscle or bone (option 2). Resonance is a hollow sound such as that produced by lungs filled with air (option 4). **Cognitive Level:** Remembering **Client Need:** Health Promotion and Maintenance **Nursing Process:** Assessment **Learning Outcome:** 3-1

2. **Answer:** 1, 2, 4, and 5 **Rationale:** A history of present illness (HPI) includes when the symptoms started (option 1), how often the problem occurs (option 2), what treatments the client has already tried (option 4), and factors that aggravate or alleviate the problem (option 5). Until there is a diagnosis and planned treatment, it is too early to determine how the problem will affect the client's future (option 3). **Cognitive Level:** Remembering **Client Need:** Health Promotion and Maintenance **Nursing Process:** Assessment **Learning Outcome:** 3-2

3. **Answer:** 4 **Rationale:** Auscultation is the process of listening to sounds produced within the body, such as by using a stethoscope that amplifies the sounds and conveys them to the nurse's ears. Sound or vibration produced when the body surface is struck occurs with percussion, not with auscultation. Four primary techniques are used in the physical examination: inspection, palpation, percussion, and auscultation (option 1). Palpation is the examination of the body using the sense of touch. The pads of the fingers are used because their concentration of nerve endings makes them highly sensitive to tactile discrimination (option 2). Inspection is visual examination, which is assessment that involves use of the sense of sight (option 3). **Cognitive Level:** Understanding **Client Need:** Health Promotion and Maintenance **Nursing Process:** Evaluation **Learning Outcome:** 3-3

4. **Answer:** 1 **Rationale:** Assessment of the abdomen involves inspection, auscultation, palpation, and percussion. The nurse performs

inspection first, followed by auscultation, palpation, and/or percussion. Auscultation is done before palpation and percussion because palpation and percussion cause movement or stimulation of the bowel, which can increase bowel motility and thus heighten bowel sounds, creating false results. **Cognitive Level:** Understanding **Client Need:** Health Promotion and Maintenance **Nursing Process:** Assessment **Learning Outcome:** 3-5o

5. **Answer:** 2 **Rationale:** Breast health guidelines vary by recommending agency but for women ages 20 to 39, the American Cancer Society recommends a clinical breast exam by a health professional every 3 years (option 2) and monthly breast self-exams, not every 3 months as incorrectly stated in option 3. A yearly screening mammogram is recommended only for women 40 or 50 years of age and older (option 1). **Cognitive Level:** Understanding **Client Need:** Health Promotion and Maintenance **Nursing Process:** Assessment **Learning Outcome:** 3-6

6. **Answer:** 3 **Rationale:** In Tanner stage 3 for an adolescent male, the pubic hair darkens, begins to curl, becomes coarser, and extends over the pubic symphysis; the penis elongates; and the scrotum shows continuing enlargement and darkening. In stages 1 and 2 there is no or only scant pubic hair, and the penis and testes are proportional to body size (options 1 and 2). In stage 4, the glans develops (option 4). **Cognitive Level:** Applying **Client Need:** Health Promotion and Maintenance **Nursing Process:** Assessment **Learning Outcome:** 3-7

7. **Answer:** 3 **Rationale:** An S_4 heart sound is considered normal in older adults. Therefore, the only action needed is to document the findings (option 3). None of the other actions are necessary at this time. **Cognitive Level:** Analyzing **Client Need:** Health Promotion and Maintenance **Nursing Process:** Diagnosis **Learning Outcome:** 3-8

8. **Answer:** 1 **Rationale:** Independent clinical judgment drives the selection of which components of an assessment are indicated. Although the nurse is able to perform a comprehensive assessment of each individual body system, more commonly the generalist nurse performs a brief screening assessment of all systems (option 2) when first encountering the client and then more detailed focused assessments of particular systems as indicated by the client's condition. An advanced practice nurse does not perform a brief screening of all systems prior to the generalist nurse's assessment (option 3). A brief, not in-depth, screening assessment is referred to as a head-to-toe assessment (option 4). **Cognitive Level:** Applying **Client Need:** Health Promotion and Maintenance **Nursing Process:** Assessment **Learning Outcome:** 3-9

9. **Answer:** 2 **Rationale:** White spots on the nails indicate zinc deficiency. There is no link between calcium deficiency and nail changes (option 1), bands across the nails may indicate protein deficiency (option 3), and spoon-shaped nails accompany iron deficiency (option 4). **Cognitive Level:** Understanding **Client Need:** Health Promotion and Maintenance **Nursing Process:** Assessment **Learning Outcome:** 3-10

10. **Answer:** 5 **Rationale:** The bases are found at the broad lower portion of the thorax (option 5). The apices are the narrow "tops" of the lungs and are found at location "A" (option 1). **Cognitive Level:** Applying **Client Need:** Health Promotion and Maintenance **Nursing Process:** Implementation **Learning Outcome:** 3-5k

Chapter 4: Diagnostic Testing

1. **Answer:** 3 **Rationale:** The test for occult (hidden) blood is often referred to as the guaiac test. An excessive amount of fat in the stool is known as steatorrhea, and can indicate faulty absorption of fat from the small intestine. None of the other answer options are indicated by the guaiac test. **Cognitive Level:** Applying **Client Need:** Physiological Integrity **Nursing Process:** Implementation **Learning Outcome:** 4-1

2. **Answer:** 1, 2, 3, 4, and 5 **Rationale:** Signs to remind staff of the test in progress should be placed in the client's room for a 24-hour urine collection (option 1). Because UAP are also caring for the client, provide

clear directions about the collection procedure, proper storage of the specimen container, and the importance of saving all of the client's urine to avoid the need to restart the collection process (option 2). The urine needs to be checked to ensure that fecal matter or toilet paper is not contaminating the specimen (option 3). The urine specimen collection begins with the first discarded specimen, and the time of that discard is documented as the start of the test (option 4). Collect all subsequent urine specimens, including the one specimen collected at the end of the period (option 5). **Cognitive Level:** Applying **Client Need:** Physiological Integrity **Nursing Process:** Implementation **Learning Outcome:** 4-2

3. **Answer:** 2 **Rationale:** Protein molecules normally are too large to escape from glomerular capillaries into the filtrate. If the glomerular membrane has been damaged, it can become "leaky," allowing proteins to escape. The urinary pH measures the relative acidity or alkalinity of the urine (option 1). The occult blood test is done to check for hidden blood in the urine (option 3). A positive glucose could indicate abnormal glucose tolerance for the client (option 4). **Cognitive Level:** Remembering **Client Need:** Physiological Integrity **Nursing Process:** Evaluation **Learning Outcome:** 4-3c

4. **Answer:** 2, 3 and 5 **Rationale:** Wearing clean gloves, not sterile, is appropriate (option 1). It is correct for the nurse to clamp the drainage tubing at least 3 inches below the sampling port for about 30 minutes (option 2) because it allows for fresh urine to collect in the catheter. Disinfecting the needle insertion site removes any microorganisms on the surface of the catheter, thereby avoiding contamination of the needle and the entrance of microorganisms into the catheter (option 3). The urine specimen is never taken from the Foley bag because this urine is considered contaminated since bacteria have had time to grow there (option 4). It is important for the specimen to be analyzed immediately (option 5). **Cognitive Level:** Applying **Client Need:** Physiological Integrity **Nursing Process:** Implementation **Learning Outcome:** 4-5e

5. **Answer:** 1 **Rationale:** Document the collection of the sputum specimen on the client's chart. Include the amount, color, consistency (thick, tenacious, watery), presence of hemoptysis (blood in the sputum), odor of the sputum, any measures needed to obtain the specimen, the general amount of sputum produced, and any discomfort experienced by the client. Options 2, 3, and 4 do not include all of the necessary elements for accurate documentation. **Cognitive Level:** Applying **Client Need:** Physiological Integrity **Nursing Process:** Evaluation **Learning Outcome:** 4-6

6. **Answer:** 1, 2, 3, and 5 **Rationale:** The nurse encourages the client to breathe normally and relax (option 1). It is the nurse's role to support and monitor the client throughout the procedure by reassuring the client and relaying what is happening at the time (option 2). The nurse also prepares the client by suggesting bladder and bowel emptying to prevent unnecessary discomfort during the procedure (option 3). A small sterile dressing is applied over the puncture site after the procedure (option 5). However, the nurse never collects the specimen. A physician is there to collect the specimen (option 4). **Cognitive Level:** Applying **Client Need:** Physiological Integrity **Nursing Process:** Implementation **Learning Outcome:** 4-7

7. **Answer:** 1, 3, and 5 **Rationale:** Serum creatinine levels help monitor the client's kidney function and can alert the health team to possible nephrotoxicity from the contrast medium (option 1). If a client is taking metformin, it should be held 6 hours before the contrast medium is given and resumed when it is certain that CIN has not occurred (option 2). Oral Mucomyst is often prescribed to prevent contrast-medium–induced nephropathy (option 3). Because the contrast medium is hypertonic, fluids are not limited. The nurse needs to monitor the client's hydration status (option 4). The contrast medium contains iodine, and it is important to check if the client is allergic to iodine

(option 5). **Cognitive Level:** Applying **Client Need:** Physiological Integrity **Nursing Process:** Implementation **Learning Outcome:** 4-8

8. **Answer:** 4 **Rationale:** It would be appropriate for the nurse to delegate the collection of a routine urine specimen to the UAP. Assisting the physician with a lumbar puncture to collect CSF (option 1), collecting a wound specimen for culture and sensitivity (option 2), and obtaining a venous blood specimen require specialized training and the use of aseptic technique and would not be appropriate to delegate to UAP (option 3). **Cognitive Level:** Analyzing **Client Need:** Safe and Effective Care Environment **Nursing Process:** Planning **Learning Outcome:** 4-4

9. **Answer:** 2 **Rationale:** The nurse should apply sterile gloves in order to avoid contaminating the wound and the specimen. Clean gloves (option 1) or no gloves (option 3) would not be appropriate when caring for a postoperative wound due to the risk of introducing pathogens into the area. It is not necessary to wear a sterile gown (option 4). **Cognitive Level:** Analyzing **Client Need:** Safe and Effective Care Environment **Nursing Process:** Implementation **Learning Outcome:** 4-5h

10. **Answer:** 3, 4, 5, 2, and 1 **Rationale:** The nurse would gather the necessary equipment (option 3), enter the client's room and perform hand hygiene (option 4), explain that a urine specimen is needed and why (option 5), teach the client how to collect the urine specimen (option 2), and label the container when the client has collected the specimen (option 1). **Cognitive Level:** Applying **Client Need:** Physiological Integrity **Nursing Process:** Implementation **Learning Outcome:** 4-5c

Chapter 5: Client Hygiene

1. **Answer:** 4 **Rationale:** Early morning care is provided to clients as they awaken in the morning. This care consists of providing a urinal or bedpan to the client confined to bed, washing the client's face and hands, and giving oral care. Providing for elimination needs, a bath or shower, perineal care, and oral, nail, and hair care (option 1) is included in morning care, which is often provided after clients have breakfast. Hour of sleep care is provided to clients before they retire for the night. It usually involves providing for elimination needs, washing face and hands, giving oral care, and possibly giving a back massage (option 2). As-needed care is provided as required by the client (option 3). **Cognitive Level:** Applying **Client Need:** Physiological Integrity **Nursing Process:** Implementation **Learning Outcome:** 5-2

2. **Answer:** 1, 2, 3, 4, and 5 **Rationale:** The different factors that influence individual hygienic practices include culture, religion, health and energy, personal preferences, and developmental level (options 1–5). **Cognitive Level:** Applying **Client Need:** Physiological Integrity **Nursing Process:** Assessment **Learning Outcome:** 5-3

3. **Answer:** 2 **Rationale:** Two categories of baths are given to clients: cleaning and therapeutic. Therapeutic baths are given for physical effects, such as to soothe irritated skin or to treat an area. Medications may be placed in the water. A therapeutic bath is generally taken in a tub one-third or one-half full. The client remains in the tub for a designated time, often 20 to 30 minutes. Option 1, a partial bath, and option 4, a bag bath, are types of cleaning baths (option 3). **Cognitive Level:** Applying **Client Need:** Physiological Integrity **Nursing Process:** Implementation **Learning Outcome:** 5-4

4. **Answer:** 1 **Rationale:** When caring for a client with dementia, focus on the person rather than the task. This includes moving slowly and letting the person know when you are going to move him or her. Using a supportive, calm approach and praising the person often is appropriate (option 2) as is stopping when the client becomes distressed and assessing the cause of the distress (option 3). Using a gentle touch is also appropriate (option 4). **Cognitive Level:** Applying

Client Need: Physiological Adaptation **Nursing Process:** Evaluation **Learning Outcome:** 5-5

5. **Answer:** 3 **Rationale:** When using a safety razor to shave facial hair, hold the skin taut, particularly around creases, to prevent cutting the skin. Option 1 is incorrect because the proper procedure is to apply shaving cream or soap and water to soften the bristles and make the skin more pliable. Hold the razor so that the blade is at a 45° angle to the skin, not at a 90° (option 2), and shave in short, firm strokes in the direction of hair growth. Option 4 is incorrect. To prevent irritating the skin, pat on lotion with the fingers and avoid rubbing the client's face. **Cognitive Level:** Applying **Client Need:** Physiological Adaptation **Nursing Process:** Evaluation **Learning Outcome:** 5-7E

6. **Answer:** 4 **Rationale:** Good foot care includes many things. When the feet are cold, use extra blankets and wear warm socks rather than using heating pads or hot water bottles, which may cause burns (option 4). To prevent burns, check the water temperature before immersing the feet or toes (option 1). To prevent or control an unpleasant odor due to excessive foot perspiration, wash the feet frequently and change socks and shoes at least daily (option 2). File the toenails rather than cutting them to avoid skin injury (option 3). **Cognitive Level:** Applying **Client Need:** Physiological Adaptation **Nursing Process:** Evaluation **Learning Outcome:** 5-7f

7. **Answer:** 4 **Rationale:** The nurse may safely delegate bathing a client diagnosed with chronic atrial fibrillation unless the client's condition is deteriorating. It would not be appropriate for the nurse to delegate bathing a client diagnosed with hemophilia (option 1) or osteogenesis imperfecta (option 2), because these clients are easily injured and require careful handling. The nurse should bathe the client scheduled for surgery that morning in order to use the opportunity to reinforce preoperative teaching as well as to assess the client's level of anxiety and provide support and reassurance if needed (option 3). **Cognitive Level:** Analyzing **Client Need:** Safe and Effective Care Environment **Nursing Process:** Planning **Learning Outcome:** 5-6

8. **Answer:** 3 **Rationale:** Bathe the child from the cleanest area to the dirtiest. Begin with the face, then bathe the abdomen (option 1) and extremities (option 4). Bathe the diaper area last (option 2). **Client Need:** Physiological Integrity **Cognitive Level:** Applying **Client Need:** Safe and Effective Care Environment **Nursing Process:** Implementation **Learning Outcome:** 5-7a

9. **Answer:** 1 **Rationale:** The nurse should accurately document the assessment findings and call the primary care provider immediately to report them. The nurse should not wait to report the assessment findings to the primary care provider (option 2). The authorities should not be notified until the primary care provider performs further assessment to determine possible physiological explanations for the bruising (option 3). If no physiological explanation is found, both the nurse and the primary care provider have a legal obligation to report suspected abuse. Documenting the assessment findings in the client's medical record is important, but it is not sufficient action in this case (option 4). **Cognitive Level:** Analyzing **Client Need:** Safe and Effective Care Environment **Nursing Process:** Implementation **Learning Outcome:** 5-8

10. **Answer:** 2 **Rationale:** The nurse would document cerumen (option 2), which is the medical term for earwax (option 3). Option 1 does not represent accurate medical terminology and should not be used by the nurse. Cerumen is normal discharge from the ear and would not be described as purulent material (option 4). **Cognitive Level:** Applying **Client Need:** Physiological Integrity **Nursing Process:** Implementation **Learning Outcome:** 5-1

Chapter 6: Bed-Making

1. **Answer:** 2 **Rationale:** An unoccupied bed (one not occupied by a client) can be either closed or open. Generally the top covers of an open

bed are folded back (thus the term open bed) to make it easier for a client to get in. Options 1 and 3 are incorrect because in both cases, the clients are occupying their beds. Option 4 is incorrect because it describes a closed bed in which the top sheet, blanket, and bedspread are drawn up to the top of the bed and under the pillows. **Cognitive Level:** Applying **Client Need:** Safe and Effective Care Environment **Nursing Process:** Planning **Learning Outcome:** 6-1

2. **Answer:** 4 **Rationale:** In a horizontal toe pleat, a fold is made in the sheet 5 to 10 cm (2 to 4 in.) across the bed near the foot. A miter or a fanfold refers to the way that a sheet is tucked in or placed, but does not allow for additional foot room (options 1 and 3). In a vertical toe pleat, a fold is made in the sheet 5 to 10 cm (2 to 4 in.) perpendicular to the foot of the bed (option 2). **Cognitive Level:** Applying **Client Need:** Safe and Effective Care Environment **Nursing Process:** Implementation **Learning Outcome:** 6-1

3. **Answer:** 4 **Rationale:** In Trendelenburg's position, the head of the bed is lowered and the foot raised in a straight incline. If the mattress is completely horizontal, the client is flat in bed (option 1). If the client is sitting in bed with the head of the bed raised 30°, this is a semi-Fowler's position (option 2). If the foot is lowered while the head of the bed is raised, this is a reverse Trendelenburg's position (option 3). **Cognitive Level:** Applying **Client Need:** Safe and Effective Care Environment **Nursing Process:** Implementation **Learning Outcome:** 6-3

4. **Answer:** 1 **Rationale:** In Fowler's position the client will be sitting with the head of the bed raised from a 45° to 60° angle. This position is used to promote lung expansion for clients with respiratory problems. Options 2, 3, and 4 are not good choices to promote lung expansion in this client. **Cognitive Level:** Applying **Client Need:** Safe and Effective Care Environment **Nursing Process:** Implementation **Learning Outcome:** 6-3

5. **Answer:** 3 **Rationale:** The linens of a surgical bed are horizontally fanfolded to facilitate transfer of the client into the bed. Do not tuck them in, miter the corners, or make a toe pleat. Flannel blankets provide additional warmth (option 1). Place the top covers on the bed as you would for an unoccupied bed (option 2). Place and leave the pillows on the bedside chair to facilitate transferring the client into the bed (option 4). **Cognitive Level:** Applying **Client Need:** Safe and Effective Care Environment **Nursing Process:** Evaluation **Learning Outcome:** 6-5b

6. **Answer:** 3, 4, and 5 **Rationale:** Soiled linen should be placed directly into a portable hamper (option 3). To avoid unnecessary trips to the linen supply area, gather all linen before starting to strip a bed (option 4). Soiled linen should not be shaken in the air because shaking can disseminate secretions and excretions and the microorganisms they contain (option 5). Soiled linen should be held away from the nurse's uniform. Linens and equipment that have been soiled with secretions and excretions harbor microorganisms that can be transmitted to others directly or by the nurse's hands or uniform (option 1). Linen for one client is never (even momentarily) placed on another client's bed (option 2). **Cognitive Level:** Applying **Client Need:** Safe and Effective Care Environment **Nursing Process:** Implementation **Learning Outcome:** 6-5a

7. **Answer:** 3 and 4 **Rationale:** The nurse could safely delegate the client with improving symptoms of Guillain-Barré and the elderly client who is chronically bedridden. The postoperative client following a lumbar laminectomy (option 1), the client who had an internal fixation (option 2), and the client in traction following a fractured cervical vertebra (option 5) require great care when moving and would require the nurse's involvement in changing the linen. **Cognitive Level:** Applying **Client Need:** Safe and Effective Care Environment **Nursing Process:** Planning **Learning Outcome:** 6-4

8. **Answer:** 2, 3, and 5 **Rationale:** Putting a "Do Not Disturb" sign on the client's door, lowering the lights, and decreasing the noise level at

change of shift can help the client to rest. Closing, rather than opening, the door would help decrease the noise level (option 1). Keeping the room temperature between 20°C and 23°C (68°F to 74°F) is comfortable for most clients (option 4). **Cognitive Level:** Applying **Client Need:** Safe and Effective Care Environment **Nursing Process:** Implementation **Learning Outcome:** 6-2

9. **Answer:** 2 **Rationale:** The nurse could make an unoccupied bed while the client was in the restroom; this would avoid the discomfort of changing the bed while the client is in it (option 1). There would be no need to make a surgical bed (option 3) or a closed bed (option 4) because the client is not postoperative and will be returning to the bed after finishing in the bathroom. **Cognitive Level:** Applying **Client Need:** Physiological Integrity **Nursing Process:** Implementation **Learning Outcome:** 6-5c

10. **Answer:** 1, 3, 4, and 5 **Rationale:** An extended-length bed promotes comfort for the tall client (option 1). Unless the client requests it, having all side rails up is considered a restraint because it restricts the client's freedom to leave the bed (option 2). Having the bed in low position (option 3) and the wheels locked (option 4) are important safety factors. Having the two top side rails up may assist the client to turn and get out of bed (option 5). **Cognitive Level:** Applying **Client Need:** Safe and Effective Care Environment **Nursing Process:** Assessment **Learning Outcome:** 6-2

Chapter 7: Infection Prevention

1. **Answer:** 2 **Rationale:** Vehicle-borne transmission involves any substance that serves as an intermediate means to transport and introduce an infectious agent into a susceptible host through a suitable portal of entry. Direct transmission involves immediate and direct transfer of microorganisms from person to person through touching, biting, kissing, or sexual intercourse (option 1). Airborne transmission may involve droplets or dust (option 3). Vector-borne transmission involves an animal or a flying or crawling insect that serves as an intermediary means of transporting the infectious agent (option 4). **Cognitive Level:** Remembering **Client Need:** Safe and Effective Care Environment **Nursing Process:** Assessment **Learning Outcome:** 7-1

2. **Answer:** 4 **Rationale:** Indirect transmission, not direct transmission, may be either vehicle-borne or vector-borne. The goal of infection prevention measures is to break the chain whenever or wherever possible so that disease is not transmitted from one person to another (option 1). Direct transmission involves immediate and direct transfer of microorganisms from person to person through touching, biting, kissing, or sexual intercourse (option 2). Droplet spread is also a form of direct transmission but can only occur if the source and the host are within 1 m (3 ft) of each other. Airborne transmission may involve droplets or dust (option 3). **Cognitive Level:** Remembering **Client Need:** Safe and Effective Care Environment **Nursing Process:** Planning **Learning Outcome:** 7-2

3. **Answer:** 1 **Rationale:** Ensure that the package is clean and dry; if moisture is noted on the inside of a plastic wrapped package or the outside of a cloth-wrapped package, it is considered contaminated and must be discarded. Placing the package in the work area so that the top flap of the wrapper opens away from you is proper technique (option 2). It is correct to place sterile items at least 2.5 cm (1 in.) from the border of the field. Items closer to the edge than 2.5 cm are considered contaminated (option 3). Always reach around the field because reaching over it could cause contamination from particles dropping from your arms (option 4). **Cognitive Level:** Applying **Client Need:** Safe and Effective Care Environment **Nursing Process:** Implementing **Learning Outcome:** 7-4a

4. **Answer:** 1, 2, and 4 **Rationale:** Place the package of gloves on a clean, dry surface. Any moisture on the surface could contaminate the gloves (option 1). Open the outer package so as not to contaminate the gloves

or the inner package (option 2). Pick up the other glove with the sterile gloved hand, inserting the gloved fingers under the cuff and holding the gloved thumb close to the gloved palm. This helps prevent accidental contamination of the glove by the bare hand (option 4). Option 3 is incorrect because the first glove should go on the dominant hand. Option 5 is incorrect because any portion of the cuff that has rolled underneath is now contaminated by contact with skin. Unrolling it would contaminate the sterile glove. **Cognitive Level:** Applying **Client Need:** Safe and Effective Care Environment **Nursing Process:** Implementation **Learning Outcome:** 7-4b

5. **Answer:** 2 and 4 **Rationale:** An N95 respirator mask (option 2) is used for clients requiring airborne precautions and is also effective against tuberculosis and other diseases. Although it is effective in this situation, it is not required and is more expensive and requires fit testing compared to surgical masks. Always perform hand hygiene before and after using gloves (option 4). Clients with tuberculosis should be cared for using standard precautions and droplet precautions. Thus, a surgical mask is only required when within 1 m (3 ft) of the client (option 1). There is no indication for gloves during all contact with such a client (option 3) or a gown during physical examination (option 5). **Cognitive Level:** Applying **Client Need:** Safe and Effective Care Environment **Nursing Process:** Planning **Learning Outcome:** 7-5

6. **Answer:** 3 **Rationale:** The nurse's action would need to be corrected if the gown were taken off outside the client's room. After a gown is worn, the nurse needs to remove it, without touching the uniform, and while still in the client's room (option 3). For contact precautions, the nurse needs to perform hand hygiene and change gloves after contact with infectious material (option 1). Also, used disposable sharps, such as needles, need to be placed directly into designated sharps containers. Sharps should not be recapped. Manipulating open sharps increases the chance of sustaining a puncture injury (option 2). Specimens to be sent to the laboratory must be placed in a plastic container with a secure lid. If the outside of the container is contaminated, the container needs to be put into a sealable plastic bag (option 4). **Cognitive Level:** Applying **Client Need:** Safe and Effective Care Environment **Nursing Process:** Evaluation **Learning Outcome:** 7-4c

7. **Answer:** 3 **Rationale:** Sterile procedures are not delegated to UAP. Care of clients requiring the different types of precautions may be delegated to UAP. UAP use standard precautions with all clients (option 1) and can care for or collect routine specimens from clients on transmission-based precautions (options 2 and 4). **Cognitive Level:** Applying **Client Need:** Safe and Effective Care Environment **Nursing Process:** Planning **Learning Outcome:** 7-3

8. **Answer:** 1 **Rationale:** Items that should be documented in the narrative notes include those that are not adequately covered by use of checklists or forms. This would include the amount, color, odor, and other characteristics of a productive cough (option 1). The nurse does not chart that care was delegated or provided by nonnursing members of the team (options 2 and 3). The actual care is documented, however, including who performed it. Chart oral and skin hygiene on a checklist (option 4). **Cognitive Level:** Applying **Client Need:** Safe and Effective Care Environment **Nursing Process:** Evaluation **Learning Outcome:** 7-6

9. **Answer:** 4 **Rationale:** This client would require standard precautions. The nurse would take care to avoid contact with blood and body fluids, as the nurse would with any client. No other special precautions would be required at this time. Droplet or airborne precautions would be used to protect visitors and staff from contracting an airborne illness, but this client does not have an airborne illness (options 1 and 3). Contact precautions would be used for someone with a wound or other infection that can be spread by direct contact (option 2). **Cognitive Level:** Applying **Client Need:** Safe and Effective Care Environment **Nursing Process:** Planning **Learning Outcome:** 7-5

10. **Answer:** 3 and 4 **Rationale:** The nurse can safely delegate vital signs and transporting the client to UAP. Teaching (option 1), whether explaining isolation requirements, helping parents follow isolation requirements (option 2), or preparing a client for discharge (option 5), should never be delegated to UAP. **Cognitive Level:** Applying **Client Need:** Safe and Effective Care Environment **Nursing Process:** Planning **Learning Outcome:** 7-3

Chapter 8: Heat and Cold Measures

1. **Answer:** 4 **Rationale:** The rebound phenomenon occurs at the time the maximum therapeutic effect of the heat or cold application is achieved and the opposite effect begins (option 4). Vasoconstriction is narrowing of the blood vessels and will not cause the rebound effect (option 1). Immobility (option 2) and compression (option 3) do not cause the client's reaction to reverse from the initial effect of the cold. **Cognitive Level:** Understanding **Client Need:** Physiological Integrity **Nursing Process:** Diagnosis **Learning Outcome:** 8-1

2. **Answer:** 3 **Rationale:** Heat relaxes muscles and increases, not decreases, their contractility (option 3). When heat is applied to stiff joints, the joint stiffness is reduced (option 1). This decrease happens by decreasing the viscosity of synovial fluid and increasing tissue distensibility. The use of cold in traumatic injury decreases bleeding by constricting blood vessels (option 2). Cold decreases pain by slowing the nerve conduction rate and blocking nerve impulses (option 4). **Cognitive Level:** Understanding **Client Need:** Physiological Integrity **Nursing Process:** Evaluation **Learning Outcome:** 8-3

3. **Answer:** 3 **Rationale:** UAP cannot design or modify treatment regimens (option 3). Application of certain heat or cold measures (i.e., baths, ice packs) may be delegated to UAP if they meet the general criteria for delegation (options 1 and 2). However, in all cases, assessment of the client and the determination that a specific measure is safe and appropriate to employ are responsibilities of the nurse. UAP may determine if basic equipment they use is functioning correctly (option 4). **Cognitive Level:** Applying **Client Need:** Physiological Integrity **Nursing Process:** Planning **Learning Outcome:** 8-4

4. **Answer:** 1 **Rationale:** Electricity in the presence of moisture can conduct a shock. A cover should be placed over the heating pad because moisture can cause the pad to short-circuit and burn or shock the client (option 2). It is appropriate to reassess the site receiving the heat after 15 minutes (option 3). A pin might strike a wire, damaging the pad and giving an electric shock to the client, thus gauze ties are safe (option 4). **Cognitive Level:** Applying **Client Need:** Physiological Integrity **Nursing Process:** Implementation **Learning Outcome:** 8-5a

5. **Answer:** 2 **Rationale:** Remove excess air by bending or twisting the device. Air inflates the device so that it cannot be molded to the body (option 2). Fill the device one-half to two-thirds full of crushed ice. Partial rather than complete filling makes the device more pliable so that it can be molded to a body part (option 1). The device should be held upside down, not upright, to check for leaks (option 3). Cover the device with a soft cloth cover (option 4). The cover absorbs moisture that condenses on the outside of the device. It is also more comfortable for the client. **Cognitive Level:** Applying **Client Need:** Physiological Integrity **Nursing Process:** Evaluation **Learning Outcome:** 8-5b

6. **Answer:** 1, 2, 3, and 4 **Rationale:** The following conditions, if present, contraindicate the use of heat: active hemorrhage, because heat causes vasodilation and increases bleeding (option 1); localized malignant tumor, because heat accelerates cell metabolism and cell growth and increases circulation (option 2); the first 24 hours after traumatic injury, because heat increases bleeding and swelling (option 3); skin disorder that causes redness or blisters, because heat can burn or cause further damage to the skin (option 4). A client with a nonbleeding open wound could receive heat because heat can increase blood

flow to an open wound (option 5). **Cognitive Level:** Applying **Client Need:** Physiological Integrity **Nursing Process:** Planning **Learning Outcome:** 8-3

7. **Answer:** 1, 2, 3, and 4 **Rationale:** When applying cold, monitor the client during the application. Assess the client in terms of circulatory status (option 1), comfort level (option 2), and skin reaction (option 4). Report any untoward reactions and remove the application. Document the method of application of the cold (option 3) and the client's response in the client record using forms or a checklist supplemented by narrative notes when appropriate. The temperature of the ice or cold pack need not be documented, and determination of the temperature is often impractical (option 5). **Cognitive Level:** Applying **Client Need:** Physiological Integrity **Nursing Process:** Implementation **Learning Outcome:** 8-6

8. **Answer:** 2 **Rationale:** For a warm heat application, such as an aquathermia pad, the temperature will be between 37°C and 40°C (98°F and 104°F) (option 2). For a tepid heat application, such as an alcohol sponge bath, the temperature will be between 27°C and 37°C (80°F and 98°F) (option 1). For a hot heat application, such as a hot compress, the temperature will be between 40°C and 46°C (104°F and 115°F) (option 3). For a very hot heat application, such as a hot water bag, the temperature will be above 46°C (115°F) (option 4). **Cognitive Level:** Applying **Client Need:** Physiological Integrity **Nursing Process:** Planning **Learning Outcome:** 8-2

9. **Answer:** 4 **Rationale:** The client should be reassured that the temperature is still warm and that increasing the temperature could cause injury. It is true that the body acclimates to heat in a few minutes and feels less warm. Turning up the temperature could cause a burn injury (option 1). Telling the client that the body adjusted without explaining the potential complication if the temperature was increased would not provide all of the necessary client information (option 2). Saying only that the compress is still warm does not teach the client anything (option 3). **Cognitive Level:** Analyzing **Client Need:** Physiological Integrity **Nursing Process:** Implementation **Learning Outcome:** 8-5c

10. **Answer:** 3 **Rationale:** The nurse's priority action is to remove the hot pack to stop the burning process. Although the primary care provider needs to be informed (option 1), and an explanation to the client might be indicated (option 4), the first and most urgent priority is to prevent further harm. Applying an ice pack could cause additional damage to injured tissues (option 2). **Cognitive Level:** Analyzing **Client Need:** Physiological Integrity **Nursing Process:** Implementation **Learning Outcome:** 8-6

Chapter 9: Pain Management

1. **Answer:** 3 **Rationale:** The nurse should state what was observed: the client's report of pain and request for pain medication. Simply stating what the client said and what you observed paints a picture of the interaction without invoking the nurse's judgment about the circumstances. The nurse should avoid use of the word *but* because this implies that the pain is not believed to be real (options 1, 2, and 4). **Cognitive Level:** Analyzing **Client Need:** Physiological Integrity **Nursing Process:** Implementation **Learning Outcome:** 9-12

2. **Answer:** 2, 3, 4, and 5 **Rationale:** These pure opioid drugs produce maximum pain inhibition, an agonist effect. Their dose can be steadily increased to relieve pain (option 2). There is also no maximum daily dose limit unless they are in compound with a nonopioid analgesic drug such as acetaminophen, which has a daily maximum limit of 2,400 to 4,000 mg (option 3). There is no ceiling on the level of analgesia from these drugs (option 4). Full agonist analgesics include morphine (e.g., Kadian, MS Contin), oxycodone (e.g., Percocet, OxyContin), and hydromorphone (e.g., Dilaudid, Palladone)—option 5. Option 1 is incorrect because full agonist analgesics are excellent

choices for clients suffering from pain as a result of terminal illness. **Cognitive Level:** Applying **Client Need:** Physiological Integrity **Nursing Process:** Planning **Learning Outcome:** 9-1

3. **Answer:** 4 **Rationale:** Behavioral changes such as confusion and restlessness may be indicators of pain in older adults. However, the nurse needs to assess if the client can report pain before intervening (option 1). Giving a sleeping pill may make the client more confused (option 2). Asking the daughter to stay and observe (option 3) may not be feasible and the nurse must still assess the client. **Cognitive Level:** Applying **Client Need:** Physiological Integrity **Nursing Process:** Assessment **Learning Outcome:** 9-6

4. **Answer:** 1 **Rationale:** Fear of addiction to narcotic analgesics is a common barrier to pain management. The other factors in options 2, 3, and 4 would not act as barriers to pain management and indicate the client is willing to participate and follow the plan of care. **Cognitive Level:** Analyzing **Client Need:** Physiological Integrity **Nursing Process:** Assessment **Learning Outcome:** 9-4

5. **Answer:** 3 **Rationale:** The nurse should acknowledge and accept the client's perception of the pain, administer the nonnarcotic analgesic, and inform the client that if the pain becomes worse or unmanageable, the nurse should be called immediately. The nurse would then reassess the client within 30 minutes to determine the need for further intervention. Administering the narcotic against the client's wishes is unethical and illegal (option 1). To meet the family member in the hall and ask them to keep the visit brief would go against the wishes of the client and endanger the trust relationship between the nurse and the client (option 2). Threatening the client that the visitor will not be allowed in if the client does not accept the nurse's strategy for pain control is not effective client care management (option 4). **Cognitive Level:** Analyzing **Client Need:** Physiological Integrity **Nursing Process:** Implementation **Learning Outcome:** 9-5

6. **Answer:** 4 **Rationale:** Research has shown that clients will often not voice their pain to the nurse unless the nurse specifically asks the question and assesses the level of pain. Therefore, the nurse should not have just accepted that the client did not complain of pain, but should have specifically asked about discomfort. Changing the client's bed linen (option 1), the need to administer an analgesic prophylactically (option 2), and getting the client out of bed and into a chair (option 3) are not indicated in the question stem and do not relate to assessing the client. **Cognitive Level:** Applying **Client Need:** Physiological Integrity **Nursing Process:** Implementation **Learning Outcome:** 9-6

7. **Answer:** 3 **Rationale:** Clients in acute pain need not be asked about how their ADLs have been affected because they are most likely not following normal daily routines. However, this is a very important question for those in chronic pain because it will contribute significantly to the pain assessment. All clients in pain should be asked about where the pain is located (option 1), the severity of the pain (option 2), and when it began (option 4). **Cognitive Level:** Analyzing **Client Need:** Physiological Integrity **Nursing Process:** Implementation **Learning Outcome:** 9-7

8. **Answer:** 1 **Rationale:** The nurse would provide the best pain control to the client with terminal cancer in severe pain if an opioid analgesic such as morphine sulfate were administered. While Demerol is an opioid analgesic, it has a short half-life, produces toxic metabolites, and has the potential to induce seizures with repeated doses (option 2). Percocet would not be a good choice for a client in severe pain, and the addition of acetaminophen would limit the maximum dosage that could be administered without creating adverse effects such as liver damage (option 3). Aspirin would not be used for severe pain in a terminal cancer client because it would be unlikely to provide adequate relief (option 4). **Cognitive Level:** Analyzing **Client Need:** Physiological Integrity **Nursing Process:** Planning **Learning Outcome:** 9-8

9. **Answer:** 3 **Rationale:** Use of a PCA avoids the roller-coaster effect of peaks of sedation and valleys of pain by allowing the client to administer less medication and maintain a more constant level of pain control. The pump is set to avoid overdosage, and the client will use less medication to control the pain, not more (option 1). PCA allows the use of less medication, not more, to achieve the same level of relief (option 2). It is never a good strategy to have someone else push the button for the client, and the family will need to be instructed that only the client should press the button to avoid the complication of overdosage (option 4). **Cognitive Level:** Analyzing **Client Need:** Physiological Integrity **Nursing Process:** Evaluation **Learning Outcome:** 9-11b

10. **Answer:** 2 **Rationale:** Nonpharmacologic interventions such as helping the client to control breathing can be very helpful in pain management. Assisting the client out of bed at this time would likely make the pain worse prior to the family's visit and would not be a good intervention (option 1). Administering morphine sulfate (option 3) and canceling visiting hours would both go against the client's wishes (option 4). **Cognitive Level:** Analyzing **Client Need:** Physiological Integrity **Nursing Process:** Implementation **Learning Outcome:** 9-9

Chapter 10: Positioning the Client

1. **Answer:** 3 **Rationale:** In the dorsal recumbent (back-lying) position, the client's head and shoulders are slightly elevated on a small pillow. In Fowler's or semisitting position, the head and trunk are raised and the knees may or may not be flexed (option 1). In the orthopneic position the client either sits in bed or on the side of the bed with an overbed table across the lap (option 2). In the prone position, the client lies on his or her abdomen with the head turned to one side (option 4). **Cognitive Level:** Applying **Client Need:** Physiological Integrity **Nursing Process:** Planning **Learning Outcome:** 10-1

2. **Answer:** 2 **Rationale:** Avoid stretching, reaching, and twisting, which may place the line of gravity outside the base of support. Before moving an object, widen your stance and flex your knees, hips, and ankles (option 1). Always face the direction of the movement (option 3). Adjust the working area to waist level and keep the body close to the area (option 4). **Cognitive Level:** Applying **Client Need:** Safe and Effective Care Environment **Nursing Process:** Evaluation **Learning Outcome:** 10-2

3. **Answer:** 2 **Rationale:** The average nurse should not lift more than 35 pounds and only under very controlled circumstances. Nurses who are physically fit are at no less risk of injury (option 1). Back belts are likely not effective in reducing back injury (option 3). Training nurses in body mechanics alone will not prevent job-related injuries (option 4). **Cognitive Level:** Applying **Client Need:** Safe and Effective Care Environment **Nursing Process:** Planning **Learning Outcome:** 10-3

4. **Answer:** 1, 2, 4, and 5 **Rationale:** Remove all pillows, and then place one against the head of the bed. This pillow protects the client's head from inadvertent injury against the top of the bed during the upward move (option 1). Elicit the client's help in lessening the workload (option 2). Ensure client comfort by elevating the head of the bed and provide appropriate support devices for the client's new position (option 4). Use a friction-reducing device to help pull the client up in bed (option 5). Option 3 is incorrect because you should face the direction of the movement, not opposite from the movement, and then assume a broad stance with the foot nearest the bed behind the forward foot and weight on the forward foot. **Cognitive Level:** Applying **Client Need:** Safe and Effective Care Environment **Nursing Process:** Planning **Learning Outcome:** 10-6b

5. **Answer:** 1 **Rationale:** A trochanter roll is usually made by rolling a towel or bath blanket. Placed from the client's iliac crest to midthigh, it prevents external rotation of the leg when the client is in a supine position. A footboard is used to prevent plantar flexion, not external rotation of the leg (option 2). A hand roll can be made by rolling a washcloth. The purpose of a hand roll is to keep the hand in a functional position and prevent finger contractures (option 3). An abduction pillow is a triangular-shaped foam pillow that maintains hip abduction to prevent hip dislocation following total hip replacement (option 4). **Cognitive Level:** Applying **Client Need:** Safe and Effective Care Environment **Nursing Process:** Planning **Learning Outcome:** 10-7

6. **Answer:** 4 **Rationale:** To support a client in the Sims' (semiprone) position (supported), it is best to use a pillow to support the head, maintaining it in good alignment unless drainage from the mouth is required. Option 1 is incorrect because a sandbag (or rolled towels) will support the feet in dorsiflexion to prevent foot drop. Option 2 is incorrect because a pillow under the upper leg will support it in alignment and prevent internal rotation and abduction of the hip and leg. Option 3 is incorrect because a pillow under the upper arm will prevent internal rotation of the shoulder and arm. **Cognitive Level:** Applying **Client Need:** Safe and Effective Care Environment **Nursing Process:** Implementation **Learning Outcome:** 10-4

7. **Answer:** 4 **Rationale:** The person lifting should rock from the front leg to the back leg when pulling, or from the back leg to the front leg when pushing to overcome inertia, counteract the client's weight, and help attain a balanced smooth motion. In moving or lifting clients, an appropriate number of staff and assistive devices should be utilized (options 1 and 2). The height of the bed should bring the client close to your center of gravity (option 3). **Cognitive Level:** Applying **Client Need:** Safe and Effective Care Environment **Nursing Process:** Implementation **Learning Outcome:** 10-2

8. **Answer:** 3 **Rationale:** The client who is in a chronic vegetative state could be safely repositioned by the UAP. Repositioning can generally be delegated to UAP, but a client who recently had a lumbar laminectomy (option 1), a client who is being evaluated for a cervical injury (option 2), and a client who was intubated and placed on a ventilator (option 4) are not considered stable enough for a UAP to reposition. **Cognitive Level:** Analyzing **Client Need:** Safe and Effective Care Environment **Nursing Process:** Planning **Learning Outcome:** 10-5

9. **Answer:** 2 **Rationale:** Explaining the procedure is an important first step in performing any procedure and is especially important when using a hydraulic lift on a client for the first time. The process may be frightening to clients. Increasing client understanding of what to expect may also help the client participate more. Positioning the client on the sling (option 1) and lifting the client gradually (option 3) occur after beginning the procedure, not before. It is not necessary to apply gloves unless the client has open wounds or the nurse may be exposed to blood or body fluids (option 4). **Cognitive Level:** Applying **Client Need:** Psychosocial Integrity **Nursing Process:** Implementation **Learning Outcome:** 10-6h

10. **Answer:** 1, 2, and 3 **Rationale:** It is important to document when the client is repositioned, the position in which the client is placed (option 1), any change in skin integrity (option 2), and the number of staff helping to reposition the client (option 3). Long-term care facilities in most areas are required to set the number of staff required for transfers and repositioning to prevent client harm, and failure to follow this procedure can result in claims of abuse. It is not necessary to document body mechanics used by the staff (option 4) or the rationale for frequent repositioning (option 5). **Cognitive Level:** Applying **Client Need:** Safe and Effective Care Environment **Nursing Process:** Evaluation **Learning Outcome:** 10-8

Chapter 11: Mobilizing the Client

1. **Answer:** 3 **Rationale:** The Lofstrand crutch is a mechanical aid that extends only to the forearm. The most frequently used crutches are the underarm crutch and axillary crutch with hand bars. The metal cuff around the forearm and the metal bar stabilize the wrists and thus

make walking safer and easier (option 1). Walkers are for clients who need more support than a cane provides (option 2). The quad cane has four feet (option 4). **Cognitive Level:** Applying **Client Need:** Physiological Integrity **Nursing Process:** Assessment **Learning Outcome:** 11-1

2. **Answer:** 2 **Rationale:** It is not safe for the client or his wife if she tries to help him stand in the shower. Wearing nonskid shoes to ambulate is correct and safe (option 1). When making a home visit, assess carefully for safety issues for ambulation. The client and family should be counseled about unfastened rugs (option 4) and loose objects on the floors (option 3). **Cognitive Level:** Applying **Client Need:** Safe and Effective Care Environment **Nursing Process:** Evaluation **Learning Outcome:** 11-2

3. **Answer:** 1 **Rationale:** The weight of the client's body should be borne by the arms rather than the axillae (armpits). Continual pressure on the axillae can injure the radial nerve and eventually cause crutch palsy, a weakness of the muscles of the forearm, wrist, and hand. The client should maintain an erect posture as much as possible to prevent strain on muscles and joints to maintain balance (option 2). The client should wear a shoe with a low heel that grips the floor. Rubber soles decrease the chances of slipping (option 3). Crutch length should be tailored for each client. The shoulder rest should be three fingerwidths below the axillae when in a standing position (option 4). **Cognitive Level:** Applying **Client Need:** Physiological Integrity **Nursing Process:** Implementation **Learning Outcome:** 11-4d

4. **Answer:** 1 and 5 **Rationale:** Always lock the brakes on both wheels of the wheelchair when the client transfers in or out of it. Recognize that the wheel locks are not brakes. They will not stop a rolling wheelchair and may not prevent sliding (option 1). Back the wheelchair into or out of an elevator, rear large wheels first. This allows the client to see the door and makes exiting the elevator easier (option 5). Option 3 is incorrect because the footplates should be raised before, not after, transferring the client into the wheelchair (option 3). Lower the footplates after, not before, the transfer, and place the client's feet on them (option 2). Ensure that the client is positioned well back in the seat of the wheelchair (option 4). **Cognitive Level:** Applying **Client Need:** Safe and Effective Care Environment **Nursing Process:** Planning **Learning Outcome:** 11-4a

5. **Answer:** 4 **Rationale:** The client who is 2 days postoperative may be more stable than the other clients in options 1, 2, and 3, who are experiencing acute issues that would negatively affect balance. **Cognitive Level:** Applying **Client Need:** Safe and Effective Care Environment **Nursing Process:** Planning **Learning Outcome:** 11-3

6. **Answer:** 1, 2, 3, and 5 **Rationale:** Document distance (option 1) and duration (option 2) of ambulation in the client record using forms or checklists supplemented by narrative notes when appropriate. Include description of the client's gait (including body alignment) when walking (option 3), pace, activity tolerance when walking (i.e., pulse rate, facial color, any shortness of breath, feelings of dizziness, or weakness), and degree of support required (option 5). Option 4 is incorrect because blood pressure should be taken after initial ambulation to compare with baseline data. **Cognitive Level:** Applying **Client Need:** Physiological Integrity **Nursing Process:** Evaluation **Learning Outcome:** 11-5

7. **Answer:** 4 **Rationale:** It is safer to use an assistive device with the appropriate number of staff than to move a client without sufficient assistance. Transferring the client without assistance (option 1) or with the help of only one other person (option 3) could result in potential injury to the client or staff, and charges of abuse for not following the assigned transfer requirement of three people. Encouraging the client to wait for additional assistance, when the client is uncomfortable, is not the best strategy because it allows the client's discomfort to continue unaddressed, and may make the client less willing to get out of bed in the future for fear of being "stuck" there (option 2). **Cognitive**

Level: Analyzing **Client Need:** Safe and Effective Care Environment **Nursing Process:** Planning **Learning Outcome:** 11-2

8. **Answer:** 2 **Rationale:** The client should be encouraged to be as independent as possible while in bed to maintain muscle strength of all extremities except the fractured leg. All other answer options would be contraindicated or impossible while the client is in traction and unable to move the restrained fractured leg. **Cognitive Level:** Analyzing **Client Need:** Physiological Integrity **Nursing Process:** Implementation **Learning Outcome:** 11-4b

9. **Answer:** 2 **Rationale:** Instead of pushing the client in a wheelchair forward into the elevator, the UAP should back into the elevator because the rear wheels are stable and larger and are less likely to tip the client out of the chair. Options 1, 3, and 4 are correct procedures for transporting a client in a wheelchair. **Cognitive Level:** Applying **Client Need:** Safe and Effective Care Environment **Nursing Process:** Evaluation **Learning Outcome:** 11-4a

10. **Answer:** 3 **Rationale:** The client should be standing upright with the elbow flexed slightly. The client should not have straight elbows (option 1) or have to stoop or flex the knees (option 2). An elbow flexed to 45° is at too great an angle (option 4). **Cognitive Level:** Analyzing **Client Need:** Safe and Effective Care Environment **Nursing Process:** Evaluation **Learning Outcome:** 11-4c

Chapter 12: Fall Prevention and Restraints

1. **Answer:** 3 **Rationale:** Electronic safety monitoring devices are available to detect clients who are attempting to move or get out of bed. Physical restraints are any manual method or physical or mechanical device, material, or equipment attached to the client's body (option 1). Chemical restraints are medications such as neuroleptics, anxiolytics, sedatives, and psychotropic agents used to control socially disruptive behavior (option 2). Seizure precautions, not a seizure monitoring device, are safety measures taken by the nurse to protect clients from injury should they have a seizure (option 4). **Cognitive Level:** Remembering **Client Need:** Safe and Effective Care Environment **Nursing Process:** Planning **Learning Outcome:** 12-1

2. **Answer:** 1, 2, 3, and 4 **Rationale:** It is important for the client to have shoes or slippers with nonskid soles that fit well (option 1), an uncluttered environment (option 2), and adequate lighting in the house (option 3) and to reduce the use of alcohol (option 4). Although a voiding routine is very helpful in minimizing the client's need to rush to the toilet and potentially fall, the schedule should be at intervals appropriate for the client and not necessarily frequent (option 5). **Cognitive Level:** Applying **Client Need:** Safe and Effective Care Environment **Nursing Process:** Planning **Learning Outcome:** 12-2

3. **Answer:** 1 **Rationale:** The purpose of restraints is to prevent the client from injuring self or others. Restraints are not indicated to prevent the nurse from having extra work (option 2), to prevent the client from being embarrassed later (option 3), or to prevent the primary care provider from having to order more medications (option 4). **Cognitive Level:** Analyzing **Client Need:** Safe and Effective Care Environment **Nursing Process:** Implementation **Learning Outcome:** 12-3

4. **Answer:** 2 **Rationale:** Belt restraints must be applied to all clients on stretchers even when the side rails are raised. If a Velcro safety belt is to be used, make sure that both pieces of Velcro are intact (option 1). Attach the belt around the client's waist, and fasten it at the back of the chair (option 3). There should be a fingerwidth between the belt and the client (option 4). **Cognitive Level:** Applying **Client Need:** Safe and Effective Care Environment **Nursing Process:** Implementation **Learning Outcome:** 12-4

5. **Answer:** 2 **Rationale:** Discuss the need to inform the Department of Motor Vehicles of the seizure disorder. Option 1 is incorrect because it is important for the nurse to discuss with the client and family factors that may precipitate a seizure, such as stress. If seizures are not well

controlled, activities that may require restriction or direct supervision by others include tub bathing, swimming, cooking, using electric equipment or machinery, and driving (option 3). When making home visits, it is important for the nurse to inspect anticonvulsant medications and confirm that clients are taking them correctly. Blood level measurements of medications may be assessed periodically, and the nurse must monitor the client for follow-through (option 4). **Cognitive Level:** Applying **Client Need:** Safe and Effective Care Environment **Nursing Process:** Implementation **Learning Outcome:** 12-6c

6. **Answer: 4 Rationale:** UAP can obtain blankets or other linens with which to pad the side rails. UAP should be familiar with establishing seizure precautions and methods of obtaining assistance during a client's seizure. Care of the client during a seizure, including careful assessment of respiratory status (option 1), determining the need to call the primary care provider (option 2), and evaluating the type and length of seizure, however, is the responsibility of the nurse. **Cognitive Level:** Applying **Client Need:** Safe and Effective Care Environment **Nursing Process:** Implementation **Learning Outcome:** 12-5

7. **Answer: 1, 2, 3, and 4 Rationale:** The nurse should monitor and document the skin status beneath the restraints (option 1), the circulatory status of the restrained limbs (option 2), the IV site because its integrity may be related to the effectiveness of the mitt (option 3), and the frequency of restraint assessment performed (option 4). Although monitoring urine output (option 5) may be indicated in the care of the client, it is not directly related to the use of restraints. **Cognitive Level:** Applying **Client Need:** Physiological Integrity **Nursing Process:** Evaluation **Learning Outcome:** 12-7

8. **Answer: 2 Rationale:** The nurse should remain at the site of the spill and send someone else to get help in order to prevent someone from slipping in the water while retrieving supplies. The nurse should not leave the site of the spill to get towels (option 1), call housekeeping (option 3), or refill the pitcher (option 4). Housekeeping personnel are the preferred personnel to clean the spill because they can place caution signs around the spill until the floor is completely dry and the nurse can resume his or her professional duties. **Cognitive Level:** Analyzing **Client Need:** Safe and Effective Care Environment **Nursing Process:** Implementation **Learning Outcome:** 12-2

9. **Answer: 4 Rationale:** The biggest risk for falls in this client is the medical diagnosis of syncope. The hospital's environment (option 1) and equipment (option 2) are monitored closely for safety and are unlikely to be this client's greatest risk. Because the client was previously healthy and vigorous, it is unlikely that prior accident history will be significant (option 3). **Cognitive Level:** Analyzing **Client Need:** Physiological Integrity **Nursing Process:** Assessment **Learning Outcome:** 12-2

10. **Answer: 1 Rationale:** The nurse would begin with the least restrictive restraint, which would be the mitt restraint, to prevent the client from being able to grasp the catheter. If the mitt restraint is not effective, it is possible the nurse may need a more restrictive restraint such as the limb restraint (option 2), but this can make the client more combative and should be avoided if possible. The waist restraint (option 3) or vest restraint (option 4) would serve no useful purpose in this scenario since the hands remain free. **Cognitive Level:** Analyzing **Client Need:** Physiological Integrity **Nursing Process:** Planning **Learning Outcome:** 12-4

Chapter 13: Maintaining Joint Mobility

1. **Answer: 1 Rationale:** Abduction is the movement of the bone away, not toward, the midline of the body. The definitions in options 2, 3, and 4 are correctly stated. **Cognitive Level:** Applying **Client Need:** Health Promotion and Maintenance **Nursing Process:** Implementation **Learning Outcome:** 13-1

2. **Answer: 4 Rationale:** When the client performs the movements systematically, using the same sequence during each session, the nurse can evaluate that the teaching was understood and is successful. When performing active ROM the client should exercise to the point of slight resistance, but never past that point of resistance in order to prevent further injury (option 1). The client should perform each exercise at least five times, not just once (option 2). The client should perform each series of exercises twice daily, not just once per day (option 3). **Cognitive Level:** Applying **Client Need:** Physiological Integrity **Nursing Process:** Evaluation **Learning Outcome:** 13-2a

3. **Answer: 3 Rationale:** The nurse is correct when stating that passive ROM exercises are useful in maintaining joint flexibility. Passive ROM requires someone else to move the joint. If the client moves independently it would be active ROM (option 1). Passive ROM does not maintain muscle strength because there is no resistance to movement (option 2). When performing passive ROM, the body parts should be moved smoothly, slowly, and rhythmically. Jerky movements cause discomfort and possibly injury. Fast movements can cause spasticity and potential injury (option 4). **Cognitive Level:** Applying **Client Need:** Health Promotion and Maintenance **Nursing Process:** Implementation **Learning Outcome:** 13-2b

4. **Answer: 2 Rationale:** The wrist should normally be flexed 80° to 90°. The elbow normally flexes 150°, and flexing it 180° would cause serious injury (option 1). The hip abducts 45° to 50°, not 90° (option 3). The knee extends no more than 120° to 130°, not 45° to 90° (option 4). **Cognitive Level:** Applying **Client Need:** Safe and Effective Care Environment **Nursing Process:** Planning **Learning Outcome:** 13-3

5. **Answer: 2, 3, and 5 Rationale:** The CPM may be safely applied for 2 hours at a time, or up to 14 hours, depending on the primary care provider's order (option 2). The nurse must carefully document the degree of flexion and extension as well as the speed of the CPM (option 3). The client is given a remote control allowing the machine to be stopped if it becomes too painful for the client to tolerate (option 5). However, once applied, the apparatus should be removed at least every 4 hours, not once per 8-hour shift, to assess skin integrity (option 1). The settings are not continuous because they will be changed to assist the joint to progress toward greater range of motion after surgery (option 4). **Cognitive Level:** Applying **Client Need:** Physiological Integrity **Nursing Process:** Implementation **Learning Outcome:** 13-6b

6. **Answer: 2 Rationale:** Performing passive ROM exercises can be delegated to unlicensed assistive personnel when the client's condition is stable, such as the client who had a cerebrovascular accident 10 days ago. Passive ROM should not be delegated to the UAP on unstable clients such as the client with a spinal cord injury due to a recent motor vehicle crash (option 1), or with increasing intracranial pressure during procedures (option 3), or the client who recently sustained an orthopedic trauma (option 4). **Cognitive Level:** Applying **Client Need:** Safe and Effective Care Environment **Nursing Process:** Planning **Learning Outcome:** 13-5

7. **Answer: 3 Rationale:** The CPM continues to be used after total joint replacement surgery. The CPM is most often used for clients requiring short-term assistance so it would not be used for a client with quadriplegia (option 1) or a client in a chronic vegetative state (option 2). CPM would not improve muscle strength in the athlete because the muscle is not actively contracting during CPM (option 4). **Cognitive Level:** Analyzing **Client Need:** Physiological Integrity: Physiological Adaptation **Nursing Process:** Planning **Learning Outcome:** 13-4

8. **Answer: 2 Rationale:** If the client's joint unexpectedly changes, such as new edema or pain, the primary care provider should be notified to determine possible new injury to the joint. Clients can be expected to be fatigued in the evening, and exercises should be initiated earlier the next day, but this does not need to be reported to the primary care provider (option 1). The client whose elbow has been resistant to movement and remains unchanged would not need to be reported

immediately, but it should be documented in the client's chart (option 3). It is not unusual for clients to prefer doing ROM when visitors are not present and this would not need to be reported to the primary care provider. **Cognitive Level:** Analyzing **Client Need:** Safe and Effective Care Environment **Nursing Process:** Evaluation **Learning Outcome:** 13-7

9. **Answer:** 3 **Rationale:** Passive range of motion should be performed in a sequential format, usually starting at the head and moving down to the feet. This leads to a more flowing process as well as ensuring that no joints are forgotten. From these choices, starting at the neck and moving down to the elbow, the hip, the knee, and then the ankle would represent the most logical and flowing sequence. The sequences presented in options 1, 2, and 4 are incorrect. **Cognitive Level:** Applying **Client Need:** Physiological Integrity: Basic Care and Comfort **Nursing Process:** Implementation **Learning Outcome:** 13-6a

10. **Answer:** 1 **Rationale:** The exercise of moving the arm laterally from the position beside the head downward laterally and across the front of the body as far as possible is adduction of the arm. External rotation would occur when the arm is held out to the side at shoulder level and the elbow is bent to a right angle with the fingers pointing down and then is moved upward so the fingers point up and the back of the hand touches the mattress (option 2). Internal rotation would be performed with the arm held out to the side at shoulder level and the elbow bent to a right angle, fingers pointing up. Bring the arm forward and down so that the palm touches the mattress (option 3). Circumduction of the arm would be moving the arm forward, up, back, and down in a full circle (option 4). **Cognitive Level:** Applying **Client Need:** Physiological Integrity **Nursing Process:** Implementation **Learning Outcome:** 13-1

Chapter 14: Drug Calculations

1. **Answer:** 3 **Rationale:** Household measures may be used when more accurate systems of measure are not required. Included in household measures are drops, teaspoons, tablespoons, cups, and glasses. The apothecaries' system, which is older than the metric system, was brought to the United States from England during the colonial period (option 1). The ratio and proportion method is considered the oldest method used for calculating dosages (option 2). The fractional equation method is similar to ratio and proportion, except that equations are written as fractions (option 4). **Cognitive Level:** Not Applicable **Client Need:** Physiological Integrity **Nursing Process:** Planning **Learning Outcome:** 14-1

2. **Answer:** 1 **Rationale:** The basic unit of weight in the apothecaries' system is the grain (gr), likened to a grain of wheat, and the basic unit of volume is the minim, a volume of water equal in weight to a grain of wheat. Basic units of measurement in the metric system are the meter (option 2), the gram (option 3), and the liter (option 4). **Cognitive Level:** Not Applicable **Client Need:** Physiological Integrity **Nursing Process:** Assessment **Learning Outcome:** 14-2

3. **Answer:** 4 **Rationale:** To convert grams to milligrams, multiply the number of grams by 1,000 or move the decimal point three places to the right: 1 gram multiplied by 1,000 equals 1,000 mg. **Cognitive Level:** Applying **Client Need:** Physiological Integrity **Nursing Process:** Implementation **Learning Outcome:** 14-3

4. **Answer:** 2 **Rationale:** 60 mg equals 1 grain (gr); 1 mg equals 1/60 grain in the apothecaries' system (option 1); 1 gram equals 15 grains (option 3); 4 grams equals 1 dram (option 4). **Cognitive Level:** Applying **Client Need:** Physiological Integrity **Nursing Process:** Planning **Learning Outcome:** 14-4

5. **Answer:** 1 **Rationale:** "1 milliliter is the same as 15 minims or 15 drops" is a correct statement. Option 2 is incorrect because 15 milliliters equals 4 drams or 1 tablespoon. Option 3 is incorrect because 500 milliliters equals 1 pint in both of the other systems. Option 4 is incorrect because 4,000 milliliters equals 1 gallon in both of the other

systems. **Cognitive Level:** Applying **Client Need:** Physiological Integrity **Nursing Process:** Planning **Learning Outcome:** 14-5

6. **Answer:** 75 kg **Rationale:** The pound is a smaller unit than the kilogram, and the nurse converts by dividing 165 lb by 2.2, which yields an answer of 75 kg. **Cognitive Level:** Applying **Client Need:** Physiological Integrity **Nursing Process:** Planning **Learning Outcome:** 14-6

7. **Answer:** 1 **Rationale:** In the ratio and proportion method of calculating dosages, the equation is set up with the known quantities on the left side (i.e., H and V). The right side of the equation consists of the desired dose (i.e., D) and the unknown amount to administer (i.e., x).

$H = 250$ mg

$V = 1$ capsule

$D = 500$ mg

250 mg: 1 :: 500 mg: x

$$\frac{250x}{250} = \frac{500}{250}$$

$x = 2$ capsules

Cognitive Level: Applying **Client Need:** Physiological Integrity **Nursing Process:** Planning **Learning Outcome:** 14-7

8. **Answer:** 1.2 mL **Rationale:** In the ratio and proportion method, the equation is set up with the known quantities on the left side (i.e., H and V). The right side of the equation consists of the desired dose (i.e., D) and the unknown amount to administer (i.e., x).

$H = 125$ mg

$V = 2$ mL

$D = 75$ mg

125: 2 :: 75: x

$125x = 150$

$$x = \frac{150}{125}$$

Cognitive Level: Applying **Client Need:** Physiological Integrity **Nursing Process:** Planning **Learning Outcome:** 14-7

9. **Answer:** 3 **Rationale:** Use dimensional analysis:

$$\frac{250 \text{ mL}}{100 \text{ mg}} \times \frac{1 \text{ mg}}{1,000 \text{ mcg}} \times \frac{20 \text{ mcg}}{1 \text{ min}} \times \frac{60 \text{ min}}{1 \text{ h}} = \frac{3 \text{ mL}}{1 \text{ h}}$$

Cognitive Level: Applying **Client Need:** Physiological Integrity **Nursing Process:** Planning **Learning Outcome:** 14-9A

10. **Answer:** 1 **Rationale:** Use the following formula:

First the nurse converts the mg in the IV bag (400) to mcg:

Cross multiply:

Next, the medication concentration (mcg/mL) needs to be determined:

Complete the formula:

Nurses using dimensional analysis would put all of the information into one formula:

$$91 \text{ kg} \times \frac{3 \text{ mcg}}{\text{kg/min}} \times \frac{1 \text{ mg}}{1,000 \text{ mcg}} \times \frac{250 \text{ mL}}{400 \text{ mg}} \times \frac{60 \text{ min}}{1 \text{ h}} = \frac{10.2 \text{ mL}}{\text{h}}$$

$x = 10.2$ mL/h if the IV pump can be set to tenths; otherwise, it would be rounded to the nearest whole number.

Cognitive Level: Applying **Client Need:** Physiological Integrity **Nursing Process:** Planning **Learning Outcome:** 14-9c

Chapter 15: Administering Oral and Enteral Medications

1. **Answer:** 3 **Rationale:** The brand name of a drug is always capitalized and is the name used by a drug manufacturer to market a drug. The generic name is not capitalized and is the name given to the drug before it becomes an officially approved medication and is used throughout

the drug's use (option 1). The chemical name is the name describing the constituents of the drug precisely (option 2). The official name is the name under which it is listed in one of the official publications (option 4). **Cognitive Level:** Applying **Client Need:** Physiological Integrity **Nursing Process:** Implementation **Learning Outcome:** 15-1

2. **Answer:** 4 **Rationale:** The nurse is equally as liable for the error as the primary care provider and pharmacist because each one of them was responsible for his or her own practice and should have caught the mistake before administering the medication to the client. Options 2, 3, and 4 are incorrect because no one in this triad was less or more responsible and each shares equally in the error. Therefore, all are legally liable. **Cognitive Level:** Analyzing **Client Need:** Physiological Integrity **Nursing Process:** Evaluation **Learning Outcome:** 15-2

3. **Answer:** 2 **Rationale:** The fastest acting route for this medication would be sublingual because of the high vascularity of the area. The drug is dissolved and absorbed into the bloodstream within a few minutes. Any of the other routes—ointment (option 1), oral (option 3), or buccal (option 4)—would be far slower acting. **Cognitive Level:** Applying **Client Need:** Physiological Integrity **Nursing Process:** Planning **Learning Outcome:** 15-3

4. **Answer:** 3 **Rationale:** The medication order for Tylenol does not have a frequency. Although it says prn there should still be an order for frequency such as every 4 hours prn or every 6 hours prn. The orders in options 1, 2, and 4 have the name of the drug, the route, the frequency, and the dosage so they would be acceptable medication orders. **Cognitive Level:** Analyzing **Client Need:** Physiological Integrity **Nursing Process:** Planning **Learning Outcome:** 15-5

5. **Answer:** 3 **Rationale:** When a drug is ordered to be administered immediately, it is a stat order. A standing order would imply the drug is to be given repeatedly based on the frequency provided by the primary care provider, but this order is a one-time order (option 1). If the drug were ordered to be given as needed, it would be a prn order (option 2). Although the medication is a single order (option 4), the fact that it is to be given immediately makes it a stat order. **Cognitive Level:** Remembering **Client Need:** Physiological Integrity **Nursing Process:** Implementation **Learning Outcome:** 15-4

6. **Answer:** 2, 3, 4, and 5 **Rationale:** The nurse types in the individual password (option 4) assigned to that nurse, chooses the client's name from a list on the screen (option 2), and then chooses the medication to be administered from an onscreen list (option 3) and compares the medication to the MAR as a safety check (option 5). The automated dispensing cabinet does not require the use of a key (option 1). **Cognitive Level:** Applying **Client Need:** Physiological Integrity **Nursing Process:** Implementation **Learning Outcome:** 15-6

7. **Answer:** 1, 2, and 3 **Rationale:** Prior to administering the medication, the nurse would check that it is the right medication (option 1), the right dosage (option 2), and the right time (option 3). Only after administering the medication would the nurse check that it is the right documentation (option 4) and the right evaluation (option 5). Drugs should never be documented until after they are administered and they cannot be evaluated until after they are administered. **Cognitive Level:** Applying **Client Need:** Physiological Integrity **Nursing Process:** Implementation **Learning Outcome:** 15-7

8. **Answer:** 3 **Rationale:** The nurse would need to clarify the right route because this is not indicated in the primary care provider's order. The right drug is morphine (option 1), the right dose is 8 mg (option 2), and the right time is every 2 hours prn (option 4); therefore, the only right missing is the route. **Cognitive Level:** Applying **Client Need:** Physiological Integrity **Nursing Process:** Evaluation **Learning Outcome:** 15-7

9. **Answer:** 5, 2, 4, 1, and 3 **Rationale:** The nurse should first determine what allergies the client may have (option 5), then check the MAR (option 2) to ensure that the allergy is recorded along with the drug name, frequency, and route of administration, and that the expiration date for

the order matches the primary care provider's order. Prior to touching medications the nurse performs hand hygiene (option 4) and then pours the medication (option 1). On entering the client's room with the medication, the nurse checks the client's ID band to ensure this is the right client (option 3). **Cognitive Level:** Analyzing **Client Need:** Physiological Integrity **Nursing Process:** Implementation **Learning Outcome:** 15-9a

10. **Answer:** 1 **Rationale:** The nurse should never crush an enteric-coated tablet because the effects of the enteric coating would be lost. It is always a safe practice to check with the pharmacy prior to crushing any tablet medication to ensure that crushing is permissible. Liquid (option 2), Tylenol tablet (option 3), and drop (option 4) medications may all be safely administered via an enteral tube. **Cognitive Level:** Applying **Client Need:** Physiological Integrity **Nursing Process:** Planning **Learning Outcome:** 15-9b

Chapter 16: Administering Topical Medications

1. **Answer:** 1, 2, 3, 4, and 5 **Rationale:** Topical skin or dermatologic preparations include ointments, pastes, creams, lotions, powders, sprays, and patches. **Cognitive Level:** Remembering: Physiological Integrity **Nursing Process:** Planning **Learning Outcome:** 16-1

2. **Answer:** 3 **Rationale:** Patches should not be applied to areas with cuts, burns, or abrasions, or on distal parts of extremities (options 2 and 3). Generally, the patch is applied to a hairless, clean area of skin that is not subject to excessive movement or wrinkling (option 1). It may also be applied on the side, lower back, or buttocks. When transdermal patches are removed, care needs to be taken as to how and where they are discarded to avoid exposure from any drug remaining on the patch (option 4). **Cognitive Level:** Applying **Client Need:** Physiological Integrity **Nursing Process:** Evaluation **Learning Outcome:** 16-3a

3. **Answer:** 2 **Rationale:** Sterile cotton balls are used to remove material from the eyelids. If not removed, material on the eyelid and lashes can be washed into the eye. Option 1 is incorrect because the first bead of ointment from a tube is considered to be contaminated. Option 3 is incorrect because cleaning toward the outer canthus prevents contamination of the other eye and the lacrimal duct. Option 4 is incorrect. Instruct the client to look up at the ceiling; the client is less likely to blink if looking up. **Cognitive Level:** Applying **Client Need:** Physiological Integrity **Nursing Process:** Evaluation **Learning Outcome:** 16-3b

4. **Answer:** 1 **Rationale:** Because in infants and children under 3 years of age, the ear canal is directed upward to administer medication, gently pull the pinna down and back, not up and back. For a child older than 3 years of age, pull the pinna upward and backward. Option 2, obtaining assistance to immobilize an infant or young child, is an appropriate action. Option 3, using cotton-tipped applicators and solution to wipe the pinna and auditory meatus, is appropriate. This removes any discharge present before the instillation so that it will not be washed into the ear canal. Option 4 is appropriate because warming the medication container in the hands or placing it in warm water for a short time makes it more comfortable for the client. **Cognitive Level:** Applying **Client Need:** Physiological Integrity **Nursing Process:** Evaluation **Learning Outcome:** 16-3c

5. **Answer:** 4 **Rationale:** Hold the tip of the dropper just above the nostril, and direct the solution laterally toward the midline of the superior concha of the ethmoid bone as the client breathes through the mouth. Option 1 is incorrect because the solution should be administered laterally not medially. Option 2 is incorrect because the client should not touch the mucous membranes of the nares. If the solution is directed toward the base of the nasal cavity, it will run down the eustachian tube. Touching the membrane with the dropper could damage the membrane and cause the client to sneeze. Option 3 is incorrect because the client should remain in the position for 5 minutes. The client remains in the same position to help the solution come in contact with

all of the nasal surface or flow into the desired area. **Cognitive Level:** Applying **Client Need:** Physiological Integrity **Nursing Process:** Evaluation **Learning Outcome:** 16-3d

6. **Answer:** 4 **Rationale:** Bronchodilators are administered first to open the airways prior to the administration of the inhaled steroid. Option 1 is incorrect because an extender or spacer may be attached to the mouthpiece to facilitate medication absorption for better results. Option 2 is incorrect because the inhaler should be shaken vigorously for 3 to 5 seconds to mix the medication evenly, holding the inhaler upright. Option 3 is incorrect because the child should hold the breath for 10 seconds or as long as possible in order for the aerosol to reach the deeper airways. **Cognitive Level:** Analyzing **Client Need:** Physiological Integrity **Nursing Process:** Evaluation **Learning Outcome:** 16-3e

7. **Answer:** 2 **Rationale:** Ask the client to remain lying in the supine position for about 5 to 10 minutes following insertion. This position allows the medication to flow into the posterior fornix after it has melted. Options 1, 3, and 4 pertain to administration of vaginal cream, jelly, or foam. **Cognitive Level:** Applying **Client Need:** Physiological Integrity **Nursing Process:** Implementation **Learning Outcome:** 16-3f

8. **Answer:** 3 **Rationale:** When administering rectal medications in an infant or a child, insert a suppository 5 cm (2 in.) or less. Options 1 and 4 are incorrect because for a child under 3 years, the mother should use the gloved fifth finger for insertion. After this age, the index finger can usually be used. The ring finger is not used. Option 2 is incorrect because the mother should obtain assistance to immobilize the client. This prevents accidental injury due to sudden movement during the procedure. **Cognitive Level:** Applying **Client Need:** Physiological Integrity **Nursing Process:** Evaluation **Learning Outcome:** 16-3g

9. **Answer:** 4 **Rationale:** Aerosolized medications are droplets suspended in a gas. Aerosolized medications are a form of nebulized medication, but there is no indication in the question as to whether they are warm mist or cool mist (options 1 and 2). Atomized medications have large droplets of medication (option 3). **Cognitive Level:** Applying **Client Need:** Physiological Integrity **Nursing Process:** Implementation **Learning Outcome:** 16-1

10. **Answer:** 1 **Rationale:** Pruritus is the symptom of itching, so asking if the client is still scratching would be an appropriate assessment question. Difficulty swallowing is dysphagia (option 2), purple spots on the arm are petechiae (option 3), and painful breathing is dyspnea (option 4). **Cognitive Level:** Applying **Client Need:** Physiological Integrity **Nursing Process:** Assessment **Learning Outcome:** 16-1

Chapter 17: Administering Parenteral Medications

1. **Answer:** 1 **Rationale:** The nurse would use a filter needle when withdrawing medication from the ampule in order to avoid potential glass shards in the medication. The gauge of the needle would be determined by the viscosity of the fluid, not the type of container the medication is removed from (option 3). There is no indication for the use of an alcohol swab (option 2) or an insulin syringe (option 4). **Cognitive Level:** Applying **Client Need:** Physiological Integrity **Nursing Process:** Implementation **Learning Outcome:** 17-1

2. **Answer:** 2 **Rationale:** For medication that is thick and viscous, a larger gauge needle would be used. The range of gauges that would be appropriate for intramuscular injection is #20 to #22, so the #20-gauge needle would be the proper choice. An #18-gauge needle (option 1) would be too large for intramuscular injection and cause a great deal of tissue trauma. A #22-gauge (option 3) or #24-gauge (option 4) needle would be too narrow to allow the fluid to pass through the needle. **Cognitive Level:** Applying **Client Need:** Physiological Integrity **Nursing Process:** Planning **Learning Outcome:** 17-2b

3. **Answer:** 5, 4, 3, 1, and 2 **Rationale:** Prior to beginning medication administration and preparation, the nurse should perform hand hygiene (option 5). After reading the label and checking that the nurse has the

correct medication, the plastic top covering the vial must be removed (option 4). The top should be cleaned with alcohol to prevent contamination from pathogens that may reside on the top of the vial (option 3). By injecting air (option 1) equal to the volume of medication to be withdrawn, the medication can be withdrawn easily (option 2) because negative pressure will not be created inside the vial. **Cognitive Level:** Applying **Client Need:** Physiological Integrity **Nursing Process:** Implementation **Learning Outcome:** 17-5a and b

4. **Answer:** 4 **Rationale:** Subcutaneous injections should be given in the abdomen for this client. Both arms should be avoided secondary to the bilateral mastectomies (option 1). The vastus lateralis (option 2) and deltoid (option 3) are muscles, and these sites are used for intramuscular injections. **Cognitive Level:** Remembering **Client Need:** Physiological Integrity **Nursing Process:** Implementation **Learning Outcome:** 17-3

5. **Answer:** 3 **Rationale:** When administering medications the fastest effects are obtained when given intravenous push. Intramuscular (option 1) is faster than subcutaneous (option 2) because of an improved blood supply in the muscle compared to the subcutaneous area, but is not as fast as the intravenous route, which enters the bloodstream immediately. Volume-controlled intravenous infusion would be the next fastest but would be slower than intravenous push because it would take longer for the medication to enter the bloodstream (option 4). **Cognitive Level:** Applying **Client Need:** Physiological Integrity **Nursing Process:** Implementation **Learning Outcome:** 17-4

6. **Answer:** 4 **Rationale:** The needle should be held at an angle of 15° when administering an intradermal injection. An angle greater than 15° increases the risk of injecting the medication into the subcutaneous space (options 1, 2, and 3). **Cognitive Level:** Applying **Client Need:** Physiological Integrity **Nursing Process:** Implementation **Learning Outcome:** 17-5d

7. **Answer:** 2 **Rationale:** Only the vastus lateralis muscle would be appropriate for a child younger than 2 years. Other sites such as the deltoid muscle (option 1), the ventrogluteal muscle (option 3), and the dorsogluteal site (option 4) are too small, have an increased risk of nerve damage, and are more likely to cause tissue trauma. **Cognitive Level:** Applying **Client Need:** Physiological Integrity **Nursing Process:** Implementation **Learning Outcome:** 17-3

8. **Answer:** 1 **Rationale:** The nurse's priority action would be to flush the line with normal saline because dextrose and Dilantin (phenytoin) create a glue-like substance that will clog the IV line. Clamping and crimping the tubing will not rid the line of dextrose and will result in the need to start a new IV site, which is not necessary if the nurse adequately flushes the catheter prior to administration (options 2 and 3). Although administering any IV push medication through the closest port is indicated, it is not the priority action in this case (option 4). **Cognitive Level:** Analyzing **Client Need:** Physiological Integrity **Nursing Process:** Implementation **Learning Outcome:** 17-4

9. **Answer:** 3 **Rationale:** The nurse should choose a #24- to #26-gauge needle, depending on the viscosity of the fluid. The smallest possible needle would be the nurse's best choice for an average-sized young adult. All other gauges in options 1, 2, and 4 would be incorrect. **Cognitive Level:** Applying **Client Need:** Physiological Integrity **Nursing Process:** Planning **Learning Outcome:** 17-2b

10. **Answer:** 3, 4, 1, 5, 2, 6, 7, and 8. **Rationale:** The nurse mixes the insulin, assesses the skin, and cleanses the skin. The nurse would then pinch the skin, insert the needle, inject the medication, count to five, and remove the syringe. **Cognitive Level:** Applying. **Client Need:** Physiological Integrity. **Nursing Process:** Implementation. **Learning Outcome:** 17-5c.

Chapter 18: Administering Intravenous Therapy

1. **Answer:** 2 **Rationale:** When a vesicant medication infiltrates the tissue, it is called an extravasation. The term infiltration would be

applied if the medication was not a vesicant (option 1). Although the extravasation might lead to phlebitis or thrombophlebitis (options 3 and 4), the majority of the trauma is on the tissues surrounding the vein, as opposed to within the vein. **Cognitive Level:** Applying **Client Need:** Physiological Integrity **Nursing Process:** Diagnosis **Learning Outcome:** 18-1

2. **Answer:** 2 **Rationale:** One reason a central venous catheter is placed is to administer multiple medications through a double- or triple-lumen catheter. Because same-day surgery clients are expected to go home at the end of the day, it would be unlikely this client would need a central catheter (option 1). A client diagnosed with myocardial infarction would be unlikely to need a central line unless the client's condition deteriorated (option 3). A client post-hernia repair would be unlikely to require a central venous line unless complications arose, which is not indicated in this answer option (option 4). **Cognitive Level:** Applying **Client Need:** Physiological Integrity **Nursing Process:** Planning **Learning Outcome:** 18-4

3. **Answer:** 4 **Rationale:** If UAP notice anything they consider abnormal, they should notify the nurse. It is the nurse's responsibility to inform the UAP of specific things to look for. Changing empty IV solution containers cannot be delegated to the UAP because the procedure requires knowledge of sterile technique (option 1). Confirming the correct IV drip rate is the nurse's responsibility (option 2). Assessment is not the responsibility of the UAP; it is the responsibility of the nurse (option 3). **Cognitive Level:** Applying **Client Need:** Safe and Effective Care Environment **Nursing Process:** Planning **Learning Outcome:** 18-5

4. **Answer:** 4 **Rationale:** If a client has an extravasation, the primary care provider should be notified as soon as possible because complications of some vesicants can be reduced by injection of specific medications, whereas others require rapid medical intervention. It is not necessary to report when you routinely initiate or complete IV therapy (options 1 and 2). Primary care providers do not need to be notified of a small infiltrate, but it should be documented in the client's medical record and your facility may require completion of an event reporting form (option 3). **Cognitive Level:** Applying **Client Need:** Physiological Integrity **Nursing Process:** Evaluation **Learning Outcome:** 18-9

5. **Answer:** 1 **Rationale:** Hypotonic solutions are administered for cellular dehydration, whereas isotonic solutions replace intravascular fluid, so these might both be appropriate for this client. Hypertonic solutions pull fluid from the extravascular spaces and would not be appropriate for this client (options 2 and 3). Whole blood is not indicated because there is no evidence of blood loss (option 4). **Cognitive Level:** Analyzing **Client Need:** Physiological Integrity **Nursing Process:** Planning **Learning Outcome:** 18-2

6. **Answer:** 3 **Rationale:** The cephalic vein is the best choice because it can accept a large-bore catheter. The metacarpal veins of the hand are too small for the administration of blood products, which are thick and frequently require a larger bore catheter (option 1). The antecubital basilic and median cubital vein would be best saved for the insertion of a peripheral intravenous central catheter or phlebotomy (options 2 and 4). **Cognitive Level:** Applying **Client Need:** Physiological Integrity **Nursing Process:** Planning **Learning Outcome:** 18-3

7. **Answer:** 13 **Rationale:** You want to deliver 80 mL per hour and it takes 10 drops to deliver 1 mL. Start by multiplying the amount to be delivered by drops per milliliter, which would be $80 \times 10 = 800$ drops per hour. You only want to count drops for 1 minute to determine you have set the proper rate, so divide the drops per hour by 60 (because there are 60 minutes in an hour). This would be 800 divided by $60 = 13.3$. Because it is impossible to have 0.3 drops, you would expect to count 13 drops per minute to deliver the proper quantity of fluid. **Cognitive Level:** Applying **Client Need:** Physiological Integrity **Nursing Process:** Planning **Learning Outcome:** 18-7

8. **Answer:** 3 **Rationale:** If the intravenous fluid is infusing four times faster than ordered, the first intervention should be to reduce the rate. Notification of the primary care provider and the charge nurse would occur after reducing the flow rate and performing an assessment of the client (options 1 and 4). Although assessing the client is vitally important, you do not want to allow the fluid to continue infusing at a rapid rate while performing the assessment (option 2). **Cognitive Level:** Analyzing **Client Need:** Physiological Integrity **Nursing Process:** Implementation **Learning Outcome:** 18-8

9. **Answer:** 4 **Rationale:** The nurse's first priority is to stop the blood transfusion. In order to keep the intravenous site patent, normal saline can be infused at a keep-open rate, but the tubing must be changed to avoid administering more blood as the saline flushes the blood from the tubing. If the tubing is not changed, additional blood will be administered and the possible transfusion reaction will increase (option 1). Notifying the charge nurse or primary care provider should be done only after assessing the client (options 2 and 3). **Cognitive Level:** Applying **Client Need:** Physiological Integrity **Nursing Process:** Implementation **Learning Outcome:** 18-6g

10. **Answer:** 33 **Rationale:** The nurse wants to deliver 1 liter (or 1,000 mL) in 5 hours; 1,000 divided by 5 is 200 mL per hour. It requires 10 drops to make 1 mL, so multiply $200 \times 10 = 2,000$ drops per hour. To calculate how many drops per minute, divide 2,000 by 60 (the number of minutes in an hour) to arrive at your answer of 33.33. Because it is impossible to deliver 0.33 of a drop, 33 drops per minute is the correct answer. **Cognitive Level:** Applying **Client Need:** Physiological Integrity **Nursing Process:** Planning **Learning Outcome:** 18-7

Chapter 19: Feeding Clients

1. **Answer:** 3 **Rationale:** Micronutrients are required in small amounts and include vitamins and minerals. Option 1 is incorrect because carbohydrates, proteins, and fats are macronutrients that are needed in large amounts. Option 2 is incorrect because although fat-soluble vitamins are micronutrients, protein is a macronutrient. Option 4 is incorrect because although minerals are micronutrients, carbohydrates are macronutrients. **Cognitive Level:** Applying **Client Need:** Health Promotion and Maintenance **Nursing Process:** Assessment **Learning Outcome:** 19-1

2. **Answer:** 2, 3, and 4 **Rationale:** Impaired pulmonary function, an incompetent immune response, and altered functional abilities are commonly seen in clients with malnutrition. Reduced cardiac output is not generally linked with this condition (option 1). A client with anorexia has a reduced appetite. The diagnosis would not indicate any difficulty in swallowing (option 5). **Cognitive Level:** Analyzing **Client Need:** Physiological Integrity **Nursing Process:** Planning **Learning Outcome:** 19-2

3. **Answer:** 2 **Rationale:** The NSI is specifically oriented to the needs of geriatric clients. A comprehensive nutritional assessment is generally performed by a nutritionist or dietitian (option 1). The PG-SGA is a tool that could be used for this client, but it is not specifically designed for assessing the nutritional status of geriatric clients, so it would not be the best option (option 3). A nutritional intake log may be part of a nutritional assessment, but it would only be one component (option 4). **Cognitive Level:** Applying **Client Need:** Health Promotion and Maintenance **Nursing Process:** Planning **Learning Outcome:** 19-3

4. **Answer:** 4, 3, 1, 5, and 2 **Rationale:** The client has most likely been kept NPO until bowel sounds returned (option 4). Once bowel sounds resume, the initial diet will be clear liquids (option 3). If clear liquids are tolerated, the client will advance to a full liquid diet (option 1), then to a soft diet (option 5), and finally to a regular diet. **Cognitive Level:** Analyzing **Client Need:** Physiological Integrity **Nursing Process:** Planning **Learning Outcome:** 19-4

5. **Answer:** 1 **Rationale:** A client who is unable to swallow due to severe acute dysphagia will require an enteral access device to provide

adequate nutrition. A client whose bowel sounds have not yet returned will remain NPO and may have no need for an enteral access device (option 2). There are less invasive strategies for the client who does not like the taste of food provided by the facility kitchen, so option 3 would be an incorrect option. The client who sustained a CVA may require an enteral access device if the ability to swallow was affected, but more information would be needed before choosing this option. **Cognitive Level:** Analyzing **Client Need:** Physiological Integrity **Nursing Process:** Planning **Learning Outcome:** 19-7

6. **Answer:** 4 **Rationale:** A jejunostomy tube would be appropriate for this client. A nasally inserted tube would be inappropriate for long-term use, which rules out options 1 and 2. A tube placed into the stomach would be inappropriate for a client with inadequate gastric emptying, which rules out options 1 and 3. **Cognitive Level:** Analyzing **Client Need:** Physiological Integrity **Nursing Process:** Planning **Learning Outcome:** 19-8

7. **Answer:** 3 **Rationale:** Bolus intermittent feedings are only administered into the stomach. This rules out options 1, 2, and 4. **Cognitive Level:** Applying **Client Need:** Physiological Integrity **Nursing Process:** Implementation **Learning Outcome:** 19-9

8. **Answer:** 3, 4, and 5 **Rationale:** Flushing the tube liberally with water before, between, and after each medication will reduce the risk of clogging (option 3), as will crushing solid medications thoroughly and mixing in water before instillation (option 5). The larger barrel (option 4) syringe exerts less pressure and reduces the risk of clogging. The rate of administering a feeding or medications is determined by the type and volume of the substance. Administering too quickly can rupture a small-bore feeding tube or cause leaking around the syringe (option 1). Mixing medications with formula is contraindicated because it increases the risk of forming a clog (option 2). **Cognitive Level:** Applying **Client Need:** Physiological Integrity **Nursing Process:** Implementation **Learning Outcome:** 19-10

9. **Answer:** 4 **Rationale:** Auscultating the epigastrium while instilling air is incorrect because this is a very unreliable indicator of tube location. Options 1, 2, and 3 are all acceptable means of assessing nasogastric tube placement although only the x-ray is truly reliable. **Cognitive Level:** Applying **Client Need:** Safe and Effective Environment **Nursing Process:** Implementation **Learning Outcome:** 19-6b

10. **Answer:** 2 **Rationale:** When feeding a client, acting as though you have all the time in the world and are enjoying your time and conversation will help to reduce the client's embarrassment. Feeding the client quickly is likely to accentuate the belief that the client is a burden (option 1). It is best to offer fluids after every three to four bites of solid food, or whenever the client requests a drink (option 3). If you minimize conversation while feeding a client, you are more likely to increase the client's feelings of embarrassment and of burdening the nursing staff (option 4). **Cognitive Level:** Applying **Client Need:** Psychosocial Integrity **Nursing Process:** Implementation **Learning Outcome:** 19-6a

Chapter 20: Assisting with Urinary Elimination

1. **Answer:** 1, 2, 4, and 5 **Rationale:** Urination (option 1), voiding (option 2), micturition (option 4), and incontinence (option 5) are all terms that are defined as the process of emptying the urinary bladder. Maturation is the process of forming gametes or spores (option 3). **Cognitive Level:** Remembering **Client Need:** Physiological Integrity **Nursing Process:** Assessment **Learning Outcome:** 20-1

2. **Answer:** 1 **Rationale:** Clients with cardiovascular system disease may be on medications that affect urine production or may have altered perfusion to the kidney, causing reduced urine production. Diseases of the integumentary system (option 2), the immune system (option 3), and the respiratory system (option 4) are less likely to influence urinary elimination. **Cognitive Level:** Analyzing **Client Need:** Physiological Integrity **Nursing Process:** Assessment **Learning Outcome:** 20-2

3. **Answer:** 2, 3, 1, 5, and 4 **Rationale:** Provide for client privacy (option 2), then apply gloves (option 3), place the urinal between the client's legs (option 1), remove the urinal when the client is finished (option 5), and rinse the urinal and return it to the client's bedside (option 4). **Cognitive Level:** Applying **Client Need:** Physiological Integrity **Nursing Process:** Implementation **Learning Outcome:** 20-4a

4. **Answer:** 4 **Rationale:** The Coudé catheter is often used for men with prostatic hypertrophy because its curved tip is somewhat stiffer than a regular catheter and can be better controlled during insertion, causing less trauma. Option 1, a Foley catheter, is a possible option, but the Coudé catheter would be the better option. Option 2, the Robinson catheter, is a straight catheter that is removed after insertion and would not be appropriate for a client who is unable to void due to hypertrophy of the prostate. Option 3, a condom catheter, is an external sheath often used for men with urinary incontinence, but would not be appropriate for this client because it would not help to resolve his urinary retention. **Cognitive Level:** Analyzing **Client Need:** Physiological Integrity **Nursing Process:** Planning **Learning Outcome:** 20-6

5. **Answer:** 2 **Rationale:** There is little risk of soiling of the surgical incision, and this risk could be eliminated through the use of a condom catheter so option 2 is not an indication for a retention catheter. Postoperatively, it is very important to accurately measure intake and output (option 1). The client usually returns from surgery heavily medicated for pain and is still under the effects of anesthesia. As a result the client cannot void normally (option 4) and is at risk for urine retention and bladder distention (option 3). **Cognitive Level:** Analyzing **Client Need:** Physiological Integrity **Nursing Process:** Implementation **Learning Outcome:** 20-5

6. **Answer:** 2 **Rationale:** When inserting a Foley catheter, the nurse must be prepared to connect tubing and a collection bag for urine to drain into (option 2). Options 1, 3, and 4 are common to the insertion of a retention catheter and a straight catheter. **Cognitive Level:** Applying **Client Need:** Physiological Integrity **Nursing Process:** Implementation **Learning Outcome:** 20-4c

7. **Answer:** 3 **Rationale:** The correct answer is to reduce the risk of infection secondary to the retention catheter, providing an open line into the sterile bladder (option 3). The client with a retention catheter does not need to maintain bed rest as long as the drainage bag is kept lower than the bladder (option 1). There is no indication that this client will be encouraged to drink fluids. It is possible the client may be on fluid restrictions as the question does not indicate the client's hydration status (option 2). The risk of skin breakdown is no greater with a retention catheter in place, and may actually be lower if the client had the catheter placed due to incontinence (option 4). **Cognitive Level:** Analyzing **Client Need:** Physiological Integrity **Nursing Process:** Planning **Learning Outcome:** 20-7a

8. **Answer:** 3 **Rationale:** Clients should be taught not to put anything into the urine collection pouch that is not specifically designed for that purpose so a client who says he or she will use baking soda needs further teaching (option 3). The use of dilute vinegar for reusable pouches (option 1), increasing fluid intake (option 2), and deodorant drops (option 4) are all appropriate options. **Cognitive Level:** Analyzing **Client Need:** Health Promotion and Maintenance **Nursing Process:** Evaluation **Learning Outcome:** 20-7c

9. **Answer:** 4 **Rationale:** UAP may empty a urinary drainage bag for a client with a retention catheter if they have been thoroughly trained and agency policy allows it. Insertion of a straight catheter (option 1) or performing bladder irrigation (option 3) requires knowledge of sterile technique and cannot be safely delegated to the UAP. Obtaining a urinary elimination history is assessment and cannot be delegated to the UAP (option 2). **Cognitive Level:** Applying **Client Need:** Safe and Effective Care Environment **Nursing Process:** Planning **Learning Outcome:** 20-3

10. **Answer:** 1 **Rationale:** The primary care provider should be notified if the client produces less than an average of 30 mL per hour of urine, because this requires further intervention (option 1). Options 2, 3, and 4 are all acceptable quantities of urine output over a 3-hour period. **Cognitive Level:** Applying **Client Need:** Physiological Integrity **Nursing Process:** Evaluation **Learning Outcome:** 20-8

Chapter 21: Assisting with Fecal Elimination

1. **Answer:** 1, 4 **Rationale:** Adding fiber and water to the diet helps to prevent constipation. Increasing foods high in fats and carbohydrates (option 2) or iron (option 3) will not treat constipation. Increasing caffeine may provide a short-term solution for some people, but it is not the healthiest approach for treating constipation (option 5). **Cognitive Level:** Applying **Client Need:** Health Promotion and Maintenance **Nursing Process:** Implementation **Learning Outcome:** 21-1

2. **Answer:** 3 **Rationale:** Ignoring the need to defecate causes expansion of the rectum to accommodate accumulated feces and eventual loss of sensitivity to the need to defecate, resulting in constipation. Bowel obstruction (option 1), rupture of the rectum (option 2), and fecal incontinence (option 4) are not the immediate concerns. **Cognitive Level:** Applying **Client Need:** Physiological Integrity **Nursing Process:** Implementation **Learning Outcome:** 21-2

3. **Answer:** 2 **Rationale:** Applying gloves is the first and most important step to avoid bacterial contamination of the nurse's hands. Only after applying gloves would the nurse remove the bedpan (option 1), change the linen (option 3), or clean the client's anal area (option 4). **Cognitive Level:** Applying **Client Need:** Physiological Integrity **Nursing Process:** Implementation **Learning Outcome:** 21-6a

4. **Answer:** 3 **Rationale:** Because the pouch and barrier are one unit, if one needs to be changed, the other must be changed as well. A one-piece ostomy appliance is no harder to apply (option 1) and is no more likely to leak (option 4). One-piece units are available in both closed and open units. An open one-piece appliance can be emptied and closed again (option 2). **Cognitive Level:** Applying **Client Need:** Health Promotion and Maintenance **Nursing Process:** Implementation **Learning Outcome:** 21-4a

5. **Answer:** 1, 2, and 5 **Rationale:** A skin barrier is placed first and then the ostomy pouch is applied (options 1 and 2). A stoma measuring guide helps the nurse to create a firm, leak-free fit for the skin barrier (option 5). A deodorant is not usually needed because the pouches are deodorized (option 3). An ostomy belt is rarely used in the early stages because it would increase client discomfort (option 4). **Cognitive Level:** Applying **Client Need:** Physiological Integrity **Nursing Process:** Planning **Learning Outcome:** 21-4b

6. **Answer:** 4 **Rationale:** When removing the bedpan, care should be taken not to contaminate the nurse. This is best achieved by holding the outside of the bedpan and keeping the bedpan level and away from the uniform. Holding the bedpan in one hand like a serving tray increases the risk of dropping or spilling it (option 1). The nurse should use care not to insert the fingers into the bedpan to avoid self-contamination (option 2). Holding the bedpan at an angle increases the risk of spilling the contents and does not reduce the odor (option 3). **Cognitive Level:** Applying **Client Need:** Physiological Integrity **Nursing Process:** Implementation **Learning Outcome:** 21-3

7. **Answer:** 1 **Rationale:** The proper position would be a left lateral position with the right leg flexed because this position facilitates the flow of solution by gravity into the sigmoid and descending colon. Options 2, 3, and 4 are incorrect. If the client is incontinent or unable to participate, position the client supine on a bedpan. **Cognitive Level:** Applying **Client Need:** Physiological Integrity **Nursing Process:** Implementation **Learning Outcome:** 21-6b

8. **Answer:** 2 **Rationale:** Administering an oil retention enema will make the procedure both more effective and less traumatic by helping the feces slide out more easily. Explaining the procedure to the client is an important step that may make the procedure less traumatic, but it will not make it more effective (option 1). Lubricating the gloved finger will make the procedure less traumatic, but it will not increase the effectiveness (option 3). Administering a cathartic suppository may cause the client to be more uncomfortable because it will cause cramping (option 4). **Cognitive Level:** Analyzing **Client Need:** Physiological Integrity **Nursing Process:** Planning **Learning Outcome:** 21-6c

9. **Answer:** 4 **Rationale:** The appliance should be changed every 24 to 48 hours if the skin is erythematous, eroded, denuded, or ulcerated to allow appropriate treatment of the skin. If the skin is intact, the appliance should be changed every 7 days (option 3) unless the client complains of discomfort at or around the stoma (option 2) so long as the appliance is snugly in place without leakage (option 1). **Cognitive Level:** Analyzing **Client Need:** Physiological Integrity **Nursing Process:** Assessment **Learning Outcome:** 21-6d

10. **Answer:** 2 **Rationale:** Children begin to have some control over their bowels before age 2 1/2, but they will still have accidents as they do not gain full control until age 2 1/2 years. The child does not need to be tested by her pediatrician because what the mother is describing is normal (option 1). Telling the mother she is approaching toilet training incorrectly is incorrect because the nurse would need to know more about what the mother is doing to make this decision, and even then it can be handled more tactfully (option 3). Diet is not related to bowel elimination accidents in this instance (option 4). **Cognitive Level:** Analyzing **Client Need:** Health Promotion and Maintenance **Nursing Process:** Implementation **Learning Outcome:** 21-2

Chapter 22: Caring for the Client with Peritoneal Dialysis

1. **Answer:** 2 **Rationale:** The solution instilled into the peritoneal cavity is called dialysate. Dialysis is the process that uses dialysate (option 1). The dialyzer is the machine equipped with a semipermeable membrane and is used for performing hemodialysis (option 3). Instillation is the administration of a liquid into a body cavity (option 4). **Cognitive Level:** Understanding **Client Need:** Physiological Integrity **Nursing Process:** Implementation **Learning Outcome:** 22-1

2. **Answer:** 2 **Rationale:** Oliguria is an inadequate production of urine. Anuria is the complete suppression of urine production (option 1). Polyuria and hydruria are defined as excessive secretion of urine, which may occur in, for example, diabetes (options 3 and 4). **Cognitive Level:** Applying **Client Need:** Physiological Integrity **Nursing Process:** Implementation **Learning Outcome:** 22-1

3. **Answer:** 3 **Rationale:** The client's status should be observed during usual care by the UAP but unusual findings must be validated and interpreted by the nurse (option 3). Assisting with peritoneal catheter insertion and conducting the peritoneal dialysis procedure require sterile technique and should not be delegated to UAP (options 1 and 2). Only nurses may assess outflow fluid (option 4). **Cognitive Level:** Analyzing **Client Need:** Safe and Effective Care Environment **Nursing Process:** Planning **Learning Outcome:** 22-2

4. **Answer:** 2, 3, and 5 **Rationale:** UAP can safely measure vital signs (option 2), obtain a daily weight (option 3), and assist the client to eat breakfast (option 5) as long as the nurse instructs the UAP when to weigh the client and what data should be immediately reported to the nurse. Changing the peritoneal catheter dressing (option 1) and instilling dialysate (option 4) are not tasks that may be delegated to UAP. **Cognitive Level:** Analyzing **Client Need:** Safe and Effective Care Environment **Nursing Process:** Planning **Learning Outcome:** 22-2

5. **Answer:** 2 and 5 **Rationale:** The nurse's role in preparing the client for the procedure includes reinforcing the key elements of client and family teaching (option 2) as well as reviewing the technique and purpose of peritoneal dialysis (option 5). Initial client and family teaching (option 1), initial explanation of the client's diagnosis and need for

peritoneal dialysis (option 2), and ensuring that the client is informed about the procedure so he can sign the informed consent (option 4) are all the physician's obligation. **Cognitive Level:** Applying **Client Need:** Safe and Effective Care Environment **Nursing Process:** Planning **Learning Outcome:** 22-3

6. **Answer: 1 Rationale:** As the physician prepares to insert the trocar, the client should be instructed to tense the abdominal muscles as if for a bowel movement to help reduce the discomfort felt by the client. Taking a deep breath does not distend the abdomen (option 2), holding the breath is not necessary and may actually cause more discomfort (option 3), and clients are kept NPO prior to and during the procedure so would not be given a drink (option 4). **Cognitive Level:** Applying **Client Need:** Physiological Integrity **Nursing Process:** Implementation **Learning Outcome:** 22-3

7. **Answer: 4 Rationale:** Heparin is added to decrease clotting within the catheter. The remaining options (1, 2, and 3) are not commonly added by the nurse because they are standard components of the solution. **Cognitive Level:** Remembering **Client Need:** Physiological Integrity **Nursing Process:** Implementation **Learning Outcome:** 22-4B

8. **Answer: −125 mL Rationale:** Add the quantity of fluid instilled (500 mL × 3) and then subtract the amount of fluid returned ($1,500 - 600 - 550 - 475 = -125$) to get the answer. If more fluid is infused than removed, the fluid balance is positive. If more fluid is removed than infused, the balance is negative. **Cognitive Level:** Applying **Client Need:** Physiological Integrity **Nursing Process:** Evaluation **Learning Outcome:** 22-4B

9. **Answer: 1 Rationale:** Although dialysate may return pink tinged on the first two to four exchanges after insertion of the dialysis catheter, on a client who has been receiving dialysis for a year pink and cloudy return would be a sign of possible peritonitis and should be reported to the primary care provider. This is not normal fluid (option 2) or a result of too much dialysate being removed at one time (option 4). Bowel perforation would be more likely if the return was brownish (option 3). **Cognitive Level:** Analyzing **Client Need:** Physiological Integrity **Nursing Process:** Assessment **Learning Outcome:** 22-4B

10. **Answer: 1 Rationale:** It is not unusual for the client's pulse rate to increase slightly during the phase when the fluid is indwelling. An elevated temperature could indicate peritoneal inflammation or infection (option 2). Normal serum potassium levels are 3.5 to 5.5 mEq/L, and a reduced level could indicate the need for more potassium to be added to the dialysate (option 3). A weight gain of 5 pounds in one day is also significant because it indicates fluid retention (option 4). **Cognitive Level:** Analyzing **Client Need:** Physiological Integrity **Nursing Process:** Assessment **Learning Outcome:** 22-4b

Chapter 23: *Promoting Circulation*

1. **Answer: 2 Rationale:** A positive Homans' sign occurs when the foot is passively dorsiflexed and pain is experienced in the calf. A positive Babinski reflex is characterized by dorsiflexion of the big toe and contraction of the extensor hallucis longus muscle when the sole of the foot is stimulated (option 1). There is no such thing as a negative Babinski sign—it is either present or it is not (option 3). A negative Homans' sign would be lack of pain when the foot is dorsiflexed (option 4). **Cognitive Level:** Analyzing **Client Need:** Physiological Integrity **Nursing Process:** Assessment **Learning Outcome:** 23-1

2. **Answer: 2 Rationale:** A blood clot alone is called a thrombus (option 2). An inflamed vein alone is called phlebitis (option 1). A clot or tissue fragment that travels is called an emboli (option 3). The term thrombophlebitis indicates both an inflamed vein and the presence of a blood clot (option 4). **Cognitive Level:** Analyzing **Client Need:** Physiological Integrity **Nursing Process:** Assessment **Learning Outcome:** 23-1

3. **Answer: 3 Rationale:** A pregnant client required to maintain bed rest due to premature labor is at increased risk for venous stasis, compounded by the fact that the weight of the baby puts pressure on the vena cava and reduces venous return still further (option 3). A client with atrial fibrillation is at risk for developing a thrombus, but this is not due to venous stasis (option 1). A client in a same-day surgery center is expected to be out of bed and able to be discharged the same day so is not at risk for venous stasis (option 2). A client with diabetes is not at risk for venous stasis unless the client develops the complication of peripheral vascular disease (option 4). **Cognitive Level:** Analyzing **Client Need:** Physiological Integrity **Nursing Process:** Assessment **Learning Outcome:** 23-2

4. **Answer: 3 Rationale:** The client on a long plane trip should be educated to ambulate hourly, walking the aisle of the plane, in order to reduce venous stasis. Drinking extra fluids when traveling is a good strategy, but will not reduce venous stasis (option 1). Elevating the legs would help, but this is not a reasonable option given the limited leg room available on most planes (option 2). Reducing sodium intake will not affect venous stasis (option 4). **Cognitive Level:** Analyzing **Client Need:** Physiological Integrity **Nursing Process:** Implementation **Learning Outcome:** 23-2

5. **Answer: 1 Rationale:** Before applying antiemboli stockings, the nurse should assess for any potential or present circulatory problems. Intake and output (option 2), alterations in vital signs (option 3), and respiratory distress (option 4) do not affect the use of antiemboli stockings. **Cognitive Level:** Analyzing **Client Need:** Physiological Integrity **Nursing Process:** Assessment **Learning Outcome:** 23-5a

6. **Answer: 3, 1, 5, 2, and 4 Rationale:** When performing the procedure of applying antiemboli stockings, the nurse should first measure the length of the legs and the circumference of the calf (option 3), then compare these measurements to the size chart to determine the proper size stocking (option 1). The next step is to apply the stockings, turning the upper portion of the stocking inside out so the foot portion is inside the leg of the stocking (option 5). Have the client point the toes (option 2), and pull the stocking over the ankle and up the leg (option 4). **Cognitive Level:** Applying **Client Need:** Physiological Integrity **Nursing Process:** Implementation **Learning Outcome:** 23-5a

7. **Answer: 4 Rationale:** The best time to apply antiemboli stockings is in the morning before arising because the veins distend when they are in a dependent position. After sitting in a chair (option 1), prior to sleep at night (option 2), or by midafternoon if the client has been out of bed (option 3), the veins have been allowed to distend and edema may have occurred. **Cognitive Level:** Analyzing **Client Need:** Physiological Integrity **Nursing Process:** Planning **Learning Outcome:** 23-5a

8. **Answer: 3 Rationale:** The client at moderate risk for DVT or PE requires antiemboli stockings and an SCD. Clients at low risk require either antiemboli stockings or an SCD (options 1 and 2). If the client is high risk, anticoagulant therapy may be needed (option 4). **Cognitive Level:** Analyzing **Client Need:** Physiological Integrity **Nursing Process:** Planning **Learning Outcome:** 23-5b

9. **Answer: 1, 2, 4, and 5 Rationale:** SCDs are contraindicated if the client has cellulitis (option 1), a DVT (option 2), arterial insufficiency (option 4), or an infected wound (option 5) of the leg. It is appropriate to apply SCDs to clients with hypertension (option 3). **Cognitive Level:** Analyzing **Client Need:** Physiological Integrity **Nursing Process:** Planning **Learning Outcome:** 23-5b

10. **Answer: 4 Rationale:** The best position for applying a sequential compression device is the semi-Fowler's or dorsal recumbent position. Although it is possible to apply a sequential compression device in the dorsal lithotomy (option 1), high-Fowler's (option 2), and prone (option 3) positions to accommodate the client's needs, they are not the best positions. **Cognitive Level:** Applying **Client Need:** Physiological Integrity **Nursing Process:** Implementation **Learning Outcome:** 23-5b

Chapter 24: Breathing Exercises

1. **Answer:** Pursed-lip breathing **Rationale:** Pursed-lip breathing is helpful for clients with COPD because it helps prevent airway collapse by maintaining positive airway pressure. **Cognitive Level:** Remembering **Client Need:** Physiological Integrity **Nursing Process:** Implementation **Learning Outcome:** 24-1

2. **Answer:** 2 **Rationale:** When huff coughing the client leans forward and exhales with a "huff" cough, so the client is properly performing the procedure. The client is working effectively to clear the airway (option 1), is not in respiratory distress (option 3), and does not require further teaching, but reinforcement for performing huff coughing correctly is in order (option 4). **Cognitive Level:** Analyzing **Client Need:** Physiological Integrity **Nursing Process:** Evaluation **Learning Outcome:** 24-1

3. **Answer:** 1, 4, and 5 **Rationale:** To promote normal respirations for this client, it is important to position the client in the orthopneic position (option 1), encourage the client to ambulate in order to mobilize pulmonary secretions (option 4), and encourage fluids to make the secretions thinner and easier to expectorate (option 5). Bed rest (option 3) and a supine or prone position (option 2) would be contraindicated. **Cognitive Level:** Applying **Client Need:** Physiological Integrity **Nursing Process:** Implementation **Learning Outcome:** 24-2

4. **Answer:** 1 **Rationale:** Teaching the client how to splint the incision with a pillow will reduce the discomfort and encourage the client to take deep breaths. Applying a binder to the chest to splint the incision will reduce the client's ability to take a deep breath (option 2) so it is contraindicated. Restricted fluids will make pulmonary secretions thicker, so reducing fluids is contraindicated (option 3). The position of choice is the orthopneic position, not the high-Fowler's position, which presses the abdominal contents into the diaphragm (option 4). **Cognitive Level:** Applying **Client Need:** Health Promotion and Management **Nursing Process:** Implementation **Learning Outcome:** 24-2

5. **Answer:** 4 **Rationale:** The sound heard by the nurse is a wheeze caused by narrowed or partially obstructed airways. Laryngeal obstruction creates a shrill harsh sound known as stridor (option 1). Fluid in the air passages and alveoli causes rales or crackles (option 2). A pleural friction rub creates a coarse, leathery, or grating sound produced by the rubbing together of inflamed pleura (option 3). **Cognitive Level:** Analyzing **Client Need:** Physiological Integrity **Nursing Process:** Assessment **Learning Outcome:** 24-3

6. **Answer:** 2 **Rationale:** Substernal retractions are seen below the breastbone. Intercostal retractions are indrawn muscles between the ribs (option 1). Suprasternal retractions are seen above the breastbone (option 3). Supraclavicular retractions are seen above the clavicles (option 4). **Cognitive Level:** Analyzing **Client Need:** Physiological Integrity **Nursing Process:** Assessment **Learning Outcome:** 24-3

7. **Answer:** 3 **Rationale:** To raise the abdomen while deep breathing, the client takes a deep breath through the nose with the mouth closed. Breathing through the mouth (option 1) is incorrect; the client should breathe in through the nose. Arching the back should be avoided (option 2). The hands should be placed on the abdomen to feel the abdominal movement, not behind the head (option 4). **Cognitive Level:** Analyzing **Client Need:** Health Promotion and Management **Nursing Process:** Evaluation **Learning Outcome:** 24-5a

8. **Answer:** 3 **Rationale:** The client should inhale deeply and hold the breath for a few seconds. If the client exhales before coughing, he or she will not have breath left to cough (options 1 and 2). Inhaling deeply is only half of the instruction (option 4). **Cognitive Level:** Applying **Client Need:** Health Promotion and Management **Nursing Process:** Implementation **Learning Outcome:** 24-5a

9. **Answer:** 1 **Rationale:** The client who uses the SMI immediately after eating needs further teaching because inhaled volume decreases when the stomach is full and presses up on the diaphragm. Taking slow deep breaths (option 2) and assuming a sitting position (option 3) are proper procedures. Exceeding the set volume level is an excellent outcome (option 4). **Cognitive Level:** Analyzing **Client Need:** Health Promotion and Management **Nursing Process:** Evaluation **Learning Outcome:** 24-5b

10. **Answer:** 1 **Rationale:** The disadvantage of the flow-oriented SMI is that the client can generate a high flow with low volume by taking a quick forceful inhalation and not meet the goal of therapy (option 1). Flow-oriented SMIs are inexpensive to use (option 2), are easy for the client to use (option 3), and allow clients to easily determine how effectively they are performing (option 4). **Cognitive Level:** Applying **Client Need:** Health Promotion and Management **Nursing Process:** Planning **Learning Outcome:** 24-5b

Chapter 25: Oxygen Therapy

1. **Answer:** 3 **Rationale:** Continuous positive airway pressure (CPAP) maintains an open airway while the client sleeps. Providing oxygen by mask or nasal cannula does not assist with obstructive sleep apnea (options 1 and 4). A Venturi mask delivers specific concentrations of oxygen and is not used for obstructive sleep apnea (option 2). **Cognitive Level:** Applying **Client Need:** Physiological Integrity **Nursing Process:** Planning **Learning Outcome:** 25-5

2. **Answer:** 3 **Rationale:** The nurse would anticipate delivering oxygen via nasal cannula at 2 liters per minute because clients with COPD require an elevated carbon dioxide level to stimulate breathing, and delivering high concentrations of oxygen could result in apnea. Oxygen via nasal cannula at 6 liters per minute would be contraindicated for the client with COPD (option 1) as would 100% via a nonrebreather mask (option 2) and 50% via a Venturi mask (option 4). **Cognitive Level:** Applying **Client Need:** Physiological Integrity **Nursing Process:** Planning **Learning Outcome:** 25-6a

3. **Answer:** 1 **Rationale:** Although oxygen is like medication and a primary care provider's order is needed in nonemergency situations, in emergency situations like that described in the question, the nurse can start oxygen without an order and then notify the primary care provider. Waiting to start oxygen until after calling the primary care provider could have serious consequences and would not be prudent (option 2). Calling the respiratory therapist would be an unnecessary delay and the therapist has no greater authority to begin oxygen in an emergency than the nurse (option 3). Returning in 15 minutes to reevaluate the client (option 4) could result in serious negative consequences and is incorrect. **Cognitive Level:** Applying **Client Need:** Physiological Integrity **Nursing Process:** Implementation **Learning Outcome:** 25-2

4. **Answer:** 3 **Rationale:** The symptoms displayed by the client are classic signs of oxygen toxicity. If the client was hypercarbic (option 1), also known as hypercapnic (option 4), the symptoms would be restlessness, hypertension, headache, lethargy, and tremor. Signs of hypoxia (option 2) are tachycardia, tachypnea, restlessness, dyspnea, cyanosis, and confusion. **Cognitive Level:** Analyzing **Client Need:** Physiological Integrity **Nursing Process:** Assessment **Learning Outcome:** 25-6a

5. **Answer:** 1 **Rationale:** Humidification of oxygen helps to prevent symptoms created by drying of the mucous membranes such as rhinorrhea and nasal irritation. A warming device would not prevent the symptoms of rhinorrhea and nasal irritation (option 2). Normal saline nose drops could interfere with oxygen delivery (option 3). The cannula should not be removed routinely to prevent these symptoms because the client could become hypoxemic as a result (option 4). **Cognitive Level:** Applying **Client Need:** Physiological Integrity **Nursing Process:** Implementation **Learning Outcome:** 25-6a

6. **Answer:** 3 **Rationale:** UAP may measure oxygen saturation (pulse oximetry) safely as long as the nurse verifies that the UAP has been

trained in the use of the equipment. Initiating oxygen therapy is similar to administering medications and is not delegated to the UAP (option 1). Determining client response is an assessment and must be performed by the nurse (option 2). The UAP should not make a decision about the client's need for more or less oxygen and should never change the flow rate without the nurse's approval and supervision (option 4). **Cognitive Level:** Applying **Client Need:** Safe and Effective Care Environment **Nursing Process:** Planning **Learning Outcome:** 25-4

7. **Answer: 4 Rationale:** The nurse needs to notify the primary care provider if the client becomes tachypneic and has an oxygen saturation that has dropped to 84% (lower than the original value on room air) while on 4 liters of oxygen per minute. The parameters in options 1 and 2 are within acceptable levels. While an oxygen saturation of 88% and respiratory rate of 26 are not as good as previously, the saturation is still better than it was on room air and the nurse should monitor the client and perform a full respiratory assessment prior to deciding to notify the primary care provider (option 3). **Cognitive Level:** Applying **Client Need:** Physiological Integrity **Nursing Process:** Planning **Learning Outcome:** 25-7

8. **Answer: 4 Rationale:** The client should sit in a chair or in bed with the chest not coming in contact with anything in order to allow full lung expansion. If a client is unable to do this, the semi-Fowler's (option 1) and high-Fowler's (option 2) positions would be the next best options. The supine position would be less effective in obtaining an accurate reading (option 3). **Cognitive Level:** Applying **Client Need:** Physiological Integrity **Nursing Process:** Implementation **Learning Outcome:** 25-6b

9. **Answer: 2 Rationale:** Noninvasive ventilation devices have the advantages of being more comfortable and reducing the complications associated with invasive ventilation (option 2). They can be used long term, which makes option 1 incorrect. If a client requires intubation, the procedure can be performed emergently and would not be scheduled for some time in the future (option 3). Although use of a noninvasive ventilation device is less expensive than invasive ventilation, that would not be a rationale for choosing this method (option 4). **Cognitive Level:** Analyzing **Client Need:** Health Promotion and Maintenance **Nursing Process:** Assessment **Learning Outcome:** 25-5

10. **Answer: 3 Rationale:** Prior to making decisions or statements about the need to use the CPAP mask every night, the nurse needs to find out why the client is not using it daily (option 3). Although options 1 and 2 are both true statements, until the nurse finds out why the client is not using the device, these statements are unlikely to have an impact. Option 4 asks why the client does not like using the device, and the nurse does not know that the client does not like using it. It may be that the client's electricity was turned off or there might be another unrelated reason other than the client "not liking" it. "Why" questions can put the client on the defensive. Health promotion is most effective when the nurse explores the client's thinking before determining the best approach to teaching. **Cognitive Level:** Analyzing **Client Need:** Health Promotion and Maintenance **Nursing Process:** Implementation **Learning Outcome:** 25-5

Chapter 26: Suctioning

1. **Answer: 2 Rationale:** A Yankauer suction tube is a hard plastic device frequently used for removing saliva and secretions from the mouth. In-line suction catheters are connected to ventilator tubing to allow suctioning without disconnecting the client from the ventilator and would not be appropriate for suctioning the mouth (option 1). A whistle-tip catheter is a flexible catheter, not a plastic tube (option 3). An open airway suction system is a suction catheter used for suctioning endotracheal or tracheostomy tubes and also would not be appropriate for a client to use independently to suction the mouth

(option 4). **Cognitive Level:** Applying **Client Need:** Health Promotion and Maintenance **Nursing Process:** Implementation **Learning Outcome:** 26-1

2. **Answer: 2 Rationale:** An oropharyngeal airway would be the best option for this client because it would hold the tongue in place and maintain a patent airway. As clients arouse from sedation, they will frequently remove the airway themselves, which is an indicator that the sedation level is lightening. A nasopharyngeal airway is a soft tube that would be less effective in holding the tongue away from the airway and more compressible than an oral airway so it would not be the best option (option 1). An endotracheal tube (option 3) or a tracheostomy (option 4) would be inserted by a primary care provider and not a nurse. **Cognitive Level:** Applying **Client Need:** Physiological Integrity **Nursing Process:** Implementation **Learning Outcome:** 26-2

3. **Answer: 4 Rationale:** Although endotracheal intubation may be used initially (option 3), for long-term airway maintenance a tracheostomy would be the best option for this client (option 4). A nasopharyngeal airway (option 1) or oropharyngeal airway (option 2) would not be effective in a client who is not breathing spontaneously. **Cognitive Level:** Analyzing **Client Need:** Physiological Adaptation **Nursing Process:** Assessment **Learning Outcome:** 26-2

4. **Answer: 4 Rationale:** Endotracheal suctioning (option 4) should always be performed using sterile technique as the catheter is entering the lungs. Although using sterile technique with any form of suctioning is suggested to prevent introducing pathogens into the airway, suctioning the nasopharynx or oropharynx may be performed using clean technique because they are not sterile cavities (options 1, 2, and 3). **Cognitive Level:** Applying **Client Need:** Physiological Adaptation **Nursing Process:** Implementation **Learning Outcome:** 26-3

5. **Answer: 3 Rationale:** Rotating the catheter prevents pulling of tissue into the opening on the catheter tip and side. Suction catheters may only be lubricated with water or water-soluble lubricant. Petroleum jelly such as Vaseline has an oil base (option 1). No suction should ever be applied while the catheter is being inserted because this can traumatize tissues (option 2). The client should be hyperoxygenated for only a few minutes before and after suctioning, and this is generally limited to clients who are intubated or have a tracheostomy (option 4). **Cognitive Level:** Applying **Client Need:** Safe and Effective Care Environment **Nursing Process:** Implementation **Learning Outcome:** 26-7a

6. **Answer: 3 Rationale:** A pressure of 80 to 120 mmHg is recommended for suctioning an endotracheal or tracheostomy tube to remove secretions while minimizing tissue trauma. Setting the suction pressure to 60 to 100 mmHg would not be strong enough to remove secretions, especially thick secretions (option 1). Pressures of 100 to 140 mmHg would increase the risk of tissue trauma (option 2), and pressures of 160 to 200 mmHg (option 4) would almost guarantee trauma. **Cognitive Level:** Applying **Client Need:** Physiological Adaptation **Nursing Process:** Implementation **Learning Outcome:** 26-7b

7. **Answer: 1, 2, 3, and 5 Rationale:** The nurse not being exposed to secretions (option 1), the client not having to be disconnected from the ventilator (option 2), the catheter being reusable (3), and not having to wear goggles (option 5) are all advantages of a closed system. The catheter on a closed system needs to be inserted to the same depth as an open system, so this is not an advantage of this system (option 4). **Cognitive Level:** Analyzing **Client Need:** Physiological Adaptation **Nursing Process:** Implementation **Learning Outcome:** 26-4

8. **Answer: 1, 2, 3, and 4 Rationale:** Suctioning is uncomfortable for the client even when properly performed and particularly painful if the client has an abdominal or chest incision because it is likely to trigger a strong cough reflex (option 1). Scheduled suctioning implies that the same amount of secretions is always produced and this is not true. More suctioning may be required if the client has been moving

about, coughing, or restless, because movement of the artificial airway increases secretion production (option 2), whereas sleeping quietly with little movement may produce fewer secretions and require less frequent suctioning (option 3). Inserting a catheter into the airway increases the risk of introducing pathogens and subsequent nosocomial infections (option 4). Although suctioning is time consuming and costly, this is not a rationale for denying the client a needed intervention (option 5). **Cognitive Level:** Applying **Client Need:** Physiological Adaptation **Nursing Process:** Planning **Learning Outcome:** 26-5

9. **Answer:** 4, 1, 2, 5, and 3 **Rationale:** Attach the catheter to the suction source (option 4), then test to ensure patency of the catheter and to make sure the pressure is set properly (option 1). Next, lubricate the tip and introduce the catheter into the naris without applying suction (option 2). When the catheter is inserted to the proper distance, determined by measuring from the tip of the client's nose to the earlobe, apply suction while withdrawing the catheter slowly for 5 to 10 seconds (option 5). Rinse and flush the catheter with sterile water or sterile saline before reintroducing if needed (option 3). **Cognitive Level:** Applying **Client Need:** Physiological Integrity **Nursing Process:** Implementation **Learning Outcome:** 26-7a

10. **Answer:** 4 **Rationale:** Hyperinflating the lungs at a volume slightly greater than the client's normal tidal volume prior to suctioning reduces the risk of hypoxemia and hypercapnia during the procedure (option 4). Suction should not be applied while introducing the catheter (option 1). Suction is usually set between 80 and 120 mmHg for an adult (option 2). Oxygen concentration should be increased, not decreased, to prevent hypoxia during the procedure (option 3). **Cognitive Level:** Applying **Client Need:** Physiological Adaptation **Nursing Process:** Implementation **Learning Outcome:** 26-7b

Chapter 27: Caring for the Client with a Tracheostomy

1. **Answer:** 2 **Rationale:** The fenestrated tube allows the client to breathe normally around the tube and to talk. A cuffed tracheostomy produces an airtight seal between the tube and trachea allowing the client, when removed from the ventilator, to breathe through the tube, but will not allow the client to talk (option 1). An uncuffed tracheostomy is often used by clients who require a tracheostomy long term because it allows the client to talk (option 3). All tracheostomy tubes are curved to fit the anatomy of the trachea (option 4). **Cognitive Level:** Analyzing **Client Need:** Physiological Integrity **Nursing Process:** Implementation **Learning Outcome:** 27-1

2. **Answer:** 3 **Rationale:** The obturator is solid and blocks the airway, providing rigidity to the tube while it is being inserted, but it must be removed as soon as the tube is in place. Some tubes have an inner cannula that can be removed for cleaning, but otherwise would remain in place (option 1). The outer cannula is inserted into the neck and remains in place until extubated (option 2). The flange rests against the neck, allowing the tube to be secured in place (option 4). **Cognitive Level:** Applying **Client Need:** Physiological Integrity **Nursing Process:** Assessment **Learning Outcome:** 27-3

3. **Answer:** 1 **Rationale:** The client with a permanent tracheostomy is likely to have an uncuffed tube (option 1) because a cuffed tube (option 2) puts pressure on the trachea and over the long term may create tissue trauma. There would be no need to use a fenestrated tube, which allows the client to talk, if the client is in a chronic vegetative state (option 3). Either a plastic or metal tube may be used so the nurse would not be able to anticipate this (option 4). **Cognitive Level:** Analyzing **Client Need:** Physiological Integrity **Nursing Process:** Assessment **Learning Outcome:** 27-2

4. **Answer:** 2 **Rationale:** Pediatric clients do not require a cuffed tube because their tracheas are resilient enough to seal the air space around the tube. An uncuffed tracheostomy tube is usually placed in children

(option 2), although a fenestrated tracheostomy tube may be used when the child is being weaned from the ventilator or the tracheostomy tube will be removed in the near future (option 3). Pediatric tracheostomies frequently have an inner cannula for easy cleaning of secretions because minimal secretions can block the smaller airway (option 4). **Cognitive Level:** Analyzing **Client Need:** Physiological Integrity **Nursing Process:** Assessment **Learning Outcome:** 27-2

5. **Answer:** 4 **Rationale:** A communication board would allow the client to point to phrases or pictures without using a great deal of strength or requiring much coordination. A client who is only 1 day postoperative after major surgery and still receiving narcotic analgesics for pain will be unlikely to have the strength or physical coordination to write using paper and pen (option 1). A fenestrated tracheostomy tube (option 2) or a speaking valve (option 3) would not be a likely option this early in the client's postoperative course. **Cognitive Level:** Applying **Client Need:** Physiological Integrity **Nursing Process:** Planning **Learning Outcome:** 27-4

6. **Answer:** 2 **Rationale:** Acknowledging the client's frustration and continuing to explore methods for the client to communicate will establish trust and show the client that you are trying to help. It is never appropriate to tell a client how to feel, so option 1 is incorrect. Telling a client not to try to talk (option 3) or to get some rest (option 4) will only frustrate the client further and destroy the development of a trusting relationship. **Cognitive Level:** Analyzing **Client Need:** Psychosocial Integrity **Nursing Process:** Implementation **Learning Outcome:** 27-4

7. **Answer:** 1 **Rationale:** Prior to starting the procedure, it is important to develop a means of communication by which the client can express pain or discomfort. The twill tape is not changed until after performing tracheostomy care (option 2). Cleaning the incision should be done after cleaning the inner cannula (option 3). Checking the tightness of the ties and knot is done after applying new twill tape (option 4). **Cognitive Level:** Applying **Client Need:** Physiological Integrity **Nursing Process:** Implementation **Learning Outcome:** 27-6a

8. **Answer:** 3, 2, 1, 5, and 4 **Rationale:** Suction the tracheostomy tube, if necessary, before beginning care (option 3). After suctioning, remove and clean the inner cannula and then replace it unless it is a disposable inner cannula, in which case you may choose to discard the inner cannula and replace it with a new one (option 2). Clean the incision site and tube flange (option 1), apply a sterile dressing (option 5), and then change the ties (option 4). **Cognitive Level:** Applying **Client Need:** Physiological Integrity **Nursing Process:** Implementation **Learning Outcome:** 27-6a

9. **Answer:** 3 **Rationale:** The best type of tube would be a fenestrated tube because of the holes in the tube that allow air to pass more easily around the tube to the vocal cords. Although a speaking valve can be used with an uncuffed tube (option 1) or with a cuffed tube as long as it is not a foam-filled cuff (option 2), they are not the optimal tubes to choose. All tracheostomy tubes are curved (option 4). **Cognitive Level:** Analyzing **Client Need:** Physiological Integrity **Nursing Process:** Assessment **Learning Outcome:** 27-6b

10. **Answer:** 4 **Rationale:** To use a speaking valve, the client needs to be alert, be responsive, and have a tracheostomy, so a client who is sleepy would not be a good candidate. Passy-Muir valves can be used with any age client (options 1 and 3) and can be used if the client is on or off the ventilator (option 2). **Cognitive Level:** Applying **Client Need:** Physiological Integrity **Nursing Process:** Assessment **Learning Outcome:** 27-6b

Chapter 28: Assisting with Mechanical Ventilation

1. **Answer:** 2 **Rationale:** When the ventilator allows clients to breathe at their own rate but still delivers a minimum number of breaths, it is called synchronized intermittent mandatory ventilation. Continuous

positive airway pressure is a continuous pressure at the end of expiration that prevents airway collapse between breaths (option 1). Pressure support ventilation indicates that a breath is given until a specific pressure is reached versus volume support that gives a preset volume of air (option 3). Assist-intermittent ventilation delivers a volume or pressure every time the client begins a breath, thereby allowing the client to set the rate while the ventilator ensures that every breath, no matter how weak the client's effort may be, will be a full breath (option 4). **Cognitive Level:** Applying **Client Need:** Physiological Integrity **Nursing Process:** Assessment **Learning Outcome:** 28-1

2. **Answer:** 1 **Rationale:** Weaning from the ventilator indicates that the amount of ventilatory support provided will be reduced. This includes reducing the time the client is on the ventilator, the pressure or volume settings, and the number of breaths supplied until the client no longer requires the ventilator. Increasing sedation to prevent the client from fighting the ventilator when he or she begins weaning will work in the client's disfavor (option 2). You want the client alert to be able to participate and report sensations. Unless the client does not tolerate weaning, settings are moved toward allowing independent breathing rather than back and forth (option 3). Weaning is a process, not an all-or-none situation such as would occur with intervals of being on and off the ventilator (option 4). **Cognitive Level:** Applying **Client Need:** Physiological Integrity **Nursing Process:** Implementation **Learning Outcome:** 28-4B

3. **Answer:** 1 **Rationale:** An important means of preventing atelectasis and pooling of secretions in the dependent area of the lungs is to reposition the client frequently because the area of the thorax that comes in contact with the bed is unable to inflate fully. Suctioning should not be done on a specific schedule, but as needed (option 2). Bathing the client daily (option 3) and monitoring the arterial blood gases (option 4) are both important interventions, but they do not affect atelectasis and pooling of secretions. **Cognitive Level:** Analyzing **Client Need:** Physiological Integrity **Nursing Process:** Implementation **Learning Outcome:** 28-2

4. **Answer:** 3 **Rationale:** The nurse's priority action is to maintain adequate ventilation for the client using a hand-controlled ventilation system. Notifying respiratory therapy of the need for a ventilator (option 1), determining ventilator settings (option 2), and assessing the client's lung sounds are all required interventions, but breathing always takes priority over these actions. **Cognitive Level:** Applying **Client Need:** Physiological Integrity **Nursing Process:** Implementation **Learning Outcome:** 28-2

5. **Answer:** 2 **Rationale:** The first thing to assess is the presence of fluid in the ventilator tubing because this will cause the high-pressure alarms to ring. Secretions in the airway significant enough to trigger high-pressure alarms would affect the oxygen saturation and breath sounds (option 1). Kinked tubing would cause hypoxia and respiratory distress (option 3). If the client is coughing, the nurse would see the client's chest movements and it would be unlikely the client would be resting quietly (option 4). **Cognitive Level:** Analyzing **Client Need:** Physiological Integrity **Nursing Process:** Assessment **Learning Outcome:** 28-2

6. **Answer:** 4 **Rationale:** The reason the tubing is secured to the bed is to prevent the weight of the tubing from pulling on the airway. If infection control was the primary goal, the tubing could be secured in any location (options 1 and 2). Telling a family member that the only reason for doing something is "hospital policy" does not give them the rationale for the action and reduces the family's trust in the nurse's knowledge of why something is done (option 3). **Cognitive Level:** Analyzing **Client Need:** Physiological Integrity **Nursing Process:** Implementation **Learning Outcome:** 28-2

7. **Answer:** 3 **Rationale:** The UAP may assist in performing routine care such as measuring vital signs and oxygen saturation for the client

who requires a mechanical ventilator, but should be taught by the nurse what parameters should be reported immediately, and the nurse should evaluate all measurements. Changes in ventilator settings (option 1), suctioning the client's airway (option 2), and tracheostomy care (option 4) should never be delegated to the UAP. **Cognitive Level:** Analyzing **Client Need:** Safe and Effective Care Environment **Nursing Process:** Planning **Learning Outcome:** 28-3

8. **Answer:** 1 **Rationale:** The nurse should first assess the client to determine if the endotracheal tube is still in the trachea by assessing breath sounds, a need for suctioning, or another problem contributing to the client's declining condition. Suctioning the airway will worsen hypoxia and should not be performed if there is no indication of a need for this procedure (option 2). Although it may be necessary to call the primary care provider, the nurse must first assess the client so that the nurse can relate the data obtained during the call (option 3). Removing the endotracheal tube before assessing placement would be contraindicated because a properly placed tube will allow better oxygenation than hand bagging without a tube in place (option 4). **Cognitive Level:** Applying **Client Need:** Physiological Integrity **Nursing Process:** Implementation **Learning Outcome:** 28-4a

9. **Answer:** 2 **Rationale:** The primary care provider needs to be notified immediately if the endotracheal tube becomes displaced in order to have a new tube inserted. An oxygen saturation of 90% may be acceptable and a respiratory rate of 28 breaths per minute might be due to the setting on the ventilator (option 1). Flecks of blood may be found in the endotracheal secretions if proper suctioning technique is not used or the client requires frequent suctioning (option 3). It should be documented, but there is no need to call the primary care provider immediately. An increased quantity of secretions may be due to client activity or frequent suctioning (option 4). It should be documented, but there is no need to call the primary care provider immediately to report. **Cognitive Level:** Analyzing **Client Need:** Physiological Integrity **Nursing Process:** Implementation **Learning Outcome:** 28-5

10. **Answer:** 1, 3, 4 **Rationale:** It is essential that the nurse document secretion appearance (option 1), ventilator settings (option 3), and vital signs, oxygen saturation, and assessment findings (option 4). The ventilator tubing should be changed every 24 to 48 hours, depending on facility policy, and will be documented by the respiratory therapist when performed. There is no need for the nurse to document this (option 2). There is no reason to record the length of the tubing from the ventilator to the client (option 5). **Cognitive Level:** Applying **Client Need:** Safe and Effective Care Environment **Nursing Process:** Implementation **Learning Outcome:** 28-5

Chapter 29: *Caring for the Client with Chest Tube Drainage*

1. **Answer:** 2. **Rationale:** Check the connections between the chest site and the drainage tube, and where the drainage tube connects to the collection chamber. Constant bubbling in the water-seal column is not a normal finding (option 1); normally the bubbling is intermittent. Constant bubbling indicates an air leak. Neither decreasing the suction (option 3) nor draining half of the water from the chamber (option 4) will correct the air leak. **Cognitive Level:** Applying **Client Need:** Physiological Integrity **Nursing Process:** Implementation **Learning Outcome:** 29-3b

2. **Answer:** 1 **Rationale:** The device described is a Heimlich chest drain valve. Pneumovax is a pneumococcal vaccine effective against 23 common strains of pneumococcus (option 2). A Pleurovac (option 3) is a brand name of a water-sealed set (option 4). **Cognitive Level:** Remembering **Client Need:** Physiological Integrity **Nursing Process:** Not Applicable **Learning Outcome:** 29-1

3. **Answer:** 2 **Rationale:** The term for the fluctuation of the water-seal chamber when the client breathes is called tidaling. Bubbling is different from tidaling because bubbling is the presence of gas moving

through the chamber, whereas tidaling is an up-and-down movement that correlates with the client's breathing (option 1). Fluttering (option 3) and alternating (option 4) reflect incorrect terminology. **Cognitive Level:** Remembering **Client Need:** Physiological Integrity **Nursing Process:** Not Applicable **Learning Outcome:** 29-1

4. **Answer: 4 Rationale:** The UAP may turn and position the client as long as the nurse ensures that the UAP understands how to manipulate the tubing safely and what signs and symptoms should be reported immediately. Care of the chest tube, including milking the tube if ordered (option 1), measuring chest tube output (option 2), and changing the chest tube drainage system (option 3), should never be delegated to UAP. **Cognitive Level:** Applying **Client Need:** Safe and Effective Care Environment **Nursing Process:** Planning **Learning Outcome:** 29-2

5. **Answer: 1 Rationale:** A blockage or kink in the tubing will inhibit pleural drainage and, in turn, prevent the lung from reexpanding or cause a mediastinal shift to the opposite side. Increasing the amount of suction cannot be done without a primary care provider's order and would not be the most appropriate initial action (option 2). The normal level for placement of the chest tube drainage system is 2 to 3 feet below heart level. Raising it can cause backflow of drainage into the client (option 3). Clamping the tube obstructs the flow of air and fluid from the pleural space and should not be done (option 4). **Cognitive Level:** Applying **Client Need:** Physiological Integrity **Nursing Process:** Implementation **Learning Outcome:** 29-3b

6. **Answer: 4 Rationale:** Drainage exceeding 100 mL/h should be reported immediately because this would be considered abnormal. Drainage would be expected to be bloody if the client has a hemothorax (option 1). The cessation of bubbling in the water seal is normal when there is no air leak (option 2). Chest tube insertion will not remove subcutaneous emphysema. The condition should be reported, documented, and monitored since it can increase if the chest tube is obstructed, but its continued presence is not an emergency (option 3). **Cognitive Level:** Analyzing **Client Need:** Safe and Effective Care Environment **Nursing Process:** Implementation **Learning Outcome:** 29-3A, 29-4

7. **Answer: 1, 3, and 4 Rationale:** Continuous bubbling in the water-seal chamber could indicate a leak in the system and should be assessed further (option 1). The presence of subcutaneous emphysema must be assessed further because it can be caused by a poor seal at the chest tube insertion site (option 3). Complaints of pain at the insertion site can be expected but should be fully assessed prior to administering analgesics (option 4). A respiratory rate of 18 breaths per minute falls within the normal range and does not, by itself, indicate a need for further assessment (option 2). A small amount of drainage on the chest tube dressing can be expected and serous drainage would be normal (option 5); however, it should be monitored for any change in appearance. **Cognitive Level:** Analyzing **Client Need:** Physiological Integrity **Nursing Process:** Assessment **Learning Outcome:** 29-4

8. **Answer: 1, 2, 3, and 4 Rationale:** The nurse should ensure that there are clamps (option 1) at the bedside to clamp the tubing in case of emergency, a plain 4×4 gauze (option 2) and sterile petroleum gauze (option 3) to make an occlusive dressing should the chest tube become dislodged, and an extra drainage system (option 4) should the current system become full. There is no need to keep a spare chest tube in most instances because it could be obtained while waiting for the primary care provider to arrive and reinsert it (option 5). **Cognitive Level:** Applying **Client Need:** Physiological Integrity **Nursing Process:** Planning **Learning Outcome:** 29-4

9. **Answer: 1 Rationale:** If bubbling stops when the chest tube is clamped between the collecting system and the body, the leak is at the insertion site or inside the client. Applying pressure to the dressing will determine which of the sites is leaking. If bubbling continues after clamping

the chest tube, the leak is below the clamp and the next step would be to move the clamp farther away from the client and reassess (option 2). Only if the bubbling never stops after moving the clamp all the way down the tubing should the collection system be replaced (option 3). Turning the suction device higher will increase bubbling in the suction chamber and will not affect bubbling in the water-seal chamber (option 4). **Cognitive Level:** Applying **Client Need:** Physiological Integrity **Nursing Process:** Implementing **Learning Outcome:** 29-3b

10. **Answer: 2 Rationale:** Placing the end of the chest tube into the bottle of sterile water will help to reestablish the water seal necessary to prevent the lung from collapsing. Notifying the primary care provider is necessary (option 1), but it is not the immediate action. Replacing the contaminated drainage system with a sterile one (option 3) should be done once the water seal has been created. Placing a sterile dressing over the chest tube insertion site (option 4) will not prevent air from reentering the pleural space. **Cognitive Level:** Applying **Client Need:** Physiological Integrity **Nursing Process:** Implementation **Learning Outcome:** 29-3b

Chapter 30: Administering Emergency Measures to the Hospitalized Client

1. **Answer: 3 Rationale:** The rapid response team would be called for the client with chest pain, hypotension, and shortness of breath to prevent a potentially life-threatening situation. A client with postoperative pain can be successfully treated by the nurse on the unit and does not require the rapid response team (option 1). If the client has no pulse and no respirations, the nurse should call the arrest team, not the rapid response team (option 2). The nurse should call the primary care provider for the client who is hypertensive (option 4). **Cognitive Level:** Applying **Client Need:** Physiological Integrity **Nursing Process:** Planning **Learning Outcome:** 30-2

2. **Answer: 4 Rationale:** A client who becomes unconscious while in ventricular tachycardia requires the intervention of the cardiac/respiratory arrest team. A hypotensive client (option 1) or a client experiencing dyspnea (option 2) requires the intervention of the rapid response team. A client in atrial fibrillation requires notification of the primary care provider (option 3). **Cognitive Level:** Applying **Client Need:** Physiological Integrity **Nursing Process:** Planning **Learning Outcome:** 30-2

3. **Answer: 1 Rationale:** The nurse's first action should be to summon the cardiac/respiratory arrest team because it will take them a few minutes to arrive and the client's best outcome depends on their rapid arrival. As soon as the team has been called, the nurse should begin CPR (option 2). If the arrest is not called over the public address system, the nurse should call a coworker for help while performing CPR or after initiating CPR (option 3). If the code is called over the public address system, coworkers will hear the call and come to the room without being summoned. Once the coworkers have been alerted, they can obtain the crash cart and summon additional support (option 4). **Cognitive Level:** Applying **Client Need:** Physiological Integrity **Nursing Process:** Implementation **Learning Outcome:** 30-3

4. **Answer: 4 Rationale:** The nurse's responsibility while awaiting the arrest team is to perform CPR, with or without assistance as available. Other team members can collect the client's records (option 1), obtain the crash cart (option 2), and notify the primary care provider (option 3). The nurse assigned to the client should stay with the client to provide the history when the team arrives. **Cognitive Level:** Applying **Client Need:** Physiological Integrity **Nursing Process:** Implementation **Learning Outcome:** 30-3

5. **Answer: 2 Rationale:** The most effective means of converting a client's electrical rhythm to normal sinus rhythm from ventricular fibrillation is to use a defibrillator. CPR should be performed until the defibrillator patches are applied, but it is not the most effective means of converting

the electrical rhythm; rather it supports life until defibrillation can be performed (option 1). Oxygen should be administered during CPR, but it is also not the means of converting the rhythm (option 3). Precordial thumps are controversial at best and would not be the most effective means of converting the rhythm (option 4). **Cognitive Level:** Applying **Client Need:** Physiological Integrity **Nursing Process:** Implementation **Learning Outcome:** 30-1

6. **Answer: 3 Rationale:** Before any intervention is begun, the nurse should assess that the client is choking and wants assistance. Performing abdominal thrusts before assessing the client could result in a life-threatening situation if the client is not actually choking (option 1). The emergency response system should not be activated until it is determined the client actually is choking (option 2). CPR would not be appropriate if the client is conscious because this indicates the client most likely has a pulse (option 4). **Cognitive Level:** Applying **Client Need:** Physiological Integrity **Nursing Process:** Implementation **Learning Outcome:** 30-5a

7. **Answer: 3 Rationale:** Establish an airway by tilting the head back and lifting the chin. An endotracheal tube should not be inserted by the nurse (option 1). It is not necessary to put tension on the tongue because the proper head tilt with chin thrust will remove the tongue from obstructing the airway (option 2). A modified jaw thrust would be used if a neck injury was suspected, but since this client collapsed in front of you that would not be a concern in this scenario (option 4). **Cognitive Level:** Applying **Client Need:** Physiological Integrity **Nursing Process:** Implementation **Learning Outcome:** 30-5b

8. **Answer: 2 Rationale:** The correct ratio of compressions to breaths is 15 chest compressions followed by 2 breaths if there are two rescuers for a child. A ratio of 30:2 would be used in adult CPR (option 1); if there are two rescuers, 1 breath is interspersed after 15 compressions but the ratio remains 30:2. Ratios of 5:2 and 5:1 (options 3 and 4) are always incorrect when performing CPR on a child. **Cognitive Level:** Applying **Client Need:** Physiological Integrity **Nursing Process:** Implementation **Learning Outcome:** 30-5c

9. **Answer: 2 Rationale:** As soon as the cable is connected, the machine begins to attempt to analyze the rhythm. First, the power should be turned on and the pads applied to the chest wall before the cable is connected to the machine. Connecting the cable, applying the pads, and then turning on the power would cause the machine to malfunction or delay analysis while it cycles on (option 1). Connecting the cable before applying the pads (options 3 and 4) could result in the rescuer being shocked. **Cognitive Level:** Applying **Client Need:** Physiological Integrity **Nursing Process:** Implementation **Learning Outcome:** 30-5d

10. **Answer: 4 Rationale:** The nurse needs to ensure that no one is touching the client while the machine is analyzing because it may interfere with correct interpretation of the client's rhythm and could put anyone touching the client at risk of being shocked. CPR may be continued up until the machine is ready to analyze, although CPR may need to be momentarily stopped to place the chest pad, and when the AED instructs the user to resume CPR. There is no risk to touching the client while the machine is plugged in (option 2), and it is not possible to apply the pads without touching the client (option 3). CPR should be performed until an AED is brought to the client, the cable is inserted into the machine with the pads already in place, and the AED is ready to analyze the rhythm (option 1). **Cognitive Level:** Applying **Client Need:** Physiological Integrity **Nursing Process:** Implementation **Learning Outcome:** 30-5d

Chapter 31: Performing Wound and Pressure Ulcer Care

1. **Answer: 2 Rationale:** Eschar is necrotic tissue found in or around a wound. Alginate is an absorbent material that can be placed in the wound to soak up drainage (option 1). Granulation is soft, pink, fleshy projections that form during the healing process in a wound (option 3). Drainage is fluid that comes from the wound (option 4). **Cognitive Level:** Remembering **Client Need:** Physiological Integrity **Nursing Process:** Assessment **Learning Outcome:** 31-1

2. **Answer: 1 Rationale:** A dry sterile dressing would be appropriate for a freshly closed surgical wound (option 1). A clean postoperative dressing would be contraindicated due to the potential for infection (option 2). Closed wounds do not require wet dressings (options 3 and 4). **Cognitive Level:** Understanding **Client Need:** Physiological Integrity **Nursing Process:** Planning **Learning Outcome:** 31-2

3. **Answer: 3 and 4 Rationale:** The best dressings for this type of wound are polyurethane foams and alginates because they will maintain moist wound healing while helping to absorb heavy amounts of exudate. Transparent films, impregnated nonadherent dressings, and hydrogels would not be used on a wound with heavy exudate (options 1, 2, and 5). **Cognitive Level:** Applying **Client Need:** Physiological Integrity **Nursing Process:** Implementation **Learning Outcome:** 31-2

4. **Answer: 1 Rationale:** Yellow wounds are characterized primarily by liquid to semiliquid slough that is often accompanied by purulent drainage from previous infection. Tissue will appear red during the late regeneration of tissue repair (option 2). Necrotic tissue will appear black in color (option 3). During the early regeneration phase of tissue repair, it is common to find minimal to moderate drainage (option 4). **Cognitive Level:** Applying **Client Need:** Physiological Integrity **Nursing Process:** Assessment **Learning Outcome:** 31-3

5. **Answer: 4 Rationale:** A category IV pressure ulcer has full-thickness skin loss with extensive destruction, tissue necrosis, or damage to muscle, bone, or supporting structures with or without sinus tracts. Category/stage I ulcers are generally red with intact skin that does not blanch (option 1). Category/stage II pressure ulcers involve partial-thickness skin loss that is superficial and looks like an abrasion or blister (option 2). Category/stage III ulcers have full-thickness skin loss with damage to the subcutaneous tissue that may go to, but not through, underlying tissues and looks like a deep crater (option 3). **Cognitive Level:** Remembering **Client Need:** Safe and Effective Care Environment **Nursing Process:** Planning **Learning Outcome:** 31-4

6. **Answer: 2 Rationale:** The UAP may be permitted to apply dry dressings to a chronic wound in most states (option 2). Skills requiring sterile technique such as a sterile postoperative dressing (option 1) and wound irrigation (option 3), or those requiring assessment such as wound packing (option 4), would not be appropriate to delegate to the UAP. **Cognitive Level:** Remembering **Client Need:** Safe and Effective Care Environment **Nursing Process:** Planning **Learning Outcome:** 31-4

7. **Answer: 1 Rationale:** The first appearance of a red area on the sacrum could be documented and reported to the primary care provider during the next visit. There would be no need to report it immediately. A postoperative wound that is draining purulent material (option 2), a new venous stasis ulcer (option 3), or a persistent red area (option 4) needs to be reported to the primary care provider today and cannot wait for the primary care provider's next visit, because the client needs to be treated quickly to avoid further complications. **Cognitive Level:** Analyzing **Client Need:** Safe and Effective Care Environment **Nursing Process:** Implementation **Learning Outcome:** 31-6

8. **Answer: 4 Rationale:** The best time to perform wound irrigation would be after medicating the client for pain, because the procedure can be uncomfortable and this would reduce the discomfort for the client. Irrigating the wound before breakfast could reduce the client's appetite (option 1). If the nurse knows when the primary care provider is arriving, it would be better to do the irrigation before the visit and be able to report wound status (option 2). The wound should be irrigated before dressing the wound, not after, because the dressing would need to be removed for irrigation

(option 3). **Cognitive Level:** Understanding **Client Need:** Safe and Effective Care Environment **Nursing Process:** Planning **Learning Outcome:** 31-5e

9. **Answer:** 3 **Rationale:** When applying an elastic bandage, the nurse should wrap the bandage above and below the joint working from distal to proximal. There would be no need to involve the knee (option 1). Bandages should be wrapped distal to proximal so the nurse should not start above the ankle (option 2) or at the heel (option 4). **Cognitive Level:** Applying **Client Need:** Physiological Integrity **Nursing Process:** Implementation **Learning Outcome:** 31-5I

10. **Answer:** 3 **Rationale:** When applying a sling, it should be fitted to provide support to the wrist and not allow the hand to hang down. A sling that stops at the wrist would need to be replaced with one that supports the wrist to maintain proper alignment and prevent complications (option 3). The straps that go from the fingers, around the lower back or waist, and around the neck are adjustable and can easily be tightened (option 1) or loosened (option 4). A sling that ends in the middle of the palm would be properly fitted (option 2). **Cognitive Level:** Analyzing **Client Need:** Physiological Integrity **Nursing Process:** Evaluation **Learning Outcome:** 31-5I

Chapter 32: Orthopedic Care

1. **Answer:** 3, 1, and 2 **Rationale:** The nurse's priority action would be to apply oxygen because the client is short of breath (option 3). After applying oxygen the nurse should summon assistance to call the primary care provider or the rapid response team (option 1) and notify the charge nurse (option 2). The nurse should not administer nitroglycerin without an order because this would be outside the nurse's scope of practice, and may not be the proper medication if this client is experiencing a pulmonary embolism (option 4). **Cognitive Level:** Analyzing **Client Need:** Physiological Integrity **Nursing Process:** Implementation **Learning Outcome:** 32-4

2. **Answer:** Plaster of paris **Rationale:** The nurse would anticipate the use of plaster of paris because of the need to cut a window to monitor healing of the wound. Plaster of paris casts are used when exact molding around a joint is desired, when serial casting is to be performed, or when a window is to be cut to monitor wound healing. **Cognitive Level:** Analyzing **Client Need:** Physiological Integrity **Nursing Process:** Planning **Learning Outcome:** 32-2

3. **Answer:** 4 **Rationale:** The nurse should assess the client every 30 minutes for 4 hours (option 4) and then every 4 hours for 24 to 48 hours. Options 1, 2, and 3 are incorrect times. **Cognitive Level:** Remembering **Client Need:** Physiological Integrity **Nursing Process:** Planning **Learning Outcome:** 32-6

4. **Answer:** 3 **Rationale:** Pale toes may indicate a reduction in circulation to the foot, and the primary care provider should be notified (option 3). If both feet are cold, the client should be given a blanket and the toes should be assessed frequently to ensure the feet warm bilaterally (option 1). A capillary refill time of 3 seconds is normal (option 2). Edema of the toes on the casted leg is to be anticipated (option 4). Any increase in edema accompanied by reduced temperature, decreased sensation, or prolonged capillary refill time should be reported to the primary care provider. **Cognitive Level:** Applying **Client Need:** Physiological Integrity **Nursing Process:** Assessment **Learning Outcome:** 32-6

5. **Answer:** 3 **Rationale:** Although synthetic casts will not be damaged if they get wet, the padding and stockinette will soak up water and dry slowly unless polypropylene material is used, so it is best to keep casts dry. If the cast gets dirty, it can be readily cleaned so the client need not come to the emergency department to have it changed (option 1). Use of a wet cloth would be appropriate (option 4), and special care such as covering the cast with a garbage bag is appropriate, making options 2 and 4 incorrect responses. **Cognitive Level:** Analyzing **Client Need:**

Health Promotion and Maintenance **Nursing Process:** Evaluation **Learning Outcome:** 32-3

6. **Answer:** 2 **Rationale:** The cast should be placed on pillows to prevent denting or misshaping of the cast, with the foot of the bed elevated. Ideally, the leg should be elevated approximately 45°, near the level of the heart. Simply raising the foot of the bed (option 1) will not provide enough elevation, especially if the head of the bed is also raised. Limbs are casted instead of, not in addition to, traction (option 3). The client can be turned once the cast is sufficiently dry but the initial drying period should occur while the leg is in anatomical position, which minimizes pressure on bony prominences (option 4). **Cognitive Level:** Applying **Client Need:** Physiological Integrity **Nursing Process:** Implementation **Learning Outcome:** 32-7a

7. **Answer:** 1 **Rationale:** The client should call the primary care provider if there are any signs of neurosensory or circulatory impairment such as reduced temperature, loss of sensation, pale color, or increase in pain. Statement 2 would indicate the need for further teaching because the leg should be elevated on pillows closer to the level of the heart, and sitting in a recliner would likely not provide sufficient height (option 2). Walking should be limited to bathroom privileges only, because holding the leg in a dependent position will increase edema (option 3). Synthetic casts dry in 10 to 15 minutes and do not require any intervention to speed up the process (option 4). **Cognitive Level:** Analyzing **Client Need:** Health Promotion and Maintenance **Nursing Process:** Evaluation **Learning Outcome:** 32-7a

8. **Answer:** 2 **Rationale:** The client should be told not to put anything into the cast but should be given other options for dealing with the issue. Option 1 is incorrect because insertion of anything into the cast can bunch the padding and cause discomfort, even if it is blunt ended. Telling the client not to use the wooden spoon, without teaching other methods of dealing with the issue, will almost guarantee noncompliance (option 3). Clients with synthetic casts often do experience itching, so telling them not to worry about it does not promote good self-care (option 4). **Cognitive Level:** Analyzing **Client Need:** Health Promotion and Maintenance **Nursing Process:** Implementation **Learning Outcome:** 32-7a

9. **Answer:** 4 **Rationale:** The nurse should reassess the area in 20 minutes. If the red area fades within 20 minutes there is no need to notify the orthotist (option 1). Lotion should be avoided because this softens the tissue and increases the risk of skin breakdown (option 2). Rubbing the area will increase the risk of further trauma and would be contraindicated (option 3). **Cognitive Level:** Applying **Client Need:** Physiological Integrity **Nursing Process:** Implementation **Learning Outcome:** 32-8

10. **Answer:** 1 **Rationale:** Parents of children wearing orthotics are taught to apply household oil to the hinges periodically to prevent stiff movement (option 1). Options 2 and 3 are incorrect because the mother acted correctly. Option 4 implies that using household oil is unusual when it is actually a necessary intervention. **Cognitive Level:** Applying **Client Need:** Health Promotion and Maintenance **Nursing Process:** Implementation **Learning Outcome:** 32-8

Chapter 33: Performing Perioperative Care

1. **Answer:** 2 **Rationale:** Dehiscence is separation of a suture line before the incision heals. The nurse would have observed purulent drainage from the wound and redness around the incision with a wound infection (option 1). Extrusion or protrusion of internal organs and tissues through the incision occurs with wound evisceration (option 3). Wound approximation is normal. It is when the incision is closed or approximated to each other (option 4). **Cognitive Level:** Remembering **Client Need:** Safe and Effective Care Environment **Nursing Process:** Implementation **Learning Outcome:** 33-1

2. **Answer:** 3 **Rationale:** The question is describing the RNFA. When the client goes into the operating room, the client is in the intraoperative

phase. During the preoperative phase, the nurse performs preoperative teaching (option 1). When the client enters the recovery room, the postoperative phase begins (option 2). All of these phases together are called the perioperative phase (option 4). **Cognitive Level:** Remembering **Client Need:** Safe and Effective Care Environment **Nursing Process:** Implementation **Learning Outcome:** 33-2

3. **Answer:** 1, 2, 3, and 5 **Rationale:** The four dimensions of preoperative teaching include information (option 1), psychosocial support (option 2), skills training (option 3), and roles of the client and support people (option 5). Physiological support is not a part of preoperative teaching (option 4). **Cognitive Level:** Applying **Client Need:** Health Promotion and Maintenance **Nursing Process:** Implementation **Learning Outcome:** 33-4

4. **Answer:** 2 **Rationale:** The use of a brush may increase the amount of skin shedding and can increase microbial counts (option 1) because of skin damage. A brush is not necessary when using alcohol-based products (option 3) and can lead to skin abrasion and dermatitis (option 4). **Cognitive Level:** Applying **Client Need:** Safe and Effective Care Environment **Nursing Process:** Planning **Learning Outcome:** 33-5

5. **Answer:** 1 **Rationale:** Option 1 is correct and states the response in terms the client can understand. Option 2 uses medical jargon such as UTI that the client may not know the meaning of, and as a result, the client will not be motivated to move. Ambulation does not prevent complications as stated in options 3 and 4, but it does help to reduce the risk. **Cognitive Level:** Applying **Client Need:** Health Promotion and Maintenance **Nursing Process:** Implementation **Learning Outcome:** 33-8

6. **Answer:** 3 **Rationale:** When providing preoperative teaching it is helpful for the nurse to know what the client knows about the surgery (option 1), the client's educational level (option 4), and what experience the client has had with surgery in the past (option 2), because all of these will affect how and what the nurse teaches. The family's agreement or disagreement with the surgery does not affect what the nurse teaches (option 3). **Cognitive Level:** Analyzing **Client Need:** Health Promotion and Maintenance **Nursing Process:** Assessment **Learning Outcome:** 33-10A

7. **Answer:** 3, 4, 1, and 2 **Rationale:** The mask (option 3) should be applied before putting on shoe covers (option 4) because the shoes are dirty and the nurse should not touch the mask after touching the shoes. After applying the mask and shoe covers, the nurse would perform surgical hand hygiene and then apply the gown (option 1), pulling on the gloves (option 2) after sliding the arms and hands into the gown. **Cognitive Level:** Applying **Client Need:** Safe and Effective Care Environment **Nursing Process:** Implementation **Learning Outcome:** 33-10c

8. **Answer:** 2 **Rationale:** The nurse would connect the tube to intermittent suction because single-lumen gastric tubes do not have a second lumen to release pressure and prevent damage to the mucous membrane near the distal port of the tube. Continuous suction is contraindicated in single-lumen tubes (option 1), as is alternating continuous and intermittent suction (options 3 and 4). **Cognitive Level:** Analyzing **Client Need:** Safe and Effective Care Environment **Nursing Process:** Implementation **Learning Outcome:** 33-10d

9. **Answer:** 4, 3, 1, 2, and 5 **Rationale:** First, place the drain on a waterproof pad to prevent soiling of the bed during the procedure (option 4). Next, open the plug prior to inverting the unit to prevent spraying contents (option 3). Slowly invert the unit over a graduated collecting container so the contents can be measured (option 1). After emptying the unit, compress the bulb to reestablish suction (option 2) and clean the end of the port before resealing it (option 5). **Cognitive Level:** Applying **Client Need:** Safe and Effective Care Environment **Nursing Process:** Implementation **Learning Outcome:** 33-10f

10. **Answer:** 1 **Rationale:** Removal of sutures in a draining wound is contraindicated. Moisture at the wound site can be dried prior to

removing sutures (option 2). A light red line marking the incision indicates good wound healing and would not contraindicate suture removal (option 3). In some circumstances, the doctor may choose to remove every other suture and this situation would not contraindicate removal of the sutures (option 4). **Cognitive Level:** Analyzing **Client Need:** Health Promotion and Maintenance **Nursing Process:** Planning **Learning Outcome:** 33-10g

Chapter 34: End-of-Life Care

1. **Answer:** 3 **Rationale:** Livor mortis is discoloration of dependent body areas due to red blood cell breakdown, so elevating the head slightly will prevent this from occurring in the facial area. None of the other options (1, 2, or 3) will prevent livor mortis of the face. **Cognitive Level:** Applying **Client Need:** Physiological Integrity **Nursing Process:** Implementation **Learning Outcome:** 34-1

2. **Answer:** 1 **Rationale:** Higher brain death occurs when the cerebral cortex is irreversibly destroyed and absence of responsiveness to external stimuli, absence of cephalic reflexes, and apnea occur. Loss of the frontal lobe does not cause brain death, and people have survived the loss of this lobe (option 2). Higher brain death involves the destruction of the cerebral cortex, not the medulla (option 3) or just the brainstem (option 4). **Cognitive Level:** Remembering **Client Need:** Physiological Integrity **Nursing Process:** Assessment **Learning Outcome:** 34-1

3. **Answer:** 3 **Rationale:** Sensory impairment is a sign of impending death. Heart rate may slow or it may increase due to reduced cardiac output (option 1). Blood pressure is more likely to decrease, not increase, as death nears (option 2). Wanting the family near does not necessarily indicate impending death (option 4). **Cognitive Level:** Remembering **Client Need:** Health Promotion and Maintenance **Nursing Process:** Assessment **Learning Outcome:** 34-3

4. **Answer:** 3 **Rationale:** Rigor mortis generally occurs 2 to 4 hours after death. Rigor mortis is unlikely to occur after only 30 minutes (option 1) or 1 hour (option 2). There would be no reason for the nurse to think the client had been dead for as long as 8 hours based on this sign alone (option 4). **Cognitive Level:** Applying **Client Need:** Physiological Integrity **Nursing Process:** Assessment **Learning Outcome:** 34-3

5. **Answer:** 2 **Rationale:** When caring for the dying client, flexing of agency rules may be required, but it is important not to put another client in danger. Therefore, the nurse would move the client to a safe space and then allow the child to visit. Allowing the child to visit with another client in the room would be unfair to the roommate and in direct violation of policy (option 1). To deny the child's visitation would not be the best option and would make the client's death more difficult for both the client and the family (option 3). Allowing the client to see the child through the window would not allow the client the opportunity to touch or talk to the child (option 4). **Cognitive Level:** Evaluating **Client Need:** Psychosocial Integrity **Nursing Process:** Implementation **Learning Outcome:** 34-5a

6. **Answer:** 3 **Rationale:** The priority information the nurse must provide to the UAP is which tubes and medical devices can be removed and which must remain in place. Bathing the body (option 1), wrapping the body (option 2), and placing identifiers on the body (option 4) are standard postmortem care in which the UAP should already be skilled. **Cognitive Level:** Applying **Client Need:** Safe and Effective Care Environment **Nursing Process:** Planning **Learning Outcome:** 34-4

7. **Answer:** 3 **Rationale:** The question specifically asks what would be documented about postmortem care so the priority documentation during this phase would be any items (such as dentures or rings) remaining on the body. Medical diagnosis (option 1) would be the responsibility of the primary care provider to put on the death certificate. Time of death (option 2) and any final words (option 4) would be

documented in the note regarding the client's death. **Cognitive Level:** Applying **Client Need:** Safe and Effective Care Environment **Nursing Process:** Implementation **Learning Outcome:** 34-6

8. **Answer:** 4 **Rationale:** Because the death occurred in the emergency department, the client will most likely be a coroner's case and the nurse should not remove dressings or tubes from the body. It is acceptable for the nurse to wash away blood (option 1), remove glass shards from the client's hair (option 2), and remove the client's clothing (option 3), although the clothing should be kept in a plastic bag and sent with the body to the morgue. **Cognitive Level:** Applying **Client Need:** Safe and Effective Environment **Nursing Process:** Implementation **Learning Outcome:** 34-5b

9. **Answer:** 1 **Rationale:** Family members should be encouraged to help with the physical care of the dying client as much as they wish, but the nurse should never require them to do so. Informing the family of what you are going to do and asking them if they would like to participate is the best option. Asking the wife if she wants to do it makes it difficult for her to say "no" (option 2). Telling the wife what she should do also does not offer her the option to say "no" (option 3). Telling the wife her husband would feel better if she bathed him requires her to perform the task without offering her the option (option 4). **Cognitive Level:** Applying **Client Need:** Psychosocial Integrity **Nursing Process:** Implementation **Learning Outcome:** 34-2

10. **Answer:** 2 **Rationale:** Acknowledging the family member's possible feelings is the correct opening. It is never correct to reprimand the family member for behavior (feeding the client) that the family member is probably regretting (option 1), or tell someone how they should feel (option 3). Option 4 is overly critical and insensitive to the family member's feelings. **Cognitive Level:** Applying **Client Need:** Psychosocial Integrity **Nursing Process:** Implementation **Learning Outcome:** 34-2

Glossary

Abbreviated bath *See* Partial bath

Abdominal (diaphragmatic) breathing Breathing that involves the contraction and relaxation of the diaphragm; permits deep, full breaths with little effort

Abdominal paracentesis A procedure to obtain a specimen of ascitic fluid for laboratory study and to relieve pressure on the abdominal organs due to the presence of excess fluid

Acid-fast bacillus (AFB) A laboratory test to identify the presence of tuberculosis (TB)

Active-assistive range-of-motion exercises Exercises in which the client, with the nurse's assistance, uses a stronger, opposite arm or leg to move each of the joints of a limb incapable of active motion

Active range-of-motion exercises Isotonic exercises in which the client independently moves each joint in the body through its complete range of movement, maximally stretching all muscle groups within each plane, over the joint

Acupressure A technique that uses the fingers to apply pressure to specific points along meridians throughout the body

Acute pain Pain that lasts only through the expected recovery period (as opposed to chronic)

Addiction A chronic, relapsing, treatable disease influenced by genetic, psychosocial, and environmental factors

Advanced cardiac life support (ACLS) A multiple-day training session appropriate for emergency medical technicians, paramedics, respiratory therapists, nurses, and other professionals who may need to respond to a cardiopulmonary emergency

Adventitious breath sounds Abnormal breath sounds that occur when air passes through narrowed airways or airways filled with fluid or mucus, or when pleural linings are inflamed

Adverse effects Severe side effects that may justify discontinuation of a drug

Aerobic Growing only in the presence of oxygen

Aerosolization A type of nebulization in which the droplets are suspended in a gas, such as oxygen, making them smaller for inhalation farther into the respiratory tract

Agonist analgesic A pure opioid drug that has no ceiling on the level of analgesia; the dose can be steadily increased to relieve pain (morphine, oxycodone, hydromorphone)

Agonist–antagonist analgesic A drug that can act like an opioid and relieve pain (agonist effect) when given to a client who has not taken any pure opioids

Airborne precautions Used for clients known to have or suspected of having serious illnesses transmitted by airborne droplet nuclei smaller than 5 microns

Alginate A highly absorbent wound dressing made from a type of seaweed

Alignment (posture) Positioning of body parts in a manner that promotes optimal balance and maximal body function whether the client is sitting, standing, or lying down

Allodynia When nonpainful stimuli (e.g., contact with linen, water, or wind) produce pain

Alopecia The loss of scalp hair (baldness) or body hair

Ambulation The act of walking

Ampule A glass container usually designed to hold a single dose of a drug

Anaerobic Growing only in the absence of oxygen

Anesthesia Loss of sensation

Angiocatheter Plastic catheter that fits over a needle (stylet) used to pierce the skin and vein wall; the needle (stylet) is then withdrawn and discarded, leaving the catheter in place

Angiogram An imaging test that allows visualization of blood vessels in many parts of the body, including the brain, heart, kidney, abdomen, and legs

Ankylosis Fusion

Anorexia Loss of appetite

Antiemboli (elastic) stockings Firm elastic hosiery that exert external pressure to compress the veins of the legs, which decreases the pooling of venous blood in the extremities and thereby facilitates the return of venous blood to the heart

Antiseptic An agent that inhibits the growth of some microorganisms

Apical pulse A central pulse located at the apex of the heart

Apical–radial pulse Measurement of both the apical and radial pulses simultaneously

Apothecaries' system An older system of measurement than the metric system, in which the basic unit of weight is the grain and the basic unit of volume is the minim

Aquathermia pad An electric device that circulates warm water through a flat case

Arrhythmias Irregular heart rhythms

Arteriogram An imaging test that specifically visualizes arteries

Artificial airway Devices inserted to maintain a patent air passage for clients whose airways have become or may become obstructed

Ascites A large amount of fluid accumulation in the abdominal cavity

Asepsis Freedom from infection or infectious material

As-needed (prn) care Hygienic care provided as required by the client

Aspiration Withdrawal of fluid that has abnormally collected (e.g., pleural cavity, abdominal cavity) or to obtain a specimen (e.g., cerebrospinal fluid)

Assist-control A ventilator setting in which there is a set volume with each client-triggered breath and a set rate

Assistive devices Client-moving lifts and devices that help avoid injury to nurses and clients

Astigmatism An uneven curvature of the cornea that prevents horizontal and vertical light rays from focusing on the retina

Asystole No heartbeat

Atelectasis Collapse of the air sacs

Atomization A type of nebulization in which a device called an atomizer produces rather large droplets for inhalation

Auscultation The process of listening to sounds produced within the body, such as with the use of a stethoscope that amplifies the sounds and conveys them to the nurse's ears

Auscultatory gap The temporary disappearance of sounds normally heard over the brachial artery when the sphygmomanometer cuff pressure is high, followed by the reappearance of sounds at a lower level

Automated external defibrillator (AED) Battery-operated device that senses the cardiac rhythm through two adhesive pads, determines the appropriateness of an electric shock to convert the rhythm to normal, and delivers the shock manually or automatically

Axillary crutch An underarm crutch with hand bars

Bag bath A commercially prepared, disposable product that contains 10 to 12 presoaked disposable washcloths for different parts of the body that contain no-rinse cleanser solution; the package is warmed in a microwave

Balance A state of equilibrium in which opposing forces counteract each other

Bandage A strip of cloth used to wrap some part of the body

Base of support The foundation on which an object rests

Basic formula Used for calculating drug dosages in which D = desired dose, H = dose on hand, and V = vehicle

Basic life support Term often used to refer to the CPR skill level required of all health care providers

Bedpan A receptacle for urine and feces

Bereaved Individuals who are mourning the dead

Bevel The slanted part at the tip of a needle

Bilevel positive airway pressure (BiPAP) A variation of the continuous positive airway pressure (CPAP) treatment for obstructive sleep apnea in which the pressure delivered during exhalation is less than the pressure delivered during inhalation

Binder A type of bandage applied to large body areas (abdomen or chest) and designed for a specific body part (e.g., arm sling); used to provide support

Biopsy Removal and examination of body tissue

Bivalve To cut a cast that appears too tight partially or completely and then wrap it with bandage material to hold it together

Blood glucose meter (glucometer) A machine that measures capillary blood glucose, frequently used in home care by clients with diabetes

Bloodborne pathogens Potentially infectious organisms that are carried in and transmitted through blood or materials containing blood

Body mechanics The efficient, coordinated, and safe use of the body to move objects and carry out activities of daily living

Bolus intermittent feedings Enteral feedings that use a syringe to deliver the formula into the stomach

Brand name (of drug) Name of the drug given by the drug manufacturer; also called the trade name

Breast self-examination (BSE) A systematic procedure for palpating one's own breast tissues in search of abnormal lumps

Buccal A medication (e.g., a tablet) that is held in the mouth against the mucous membranes of the cheek until the drug dissolves

Buck's extension A type of skin traction used to immobilize fractures of the hip

Butterfly (wing-tipped) needle A needle used for intravenous infusions that has plastic flaps that are held tightly together to hold the needle securely during insertion

Canes Mechanical walking aids

Cannula A tube with a lumen (channel) that is inserted into a cavity or duct and is often fitted with a trocar during insertion for abdominal paracentesis

Capillary blood glucose (CBG) A specimen taken to measure the current blood glucose level

Cardiac catheterization An imaging test performed to visualize heart structure, coronary arteries, and blood flow

Cardiopulmonary resuscitation (CPR) The techniques of providing rescue breathing and effective chest compressions in an attempt to restore oxygenation and circulation

Carminative enema An enema given primarily to help relieve abdominal distention by expelling flatus

Cataract An opacity of the eye lens or its capsule that blocks light rays

Catheter A hollow flexible tube introduced into the body to deliver or remove fluid (e.g., through the urethra into the urinary bladder for urinary catheterization)

Center of gravity The point at which all of the mass of an object is centered

Central neuropathic pain Pain that results from malfunctioning nerves in the central nervous system (e.g., spinal cord injury pain, poststroke pain, or multiple sclerosis pain)

Central venous access device (CVAD) A device defined by the location of a catheter tip in a central vein, in the lower one third of the superior vena cava, above the right atrium

Cerebral death Occurs when the cerebral cortex is irreversibly destroyed

Cerumen Earwax

Chemical name The name by which a chemist knows a drug; describes the constituents of the drug precisely

Chemical restraints Medications used to control socially disruptive behavior

Chronic obstructive pulmonary disease (COPD) A disease process that decreases the ability of the lungs to perform ventilation

Chronic pain Prolonged pain, usually recurring or persisting over 3 months or longer, that interferes with functioning

Chyme Contents of the colon

Circulating nurse Coordinates activities and manages client care by continually assessing client safety, aseptic practice, and the environment (e.g., temperature, humidity, and lighting); with the scrub nurse, is responsible for accounting for all sponges, needles, and instruments at the close of surgery

Clean-catch urine specimen A type of urine specimen that is collected when a urine culture is ordered to identify microorganisms causing urinary tract infection; care is taken to ensure that the specimen is as free as possible from contamination by microorganisms around the urinary meatus; the specimen is collected in a sterile container with a lid

Cleaning bath A bath given for hygienic purposes

Cleansing enema Intended to remove feces; given chiefly to prevent the escape of feces during surgery, prepare the intestine for certain diagnostic tests, or remove feces in instances of constipation or impaction

Clear liquid diet Limited to water, tea, coffee, clear broths, ginger ale or other carbonated beverages, strained and clear juices, and plain gelatin

Closed bed An unoccupied bed with the top sheet, blanket, and bedspread drawn up to the top of the bed and under the pillow

Closed suction system A method for suctioning an endotracheal tube or tracheostomy in which the suction catheter, enclosed in a plastic sheath, attaches to the ventilator tubing, and the client does not need to be disconnected from the ventilator

Closed system Enteral feedings that consist of a prefilled container that is spiked with enteral tubing and attached to the enteral access device

Closed wound drainage system Consists of a drain connected to either an electric suction or a portable drainage suction

Coanalgesic A medication that is not classified as a pain medication but has properties that may reduce pain alone or in combination with other analgesics, relieve other discomforts, potentiate the effect of pain medication, or reduce the pain medication's side effects

Code Blue Term used by an agency such as a hospital to indicate a medical emergency such as a cardiac or respiratory arrest

Colostomy An opening into the colon (large bowel) to divert and drain fecal material

Commode A portable chair with a toilet seat and a removable collection receptacle beneath the seat that can be emptied; often used for the adult client who is able to get out of bed but is unable to walk to the bathroom

Compartment syndrome A serious complication that can result when swelling and pressure within a closed fascial compartment build to dangerous levels, preventing nourishment from reaching nerve and muscle cells

Complete bed bath A bath in which the entire body of a dependent client is washed while the client is in bed

Compress A damp dressing applied with pressure

Condom catheter A condom attached to a urinary drainage system to prevent complications and inconveniences associated with incontinence in males

Conjunctivitis An inflammatory process of the bulbar and palpebral conjunctiva, resulting from foreign bodies, chemicals, allergenic agents, bacteria, or viruses

Constipation Passage of small, dry, hard stool or passage of no stool for a period of time

Contact precautions Used for clients known to have or suspected of having serious illnesses easily transmitted by direct client contact or by contact with items in the client's environment (GI, respiratory, skin or wound infections, etc.)

Continuous ambulatory peritoneal dialysis (CAPD) Technique performed by clients that allows them to go home with a peritoneal catheter in place and perform the dialysis exchange on themselves

Continuous cycling (or cycler-assisted) peritoneal dialysis (CCPD) Technique that involves the cycling of dialysate infused through a mechanical cycler and warmer

Continuous feedings Enteral feedings administered over a 24-hour period using an infusion pump that guarantees a constant flow rate

Continuous passive motion (CPM) An electric device used to promote recovery after joint surgery; provides joint motion passively

Continuous positive airway pressure (CPAP) A treatment for obstructive sleep apnea in which a mask is fitted over the client's nose during sleep, providing air under pressure during inhalation and exhalation so that the airway is kept open and cannot collapse

Continuous suction Used for clients returning from surgery with a gastric or intestinal tube in place; may be applied if a double-lumen tube (Salem sump tube) is in place

Continuous sutures A method of suturing in which one thread runs in a series of stitches and is tied only at the beginning and at the end of the run

Contracture Permanent shortening of a muscle

Contrast medium A solution (dye) that is injected intravenously during certain x-ray tests (e.g., angiogram, cardiac catheterization) to make blood vessels or the heart visible

Core temperature The temperature of the deep tissues of the body (e.g., abdominal cavity, pelvic cavity); when measured orally, the average body temperature of an adult is between 36.7°C and 37°C (98°F and 98.6°F)

Coroner A physician who is authorized by a county or other government agency to determine causes of deaths under unusual circumstances

Costal (thoracic) breathing Movement of the chest upward and outward

Countertraction In traction, the second force that pulls opposite to the pulling force applied to a part of the body

CPR *See* Cardiopulmonary resuscitation

Cross contamination The transfer of microorganisms from one surface to another

Crutchfield tongs Metal device inserted into each side of the skull to which traction is applied

Cuffed tracheostomy tube Tracheostomy tube that is surrounded by an inflatable cuff that produces an airtight seal between the tube and the trachea, which prevents aspiration of oropharyngeal secretions and air leakage between the tube and the trachea

Cutaneous stimulation A physical intervention such as massage, acupressure, and contralateral stimulation that can provide temporary pain relief by distracting the client as it focuses attention on tactile stimuli, away from the painful sensations, thus reducing pain perception

Cyanosis A bluish tinge of skin color

Cyclic feedings Continuous feedings that are administered in less than 24 hours (e.g., 12 to 16 hours)

Dandruff A diffuse scaling of the scalp, often accompanied by itching

Debridement Removal of infected and necrotic material

Deep venous thrombosis (DVT) Condition that occurs when venous stasis (decreased blood movement) allows clots (venous thrombosis) to develop in a deep vein, often in the thigh or calf

Defecation Expulsion of feces from the anus and rectum

Delegation Transference of responsibility and authority for an activity to a competent individual

Deltoid site Site of the deltoid muscle, found on the lateral aspect of the upper arm; sometimes considered for use in adults because of rapid absorption from the deltoid area, but no more than 1 mL of solution can be administered

Dentifrice Toothpaste

Dermatologic preparations Medications that are applied topically to the skin

Desired effect A drug's primary intended effect; that is, the reason a drug is prescribed

Dialysate The solution used in peritoneal dialysis

Dialysis The technique by which blood is filtered for the removal of body wastes and excess fluid

Diaphragmatic (abdominal) breathing Breathing that involves the contraction and relaxation of the diaphragm, as observed by the movement of the abdomen

Diastolic In measuring blood pressure, the pressure when the ventricles are at rest

Diet as tolerated (DAT) A diet that is ordered when the client's appetite, ability to eat, and tolerance for certain foods may change

Diluent A liquid agent that is added to a powdered medication before the medication can be injected

Dimensional analysis method A method of calculating dosages in which a quantity in one unit of measurement is converted to an equivalent quantity in a different unit of measurement by canceling matching units of measurement

Disinfectant Agent that destroys microorganisms other than spores

Divided colostomy Consists of two edges of bowel brought out into the abdomen but separated from each other

Do not resuscitate (DNR; no Code Blue) A designation made on the client record, after discussion with the primary care provider and following agency policies, that should the client arrest, the client will not be resuscitated

Documenting The process of making an entry in a client record; recording; charting

Dorsal recumbent (back-lying) position A supine position with the head and shoulders slightly elevated

Double-barreled colostomy A colostomy in which the proximal and distal loops of bowel are sutured together and both ends are brought up onto the abdominal wall

Drains Devices that are inserted and sutured through the surgical incision line or through drain incisions a few centimeters away from the incision line to permit the drainage of excessive serosanguineous fluid and purulent material and to promote healing of underlying tissues

Dressings Materials used to protect a wound, provide humidity to the wound surface, absorb drainage, prevent bleeding, immobilize, and hide the wound from view

Drop factor The number of drops that equal 1 mL as specified on the package of IV tubing

Droplet nuclei Residue of evaporated droplets emitted by an infected host, such as someone with tuberculosis, that can remain in the air for long periods of time

Droplet precautions Used for clients known or suspected to have serious illnesses transmitted by particle droplets larger than 5 microns (diphtheria, mycoplasma pneumonia, etc.)

Drug (medication) A substance administered for the diagnosis, cure, treatment, or relief of a symptom or for prevention of disease

Dullness A thudlike sound heard with percussion over dense tissue such as the liver, spleen, or heart

Duration The length (long or short) of a sound during auscultation

Dwell In peritoneal dialysis, when the dialysate is allowed to remain in the abdomen for 4 to 6 hours, three to four times each day and overnight

Dysesthesia An unpleasant abnormal sensation that mimics the pathology of a central neuropathic pain disorder, such as pain that follows a stroke or spinal cord injury

Dysphagia Difficulty swallowing

Dysuria Painful or difficult voiding

Early morning care Hygienic care provided to clients as they awaken in the morning

Earmold The part of a hearing aid that directs the sound into the ear

Edema The presence of excess interstitial fluid in the body that makes skin appear swollen, shiny, and taut, and tends to blanch skin color

Emesis Nausea and vomiting

Empyema A collection of pus in the pleural space, usually associated with a lung infection

End-of-life care The care provided in the final weeks before death

Endotracheal tube (ETT) A tube that is inserted through the mouth or nose and into the trachea with the guide of a laryngoscope; used for clients who have had general anesthetics or for those in emergency situations in which mechanical ventilation is required

End-stage renal disease (ESRD) A condition that requires dialysis to provide the functions no longer possible by kidneys that have permanently failed

Enema A treatment for constipation that distends the intestine and sometimes irritates the intestinal mucosa, thereby increasing peristalsis and the excretion of feces and flatus

Enteral Through the gastrointestinal system

Epidural The injection of an anesthetic agent into the epidural or intrathecal (subarachnoid) space

Equianalgesia The relative potency of various opioid analgesics compared to a standard dose of parenteral morphine

Erythema A reddish tinge to skin color

Erythematous Reddened

Eschar Black or brown necrotic tissue

Exhalation (expiration) Breathing out, or the movement of gases from the lungs to the atmosphere

Exophthalmos A protrusion of the eyeballs with elevation of the upper eyelids, resulting in a startled or staring expression

Expectorate Cough up

Expiration (exhalation) The outflow of air from the lungs to the atmosphere

External catheter *See* Condom catheter

Extravasation Infiltration that involves a vesicant drug

Extubation The removal of an endotracheal tube

Exudate Purulent drainage

Face mask A mask covering the client's nose and mouth; used to deliver oxygen

Face tent An open-topped device that covers the face; used to deliver oxygen when clients poorly tolerate face masks

Fasciculation An abnormal contraction of a bundle of muscle fibers that appears as a twitch

Febrile Pertaining to a fever; feverish

Feces (stool) Excreted waste products

Fenestrated tracheostomy tube A tracheostomy tube that has holes in the outer cannula

Fever Body temperature above the usual range

Fifth vital sign Pain assessment, as viewed by many health facilities

Filter needle When accessing a medication in an ampule, a needle that prevents glass particles from being withdrawn with the medication into the syringe

Filter straw When accessing a medication in an ampule, a flexible, clear, plastic tube that prevents glass particles from being withdrawn with the medication into the syringe

Flange The part of the outer cannula of a tracheostomy tube that rests against the neck and allows the tube to be secured in place with twill ties or a Velcro collar

Flatness An extremely dull sound heard when percussing over very dense tissue, such as muscle or bone

Flow-oriented SMI A device that consists of one or more clear plastic chambers containing movable colored balls or disks that the client is asked to keep elevated as long as possible with a maximal sustained inhalation; the longer the inspiratory flow is maintained, the larger the volume

Foley catheter A double-lumen retention catheter in which the smaller lumen is used to inflate a balloon near the tip of the catheter to hold the catheter in place within the bladder

Foreign body airway obstruction (FBAO) Obstruction of the airway caused by aspirated food, mucous plug, or foreign bodies, such as dentures

Fowler's position A semisitting position in which the head of the bed is raised to an angle between 45° and 60°, typically at 45°

Fraction of inspired oxygen (FiO$_2$) The total concentration of oxygen in the inspired air

Fractional equation method A method of calculating dosages that is similar to ratio and proportion except it is written as a fraction

Fremitus The faintly perceptible vibration felt through the chest wall when the client speaks

Friction A force acting parallel to the skin surface that may cause skin abrasion

Full liquid diet A diet containing only liquids or foods that turn to liquid at body temperature such as ice cream

Gait belt A safety device used for moving or transferring a person

Gastrocolic reflex Increased peristalsis of the colon after food has entered the stomach

Gastrostomy A tube that is placed surgically or by laparoscopy through the abdominal wall into the stomach for long-term nutritional support

Gauge The diameter of the shaft of a needle; the larger the gauge number, the smaller the diameter of the shaft

Generic name (of drug) The name given before a drug officially becomes an approved medication; generally used throughout the drug's lifetime

Gingivitis Red, swollen gingiva (gum)

Glaucoma A disturbance in the circulation of aqueous fluid, which causes an increase in intraocular pressure

Glossitis Inflammation of the tongue

Goniometer A handheld device used to measure the angle of a joint movement in degrees

Gtts Abbreviation used for drops per milliliter in an infusion set

Guaiac test A test performed for occult (hidden) blood in the stool to detect gastrointestinal bleeding not visible to the eye

Health care–associated infection (HAI) An infection that may have originated in any health care setting

Hearing aid A battery-powered, sound-amplifying device used by persons with hearing impairments

Heart-lung death The traditional clinical signs of death: cessation of the apical pulse, respirations, and blood pressure

Heimlich chest tube drain valve A one-way flutter valve that allows air to escape from the chest cavity, but prevents air from reentering; used in chest tube drainage systems instead of a full collection system for clients who are ambulatory

Heimlich maneuver Abdominal thrusts used to clear an obstructed airway

Hematomas Contusions commonly called "black eyes" resulting from injury

Hematuria The presence of blood in the urine

Hemiplegia Loss of movement on one side of the body

Hemothorax The accumulation of blood in the pleural cavity

Hemovac A portable drainage suction device used in closed wound drainage systems

High-Fowler's position A bed-sitting position in which the head of the bed is elevated 60° to 90°

Higher brain death *See* Cerebral death

Hirsutism The growth of excessive body hair

Homans' sign Pain in the calf with passive dorsiflexion of the foot

Hordeolum (sty) Redness, swelling, and tenderness of the hair follicle and glands that empty at the edge of the eyelids

Hospice Care that focuses on support and care for the dying person and family, with the goal of facilitating a peaceful and dignified death

Hour of sleep care Hygienic care provided to clients before they go to sleep for the night

Household measures Used when more accurate systems of measurement are not required; consists of drops, teaspoons, tablespoons, cups, and glasses

Hub The part of the needle that fits onto the syringe

Huber needle A noncoring needle used to access implantable vascular access devices

Huff coughing After inhaling deeply the client exhales through pursed lips with a "huff" sound in mid-exhalation to help keep the airways open while moving secretions up and out of the lungs; performed by clients with chronic obstructive lung disease

Humidifier A device that adds water vapor to inspired air

Hydrocolloid A substance that forms a gel with water

Hyperalgesia A heightened response to painful stimuli

Hyperalimentation See Total parenteral nutrition (TPN)

Hypercarbia (hypercapnia) Elevated carbon dioxide levels in the blood

Hyperesthesia More-than-normal sensation

Hyperinflation Giving a client breaths that are greater than the client's normal tidal volume set on the ventilator through the ventilator circuit or via a manual resuscitation bag

Hyperopia Farsightedness

Hyperoxygenation Increasing the oxygen flow before suctioning and between suction attempts to avoid suction-related hypoxemia

Hyperpigmentation Increased pigmentation of the skin caused by changes in the distribution of melanin in the epidermis

Hyperpyrexia An extremely high body temperature (e.g., 41°C [105.8°F])

Hyperresonance An abnormal booming sound heard with percussion of an emphysematous lung

Hypertension Blood pressure that exceeds a certain range; over 140 mmHg systolic and/or 90 mmHg diastolic

Hyperthermia A body temperature above the usual range; fever

Hyperventilation Very deep, rapid respirations; in endotracheal and tracheostomy suctioning, increasing the number of breaths the client is receiving through the ventilator or using a manual resuscitation bag

Hypoesthesia Less-than-normal sensation

Hypopigmentation Decreased pigmentation of the skin caused by changes in the distribution of melanin in the epidermis

Hypotension Blood pressure that is lower than the usual range; less than 100 mmHg systolic in an adult

Hypothermia A core body temperature below the lower limit of normal

Hypoventilation Very shallow respirations

Hypoxemia Decreased oxygen concentration in the arterial blood

Ileal conduit (ileal loop) Urinary diversion in which the client must wear an external pouch over the stoma to collect the continuous flow of urine

Ileostomy A colostomy that generally empties from the distal end of the small intestine

Impaction A mass or collection of hardened feces in the rectum

Implanted venous access device (IVAD) A port that is designed to provide repeated access to the central venous system, avoiding the complications of multiple venipunctures

Incentive spirometer (sustained maximal inspiration device, SMI) A device that measures the flow of air inhaled through a mouthpiece

Incontinence Loss of control of expulsion of feces

Infiltration A condition that occurs when the tip of the IV is outside the vein and the fluid is entering the tissues instead; manifested by local swelling, coolness, pallor, and discomfort at the IV site

Infusion The instillation of fluid, electrolytes, medications, blood, or nutrient substances into a vein by means of venipuncture

Inhalation (inspiration) The intake of air into the lungs

In-line suctioning See Closed suction system

Inner cannula A tube (i.e., cannula) that is inserted into some tracheostomy tubes (i.e., outer cannula) and locked into place; it is in place when a client is on mechanical ventilation and is removed and deflated when the client is being weaned

Inspection Visual examination, which is assessing by using the sense of sight

Inspiration (inhalation) See Inhalation

Instillations Applications of medication into the eye by slowly pouring or dropping a liquid on a surface

Insulin syringe Syringe that has a scale specially designed for insulin and is the only syringe that should be used to administer insulin

Intensity (amplitude) The loudness or softness of auscultated sound

Intermittent feedings Administration of 300 to 500 mL of enteral formula several times per day

Intermittent pneumatic compression devices (IPCDs) See Sequential compression device (SCD)

Intermittent suction For clients with a gastric or intestinal tube in place, type of suction that may be applied when a single-lumen tube (Levin tube) is used to reduce the risk of damaging the mucous membrane near the distal part of the tube

Interrupted sutures A method of suturing in which each stitch is tied and knotted separately

Intradermal (ID) injection The administration of a drug into the dermal layer of the skin just beneath the epidermis

Intramuscular (IM) injections The administration of a drug into the muscle tissue

Intraoperative phase The phase of surgery that begins when the client is transferred to the operating room table and ends when the client is admitted to the postanesthesia care unit

Intravenous (IV) Within or into a vein

Intravenous push (IVP) The intravenous administration of an undiluted drug directly into the systemic circulation; a bolus

Iritis Inflammation of the iris caused by local or systemic infections

Irrigation Administration of a specified solution to flush or wash out (e.g., eye, ear, bladder)

Jackson–Pratt A portable drainage suction device used in closed wound drainage systems

Jaundice A yellowish tinge to skin color

Jejunostomy A tube that is placed surgically or by laparoscopy through the abdominal wall into the jejunum for long-term nutritional support

Korotkoff's sounds The five phases of blood pressure sounds

Lancet A sharp device used to puncture the skin

Lancet injector A spring-loaded mechanism that holds the lancet

Lateral (side-lying) position Position in which a person lies on one side of the body

Level of consciousness (LOC) Varying degrees of alertness and awareness

Lifting devices Used primarily for clients who are heavier than 16 kg (35 lb) (when solo lifting is necessary) and who cannot assist health care personnel in moving or transferring themselves

Light diet A diet designed for postoperative and other clients who are not ready for the regular diet; contains foods that are plainly cooked

Limb restraints Protective devices generally made from cloth; may be used to immobilize a limb, primarily for therapeutic reasons

Line of gravity An imaginary vertical line drawn through an object's center of gravity

Livor mortis The discoloration of surrounding tissues that occurs after blood circulation has ceased and the red blood cells break down, releasing hemoglobin

Lofstrand crutch A type of crutch with a metal cuff that goes around the forearm and a metal bar that stabilizes the wrists

Logrolling A technique used to turn a client whose body must at all times be kept in straight alignment

Loop colostomy A colostomy in which a loop of bowel is brought out into the abdominal wall and supported by a plastic bridge or a piece of rubber tubing

Lumbar puncture (LP) Procedure in which cerebrospinal fluid is withdrawn through a needle inserted into the subarachnoid space of the spinal canal between the third and fourth lumbar vertebrae, or between the fourth and fifth lumbar vertebrae; also called a spinal tap

Macrodrip A term that refers to the drip chamber in an infusion administration set that delivers between 10 and 20 drops per milliliter of solution

Macrodrip infusion set Intravenous tubing that delivers 10, 15, or 20 drops/mL in the drip chamber

Macronutrients Carbohydrates, fats, and protein that are needed in large amounts to provide energy

Magnetic box mobility monitor A safety monitoring device that mounts on a bed or chair and connects with a clip to clothing

Malnutrition The lack of necessary or appropriate food substances; includes both undernutrition and overnutrition (obesity)

Manometer A glass or plastic tube calibrated in millimeters that is used to take cerebrospinal fluid pressure readings

Massage A comfort measure that can aid relaxation, promote blood and lymph circulation, decrease muscle tension, and ease anxiety

Mean arterial pressure (MAP) Represents the blood pressure actually delivered to the body organs

Meatus The urinary meatus, which is the external opening from the urethra to the surface of the body

Meconium The first fecal material passed by a newborn, normally up to 24 hours after birth

Medical asepsis All practices intended to confine a specific microorganism to a specific area, limiting the number, growth, and spread of microorganisms

Medication (drug) A substance administered for the diagnosis, cure, treatment, or relief of a symptom or for prevention of disease

Medication history Information about the drugs a client is taking currently or has taken recently

Medication reconciliation The process of creating the most accurate list possible of all medications a client is taking—including drug name, dosage, frequency, and route—and comparing that list against the physician's admission, transfer, and/or discharge orders, with the goal of providing correct medications to the client at all transition points within the hospital

Meniscus The crescent-shaped upper surface of a column of liquid

Metered-dose inhaler (MDI) A handheld nebulizer that is a pressurized container of medication that can be used by the client to release the medication through a mouthpiece

Metric system A decimal system of measurement that is logically organized into units of 10

Microdrip A term that refers to the drip chamber in an infusion administration set that delivers 60 drops per milliliter of solution

Microdrip infusion set Intravenous tubing that delivers 60 drops/mL in the drip chamber

Micronutrients Those vitamins and minerals required in small amounts to metabolize the energy-providing nutrients

Micturition *See* Urination

Midstream urine specimen *See* Clean-catch urine specimen

Miosis Constricted pupils

Mitt (hand) restraint A device used to prevent clients of any age from using their hands or fingers to scratch and injure themselves

Morning care Hygienic care provided after clients have had breakfast, although it may be provided before breakfast

Mucus clearance device A small handheld device with a steel ball sitting inside that has a hard plastic mouthpiece at one end and a perforated cover at the other end; the client inhales slowly and then, keeping the cheeks firm, exhales quickly through the device, causing the steel ball to move up and down, resulting in vibrations that loosen mucus and assist its movement up the airways to be expectorated

Mydriasis Enlarged pupils

Myopia Nearsightedness

Nares The nostrils

Naris A single nostril

Nasal cannula A low-flow device used to administer oxygen; also called nasal prongs

Nasogastric (NG) tube A tube inserted through one of the nostrils by way of the nasopharynx or the oropharynx; it is placed into the stomach for the temporary purpose of feeding the client or to remove gastric secretions

Nasopharyngeal airway A device used to keep the upper air passages open if they become obstructed by secretions or the tongue

Nasopharyngeal culture A sample collected from the mucosa of the nasopharynx using a culture swab

Nasopharyngeal suctioning Removal of secretions from the upper respiratory tract

Nebulizers Devices used to deliver a fine spray of medication or moisture to a client through the inhaled route

Negative pressure wound therapy (NPWT) Refers to the use of suction equipment to apply negative pressure to a variety of wound types. Also termed vacuum-assisted closure (VAC), wound V.A.C., vacuum sealing, and topical negative pressure

Neuropathic pain Pain experienced by people who have damaged or malfunctioning nerves as a result of illness, injury, or undetermined reasons

Nociceptive pain Pain experienced when an intact, properly functioning nervous system sends signals that tissues are damaged, requiring attention and proper care

No Code Blue *See* Do not resuscitate (DNR)

Noninvasive positive pressure ventilation Delivery of air or oxygen under pressure but without the need for an invasive tube such as an endotracheal or tracheostomy tube; used in clients with acute and chronic respiratory failure, pulmonary edema, chronic obstructive pulmonary disease, and obstructive sleep apnea

Nonrebreather mask An oxygen delivery device that covers the mouth and nose and delivers the highest oxygen content possible by means other than intubation or mechanical ventilation; one-way valves on the mask and between the reservoir bag and the mask prevent the room air and the client's exhaled air from entering the bag

Nonsteroidal anti-inflammatory drugs (NSAIDs) Drugs such as aspirin and ibuprofen that have anti-inflammatory, analgesic, and antipyretic effects

Normocephalic Normal head size

Nose culture A specimen collected from the mucosa of the nasal passages using a culture swab

Nosocomial infections Infections that originate in the hospital

Nothing by mouth (NPO) Fasting; literally, "nil per os"

Nutrients Organic and inorganic energy-producing substances found in foods and required for body functioning

Nutrition What a person eats and how the body uses it

Nutritive value The nutrient content of a specified amount of food

Nystagmus Rapid involuntary rhythmic eye movement

Obstructive sleep apnea (OSA) A condition that consists of periods of nonbreathing due to closure of the upper airway while sleeping

Obturator The part of a tracheostomy tube that is used in the insertion of the outer cannula and is kept at the client's bedside in case the tube or outer cannula becomes dislodged and needs to be reinserted

Occult Hidden

Occupied bed A bed currently being used by a client

Official name (of drug) The name under which a drug is listed in one of the official publications (e.g., the *United States Pharmacopeia*)

Open bed An unoccupied bed with the top covers folded down toward the bottom of the bed

Open suction system The traditional method for suctioning an endotracheal tube or tracheostomy in which, if a client is connected to a ventilator, the nurse disconnects the client from the ventilator, suctions the airway, reconnects the client to the ventilator, and discards the suction catheter; also called an open airway suction system

Open system Administration of enteral feedings using an open-top container or syringe

Open-tipped catheter A flexible, plastic suction catheter that has an opening at the end of the catheter and may be more effective than a whistle-tipped catheter for removing thick mucous plugs

Ophthalmic Pertaining to medications for the eye

Opioids Narcotics

Oral A method of drug administration in which a drug is swallowed

Orogastric (OG) tube A nasogastric tube that is inserted through the mouth; used in infants and children

Oropharyngeal airway A device used to keep the upper air passages open when they may become obstructed by secretions or the tongue

Oropharyngeal suctioning Removal of secretions from the upper respiratory tract

Orthopneic position A position to relieve respiratory difficulty in which the client sits either in bed or on the side of the bed, leaning over an overbed table across the lap; an adaptation of the high-Fowler's position

Orthoses Orthotic devices that provide musculoskeletal support, balance, stretch, and comfort

Ostomy An opening on the abdominal wall for the elimination of feces or urine

Ostomy appliance Consists of a skin barrier and a pouch that are used to protect the skin, collect stool, and control odor

Otic Refers to instillations or irrigations of the external auditory canal

Otoscope A lighted instrument used to view the ear

Outer cannula The part of the tracheostomy tube that is inserted into the trachea

Ova and **parasites** Intestinal organisms such as protozoa and worms and their eggs

Overnutrition A caloric intake in excess of daily energy requirements, resulting in storage of energy in the form of increased adipose tissue

Oxygen concentrator An electrically powered system that manufactures oxygen from room air

Oxygen saturation (SaO$_2$) The amount of hemoglobin fully saturated with oxygen; given as a percentage

Pain An unpleasant and highly personal experience that may be imperceptible to others, while consuming all parts of a person's life

Pain threshold The least amount of stimuli that is needed for a person to label a sensation as pain

Pain tolerance The maximum amount of painful stimuli that a person is willing to withstand without seeking avoidance of the pain or relief

Palliate To ease, reduce, or allay pain without curing

Palliative care The prevention and relief of suffering by means of early identification and impeccable assessment and treatment of pain and other problems, physical, psychosocial, and spiritual

Pallor Paleness

Palpation The examination of the body using the sense of touch

Parenteral Administration of a medication using a route other than topically or via the alimentary or digestive tract; injected into the body intradermally, subcutaneously, intramuscularly, or intravenously

Paresthesia An abnormal sensation such as burning, pain, or electric shock

Parotitis Inflammation of the parotid salivary gland

Partial bath (abbreviated bath) A bath in which only parts of the client's body that might cause discomfort or odor, if neglected, are washed

Partial rebreather mask An oxygen delivery device that covers the mouth and nose and has a reservoir bag attached that allows the client to rebreathe about the first third of the exhaled air in conjunction with oxygen

Passive range-of-motion exercises Exercises in which another person moves each of the client's joints through their complete range of movement, maximally stretching all muscle groups within each plane over each joint

Patient-controlled analgesia (PCA) An interactive method of pain management that permits clients to treat their pain by self-administering doses of analgesics

Peak expiratory flow rate (PEFR) The maximum amount of air that the client can expire from the lungs

Pearson attachment A sling appliance that joins the Thomas leg splint at knee level to support the lower leg off the bed and permit the knee to be flexed; used for fractures of the femur

Pediatric advanced life support (PALS) A multiple-day training session appropriate for emergency medical technicians, paramedics, respiratory therapists, and other professionals who may need to respond to an emergency involving a child

Pediculosis (lice) Infestation with head lice, *Pediculus capitis*; body lice, *Pediculus corporis*; or crab lice, *Pediculus pubis*

Penrose drain A flat, thin, rubber tube inserted into a wound to allow for fluid to flow from the wound; it has an open end that drains onto a dressing

Percussion A method in which the body surface is struck to elicit sounds that can be heard or vibrations that can be felt

Percutaneous endoscopic gastrostomy (PEG) A procedure in which a PEG catheter is inserted into the stomach through the skin and subcutaneous tissues of the abdomen; used as a feeding tube

Percutaneous endoscopic jejunostomy (PEJ) A procedure in which a PEJ catheter is inserted into the jejunum through the skin and subcutaneous tissues of the abdomen; used as a feeding tube

Perineal (peri-) care Cleansing of the perineum (genitalia)

Perioperative period The three phases of surgery: preoperative, intraoperative, and postoperative

Peripheral neuropathic pain Phantom pain, post-herpetic neuralgia, or carpal tunnel syndrome that follows damage and/or sensitization of peripheral nerves

Peripheral parenteral nutrition (PPN) Intravenous nutrition administered through a peripheral (rather than a central) vein

Peripheral pulse A pulse located in the periphery of the body (e.g., foot, hand, or neck)

Peripherally inserted central catheter (PICC) A long venous catheter inserted in an arm vein and extending into the distal third of the superior vena cava

Peritoneal dialysis The technique of instillation and drainage of a solution (dialysate) into the peritoneal cavity to filter impurities, excess fluid, and electrolytes from the blood that would normally be excreted through the kidneys

PERRLA Pupils equally round and react to light and accommodation; abbreviation used to record normal assessment of the pupils

Persistent vegetative state (PVS) State in which an individual has lost cognitive function and awareness, but respiration and circulation remain

Personal hygiene The self-care by which people attend to such functions as bathing, toileting, general body hygiene, and grooming

Personal protective equipment (PPE) Barriers such as gloves, gowns, eyewear, and mask used to protect persons from contact with potentially infective materials

Petal The application of strips of tape or moleskin around the edges of a cast

Phlebitis Inflammation of a vein

Physical dependence Expected physical response of withdrawal symptoms when a client who is on long-term opioid therapy has the opioid significantly reduced or withdrawn

Physical restraints Any manual method or physical or mechanical device, material, or equipment attached to a client's body that cannot be removed easily and that restricts the client's movement

Piggyback A secondary IV setup that connects a second container to the tubing of a primary container at the upper port; used solely for intermittent drug administration

Pitch The frequency (number of the vibrations per second) heard during auscultation

Pivot A technique in which the body is turned in a way that avoids twisting of the spine

Placebo Any medication or procedure that produces an effect in a client because of its implicit or explicit intent, and not because of its specific physical or chemical properties

Plaque An invisible soft film consisting of bacteria, molecules of saliva, and remnants of epithelial cells and leukocytes that adheres to the enamel surface of teeth

Pleural effusion Excessive fluid in the pleural space

Pleximeter In percussion, the middle finger of the nondominant hand that is placed firmly on the client's skin

Plexor In percussion, the middle finger of the dominant hand or a percussion hammer used to strike the pleximeter

Pneumothorax Accumulation of air in the pleural space

Point of maximal impulse (PMI) The point where the apex of the heart touches the anterior chest wall and heart movements are most easily observed and palpated

Positive affirmation A positive statement such as "I am focused and caring" that helps a person to focus attention and intention to remain mindful

Positive end-expiratory pressure (PEEP) Pressure that may be added to the ventilator settings to keep alveoli open and facilitate diffusion of oxygen into the blood

Postanesthesia care unit (PACU) Unit to which the client is admitted after surgery

Postanesthesia room (PAR) *See* Postanesthesia care unit (PACU)

Postmortem care Care of the body after death

Postoperative phase The period of surgery that begins with the admission of the client to the postanesthesia area and ends when healing is complete

Postural drainage Positioning of a client to allow gravity to facilitate drainage of secretions from the lungs

Posture The bearing and position of the body; the relative arrangements of the various parts of the body

Preemptive analgesia The administration of analgesics before surgery to decrease or relieve pain after surgery

Prefilled unit-dose systems Disposable units that supply injectable medications that are available as prefilled syringes ready for use, or as prefilled sterile cartridges and needles that require the attachment of a reusable holder before use

Preoperative phase The period of surgery that begins when the decision to have surgery has been made and ends when the client is transferred to the operating room table

Presbycusis Generalized loss of hearing related to aging

Presbyopia Loss of elasticity of the lens and thus loss of ability to see close objects as a result of the aging process

Prescription The written direction for the preparation and administration of a drug

Pressure ulcer Reddened areas, sores, or ulcers of the skin occurring over bony prominences

Primary port The port on the IV tubing that is farthest from the client

prn order An *as-needed* order that permits the nurse to give a medication when, in the nurse's judgment, the client requires it; literally, "pro re nata"

Prone position Position in which a client lies on his or her abdomen with the head turned to one side

Protein-calorie malnutrition (PCM) An imbalance between nutritional intake and the body's protein requirements

Pruritus Itching

Pseudoaddiction Condition that results from the undertreatment of pain in which the client may become so focused on obtaining medications that he or she may become angry and demanding, may "clock watch," and may otherwise seem inappropriately "drug seeking"

Pulmonary embolism (PE) In deep venous thrombosis, when a thrombus (blood clot) breaks free and travels to where it blocks a pulmonary artery or one of its branches

Pulse deficit The difference between the apical pulse and the radial pulse rates

Pulse oximeter A noninvasive device that measures the arterial blood oxygen saturation by means of a sensor attached to the finger or other location

Pulse pressure The difference between the systolic and the diastolic blood pressures

Pureed diet A modification of the soft diet wherein liquid may be added to the food, which is then blended to a semisolid consistency

Purosanguineous Exudate containing pus and blood; often seen in a new wound that is infected

Pursed-lip breathing Pursing the lips as if about to whistle, and breathing out slowly and gently, tightening the abdominal muscles to exhale more effectively; exhalation of air against the resistance of pursed lips to the air flowing out of the lungs prolongs exhalation and prevents airway collapse by maintaining positive airway pressure

Purulent Thick exudate containing pus, and varying in color depending on the causative organism

Pus Pooled exudates

Pyorrhea Advanced periodontal disease in which teeth are loose and pus is evident when the gums are pressed

Pyrexia A body temperature above the normal range; fever

Quad cane A mechanical walking aid that has four feet

Quality A subjective description of an auscultated sound (e.g., whistling, gurgling, or snapping)

Radiate Spread or extend as in pain

Range of motion (ROM) The maximum degree of movement possible for each joint

Rapid response team (RRT) A special team of health care providers that provides support when requested by the general floor nurses for clients experiencing potential life-threatening changes in their condition

Ratio and proportion method Used for calculating dosage problems in which the equation is set up with the known quantities on the left side and the desired dose and the unknown amount to administer on the right side

Reagent A substance used to produce a chemical reaction to detect or measure other substances

Rebound phenomenon The time when the maximum therapeutic effect of a hot or cold application is achieved and the opposite effect begins

Reconstitution The technique of adding a diluent to a powdered drug to prepare it for administration

Recovery room (RR) *See* Postanesthesia care unit (PACU)

Rectus femoris site The rectus femoris muscle, situated on the anterior aspect of the thigh; used only occasionally for intramuscular injections

Referred pain Pain perceived to be in one area but whose source is another area

Registered nurse first assistant (RNFA) A nurse who has had additional education and training from the scrub person and assists the surgeon by controlling bleeding, using instruments, handling and cutting tissue, and suturing during the procedure

Regular (standard or house) diet A balanced diet that supplies the metabolic requirements of a sedentary person

Regulator A device that releases oxygen at a safe level and at a desirable rate that must be attached before the oxygen supply is used

Resonance A hollow sound heard with percussion over lungs filled with air

Respiration The act of breathing; includes the intake of oxygen and the output of carbon dioxide from the cells to the atmosphere

Respiratory arrest The absence of breathing

Respiratory hygiene/cough etiquette Covering the mouth and nose when sneezing or coughing, proper disposal of tissues, and separating potentially infected persons from others by at least 3 feet, or having them wear a surgical mask

Restraint-free environment Using means other than restraints for controlling behaviors that may pose a threat to self or others

Restraints Protective devices used to limit the physical activity of a client or a part of the body

Retention enema An enema that introduces oil or medication into the rectum and sigmoid colon, where it is held to soften the feces or to deliver a medication

Retention sutures Large sutures used in addition to skin sutures to attach underlying tissues of fat and muscle as well as skin; used to support incisions in individuals who are obese or when healing may be prolonged

Return-flow enema Used occasionally to expel flatus by alternating flow of fluid into and out of the rectum to stimulate peristalsis

Reverse Trendelenburg's position A position with the head of the bed raised and the foot lowered

Rh factor Antigens that are either present or absent on the surface of red blood cells; persons without the factor (Rh negative) may have a serious reaction if exposed to blood with the factor (Rh positive)

Rigidity Resistance of a relaxed limb to passive movement

Rigor mortis Stiffening of the body that occurs 2 to 4 hours after death

Robinson catheter A straight catheter, single-lumen tube with a small eye or opening about 1.25 cm (0.5 in.) from the insertion tip

Safety monitoring device An electronic sensor or monitor that detects when clients are attempting to get out of a bed or a chair and triggers an alarm

Salem sump tube A nasogastric tube with a double lumen that allows delivery of liquids to the stomach or removal of gastric contents

Saline lock The sterile injection cap attached to an existing intravenous catheter that requires periodic injection with saline to keep blood from coagulating within the tubing

Saliva The clear liquid secreted by the salivary glands in the mouth

Sanguineous Hemorrhagic exudate that may be bright or dark red; bright red indicates fresh bleeding, and dark red indicates older bleeding

Scabies A contagious skin infestation by the itch mite that produces intense itching, especially at night

Scrub person Usually UAP but can be an RN or LPN; assists the surgeons by draping the client with sterile drapes and handling sterile instruments and supplies; with the circulating nurse, is responsible for accounting for all sponges, needles, and instruments at the close of surgery

Seclusion Involuntary confinement of a client alone in a room or area from which the client is physically prevented from leaving

Second-voided specimen The client is asked to void and, in 30 minutes, to void again; the second voiding is used for testing because it more accurately reflects the present condition of the body

Secondary port The port on the IV tubing that is closest to the client

Seizure An uncontrolled electrical neuronal discharge of the brain resulting in an interruption of normal brain function

Seizure precautions Safety measures taken to protect clients from injury should they have a seizure

Self-care Care that includes engaging in a regular movement or exercise discipline, paying attention to healthy nutrition, practicing clear communication, cultivating positive relationships, and taking regular meal and rest breaks while on the job

Self-help bed bath Bath that clients confined to bed give themselves with help from the nurse for washing the back and perhaps the feet

Semi-Fowler's position A bed-sitting position in which the head of the bed is raised 15° to 45°, typically at a 30° angle; sometimes called low-Fowler's position

Sepsis An acute organ dysfunction secondary to infection

Sequential compression device (SCD) A device used to promote venous return in the legs by alternately inflating and deflating disposable sleeves wrapped around the legs

Serosanguineous Clear and blood-tinged drainage that is commonly seen in surgical incisions

Serous Watery, clear exudate

Shaft The part of the needle that is attached to the hub

Shearing force A combination of friction and pressure that occurs commonly when a client sitting in bed tends to slide downward toward the foot of bed, and can damage the blood vessels and tissues in the area

Shower Ambulatory clients use shower facilities for cleansing purposes; clients in long-term care settings are often given showers with the use of a shower chair

Shroud A large piece of plastic or cotton material used to enclose a body after death

Side effect Secondary effect of a drug that is unintended

Sims' (semiprone) position A position halfway between the lateral and the prone positions, with the lower arm behind the body and the upper arm flexed at the shoulder and the elbow, with the legs flexed in front

Single (end) colostomy A colostomy that has only one stoma, which is created when one end of bowel is brought out through an opening onto the anterior abdominal wall

Single order An order that medication is to be given once at a specified time

Situation, Background, Assessment, and Recommendation (SBAR) process An approach to documentation that can enhance safety in situations where nurses communicate with primary care providers and other nurses about client status

Sitz bath A bath in which the client sits in warm water to help soothe and heal the perineum

Skull tongs Metal device inserted into each side of the skull to which traction is applied

Sling A binder bandage shaped to support the elbow, lower arm, and hand

Small-bore feeding tube (SBFT) A tube that is softer, more flexible, and less irritating than a large-bore nasogastric tube, ranging from 8 to 12 Fr in diameter

Soft diet A diet that is easily chewed and digested and is often ordered for clients who have difficulty chewing and swallowing

Somatic pain Pain that originates in the skin, muscles, bone, or connective tissue

Sordes Accumulation of foul matter (food, microorganisms, and epithelial elements) on the teeth and gums

Spasticity Sudden prolonged involuntary muscle contraction

Specimens Small samples of urine, blood, stool, sputum, and wound drainage taken for laboratory examination to provide important information for diagnosing health problems as well as measuring a response to therapy

Sphygmomanometer A blood pressure measuring device consisting of a cuff and gauge

Spica Any bandage that is applied in successive V-shaped crossings and is used to immobilize a limb, especially at a joint

Splint A partial cast that does not extend all the way around the limb and is commonly used for injuries of the finger, wrist, foot, and ankle

Sputum Mucous secretion from the lungs, bronchi, and trachea

Standard precautions (SP) Those actions appropriate for infection control in all situations; the risk of caregiver exposure to client body tissues and fluids rather than the suspected presence or absence of infectious organisms determines the use of clean gloves, gowns, masks, and eye protection

Standing order An order that may be carried out indefinitely until an order is written to cancel it, or that may be carried out for a specified number of days

Staples Wire clips used to sew body tissues together

Stat order An order that is to be carried out immediately and only once

Steatorrhea Excessive amount of fat in the stool

Sterile field A microorganism-free area

Stockinette A soft, flexible, tubular, cloth material that is placed over a body part before cast material is applied

Stoma The opening created in the abdominal wall by an ostomy

Stomatitis Inflammation of the oral mucosa

Stool *See* Feces

Strabismus Cross-eye

Sublingual A method of drug administration in which the drug is placed under the tongue

Suctioning The aspiration of secretions through a catheter connected to a suction machine or wall suction outlet

Sulcular technique A technique of brushing the teeth that removes plaque and cleans under the gingival margins

Suppositories Solid medicated substances inserted into the rectum, vagina, or urethra

Suprapubic catheter An indwelling catheter that has been surgically placed in the bladder through the abdominal wall

Surgical asepsis Practices that keep an area or object free of all microorganisms; also called sterile technique

Surgical hand antisepsis The antiseptic surgical scrub or antiseptic hand rub that is performed before applying (i.e., putting on) sterile gloves and gowns preoperatively

Surgical bed A bed with the linens horizontally fanfolded to facilitate transfer of the client into the bed; used for a client who is having surgery and will return to the bed for the postoperative phase

Suture A thread used to sew body tissues together

Sympathetically maintained pain Pain that occurs occasionally when abnormal connections between pain fibers and the sympathetic nervous system perpetuate problems with both the pain and sympathetically controlled functions (e.g., edema, temperature, and blood flow regulation)

Synchronized intermittent mandatory ventilation (SIMV) A ventilator setting in which there is a set number of breaths and tidal volume while also allowing the client to take spontaneous breaths with a client-determined tidal volume and rate

Syringe pump A method of intermittently administering an IV medication wherein the medication is mixed in a syringe that is connected to the primary IV line via a mini-infuser

Systolic In measuring blood pressure, the pressure of the blood when the ventricles contract

Tandem A secondary IV setup in which a second IV container is attached to the line of the first container at the lower, secondary port to permit medications to be administered intermittently or simultaneously with the primary solution

Tartar A visible, hard deposit of plaque and dead bacteria that forms at the gum lines

Therapeutic bath A bath given for physical effects, such as to soothe irritated skin or to promote healing of an area (e.g., the perineum); two common types are the sitz bath and the medicated bath

Therapeutic effect A drug's primary intended effect; that is, the reason a drug is prescribed

Therapeutic presence Deep listening, compassion, focus, self-awareness, finding meaning, and using the imagination

Thomas leg splint With the Pearson attachment, a method of traction in which a pin or wire drilled through bone is attached to a spreader, which in turn is attached to ropes, pulleys, and weights; used for balanced suspension skeletal traction

Thoracentesis A procedure to remove excess fluid or air from the pleural cavity to ease breathing or to introduce chemotherapeutic drugs intrapleurally

Thoracostomy A chest tube in place

Throat culture A specimen collected from the mucosa of the oropharynx and tonsillar regions using a culture swab

Tidaling In a water-seal drainage system, if a "wet" water seal is used, the action in which the level of water fluctuates with the client's respirations

Tolerance Occurs when the client's opioid dose, over time, leads to a decreased sensitivity of the drug's analgesic effect

Total parenteral nutrition (TPN) The intravenous infusion of water, protein, carbohydrates, electrolytes, minerals, and vitamins into high-flow central veins through a central venous catheter or a peripherally inserted central catheter; also referred to as hyperalimentation

Towel bath Similar to a bag bath, but uses regular towels

Tracheostomy A surgical incision in the trachea just below the larynx

Traction A means of immobilization using a pulling force applied to a part of the body while a second force, called countertraction, pulls in the opposite direction

Trade name (of drug) Name of a drug given by the drug's manufacturer; also known as a brand name

Transcutaneous electric nerve stimulation (TENS) A method of applying low-voltage electrical stimulation directly over pain areas

Transdermal patch A dermatologic medication delivery system that administers sustained-action medications via multilayered films containing the drug and an adhesive layer

Transfer belt *See* Gait belt

Transfusion (blood) The introduction of whole blood or its components into the venous circulation

Transmission-based precautions Actions taken in addition to standard precautions when those precautions do not completely block the chain of infection, and the infections are spread by airborne transmission, by droplet transmission, or by contact

Transparent wound barrier A see-through semipermeable membrane dressing that helps retain wound moisture while allowing gases (oxygen, carbon dioxide) to pass into and away from the wound

Transtracheal catheter A small plastic cannula placed through a surgically created tract in the lower neck directly into the trachea; used to deliver oxygen therapy

Tremor An involuntary trembling of a limb or body part

Trendelenburg's position Position in which the head of the bed is lowered and the foot of the bed is raised in a straight incline

Tripod position Position often assumed by people in respiratory distress in which they sit upright and lean on their arms or elbows

Trocar A sharp, pointed instrument

Tub bath Use of a tub for a cleaning or therapeutic bath

Tuberculin syringe A narrow syringe, calibrated in tenths and hundredths of a milliliter on one scale and in sixteenths of a minim on the other scale, that can be useful in administering other drugs, particularly when small or precise measurement is indicated

Tympany A musical or drumlike sound produced when percussing an air-filled organ such as the stomach

Uncuffed tracheostomy tube A plastic or metal tracheostomy tube that allows for air to flow around the tube

Undernutrition Intake of nutrients insufficient to meet daily energy requirements as a result of inadequate food intake or improper digestion and absorption of food

Unlicensed assistive personnel (UAP) Personnel such as certified nursing assistants, hospital attendants, nurse technicians, and orderlies who work in health care settings and are responsible for nursing activities that require less technical skill (e.g., bathing, feeding, specimen collection, hygiene) than the skills an RN has and that do not require nursing judgment

Unoccupied bed A bed not occupied by a client

Urinary incontinence (UI) A temporary or permanent inability of the external sphincter muscles to control the flow of urine from the bladder

Urinary retention The accumulation of urine in the bladder and inability of the bladder to empty itself

Urinary sheath *See* Condom catheter

Urination (micturition, voiding) The process of emptying the bladder

Vasoconstriction Constricted blood vessels

Vasodilation An increase in the diameter of blood vessels

Vastus lateralis site Situated on the anterior lateral aspect of an infant's thigh, the middle third of the muscle is the recommended site of choice for intramuscular injections for infants 1 year and younger

Vector-borne transmission Transport of an infectious agent from an animal or flying or crawling insect that serves as an intermediate means via biting or depositing feces or other materials on the skin through the bite wound or a traumatized skin area

Vehicle-borne transmission Transport of an infectious agent into a susceptible host via any intermediate substance (e.g., fomites, food, or water)

Venogram An imaging test that studies the veins

Venous thromboembolism (VTE) The collective name for deep venous thrombosis (DVT) and pulmonary embolism (PE)

Ventilation The movement of air in and out of the lungs; the process of inhalation and exhalation

Ventilator A mechanical device that controls or assists with breathing

Ventilator-associated event (VAE) Situation in which the client's condition worsens because of the use of a ventilator

Ventilator bundle Interventions created by the Institute of Healthcare Improvement that, when all are implemented simultaneously, can significantly reduce VAP

Ventricular fibrillation (VF) A quivering, nonperfusing, nonfunctional heartbeat rhythm that, if untreated, converts to asystole; VF is the most common arrhythmia in cardiac arrest

Ventrogluteal site The preferred site for intramuscular injections is in the gluteus medius muscle, which lies over the gluteus minimus

Venturi mask A special mask that delivers oxygen at varying concentrations

Vesicant Medication or fluid with the potential for causing blisters, severe tissue injury, or necrosis if it escapes from the vein

Vest restraints Sleeveless jackets or vests with straps (tails) that can be tied to fixed parts of the bed frame under the mattress or wheelchair frame

Vial A small glass bottle with a sealed rubber cap used for single or multiple doses of medication

Visceral pain Pain arising from organs

Visual acuity The degree of detail the eye can discern in an image

Visual field The area an individual can see when looking straight ahead

Vital signs Body temperature, pulse, respiration, and blood pressure; many agencies have designated pain as the fifth vital sign

Vitiligo Patches of hypopigmented skin, caused by the destruction of melanocytes in the area

Void Urinate

Voiding *See* Urination

Volume-control infusion set A method of administering intermittent medications in which a small fluid container is attached below the primary infusion container so that the medication is administered through a client's IV line

Volume expanders Substances used to increase the blood volume following severe loss of blood or plasma

Volume-oriented sustained maximal inspiration device (SMI) A device that measures the inhalation volume maintained by a client

Walker A metal rectangular frame that usually has four legs, but may have wheels; used as an aid to ambulation

Water-seal drainage system A chest tube drainage system in which water in the bottom of the container prevents air from entering the chest tube and pleural cavity during inspiration

Wean Gradual discontinuation of mechanical support

Wheal A small raised area like a blister

Whistle-tipped catheter A flexible, plastic suction catheter that has an angle opening at the end of the tip and is less irritating to respiratory tissues than an open-tipped catheter

Wound The injured body area that results when the skin or underlying tissues are damaged

Wound dehiscence Separation of a suture line before an incision heals

Wound evisceration Extrusion of internal organs and tissues through an incision

Xerostomia Dry mouth as a result of a reduced supply of saliva

Yankauer suction tube A rigid, plastic tube used to suction the oral cavity

Z-track technique The recommended technique for administering intramuscular injections because it has been found to be less painful than the traditional injection technique and decreases leakage of irritating and discoloring medications into the subcutaneous tissue

Index

Page numbers followed by *f* indicate figures and those followed by *t* indicate tables, boxes, or special features.

PRACTICE GUIDELINES

SKILLS